OXFORD MEDICAL PUBLICATION

Oxford Desk Reference
Oncology

Oxford Desk Reference
Oncology

Thankamma Ajithkumar
Consultant Clinical Oncologist
Norfolk and Norwich University NHS Foundation Trust
Norwich, UK

Ann Barrett
Emeritus Professor of Oncology
University of East Anglia
Norwich, UK

Helen Hatcher
Senior Lecturer and Honorary Consultant Medical Oncologist
University of Cambridge
Cambridge, UK

Natalie Cook
Specialist Registrar in Medical Oncology
Addenbrookes Hospital
Cambridge, UK

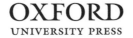

OXFORD
UNIVERSITY PRESS

OXFORD
UNIVERSITY PRESS

Great Clarendon Street, Oxford OX2 6DP

Oxford University Press is a department of the University of Oxford.
It furthers the University's objective of excellence in research, scholarship,
and education by publishing worldwide in

Oxford New York

Athens Auckland Bangkok Bogotá Buenos Aires Cape Town
Chennai Dar es Salaam Delhi Florence Hong Kong Istanbul Karachi
Kolkata Kuala Lumpur Madrid Melbourne Mexico City Mumbai Nairobi
Paris São Paulo Shanghai Singapore Taipei Tokyo Toronto Warsaw

with associated companies in Berlin Ibadan

Oxford is a registered trade mark of Oxford University Press
in the UK and in certain other countries

Published in the United States
by Oxford University Press Inc., New York

British Library Cataloguing in Publication Data

Data available

Library of Congress Control Number: 2011922686

ISBN 978-0-19-923563-6

10 9 8 7 6 5 4 3 2 1

Typeset in GillHandbook
by Glyph International, Bangalore, India
Printed in Great Britain
on acid-free paper by
CPI Antony Rowe, Chippenham, Wiltshire

Preface

This book forms part of the Oxford Desk Reference series and is designed to bridge the gap between the *Oxford Handbook of Oncology* and the substantial *Oxford Textbook of Oncology*. We hope this book will be on the desk of every oncologist to provide an easily accessible and succinct source of information on the common situations encountered within a normal oncology practice. The layout over 2–4 pages is designed to make it quick and easy to find relevant tumour and treatment details. Many international contributors have ensured this represents global philosophies of cancer management. English spelling is used in chapters contributed from Europe and American spelling for contributors from the USA. Up-to-date details of relevant clinical trials are included and useful Internet addresses where continuing treatment updates may be found. Blank pages are included throughout the book to provide space for your own notes from journals, guidelines, seminars, and lectures. The editors take responsibility for any mistakes but particular care should be taken to check drug and radiotherapy doses before treating individual patients. We will be glad to receive any feedback on the usefulness of this volume.

Acknowledgements

Any book of this size involves hard work by many contributors and we are grateful to them all. Valuable assistance has been received from Oxford University Press. The editors are grateful for the continuing support and encouragement of colleagues, family, and friends.

Contents

Contents

Detailed contents

List of abbreviations

±	with or without
<	less than
>	greater than
5-FU	Fluorouracil
AAO–HNS	American Academy of Otolaryngology – Head and Neck Surgery
ABVD	doxorubicin (Adriamycin®), bleomycin, vinblastine, dacarbazine
AC	atypical carcinoid
ACC	adenoid cystic carcinoma
ACCP	American College of Chest Physicians
ACE	angiotensin-converting enzyme
AD	autosomal dominant
ADCC	antibody dependent cell-mediated cytotoxicity
ADH	antidiuretic hormone
AED	antiepileptic drug
AFP	alpha-fetoprotein
AHP	allied health professional
AI	aromatase inhibitor
ALA	5-aminolevulinic acid
ALL	acute lymphoblastic leukemia
AML	acute myeloid leukaemia
APTT	activated partial thromboplastin time
ASCO	American Society of Clinical Oncology
ASCT	autologous stem cell transplantation
ATP	adenosine triphosphate
β-hCG	beta-human chorionic gonadotropin
BAC	bronchioloalveolar carcinoma
BBB	blood–brain barrier
BCC	basal cell carcinoma
BCG	bacillus Calmette–Guérin
BCLC	Barcelona Clinic Liver Cancer
BCNU	carmustine
BCT	breast conservation therapy
BEP	bleomycin, etoposide, cisplatin
BSC	best supportive care
BSO	bilateral salpingo-oophorectomy
CA	carbohydrate antigen
CAF	cyclophosphamide, doxorubicin, fluorouracil
CBC	complete blood count
CCA	cholangiocarcinoma
CCNU	Lomustine
CC-RCC	clear-cell renal cell carcinoma
CCyR	complete cytogenetic response
CDC	complement dependent cytotoxicity
CEA	carcinoembryonic antigen
CE-CT	contrast-enhanced computed tomography
CEF	cyclophosphamide, epirubicin, fluorouracil
CEUS	contrast-enhanced ultrasound
CHART	continuous hyperfractionated accelerated radiotherapy
CHM	complete hydatidiform mole
CHOP	cyclophosphamide, hydroxydaunorubicin (doxorubicin), Oncovin® (vincristine), and prednisone
CI	confidence interval
CIN	cervical intraepithelial neoplasia
CLL	chronic lymphocytic leukaemia
cm	centimetre(s)
CMF	cyclophosphamide, methotrexate, fluorouracil
CMFVP	cyclophosphamide, methotrexate, fluorouracil, vincristine, prednisone
CML	chronic myeloid leukaemia
CMV	cytomegalovirus
CNS	central nervous system
COPD	chronic obstructive pulmonary disease
COX	cyclo-oxygenase
CPC	choroid plexus carcinoma
CPP	choroid plexus papilloma
CR	complete remission
CRC	colorectal cancer
CRM	circumferential resection margin
CRT	chemoradiotherapy
CS	carcinosarcoma
CSF	colony-stimulating factor or cerebrospinal fluid
CSRT	craniospinal radiotherapy
CT	computed tomography
CTCAE	common terminology criteria for adverse events
CTPA	computed tomography pulmonary angiogram
CTV	clinical target volume
CUP	cancer of unknown primary
CVD	cardiovascular disease
CXR	chest X-ray
CyR	cytogenetic response
DCIS	ductal carcinoma in situ
DEC-MRI	dynamic contrast-enhanced magnetic resonance imaging
DFS	disease-free survival
DHFR	dihydrofolate reductase
DI	diabetes insipidus
DIC	disseminated intravascular coagulation
DLCL	diffuse large cell lymphoma
DLCO	diffusion lung capacity for carbon monoxide
DNA	deoxyribonucleic acid

DOH	Department of Health		GBM	glioblastoma multiforme
DRE	digital rectal examination		G-CSF	granulocyte colony stimulating factor
DVH	dose–volume histogram		GCT	granulosa cell tumour
DVT	deep vein thrombosis		GFR	glomerular filtration rate
EAC	external auditory canal		GI	gastrointestinal
EBRT	external beam radiotherapy		GIST	gastrointestinal stromal tumour
EBUS	endobronchial ultrasound		GM-CSF	granulocyte-macrophage colony stimulating factor
EBV	Epstein–Barr virus			
EC	epirubicin and cyclophosphamide		GOJ	gastro-oesophageal junction
ECOG	Eastern Cooperative Oncology Group		GORD	gastro-oesophageal reflux disease
EFRT	extended-field radiotherapy		GP	general practitioner
EFS	event-free survival		GTD	gestational trophoblastic disease
EFT	Ewing's sarcoma family of tumours		GTN	gestational trophoblastic neoplasia
EGC	early gastric cancer		GTT	gestational trophoblastic tumour
EGFR	epidermal growth factor receptor		GTV	gross target volume
EGGCT	extragonadal germ cell tumours		HAART	highly active antiretroviral therapy
EHCCA	extrahepatic cholangiocarcinoma		HADS	Hospital Anxiety and Depression Scale
EIAED	enzyme-inducing antiepileptic drug		HBIG	hepatis B immune globulin
ENT	ear, nose, and throat		HBOS	hereditary breast/ovarian cancer syndromes
EORTC	European Organisation for Research and Treatment of Cancer			
			HBV	hepatitis B virus
EPP	extrapleural pneumonectomy		HCC	hepatocellular cancer
ER	oestrogen receptor		HCD	heavy-chain disease
ERCP	endoscopic retrograde cholangiopancreatography		HCS	hereditary cancer syndrome
			HCV	hepatitis C virus
ESA	erythropoiesis stimulating agent		HD	Hodgkin disease
ESMO	European Society for Medical Oncology		HDCT	high-dose chemotherapy
ESR	erythrocyte sedimentation rate		HER	human epidermal growth factor receptor
ESS	endometrial stromal sarcoma		HIF	hypoxia-inducible factor
ES-SCLC	extensive-stage small-cell lung cancer		HIFU	high intensity frequency ultrasound
EUA	examination under anesthesia		HIT	heparin-induced thrombocytopenia
EUS	endoscopic ultrasound or endoluminal ultrasound		HIV	human immunodeficiency virus
			HNPCC	hereditary non-polyposis colorectal cancer
Fab	fragment antigen binding		HNSCC	head and neck squamous cell carcinoma
FAB	French–American–British		HPF	high power field
FAP	familial adenomatosis polyposis		HPV	human papilloma virus
FBC	full blood count		HR	hazard ratio
FDA	Food and Drug Administration		H-RS	Hodgkin and Reed–Sternberg
FDG	fludeoxyglucose (^{18}F)		HRPC	hormone resistance prostate cancer
FEV1	forced expiratory volume in 1 second		HRT	hormone replacement therapy
FFTF	freedom from treatment failure		HSCT	haematopoietic stem cell transplantation
FIGO	International Federation of Gynecology and Obstetrics		HSIL	high-grade squamous intraepithelial lesion
			HVA	homovanillic acid
FISH	fluorescent in situ hybridization		IASLC	International Association for the Study of Lung Cancer
FLIPI	Follicular Lymphoma International Prognostic Index			
			IBC	inflammatory breast cancer
FMTC	familial medullary thyroid cancer		IBD	inflammatory bowel disease
FN	febrile neutropenia		IFN	Interferon
FNA	fine needle aspiration		IFRT	involved-field radiotherapy
FNAC	fine needle aspiration cytology		Ig	immunoglobulin
FOB	faecal occult blood		IgH	immunoglobulin heavy chain
FOBT	faecal occult blood test		IGRT	image guided radiotherapy
FSH	follicle stimulating hormone		IHC	immuno-histo-chemistry
g	gram(s)			

IHCCA	intrahepatic cholangiocarcinoma		MMR	measles, mumps, rubella or mismatch repair
IJV	internal jugular vein		MMS	Mohs micrographic surgery
IL	Interleukin		MOGT	malignant ovarian germ cell tumour
IM	intramuscular		MPE	malignant pleural effusion
IMRT	intensity-modulated radiotherapy		MPM	malignant pleural mesothelioma
IMWG	International Myeloma Working Group		MPNST	malignant peripheral nerve sheath tumour
INR	international normalized ratio		MRC	Medical Research Council
IPI	International Prognostic Index		MRCP	magnetic resonance cholangiopancreatography
IPMN	intraductal papillary mucinous neoplasm		MRD	minimal residual disease
IV	intravenous		MRI	magnetic resonance imaging
IVC	inferior vena cava		MRS	magnetic resonance spectroscopy
IVF	in vitro fertilization		MSI	microsatellite instability
J	joule(s)		MRSA	Methicillin Resistant Staphylococcus Aureus
kg	kilogram(s)		MSS	microsatellite stable
KPS	Karnofsky performance status		MTC	medullary thyroid cancer
L	litre(s)		NAFLD	non-alcoholic fatty liver disease
LABC	locally advanced breast cancer		NASH	non-alcoholic steatohepatitis
LCC	large cell carcinoma		NaSSA	noradrenaline and specific serotonin antagonist
LCIS	lobular carcinoma in situ		NCCN	National Comprehensive Cancer Network
LCNEC	large-cell neuroendocrine carcinoma			
LCP	Liverpool Care Pathway for the Dying Patient		NCRI	National Cancer Research Institute
			NET	neuroendocrine tumour
LDH	lactate dehydrogenase		NF	neurofibromatosis
LEEP	loop electrosurgical excision procedure		NHL	non-Hodgkin lymphoma
LFS	Li–Fraumeni syndrome		NICE	National Institute for Health and Clinical Excellence
LH	luteinizing hormone			
LHRH	luteinizing hormone-releasing hormone		NK	natural killer
LMWH	low-molecular-weight heparin		NMDA	N-methyl-D-aspartate
LOH	loss of heterogeneity		NNT	number-needed-to-treat
LSIL	low-grade squamous intraepithelial lesion		nocte	at night
LS-SCLC	limited-stage small-cell lung cancer		NOS	not otherwise specified
MA	monoclonal antibody		NPC	nasopharyngeal carcinoma
MALT	mucosa-associated lymphoid tissue		NS	nodular-sclerosing
MBC	male breast cancer		NSAID	non-steroidal anti-inflammatory drug
MBO	malignant bowel obstruction		NSCLC	non-small cell lung cancer
MC	mixed-cellularity		NSCLC-ND	non-small cell lung carcinoma with neuroendocrine differentiation
MCC	Merkel cell carcinoma			
mcg	microgram(s)		NST	no special type
MDR	multidrug resistance		NTCP	normal tissue complication probability
MDS	myelodysplastic syndrome		OAR	organs at risk
MDT	multidisciplinary team		OD	once daily
MDU	Medical Defence Union		OGCT	ovarian germ cell tumour
MEDD	morphine equivalent daily dose		OGD	oesophago-gastro-duodenoscopy
MEN	multiple endocrine neoplasia		ONS	Office for National Statistics
MF	mycosis fungoides		OPG	optic pathway glioma
MG	myasthenia gravis		OPSI	overwhelming postsplenectomy infection
MGCT	malignant germ cell tumour		OR	odds ratio
MGUS	monoclonal gammopathy of undetermined significance		OS	overall survival
			PARP	poly (ADP-ribose) polymerase
MIBG	metaiodobenzylguanidine		PCI	prophylactic cranial irradiation
mL	millilitre(s)		PCNSL	primary malignant central nervous system lymphoma
mm	millimetre(s)			
MMC	mitomycin-C			

PCR	polymerase chain reaction		SMI	small molecular inhibitor
PCV	procarbazine, CCNU, and vincristine		SMM	smouldering multiple myeloma
PD	pharmacodynamic *or* progressive disease		SMR	standardized mortality ratio
PDGFR	platelet-derived growth factor receptor		SNB	sentinel node biopsy
PDT	photodynamic therapy		SNRI	serotonin-noradrenergic reuptake inhibitor
PE	pulmonary embolism		SNUC	sinonasal undifferentiated carcinoma
PEG	percutaneous endoscopic gastrostomy		SS	Sézary syndrome
PET	positron emission tomography		SSI	selective serotonin antagonist
PFS	progression-free survival		SSRI	selective serotonin reuptake inhibitor
PG	pepsinogen		STI	signal transduction inhibitor
PgR	progesterone receptor		SVC	superior vena cava
PICC	peripherally inserted central catheter		TACE	transarterial chemoembolization
PK	pharmacokinetic		TAE	transarterial embolization
PKC	protein kinase C		TAH	total abdominal hysterectomy
PNET	primitive neuroectodermal tumor		TC	testicular cancer *or* typical carcinoid
PO	by mouth (per os)		TCC	transitional cell carcinoma
PR	partial remission		TCP	tumour control probability
PRN	as required		TDS	three times daily
PS	performance status		TENS	transcutaneous electrical nerve stimulation
PSA	prostate-specific antigen		TIN	testicular intraepithelial neoplasia
PSC	primary sclerosing cholangitis		TK	tyrosine kinase
PSTT	placental site trophoblastic tumour		TNF	tumour necrosis factor
PT	prothrombin time		TRAM	transverse rectus abdominis myocutaneous
PTD	persistent trophoblastic disease		TRUS	transrectal ultrasound
PTHrP	parathyroid hormone-related peptide		TSH	thyroid stimulating hormone
PTL	primary thyroid lymphomas		TTP	time-to-progression
PTSD	post-traumatic stress disorder		TURB	transurethral resection of the bladder
PTV	planning target volume		TURP	transurethral resection of the prostate
QDS	four times daily		UC	ulcerative colitis
QoL	quality of life		UFH	unfractionated heparin
RCC	renal cell carcinoma		UICC	International Union against Cancer
RF	radiofrequency		UK	United Kingdom
RFA	radiofrequency ablation		USA	United States of America
RIC	reduced-intensity conditioning		USO	unilateral salpingo-oophorectomy
RIT	radioimmunotherapy		UV	ultraviolet
RP	radical prostatectomy		VAD	vascular access device
RR	relative risk		VATS	video-assisted thoracoscopic surgery
RT-PCR	reverse transcriptase polymerase chain reaction		VEGF	vascular endothelial growth factor
SaO2	arterial oxygen saturation		VHL	von Hippel–Lindau
SAR	specific absorption rate		VIN	vulval intraepithelial neoplasia
SBA	small bowel adenocarcinoma		VMA	vanillylmandelic acid
SC	subcutaneous		VRE	vancomycin-resistant enterococci
SCC	squamous cell carcinoma		VTE	venous thromboembolism
SCM	sternocleidomastoid		WBC	white blood cell
SCST	sex cord-stromal tumour		WBRT	whole brain radiotherapy
SCTAT	sex cord tumour with annular tubules		WCC	white cell count
SD	stable disease		WE	wide excision
SEER	Surveillance, Epidemiology, and End Results		WHO	World Health Organization
SERM	selective oestrogen receptor modulator		WLE	wide local excision
SFT	solitary fibrous tumour			

List of contributors

Dr T. Ajithkumar
Consultant Clinical Oncologist
Norfolk and Norwich University Hospital
Norwich, UK

Mr M. Alazzam
Subspecialty Fellow in
Gynaecological Oncology
Sheffield Gynaecological Cancer Centre, Royal
Hallamshire Hospital, Sheffield, UK

C. Ang
Northern Gynaecological Oncology Centre, Queen
Elizabeth Hospital, Gateshead, UK

Professor A. Barrett
Emeritus Professor of Oncology,
University of East Anglia,
Norwich, UK

Dr M. Beresford
Consultant Clinical Oncologist
Bristol Haematology and
Oncology Centre, Bristol, UK

Dr S. Biswas
Clinical Senior Lecturer and Honorary Consultant in
Medical Oncology
Newcastle University & Northern
Centre for Cancer Care (NCCC),
Sir Bobby Robson Clinical Trials Unit, Freeman Hospital,
Newcastle-Upon-Tyne, UK

Dr T. Branson
Consultant Clinical Oncologist,
Northern Centre for Cancer Care,
The Freeman Hospital,
Newcastle upon Tyne, UK

Dr P. Brock
Consultant Paediatric Oncologist
Great Ormond Street Hospital for Children NHS Trust
and Institute of Child Health
Great Ormond Street, London, UK

Dr N. Cook
Specialist Registrar in Medical Oncology,
Addenbrookes Hospital,
Cambridge, UK

R. Cooper
Consultant Clinical Oncologist
St James's Institute of Oncology, Leeds, UK

Dr E. Copson
Consultant Medical Oncologist
Southampton Oncology Centre, Southampton General
Hospital,
Southampton, UK

B. Davidson
Consultant Surgeon,
Royal Free Hospital
And
Professor of Surgery, UCL, London, UK

J. Davies
Consultant Colorectal Surgeon
Bradford Royal Infirmary
Bradford, UK

Dr B. Dezube
Beth Israel Deaconess Medical Centre
Boston, MA, USA

K. Dinshaw
Tata Memorial Hospital,
Mumbai, India

M. Eadens
Division of Medical Oncology
Mayo Clinic
Rochester, Minnesota, USA

E. Edwards
Cancer Genetic Counsellor
Wessex Clinical Genetics Service,
Princess Anne Hospital,
Southampton, UK

Professor T. Eisen
Professor of Medical Oncology
University of Cambridge
Department of Oncology,
Addenbrooke's Hospital,
Cambridge, UK

Professor A. Engert
German Hodgkin Study Group/
Dept. I of Internal Medicine,
University Hospital Cologne, Germany

Professor E. Ernst
Laing Chair of Complementary Medicine
Complementary Medicine, Peninsula Medical School,
University of Exeter,
Devon, UK

Professor M. Fallon
St Columba's Hospice Chair of
Palliative Medicine
University of Edinburgh, Edinburgh Cancer Research
Centre (CRUK), Western General Hospital,
Edinburgh, UK

Dr D. Ford
Consultant Clinical Oncologist
Cancer Centre, Queen Elizabeth Hospital,
Birmingham, UK

Professor S. D. Fosså
Professor, Senior consultant
Department of Oncology,
Oslo University Hospital and
University of Oslo,
Montebello, Norway

Dr I. Geh
Consultant Clinical Oncologist
Cancer Centre, Queen Elizabeth Hospital,
Birmingham, UK

Dr P. Ghaneh
Clinical Senior Lecturer
Division of Surgery and Oncology, University of Liverpool,
Liverpool, UK

Dr N. Goulden
Consultant Haematologist
Great Ormond St Hospital,
London, UK

I. Gounaris
Specialist Registrar in Medical Oncology
Department of Oncology,
Cambridge University NHS Trust,
Addenbrookes Hospital, Cambridge, UK

Dr D. Gregory
Consultant Clinical Oncologist
Addenbrookes Hospital, Cambridge, UK

J. Griffin
Specialist Registrar in Haematology
Bristol Haematology and Oncology Centre,
Bristol, UK

Professor B.W. Hancock
Emeritus Professor of Medical Oncology
Weston Park Hospital, Sheffield, UK

Dr H. Hatcher
Senior Lecturer and Honorary Consultant Medical
Oncologist,
University of Cambridge,
Cambridge, UK

P. Hatfield
Consultant Clinical Oncologist
St James's Institute of Oncology, Leeds, UK

M. Hingorani
Consultant Clinical Oncologist,
Castle Hill Hospital, Hull, UK

Dr C. Holland
Clinical Lecturer
University of Manchester,
Academic Unit of Gynaecology, School of Cancer and
Enabling Sciences, and
Honorary Consultant in Gynaecological Oncology
St Marys Hospital, Manchester, UK

J. Hook
Specialist Registrar in Medical Oncology
St James's Institute of Oncology, Leeds, UK

Dr S. Jefferies
Consultant Clinical Oncologist
Addenbrooke's Hospital, Cambridge, UK

Professor I. Judson
Consultant Medical Oncologist
Head of Sarcoma Unit, Royal Marsden Hospital,
London, UK

Professor S. Kaye
CRUK Professor of Medical Oncology,
Head, Section of Medicine,
Institute of Cancer Research,
Head, Drug Development Unit, Royal Marsden Hospital,
Royal Marsden Hospital, Surrey, UK

Dr B. Klimm
German Hodgkin Study Group/
Dept. I of Internal Medicine,
University Hospital Cologne,
Germany

Dr B. Laird
Clinician Scientist in Palliative Medicine,
University of Edinburgh, Honorary Consultant in
Palliative Medicine, Beatson West of Scotland
Cancer Centre, Glasgow and the Edinburgh
Cancer Centre, Edinburgh, UK

G. Lehne
Senior Consultant
Department of Oncology, Norwegian Radium Hospital,
Oslo University Hospital, Montebello, Norway

Dr E. Macdonald
Consultant Clinical Oncologist
Consultant Emeritus Guys Hospital
London, UK

Dr U. Mahantshetty
Assistant Professor,
Department of Radiation Oncology,
Member: Gynae Working Group,
Tata Memorial Hospital, India

Professor D. Marks
Professor of Haematology and Stem cell transplantation
Bristol BMT Unit, University Hospitals Bristol,
Bristol, UK

Dr P. Mehta
Consultant Haematologist
University Hospitals Bristol NHS Foundation Trust,
Bristol, UK

C. Messina
Specialist Registrar in Medical Oncology
San Camillo Forlanini Hospital,
Rome, Italy

Dr R. Muirhead
Clinical Research Fellow in Clinical Oncology
Beatson West of Scotland Cancer Centre,
Glasgow, UK

Mr R. Naik
Consultant & Clinical Director,
Northern Gynaecological Oncology Centre,
Queen Elizabeth Hospital, Gateshead, UK

Professor J. Neoptolemos
The Owen and Ellen Evans Chair of Cancer Studies
The Liverpool Cancer Research UK Centre, Head of
School of Cancer Studies, Head Division of Surgery and
Oncology, Liverpool, UK

Dr S. Neumann
Specialist Registrar
Hematology and Oncology, University of Goettingen,
Goettingen, Germany

Dr S. Nicum
Consultant Medical Oncologist
University of Oxford Department of Medical Oncology,
Oxford, UK

J. Oldenburg
Department of Oncology, Oslo University Hospital,
Oslo, Norway

V. Pamecha
University Department of Surgery,
Royal Free Hospital, London, UK

Dr L. Pantanowitz
Assistant Professor of Pathology
Tufts University School of Medicine,
Department of Pathology, Baystate Medical Centre,
Springfield, MA, USA

A. Pardanani
Consultant
Division of Hematology, Mayo Clinic,
Rochester, Minnesota, USA

Dr C. Parkinson
Clinical Lecturer in Medical Oncology
Addenbrooke's Hospital, Cambridge, UK

Professor N. Pavlidis
Professor of Medical Oncology
Department of Medical Oncology, Medical School,
University of Ioannina, Greece

Dr A. Pender
Clinical Fellow
Tuveson Laboratory, CRUK Cambridge Research
Institute, Cambridge, UK

G. Pentheroudakis
Assistant Professor in Medical Oncology
School of Medicine, University of Ioannina, Greece

Dr B. Pizer
Consultant Paediatric Oncologist
Oncology Unit, Alder Hey Children's Hospital,
Liverpool, UK

Dr R. Protheroe
Consultant in Haematology and Bone Marrow
Transplantation
Department of Adult Bone Marrow Transplantation
Bristol Royal Hospital for Children, Bristol,
UK

Dr A. Qureshi
Consultant Paediatric Haematologist
Children's Hospital, John Radcliffe Infirmary,
Oxford, UK

Dr K. Raj
Consultant Haematologist
Guys and St Thomas' NHS Foundation Trust,
London, UK

S.V. Rajkumar
Professor of Medicine
Chair, Myeloma Amyloidosis Dysproteinemia Group
Division of Hematology, Mayo Clinic, Rochester,
Minnesota, USA

Professor R. Rampling
Beatson West of Scotland Cancer Centre
Glasgow, UK

Dr D. Sebag-Montefiore
Professor of Clinical Oncology,
St James's Institute of Oncology, Leeds, UK

Professor S. Senan
Professor of clinical experimental radiotherapy
Department of Radiation Oncology
VU University Medical Center, Amsterdam
The Netherlands

Dr N. Slevin
Consultant Clinical Oncologist
The Christie, Manchester, UK

S.K. Srivastava
Professor & Head of Department of Radiation Oncology
Tata Memorial Hospital
Mumbai, India

C. Sternberg
Chief, Department of Medical Oncology,
San Camillo Forlanini Hospital,
Rome, Italy

D. Swinson
Consultant Medical Oncologist
St James's Institute of Oncology
St James's University Hospital
Leeds, UK

Professor R. Thomas
Visiting Professor
Cranfield University, Consultant Clinical Oncologist
Bedford and Addenbrooke's Hospitals, Addenbrooke's
Hospital Cambridge University Trust, Cambridge, UK

X. Thomas
Praticien Hospitalier
Hematology Department, Leukemia Unit, Edouard
Herriot Hospital, Hospices Civils de Lyon
Lyon, France

H.B. Tongaonkar
Professor & Head Urologic and Gynaecologic Services
Department of Surgical Oncology
Tata memorial Hospital
Mumbai, India

Professor L. Trümper
Consultant, Head of Department
Hematology and Oncology,
University of Goettingen, Goettingen, Germany

Dr N. Walji
Consultant Clinical Oncologist
University Hospitals Coventry
Warwickshire NHS Trust, Coventry, UK

Chapter 1

Introduction

An approach to the oncology consultation

It is important to have a good structure for the oncological consultation to ensure holistic care for the patient and efficient completion of administrative tasks.

Assess starting position

Patients may have been seen already by other healthcare professionals and have undergone a number of investigations. They may or may not have received the results of these. They may have some knowledge of the diagnosis, prognosis, and treatment options. Following appropriate introductions it is important to assess the patient's current understanding of the situation.

Establish rapport

For most patients the initial consultation is the beginning of a long-term relationship with the oncologist, and it is therefore essential to make the patient feel that their ideas, concerns, and expectations have been understood clearly. Adequate time must therefore be invested in this first meeting.

Collect information

Although the patient has already told their story to others, it is useful for them to say again in their own words what took them to the doctor and what has happened subsequently. Patients' recall of facts may be impaired at presentation because of anxiety and they may remember relevant facts which can contribute to further decision making (e.g. growth rate of the tumour may be deduced from the pattern of development of symptoms).

Clinical examination

Findings from previous examination should be confirmed, since changes may have occurred since presentation. Systematic examination is important to help to decide appropriate treatment and to act as a baseline, since cancer treatment can affect normal organ function.

Review imaging, staging information, and risk factors

Before treatment decisions can be made, investigations should be reviewed and any additional staging tests carried out. Stage of tumour, histological findings including any prognostic factors, and performance status should be recorded.

Consider relevant protocols and trials

Taking into account stage, prognosis, performance status, and comorbidities, treatment options as specified in departmental or national protocols or randomized trials should be considered.

Agree treatment plan

Treatment options should be presented to the patient with the benefits and risks of treatment and expected outcomes. Where there are treatments of proven benefit, a clear recommendation from the doctor is helpful. Where a number of equally effective treatments are available and urgent treatment is not essential, further written information may be given and discussion continued at a subsequent consultation. Although family and friends may be involved in the discussion, the final decision must rest with the patient.

Obtain consent

Written consent for the agreed treatment should be obtained prior to starting treatment.

Discuss patient concerns

Time to discuss any concerns or anxieties should be made in the first and every subsequent consultation. Patients should be encouraged to express their concerns in spite of pressures of consultation time and reluctance to bother the doctor.

Signpost to other sources of support

Since patient need for information and psychological support cannot be met in a single consultation, written information should be given to supplement that given verbally. It is helpful to indicate other sources of support especially for practical issues such as finance, work, and housing (see Chapter 6.5).

Carers and family members may also need access to these sources of support.

Communicate to relevant others

Good documentation of the consultation should be shared with the patient's general practitioner and other involved health professionals. A letter to the patient summarizing the discussion with the doctor is helpful for some patients and should be offered.

Useful resources

General information for patients can be found in sections in Chapter 6, Special situations in oncology. Resources for clinicians are detailed in site-specific chapters.

Chapter 2

Clinical approach to suspected cancer

Lung cancer

Risk factors
- Smokers—current, previous, and those with smoking associated chronic obstructive pulmonary disease (COPD)
- Exposure to asbestos
- Previous head and neck or lung cancer

Warning features
- Persistent chest symptoms lasting >3 weeks
- Unexplained weight loss
- Haemoptysis

Indication for emergency referral
Acute admission and evaluation is recommended for the following:
- Stridor
- Features of superior vena caval obstruction

Indications for urgent referral
National Institute for Health and Clinical Excellence (NICE) recommendations for urgent referral for a chest X-ray (CXR) and/or further evaluation to rule out lung cancer include:
- Haemoptysis—persistent in a smoker or ex-smoker >40 years old
- The following unexplained features lasting for >3 weeks:
  - Respiratory features—cough, chest signs, dyspnoea
  - Pain—chest and/or shoulder

- Weight loss
- Hoarseness
- Lymphadenopathy—neck or supraclavicular nodes
- Finger clubbing
- Features of metastatic disease (brain, bone, liver, etc.)

Investigations of suspected lung cancer
CXR is the initial investigation of choice for all patients with suspected lung cancer. It is also indicated in patients with chronic chest problems with changes in existing symptoms. All patients with abnormal CXR should be referred to a chest physician for further evaluation. Patients with normal CXR but with a high suspicion of lung cancer need computed tomography (CT) scan of the chest and upper abdomen.

All patients with chest infection with an associated radiological abnormality need a further CXR 6 weeks after completion of antibiotic treatment to confirm resolution of the abnormality. This is because infection can sometimes be due to an obstructive growth.

Internet resources
NICE: The diagnosis and treatment of lung cancer—available at: http://www.nice.org.uk/nicemedia/pdf/cg024fullguideline.pdf

NICE referral guidelines for suspected cancer—available at: http://guidance.nice.org.uk/CG27/NICEGuidance/pdf/English

Breast cancer

Indications for urgent referral

NICE recommendations for urgent referral for suspected breast cancer are as follows:
- Discrete breast lump in postmenopausal women
- Discrete lump persisting after next menstrual period in women aged ≥30 years
- Lump with fixation with or without skin tethering or ulceration
- Spontaneous unilateral bloody nipple discharge
- Recent nipple retraction or distortion (within 3 months)
- Nipple eczema
- New breast lump in women who have previous history of breast cancer
- Men aged ≥50 years with firm subareolar mass with or without skin changes or nipple distortion

Indications for non-urgent referral

NICE recommends non-urgent referral for women aged <30 years presenting with:
- Enlarging breast lump
- Hard and fixed breast lumps

Indications for emergency referral
- Patients presenting with features of impending or actual spinal cord compression
- Patients presenting with features of brain metastasis

Investigations of suspected breast cancer

All patients with suspected breast cancer should undergo 'triple' assessment in a one-stop clinic. Triple assessment consists of clinical, radiological (mammogram and/or ultrasound), and pathological assessment (core biopsy).

Internet resource

NICE referral guidelines for suspected cancer—available from: http://guidance.nice.org.uk/CG27/Guidance/pdf/English

Urological cancer

Warning features
Warning features of urological cancers include:
- Lower urinary tract symptoms
- I laematuria
- Suspicious lumps
- Bone pain

Indication for emergency referral
All patients presenting with features of impending or actual spinal cord compression, a presentation common in disseminated prostate cancer, need emergency evaluation (within 24 hours).

Indications for urgent referral
Renal and urinary bladder cancer
Patients presenting with the following features need urgent referral to rule out renal and bladder cancers:
- Macroscopic haematuria with or without associated urinary infection
- Microscopic haematuria in adults aged ≥50 years
- Recurrent or persistent urinary infection with haematuria in adults aged ≥40 years
- Clinical or radiological evidence of an abdominal mass suggesting renal or bladder cancer

Prostate cancer
- Patients presenting with obstructive or low urinary tract symptoms suggesting prostate cancer
- Progressive rise in prostate-specific antigen (PSA) or raised PSA
- Symptomatic patients with high PSA (>50)
- Men with hard and irregular prostate on rectal examination
- Patients with any of the following unexplained symptoms:
  - Haematuria
  - Erectile dysfunction
- Lower back and bone pain
- Weight loss

Testicular cancer
- Any patient with swelling or lump in the body of testis
- Any scrotal swelling which is not diagnostic of hernla and/or when the body of the testis cannot be distinguished
- Unexplained persistent lower thoracic/upper lumbar pain in a young man (arising from lymph node enlargement)

Penile cancer
Progressive ulceration or a mass in the glans or prepuce.

Indications for non-urgent referral
Patients with features of lower urinary tract infection, especially recurrent, need evaluation to rule out urological cancer.

Investigations of suspected urological cancer
Patients presenting with features suggestive of lower urinary tract infection should have investigations to rule out infection. In those with infection, serum PSA is only estimated at least 1 month after treatment of the infection. Initial investigations for suspected prostate cancer include serum PSA estimation and digital rectal examination.

Evaluation for haematuria includes clinical examination, urine testing, flexible cystoscopy, ultrasound, and intravenous urography.

Patients with a testicular mass on clinical examination and ultrasound need assays for serum alpha-fetoprotein (AFP), beta-human chorionic gonadotropin (β-hCG), and lactate dehydrogenase (LDH). Abdominal CT scan will show lymphadenopathy. Studies have shown that delay in instituting appropriate treatment for testicular cancer, especially in those with metastatic disease, can compromise survival.

Internet resource
NICE referral guidelines for suspected cancer—available from: http://guidance.nice.org.uk/CG27/Guidance/pdf/English

Nervous system tumours

Warning signs of brain tumours

For primary brain tumours these features include:

1. Central nervous system (CNS) symptoms such as:
- Any progressive neurological deficit
- Seizure of recent onset
- New onset of severe headaches for which there is no obvious other explanation
- Changes in personality or behaviour
- Cranial nerve palsies
- Unilateral deafness
2. Headaches of recent onset with features of raised intracranial pressure such as vomiting, or positional exacerbation, such as being worse in the morning.
3. Ataxia and head tilt can be associated with posterior fossa tumours in children.

Risk factors

High-grade tumours may present with rapidly deteriorating symptoms but in other cases, the onset of symptoms may be more insidious.

Patients with rapid progression of any of these symptoms and no known cancer diagnosis should be referred urgently to a neurologist for full neurological examination and investigation which will include CT and/or magnetic resonance imaging (MRI) scanning. Lesions in the posterior fossa are more readily seen with MRI than CT.

Patients who present with seizures should have a full history taken and an account of the seizures should be sought from an eyewitness. Physical examination should exclude cardiac, neurological, and mental state abnormalities. A referral to a neurologist urgently or electively depending on other clinical findings is appropriate.

Neurosurgical services are centralized and will be accessed by the CNS multidisciplinary team (MDT) after appropriate imaging and discussion. Biopsy is undertaken only by the neurosurgeon.

Direct referral to an oncologist

Patients who have previously been treated for cancers at other sites may present with the same symptoms if they develop metastatic disease and direct referral to the oncologist who has previously treated them may be appropriate for consideration of palliative radiotherapy.

Warning features of spinal cord compression

Patients with a history of cancer, especially those with a high risk of bone metastases (e.g. prostate, breast cancer etc.) and those with primary spinal cord tumours can present with the following features suggestive of spinal cord compression which needs urgent evaluation (within 24 hours):

- Pain in the thoracic or cervical spine region
- Progressive or severe unremitting pain in the lumbosacral region
- Spinal pain aggravated by straining
- Nocturnal spinal pain preventing sleep
- Pain associated with weakness, sensory symptoms, or sphincter dysfunction

Patients with known or suspected cancer with the following features suggestive of spinal cord compression need emergency evaluation:

- Radicular pain
- Limb weakness
- Sensory symptoms
- Bladder or bowel dysfunction
- Signs of cauda equina or spinal cord compression

The aim after emergency evaluation is to start appropriate treatment of spinal cord compression within 24 hours of referral which offers the best chance of maintaining the ability to walk and functional independence.

Internet resources

Brain and CNS cancer: NICE quick reference guide for suspected cancer, pp.21–2—available at http://guidance.nice.org.uk/CG27/QuickRefGuide/pdf/English

CancerHelp UK: types of brain tumour—available at http://www.cancerhelp.org.uk/type/brain-tumour/index.htm

NICE guideline: metastatic spinal cord compression—available at: http://guidance.nice.org.uk/CG75/NICEGuidance/pdf/English

NICE referral guidelines for suspected cancer—available at: http://guidance.nice.org.uk/CG27/NICEGuidance/pdf/English

Upper gastrointestinal cancer

Risk factors
- Barrett's oesophagus
- Known dysplasia, atrophic gastritis, or intestinal metaplasia
- Peptic ulcer surgery >20 years ago
- Achalasia
- Family history of upper gastrointestinal (GI) cancer in more than one first-degree relative
- Smoking
- Alcohol

Warning features
- Dysphagia
- Dyspepsia combined with one or more of these alarm symptoms:
  - Weight loss
  - Anaemia
  - Anorexia

Indication for urgent referral/endoscopy
NICE have laid down recommendations for urgent referral (<2 weeks) of patients based on common presenting symptoms. *Helicobacter pylori* status should not affect the decision to refer for suspected cancer. In patients aged <55 years, endoscopic investigation of dyspepsia is not necessary in the absence of warning symptoms.

An urgent referral for endoscopy or to a specialist with expertise in upper GI cancer should be made for patients of any age with dyspepsia who present with any of the following:
- Chronic GI bleeding
- Dysphagia
- Progressive unintentional weight loss
- Persistent vomiting
- Iron deficiency anaemia
- Epigastric mass
- Suspicious barium meal result
- Jaundice

In patients 55 years of age and older with unexplained and persistent recent-onset dyspepsia alone, an urgent referral for endoscopy should be made.

In patients without dyspepsia, but with unexplained weight loss or iron deficiency anaemia, the possibility of upper GI cancer should be recognized and an urgent referral for further investigation considered.

An urgent referral should be made for patients presenting with either:
- Unexplained upper abdominal pain and weight loss, with or without back pain, or
- An upper abdominal mass without dyspepsia

Patients being referred urgently for endoscopy should ideally be free from acid suppression medication, including proton pump inhibitors, for a minimum of 2 weeks.

Investigations of suspected upper GI cancer
All patients with new-onset dyspepsia should be considered for a full blood count in order to detect iron deficiency anaemia.

Flexible oesophago-gastro-duodenoscopy (OGD) is the diagnostic procedure of choice

Double contrast barium studies have a continuous but limited role in detecting malignant lesions and some early gastric cancers when endoscopy is not feasible

Endoscopic ultrasound (EUS) combines high-frequency ultrasonography with OGD and provides a more accurate prediction of depth of tumour invasion, particularly in early cancers.

A staging CT scan of the thorax, abdomen, and pelvis is recommended routinely in all patients to demonstrate the size of the primary tumour and its relationship with adjacent organs as well as any enlarged lymph nodes.

Patients should have endoscopic-guided biopsy to establish a diagnosis of upper GI cancer.

Indications for urgent referral
Patients should be discussed in the MDT meetings and referred for an oncology opinion when radiology and histology have been reviewed.

Further reading
Allum WH *et al.* Guidelines for the management of oesophageal and gastric cancer. *Gut* 2002; **50**(suppl V): v1–v23

Internet resource
NICE referral guidelines for suspected cancer—available at: http://guidance.nice.org.uk/CG27/NICEGuidance/pdf/English

Lower gastrointestinal cancer

Risk factors
- Familial adenomatosis polyposis (FAP)
- Hereditary non-polyposis colorectal cancer (HNPCC)
- Personal or family history of sporadic cancers or adenomatous polyps
- Inflammatory bowel disease
- Alcohol
- Obesity
- Cigarette smoking
- Ureterocolic anastomoses
- Acromegaly

Warning features
- Abdominal pain
- Change in bowel habit
- Haematochezia or melaena
- Weakness
- Anaemia without other GI symptoms
- Weight loss

Indications for urgent referral
NICE and the Department of Health have laid down guidelines for urgent referral (<2 weeks) of patients based on common presenting symptoms (NICE 2004). When these symptom and sign combinations occur for the first time in any patient, he or she should be referred to a colorectal cancer diagnostic service as an urgent case under the 2-week standard:
- Rectal bleeding with a change in bowel habit
- Looser stools and/or increased frequency of defaecation persistent for 6 weeks
- A definite palpable right-sided abdominal mass
- A definite palpable rectal (not pelvic) mass
- Rectal bleeding and persistent anal symptoms in those >60 years
- Change of bowel habit to looser stools and/or increased in those >60 years
- Frequency of defaecation, without rectal bleeding, persistent for 6 weeks
- Iron deficiency anaemia without an obvious cause, no age criterion

Regular colonoscopy is recommended for people in high-risk groups (FAP, HNPCC, long-standing history of inflammatory bowel disease, previous colorectal cancer, and polyps), but the frequency with which this should be carried out depends on the particular condition.

Indication for non-urgent referral
Patients with the following symptoms and no abdominal or rectal mass are at low risk of cancer:
- Rectal bleeding with anal symptoms
- Change in bowel habit to decreased frequency of defaecation and harder stools
- Abdominal pain without clear evidence of intestinal obstruction

Investigations of suspected lower GI cancer
- Endoscopy (flexible sigmoidoscopy or colonoscopy)
- Imaging (barium enema and CT, including CT colonography)
- If suspected rectal cancer then MRI is also required
- Patients require bowel preparation for any of these methods to produce accurate results
- Patients should have endoscopic-guided biopsy to establish a diagnosis of colon cancer

Referral to oncology
Patients should be discussed in the MDT meetings and referred for oncology opinion when radiology and histology have been reviewed.

Internet resource
NICE (2004). Improving Outcomes in Colorectal Cancers. Manual Update—available at: http://www.nice.org.uk/Guidance/CSGCC/Guidance/pdf/

Gynaecological cancer

Warning symptoms

The following warning symptoms necessitate a full pelvic examination (including a speculum examination):

- Postmenopausal bleeding
- Postcoital bleeding
- Intermenstrual bleeding
- Vaginal discharge
- Alterations in the menstrual cycles
- Persistent unexplained non-specific abdominal or urinary symptoms

Indications for urgent referral

NICE recommendations for urgent referral for suspected gynaecological cancer are as follows:

- Suspicious cervical lesion on speculum examination
- Ultrasound examination suggestive of abdominal or pelvic mass of gynaecological origin
- Palpable abdominal or pelvic mass not suggestive of fibroid

- Postmenopausal bleeding in a woman who is not on hormone replacement therapy (HRT)
- Postmenopausal bleeding persisting 6 weeks after cessation of HRT
- Postmenopausal bleeding in a woman taking tamoxifen
- Unexplained vulval lump or vulval ulceration with bleeding

Indication for emergency referral

- Patient presenting with acute abdomen

Investigations of suspected gynaecological cancer

All patients with suspected gynaecological cancer should have full examination including pelvic examination and speculum examination.

Internet resource

NICE referral guidelines for suspected cancer—available at: http://guidance.nice.org.uk/CG27/NICEGuidance/pdf/English

Haematological cancer

Warning features

A number of features or combinations of features suggest the possibility of a haematological malignancy that requires further investigation. These features are the consequence of bone marrow suppression, or extramedullary haematopoiesis, lymphadenopathy, and hepato- or splenomegaly.

- Features of bone marrow suppression:
  - Fatigue, breathlessness (anaemia)
  - Recurrent infection (white cell abnormality)
  - Bruising and bleeding (low platelets)
- Extramedullary haemopoiesis:
  - Splenomegaly and hypersplenism
- Lymphadenopathy (>1cm) particularly with the following features:
  - Persists for ≥6 weeks
  - Generalized in nature
  - Size >2cm
  - Increasing in size
  - Associated with B symptoms (fever, night sweats, and weight loss)
  - Associated with hepatomegaly, and/or splenomegaly
- General features:
  - B symptoms (fever, drenching night sweats, and weight loss)
  - Generalized itching
  - Bone pain
  - Alcohol induced pain in lymph nodes

Indications for immediate referral

Patients with a blood count or blood film suggesting acute leukaemia, and spinal cord compression or renal failure (which occurs in myeloma) require immediate referral for further evaluation.

Indications for urgent referral

All patients with persistent unexplained splenomegaly need urgent referral. In other patients, the urgency of referral depends on the severity of symptoms and the findings of initial investigations. In general the following features suggest the need for urgent referral:

- Lymphadenopathy persisting for >6 weeks
- Hepatosplenomegaly
- Bone pain associated with anaemia and raised erythrocyte sedimentation rate (ESR)
- Bone X-ray suggesting myeloma (widespread lytic changes)
- Any feature suggesting bone marrow suppression

Investigations of suspected haematological cancer

Initial investigations of patients with unexplained fatigue, unexplained lymphadenopathy, bleeding manifestations, and unexplained persistent bone pain should include a full blood count, blood film, and ESR, plasma viscosity or C-reactive protein. Patients with bleeding manifestations need a clotting screen. Patients with bone pain also need estimation of urea and electrolytes, liver function tests, bone profile, and in males serum PSA.

Internet resource

NICE referral guidelines for suspected cancer—available at: http://guidance.nice.org.uk/CG27/NICEGuidance/pdf/English

Head and neck cancer

Warning features

Warning features of head and neck cancers include:
• Neck swelling persisting for >6 weeks
• Oral symptoms persisting for >3–6 weeks
• Hoarseness persisting for >3 weeks
• Unexplained and persistent (>4 weeks) unilateral pain

Indication for emergency referral

All patients presenting with acute shortness of breath suggesting stridor or tracheal obstruction need emergency evaluation (within 24 hours).

Indications for urgent referral

NICE recommendations for urgent referral are as follows:
• Oral cavity symptoms or signs persisting for >6 weeks
• Patients with unexplained red and white oral mucosal patches associated with pain, bleeding, or swelling.
• Unexplained persistent (>3 weeks) mass or ulcer of oral mucosa
• Hoarseness of voice persisting for >3 weeks particularly in heavy drinkers and smokers aged ≥50 years
• Unexplained persistent (>3 weeks) loose tooth
• Recent lump in the neck or a previous lump which has changed over the preceding 3–6 weeks
• Unexplained persistent throat pain, unilateral head and neck pain (of >4 weeks), and/or earache

• Unexplained persistent parotid swelling or swelling in the submandibular region
• Dysphagia persisting for >3 weeks
• Unilateral nasal obstruction particularly with purulent discharge
• Cranial nerve paralysis
• Orbital swelling

Indications for non-urgent referral

Patients who present with red and white oral mucosal patches without associated pain, swelling, or bleeding need non-urgent referral for further evaluation. Those with confirmed oral lichen planus need routine monitoring to rule out oral cancer.

Investigations of suspected head and neck cancer

Investigations of patients with suspected head and neck cancer are undertaken by a multidisciplinary head and neck team. Investigations depend on the site of suspected disease and include clinical examination, flexible or rigid endoscopy, and imaging. All patients with hoarseness of voice need urgent CXR.

Internet resource

NICE referral guidelines for suspected cancer—available at: http://guidance.nice.org.uk/CG27/NICEGuidance/pdf/English

Thyroid cancer

Indication for emergency referral

Patients presenting with features of stridor due to thyroid swelling need emergency evaluation and management.

Indications for urgent referral

NICE recommends urgent referral for all patients presenting with a thyroid swelling associated with any of the following features:
• Enlarging solitary nodule
• Unexplained hoarseness
• Associated neck node enlargement
• Those with family history of endocrine tumour(s)
• Prepubertal patients
• Patients aged ≥65 years
• Patients with previous history of neck irradiation

Investigations of suspected thyroid cancer

The initial investigations include thyroid function tests and estimation of serum thyroglobulin. Further investigations are undertaken by a MDT and these include ultrasound, isotope scanning, and CT and/or MRI scans.

Internet resource

NICE referral guidelines for suspected cancer—available at: http://guidance.nice.org.uk/CG27/NICEGuidance/pdf/English

Bone cancer and sarcoma

Warning features

For primary bone tumours, these features include:
- Bone pain at rest, especially if worsening or no improvement over a number of weeks
- Pain not responding to simple analgesia and limiting normal activities in a young person under 25
- Strong family history of cancers, especially breast and sarcomas
- Bone pain in combination with systemic features
- Hot swollen area overlying bone or close to a joint

For soft tissue sarcomas the risk factors are:
- >5cm in size
- Rapid growth in size
- Deep to the deep fascia
- Painful

Indication for urgent X-ray

Any of the warning features noted earlier. These must be clearly stated in the request.

Extreme care must be taken to ensure the correct bone(s) and joint are included in the X-ray. A significant number of delays in diagnosis are due to inappropriately reported 'normal' X-rays, either because the incorrect area was imaged or it was viewed without appropriate clinical information or by someone inexperienced in the imaging of bone tumours.

Remember when deciding upon which area to X-ray to consider that the pain may be felt in one part of the bone but referred from another area.

Indications for urgent referral

Any isolated bone lesion or clinically detectable bone mass which is unlikely to be due to another cause. For example, in an elderly man non-isolated lesions are far more likely to be due to metastatic prostate cancer than a primary bone tumour. Conversely in an adolescent man even with a history of sports injury, an abnormal area on X-ray should always be assessed.

If the centre has significant sarcoma experience, an MRI may be performed in the case of an isolated bone lesion before referral to the surgical sarcoma centre to give more information.

All suspected bone tumours which meet these criteria should be biopsied only at a surgical sarcoma centre. This is to allow planning of future surgery, ensure adequate drainage of the biopsy site, and aims to prevent tumour seeding.

Investigations of suspected bone cancer and sarcoma

In young people <40 years old, metastatic disease is unlikely and they should be referred for an urgent biopsy at a sarcoma surgical centre.

For those aged >60 years, unless the X-ray looks like a classic bone sarcoma, they may undergo additional screening (breast, prostate) to exclude metastatic disease. This could include tumour markers (PSA, thyroid-stimulating hormone [TSH], thyroglobulin, carcinoembryonic antigen [CEA], AFP, HCG, CA-125), a bone scintigram and possibly a body CT scan.

For those between these ages, imaging and clinical judgement should guide the physician but referral to a sarcoma centre is advised if a primary sarcoma is suspected.

For those with a likely bone or soft tissue sarcoma, an MRI scan of the primary site and the remainder of that bone is mandatory to examine for intramedullary metastases. Staging should also include a CT scan of the chest and a bone scintigram in the majority of cases. Bone marrow aspiration may be useful in some tumours such as Ewing's sarcomas.

In individual sarcomas (see p.408, 420) further investigations may be required or have prognostic value.

Indications for urgent oncology referral

- Impending or actual spinal cord compression for treatment with neurosurgery and/or radiotherapy
- Other significant neurological or vascular impairment due to a rapidly expanding mass
- After a biopsy has shown a tumour which will need neoadjuvant chemotherapy, e.g. osteosarcoma, Ewing's sarcomas (see Fig 2.11.1)
- An X-ray or ultrasound which shows a likely sarcoma for a decision on immediate further management by a sarcoma service.

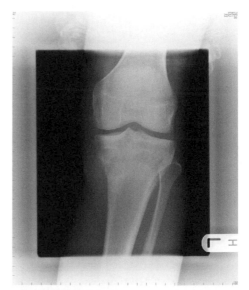

Fig. 2.11.1 X-ray of the femur showing an osteosarcoma in the proximal medial left tibia. Note the bone expansion with lifting of the periosteum and overlying soft tissue reaction

Internet resources

Bone cancer Research Trust provides information, support and counselling services for those with primary bone cancer and their families: http://www.bonecancerresearch.org.uk

Memorial Sloan Kettering Cancer Center in New York has a series of nomograms to predict survival for sarcomas: http://www.mskcc.org/mskcc/html/443.cfm

Sarcoma UK offers information and access to a growing support network for sarcoma patients and their carers: http://www.sarcoma-uk.org

Skin cancer—melanoma

Warning features

Any change in a pre-existing naevus should be assessed to rule out melanoma. A weighted 7-point checklist is used to assess pigmented lesions. Major features score 2 points each and minor features score 1 point each.

Major features:
• Change in size
• Irregular shape
• Irregular colour

Minor features:
• Largest diameter ≥7mm
• Inflammation
• Change in sensation
• Oozing

Lesions with a score of ≥3 points are suspicious of melanoma. Low-scoring lesions may be monitored for 8 weeks unless there is a strong suspicion of melanoma.

Indications for urgent referral

All patients with lesions with a strong suspicion of melanoma should be referred urgently for further assessment. Excision in primary care setting is not advised.

Internet resource

NICE referral guidelines for suspected cancer—available at: http://guidance.nice.org.uk/CG27/NICEGuidance/pdf/English

Skin cancer—non-melanoma

Indications for urgent referral

NICE recommends that patients with skin lesions suggesting squamous cell carcinoma need urgent evaluation. The following are the indications for urgent referral:

- A non healing skin lesion of >1 cm size with significant palpable induration occurring on the face, scalp or back of the hand with a progressive increase in size during the previous 8 weeks
- All immunocompromised patients who develop new or growing skin lesions
- Patients with a histological diagnosis of squamous cell carcinoma

All patients with suspected Merkel cell carcinoma should also be referred for urgent evaluation and management.

Indications for non-urgent referral

Skin lesions that are slow-growing and suggestive of basal cell carcinoma need non-urgent referral.

Web resources

Referral for suspected cancer – Available from: http://guidance.nice.org.uk/CG27/Guidance/pdf/English

Concepts of multidisciplinary management

Cancer prevention

Carcinogenesis is a multistep process consisting of progressive molecular and cellular changes leading to early invasive cancer and finally to distant metastasis and death. The initiation and progression of cancer usually takes years. Attempts are being made to reverse the molecular and cellular changes at an early state of cancer initiation or progression. The World Health Organization (WHO) estimates that at least one-third of all cancers are preventable and cancer prevention is the most cost-effective long-term strategy for the control of cancer.

Risk and protective factors of cancer

Smoking, infection, and radiation have been shown to increase the risk of various cancers. A number of lifestyle factors such as diet, alcohol, and physical activity have been studied. These factors have an uncertain association with cancer. Obesity is being increasingly recognized as a risk factor.

Smoking and cancer

Smoking is the single largest preventable cause of cancer worldwide. It causes 30% of all cancer deaths. Smoking increases the risk of lung, head and neck, oesophageal, stomach, pancreas, cervical, and bladder cancer. Smoking is responsible for 90% of lung cancer deaths.

Passive smoking (defined as the inhalation of the smoke coming from the end of a lighted cigarette, pipe, or cigar and the smoke that is exhaled by a smoker) also increases the risk of cancer. It has been estimated that workplace smoking increases the risk of lung cancer by 16%. Many developed countries have now implemented a non-smoking policy in public places.

Infectious diseases

Infectious agents are responsible for 6% of cancer deaths in developed countries and 22% in developing countries (Table 3.1.1). Preventive measures include vaccination and prevention of infection.

Radiation exposure

Ultraviolet (UV) radiation increases the risk of all types of skin cancers. Preventive measures include avoidance of exposure, use of sunscreen, and protective clothing.

Exposure to ionizing radiation increases the risk of haematological cancers and breast and thyroid cancer.

Environmental hazards

Radon is a naturally occurring carcinogen found in soil and rock which can act synergistically with smoking, leading to an increased risk of lung cancer. It has been estimated that approximately one-third of radon-induced lung cancer could be prevented by keeping the radon concentration at home to a level below 4pCi/L.

Prolonged exposure to diesel exhaust probably increases the risk of lung cancer.

Obesity, diet, and alcohol

Overweight and obesity are linked to cancers of the breast, colorectum, endometrium, pancreas, kidney, and oesophagus. Obesity is also a probable risk factor in gall bladder cancer.

Based on systematic reviews by the World Cancer Research Fund/American Institute for Cancer Research, fruits and non-starchy vegetables are associated with 'a probable decreased risk' of cancers of mouth, oesophagus, and stomach. Fruit consumption is associated with 'a probable decreased risk' of lung cancer.

Alcohol is the strongest dietary factor associated with cancer. Alcohol increases the risk of cancers of the mouth, oesophagus, breast, and colorectum. It may also increase the risk of liver cancer.

Physical activity

There is increasing evidence that physical activity is protective, particularly in colorectal cancer. Physical activity probably also decreases the risk of postmenopausal breast cancer and endometrial cancer.

Table 3.1.1 Risk factors of carcinogenesis

Cause	Type of cancer	Preventative measures
Viruses:		
HPV	Cervical cancer Anogenital cancer	HPV vaccine
EBV	Burkitt's lymphoma and Hodgkin disease	
HBV and HCV	Liver cancer	
HIV	Anal cancer, lymphoma, lung cancer, etc.	Measures to prevent acquisition of HIV infection
HHV-8	Kaposi's sarcoma	
HTLV-1	Adult T-cell leukaemia/lymphoma	
Bacteria:		
Helicobacter pylori	Stomach cancer and lymphoma	
Parasites:		
Clonorchis sinensis and *Opisthorchis viverrini*	Liver cancer	
Schistosoma haematobium	Bladder cancer	

Hormone replacement therapy (HRT)

HRT using oestrogen and progesterone or oestrogen alone is used in postmenopausal women to prevent menopausal symptoms. This can be given either systemically or topically.

HRT increases the risk of endometrial cancer, and therefore oestrogen-alone HRT is not given in patients with an intact uterus. Patients with an intact uterus are treated with combined HRT as progestin is thought to be protective.

HRT has also been shown to increase the risk of breast and ovarian cancer.

Cellular phone

Cellular phones operate at the radiofrequency (RF) level of the electromagnetic spectrum (non-ionizing) and the radio waves have a very low energy (one millionth of an electron volt). Radio waves from cellular phones are unlikely to cause molecular changes at a cellular level. Studies so far have not suggested any increased risk of cancer with the use of cellular phones. However, many of these are case–control studies (limited by recall bias) with only a limited period of follow-up and the effect of cellular phones has not been evaluated in children. A number of ongoing studies (e.g. INTERPHONE study) will help to address these issues.

It is recommended to minimize the RF exposure by using cell phones with a low SAR (specific absorption rate) value. The SAR is the amount of energy absorbed from the phone into the user's local tissue. The upper limit of SAR allowed is 1.6W/ kg body weight in 1g of tissue in North America and 2W/kg in 10g in tissue in Europe. Use of hand-free devices (corded ear pieces have 0 RF value and Bluetooth® earpieces have a SAR value of 0.001W/kg), and limiting cell phone use by children are also recommended.

Prevention of cancer

Chemoprevention and vaccination have been shown to prevent cancer. There is no consistent evidence that vitamins and dietary supplements prevent cancer.

Chemoprevention

Cancer chemoprevention is the use of natural or synthetic biological or chemical agents to reverse, suppress, or prevent carcinogenic progression to invasive cancer. Cancer chemoprevention is based on the concepts of multifocal field carcinogenesis (development of multiple areas of genetically distinct clones) and multistep carcinogenesis (progressive changes with accumulation of somatic mutations in a single clone). Chemoprevention may interrupt these processes and reduce the incidence of cancer. Clinical trials of chemopreventive agents, however, take years to assess benefit, and there is therefore a need for intermediate markers to allow a more expeditious evaluation of potential benefits of experimental agents. Premalignant lesions (e.g. intraepithelial neoplasia) are good intermediate markers and disappearance of these lesions can correlate with a reduction in cancer incidence.

Daily use of tamoxifen or raloxifene (selective oestrogen receptor modulators) for up to 5 years has been shown to reduce the incidence of breast cancer by 50% in high-risk women. Other agents used for chemoprevention include finasteride (an alpha-reductase inhibitor) for prostate cancer and COX-2 inhibitors for the prevention of colon and breast cancer.

Chemoprevention in breast cancer

A number of lesions in the breast, such as atypical ductal hyperplasia, atypical lobular hyperplasia, and carcinoma in situ, have been associated with an increased risk of breast cancer. The Breast Cancer Prevention Trial (BCPT), a placebo controlled trial of tamoxifen in 13,000 women at high risk of breast cancer has shown that tamoxifen resulted in a 49% reduction in incidence of invasive breast cancer (p <0.00001). A meta-analysis of chemopreventive studies in breast cancer also showed a reduction in oestrogen receptor (ER) positive tumours but not ER negative. There was also an increase in endometrial cancer (2.5 times greater risk) and thrombotic events especially in women aged ≥50 years. The highest benefit was seen particularly in premenopausal women with lobular carcinoma and atypical ductal hyperplasia. These studies suggest that the benefit of tamoxifen in chemoprevention is not consistent.

The NSABP-P2 study has compared tamoxifen with raloxifene and the initial results have shown that both drugs have reduced the risk of development of invasive cancer by 50% and the risk of uterine cancer and thrombotic events were less with raloxifene. Raloxifene did not prevent non-invasive carcinoma whilst tamoxifen decreased the incidence of non-invasive cancer by 50%. However tamoxifen is not routinely used as a chemopreventive agent in breast cancer due to the increased risk of endometrial cancer and thrombotic events.

Other agents being investigated in breast cancer prevention include aromatase inhibitors, COX-2 inhibitors, and retinoids.

Chemoprevention in colorectal cancer

A number of agents such as COX-2 inhibitors, vitamin D, selenium, folic acid, HRT, etc. have been investigated in the prevention of colorectal cancer. Studies have reported potential benefits in terms of reduction in colorectal cancer incidence with selenium (58% reduction in the Nutritional Prevention of Cancer Trial), HRT (a meta-analysis showing 20% reduction in risk), and aspirin (reduction in adenoma and colorectal recurrence).

Vaccination

The role of hepatitis B virus (HBV) vaccination in preventing hepatocellular carcinoma is not clearly defined. Early studies from HBV endemic areas show that vaccination can reduce the risk of childhood hepatocellular carcinoma.

Human papilloma virus (HPV) types 16 and 18 together account for about 70% of cervical cancers. Two types of HPV vaccines are available: one protects against HPV 16 and 18 (Cervarix®) and other against HPV 6, 11, 16, and 18 (Gardasil®). A phase III study of Cervarix has shown that it reduces the overall burden of precancerous cervical lesions (CIN2+) by 70% in HPV naïve young girls. Gardasil® also has shown similar benefit. Recent data indicate that Cervarix® also offers cross protection against HPV 31, 33, and 45 which might give an additional 11–16% protection against cervical cancer, including adenocarcinoma. Cervarix® is effective for 6.4 years and Gardasil® for 5 years.

The current recommendation for HPV vaccination is for girls aged 11–13 years and females up to 18 years old (to catch up on those who missed vaccination or to complete the series). The role of vaccination in females aged 19–25 years is unknown. In the UK, cervical cancer screening starts at the age of 25 years.

Vitamins and dietary supplements

Based on the hypothesis that oxidative damage to DNA leads to carcinogenesis, a number of antioxidants have been evaluated for cancer prevention. Beta carotene was thought to prevent smoking related cancer. However, two prospective placebo-controlled studies found that beta carotene supplements increased lung cancer incidence and mortality.

Studies of use of selenium, vitamin C, and vitamin E have not shown a reduction in the incidence of prostate cancer. The Women's Antioxidant Cardiovascular Study showed that supplementation with vitamin C, vitamin E, or beta carotene did not offer any benefit in the primary reduction in total cancer incidence or cancer mortality. The same study also showed that daily supplements of folic acid, vitamin B6, and vitamin B12 had no effect on overall risk of total invasive cancer or breast cancer.

Surgical prevention

One of the common approaches of prevention in high-risk people with genetic disorders is prophylactic surgery such as mastectomy and oophorectomy in BRCA-positive people (p.24, 39). However, a decision to pursue such extensive surgery is difficult.

Further reading

Fisher B, Jeong JH, Dignam J, et al. Findings from recent National Surgical Adjuvant Breast and Bowel Project adjuvant studies in stage I breast cancer. J Natl Cancer Inst Monogr 2001; 30:62–6.

Lin J, Cook NR, Albert C, et al. Vitamins C and E and beta carotene supplementation and cancer risk: a randomized controlled trial. J Natl Cancer Inst 2009; 7; 101(1):14–23.

Lippman SM, Hawk ET. Cancer prevention: from 1727 to milestones of the past 100 years. Cancer Res 2009; 69(13):5269–84.

Saslow D, Castle PE, Cox JT, et al. American Cancer Society guideline for human papillomavirus (HPV) vaccine use to prevent cervical cancer and its precursors. CA Cancer J Clin 2007; 57:7–28.

Tsao AS, Kim ES, Hong WK. Chemoprevention of cancer. CA Cancer J Clin 2004; 54(3):150–80.

William WN Jr, Heymach JV, Kim ES, et al. Molecular targets for cancer chemoprevention. Nat Rev Drug Discov 2009; 8(3):213–25.

Internet resources

American Cancer Society: http://www.cancer.org

Canadian Task Force on Preventive Health Care: http://www.ctfphc.org/

National Cancer Institute: http://www.cancer.gov

NHS immunization information: http://www.immunisation.nhs.uk

World Cancer Research Fund: http://www.wcrf-uk.org

World Cancer Research Fund/American Institute for Cancer Research: Food, Nutrition, Physical Activity and the Prevention of Cancer: a Global Perspective—available at http://www.dietandcancerreport.org

World Health Organization: http://www.who.org

Cancer screening

Introduction

The aim of cancer screening is to detect a tumour at a very early stage when treatment is most likely to be effective and to thereby produce a reduction in disease specific mortality.

Criteria for effective screening programmes have been defined by WHO (Wilson and Junger 1968). These are that

1. The condition should be an important health problem
2. Its natural history should be well understood
3. It should be recognizable at an early stage
4. Treatment should be better at an early stage
5. A suitable test for the cancer must exist
6. The test must be acceptable to the public
7. Adequate facilities must exist to cope with any abnormalities detected
8. Screening can be done at repeated intervals when the onset of cancer is insidious
9. The chance of harm must be less than the chance of benefit
10. The cost–benefit analysis must be satisfactory

Screening tests must have both high sensitivity—that is, a good chance of successfully diagnosing a cancer which is present—and high specificity—a high chance that a positive result is due to cancer. The rate of false positive and negative results must be low.

Coverage is defined as the percentage of people in the population eligible for screening at a given point in time, who were less than the specified period since their last test, in whom an adequate test result is produced. It is an important measure of the success of a screening programme.

In the UK only screening programmes for cervical, breast, and bowel cancers are considered to meet these criteria, although there is a continuing search for an effective screening method for lung, prostate, and ovarian cancers.

Cervical screening

In the UK, women are invited for screening between the ages of 25–64: those aged 25–49 every 3 years and those aged 50–64 every 5 years to correspond with patterns of sexual activity. With 3-yearly screening, 41% of cancers are preventable in those aged <40 years and 69% of cancers are preventable in those aged 40–54 years. In women aged 55–69 years, 3- and 5-year screening prevents equal proportion of cancers (73% each). Studies show that screening women <25 years old is less effective in preventing cancer including advanced stage cancer than screening women aged ≥25 years.

About 80% of eligible patients in fact attend for screening which reduces the long-term death rate by approximately 95%. There has been difficulty in attracting the younger, most at-risk population, but recent statistics have shown that an increasing number of these are now being seen. Approximately 4 million screening tests are carried out each year in the UK. The introduction of screening has reduced the incidence of invasive cervix cancer by >50%.

Screening is based on cytological examination of cells obtained from the cervix using a curette under direct vision (the Pap smear—Table 3.2.1), liquid-based cytology, or HPV testing (which has a high sensitivity but low specificity).

Of those showing an abnormal result, approximately 0.1% turn out to have cervical cancer, 7% CIN3 or adenocarcinoma *in situ*, 10.7% CIN2, and 25% CIN1. An abnormal smear test is followed by colposcopy and in those attending for colposcopy, 64% go on to have treatment or another procedure, although this rate is higher in those with high-grade abnormalities (83%).

The US Food and Drug Administration (FDA) has recently approved HPV DNA testing as an adjunct to cytology for cervical cancer. Studies show that HPV testing is more sensitive than cytology (96.1% vs. 53%) and with HPV testing, screening intervals can be 6 years or more.

Many countries have recently implemented HPV immunization (p.19) for girls aged 12–13 years. The potential impact on cervical screening of the HPV vaccination programmes will take some time to elucidate.

Breast

Currently women between the ages of 50–65 years are invited for screening every 5 years but there is a plan to extend the age range to 45–73 years. Nearly 2 million women are screened per year in the UK. Survival rates for screen detected cancer are 85% at 15 years. Studies show that breast cancer screening results in a 35% reduction in breast cancer mortality. Digital mammography is gradually replacing film mammography and has particular advantages in detecting cancer in younger patients with more dense breast tissue.

There has been considerable controversy recently about the overall benefit of breast screening. Problems arise from the increased frequency of detection of ductal carcinoma *in situ* (DCIS) and from changes in incidence of breast cancer believed to be due to lifestyle factors. A recent publication has suggested overdiagnosis and overtreatment, but these findings are questioned by others.

DCIS is diagnosed in >3000 women each year in the UK. The incidence of this early form of breast cancer has been increasing over the last few years but the best treatment choice for an individual woman is much more difficult than it is for clearly invasive cancer since the natural progression of disease is poorly understood. High-grade disease is known to progress to invasive cancer, but the outcome for medium- and low-grade disease is less clear. Thirty per cent of screen-detected DCIS is treated by mastectomy and for some of these, the changes detected might not have shown progression.

Changes in women's lifestyle have increased breast cancer incidence in the UK, where the screening programme results show one in eight cancers diagnosed through the programme would not have been diagnosed otherwise. The result of this screening is estimated to be one extra survival for every eight women diagnosed with breast cancer. Around one in six women have an abnormality on routine screening and of these 20% have DCIS. Uptake is around 73% and is influenced by wealth but not by education or ethnicity.

Bowel

One in 20 people will develop bowel cancer during their lifetime and it is the third commonest tumour in the UK and the second leading cause of cancer deaths with overall

Table 3.2.1 Cervical screening

Bethesda classification	Pap	Description	Treatment
Low-grade squamous intraepithelial lesion (LSIL)	CIN1	This carries the lowest risk. Represents mild dysplasia confined to the basal 1/3 of the epithelium. Infection with HPV will typically be cleared by immune response within a year	Observation/colposcopy and biopsy
High-grade squamous intra-epithelial lesion (HSLI)	CIN2	Moderate dysplasia confined to the basal 2/3 of the epithelium	Loop electrosurgical excision procedure (LEEP) cryotherapy or laser
HSLI	CIN3	Severe dysplasia involving >2/3 of the epithelium, or up to full thickness carcinoma *in situ*	

16,000 people dying each year. Bowel cancer screening aims to detect cancer at an asymptomatic stage when treatment is more likely to be effective. It is based on the detection of faecal occult blood from a stool sample and as well as cancers, polyps will also be detected. Their removal will prevent any risk of subsequent bowel cancer development. Screening is offered every 2 years to all men and women aged 60–69. Screening will reduce the risk of death from bowel cancer by 16%.

Out of every 1000 people with a normal result <1 will be diagnosed with bowel cancer within the next 2 years. Uptake has been around 60% in pilot studies and the overall rate of positive abnormal results was 1.9%. The rate of cancer detection was 1.62 per 1000 screened. These values were higher in men and with increasing age. The positive predictive value was 10.9% for cancer and 35% for adenoma. Sixteen per cent of detected cancers arose in polyps, 48% were Dukes stage A and only 1% had metastasized at the time of diagnosis. The annual cost of the bowel screening programme in the UK is £76.2 million. Those with abnormal results are offered colonoscopy.

Prostate

There is no national screening programme in the UK yet because there is no evidence that early treatment of small volume disease leads to an improved outcome and only criterion 1 for screening programmes is met. Measurement of PSA for screening for prostate cancer fulfils many of the criteria for a successful screening programme in terms of acceptability and feasibility, but it is not sensitive or specific enough to be routinely recommended and there is still no clear evidence of proven benefit for early cancers detected in this way. Men with prostate cancer may not have a raised PSA and two out of three men with a raised PSA do not have prostate cancer

Early-stage disease may have an extremely long natural history and the patient may survive longer than the time which it would take for the tumour to progress. There is also considerable uncertainty as to the best type of treatment for early stage disease. There is evidence from a prostate screening trial in Europe, of a reduction in mortality by 20% but this was achieved at the cost of a high level of complications from overtreatment in the rest of the group. Forty-eight additional cases of prostate cancer were treated to result in one additional survival.

In view of the demand from many men for this test the UK has introduced a programme of Informed Choice to help men to decide whether they do wish to be tested and what decisions may then be required with information given about the benefits and risks of the various treatment options.

Lung

Lung cancer screening with annual CXRs has been evaluated in the US Prostate, Lung, Colorectal and Ovarian Cancer Screening Trial but has not shown a benefit. Studies are now underway using CT scanning but no screening outside a clinical trial is appropriate yet.

Ovary

A suitable screening method for ovarian cancer would be very advantageous as the lack of symptoms of early disease and the non-specific nature of symptoms in the late stages lead to many presentations with stage III/IV disease where treatment outcomes are relatively poor. Ultrasound would be an acceptable test but there are still no clear trial data showing a benefit for this approach.

Screening women at higher risk

Higher than average risk means having two or more relatives on the same side of the family diagnosed with ovarian cancer or breast cancer at a young age. In this group, early mammography may be replaced by MRI breast screening and regular US may be undertaken, although prophylactic organ removal may also be advised.

Further reading

Cuzick J, Clavel C, Petry KU, et al. Overview of the European and North American studies on HPV testing in primary cervical cancer screening. *Int J Cancer* 2006; **119**:1095–101.

Hassan MA, Fagerstrom RM, Kahane DC, et al. Prostate, Lung, Colorectal and Ovarian Cancer Screening Trial Project Team. Design and evolution of the data management systems in the Prostate, Lung, Colorectal and Ovarian (PLCO) Cancer Screening Trial. *Control Clin Trials* 2000; **21**(6 suppl):329S–348S.

Papanicolaou GN, Traut HF. The diagnostic value of vaginal smears in carcinoma of the uterus. *Am J Obstet Gynae* 1941; **42**:193–206.

Wilson JMG, Junger G. *Principles and practice of screening for disease.* Public Health Papers 34. Geneva: World Health Organization, 1968.

Internet resources

NHS Cancer Screening Programmes: http://www.cancerscreening.nhs.uk/

UK Collaborative Trial of Ovarian Cancer Screening (UKCTOCS): http://www.instituteforwomenshealth.ucl.ac.uk/academic_research/gynaecologicalcancer/gcrc/ukctocs

Cancer genetics

The vast majority of cancers are caused by a number of interacting factors including environmental and hormonal risk factors, random genetic events, and low-risk inherited genetic variants, (polymorphisms). However, 5–10% of cancers are due to inheritance of alterations in genes that confer a high lifetime risk of certain malignancies. These genetic variations can increase both the risk of common cancers, such as breast and colorectal cancer, and very rare tumours (Foulkes 2008). Most of these so-called 'hereditary cancer predisposition syndromes' are due to mutations within a single allele (copy), of a tumour suppressor gene inherited in an autosomal dominant fashion

Mechanisms of inherited cancer

Tumourigenesis involves two classes of genes. Oncogenes act to control cell growth and proliferation under normal circumstances, but once inappropriately activated or over-expressed can promote rapid clonal expansion. Tumour suppressor genes normally inhibit abnormal cell proliferation; reduced expression of these genes can result in uncontrolled cell division.

Most hereditary cancer predisposition syndromes are due to the inheritance of a germline mutation in a tumour suppressor gene. The inherited mutation inactivates one copy of the gene and the subsequent development of a mutation in the remaining 'normal' copy of the gene results in failure of a cell to produce the tumour suppressor protein (Garber and Offit 2005). Inheritance of two alleles each carrying a mutation within the same tumour suppression gene is extremely rare and can result in a different and more severe phenotype than monoallelic mutation inheritance

Diagnosis

An underlying hereditary predisposition towards developing a malignancy is typically characterized by:
- Young age at presentation
- Increased incidence of bilateral tumours
- More than one primary tumour site
- Family history of specific cancers

Although most cancer predisposition syndromes are inherited in an autosomal dominant fashion with affected individuals in each generation, penetrance (the likelihood of a mutation carrier developing clinical manifestations of the syndrome) can vary.

Analysis of DNA for mutations in known cancer predisposition genes is performed using DNA derived from a peripheral blood sample. A full screen for unknown mutations will take several weeks to process. 'Predictive testing', in which genetic testing is directed at establishing whether or not an individual has a specific mutation carried by another family member, is, however, much faster. It is essential that any individual considering undergoing genetic screening for an inherited cancer predisposition syndrome receives expert counselling both prior to being tested and on receiving their result.

Inherited breast cancer

A positive family history is reported by 20–30% of breast cancer patients. Approximately 5% of all breast cancer cases are thought to be due to highly penetrant autosomal dominant cancer predisposition syndromes. The two most frequent highly penetrant breast cancer susceptibility genes are BRCA1 and BRCA2. Much rarer syndromes including Li–Fraumeni, Cowden, Peutz–Jeghers, and hereditary diffuse gastric cancer syndromes are associated with lifetime breast cancer risk in the order of 20–100%. It is likely that most familial clusters of breast cancer are the consequence of multiple low-penetrance cancer susceptibility genes acting in conjunction with environmental factors. A number of large case–control studies have recently identified variants in DNA repair genes (e.g. CHEK2, ATM, BRIP1, and PALB2), which double the risk of breast cancer. The population prevalence of these variants seems to be only in the order of 1–5%.

Hereditary breast/ovarian cancer syndromes (HBOS)

Clinical features

HBOS are caused by mutations of the BRCA1 or BRCA2 genes and are associated with a lifetime breast cancer risk of 40–80% and an increased lifetime risk of ovarian cancer (40–60% for BRCA1 mutation carriers and 10–20% for BRCA2 mutation carriers). BRCA1 mutation carriers additionally have an increased risk of pancreatic cancers whilst male breast cancer, pancreatic, and prostate cancer all occur at an increased frequency in BRCA2 mutation carriers.

BRCA1-associated breast tumours are typically high grade with lymphocytic infiltrate and pushing tumour margins, and ER, PR, and HER-2 negative. There is no distinct phenotype associated with BRCA2 tumours.

Incidence

The population frequency of BRCA1/2 mutation carriers is 1 in 400, increasing to 1 in 50 in Ashkenazi Jews.

Inheritance pattern

Autosomal dominant

Genetics and pathology

BRCA1 and BRCA2 are located on chromosomes 17 and 13 respectively and are classical tumour suppressor genes. The precise functions of the BRCA1 and BRCA2 gene products remain unclear but these proteins are involved in DNA repair and transcription regulation, with additional roles in cell cycle checkpoint control.

Diagnosis

High throughput genetic analysis systems can now achieve screening of all coding regions of the BRCA1 and BRCA2 genes for nonsense mutations within approximately 8 weeks. Predictive testing for known mutations can be accomplished within a week. Prenatal and preimplantation genetic diagnosis is now available.

Clinical management

Primary prevention

For individuals with known BRCA1 or BRCA2 mutations, prophylactic double mastectomy reduces the risk of breast cancer by up to 90%. More acceptable to many women is prophylactic bilateral oophorectomy which reduces breast cancer rates by 60% and ovarian cancer rates by 95% (Guillem et al. 2006). The use of chemoprevention with tamoxifen remains controversial.

Secondary prevention

Yearly MRI offers improved sensitivity for the detection of malignancy in high-risk women and detects tumours at an earlier stage than mammography. The 2006 NICE guidelines for the management of familial breast cancer therefore recommended annual MRI surveillance of all BRCA1/2 mutation carriers aged 30–49. Regular breast screening by mammography, together with clinical breast examinations, is also recommended for all patients with known BRCA1 or BRCA2 mutations. Screening for ovarian cancer remains under investigation.

Treatment of BRCA-associated breast cancer
Comparisons with age-matched controls suggest that local recurrence rates of BRCA-related breast tumours treated by breast conserving surgery are similar to those of sporadic cancer, providing the BRCA mutation carriers have undergone prophylactic oophorectomy. Risk of contralateral breast cancer remains significantly higher in BRCA mutation carriers than controls, (approximately 30% at 10 years). Concerns that healthy cells carrying BRCA1/2 mutations are at increased risk of malignant transformation following irradiation have not been verified by clinical studies of contralateral breast cancer rates in patients receiving chest wall radiotherapy.

In vitro studies suggest that BRCA-associated breast tumours are particularly vulnerable to cytotoxic agents that promote cross-linking of DNA but show resistance to the mitotic spindle poisons. A national study of docetaxel versus carboplatin as first-line therapy for metastatic BRCA-related breast cancer is currently in progress. Recognition that poly (ADP-ribose) polymerase-1 (PARP) inhibitors may offer a selective method of killing tumour cells with underlying BRCA deficiencies has also led to clinical trials of these agents.

Hereditary colorectal cancer
Approximately 5% of cases of colorectal cancer are due to an underlying hereditary cancer syndrome. Most familial cases are due to either hereditary non-polyposis colon cancer (HNPCC or Lynch syndrome), which accounts for an estimated 2–3% of all colorectal cancers, or FAP, which accounts for <1% of all colorectal cancers. There is also an increased risk of GI cancer in Peutz–Jeghers syndrome, caused by the inheritance of mutations in STK11. Features that suggest a familial colorectal cancer syndrome include:
- Early-age onset (<50 years) colorectal cancer or endometrial cancer
- Multiple colorectal carcinomas or >10 adenomatous polyps in same individual
- Individuals with an HNPCC related tumour who have either:
  - One first-degree relative with an *HNPCC-related cancer at 50 years *or*
  - ≥Two first- or second-degree relative with an *HNPCC-related cancer at any age
- History of multiple *HNPCC related tumours in same individual

(*HNPCC-related cancers: endometrial, ovarian, gastric, duodenal, and urological malignancies.)

Familial adenomatous polyposis
Clinical features
FAP is characterized by the development of hundreds of colonic adenomatous polyps by the age of 20, with a risk of malignant transformation of almost 100%. The average age of diagnosis of colon cancer is 39 years. Patients are also at increased risk of rectal and duodenal adenomas and carcinomas, as well as desmoid tumours, osteomas, thyroid

carcinomas, and hepatoblastomas. In the attenuated FAP syndrome the risk of colon cancer is 80% by age 70.

Incidence
The carrier frequency is 1 in 8000.

Genetics and pathology
Mutations within the APC gene on chromosome 5 are found in >90% of FAP cases. The APC protein binds numerous proteins including members of the Wnt signalling pathway and cytoskeleton regulators. Loss of the APC protein results in chromosomal instability due to loss of cytoskeleton control and activation of the Wnt pathway which promotes tumourigenesis. The attenuated form of FAP is associated with mutations at the very ends of the APC gene.

Diagnosis
A clinical diagnosis of FAP can be made by flexible sigmoidoscopy at an early age. Genetic screening for APC mutations is recommended from the age of 10–12 years, with the aim of sparing children carrying the wild type APC gene from invasive surveillance.

Primary prevention
Carriers of APC mutations should undergo surveillance colonoscopy annually from the age of 10 up to 15 years. Prophylactic colectomy by the age of 20 years is recommended for those found to have multiple adenomas on surveillance. The COX2 inhibitor celecoxib and non-steroidal anti-inflammatory agent sulindac may both reduce duodenal adenoma formation but severe duodenal polyposis will require a Whipple's resection.

Secondary prevention
Long-term surveillance of the small intestine by upper endoscopy, starting from age 25–30 years, is required as periampullary carcinoma is the commonest cause of death in FAP patients who have undergone prophylactic colectomy. Regular abdominal examination and/or imaging should also be considered it there is a family history of desmoids or hepatoblastoma.

Management of colonic carcinoma
FAP patients who do develop invasive cancers should be managed in the same way as the general population.

Hereditary non-polyposis colorectal cancer
Clinical features
HNPCC is an autosomal dominant pattern hereditary cancer syndrome consisting of a high risk of early onset colorectal cancer with an increased frequency of endometrial, ovarian, gastric, duodenal, and urological malignancies. Pancreatic and brain tumour and sebaceous adenomas/carcinomas are also associated. Characteristically, the colonic tumours are predominantly right sided (70%) and there is an increased rate of synchronous and metachronous tumours.

Incidence
The carrier frequency is 1 in 1700.

Genetics and pathology
In up to 70% of patients with HNPCC, the underlying genetic defect is a germline mutation in one of three genes: hMLH1, hMSH2, hMSH6. These genes all encode DNA mismatch repair proteins. Defective mismatch repair promotes malignant transformation by permitting rapid accumulation of mutations in other genes, such as those that regulate the cell cycle. Deficiency of mismatch repair is

characterized by the presence in tumour cells of microsatellites (DNA sequences that contain a short motif repeated several times), that have changed in length due to nucleotide insertions or deletions. This phenomenon is termed 'microsatellite instability'.

Diagnosis
The National Comprehensive Cancer Network guidelines state that for a clinical diagnosis of HNPCC, at least three relatives must have a tumour associated with HNPCC and all of the following criteria should be present:
- One must be a first-degree relative of the other two
- At least two successive generations must be affected
- At least one of the relatives should have the relevant cancer diagnosed before the age of 50 years
- FAP should be excluded

Analysis of tumour tissue for high microsatellite instability (MSI), using a panel of five or six polymorphic markers, is positive in >80% of patients fulfilling the clinical criteria for HNPCC. Patients with evidence of MSI should be offered genetic screening for germline mutations of hMLH1, hMSH2, and hMSH6. Alternatively, immunohistochemical staining of colorectal tumours for the hMLH1, hMSH2, and hMSH6 proteins is highly sensitive and specific in predicting an underlying mismatch repair gene defect.

Primary prevention
The role of prophylactic colectomy in the management of patients with HNPCC remains controversial. Some specialists recommend prophylactic hysterectomy and bilateral salpingo-oophorectomy on completion of child-bearing for female carriers of HNPCC-associated gene mutations.

Secondary prevention
Annual colonoscopy screening from the age of 20–25 years is recommended for carriers of HNPCC-associated gene mutations. Regular upper endoscopy screening should also be considered for HNPCC families with a history of gastric cancer and urine cytology for patients with a family history of urological tumours.

Female HNPCC mutation carriers should be screened for ovarian and endometrial tumours by pelvic ultrasonography with annual transvaginal measurements of endometrial thickness and/or endometrial aspirates.

Management of colonic carcinoma
Subtotal colectomy can be offered to HNPCC patients presenting with a colonic carcinoma, because of the high rate of synchronous tumours in these patients.

Li–Fraumeni syndrome (LFS)
Clinical features
Classic LFS is a rare cancer susceptibility syndrome characterized by a predominance of soft tissue sarcomas, osteosarcoma, and breast cancer, and an excess of brain tumours, leukaemia, and adrenocortical carcinomas in children and young adults (Gonzalez et al. 2009). Many additional tumours have also been reported including leukaemia, lung carcinomas, GI, and ovarian tumours, lymphomas, and a variety of paediatric tumours.

Inheritance pattern
Autosomal dominant
Genetics and pathology
Germline mutations of the TP53 gene (chromosome 17), are found in approximately 70% of families meeting the criteria for classic LFS criteria. The detection rate drops as the criteria become less stringent. The protein product of TP53 is a regulator of the cell cycle and apoptosis. Loss of p53 results in cells with mutated DNA dividing in an uncontrolled fashion to form tumours.

Incidence
The estimated incidence of TP53 germline mutations is 1 in 5000. Penetrance is at least 50% by age 50.

Diagnosis
TP 53 mutations are detected by direct sequencing of the TP53 gene.

Clinical management
Females with a proven TP53 mutation should be screened for breast cancer according to the NICE guidelines, with annual breast MRI from age 30 for high-risk women and regular breast MRI from as young as 20 years for very high-risk individuals. Exposure to ionizing radiation should be minimized and mammography is not recommended currently in the UK for breast screening in LFS.

Von Hippel–Lindau (VHL) syndrome
Clinical features
VHL is a rare hereditary cancer syndrome consisting of:
- Haemangioblastomas of the retina and CNS (particularly cerebellar, medullary, and spinal sites)
- Phaeochromocytomas
- Clear cell renal carcinomas

Inheritance pattern
Autosomal dominant

Genetics and pathology
The VHL gene is sited on chromosome 3. It encodes an ubiquitin ligase that downregulates hypoxia-inducible mRNAs in the presence of oxygen (Kim and Kaelin 2004). Cells lacking pVHL fail to break down the transcription factor complex HIF (hypoxia-inducible factor) which is then able to induce the transcription of genes promoting cell growth, survival, and angiogenesis. Mutations or deletions of the VHL gene are found in virtually all clinically diagnosed VHL families using modern genetic diagnostic methods.

Incidence
VHL syndrome is estimated to affect 1 in 35,000.

Clinical management
Screening for retinal tumours should begin at the age of 5 years together with annual blood pressure monitoring and analysis of urinary or plasma catecholamine metabolites. Annual renal imaging should be commenced before the age of 20 and consideration should also be given to regular screening for CNS tumours using CT or MRI. Prenatal and preimplantation genetic diagnosis is now available for VHL when a mutation has been identified in a family.

Multiple neuroendocrine neoplasia (MEN) syndromes
Clinical features
The MEN syndromes are characterized by the development of multiple benign and malignant tumours of endocrine glands.

MEN1
- Parathyroid adenomas (up to 95% of cases)
- Pancreatic islet cell tumours (50–75% of cases)

- Pituitary adenomas (25–65% of cases)
- Carcinoid tumours
- Thyroid tumours

MEN2A
- Medullary thyroid carcinoma (up to 100% of cases)
- Phaeochromocytoma (40% of cases)
- Parathyroid hyperplasia (10–35% of cases)

MEN2B
- Medullary thyroid carcinoma (up to 100% of cases)
- Gangliomas (up to 100% of cases)
- Phaeochromocytoma
- Skeletal abnormalities
- Megacolon

Inheritance
Autosomal dominant

Genetics and pathology
MEN1 is caused by mutations in the menin gene located on chromosome 11. Menin is a tumour suppressor gene which interacts with a number of nuclear proteins including transcription factors.

MEN2A and MEN2B are associated with mutations of the chromosome 10 proto-oncogene RET which codes for a transmembrane receptor tyrosine kinase. Activating mutations in RET upregulate cell proliferation resulting in tissue hyperplasia with a high rate of malignant transformation. The position of the mutation within the RET gene determines whether the clinical features of MEN2A or MEN2 develop.

Incidence
The incidence of MEN is between 0.2–2 per 100,000

Diagnosis
Direct mutation detection is now available for both the MEN and RET genes.

Clinical management
Regular screening of individuals from MEN1 families or known MEN mutation carriers should commence before the age of 10 and should consist of serum calcium and prolactin measurements as a bare minimum. Consideration should also be given to measurements of pituitary, parathyroid, and pancreatic hormones as well as imaging of the pituitary gland. RET mutation carriers benefit from prophylactic thyroidectomy performed between the ages of 3–5 years. Screening for phaeochromocytomas should be performed from adulthood through to the age of 35 years (Callender et al. 2008).

Further reading
Callender GG, Rich TA, Perrier ND. Multiple endocrine neoplasia syndromes. *Surg Clin North Am* 2008; **88**:863–95.

Foulkes WD. Inherited susceptibility to common cancers. *N Eng J Med* 2008; **359**:2143–53.

Garber JE, Offit K. Hereditary cancer predisposition syndromes. *J Clin Oncol* 2005; **23**:276–92.

Gonzalez KD, Noltner KA, Buzin CH, et al. Beyond Li Fraumeni syndrome: clinical characteristics of families with p53 germline mutations. *J Clin Oncol* 2009; 27:1250–6.

Guillem JG, Wood WC, Moley JF, et al. ASCO/SSO review of current role of risk-reducing surgery in common hereditary cancer syndromes. *J Clin Oncol* 2006; **24**:4642–60.

Kim WY, Kaelin WG. Role of VHL gene mutation in human cancer. *J Clin Oncol* 2004; **22**:4991–5004.

Internet resources
NCCN clinical practice guidelines in oncology: *Colorectal cancer screening*—available at http://www.nccn.org

NCCN clinical practice guidelines in oncology: *Genetic/familial high-risk assessment: breast and ovarian*—available at http://www.nccn.org

NICE clinical guideline 41: *Familial breast cancer* (issue date October 2006)—available at http://www.nice.org

Genetic counselling

Genetic counselling is the process by which individuals at possible risk of an inherited medical disorder are advised about:
• The natural history of the condition
• Their personal risk of developing or transmitting the condition
• The methods available to test for the inherited condition
• The advantages and disadvantages of undergoing testing
• The management options available if tests confirm that they are carrying the inherited condition

In the UK, genetic counselling is provided by specially trained professionals, most of whom have a background in nursing, medical, or scientific disciplines. Genetic counsellors work within MDTs and are attached to regional clinical genetics services.

It is essential that any individual considering undergoing genetic screening for an inherited cancer predisposition syndrome is seen by a genetic counsellor both prior to being tested and on receiving their result.

Who should be referred for genetic counselling?

Cancer patients and/or their relatives should be referred to their regional clinical genetics unit for genetic counselling when a suspicion arises that a family or individual history of cancer may be due to an inherited predisposition. Suspicious features include:
• Unusual age of onset for the type of cancer
• Numerous affected family members with the same type of cancer
• Numerous affected family members with cancers within characteristic groups, e.g. breast and ovarian cancers, colorectal and endometrial tumours
• History of multiple primary cancers in a single individual

When referring an individual to a clinical genetics unit for consideration of genetic counselling it is important to state whether they have had cancer personally and if so, to provide the clinical details of their diagnosis and treatment. The pathology report should also be included in the referral.

The genetic counselling process

Genetic counselling of an individual or family who potentially has a hereditary cancer predisposition syndrome should consist of a number of key stages:
• Determining the patient's perception and experience
• Explaining the difference between sporadic and inherited cancer risk
• Documenting and verifying the family history of malignancies
• Identifying the most likely underlying genetic fault
• Assessing the genetic risk to the patient and other family members
• Discussing whether genetic testing is appropriate
• Explaining alternative options to genetic testing, i.e. research
• Approximation of personal risk on basis of family history
• Identifying the most appropriate family member to undergo genetic testing
• Ensuring individuals understand the implications of a positive, negative, and ambiguous genetic result

• Helping to communicate test results to other members of the family

Eliciting the patient issues at the outset is an important step in building rapport and trust and setting up successful communication. The patient's experience of cancer within the family, such as whether people have survived or not and how old the patient was when a parent was affected, can play a huge role in their risk perception.

Taking a family history: key points
• Confirm whether patient has had cancer personally
• Construct a three-generation family tree (i.e. parents, grandparents, aunts/uncles, siblings, and children)
• Include both affected and unaffected individuals
• Identify all relatives affected by malignancy including type of cancer and age of diagnosis
• Obtain details of treatments given for cancer
• Confirm whether anyone in the family has previously been assessed by a clinical genetics service. If they have, determine whether genetic testing has been performed.

Unlike other medical referrals, a referral for genetic counselling often involves the whole family. Unaffected individuals who are seeking advice may find it difficult to approach a family member who has only recently been diagnosed with a malignancy or who has terminal cancer. The relationship between counsellor and patient is therefore critical in acknowledging family dynamics or allowing time for the referred patient to 'find the right time' to approach different members of the family.

Verifying the family history

It is well documented that individuals often misreport their family's history of malignancies. In particular, there is frequently confusion about the site of the primary tumour versus metastases, e.g. breast cancer with hepatic metastases may be described as a 'liver cancer'. Abdominal tumours are also frequently misidentified whilst reports of breast cancers are rarely incorrect (Douglas et al. 1999). Several studies also suggest that accuracy decreases in the reporting of cancers in more distant relatives (Eerola et al. 2000; Sijmons et al. 2000). Pathology plays a key role in genetic assessment as some cancers, such as ovarian cancer, may feature in more than one cancer syndrome. Pathology can also help to determine the likelihood of identifying a mutation within a cancer predisposition gene; a family history consisting of high grade breast cancer is more likely to be associated with BRCA1/2 than a similar family history consisting of low grade breast cancer. Genetic centres therefore seek to confirm the pathology of all reported affected individuals within a family tree. This can take some time while consent from affected family members is sought.

Verification of pathology can be obtained from several sources:
• Pathology laboratory reports—gold standard
• Hospital discharge summaries
• General practitioner (GP) records
• Cancer registries
• Death certificates

Identifying the potential genetic fault

The location of a potential inherited genetic fault can usually be narrowed down to a small number of genes by examining the pattern of inheritance and the type of malignancies present in a family.

Pattern of inheritance

Autosomal dominant

Most of the single high-risk genes that predispose to cancer when a mutation is present are inherited in an autosomal dominant fashion. When a condition is dominantly inherited an individual who has one normal copy and one faulty copy of a particular cancer gene is said to be a 'gene carrier', and has an increased risk of developing cancer. They also have a 50% chance of passing the faulty copy on to their offspring. An individual's risk of developing cancer if they are a 'carrier' of a dominantly inherited gene is related to the 'penetrance' of that gene.

Penetrance:
• Is the risk of an individual developing the disease
• May vary depending on age and gender
• 100% penetrance = all individuals will develop symptoms
• 50% penetrance = half will develop symptoms

Autosomal recessive

A small number of cancer syndromes are inherited in an autosomal recessive fashion, whereby an individual requires two faulty copies of the particular cancer gene to express the condition. As this person has no normal copies of the gene, they will always pass on one faulty copy to each of their children. Typically, individuals with only one faulty copy of a recessively inherited gene will not be at increased risk of developing cancer.

Type of malignancies

Different hereditary cancer predisposition syndromes are caused by mutations in specific genes and are characterised by the coassociation of groups of tumours, as detailed in Table 3.4.1.

Risk assessment models

A number of different algorithms exist to predict the probability that an individual/family carries a mutation in a specific cancer predisposition gene based on their family history and and/or pathological details. Examples include models for predicting mutations in Lynch syndrome genes (reviewed by Chen, 2008) and the BRCAPRO and the Manchester score for familial breast cancer (Evans et al. 2004). NICE guidance for familial breast cancer recommends that women from families with a 20% or greater chance of carrying a mutation such as BRCA1, BRCA2, or TP53 should have access to genetic testing.

Who should be tested?

Ideally genetic mutation analysis needs to be performed initially in an affected individual. This gives the highest chance of identifying a mutation within a family. The best person to test is generally the youngest affected individual whose pathology matches the type of cancer that fits the pathology seen in the predisposition syndrome being tested for. Testing unaffected individuals poses multiple problems. If a mutation has not been sought within an affected individual a negative result in an unaffected family member does not necessarily negate the family history, as a mutation may not be identified if testing was performed in an affected member of the family.

When arranging genetic testing, care is taken to ensure that the individual is aware of the possible results and implications of the result and has thought through how they might handle this information. Discussions are also held about informing the wider family.

Genetic testing

Analysis of DNA for mutations in known cancer predisposition genes is performed in a limited number of specialist molecular genetics laboratories using DNA derived from a peripheral blood sample.

Full mutation screen

The gold standard for mutation screening is direct sequencing of the entire gene to look for single base changes and rearrangements, but this is generally not commercially viable for very large genes such as BRCA1/2. Some molecular genetics laboratories therefore now use high-throughput technology to detect possible potential mutation sites. The exact position and nature of the mutation is then confirmed by direct sequencing of a limited region of the gene only. Additional technologies are required to detect exonic deletions and duplications. A full screen for unknown mutations will take a number of weeks to process.

Partial mutation screen

Some cancer predisposition genes cannot be screened due to limitations in technology. In these cases mutation testing is limited to a restricted region of the gene. Other cancer predisposition genes contain 'hot spots' where mutations commonly occur, permitting genetic analysis of a limited portion of the gene only.

Predictive testing

Once a causative genetic mutation has been identified within a family, 'predictive testing' can be offered to other family members to establish whether or not they carry the same specific mutation. This is a much faster process than mutation screening and can be offered to individuals both affected and unaffected by cancer. Genetic counselling is critical within these families in giving an individual at risk of having a faulty cancer predisposition gene the opportunity to explore how having this information may impact medically, emotionally, and psychosocially. Individuals at a 50% risk of inheriting a cancer predisposition gene will be counselled about the chance of having the faulty gene, cancer risks associated with this faulty gene, screening recommendations, possible surgical management, implications for current/future offspring, insurance, coping ability, sharing information within the family, and how they think this information would affect them.

Explaining genetic test results

The result of genetic testing is given by a member of staff with whom the patient has built a rapport during pre-test counselling and ongoing support is offered following receipt of the result. Research shows that patients retain little information after being given a 'bad' news result. Discussions are therefore often kept short and simple at this appointment and a follow-up is arranged shortly after to have a more in-depth discussion about future health care plans.

Mutation screening

This can result in one of three results:
1. *Positive result:* a mutation with definite pathogenic potential is identified within the cancer predisposition gene screened. Carriers will be advised of the implications of

Table 3.4.1 Inherited cancer syndromes

Cancer syndrome	Gene	Inheritance	Clinical features and associated cancers
Cowden syndrome (PTEN hamartoma tumour syndrome)	PTEN	Autosomal dominant	Macrocephaly, trichilemmomas, papillomatous papules Breast cancer, thyroid cancer (usually follicular), endometrial cancer
Familial adenomatous polyposis Including: Gardner syndrome Turcot syndrome	APC	Autosomal dominant	100+ colorectal adenomas, colorectal cancer, duodenal polyps/cancer, thyroid cancer, hepatoblastoma + dental cysts, desmoid tumours + CNS tumours (medulloblastoma)
Familial medullary thyroid cancer	RET	Autosomal dominant	Medullary thyroid cancer
Hereditary breast and ovarian cancer	BRCA1, BRCA2	Autosomal dominant	Breast cancer, epithelial ovarian cancer, prostate cancer, pancreatic cancer (BRCA2)
Hereditary leiomyomatosis and renal cell cancer	FH	Autosomal dominant	Cutaneous leiomyomata, uterine leiomyomata, renal cancer
Hereditary paraganglioma–phaeochromocytoma syndrome	SDHB, SDHC, SDHD	Autosomal dominant	Paraganglioma, phaeochromocytoma
Juvenile polyposis syndrome	SMAD4, BMPR1A	Autosomal dominant	GI hamartomatous polyps (colon, stomach, small intestine, rectum), colon cancer, other GI cancers
Li–Fraumeni syndrome	TP53	Autosomal dominant	Breast cancer (premenopausal), soft tissue sarcoma (childhood), malignant brain tumours, adrenal cortical tumours (childhood), osteosarcoma (teenage), other cancers (including leukaemia, melanoma, stomach, colon, pancreatic, oesophageal, Wilms' tumour, gonadal germ cell tumours)
Lynch syndrome/hereditary non-polyposis colon cancer Including: Muir–Torre syndrome	MLH1, MSH2, MSH6, PMS2	Autosomal dominant	Colorectal cancer, endometrial cancer, ovarian cancer GI cancer, pancreatic cancer, renal pelvis tumours, brain tumours + sebaceous carcinoma, keratocanthomas
Multiple endocrine neoplasia type 1	MEN1	Autosomal dominant	Endocrine tumours (parathyroid, pituitary, gastro-entero-pancreatic, carcinoid, adrenocortical), skin tumours (facial angiofibromas, collagenomas), lipomas CNS tumours (meningiomas, ependymonas), leiomyomas
Multiple endocrine neoplasia type 2A	RET	Autosomal dominant	Medullary thyroid cancer, phaeochromocytoma, parathyroid adenoma or hyperplasia
Multiple endocrine neoplasia type 2B	RET	Autosomal dominant	Medullary thyroid cancer, phaeochromocytoma Mucosal neuroma of lips and tongue, ganglioneuromatosis of GI tract, Marfanoid habitus
MutYH associated polyposis	MYH	Autosomal recessive	Colorectal adenomas, colorectal cancer
Neurofibromatosis type 2	NF2	Autosomal dominant	Bilateral vestibular schwannomas, peripheral schwannomas, meningiomas, ependymomas, astrocytomas
Peutz–Jeghers syndrome	STK11	Autosomal dominant	GI polyposis/cancer, mucosal pigmentation Breast cancer, sex cord tumours of the ovary with annular tubules (SCTAT), calcifying Sertoli cell tumours
Von Hippel–Lindau syndrome	VHL	Autosomal dominant	Hemangioblastomas of the brain, spinal cord, and retina, renal cysts, clear cell renal cell carcinoma, pancreatic cysts, pheochromocytoma, endolymphatic sac tumours

this result including lifetime risk of malignancies, current recommendations for screening, and other management options including prophylactic surgery.

2. *Negative result:* no mutation is found within the regions of the gene examined. Patients must be advised that failure to detect a mutation does not always mean that no mutation is present and that further results may become available in the future as genetic testing becomes more sophisticated.

3. *Ambiguous result:* a DNA sequence variation is identified but it is not clear whether this is pathogenic or not. The uncertain implications of this result must be communicated carefully to the patient with the advice that further information about their specific DNA alteration may become available in the future. Recommendations for screening and other management strategies should be based upon individual circumstances.

Advantages and disadvantages of mutation screening
- May provide an explanation for the family history
- If positive, allows planning of medical intervention or risk reducing surgery
- May identify an increased risk of other cancers that the patient had not previously been concerned about
- If negative, may permit reduction of screening
- In some cases may reassure that there is not a single high-risk genetic factor, but if the family history looks very suspicious it can be difficult to explain that someone may still be at risk despite a 'negative result'
- Genetic testing cannot give all the answers

Predictive testing
This will result in one of two results:

1. *Positive result:* the tested individual is carrying the same pathogenic mutation previously identified in another family member. Carriers will be advised of the implications of this result including lifetime risk of malignancies, current recommendations for screening, and other management options including prophylactic surgery.

2. *Negative (normal) result:* the tested individual has not inherited the pathogenic mutation found in other family member(s). Their risk of developing the malignancy in question is therefore the same as the population risk.

Advantages and disadvantages of predictive testing
Advantages
- Provides definitive answer
- If negative, no additional screening is required
- If positive, allows planning of medical intervention or risk-reducing surgery
- Possible relief that fears were justified
- Ability to warn children

Disadvantages
If negative:
- Feelings of guilt if other close family members are positive
- Readjustment of risk perception
- Increased screening will cease (note: this is not necessarily a negative for all people but is related to readjustment of risk)

If positive:
- Definitive answer versus loss of hope of a normal result
- Emotional consequences (guilt that they may have passed this on to children, concerns about their own risk of cancer now confirmed, anger, fear)
- Surgical options may now need to be considered
- How to inform family
- Possible insurance implications in the future

Confidentiality
Unlike other medical conditions about which individuals seek advice, a referral to clinical genetics may have implications not only for the individual referred, but also for the wider family. A family tree will have information on the whole family collected from one or more individuals, who on their own may not know certain pieces of information. Confidentiality is therefore critical. However, problems with duty to inform can also become an issue if individuals do not want a positive mutation result to be shared within the wider family. This could result in other family members assuming incorrectly that they are not at risk of inheriting a cancer predisposition syndrome and prevent them from seeking genetic testing or appropriate screening themselves.

The General Medical Council (2009, p.21) and Human Genetics Commission (2002 p.10) recognize that the doctor's duty of confidentiality to the individual may be breached in exceptional circumstances where the patient refuses consent of disclosure. This may include where failure to disclose may expose others to a risk of death or serious harm.

Further reading
Chen, S, Euhus, DM, Parmigiani G. Quantitative models for prediction of mutations in Lynch syndrome genes. *Curr Col Ca Rep* 2007; 3:206–211.

Douglas FS, O'Dair LC, Robinson M, et al. The accuracy of diagnoses as reported in families with cancer: a retrospective study. *J Med Genet* 1999; 36(4):309–12.

Eerola H, Blomqvist C, Pukkala E, et al. Familial breast cancer in southern Finland: how prevalent are breast cancer families and can we trust the family history reported by patients? *Eur J Cancer* 2000; 36(9):1143–8.

Evans DG, Eccles DM, Rahman N, et al. A new scoring system for the chances of identifying a BRCA1/2 mutation outperforms existing models including BRCAPRO. *J Med Genet* 2004; 41(6):474–80.

Sijmons RH, Boonstra AE, Reefhuis J, et al. Accuracy of family history of cancer: clinical genetic implications. *Eur J Hum Genet* 2000; 8(3):181–6.

Internet resources
General Medical Council. Guidance for doctors: *Confidentiality* (2009), p.27—available at http://www.gmc-uk.org/guidance/ethical_guidance/confidentiality.asp

Human Genetics Commission. *Inside information—balancing interests in the use of personal genetic data*, p.10. London: Human Genetics Commission, 2002—available at http://www.hgc.gov.uk/UploadDocs/DocPub/Document/insideinformation_summary.pdf

NICE guidance: *CG41 Familial breast cancer*—available at http://guidance.nice.org.uk/CG41

Principles of cancer diagnosis and management

Introduction

Cancer is a global healthcare problem. In the year 2000, cancer accounted for 12% of approximately 56 million deaths worldwide from all causes. It is estimated by 2050 that more than 27 million cancer cases per year will be diagnosed and result in 17·5 million deaths. In the UK, 1 in 3 adults will develop some form of cancer during their life time and 1 in 4 die from cancer.

Patients presenting to their primary care physician with warning signs of cancer (see sections in Chapter 2) should be referred to a specialist centre for urgent evaluation. In the UK and many parts of the world, cancer treatment is organized around a MDT (see later in this section) which consists of physicians, surgeons, cancer specialists, radiologists, pathologists, and clinical nurse specialists. Many investigations for suspected cancer are done either in 'one-stop' (e.g. for breast cancer) or 'two-stop' clinics (e.g. lung cancer) to expedite diagnosis and treatment.

Investigations for a suspected cancer

Initial investigations are to establish a histological diagnosis of cancer, to assess the extent of local disease, and to look for metastatic disease. Further investigations are done to evaluate suitability for standard or trial treatment and to assess the severity of any comorbid medical conditions.

Diagnostic investigations

Diagnostic investigations are usually undertaken in a logical order beginning with blood tests, including relevant tumour markers, and simple imaging such as CXR as appropriate. After this the diagnostic imaging of choice for particular tumour types is undertaken. Histological confirmation of tumour type is often needed to determine appropriate specialized investigations.

Blood tests

Baseline blood tests include full blood count, and liver and renal function tests. Further blood tests will depend on the type of cancer, e.g. LDH for melanoma and lymphoma, beta2-microglobulin for myeloma.

Serum tumour markers

There are a number of tumour markers currently used for diagnosis, monitoring of treatment, assessing prognosis, and follow-up. Table 3.5.1 lists the clinical use of some of the common tumour markers.

Imaging

Imaging helps to determine the extent of local and distant metastatic spread of disease.

CT scan is the diagnostic imaging of choice for most cancers. Additional information may be gained by MRI scan, isotope scans, and functional imaging depending on the site and type of tumour and proposed management plan.

Endoscopy

Direct visualization of the tumour is important for many tumours in body cavities or hollow organs. Endoscopic ear, nose, and throat (ENT) examination; OGD for cancers in the oesophagus, stomach, and duodenum; colonoscopy for bowel tumours; endoscopic retrograde cholangiopancreatography (ERCP) for pancreatic and gall bladder tumours; and cystoscopy for bladder lesions permit the examining clinician to estimate extent of local disease and assess operability. Careful drawings or photos make this information available to other treating clinicians subsequently.

Table 3.5.1 Commonly used tumour markers

Tumour marker	Type of cancer	Clinical use
βhCG	Germ cell tumours of testis and ovary and choriocarcinoma	Diagnosis, monitoring of treatment, detection of recurrence and prognosis
AFP	Germ cell tumours, hepatocellular carcinoma	Diagnosis, monitoring of treatment, detection of recurrence and prognosis
CA-125	Ovarian cancer	Diagnosis, monitoring of treatment, detection of recurrence and prognosis
CA-15-3	Breast cancer	Monitoring of treatment and detection of recurrence
CEA	Colorectal cancer	Diagnosis, monitoring of treatment, detection of recurrence and prognosis
PSA	Prostate cancer	Diagnosis, monitoring of treatment, detection of recurrence and prognosis
Calcitonin	Medullary carcinoma thyroid	Diagnosis, monitoring of treatment, and prognosis
Thyroglobulin	Well differentiated thyroid cancer	Monitoring of treatment and detection of recurrence

Histology

Confirmation of the diagnosis can be obtained by cytology obtained by fine needle aspiration or by tru-cut biopsy. Many tumours subsequently require open biopsy for further characterization and immunohistochemical assessment. Biopsies can be obtained by direct vision, or guided by ultrasound, CT, or MRI or endoscopic visualization.

All patients need a definite histological diagnosis if specific cancer treatment is contemplated. Rarely, treatment can be undertaken when the radiological appearance and tumour markers are typical (e.g. choriocarcinoma, germ cell tumours).

Staging investigations

Once the histological diagnosis is established, further investigations are undertaken to stage the cancer, assess degree of comorbidities, and evaluate prognostic factors. The choice of investigation depends on the primary tumour and pattern of metastasis. For example, the common sites of metastasis in lung cancer are regional lymph nodes, adrenals, and liver and hence all patients with a lung cancer require a CT scan of chest and abdomen.

All patients for whom curative treatment is planned, particularly if this is an extensive surgical resection, need additional investigations to assess their suitability for radical treatment. EUS and thoracoscopy and laparoscopy are also used in staging in appropriate situations.

Functional and molecular imaging

Functional imaging is more sensitive than anatomical imaging in detecting distant metastasis (e.g. positron emission tomography [PET] scan staging alters conventional staging in up to 25% of patients). Imaging based on molecular markers is still at a preliminary stage of development but is likely to become of increasing significance.

Pretreatment assessment

As cancer is often a disease of the elderly, as well as determining all the tumour characteristics, full assessment of the patient's general condition and any comorbidities is essential to determine whether treatment should be undertaken with the aim of cure or whether the aim should be relief of symptoms and improvement in quality of life. Good palliation may, however, still require optimal use of surgery, radiotherapy, or chemotherapy. Diseases such as cardiovascular impairment, diabetes, and renal dysfunction will affect the tolerance and efficacy of treatment and appropriate history, clinical examination, and investigations should inform treatment decisions. Specialist advice should be sought as appropriate.

Standard internationally agreed scales such as Karnofsky or WHO (see following sections) are used to grade performance status and baseline assessment of quality of life using agreed criteria is commonly carried out for patients eligible for treatment in a clinical trial.

Staging

The purpose of staging is to assess the extent of disease, choose the appropriate treatment, and to assess the likely outcome. Staging is also important to enable comparison of results between treatment centres.

The TNM system has been developed for many cancers. TNM staging denotes **t**umour, **n**ode, and **m**etastatic status. T staging is generally based on the size of the tumour (usually according to defined size criteria, e.g. in breast cancer) or depth of invasion in hollow organs (e.g. oesophageal cancer, bladder cancer) or local spread to neighbouring organs or subsites (e.g. supraglottic cancer).

N staging is based on pattern of spread along the lymphatic chain, or number of nodes involved or size of nodes involved. It may be defined as clinical (from examination or imaging) or pathological (from histology).

M1 denotes distant metastasis. Composite staging involves grouping various T, N, and M combinations into four stages. Each tumour site has a different stage grouping. Other descriptors of TNM staging are shown in Table 3.5.2. Other cancers are staged by slightly different systems such as FIGO which is used for many gynaecological cancers.

Prognostic factors

Many factors influence the prognosis of cancer apart from staging. Two generally important prognostic factors are performance status (PS, discussed in 'Decision about the most appropriate treatment' section) and significant weight loss ($\geq$10% weight loss in last 3 months). A poor performance status WHO 3–4 and significant weight loss suggest poor prognosis for many solid tumours.

Multidisciplinary management

In the UK, all patients with suspected cancer are managed within the MDT. This journey starts from the referral with suspected cancer to the end of the treatment and into follow-up or death. The MDT is constituted by people from different disciplines who can contribute independently to the diagnostic and treatment decisions about patients. The role of multidisciplinary management is to

- Standardize the treatment, minimizing the influence of bias and personal anecdotal experience
- Improve continuity of care and avoid delays in the management by choosing the most appropriate investigations and treatment
- Improve communication between health professionals
- Improve recruitment to clinical trials
- Improve educational opportunities

There are a number of barriers to achieving these intentions. Over the years, the logistics of MDT meetings have become more complicated and there is a risk, particularly where common cancers and therefore large numbers of patients are being discussed, that the meeting may become a simple box ticking exercise. Personality conflicts between team members rather than intellectual or clinical disagreements can make team working ineffectual or unsatisfactory.

The main limitations of centralized decision making are the lack of knowledge of patient circumstances and preferences, and the risk of taking a decision without proper assessment of comorbidities. Occasionally these limitations necessitate a deviation from the recommended 'gold standard' treatment.

Though there are sufficient data to show that multidisciplinary management has improved the consistency of care,

Table 3.5.2 TNM staging descriptors

Prefix	• c: clinical staging—based on physical examination, imaging, and endoscopy
	• p: pathological staging—after surgery and histopathological examination. Some tumours have different c and p staging (e.g. breast cancer) whereas others have only p staging (e.g. colon cancer)
	• y: denotes staging after neoadjuvant therapy
	• r: recurrent tumour: restaging following a disease free interval
	• a: autopsy staging
Grading (G)	• Gx: cannot be assessed
	• G1: well differentiated
	• G2: moderately differentiated
	• G3: poorly differentiated
	• G4: undifferentiated
L—lymphatic invasion	• Lx: cannot be assessed
	• L0: no lymphatic invasion
	• L1: lymphatic invasion
V—venous invasion	• Vx: cannot be assessed
	• V1: microscopic invasion
	• V2: macroscopic invasion
R—residual tumour after surgery	• R0: no residual tumour
	• R1: microscopic residual tumour
	• R2: macroscopic residual tumour
Multiple tumours	• Multiple tumours in one organ, the tumour with highest T category should be identified and the multiplicity of the number of tumours is indicated in parentheses, e.g. T1 (m) or T1 (3)
	• In simultaneous bilateral cancers of paired organs, each tumour is classified independently

evidence showing an improvement in the treatment outcome is still weak.

If medical litigation should arise as a result of an MDT decision, all those present at the meeting would be personally accountable for the decisions related to their expertise, irrespective of whether they have spoken or not in the meeting.

More work is needed to ensure that the undoubted advantage to the patient and clinician of proper multidisciplinary treatment planning is undertaken in the most relevant and effective way, considering the need for informed input about each individual patient and the time constraints of the involved clinicians.

Initial consultation and breaking the news

When patients attend oncology clinics, many of them already have some idea about the details of their cancer and an outline of the further management possibilities. However most patients are still in shock and may take a long time to come to terms with a diagnosis of cancer. The clinician's role is to help the patient to cope with the situation, to give them clear advice on further management, and to explain the intent of treatment.

Decision about the most appropriate treatment

The decision about the appropriate treatment for an individual patient depends on the type of cancer, stage, fitness of the patient, comorbidities which might necessitate modification of standard treatment, and the patient's preference.

Assessing fitness for treatment is an important part of decision making. It is mainly based on the PS of patient, active comorbidities at diagnosis, likely responsiveness of the particular tumour type and an assessment of the likely tolerance of the patient to any planned treatment.

PS helps to quantify the physical well-being of patients and to determine optimal treatment, make treatment modifications (including dose modification of chemotherapy), and to measure the intensity of supportive care required. It should be clearly documented before and throughout treatment. There are a number of scoring systems but the two most commonly used are Karnofsky performance status (KPS) and WHO score (Table 3.5.3). Patients are generally eligible for curative treatment only if PS is 0–1, palliative anticancer treatment if PS is 0–2, and generally no anticancer treatment is given if PS 3–4. However, in certain situations, when the disease is very responsive to treatment and rapid deterioration is due to the current disease process, modified curative treatment is considered (e.g. for germ cell tumours, lymphomas). If performance status deteriorates rapidly during anticancer treatment, treatment is either stopped or modified.

A proper assessment of active comorbidities is important in predicting side effects from the proposed cancer treatment. For example, patients with severe COPD with poor pulmonary function tests (FEV_1 <1) are not considered for surgery or radical radiotherapy even if the tumour is very small and potentially curable. Similarly, many chemotherapy drugs have systemic organ effects which need to be taken into account when planning anticancer treatment.

Intent of treatment

With the recent progress in multimodality treatment, the distinction in treatment intent between cure and palliation is becoming increasingly difficult. This is because with multiple lines of treatment a significant number of cancer patients may live for years. However, in the majority of cases, after initial assessment, it is possible to clearly define the intent of treatment. In the rest of the patients a proper assessment of the expected benefit versus cure ratio, and the patient's own views are of major importance in devising a plan for treatment.

Palliation

Relief of symptoms and prolongation of good quality of life determine the choice of treatment for those for whom cure cannot be achieved .This may be obtained by drugs appropriate for pain control, treatment of nausea and vomiting, etc. but oncological treatments such as, for example, radiotherapy for relief of bone pain or surgery for spinal cord compression, may be very effective. Multidisciplinary input by palliative care physicians, oncologists, and surgeons may be appropriate and a clear management plan with well-defined responsibilities is needed to ensure that the patient is well cared for.

Internet and information overload

Patients who are anxious for more information may search the Internet. If they do not have the knowledge to sift this information appropriately, their anxiety may be increased and their need for medical time paradoxically may therefore be increased. With inappropriate information overload many patients suffer a phase which is like being on an emotional roller coaster. Information sources, such as those available through the national programme in the UK (Macmillan), are helpful but often considered inadequate by patients consciously or subconsciously seeking to know that they will be cured. Valuable additional support is given by specialist nurses and through support and information centres where facilities such as counselling, relaxation, and alternative treatments are valued by many.

Implementing planned treatment

For many early stage cancers, delay in treatment is proven to compromise the chances of cure (e.g. germ cell tumours) and in tumours with rapid proliferation (e.g. Burkitt's lymphoma which has a doubling time of <24 hours) even a few days delay in initiating treatment can be detrimental. Hence it is important to start curative treatment as soon as possible.

There is good evidence that interruptions in radical radiotherapy treatments for some cancers, such as those in the head and neck, also lead to poorer control rates and adjustment using twice-daily treatments is therefore made if a gap in treatment occurs. It is not clear how important is initial delay for tumours that are not growing very quickly relative to other tumour prognostic factors but with the introduction of cancer treatment time targets as in the UK any risk is minimized.

Follow-up during treatment

Follow-up during treatment is undertaken to assess response to treatment, monitor toxicity, and modify further treatment. Toxicity should be monitored alongside treatment so that patients receiving a 3-weekly cycle of chemotherapy will be seen every 3 weeks before each treatment to modify the dose or adjust supportive treatments. Patients who have had significant toxicities with a previous cycle may be seen in between the cycle dates. Patients undergoing radiotherapy will often be seen at least once weekly throughout their treatment to assess acute toxicities and prescribe supportive measures as necessary.

Table 3.5.3 Karnofsky performance status (KPS) and WHO score

KPS		WHO (KPS)	
Score (%)	Description	Score	Description
100	Normal, no signs of disease	0 (90–100)	Asymptomatic, fully active and able to carry out all pre-disease activities without restriction
90	Capable of normal activity, a few symptoms or signs of disease	1 (70–90)	Symptomatic, restricted in physically strenuous activity but ambulatory and able to carry out light or sedentary work
80	Normal activity with some difficulty. Some symptoms or signs		
70	Self-caring, not capable of normal activity or work	2 (50–70)	Capable of all self-care but unable to carry out any work activities; <50% in bed during day
60	Needs some help with care, can take care of most personal requirements		
50	Help required often, frequent medical care needed	3 (30–50)	Capable of only limited self-care; >50% in bed during the day
40	Disabled, requires special care and help		
30	Severely disabled, hospital admission needed but no risk of death	4 (10–30)	Completely disabled and cannot do any self-care. Totally confined to bed or chair
20	Very ill, needs urgent admission and requires supportive care		
10	Moribund, rapidly progressive fatal disease		
0	Death	5	Death

The optimal timing to assess tumour response to treatment varies depends on the type of cancer treatment. For example, radiotherapy and hormonal agents generally take 3–4 months to show any response to treatment whereas chemotherapy response is faster (6–9 weeks). Hence, investigations to assess response to treatment should be planned according to the appropriate timescale. However, if there is any clinical suspicion of progression during treatment, prompt investigations are required without waiting for any planned investigations.

Second opinions

A second opinion about treatment options may be sought by the clinician in the case of very rare tumours where there is no local expertise. Formalized referral patterns for specialized surgery have been developed in the UK (e.g. surgery for osteosarcoma is centralized to a few units). A well-functioning MDT will also fulfil this need for clinicians.

Patients may seek a second opinion if they are unsure of the expertise of the person to whom they have been referred, particularly if they are privately insured or have medical connections. Facilitation of such a request by the person to whom the patient has first been referred can be helpful in enabling them to confidently pursue treatment locally. People giving second opinions have a duty to advise constructively and within any unavoidable constraints. They should avoid undermining other clinicians and work collaboratively.

However, patients in the UK should be clearly informed, when there are national protocols or agreed practices and the diagnosis and treatment are uncontroversial, that a second opinion is unlikely to be useful. Healthcare resources within a publicly funded service must be used in a cost-effective way and seeking second opinions should be limited wherever possible to difficult situations or where patient–doctor relations will preclude good care.

Support during treatment

From the moment of diagnosis of cancer a person's life is changed forever. It affects not only their physical health but their mental health is also challenged. Different individuals deal with this process in different ways but each should be offered appropriate support for their needs. This may involve psychological support or something more practical such as directing them to possible sources of financial support. Many people are working at the time of diagnosis and their future employment may be affected depending on their job and employer. Laws exist to protect individuals but those who are self-employed will only be protected if they had pre-existing insurance. Relationships are frequently challenged by the diagnosis of cancer and the journey through treatment and it is not uncommon for couples to separate at this time. Financial worries may continue after treatment is completed as the diagnosis of cancer affects the ability to gain new life insurance or a mortgage. Those living in countries which require health insurance will notice an increase in premiums or difficulty obtaining further health insurance. Holiday planning may be affected by difficulty in getting insurance cover (p.618).

Local health providers such as GPs will have a key role in coordinating some of the aftercare for patients and providing additional necessary services such as physiotherapy and occupational therapy.

At the time of diagnosis, an individual should therefore be provided with sources of information to help them through all these areas to facilitate their treatment and return to health. The key areas are:
• Psychosocial support
• Income support
• Macmillan team
• Cancer care In the community

The potential sources of this support can be in the form of documentation of helpful websites (p.615, 626) or organizations, local cancer support groups, and named key workers such as specialist nurses or Macmillan nurses. It should be emphasized at the start of diagnosis and treatment that it is natural to require the help of others at some point in the journey and that this will help their overall outcome. The special needs of children diagnosed with cancer and their family require expert consideration.

Follow-up after treatment and management of recurrence

Almost all patients who have been treated with curative intent need some regular follow-up to detect an early potentially curable recurrence or a second cancer. The frequency and mode of follow-up depend on the pattern of recurrence of individual cancers, which are dealt with for each cancer in the appropriate chapter. It is still debatable whether early detection of a metastatic recurrence improves overall survival in most cancers but continuing care and support of the patient are always important for their overall well-being.

Beyond cure and survivorship

For many patients treatment will be possible and they will succeed in climbing the mountain of diagnosis, treatment, and its complications. However the long-term impact of this on their lives must not be underestimated and many patients feel at their most lost at the end of treatment or when follow-up is discontinued (see also Chapter 6, Late effects, p.610). An understanding of this process will help facilitate any further care that is necessary to return them to a functional life.

Further reading

Sidhom MA, Poulsen MG. Multidisciplinary care in oncology: medicolegal implications of group decisions. *Lancet Oncol* 2006; **7**:951–54.

Internet resources

Macmillan Cancer Support charity: http://www.macmillan.org.uk
TNM staging: http://www.uicc.org

Principles of surgical oncology

Introduction

Surgery accounts for approximately 60% of all cancer cures. It also has a significant role in the prevention, diagnosis, palliation, and rehabilitation of the cancer patient. After extensive curative surgery, the resultant impairment of appearance and function can be corrected to a certain extent by reconstructive surgery (oncoplastic surgery) to restore body image and to enable the patient to return to a normally functioning life.

Role of surgery in diagnosis and staging

Diagnosis

Obtaining a histological diagnosis is an essential step in the management of cancer. The various techniques used to obtain a histological diagnosis include fine needle aspiration (FNA) cytology, core biopsy, incisional biopsy, and excisional biopsy. The choice of a particular technique is based on the location of tumour, anticipated type of tumour, and the reliability of the method to make a definite diagnosis.

FNA yields a quick result and shows cellular characteristics but not architecture. FNA serves as a good screening tool prior to more definitive diagnostic methods. FNA is useful for diagnosis of enlarged lymph nodes, aspiration of cysts, diagnosis of thyroid nodules, and confirmation of recurrent or metastatic disease.

In needle biopsy, a core of tissue is obtained which helps to visualize architecture as well as to perform immunohistochemical studies. It is useful in the diagnosis of most solid tumours. However, core biopsy should not be used in lymphoma (a whole lymph node is needed to evaluate the architectural pattern and for further immunohistochemical studies to accurately identify the subtype of lymphoma).

Incisional biopsy involves removal of a small wedge of tissue from a large tumour and is indicated when core biopsy is non-diagnostic and an excision biopsy is inappropriate. A common situation is a suspected sarcoma. Care should be taken when planning incision biopsy to ensure that the site of biopsy is within the area of definite surgery and preferably is undertaken by surgeons who will undertake the final surgery. A poorly planned incision biopsy can lead to unnecessary morbid surgery.

Excision biopsy involves removal of the entire mass or skin lesion. It is important to make sure that this procedure does not compromise a later wider excision if necessary. The specimen needs to be oriented in three dimensions and marked for the pathologist to determine surgical margins.

Frozen section is occasionally used perioperatively to confirm the diagnosis when previous histological diagnosis is not available (e.g. solitary lung lesions), to decide need for further surgery (e.g. lymph node dissection), and ensure adequate surgical margins.

A number of precautions should be taken when performing a surgical procedure for histological diagnosis. These include:
- Needle tracks or incisions should be placed in such a way that they can be removed, if indicated, during the definitive surgery without unwanted morbidity
- Care should be taken to avoid contamination of unaffected tissue planes
- After biopsy, haemostasis should be ensured to avoid haematoma formation which otherwise can lead to local tumour spread
- An adequate tissue sample should be obtained for all necessary diagnostic tests
- After an excision biopsy, the specimen should be properly orientated and marked with ink to identify all the margins
- Placement of surgical clips during the biopsy is useful in patients who will undergo neoadjuvant chemotherapy (helps to identify the site of primary tumour during later surgery in cases of complete response) and in those who need definitive radiotherapy to a localized area

Staging

Various surgical procedures such as endoscopy and laparoscopy help to define the extent of disease as well as obtaining histological confirmation of metastatic disease (see later in section).

Role of surgery in treatment

Curative surgery

Surgery plays an important role in achieving a cure when the cancer is confined to the site of origin. A decision regarding curative surgery is made after careful consideration of various patient- and tumour-related characteristics at a multidisciplinary meeting with surgeons, oncologists, radiologists, and pathologists. Patient-related factors which influence the choice of curative surgery include age, performance status, and comorbidities. Tumour-related factors include the chances of long-term benefit and potential surgical risks and complications.

Surgery of the primary tumour

Curative surgery is aimed at removal of the tumour with a clear margin of normal tissue ('R0' resection) with reconstruction of the surgical defect if appropriate. The margin of normal tissue removed depends on the type of malignancy and pattern of local spread. An adequate gross margin helps to ensure an adequate microscopic margin of resection. The tumour should be orientated and marked at the time of surgery so that any positive margins can be identified anatomically should the need for re-excision arise.

Based on the extent of removal of cancer, resections are classified as follows as part of the TNM staging:
- R0: all margins are histologically free of tumour
- R1: microscopic residual disease after resection
- R2: gross residual disease after resection

At the time of surgery, exposure of tumour with the risk of shedding viable tumour cells should be avoided if possible. Certain tumours have a propensity to recur along surgical incision lines or drainage sites, e.g. sarcoma.

Depending on the type of cancer and anatomical site, curative surgery can be:
- Wide excision—the tumour is removed with a margin to account for microscopic spread
- Removal of part of an organ and surrounding tissue at risk of spread (e.g. partial gastrectomy)
- Removal of an entire organ with or without important adjacent structures (e.g. total abdominal hysterectomy with bilateral salpingo-oophorectomy)

Recent advances in multimodality treatment have influenced the surgical approach to many cancers. The use of radiotherapy, chemotherapy, or both has led to the use of less radical procedures with an improvement in quality of life.

Surgery of regional lymph nodes

In some tumours, regional lymph node spread occurs in a predictable fashion. In such situations, the regional lymph nodes in continuity with lymphatics are removed along with the primary tumour. The removal of lymph nodes provides important staging information and if there is nodal involvement often results in a therapeutic gain, in terms of reducing the risk of a regional recurrence and thus preventing further morbidity.

In patients with an unknown or low risk of lymph node involvement, various methods are used to screen for pathological involvement of lymph nodes before extensive lymph node dissection is undertaken. These methods include

- FNA of enlarged regional lymph nodes
- Node sampling—involves cherry picking of 4–5 regional lymph nodes (e.g. breast cancer)
- Sentinel node biopsy (SNB)—SNB is based on the principle that the tumour spreads to a single (sentinel) node before spreading to other nodes in an 'ordered' fashion. Sentinel lymph nodes can be identified by using blue dye or radioisotopes

In many clinical situations the role of lymph node dissection in overall survival remains controversial. In practice, patients with positive sentinel lymph nodes undergo a complete node dissection whereas the role of elective lymph node dissection is dependent on the site of cancer, type of cancer, and other prognostic factors. Benefits of nodal dissections in different cancers are discussed in the relevant chapters.

Debulking surgery

In certain situations, debulking surgery is useful in improving the ability of other treatments to control the residual tumour (e.g. ovarian cancer) and in some cancers maximal cytoreduction is associated with a better outcome (e.g. ovarian cancer and glioblastoma multiforme).

Metastatectomy

Resection of a single metastatic lesion results in better survival for a selected group of patients with certain cancers (Table 3.6.1). Metastatectomy is also an option for patients with a limited number of metastases (oligometastasis). This approach is especially suitable for a patient with good PS who has limited disease which does not respond well to systemic treatment, has surgically resectable metastatic disease at presentation or recurs with limited disease a long time (at least 12 months) after successful treatment of the primary tumour.

In the absence of proper randomized studies it is not known whether the observed therapeutic benefit of metastatectomy is real or due to the strict selection process (selection bias). Studies show that resection of isolated or limited liver metastases in colorectal cancer results in 20–40% 5-year survival. Pulmonary metastatectomy in sarcomas leads to a 5-year survival of 20–30%. An alternative to metastatectomy is the evolving use of RF ablation.

Salvage surgery

Surgery is useful as a salvage measure after primary treatment failure or recurrence after definitive treatment. It is only appropriate for fit patients with a good chance of prolonged survival. Examples include abdomino-perineal resection after chemoradiotherapy for anal cancer, and exenteration in cervical cancer after chemoradiotherapy.

In patients with prior limited surgery or chemoradiotherapy, a second chance of cure is aimed at with salvage surgery. Examples include mastectomy for local recurrence

Table 3.6.1 Role of metastatectomy

Liver	Selected patients with colorectal cancer
Lung	Selected patients with colorectal, renal, and testicular cancers and sarcoma
Adrenal	Selected patients with resectable lung cancer and isolated adrenal disease
Brain	Solitary metastasis with controlled/potentially curable systemic disease

after conservative surgery for breast cancer and neck node dissection for isolated nodal recurrence after chemoradiotherapy for head and neck cancer.

Palliative and emergency surgery

The aim of palliative surgery is to improve or prevent significant symptoms (e.g. pain, bleeding, and obstruction) which are likely to occur without intervention.

Emergency surgery has a role in life-threatening bleeding, perforation and obstruction of an abdominal viscus, and neurological compression.

Reconstructive (oncoplastic) surgery

Extensive resection often results in the disruption of normal anatomy with subsequent impaired cosmesis and function. Plastic surgical techniques are useful in correcting the anatomical defects and improving cosmesis (e.g. reconstructive breast surgery) and function (e.g. in head and neck surgery).

Risk reduction surgery

Fewer than 5% of patients have a genetic component to their cancer. Increasing understanding of the development of genetically associated cancers has led to prophylactic surgery for some patients. Table 3.6.2 shows the indications for common prophylactic surgeries. Appropriate genetic testing and counselling is, however, an absolute prerequisite before any prophylactic surgery. Women with BRCA1 and BRCA2 mutations have a high risk of breast cancer which is reduced by 90–95% with bilateral mastectomy. However, the decision to undergo prophylactic mastectomy should be made after careful discussion, exploring future quality of life, potential surgical risks, and wishes of the patient. Alternative risk reduction methods such as use of tamoxifen and prophylactic oophorectomy after completion of family should also be considered.

Table 3.6.2 Potential indications for risk reducing surgery

Surgery	Indication
Bilateral mastectomy	BRCA1/2 mutations Familial breast cancer Unilateral breast cancer in <40 years
Bilateral oophorectomy	BRCA1/2 mutations Familial ovarian cancer
Total proctocolectomy	FAP or APC mutations HNPCC—germline mutations
Thyroidectomy	RET oncogene mutation MEN2

Minimal access surgery

The role of minimal access surgery is being increasingly studied in the management of solid tumours.

Laparoscopy has an established role in the staging of many abdominal malignancies. It is useful in identifying peritoneal metastases which are easily missed on anatomical imaging. It is also helpful to correctly stage patients who might otherwise have been overstaged with anatomical imaging. Preoperative laparoscopy has significantly reduced the rates of 'open and close' laparotomies. An example is the use of laparoscopy to detect small peritoneal and liver metastases which reduces the number of 'open and close' laparotomies to <5% in stomach cancer. Laparoscopy has an established role in the staging of oesophageal and stomach cancer. It has a limited role in the staging of pancreatic and liver cancers. Its role in the staging of gynaecological and testicular cancers is evolving.

Laparoscopy has also been evaluated as a treatment option for abdominal malignancies and studies show that laparoscopic surgery results in the same long-term survival as that of open surgery, with no increased risk of abdominal wall recurrence, less surgical morbidity, and faster return to normal function. Laparoscopic surgery is an accepted surgical treatment for gastric, renal, adrenal, and colorectal cancers.

Laparoscopic stapled gastrojejunostomy is a treatment option for the palliation of gastric outlet obstruction in gastric and pancreatic cancer. In intestinal obstruction, a laparoscopic bypass procedure or intestinal stoma creation procedure results in prompt relief of symptoms.

Video-assisted thoracic surgery for stage I lung cancer has been studied recently as an attractive option for the treatment of elderly patients with lung cancer.

Robotic surgery

Robotic assisted surgery is being studied in prostate and renal cell cancers. This technique may result in minimal surgical trauma with a better toxicity profile.

Further reading

Hagiike M and Lefor AT. Laparoscopic surgery. In: DeVita VT, Lawrence TS, Rosenberg SA (eds) *Cancer: Principles and Practice of Oncology*, Volume 8, pp.293–305. Philadelphia: Lippincott Williams & Wilkins, 2008.

Radiotherapy

Role in the treatment of cancer

Radiotherapy is an extremely effective local treatment for cancer and is used in at least 50% of patients in whom cure is achieved. As well as treatment given with the aim of local control and cure, radiotherapy is widely used to palliate symptoms of advanced cancer. It may be given as the sole curative treatment as for carcinoma of the cervix, as adjuvant therapy after surgery, e.g. for breast cancer, or in combination with chemotherapy, as in head and neck cancer.

Mode of action

Radiotherapy uses electromagnetic radiation (X-rays, gamma rays, or electrons) at the high-energy end of the spectrum. The unit of dose is Gy which is defined as 1Joule of energy deposited in 1kg of tissue. Energy deposition in the tissues through which the X-rays pass causes ionization, which in turn produces free radicals, fragments of molecules with an unpaired electron which interact either directly or indirectly to produce DNA damage. This damage can manifest as single- or double-strand breaks, base damage, DNA or protein cross links, protein–protein cross links, and intra- or interstrand cross links.

One unrepaired double-strand break is enough to kill the cell. Mitotic cell death is the main mechanism of cell death following irradiation. Cells do not generally show evidence of damage until they divide.

The effects of radiation on tissues depend on dose as shown in the diagram for tumour control probability (TCP) and normal tissue complication probability (NTCP) (Fig. 3.7.1). The effects of radiotherapy on normal tissue irradiated depend on the volume treated, total dose given, and fractionation schedule used, and whether the tissue has a large functional reserve capacity (parallel organization) such as lung and kidney, or like the spinal cord or gut a serial organization, which means that damage to a small segment only may result in severe injuries such as paralysis. When there is little or no functional reserve, dose is more important than volume.

The ability to give high enough doses to local tumours to cure them is dependent on fractionation of total dose to exploit underlying biological factors. Recovery of radiation damage between fractions of treatment occurs more readily in normal tissues than in tumour. Between fractions, cells may redistribute into a more radiosensitive phase of the cell cycle, or hypoxic radiation-resistant cells become re-oxygenated and more sensitive as surrounding well-oxygenated cells are killed. The amount of cell kill can also depend on the radiosensitity of the tumour—for example, lymphomas are very radiosensitive while melanoma is resistant. The overall time in which treatment is given is also important and shorter treatment times allow less repopulation by tumour cells.

Various fractionation schemes are used. Classically, doses of 45–60Gy in 2Gy/ fraction treating five times weekly are used for radical treatments of squamous carcinomas. Different schedules using shorter treatment times (acceleration), several smaller doses per day (hyperfractionation), or fewer large fractions (hypofractionation) can be useful in specific situations.

Types of radiotherapy treatment

Superficial X-rays (orthovoltage)

Low-energy X-rays can be produced by an orthovoltage machine (formerly known as deep X-rays or DXT). The mode of interaction with tissues is by the photoelectric effect rather than by Compton scattering as occurs with high-energy X-rays. This effect depends on the density of tissue and there is therefore maximum absorption of the X-rays in the skin because of their low penetration and in bone because of its high density. They are therefore used to treat skin tumours and to palliate metastasis in superficial bones such as the ribs. Erythema of the skin is seen as an acute reaction, and telangiectasia may develop later.

Brachytherapy

Sources of radioactive material may be inserted directly into body cavities such as the uterus and vagina. The dose distribution from such sources gives a very conformal treatment, with very high doses close to the surface of the source and rapid falloff of dose thereafter. Normal tissues are therefore better protected, although great care must be taken to avoid hotspots where high doses in a small area may produce damage, for example, in pelvic treatments and care must be taken that there are no small bowel loops adjacent to the high-dose region. Originally, radium was used for brachytherapy, but has now been replaced with caesium, cobalt, or iridium. After loading techniques, in which hollow source carriers are placed *in situ* and their position checked before loading with the active source, have helped to reduce doses to personnel. Doses much higher than can be delivered by external beam radiotherapy can be used to control local disease.

Melanoma of the choroid may be treated with iodine-125 or ruthenium-106 plaque brachytherapy. Brachytherapy with iridium wire may be used in conjunction with external beam therapy to deliver a high local dose for some soft tissue sarcomas, to treat recurrent disease in neck nodes and to give a local boost in breast cancer. Localized prostate cancer may be treated by permanently implanting iodine-125 seeds or with iridium wire loaded temporarily into flexible catheters.

Radio isotopes

These are most commonly used in the treatment of well-differentiated thyroid cancer with iodine-131 which is specifically taken up by the thyroid, thyroid cancer, and its metastases. An initial dose is given to ablate normal thyroid tissue which takes up the isotope most avidly, and this is followed by therapeutic doses to treat the cancer. Strontium-89 and samarium-153 are used for the relief of cancer-induced bone pain, particularly from prostate cancer. Phosphorus-32 can be used in the treatment of polycythemia rubra vera.

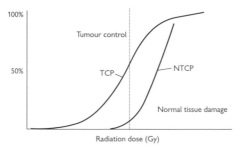

Fig. 3.7.1 TCP and NTCP.

Megavoltage radiotherapy

Modern linear accelerators accelerate electrons by subjecting them to a series of oscillating electrical potentials in a wave guide. These accelerated electrons can be used directly for therapy, or they can be made to hit a target which produces high-energy X-rays. A series of collimators are used to produce a focused beam which can be further shaped with a series of lead rods in the head of the machine known as a multileaf collimator. Energies in the range of 6–16MV or MeV are commonly used for external beam therapy.

Protons

Protons have a pattern of dose distribution which shows a sharply defined range of energy deposition rather than the attenuation pattern of photons. This can be favourable for treatment of some tumour types such as skull-based tumours, spinal chondrosarcoma, and some paediatric tumours.

Stereotactic radiotherapy

This technique, using multiple highly collimated (focused) beams, can be used to deliver very high doses to small volumes as either single dose or fractionated treatments. A high degree of immobilization with a stereotactic frame is essential (1mm).

The radiotherapy process

The process of radiotherapy planning can be divided into several phases.

Collection of relevant data

Clinical assessment and decision for radical or palliative treatment, taking into account the extent of disease and any comorbidities is critical.

Collection of data from appropriate imaging techniques is necessary for target volume definition using internationally standardized criteria. Planning of treatment and estimation of dose distribution relies on electron density measurements and therefore a CT scan is essential. This must be done with the patient in the treatment position using any immobilization devices appropriate.

Techniques for fusing information from CT and MRI scans give the best definition of tumour volume for a number of disease sites and PET scanning may contribute as well.

Several volumes must be defined using the criteria of the International Commission on Radiation Units (ICRU; Report 58 [See Fig. 3.7.2]). The gross target volume (GTV)

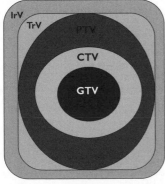

Fig. 3.7.2 ICRU recommendations for target volume definition. IrV, irradiated volume; TrV, treatment volume.

is the macroscopic extent of tumour determined from imaging the entire tumour mass or as defined surgically and pathologically.

The clinical target volume (CTV) includes a margin around the GTV to encompass any subclinical or microscopic disease. A planning target volume (PTV) is then defined to ensure that the CTV remains within the volume that is actually treated each day, taking into account any movement that occurs physiologically, by the patient changing their position, or from errors in setting up the treatment in the same way each day.

These errors can be minimized by the use of immobilization devices to help the patient to maintain the same position for treatment each day. They include the use of arm supports, foot restraints, vacuum bags which can be moulded to support the area being treated, or customized shells made individually using thermoplastic materials (particularly used for head and neck and brain treatments).

Another source of day-to-day variability arises from physiological changes which may be predictable, such as those with respiration, in which case radiation delivery can be gated to a particular phase of respiration to ensure the tumour is always included in the treatment volume. Physiological movements of bowel and bladder are unpredictable and although a number of studies have explored ways of reducing them, such as by use of bladder filling protocols or routine enemas, there is at present no satisfactory solution. Implanted fiducial markers such as gold grains or clips may be helpful in ensuring reproducibility of treatment set up.

Devising of an optimal treatment plan/calculation of dose distributions

This is usually done by a physicist or radiation technologist. As the dose from each beam of radiation from the linear accelerator is attenuated as it passes through tissue, the dose in tissues outside the tumour will be greater than that to a deep-seated tumour. Multiple beams are therefore used to deliver a homogeneous dose throughout the tumour while minimizing dose to other normal tissues through which each beam must pass. Conventional plans often use three beams but intensity modulated radiotherapy (see later in section) may use as many as seven. The distribution of dose may also be modified by insertion of a wedge of absorbing material into the beam so that less dose is delivered through the thick end of the wedge. Beams can be shaped to conform to the tumour using the multileaf collimator in the head of the linear accelerator.

Dose–volume histograms (DVHs) are used to help choose the best plan. A DVH is a plot of the radiation dose against the volume of the structure of interest and the shape and area under the curve is used to ensure that the target volume is covered with a homogeneous dose and that dose to normal structures is within acceptable limits (Table 3.7.1).

With intensity modulated radiotherapy (IMRT), multiple beam segments of variable intensity are defined. These are used to modulate dose and ensure maximum tumour conformality. It also makes it possible to limit dose to normal organs more effectively. As acute side effects are therefore reduced, dose escalation, leading to improved tumour control, may be achieved.

Delivery of treatment and verification of accuracy

Radical treatments (other than those for superficial skin tumours where low-energy X-rays are used) are given using a linear accelerator with high energy photons or

Table 3.7.1 Radiation tolerance dose (treated with 2Gy per fraction)

Organ	Tolerance dose for 5% chance of dose limiting toxicity in 5 years			Dose limiting toxicity
	Whole organ	2/3 organ	1/3 organ	
Brain	45	50	60	Necrosis
Brain stem	50	53	60	Necrosis
Colon	45	–	55	Obstruction, perforation, and ulceration
Heart	40	45	60	Pericarditis
Kidney	23	30	50	Renal failure
Lens	10	–	–	Cataract
liver	30	35	50	Hepatitis
Lung	17.5	30	45	Pulmonary fibrosis
Oesophagus	55	58	60	Stricture
Optic apparatus	50	–	–	Blindness
Parotid	32	32	–	Xerostomia
Rectum	60	–	–	Necrosis, fistula, stenosis
Retina	45	–	–	Blindness
Small intestine	40	–	50	Obstruction, perforation
Spinal cord	47	50	50	Myelitis
Stomach	50	55	60	Ulceration, perforation

electrons (6–16 MV linear accelerator). The multileaf collimator is adjusted to conform to the tumour shape in three dimensions. Accuracy of treatment delivery is checked in various ways including measurement of exit doses by in vivo dosimetry using thermoluminescent dosemeters or diodes and analysis of images taken during treatment.

Special techniques

Image guided radiotherapy (IGRT) uses images obtained during treatment to check that the actual treatment delivered corresponds to that which was planned by gating it to a specific phase of respiration. Adaptive radiotherapy involves changing treatment on a daily or less frequent basis by comparison of planning scans with images taken during treatment.

Tomographic devices can be use to deliver gated rotational IMRT using a multileaf collimator and a machine mounted CT scanner. Images taken during treatment are used to gate dose delivery to the correct body slice.

Monitoring treatment effects

Side effects of radiation are classified as early (occurring at <90 days) or late (>90 days). Late effects are much more dependent on dose per fraction, being more severe with high doses per fraction. Overall treatment time affects acute responses, which are increased when treatment times are short and which, in contrast with late effects, are reversible. Unlike the side effects of chemotherapy which are systemic, radiotherapy side effects are local or regional, manifested in the irradiated area only. Acute effects include skin and mucosal damage predominantly. Late effects are the result of vascular damage and fibrosis. They are modified by pre-existing comorbidities such as hypertension or diabetes mellitus, where end-vessel disease may occur.

Other factors which are important include individual radiosensitivity, smoking, age, dose delivered, volume treated, dose per fraction, overall treatment time, type of radiation, concomitant chemotherapy, radiotherapy technique, type of tumour, proximity of any organs at risk, tumour size, tissue type, and structural organization. The effectiveness of any new technique with combinations of drugs with radiation must be assessed in terms of improved therapeutic ratio and the pattern of relapse, whether within or outside the radiation treatment volume, as well as in overall or disease-free survival.

Tables of maximum tolerated doses to various organs have been devised and are shown in Table 3.7.1. Long-term follow-up of patients treated with radiotherapy is important as data on late effects always reflects treatments given some time previously. The use of different combinations of chemotherapy or other novel biological agents may alter the pattern of radiation late effects which are seen and necessitate changes in treatment approach.

Further reading

Barrett A, Dobbs J, Morris S, et al. Practical Radiotherapy Planning (4th edition). London: Hodder Arnold, 2009.

International Commission on Radiation Units and Measurements. Prescribing, Recording and Reporting Photon Beam Therapy. ICRU Report 50, Bethesda, MD: Nuclear Technology Publishing, 1993.

Joiner M, Van der Kogel A (eds). Basic Clinical Radiobiology (4th edition). London: Hodder Arnold, 2009.

The Royal College of Radiologists. Radiotherapy Dose-Fractionation. London: The Royal College of Radiologists, 2006.

World Health Organization. Quality Assurance in Radiotherapy. Geneva: WHO, 1988.

Principles of systemic therapy

Introduction
The effective use of cancer systemic therapies requires an understanding of the principles of tumour biology, cellular kinetics, pharmacology, and drug resistance. There are major biological and histological differences even within a single cancer, with complex interactions occurring between the cancer cells, stromal cells, blood vessels, extracellular matrix, and parenchymal cells.

For systemic therapy to be effective several features must be present:
- The drug must reach the cancer cells
- Sufficient toxic amounts of the drug (or its active metabolites) must enter the cells and remain there for a long enough period of time to have an effect
- Cancer cells must be sensitive to the effect of the drug

All of this must occur before resistance emerges and the patient must be able to tolerate the adverse effects of treatment. Optimal anticancer drug treatment, whether it involves the use of classical cytotoxic agents or novel molecularly targeted anticancer drugs, will require oncologists to incorporate their therapeutic decisions with up-to-date knowledge of the factors that contribute to the variability in human drug response.

Pharmacokinetic (PK) and pharmacodynamic (PD) measurements
These are both important parts of pharmacological studies and are being increasingly recognized as an integral part of drug development and clinical trial design. PK studies, very broadly, refer to 'what the body does to the drug' and PD studies describe 'what the drug does to the body'. With regard to cytotoxic chemotherapy, studies have mainly focused on the pharmacokinetics of the drug, but with the era of molecularly targeted therapies, equal emphasis is now being placed on PD measurements. Preclinical PK information on drug distribution, absorption, metabolism, and excretion can provide very helpful data for the design of early stage clinical trials. Preclinical and clinical data on PD parameters, and the development of PD assays, will indicate whether a drug is having the desired effect on the tissue being examined. Increasingly, it is being acknowledged that assessing PD endpoints in tumour tissue, whether by molecular or imaging techniques, is very important to be able to relate back to the intended biological effect. These PK–PD relationships may help support subsequent drug development and clinical trial design for new compounds.

Chemotherapy
Classical cytotoxic chemotherapy is treatment involving agents that have a non-specific effect on cell division or cause cell death by means of damaging DNA, directly or indirectly. Cytotoxic agents can be classified by:
- Chemical properties or mechanism of action
- Source (natural products)
- Cell cycle- or phase-specific activities

Chemotherapeutic agents are preferentially toxic to actively proliferating cells, although they also kill non-proliferating cells; therefore understanding the growth and cell cycle kinetics of cancer cells is important.

Cellular kinetics
Most cancer cells are not characterized by rapid growth. The growth and division of cells occurs through the cell cycle, which is divided into several different phases, during which the cell prepares for and undergoes mitosis:
- G_0: resting phase (non-proliferation of cells)
- G_1: pre-DNA synthetic phase
- S: DNA synthesis
- G_2: post-DNA synthesis
- M: mitosis

The cell then divides and produces two daughter cells which consist of three subpopulations:
- Non-dividing and terminally differentiated cells
- Cells that are continually proliferating
- Cells that are resting but may be recruited into the cell cycle

All three populations exist simultaneously in tumours. Also located within the cell cycle are checkpoints that can be activated during the cell cycle process. They can prevent the cell from moving forward to the next phase if adverse genetic conditions have occurred. Many cancer cells have lost these checkpoints. Chemotherapeutic agents can be classified according to the phase of the cell cycle in which they are active (Table 3.8.1).

The growth of a tumour depends on several different factors. It is a reflection of the proportion of actively dividing cells (the growth fraction), the length of the cell cycle (doubling time), and the rate of cell loss. Chemotherapeutic agents are most effective during the period of logarithmic growth (the exponential phase of rapid growth) (Fig. 3.8.1), which is the basis for the addition of chemotherapy to other treatments, such as surgery and radiotherapy. If the cell population is reduced by these methods, a higher fraction of the remaining cells would be in logarithmic growth, potentially making chemotherapy more effective. A higher growth fraction causes more cancer cells to be killed when they are exposed to cell cycle specific drugs. Tumours with a greater fraction of cells in G_0 are more sensitive to cell cycle non-specific agents.

Combination chemotherapy
Combination chemotherapy can provide important objectives not possible with single-agent therapy. They can provide maximum cell kill within a range of toxicity tolerated by the host for each drug, offer a broader range of coverage of resistant cell lines in a heterogeneous tumour population, and prevent or slow the development of new drug-resistant

Table 3.8.1 Examples of cell cycle phase-specific drugs

Phase of cell cycle	Class	Characteristic agents
S phase	Antimetabolites	Methotrexate Gemcitabine Fluorouracil Doxorubicin
M phase	Natural products	Vinca alkaloids
G_1 phase	Hormone Natural product	Corticosteroids Asparaginase
G_2 phase	Natural products	Bleomycin, topotecan

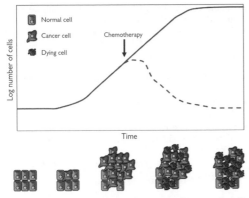

Fig. 3.8.1 Growth curve depicting the growth of cancer cells and the impact chemotherapy can have (see also colour plate section).

cell lines. The following principles should be adhered to when selecting chemotherapy combinations:
• Drugs should show activity as single agents in the specific tumour type
• Each drug should have a different mechanism of action to allow for additive or synergistic effects on the tumour
• Drugs that work in different phases of the cell cycle are preferable
• Drugs with differing dose-limiting toxicities are preferred to allow each to be given at an optimal dose and schedule
• Drugs should not share the same mechanism of resistance

Other factors that should be considered when selecting a combination regimen include schedule and frequency of administration and possible PK and PD interactions.

Drug resistance
The single biggest obstacle to efficacy of chemotherapy is the development of resistance. Various mechanisms are now understood and these are normally classified into either natural or acquired resistance. Natural resistance refers to the initial unresponsiveness of a tumour to a given drug, and acquired resistance refers to the unresponsiveness that emerges after initially successful treatment. Cells may exhibit reduced degrees of sensitivity to drugs because of their position in the cell cycle. Cells that are in the G_0 phase are generally resistant to all drugs active in the S phase. Cells may also exhibit pharmacological resistance, in which failure to kill cells is also a function of insufficient drug concentration. In general this can be due to:
• Decreased drug-activating enzymes
• Increased drug-inactivating enzymes
• Increased DNA repair
• Mutations in drug targets
• Excretion of drug out of the cells

Repeated exposure of a tumour to a single chemotherapy agent will generally result in cross resistance to some agents of the same drug class as the original. This can be due to expression of the multidrug resistance (MDR) gene, which encodes a transmembrane P-glycoprotein. MDR is commonly mediated by an enhanced energy-dependent drug efflux mechanism that results in lower intracellular drug concentrations. A high level of MDR expression is reliably correlated with resistance to cytotoxic agents.

Tumours that intrinsically express the MDR1 gene before chemotherapy characteristically display poor or short lived responses.

Classification of chemotherapy agents
There are several ways of classifying chemotherapy agents; one is by their mechanism of action. Table 3.8.2 shows some common chemotherapeutics classified in this way.

Alkylating agents
Alkylating agents form adducts with DNA bases that disrupt DNA synthesis. They can react with one or both strands of DNA (monofunctional or bifunctional agents). Most alkylating agents are bifunctional, and form cross-links within the DNA double helix, which prevent replication of DNA and transcription of RNA. The most common sites of alkylation are the N^7 and O^6 positions of guanine. These links can be formed at any stage of the cell cycle, so alkylating agents are not phase-specific. Although most of these drugs have similar mechanisms of action, there are differences in the spectrum of activity, PK parameters, and toxicity. They play a major role in the treatment of breast cancer, ovarian cancer, and the haematological malignancies, and can be incorporated into transplant regimens.

Antimetabolites
These are so called because they exert their effects mostly in the synthetic phase of the cell cycle, and have little effect on cells in G_0. Consequently, these drugs are most effective in tumours that have a high growth fraction. Some antimetabolites are structural analogues of the naturally occurring metabolites involved in DNA and RNA synthesis. They exert their cytotoxic activity either by competing with normal metabolites for the catalytic or regulatory site of a key enzyme or by substituting for a metabolite that is normally incorporated into DNA and RNA. Other antimetabolites inhibit enzymes that are necessary for the synthesis of vital compounds.

The antimetabolites can be divided into:
• Antifolates: e.g. methotrexate, competitively inhibits the enzyme dihydrofolate reductase (DHFR), essential for purine and pyrimidine production and therefore DNA synthesis
• Fluorinated pyrimidines: e.g. fluorouracil (5-FU); prodrugs that are intracellularly activated and whose products inhibit pyrimidine synthesis (inhibition of thymidylate synthase)
• Antipurines: e.g. mercaptopurine; these inhibit purine synthesis and the nucleotide product is incorporated into DNA
• Ribonucleotide reductase inhibitors: e.g. hydroxyurea; reduce availability of all deoxynucleotides

Table 3.8.2 Classification of chemotherapeutic agents according to mechanism of action

Alkylating agents	Antimetabolites	Natural products
Cisplatin	Fluorouracil	Bleomycin
Cyclophosphamide	Methotrexate	Doxorubicin
Melphalan	Cytarabine	Mitomycin C
Chlorambucil	Capecitabine	Vinca alkaloids
Ifosfamide	Gemcitabine	Taxanes

- Cytosine analogues: e.g. gemcitabine; also inhibit ribonucleotide reductase, and compete with cytidine triphosphate for incorporation into DNA.
- Adenosine analogues: e.g. pentostatin; interact with adenosine deaminase, inhibit both DNA synthesis and repair

Natural products
A wide variety of compounds fall into this class. Drugs possessing antitumour activities have been isolated from natural substances such as plants, fungi and bacteria. They are separated into the following categories:
- *Antitumour antibiotics*: drugs that are derived from microorganisms are termed antitumour antibiotics. Included in this group are the anthracyclines, bleomycins, mitoxantrone, and mitomycin c. They are useful in treating many solid tumours and haematological malignancies. Recently, liposomal formulations have entered clinical practice. Several of these drugs interfere with DNA through intercalation, a reaction whereby the drug inserts itself between DNA base pairs. Some of the antitumour antibiotics have other mechanisms of action, such as inhibition of the enzyme topoisomerase (see later in list), antimitotic effects, and alteration of cellular membranes. Oxygen free radical formation from reduced doxorubicin intermediates is thought to be a mechanism associated with cardiotoxicity. Most of the drugs in this group are not cell cycle specific.
- *Mitotic inhibitors*: the vinca alkaloids (vincristine, vinblastine, vinorelbine) are derived from the periwinkle plant, *Vinca rosea*. They exert their effects by binding to tubulin and preventing polymerization. As polymerized tubulin forms the spindles that retract chromosomes into daughter cells at mitosis, this disrupts the formation of microtubules causing metaphase arrest. Their mechanisms of action and metabolism are similar, but their antitumour spectrum, dose, and clinical toxicities are very different. Paclitaxel and docetaxel are semisynthetic derivatives of extracted precursors from the needles of yew plants. These drugs have a novel 14-member ring, the taxane. They differ from the vinca alkaloids, in that they enhance microtubule formation. As a result, a stable and non-functional microtubule is produced.
- *Topoisomerase inhibitors*: topoisomerases are enzymes that break and reseal DNA strands. There are two forms of this enzyme, named topoisomerase I (topo I) and topoisomerase II (topo II). The plant alkaloid camtothecin and its analogues are non-classic enzyme inhibitors of topo I. Inhibitors of topo II include etoposide, and agents from other classes, such as doxorubicin. Topo I binds to double-stranded DNA, then cleaves and demotes one strand of duplex DNA. The supercoiled DNA reduction is then used during the process of replication and transcription. Topo II creates transitory double-stranded breakage of DNA, permitting subsequent passage of an intact DNA duplex through the break.
- *Enzymes*: asparaginase is an example of this type of compound. It catalyses the hydrolysis of asparagines to aspartic acid and ammonia and deprives selected malignant cells of an amino acid essential to their survival.

Recent advances in chemotherapy
We now have more active and better tolerated drugs, although, despite better understanding of cancer as a disease, the basic principles of treatment and drug resistance remain the same. The future presents the challenge of designing clinical trials with targeted drugs and cytotoxics

in rational combinations. These trials will certainly be aided by the advances in the following areas:
- Plasma and tumour pharmacokinetics: measuring drug and metabolites in the blood and tumour tissue with advancements in analytical methodology, and modelling of data
- PD endpoints: measuring the action of the drug in blood, tumour tissue, and other surrogate tissues
- Mathematical techniques applied to PK modelling and PD response
- Pharmacogenetic and gene regulatory determinants of response and toxicity, including the influence of epigenetics
- Novel imaging techniques for drug, metabolites, and surrogate markers

Hormonal therapy
Principles of hormone therapy
Hormones have been implicated in the development and behaviour of many malignant tumours. Hormones and hormone antagonists that are clinically active against cancer include steroid oestrogens, progesterones, androgens, corticosteroids, and thyroid hormones. The strongest evidence that hormones can maintain the growth of tumours relates to the sex steroid hormones (oestrogens and progestogens in breast and endometrial cancer and androgens in prostate cancer). Treatment of hormone-sensitive cancers is based on the principle of depriving them of the mitogenic hormone, which can be achieved by either preventing steroid synthesis or blocking their effects at the target cell level. The comparative roles of the actions of hormones and hormone antagonists are only partially understood and vary between different malignancies.

Hormone therapy is normally better tolerated than chemotherapy due to the effect of treatment being primarily localized to its target organ. However, many tumours appear resistant to hormone therapy, and more become insensitive during treatment and at progression. Thus, even patients who start with hormone dependent cancers, particularly breast and prostate cancer, die with hormone-independent disease.

Types of hormone therapy
Disruption of steroid synthesis
This was originally achieved by removing the major sites of steroid hormone synthesis—ovary and testis, and less so, adrenal and pituitary (in postmenopausal women). These procedures were associated with significant morbidity, were irreversible, with no specificity, and could not be guaranteed to work. Therefore medical rather than surgical ablation is now the method of choice. An example of this is the use of goserelin (Zoladex®), a luteinizing hormone-releasing hormone (LHRH) analogue (see later)), to prevent oestrogen production in the ovaries in the treatment of hormone receptive positive breast cancer rather than undertaking surgical removal of ovaries.

In breast cancer, oestradiol is the main oestrogen and is mostly synthesized in the ovary. Its function is regulated by hormones produced by the anterior pituitary gland—luteinizing hormone (LH) and follicle stimulating hormone (FSH). LHRH, synthesized in the hypothalamus, controls the release of LH and FSH from the pituitary.
- *Agonists of hormones*: agonists have been synthesized that act against LHRH. In the short term, the synthetic analogues of LHRH cause a rapid release of gonadotrophins,

but then they bind to the LHRH receptors and down-regulate them. This desensitizes the pituitary gland, causing decreased oestradiol production in the ovary. Depot formulations of LHRH agonists are available, allowing effective medical ablation of the sex steroid hormones over prolonged periods. These agonists are also effective against prostate cancer because the same hypothalamic–pituitary axis occurs in men.

- *Inhibitors of steroid synthesis:* drugs that can block steroid biosynthesis are also used to decrease oestradiol production. The last step in this pathway requires an aromatase enzyme that converts testosterone to oestradiol. Two types of aromatase inhibitor have been developed. Steroidal aromatase inhibitors act irreversibly to inactivate the enzyme by interfering with the attachment of androgen substrate to the catalytic site. These are also known as type 1 inhibitors, an example being exemestane. Non-steroidal, or type 2, aromatase inhibitors are reversible and interfere with the enzymes cytochrome p450 prosthetic group. Selective type 2 aromatase inhibitors, such as the triazole drugs, anastrozole and letrozole, block the conversion of adrenally generated androstenedione to oestrone by aromatase in peripheral tissues without inhibition of progesterone or corticosteroid synthesis. Both can also block extraglandular oestrogen synthesis (p.163).

- Steroid receptor antagonists: these therapies block hormone-mediated effects, usually at the level of their receptors. The commonest, and most researched type of steroid receptor antagonist, is the antioestrogen agent tamoxifen, although antagonists have been developed for progestins and androgens. Antioestrogens bind to the oestrogen receptor but do not activate gene transcription. Receptor binding by the antagonist prevents oestradiol binding and blocks its effect. Tamoxifen is a derivative of the non-steroidal oestrogen diethylstilboestrol. The main toxic effect of this type of hormone therapy is interference with sexual functions such as ovulation, but it can also cause secondary endometrial cancers. Prostate cancer growth is driven by androgens from the testis. Antiandrogen therapies, such as flutamide and casodex, have also shown clinical efficacy, and will inhibit nuclear androgen binding (p.284).

- *Others*:
  - Corticosteroids: these can cause lysis of specific tumours, particularly lymphoid derived tumours that are rich in specific cytoplasmic receptors.
  - Thyroid hormones: these inhibit the release of TSH, thus potentially inhibiting the growth of well-differentiated thyroid tumours.

Molecularly targeted therapy

We now have an increased understanding of the molecular and cellular biology of cancer and the current generation of molecularly targeted agents in development utilize that knowledge. Traditional cytotoxic chemotherapy works primarily through the inhibition of cell division in rapidly dividing cancer cells. Unfortunately, other rapidly dividing cells (e.g. hair and bone marrow) are also affected by these drugs. In contrast, targeted therapy blocks the proliferation of cancer cells by interfering with specific molecules required for tumour growth. Targeted therapies can be defined as drugs developed against a specific target based on its principal biological function in cancer. They are designed to selectively inhibit a target that is not present in normal tissues, but is often mutated or overexpressed in cancerous tissues.

Target and agent development

Developing molecularly targeted agents requires an integrated approach from many different disciplines in oncology; genomics, proteomics, and protein engineering facilities are required to give biologists, chemists, and clinicians to ability to accelerate the development of increasingly selective and effective targeted therapies. Once a potential new target is recognized, high-throughput *in vitro* screening assays, often involving thousands of compounds, are undertaken to find a lead compound that inhibits the reaction. Preliminary compounds are often active at very low doses, although further analogue manufacturing is required to develop potential therapies with other desirable properties such as prolonged half-life or oral bioavailability. To enable a compound to proceed through cell culture experiments, animal model work, including toxicity work and different animal model systems, into clinical trials, requires many years of work, and countless individuals' efforts.

Preclinically, biological effects need to be reproduced in experimental systems at concentrations of drug comparable to those achievable clinically. PK and toxicity analysis must still be undertaken, as toxicity or even antagonism may result from off-target effects of the drugs. Early clinical trial design must include assays that prove the agent is actually hitting its target and having the desired biological effect. Conventional methods of assessing tumour response, such as CT scans, may not show changes to these new cytostatic agents, and therefore newer methods of assessing response to treatment are also required, both radiological and histological.

Finally, these therapies have expanded the concept of individually customized cancer treatment because some of these drugs may only be helpful in a subpopulation of cancers with a particular molecular change, and not effective in the absence of such a target. This distinction may be influenced by patient sex and ethnicity, as well as by tumour pathology. Accordingly, it will be critical to stratify patients for treatment based on the propensity of their tumours to respond.

Few compounds survive this arduous journey, but several have now been used in large clinical trials with variable results. The cost of these therapies is already an important issue in healthcare economics.

Functional and molecular imaging studies

Clear guidelines exist for assessing conventional treatment responses radiologically. The most widely used are the RECIST criteria (Therasse et al. 2000). With the newer targeted agents, it is becoming increasingly important to develop more effective ways to assess responses to treatments that may have a cytostatic, rather than a cytotoxic effect. Multiple functional imaging techniques now exist, and are being incorporated into clinical trial design. These include dynamic contrast enhanced magnetic resonance imaging (DCE-MRI), PET, and dynamic CT. These more dynamic imaging techniques can be used to study drug distribution, changes in tumour metabolism, and alterations in blood flow to the tumour, although there are still major challenges involved in the development, interpretation, standardization, and integration of some of these techniques into routine clinical practice.

Types of molecularly targeted agents

The two main forms of targeted therapy are monoclonal antibodies and small molecule inhibitors (SMIs). Tables 3.8.3 and 3.8.4 give an overview of commonly used agents

Table 3.8.3 Examples of biological therapy—small molecules

Agent	Trade name	Mechanism of action	Potential indications
Imatinib mesylate	Gleevec®	Inhibits Bcr-Abl tyrosine kinase, the constitutive abnormal gene product of the Philadelphia chromosome in chronic myeloid leukaemia (CML). Inhibition of this enzyme blocks proliferation and causes apoptosis in fresh leukaemic cells in Philadelphia chromosome positive CML. Also inhibits tyrosine kinase for platelet-derived growth factor (PDGF), stem cell factor (SCF), c-KIT, and cellular events mediated by PDGF and SCF	Gastrointestinal stromal tumours (GISTs) CML (see text)
Dasatinib	Sprycel®	Multi-targeted tyrosine kinase inhibitor; targets most imatinib-resistant BCR-ABL mutations. Kinase inhibition halts proliferation of leukaemia cells. Also inhibits SRC family, c-KIT, EPHA2, and PDGF receptor	CML ALL
Nilotinib	Tasigna®	Tyrosine kinase inhibitor that targets BCR-ABL kinase, c-KIT and PDGFR	CML
Gefitinib	Iressa®	This small-molecule drug inhibits the tyrosine kinase (TK) activity of the epidermal growth factor receptor (EGFR), which is overproduced by many types of cancer cells. TK activity appears to be vitally important to cell proliferation and survival	Non-small cell lung cancer (NSCLC)
Erlotinib	Tarceva®	Inhibits overall EGFR-TK activity. Active competitive inhibition of adenosine triphosphate inhibits downstream signal transduction of ligand dependent EGFR activation	NSCLC Pancreatic cancer
Lapatinib	Tykerb®	Inhibits several tyrosine kinases, including the tyrosine kinase activity of EGFR and Her-2, blocking phosphorylation and activation of downstream second messengers (Erk1/2 and Akt) and regulating proliferation and survival in EGFR and Her-2 expressing tumours	Advanced breast cancer
Temsirolimus	Torisel®	Specific inhibitor of a kinase called mTOR (mammalian target of rapamycin) that is activated in tumour cells and stimulates their growth and proliferation. Binds to FKBP-12, an intracellular protein, to form a complex which inhibits mTOR signalling. In renal cell carcinoma also exhibits activity by reducing levels of hypoxia inducible factors and vascular endothelial growth factor (VEGF)	Advanced renal cell carcinoma
Bortezomib	Velcade®	Interferes with the action of large enzyme complexes called proteasomes causing cancer cells to undergo cell cycle arrest and apoptosis (normal cells can be affected to a lesser extent)	Multiple myeloma Mantle cell lymphoma
Sorafenib	Nexavar®	Inhibits intracellular Raf kinases (CRAF, BRAF, and mutant BRAF), and cell surface kinase receptors (VEGFR-2, VEGFR-3, PDGFR-beta, cKIT, and FMS-like tyrosine kinase-3 [FLT-3]), thereby inhibiting tumour growth and angiogenesis	Renal cell carcinoma Hepatocellular carcinoma
Sunitinib	Sutent®	Multi-targeted receptor tyrosine kinase inhibitor, whose targets include; PDGFRα and PDGFRβ, VEGFR1, VEGFR2, and VEGFR3, FLT3, colony-stimulating factor type 1 (CSF-1R), and glial cell-line-derived neurotrophic factor receptor (RET)	Renal cell carcinoma GISTs not responding to imatinib

in these classes. The molecular pathways most often targeted in the treatment of solid tumours are those of the epidermal growth factor receptor (EGFR or HER1), vascular endothelial growth factor (VEGF), and HER2/neu, a molecular target related to EGFR.

These pathways can be inhibited at various levels:
• Binding and neutralizing ligands—molecules that bind to specific receptor sites on cells
• Occupying receptor-binding sites—preventing ligand binding by blocking receptor signalling
• Interfering with downstream intracellular molecules

EGFR is present in many tumour types and contributes to cancer cell proliferation and invasion. It is also present in normal epithelial tissue and inhibition of this pathway can lead to significant dermatological and GI toxicities. Several mechanisms can lead to abnormal EGFR activation, including receptor overexpression, activating mutations, amplification of the gene, and overexpression of the receptor ligands.

Targeting of VEGF limits cancer growth by preventing angiogenesis (the formation of new blood vessels). This is thought to be a key process in cancer development

Table 3.8.4 Examples of monoclonal antibodies

MAb	Trade name	Mechanism of action	Potential indications
Cetuximab	Erbitux®	This binds specifically to the EGFR and competitively inhibits the binding of EGF and other ligands. Binding to the EGFR blocks phosphorylation and activation of receptor-associated kinases. EGFR signal transduction results in KRAS wild-type activation; cells with KRAS mutations appear to be unaffected by EGFR inhibition.	Colorectal cancers Head and neck cancers
Trastuzumab	Herceptin®	Binds to the extracellular domain of the human epidermal growth factor receptor 2 (HER-2). The likely mechanism of action involves binding HER-2 on the surface of tumour cells that express high levels of HER-2, thereby preventing HER-2 from sending growth-promoting signals and inhibiting proliferation of cells which over-express HER-2 protein.	Breast cancer
Rituximab	Rituxan®	Recognizes the CD20 molecule that is found on B cells. When it binds to these cells, it activates complement-dependent B-cell cytotoxicity, mediating cell killing through an antibody-dependent cellular toxicity	Non-Hodgkin lymphoma
Bevacizumab	Avastin®	Binds to VEGF preventing it from interacting with its receptors on endothelial cells, Flt-1 and KDR, thereby inhibiting new blood vessel growth and potentially cancer growth	Colorectal cancer NSCLC Breast cancer GBM Kidney cancer
Panitumumab	Arzerra®	Attaches to EGFR and prevents it from sending growth signals	Chronic lymphocytic leukaemia (CLL) Colorectal cancer
Tositumomab	Bexxar®	Recognizes the CD20 molecule. Some of the antibodies are linked to a radioactive iodine. The radioactive component delivers radioactive energy to CD20-expressing B cells. In addition, the binding of tositumomab to the CD20-expressing B cells triggers the immune system to destroy these cells	B-cell lymphoma

and progression. Inhibiting VEGF is also thought to normalize the vasculature within a tumour, potentially improving drug delivery to the cancer cells. VEGF is also present on normal endothelial cells and effects on normal blood vessels can occur, including bleeding, thrombosis, and hypertension.

A targeted therapy that has lead to a dramatic change in treatment and prognosis for certain breast cancer patients is trastuzumab (Herceptin®). This is a monoclonal antibody which binds with high affinity and specificity to the extracellular domain of the HER2 receptor. Amplification of HER2 occurs in around 25% of patients with breast cancer, and is associated with a poor prognosis. The patients whose tumours overexpress HER2 will receive treatment with trastuzumab, and when combined with chemotherapy, this can lead to significantly increased survival rates compared with chemotherapy alone. (p.163).

Monoclonal antibodies, which are usually water soluble with large molecular weights, target the extracellular components of these pathways, such as ligands and receptor-binding sites (see immunotherapy section for more information). Small molecule inhibitors differ in the fact that they have much lower molecular weights and can enter cells, thereby blocking receptor signalling and interfering with downstream intracellular molecules.

Small molecule inhibitors

SMIs typically interrupt cellular processes by interfering with the intracellular signalling of tyrosine kinases

(enzymes that transfer phosphate groups from adenosine triphosphate to tyrosine amino acid residues in proteins). This signalling leads to a cascade of enzymatic and biochemical reactions that can initiate cell growth, proliferation, and migration signals transmitted from the cell surface through the cytoplasm to the nucleus. EGFR, HER2, and VEGF receptors are tyrosine kinases. Common to the structure of all tyrosine kinases is a substrate binding domain, an ATP binding domain, and a catalytic or kinase domain.

The first major success of this type of tyrosine kinase inhibitor was imatinib mesylate (Gleevec®), a competitive inhibitor of several cellular Abl-kinases, including the Bcr-Abl kinase fusion protein. Most cases of chronic myeloid leukaemia (CML) are caused by the formation of a gene called BCR-ABL, which results from a reciprocal translocation between chromosomes 9 and 22. The protein normally produced by the ABL gene (Abl) is a signalling molecule that plays an important role in controlling cell proliferation and usually must interact with other signalling molecules to be active. However, Abl signalling is constitutively active in the protein produced by the BCR-ABL fusion gene, promoting the continuous proliferation of CML cells. Imatinib can prevent this by inhibiting the phosphorylation and activation of downstream proteins of the tyrosine kinases associated with Abl.

As is often the case though, resistance occurs. A mutation in the BCR-ABL gene has arisen that changes the shape of the protein so that it no longer binds imatinib, ultimately leading to resistant disease in a number of patients with CML. However, imatinib is also active in inhibiting other tyrosine kinases, including KIT, and has become the standard of care for patients with gastrointestinal stromal tumours (GIST), as these patients have frequent gain of function mutations in KIT.

General differences between small molecule inhibitors and monoclonal antibodies

- SMIs are normally administered orally; monoclonal antibodies are administered intravenously
- SMI achieve less specific targeting than monoclonal antibodies
- Unlike monoclonal antibodies, most SMIs are metabolized by cytochrome P450 enzymes, which may result in interactions with certain medications, such as warfarin, St. John's wort, and certain antifungal agents and antibiotics
- monoclonal antibodies have half-lives ranging from days to weeks, and are usually administered once every 1–4 weeks; most SMIs have half-lives of only hours and require daily dosing

The future of molecularly targeted agents

As we learn more about tumours, many new potential targets are being realized. Drugs are being developed that target the pathways and processes of:

- Cell cycle regulation, including cyclin-dependent kinase, survivin, and agents that target mitosis (auroro kinases)
- Apoptotic pathways, including death receptor pathways
- Signalling pathways, including Ras and its downstream effectors, insulin growth factor receptors and Src family kinases
- Epigenetic agents, including histone deacetylase inhibitors
- Senescence
- Telomerase instability
- Inhibitors of the DNA repair mechanisms—poly (ADP-ribose) polymerase (PARP) inhibitors
- Ubiquitin-proteosome system
- Matrix metalloproteinase inhibitors
- Developmental pathway inhibitors, such as Notch and Hedgehog pathway inhibitors

Greater understanding of these targets, and their roles in cancer biology, has great potential to generate therapies that significantly impact on patient outcomes.

Immunotherapy

Principles of immunotherapy

Cancer immunotherapy encompasses all the therapeutic manipulations of the immune system, utilizing immune-related agents such as cytokines, vaccines, cellular and humoral therapies, and transfected agents, with or without immune-potentiation by drugs or other agents. These reagents act through one of several mechanisms:

- Stimulating the antitumour response
- Decreasing suppressor mechanisms
- Improving tolerance to chemo- or radiotherapy
- Altering tumour cells to increase their immunogenicity

The immune system is comprised of innate cells, that mediate immediate short-lived responses (non-specific immunity) and adaptive cells that develop long-standing responses and memory (specific immunity).

The innate immune system is comprised of:

- Anatomical barriers (e.g. skin, tears, saliva, and cilia in the intestinal and respiratory tract)
- Humoral and chemical barriers: the complement system and inflammation (cytokines and chemokines)
- Cellular barriers: phagocytes (macrophages, dendritic cells, and neutrophils), mast cells, eosinophils, basophils, and natural killer cells

The adaptive immune response is antigen specific and requires recognition of specific 'non-self' antigens during antigen presentation. The main cell type responsible for acquired immunity is the lymphocyte. Dendritic cells, cytokines, and the complement system (which enhances the effectiveness of antibodies) are involved to a lesser extent. In the humoral response, B-lymphocytes recognize and attach to the antigen. Plasma cells are then formed that produce antibodies against the antigen. In the cell-mediated response, T-lymphocytes (killer and helper T cells) recognize the antigen and either directly kill it or elicit the production of antibody from plasma cells. Suppressor (regulatory) T cells are a subpopulation of T cells that suppress activation of the immune system and maintain immune system homeostasis and tolerance to self-antigens.

Today research into immunotherapeutic strategies for the treatment of cancer focuses on several areas. They include:

- Cancer vaccines
- Monoclonal antibodies
- T-cell-based adoptive therapy
- Employment of cytokines to enhance immunity

Cancer vaccines

These can be used to induce and/or augment the immune response to tumour cells, to prevent infections with cancer-causing viruses (Gardasil®, against HPV), or prevent the development of cancer in certain high-risk individuals (vaccines against HBV lowering the risk of liver cancer). They can also be used therapeutically in patients with existing cancer. This approach is currently being tested in cancers such as melanoma, renal cell, ovarian, colorectal, and prostate cancer. Patient-specific cancer vaccines include dendritic cell and tumour antigen vaccines. There are also tumour antigen-specific vaccines, such as NY-ESO-1. This is a protein that is produced by several types of tumours (e.g. melanoma and lung cancer) but is not expressed by normal cells.

Monoclonal antibodies

Monoclonal antibodies are made by injecting human cancer cells or proteins from cancer cells into mice so that their immune systems create antibodies against foreign antigens. The plasma cells that produce the antibodies are then removed and fused with cells grown in the laboratory to create hybrid cells (hybridomas). Hybridomas can indefinitely produce large quantities of these pure antibodies. The fragment antigen binding (Fab) of a monoclonal antibody recognizes and binds to antigens. This is responsible for the highly specific targeting that is possible with these treatments.

Recently developed monoclonal antibodies contain an increased proportion of human components and a decreased proportion of murine (mouse) components; chimeric antibodies are 65% human and humanized antibodies are 95% human. The type of antibody can often be identified by the suffix of the drug name: -momab (murine), -ximab (chimeric), -zumab (humanized), or -mumab (human).

Monoclonal antibodies can be used in diagnosing, monitoring, and treating cancer. They can have direct effects by inducing apoptosis and blocking growth factor receptors, thereby halting proliferation, and indirect effects by recruiting cells that have cytotoxicity (monocytes and macrophages).

See Table 3.8.4 for a list of commonly available monoclonal antibodies.

T-cell based adoptive therapy
T cells that have a natural or genetically engineered reactivity to a patient's cancer are cultured with IL-2 and other cytokines and then adoptively transferred back to the patient. These methods are used to increase the number of reactive T cells and provide long-term immune protection with minimal autoimmune responsiveness. These can directly attack tumour cells and this approach has been used successfully in the treatment of metastatic melanoma. Unfortunately this approach has been limited due to the need for specialized cell culture equipment and the requirements of intensive cell preparations.

Cytokines
Cytokines are soluble proteins that mediate the interactions between the cells and their extracellular environment, both in a cell autonomous and non-cell autonomous manner. Several cytokines appear to be of therapeutic importance, amongst them:
- Interleukins (ILs)
- Tumour necrosis factor (TNF)
- Colony-stimulating factor (CSF)
- Interferons (IFNs)

IL-2, a lymphokine produced by activated T cells, was the first interleukin discovered. Recombinant IL-2 was shown subsequently to have potent immunomodulatory and antitumour activity in a number of murine tumour models. It has been widely used the management of patients with advanced malignancy, particularly renal cell carcinoma and melanoma (p.262, 400). The use of high dose IL-2 is limited by the severe toxicity it can cause and the fact that only a minority of patients will respond to treatment. Lower doses and different dosing schedules have been used but have not proven to be as effective as high dose IL-2.

CSFs are defined by their ability to support colony formation *in vitro*. They are glycoproteins that bind to specific cell surface receptors and stimulate the proliferation and activation of blood cells from primitive haematopoietic stem and progenitor cells, as well as cause functional activation of some mature cells. There are various CSFs in use and these include:
- Granulocyte colony stimulating factor (G-CSF)
- Erythropoietin
- Granulocyte-macrophage colony-stimulating factor (GM-CSF)
- Thrombopoietin

The goal of treatment with CSFs is to increase the number of functional blood cells so that host defence mechanisms can be maintained. Recombinant CSFs are administered in a number of clinical settings including:
- Transient bone marrow failure following chemotherapy
- Bone marrow transplantation
- Myelodysplastic syndrome
- Aplastic anaemia
- Chronic bone marrow failure
- Anaemia of chronic disease
- Stem cell and progenitor cell mobilization

The success of treatment with CSFs can be measured in terms of decreased neutropenia, infection, decreased length of hospital stay, and reduced treatment costs.

The IFNs (α, β, and γ) are a family of related proteins produced by the immune system in response to viral infection. Their effects include antiviral activity, antiproliferative properties, inhibition of angiogenesis, regulation of cell differentiation, enhancement of major histocompatibility complex antigen expression, and a wide variety of immunomodulatory activities. Most cells have receptors for and respond to IFNs. The IFNs have been used successfully in the treatment of many cancers, particularly the haematological malignancies. When used as a systemic therapy, IFNs are mostly administered by intramuscular injection. The most frequent adverse effects are flu-like symptoms.

Non-specific immunomodulating agents are substances that stimulate or indirectly augment the immune system. Often, these agents target key immune system cells and cause secondary responses such as increased production of cytokines and immunoglobulins. Two non-specific immunomodulating agents that have not yet been mentioned are bacillus Calmette—Guérin (BCG) and levamisole. BCG is used in the treatment of patients with superficial bladder cancer. It activates macrophages, T and B lymphocytes and NK cells, and can also induce local immunological responses via ILs. Levamisole has been used with fluorouracil (5-FU) chemotherapy in the treatment of colorectal cancer.

The future of immunotherapy in oncology
This area has the potential to enhance current cancer therapies and to provide new therapeutic options for traditionally refractory cancers. It is not likely to eliminate cancer alone, but combination therapies that incorporate immunotherapeutic agents offer promise for clinical success in treating cancer in the future.

Further reading

Chabner B, Roberts TG Jr. Chemotherapy and the war on cancer. *Nat Rev Cancer* 2005; **5**(1):65–72.

Boddy AV. Recent developments in the clinical pharmacology of classical cytotoxic chemotherapy. *Br J Clin Pharmacol* 2006; **62**(1):27–34.

Eisenhauer EA, Twelves C, Buyse M. *Phase 1 cancer clinical trials. A practical guide.* Oxford: Oxford University Press, 2006.

Finn OJ. Cancer immunology. *N Engl J Med* 2008; **358**(25):2704–15.

Gutierrez ME, Kummar S, Giaccone G. Next generation oncology drug development.: opportunities and challenges. *Nat Rev Clin Onc.* 2009; 6(5): 259–65.

Therasse P, Arbuck SG, Eisenhauer EA, *et al.* New guidelines to evaluate the response to treatment in solid tumours (RECIST guidelines). *J Nat Cancer Inst* 2000; **92**:205–16.

Site-specific cancer management

Principles of management for cancer of the head and neck

The head and neck region encompasses anatomical sites below the brain and above the clavicles, excluding skin and thyroid. The sites most commonly involved with cancer are the oral cavity, larynx, and pharynx. Overall 5-year survival rates for head and neck cancer have improved only slightly over the past two decades remaining at just over 50%. This figure in part reflects the population who present with this disease in terms of age and comorbidity (typically about 15% intercurrent death rates at 5 years), as well as the tendency to develop second primaries and metastases. The poor long-term survival rates may also reflect the fact that 60% of patients with head and neck cancer have advanced disease at the time of presentation (stage III/IV disease). The dominant treatment failure in head and neck cancer is locoregional relapse and this remains the main focus for clinicians involved in the management of these patients.

About 90% of head and neck cancers are squamous cell carcinomas, with the remainder being lymphoma, salivary cancers, mucosal melanomas, and sarcomas. Histology is most diverse in the nasal passages and salivary glands. Management of head and neck squamous cell carcinomas (HNSCC) depends largely on clinical parameters, in particular the stage of the tumour. The TNM staging system as laid out by the UICC (International Union against Cancer) describes the anatomical extent of the tumour. T describes the two-dimensional size of the primary tumour, and is dependent on the subsite within the head and neck from which the primary tumour is arising. N defines the presence of any regional nodal disease and again represents a two-dimensional measurement of nodal size as well as number of nodes. M denotes the presence of any distant metastases. Classification of tumours by the TNM system allows a fairly precise description of the anatomical extent of the disease. Tumour with four degrees of T, three degrees of N, and two degrees of M, will have 24 TNM categories; these can be condensed into four stage groups (I–IV), which aim to classify them into homogeneous clusters with similar survival rates which are distinctive for each anatomical subsite. In reality, identically staged tumours often have different survival rates due to diversity in biological characteristics of tumour and variable patient performance status.

Early stage disease

Early head and neck cancer (stage I–II) is generally managed with single modality therapy. The choice of surgery or radiotherapy is determined by the location of the tumour and the likely morbidity, i.e. the anticipated structural, functional, and cosmetic preservation. With the advent and popularization of conservative techniques, including transoral laser microsurgery, patients with early stage tumours at sites within the larynx and mouth can now be treated with organ-preserving surgery. The determinants of choice between surgery and radiotherapy are complex and multifactorial. (For tumours where radiotherapy is the favoured modality, the consequences of failing to detect radioresistant tumours can be disastrous. Salvage surgery usually has to be radical with no option for conservation of normal tissues and may be associated with a poor outcome.) The probability of eradicating tumour with radiotherapy is related to tumour volume; for T1 tumours, the primary local control rate is 85–95% and for T2, 70–85%. Small accessible tumours within the oral cavity (T1–T2) can be considered for brachytherapy, permitting full-dose external beam irradiation should a second primary arise. Nevertheless, surgery is the most frequent approach for early stage oral cancers.

Locally advanced disease

The management of locally advanced disease requires a multidisciplinary approach since the choice of radical treatment involves different combinations of surgery, radiotherapy and systemic treatment. The three commonest approaches are:
- Surgery with postoperative (chemo) radiotherapy
- Chemoradiotherapy
- Nodal dissection followed by chemoradiotherapy

Decisions are often based on clinical intuition, taking into account tumour stage, patient PS, and sound support. The main determinants are the likelihood of tumour control and the functional outcome. However the significance of getting this decision wrong is monumental. A patient who develops a local recurrence following treatment with chemoradiotherapy may be unfit for salvage surgery, and when resection is possible, the functional and survival outcome is poorer than for primary surgery. On the other hand, the use of surgery to treat a tumour which might have been cured with chemoradiotherapy exposes a patient to the potential mutilating effects of surgery. Hence, the ability of the MDT to ensure the patient receives the most appropriate treatment is crucial.

Until 20 years ago, suitably fit patients with locally advanced disease (stage III–IV) tended to receive radical surgery and postoperative radiotherapy. However, the Veterans Administration Laryngeal Cancer Study in the 1980s and the EORTC 24891 trial of hypopharyngeal cancers demonstrated that induction chemotherapy followed by radiotherapy resulted in survival rates comparable to those with surgery and postoperative radiotherapy. Their work showed that organ preservation was possible without detriment to overall survival. Furthermore, the simultaneous administration of chemotherapy and radiotherapy (concurrent chemoradiotherapy) has been shown to be superior to radiation alone in terms of overall survival and organ preservation. Cisplatin-based regimens are the standard for concurrent chemotherapy. In addition, modified fractionation schedules have been and continue to be explored, and can involve acceleration and hyper-fractionation.

Tumour volume delineation for three-dimensional conformal radiotherapy

Expert assessment of the patient is critical to the interpretation of radiological images in defining target volumes on radiotherapy computer planning systems. For a detailed definition of various radiotherapy volumes see p.43. In short, gross tumour volume (GTV) denotes macroscopic tumour, clinical target volume (CTV) describes area at risk of microscopic disease, and planning target volume (PTV) takes into account potential organ and patient movement which for immobilized patients with head and neck tumours usually entails a transaxial margin of 3–5mm around CTV. Organs at risk (OAR) need to be outlined and may include spinal cord, brain stem, salivary glands, and visual pathway. The conformation of beams is achieved by multileaf collimators which can produce any shape of field within the limits of blade width (usually 0.5–1cm). The treatment planning system using CT images will generate a full three-dimensional plan with dose distributions displayed in axial, sagittal, and coronal planes.

Fractionation regimens
The effectiveness of a radiotherapy 'dose' is related to a whole package of fractionation parameters including over-all treatment time and fraction size, as much as the total dose. Myriad permutations of dose/fractionation have been trialled to seek a therapeutic gain, i.e. improvement in local control without an increase in normal tissue morbidity, particularly in late (enduring) effects. 'Conventional' fractionation is defined as 2Gy per day, 5 days a week. For definitive head and neck cancer treatment, 70Gy are used whilst for postoperative therapy, 60–66Gy are given. A different approach used in many UK centres uses 55Gy in 20 fractions which provides good outcomes at least for some patients with larynx cancer (Wiernik et al. 1991). Other modifications to conventional fractionations include hyperfractionation (use of >5 smaller fractions per week while maintaining a conventional overall treatment time to deliver an increased total dose) and modest acceleration (use of >5 fractions per week while maintaining a conventional total dose delivered in a shorter overall treatment time). The rationale behind hyperfractionation is to manipulate the two parameters which most influence late effects of radiotherapy, i.e. total dose and fraction size. By reducing fraction size, total dose can be increased to improve tumour control without exacerbating late effects. An example of pure hyperfractionation is 80.5Gy in 70 fractions over 7 weeks (Horiot et al. 1992). The radiobiological rationale of modest acceleration is to manipulate the two parameters which most influence local control of squamous cancer, i.e. total dose and overall treatment time; reducing treatment time combats accelerated repopulation of tumour clonogens as a potential cause of treatment failure. Examples include 68Gy in 34 fractions over 5.5 weeks (6 fractions a week) and 72Gy in 42 fractions over 6 weeks (concomitant boost over 2.5 weeks) (Fu et al. 2000; Overgaard et al. 2003). All these intensified regimens have demonstrated improved local control with an associated increase in mucositis compared with conventional fractionation. These modified fractionation schedules have not been adopted into routine practice because the alternative practice of chemoradiotherapy has developed, which also improves local control with increased mucositis and which may have some advantages in logistics and patient convenience.

Whilst it is clear that there are modest benefits to be gained from altered fractionation regimens, this is not the case with all squamous carcinomas. This reflects the heterogeneity in tumour biology and treatment response. It has led to a drive to try and identify those tumour characteristics most likely to predict response to radiotherapy and its various modifications.

Systemic treatments
Radical
Meta-analysis demonstrates an absolute improvement in 5-year survival of about 10% when cisplatin is added synchronously to radiotherapy (Pignon et al. 2000).

Other cytotoxic agents currently being studied include 5-FU analogues and taxanes.

The value of chemoradiotherapy in these patients can be hindered by the increased and prohibitive toxicity of the treatment, which may be enhanced by the associated comorbidities suffered by these patients. This has led to interest in novel non-cytotoxic targeted therapies such as cetuximab (monoclonal antibody targeting EGFR). A recent finding is that synchronous cetuximab improves survival when compared with radiotherapy alone. It is not clear how this magnitude of benefit compares with that afforded by cytotoxic therapy (Bonner et al. 2006). If induction chemotherapy before radiotherapy is deemed appropriate, the three-drug combination of docetaxel, cisplatin, and 5-FU improves outcome relative to the previous standard of cisplatin, 5-FU (Vermorken et al. 2007). Further studies are required to clarify whether induction chemotherapy can be used with full-dose chemoradiotherapy or is better applied with the pairing of biological targeting agents added to radiotherapy. One study has shown an improved response rate for advanced larynx and hypopharynx cancer when docetaxel has added to cisplatin and 5-FU (Pointreau et al. 2009)

Palliative
Palliative chemotherapy provides a modest benefit overall in advanced head and neck cancer with objective response rates of 30–40%. Cisplatin/5-FU combinations are most commonly used though capecitabine, taxanes, and biological targeting agents are all being studied. Patients who fail to respond to first-line chemotherapy should be considered for phase 2 experimental studies. Head and neck cancer provides an ideal situation for the study of novel agents as its accessibility permits scrutiny of both tumour control and normal tissue effects.

The EXTREME study has shown that patients with untreated recurrent/metastatic head and neck cancer who received cetuximab with cisplatin and fluorouracil showed improved overall survival (10.1 vs. 7.4 months) and 46% increase in progression free survival (5.6 vs. 3.3 months) compared with patients who received chemotherapy alone. Toxicity was increased in the cetuximab group but treatment related deaths are increased in the chemotherapy group (Vermorken et al. 2008)

Intensity modulated radiotherapy
Radiation therapy has evolved over the past two decades from two-dimensional therapy to a conformal three-dimensional treatment, which aims to spare surrounding normal tissue whilst delivering radiation to the tumoural target. Intensity modulated radiotherapy (IMRT) is an advanced form of treatment delivery which not only delivers conformally shaped beams but also produces non-uniform beam intensities (fluence profiles). The dosimetric advantages of IMRT can essentially be ascribed to better conformation of dose to target volume or use of differential doses to areas at different risk of harbouring tumour deposits. Additional benefits include avoidance of matching field junctions as well as ease of set up using a single isocentre. Typical doses would be 65Gy in 30 fractions to macroscopic disease; 60Gy in 30 fractions for high-risk areas; and 55Gy in 30 fractions to moderate risk areas (so-called 'elective' RT) (see Fig. 4.1.1). The potential clinical advantages relate to reducing normal tissue toxicity or escalating dose to macroscopic disease.

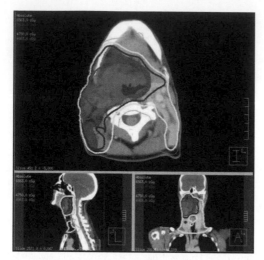

Fig. 4.1.1 IMRT contours (see also colour plate section).

Principles of patient management

In management of patients with head and neck cancer, there are at least 'ten commandments' which need to be addressed before treatment:

1. Performance status: weight loss; associated comorbidities (all central to management plan).
2. Smoking status: smoking cessation programme; smoking during radiotherapy reduces local tumour control and increases late toxicity.
3. Dental status: post-RT extraction may precipitate osteoradionecrosis.
4. Nutritional status: consider elective gastrostomy in patients where oral intake is likely to become impaired, or is already poor.
5. Bite block ± tongue depressor for radiotherapy for oral/nasal cancer.
6. Routine bloods: consider transfusion if moderate anaemia; caution in patients with deranged renal/liver function receiving cytotoxic therapy.

7. Imaging of chest: to exclude synchronous lung primary—or metastases, particularly if N2/3 disease.
8. Alcohol intake needs to be stopped/moderated if possible during radiotherapy.
9. Close scrutiny of concomitant medications.
10. Fully informed consent.

Further reading

Bonner JA, Harari PM, Giralt J, et al. Radiotherapy plus cetuximab for squamous-cell carcinoma of the head and neck. *N Eng J Med* 1006; **354**(6):567–78.

Fu KK, Pajak TF, Trotti A, et al. A Radiation Therapy Oncology Group (RTOG) phase III randomised study to compare hyperfractionation and two variants of accelerated fractionation to standard fractionation radiotherapy for head and neck squamous cell carcinomas: first report of RTOG 9003. *Int J Radiat Oncol Biol Phys* 2000; **48**(1):7–16.

Horiot JC, Le Fur R, N'Guyen T, et al. Hyperfractionation versus conventional fractionation in oropharyngeal carcinoma: final analysis of a randomised trial of the EORTC cooperative group of radiotherapy. *Radiother Oncol* 1992; **25**(4):231–41.

Overgaard J, Hansen HS, Specht L, et al. Five compared with six fractions per week of conventional radiotherapy of squamous-cell carcinoma of head and neck: DAHANCA 6 and 7 randomised controlled trial. *Lancet* 2003; **362**(9388):933–40.

Pignon JP, Bourhis J, Domenge C, et al. Chemotherapy added to locoregional treatment for head and neck squamous-cell carcinoma: three meta-analyses of updated individual data. *Lancet* 2000; **355**(9208):949–55.

Pointreau Y, Garaud P, Chaper S, et al. Randomised trial of induction chemotherapy with cisplatin and 5-fluorouracil with or without docetaxel for larynx preservation. *J Natl Cancer Inst* 2009; **101**:498–506.

Vermorken JB, Remenar E, van Herpen C, et al. Cisplatin fluorouracil, and docetaxel in unresectable head and neck cancer. *N Eng J Med* 2007; **357**(17):1695–704.

Vermorken JB, Mesia R, Rivera F, et al. Platinum based chemotherapy plus cetuximab in head and neck cancer. *N Eng J Med* 2008; **359**:1116–27.

Wiernik G, Alcocok CJ, Bates TD. Final report on the second British Institute of Radiology fractionation study: short versus long overall treatment times for radiotherapy of carcinoma of the laryngo-pharynx. *Br J Radiol* 1991; **64**(759):232–41.

Tumours of the eye, orbit, and ear

Tumours of the eye

Introduction

Malignant tumours of the eyelids include basal cell carcinoma (BCC) and squamous cell carcinoma (SCC). The more common BCC accounts for 90% of tumours of the eyelid and often occurs as a result of sun damage to the skin. Typically it affects the lower eyelids, followed by the canthal area and less frequently the upper lid. SCCs account for <10% of malignant eyelid tumours, but are capable of metastases. Within the eyelid, the meibomian glands in the tarsal plate, and the sweat and sebaceous appendages adjacent to the cilia can give rise to adenocarcinomas, which may present as slowly expanding nodules.

SCC is the commonest malignancy affecting the conjunctiva. Lymphocytic proliferative disorders can also affect the conjunctiva. Melanocytic lesions of the conjunctiva have varying degrees of malignant potential.

Clinical features

BCCs often develop as a small indurated, well-demarcated nodule which may have some degree of pigmentation. The overlying skin may break down with resultant painless ulceration. As with other cutaneous BCCs they are usually locally invasive, but rarely metastasize. SCCs can also present in a similar fashion, which may make them difficult to distinguish. Conjunctival SCCs may present as a fleshy vascular mass at the limbus, melanomas may present as a raised pigmented or non-pigmented area on the conjunctiva.

Management

Punch biopsy will confirm diagnosis in diffuse eyelid tumours. Treatment usually comprises complete surgical excision with frozen section control of margins for localized tumours. Dependent on the extent of surgical excision, reconstruction of the eyelids may be required, using sliding skin flaps, rotational flaps, and free skin grafts.

Conjunctival tumours are similarly treated with complete surgical excision with frozen section to confirm margins, with cryotherapy to the tumour bed. Reconstruction may involve grafting of the area. In radiosensitive tumours such as lymphoma, external beam radiotherapy, or plaque brachytherapy can be used.

Tumours of the globe

Introduction

Malignant melanoma is the most common primary intraocular tumour in adults, commonly affecting adults in the fifth and sixth decades of life. There is no significant difference in the incidences between genders; however it is more common in Caucasians than non-Caucasians. It may arise from any portion of the uveal tract but commonly affects the choroid, then the ciliary body, and least often the iris. Usually slow to grow and metastasize, it generally affects one eye only and may develop spontaneously or from a mole within the eye. Development of distant metastases rather than local failure determines survival. Common metastatic sites include the liver, lung, and bones.

Retinoblastoma is the most common type of malignant intraocular tumours found in children, though it occurs with less frequency than malignant melanomas. There is no gender or racial predilection. Retinoblastomas may be hereditary or develop sporadically. The less common hereditary type is usually present at birth and has its onset near 1 year of age. In both types, the condition is almost always expressed by the age of 5 years and is bilateral in 30–50% of patients. Although hereditary retinoblastomas are not always present in family histories, any occurrence of bilateral retinoblastoma should be considered indicative of being hereditary in origin. Other tumours include intraocular lymphomas. These are typically a diffuse large B cell non-Hodgkin lymphoma arising in immunocompromised individuals, although the incidence in both immunocompetent and immunocompromised individuals is on the rise.

Diagnosis

This is often based on the clinical assessment of the patient. However, ultrasonography can aid diagnosis and staging of disease. Fine needle biopsies, although not usually required, may be helpful in difficult diagnostic cases.

Malignant melanoma

Malignant melanomas are often detected incidentally, when the patient seeks medical help, following deterioration in vision. These tumours often cause an exudative detachment of the retina. The displacement of the retina may move the lens forward, creating a pupillary block and angle-closure glaucoma with a resultant painful eye.

Retinoblastoma

Retinoblastomas may present in the first week of life, and are usually evident by the age of 2, manifesting as a white mass visible in the pupil as a result of tumour growing forward into the vitreous, and obstructing the retina, with the red pupillary reflex replaced by a white reflex (leucocoria). Other presentations include strabismus, glaucoma with a painful red eye, poor vision, and enlargement of the globe.

Management

The main aim in the management of these patients is clearance of disease, attempting to preserve useful vision, whilst also taking into consideration the morbidity of any treatment. Management decisions will depend on the stage of the disease, and should be made in a multidisciplinary forum.

The choice of treatment of malignant melanoma remains controversial in many respects. Enucleation has been the favoured approach in the past; however, various vision-sparing approaches have been shown to confer similar locoregional control rates. These include plaque brachytherapy, external beam irradiation, and block excision with most patients retaining some useful vision.

Tumours of the orbit

Introduction

Malignant tumours of the orbit have no gender predilection and may present at any age. They may be derived from mesenchymal elements within the orbit, the lacrimal glands, the reticuloendothelial system, the optic nerve and rarely may even be a manifestation of the anaplastic degeneration of a hamartoma and choristoma.

Rhabdomyosarcoma is the most common malignant orbital tumour in childhood, arising from the mesenchymal tissue within the orbit, usually presenting in the first or second decades of life. The tumour spreads rapidly, but can be detected by a biopsy taken through the eyelid.

Adenoid cystic carcinomas can arise within the lacrimal gland of the eye, and are aggressive tumours capable of local invasion and metastases. They usually present in adult life.

Clinical features

Typical symptoms are of rapidly developing proptosis, as a result of the mass effect; however other symptoms may occur, including pain, diplopia, and decreased vision. Lid dysfunction or lagopthalmos may result in exposure keratitis and corneal ulceration.

Management

Treatment is usually in the form of exenteration of the eye, with adjuvant radiotherapy

Tumours of the ear

Introduction

The most common malignancies of the external ear are cutaneous BCCs and SCCs, the greatest risk factor being chronic long-term exposure to sun, specifically with UVB radiation. (See Fig. 4.1.2 for an example of SCC of the pinna.) Other risks include fair skin pigmentation. These malignancies tend to be locally invasive with low incidences of metastases. Unlike BCCs, SCCs occur far less commonly, but however are much more aggressive, with risk of locoregional spread. They occur more commonly in males. Along with exposure to UV radiation, other risks include advancing age, immunosuppression, and non-healing ulcers. In the pinna, BCCs are about four times more common than SCCs; however, in the external auditory canal the ratio is reversed, with SCCs being more common than BCCs.

Malignant melanomas can affect the ear, typically the helix and antihelix. The external ear accounts for about 10% of all head and neck melanomas. These tumours are aggressive, and can spread to regional lymph nodes early in the course of disease. Adenoid cystic tumours can also affect the external auditory canal. They have a low tendency for regional spread, but can demonstrate perineural spread.

Clinical features

Patients often present with an ulcerated area typically occurring on the posterior surface of the pinna, and in the pre-auricular area. Lesions may be painless, but are prone to bleeding. Occasionally depending on the pathology, the patients may have disease in neck nodes.

Investigations

Tissue diagnosis is easily obtained via a punch biopsy which can be taken in clinic. In squamous tumours, spread to adjacent structures such as the temporal bone can be identified with MRI scanning, facilitating proper planning of surgery.

Management

For small cutaneous tumours of the pinna, local excision with an adequate margin of at least 4mm can be performed. Mohs surgery can also be used, which involves complete micrographic excision of the tumour, with the use of intra-operative histopathology to assess the margins. For those patients not fit for surgery, radiotherapy can be used. Definitive radiotherapy for pinna cancer often utilizes electrons with covered lead behind the pinna.

In those tumours arising from the external canal (or middle ear), treatment needs to be more aggressive. This is often because of their high chance of local recurrence if less aggressive treatment is used. It is increasingly suggested that these tumours be treated primarily by a lateral or subtotal temporal bone resection, dependent on the stage, combined with a parotidectomy as well as a neck dissection. Following a temporal-bone resection, a regional myocutaneous flap or a free flap can be used to repair any residual defect. Even in early stage tumours of the external auditory

canal (EAC), local resection of the EAC is not sufficient. The most important survival factor is removal of the primary tumour with histologically clear margins; this combined with adjuvant radiotherapy has been proven to improve local control rates. Prognosis is dependent on the stage of the tumour and the histological subtype. In these cases, depending on stage of disease and treatment protocols, 5-year survival rates range from 10% for advanced disease to 83% for early disease.

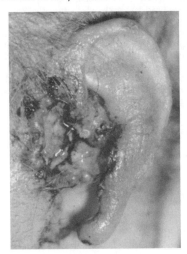

Fig. 4.1.2 Squamous cell carcinoma of the pinna.

Tumours of the middle ear

Introduction

Malignant tumours of the middle ear are extremely uncommon, and histologically are usually SCCs.

Other rare tumours include metastatic tumours (usually adenocarcinomas), and rhabdomyosarcomas. Chronic otitis media and cholesteatoma have been implicated as aetiological factors. Chronic suppurative otitis media and the resulting chronic inflammation may lead to squamous metaplasia. As a consequence the disease is often advanced at time of presentation.

Clinical features

Advanced disease at presentation may be because it may have been mistaken as benign disease initially. Features that should raise the index of suspicion include the presence of significant pain, which may appear out of proportion to the clinical findings and bleeding.

Investigations

Biopsy of any suspicious tissue identified through a tympanic membrane perforation or at the time of mastoid surgery, should be submitted for pathological analysis.

Imaging in the form of high-resolution CT scanning will aid in staging the disease and planning the treatment.

Management

Effective treatment of these tumours is by radical surgery with the aim of tumour-free resection margins, with post-operative radiotherapy. This once again usually involves some form of temporal bone resection dependent on the stage, along with a parotidectomy and neck dissection. Radical radiotherapy is effective for small tumours and must encompass the full extent of the disease whilst sparing the contralateral parotid.

Salivary gland cancers

Introduction

Salivary gland malignancies are uncommon with an incidence of about 1 per 100,000 per year. They represent a diverse group, often posing diagnostic and management challenges. The majority typically occur in the sixth decade of life with an equal sex incidence. Unlike other cancers within the head and neck, which are usually related to smoking and alcohol consumption, the aetiology in salivary malignancies is less clear. History of previous irradiation has been shown to increase the risk of tumour development, as demonstrated in patients who received radiotherapy for benign conditions, as well as studies of atomic bomb survivors. Other purported risks include chemical exposure to silica dust and kerosene and a possible link between Epstein–Barr virus and undifferentiated carcinomas.

Anatomy

Salivary glands within the head and neck can be classified into major and minor glands. The major glands refer to the paired parotid, submandibular, and sublingual. The minor glands refer to the 600–1000 predominantly mucous secreting glands located throughout the upper aerodigestive tract submucosa (i.e. mouth, lip, pharynx, larynx, parapharyngeal space).

Pathology

In 1991, the WHO classified salivary tumours into carcinomas, non-epithelial tumours, lymphomas, metastatic tumours, and unclassified tumours. The classification (18 types) is based on the clinical characteristics, histological features, and immunohistochemical staining. Histologically, salivary gland tumours represent the most heterogeneous group of tumours of any tissue in the body.

Approximately 20% of parotid tumours are malignant. In the submandibular gland this rises to approximately 50% and within the sublingual and minor glands approximately 80% are malignant. The most common malignant major and minor salivary gland tumours are the mucoepidermoid carcinomas, which comprise about 10% of all salivary gland neoplasms and approximately 30% of malignant salivary gland neoplasms. This neoplasm occurs most commonly in the parotid gland.

In order of decreasing frequency, the commonest histological types are:

Mucoepidermoid >adenoid cystic >adenocarcinoma >acinic cell carcinomas >SCC, undifferentiated carcinomas, and carcinoma ex pleomorphic adenoma (all <1%).

A division into low and high aggressiveness can be made:

Low

- Acinic
- Adenocarcinoma (some)
- Mucoepidermoid (some)

High

- Squamous
- Undifferentiated
- Carcinoma ex pleomorphic adenoma
- Adenocarcinoma (some)
- Mucoepidermoid (some)

Clinical features

Major glands

Most patients present with an incidental painless swelling of the affected gland. Occasionally deep lobe tumours of the parotid may present as an oropharyngeal mass with no external abnormality.

Features suggestive of malignancy include: pain, nerve palsies (usually the facial nerve in parotid tumours, although the hypoglossal and lingual nerves can be affected in sublingual and submandibular tumours), presence of associated lymphadenopathy, fixation of the tumour to deep structures or overlying skin, and rapid growth.

Minor glands

Presentation will depend on the site, but tumours are often painless submucosal swellings, which may ulcerate following trauma.

Investigations

Clinical examination of these patients must include a thorough assessment of the salivary mass, peroral examination with assessment of the salivary duct orifice, oropharyngeal examination to check for parapharyngeal involvement, facial nerve assessment, and palpation for cervical lymphadenopathy.

Fine needle aspiration cytology (FNAC)

Tumours are usually accessible for cytological assessment, with the risk of tumour seeding being negligible. However, analysis can prove challenging for the cytologist and depends on local experience. In those tumours which are cystic, aspiration of fluid may prove to be undiagnostic, and unhelpful. Generally as a rule, if the FNA is in contradiction to other findings clinical judgement should prevail.

Imaging

Diagnostic imaging is useful in certain situations. In those tumours arising from the parapharyngeal space, it may help identify the site of origin. For malignant tumours, it may also help in determining the anatomical extent of the tumour, relationship to other structures, and lymph node status. CT and MRI are complementary modalities.

Management

The main aim of any treatment is complete removal of the tumour, with an adequate margin of normal tissue, whilst ensuring minimal morbidity. Surgery is the mainstay of treatment, which depending on the site can result in significant morbidity.

Major salivary glands

Advanced parotid cancers require a total parotidectomy, with sacrifice of the facial nerve if this is involved. If the deep lobe of the parotid is involved with parapharyngeal space involvement, then this area needs to be dissected. This can be approached via a cervicoparotid approach or a paramedian mandibulotomy. In tumours of the submandibular or sublingual glands, excision of the gland is performed in combination with clearance of the nodes at level I. Once again, sacrifice of the hypoglossal or lingual nerves may be required if these are involved.

Minor salivary glands

In minor salivary gland tumours, wide surgical excision is recommended, which depending on the site and size can imply extensive resection.

Those tumours of the paranasal sinuses or nasal cavity may require a partial or total maxillectomy with possible orbital exenteration, and craniofacial resection depending on the extent of the tumour. Tumours arising from the larynx or trachea may be amenable to conservation surgical procedures.

Neck disease
Clinically palpable neck disease is treated by a neck dissection. In carefully selected patients, a selective dissection may be adequate, whilst those with extensive disease require a modified radical neck dissection with attempts to preserve non lymphatic structures such as the accessory nerve. In the node negative neck, the risk of occult regional disease is low, and therefore elective neck dissection is not routinely warranted. For cancers of <4cm, 5-year survival is >50%. Occult neck disease is uncommon and distant metastases rare. However in patients with high grade aggressive tumours this may not be the case, and a selective neck dissection of those levels at greatest risk should be carried out.

Radiotherapy
In patients with contraindications to surgery, radiotherapy can be used with enduring local control in at least two-thirds of cases.

The use of radiotherapy in the adjuvant setting has been shown to improve locoregional control rates. The target volume should encompass the salivary gland bed and adjacent lymph node areas; for parotid radiotherapy, the beams are angled away from the eyes and contralateral parotid. It is particularly indicated in patients with advanced stage disease, in high grade tumours, where the resection margins are close or involved, and where there is evidence of bone, cartilage, muscle, or perineural involvement. There is evidence that postoperative radiotherapy increases overall survival in advanced stage disease, though no randomized trials have been performed to demonstrate this.

Prognosis
Many salivary gland malignancies have an indolent clinical course, warranting long-term follow-up. Overall survival at 5 years is 60–75% with local control in T1/T2 tumours of 90% and T3/T4 tumours of <50% if postoperative radiotherapy is used.

Outcomes following treatment are dependent on the specific histological subtype. High grade tumours carry a poorer prognosis, often presenting with locoregional advanced disease. Other poor prognosticators include presence of neck nodes, perineural involvement, and involvement of extra-salivary tissue. Overall up to 30% of salivary cancers demonstrate distant metastases at 5 years. In adenoid cystic tumours, there is a marked propensity for local recurrence which is often many years after primary treatment. Systemic spread is also common in adenoid cystic carcinoma with lung being the commonest site.

Pleomorphic adenoma
This is a common benign tumour of the parotid gland usually arising in the superficial lobe and often arising in close proximity to the facial nerve. Treatment is by surgical removal with excellent local control rates up to 98%. Causes of local recurrence include extension of 'pseudo-pods' of tumour beyond an incomplete capsule, rupture of capsule during dissection, or tumour adherent to facial nerve.

If radiotherapy is given after the first operation for presumed residual disease, local recurrence is rare. Use of adjuvant radiotherapy should, however, be tempered by the knowledge of the typical long natural history, the ability of re-operation to control unifocal recurrence as well as the risk of radiation induced malignancy.

Nose, nasal cavity, and paranasal sinuses

Introduction
Malignant lesions of this region are diverse and rare. They account for approximately 3% of all head and neck cancers. There is a slight male preponderance, with peak incidences in the fifth to sixth decades of life. Tumours of the nasal cavity are equally divided between benign and malignant types, while most paranasal sinus tumours are malignant. Approximately 50% of sinonasal tumours arise from the maxillary sinus, the remainder arising from the ethmoids (25%) and nasal cavity (25%). In large tumours the site of origin is often difficult to identify.

Pathology
SCC is the most common histological type, accounting for >50% of cancers. The remainder include adenocarcinoma, adenoid cystic carcinoma, malignant melanoma, olfactory neuroblastoma, and undifferentiated sinonasal carcinoma. Other malignancies include a variety of lymphomas, plasmacytoma, and sarcomas.

The glands within the sinonasal tract can give rise to adenoid cystic tumours. These are clinically locally aggressive usually typified by perineural spread making local control difficult to achieve. Distant metastases and local recurrence may manifest in a delayed fashion several years after primary treatment.

Melanomas comprise <1% of sinonasal malignancies, originating from the neural crest-derived melanocytes present in the submucosa and mucosa, particularly the septum and lateral nasal wall. The aetiology of these tumours is unclear; however, smoking may play a role in metaplastic activation of pre-existing melanocytes. They tend to be more aggressive than their cutaneous equivalent.

Olfactory neuroblastomas arise from the neural crest stem cells, the precursors of the olfactory cells. There is a bimodal age distribution, with a peak in the younger population in the first and second decades and a second peak in the fifth and sixth decades. Tumours are usually locally aggressive involving the cribriform plate and tending to invade adjacent structures such as the orbit and anterior cranial fossa.

Sinonasal undifferentiated carcinomas (SNUCs) are highly aggressive locally invasive tumours thought to be part of the spectrum of neuroendocrine tumours. They frequently involve the nasal cavity and multiple sinuses, and carry a poor prognosis as a result of their local invasion, with mean survival times of <12 months. Prognosis has improved with greater use of chemotherapy.

Metastatic deposits from other locations are rare; however, the most common tumour described is metastatic renal cell carcinoma, which may be the only clinical manifestation.

Aetiology
Whilst smoking and alcohol are recognized risk factors in the pathogenesis of other head and neck cancers, this is not the case with sinonasal tumours. Occupational exposure to nickel and chrome dust have been associated with development of SCCs.

The association between hardwood workers and adenocarcinomas is well documented. The commonest site is within the superior nasal cavity and ethmoidal sinuses. There are three basic histological types: papillary, sessile, and alveolar-mucoid. It is the papillary form which is associated with wood workers, and carries the better prognosis. The other two are more aggressive and carry a poorer prognosis. Adenocarcinomas account for 40–68% of ethmoidal malignancies.

Presentation
These tumours often mimic benign inflammatory conditions in the early stages, often resulting in advanced disease at presentation. An appreciation of the complex anatomy in this region is helpful in understanding the various ways in which these tumours may present.

Symptoms will usually depend on the site of origin, although this is often difficult to identify when the presentation is late. Initial presentation is often insidious. Nasal cavity tumours may present with epistaxis and nasal obstruction. In addition, ethmoidal tumours may present with eye signs, such as proptosis, diplopia, or epiphora if there is breach of the lamina papyracea. Antral tumours may present with a unilateral cheek swelling if the anterior antral wall is breached. Other symptoms may include trismus, oro-antral fistulas and problems wearing dentures. Unlike paranasal sinus tumours, those of the nasal cavity tend to be diagnosed earlier, because of the development of earlier obstructive symptoms. Five per cent of patients may have a neck node on presentation, which portends a poor prognosis.

Generally patients presenting with unilateral symptoms should be investigated thoroughly with a high index of suspicion.

Investigations
A thorough history and examination of these patients should be performed; anterior rhinoscopy along with flexible or rigid nasal endoscopy should be performed to gain a thorough assessment of the nasal cavity and nasopharynx and any mass within. Ocular examination should check for diplopia, visual acuity, and pupillary response along with signs of proptosis. Peroral examination may identify abnormalities of the hard palate and upper alveolus from a maxillary tumour. Neurological examination should concentrate on the cranial nerves I–VI, which may be involved in sinonasal tumours.

Imaging allows delineation of the extent of disease mapping the extent of any bony or skull base erosion, and facilitating surgical planning. MRI scanning is superior in determining anterior skull base and orbital involvement and differentiating between tumour and adjacent soft tissue; however, the use of CT scanning may complementary with demonstration of invasion of fine bony structures.

In order to obtain a tissue diagnosis, biopsy of the lesion is warranted to confirm the diagnosis. This is usually easily performed endoscopically. On occasion if accessible, biopsy may be performed in the clinic setting, however it is important to ensure the tumour is not highly vascular, or indeed contiguous with intracranial contents. The use of radiological imaging prior to biopsy should reduce the risk of inadvertent surprises.

Management
The management of such patients is often complex and any decisions should be made within a multidisciplinary forum. Factors to consider include: tumour and patient related

factors; tumour histology and stage, the associated treatment morbidity and risks associated with surgical treatment, and ultimately the patient's wishes.

Treatment for most sinonasal malignancies generally involves dual modality treatment in the form of total surgical excision combined with postoperative radiotherapy. The details of the surgical excision are dependent on the site and size of the tumour and the ease of access.

For tumours limited to the lateral nasal wall, nasal cavity and ethmoid sinuses, a lateral rhinotomy approach may allow adequate access for excision. In the case of maxillary tumours, a total maxillectomy may be required with suitable reconstruction of any residual defect, which may involve microvascular free tissue transfer.

In those tumours involving the cribiform plate, a craniofacial resection is required, and may also involve orbital exenteration if the tumour has breached the periosteum of the orbit to involve the orbital fat.

Clinically positive neck disease is generally managed surgically with a neck dissection, usually with attempts at preservation of non-lymphatic structures such as the accessory nerve, if not involved with tumour. Treatment of the N0 neck is contentious, with some centres only advocating neck dissection if the primary tumour involves sites with increased risk for regional spread such as the nasopharynx, or soft palate.

In those patients where surgical resection of the primary tumour is not considered appropriate, radiotherapy can be used. Modern conformal techniques permit sparing of normal tissue such as the visual pathway. A bite block with tongue depressor excludes the lower oral cavity and shielding of the lacrimal gland can prevent xerophthalmia.

Prognosis

The combined treatment of surgery with postoperative radiotherapy markedly improves survival rates, with figures for 5-year survival rates of 30–50% being quoted. The difficulties with local control are also linked to the complex anatomy of this region, the often advanced disease at initial presentation, and the histological subtype.

Nasopharynx

Introduction

The majority (80–95%) of all malignant nasopharyngeal tumours arise from the epithelium and should be considered variants of SCC. The WHO has classified nasopharyngeal carcinoma (NPC) into three subtypes on the basis of light microscopy findings:

- Type 1: keratinizing SCC
- Type 2: non-keratinizing SCC
- Type 3: undifferentiated carcinoma

A variety of other malignant tumours develop in the nasopharynx and include lymphomas and sarcomas.

Cancers of the nasopharynx are rare in most countries of the world; however they are common in south-east Asia, especially in people from the Kwantung, Kwangsi, and Fukien regions. In North America, WHO types 1, 2, and 3 account for 20%, 10%, and 70% of all NPCs, respectively. In Hong Kong, the respective rates are 3%, 9%, and 88%. Typical presentation is in the fourth and fifth decades, although a bimodal peak is seen with a presentation also seen in late adolescence. The male to female ratio is approx 2–3:1.

Aetiology

There are three main aetiological factors:

- *Environmental*: diets of salty fish, a common staple diet in certain parts of south-east Asia have been associated consistently with an increased risk of NPC.
- *Viral*: latent Epstein–Barr virus (EBV) infection is also endemic in this population, and has been implicated in the transformation of epithelial cells. Viral genomes are detectable in the majority of NPC tumours from high incidence areas.
- *Genetic*: predisposition for NPC may also exist, as evidenced in the almost 100-fold increase in incidence in a relatively homogeneous genetic group of southern Chinese individuals compared with the incidence in a comparable group of white persons.

Studies have also demonstrated a significantly increased risk of NPC, in particular type I tumours in long-term smokers.

Clinical features

Tumours typically arise from the fossa of Rosenmüller behind the Eustachian tube cushion, with clinical presentation dependent on the pathway taken. The majority of patients have a metastatic neck node at presentation (70%). Other common symptoms include epistaxis, nasal obstruction, or referred otalgia.

Anterior spread via the Eustachian tube can result in a unilateral middle ear effusion, with the patient complaining of otalgia, or reduced hearing.

Posterolaterally, parapharyngeal spread can occur through the pharyngobasilar fascia, resulting in cranial nerve involvement. Involvement of the mandibular division of the trigeminal can result in the initial development of facial pain which usually precedes motor involvement.

Posterior invasion to the skull base can affect the sympathetic plexus resulting in a Horner's syndrome as well as affecting cranial nerves IX–XII. Tumour infiltration can also occur superiorly through the foramen lacerum into the cavernous sinus, affecting cranial nerves III, IV, and VI as well as the upper divisions of the trigeminal nerve.

Investigations

A comprehensive history and examination along with specific investigations should raise the suspicion of a nasopharyngeal tumour. The submucosal spread of NPC may result in no abnormality noted on endonasal examination.

Tissue diagnosis is required to confirm the diagnosis, and can be obtained under local or general anaesthesia via endoscopic guidance.

Imaging should be obtained to stage both the primary site as well as any neck disease. The ideal imaging modality is MRI, which is superior in demonstrating soft tissue involvement and the extent of any submucosal involvement (Fig. 4.1.3).

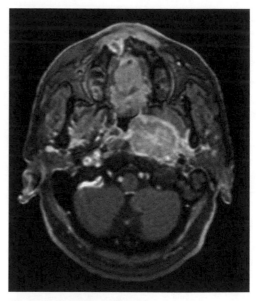

Fig. 4.1.3 T1 postcontrast MRI with fat suppression demonstrating nasopharyngeal carcinoma.

Management

Radiation therapy is the treatment of choice. The target volume encompasses both the primary tumour site and the neck. Neck dissection is usually only indicated for radiotherapy failures.

Concurrent chemoradiotherapy with induction or subsequent chemotherapy has been shown to confer improved survival and is now the standard of care. EBV vaccination is now being explored.

Poststyloid parapharyngeal spread needs a conformal technique to encompass the tumour. Involvement of the cavernous sinus with proximity of the visual pathway dictates the dose of radiotherapy that can be delivered. Typical dose constraints in treatment planning are:

At 2Gy/fraction:	
Spinal cord:	45–48
Brain stem:	50–54
Optic chiasm:	50–54
Optic nerve (whole):	50
Retina:	46–48

Serious late effects from radiotherapy to the nasopharynx are unusual but may include:
• Xerostomia/dental caries/osteoradionecrosis of jaw
• Fibrosis/stiffness of neck
• Hypopituitarism/hypothyroidism
• Trismus

• Dysphagia/aspiration
• Deafness/vestibular dysfunction
• Carotid artery stenosis/premature cerebrovascular accident
• Temporal lobe epilepsy
• Blindness
• Radiation induced malignancy
• Spinal cord/brain stem damage

Prognosis

Stage is the most important prognostic factor in terms of survival, with overall survival rate of 80% for stage I disease dropping down to 30% for stage IV disease. The overall 5-year survival has improved to about 60% depending on geography and stage. Adverse prognostic features include cranial nerve palsies, involvement of the skull base, advanced age, male sex, and involvement of the lymph nodes in the supraclavicular fossa.

Lip and oral cavity

Introduction

This is the sixth most common cancer worldwide accounting for an estimated 4% of all cancers and approximately 30% of all head and neck cancers, with >20,000 diagnosed in the US each year. Globally the highest rates are generally seen within the Indian subcontinent, where the disease accounts for up to 40% of all malignancies, and represents the most common malignancy amongst men.

A recent descriptive epidemiological study of oral cancer from 12 UK cancer registries showed 32,852 oral cancer cases were registered between 1990–1999, with a statistically significant increase in incidence over this period. Figures are higher in men than women, in older compared with younger groups, and in northern regions of the UK.

The majority (90%) are SCCs, the remainder include non-Hodgkin lymphoma, minor salivary gland carcinomas, and other rare tumours such as rhabdomyosarcomas. The commonest sites in order of decreasing frequency are (lip >lateral border of tongue >anterior floor of mouth >soft palate). Multifocal lesions are not unusual and may be synchronous or metachronous.

Anatomy

The oral cavity extends from the skin—vermilion junctions of the anterior lips to the junction of the hard and soft palates above and to the line of circumvallate papillae below and is divided into the following specific areas:
- Lip
- Anterior two-thirds of tongue
- Buccal mucosa
- Floor of mouth
- Lower gingiva
- Retromolar trigone
- Upper gingiva
- Hard palate

Aetiology and pathology

The major risk factors for the development of oral cancers are smoking and alcohol with at least 80% of oral cancers being attributable to alcohol and tobacco exposure. The effect of alcohol and smoking together is synergistic. As an example of this synergistic effect, the risk of oral cancer with joint consumption of high amounts of alcohol (>5 drinks per day) and cigarettes (>20 per day) is 13-fold greater than expected based upon the independent effects of the same amount of alcohol or tobacco alone. The most significant risk factors for oral cancers among the current non-smoker and non-drinker are previous use of alcohol and tobacco. Other risk factors include the practice of betel nut chewing. Unfortunately chronic carcinogen exposure creates a field change, which places the entire mucosa at risk. This also increases the chances of developing a second primary.

Other suspected but not confirmed aetiological agents include human papilloma virus (HPV subtypes 16 and 18), which have been associated with the development of verrucous squamous carcinomas, poor oral hygiene, and chronic irritation. Premalignant conditions include submucosal fibrosis and lichen planus with reported transformation rate of 0.5–3% and 0.5 % respectively.

Clinical features and natural history

The clinical features of oral cavity malignancies can be quite variable. Early cancers may simply present as a white or red patch which is non-ulcerated. Advanced presentation may vary from a predominantly submucosal lesion to an ulcerative, fungating mass. Other presentations include a non-healing painful ulcer, halitosis, difficulty in eating, or ill-fitting dentures. Dental practitioners often make the clinical diagnosis, but unfortunately many patients with oral cancer do not attend for dental checks.

A malignancy may arise within a premalignant lesion such as leucoplakia or erythroplakia. Usually the clinical characteristics of the lesion are sufficient to provide a low threshold to obtain a tissue diagnosis by biopsy. Assessment of patient risk factors may help to further stratify the risk of malignancy and determine fitness for any treatment. Features in the examination which may bode a poor prognosis include the presence of trismus (suggesting pterygoid involvement), cranial nerve involvement, including hypoglossal, facial nerve function and gag and palatal elevation, and the presence of palpable neck nodes.

Management

Early cancers (stages I and II) of the lip and oral cavity are highly curable by surgery or by radiation therapy, and the choice of treatment is dictated by the anticipated functional and cosmetic results of treatment and by the availability of the particular expertise required of the surgeon or radiation oncologist for the individual patient. The presence of a positive margin or a tumour depth >5mm significantly increases the risk of local recurrence and suggests that combined modality treatment may be beneficial. The use of the CO_2 laser has been shown to be effective in the treatment of carefully selected early stage tumours. Brachytherapy, either alone, or with a neck dissection has a role in oral cavity carcinomas. The success of brachytherapy techniques is in part dependent on the experience of the implant team.

Advanced cancers (stages III and IV) of the lip and oral cavity present a wide spectrum of challenges for the surgeon and radiation oncologist. In the majority of patients with stage III or IV tumours, treatment is often a combination of surgery and radiation therapy.

One of the most important advances in head and neck surgery which has greatly transformed the surgical management of advanced disease has been the safe and effective use of single-stage free tissue transfer for reconstruction. This includes the use of bone flaps from areas such as the fibula, iliac crest, and scapula, and soft tissue from the radial forearm, trapezius, and anterolateral thigh. The availability of such techniques has made a dramatic impact on the functional outcome of such patients. Access for free flap transfer is via the neck such that neck dissection is routinely done in association. Loss of free flap viability is usually reported to be <5%, depending on which series are examined. Factors determining choice of surgical treatment include the size, site, and proximity of the tumour to the mandible or maxilla.

The rehabilitation of patients after oral surgery remains a crucial element in determining outcome. Patients need the support of an MDT for rehabilitation of speech, swallow, dentition, and cosmesis.

Radiotherapy

Definitive radiotherapy can be used for small cancers in the oral cavity with excellent local control rates. The dominant role of surgery is related more to the risk of mandibular necrosis associated with radiotherapy. This risk is increased by concomitant chemotherapy, continuation of smoking, and post-treatment dental extraction. Radiotherapy should be ipsilateral where possible and target volumes minimized by use of bite block and tongue depressor if appropriate.

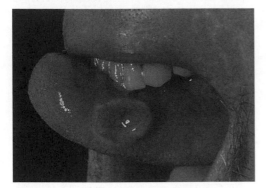

Fig. 4.1.4 Squamous cell carcinoma of the lateral border of tongue.

Prognosis

Prognosis of these tumours is largely dependent on the stage and specific site of the tumour. Early lip cancers are usually highly curable by surgery or radiotherapy with rates of 90–100%. Similar local control rates can be achieved for small tumours within the oral cavity.

In advanced tumours of the oral cavity, effective control rates can be achieved with dual modality treatment. The choice of treatment is generally dictated by the anticipated functional and cosmetic results of the treatment. Moderately advanced lesions of the retromolar trigone without evidence of spread to cervical lymph nodes are usually curable and have shown local control rates of as much as 90%; such lesions of the hard palate, upper gingiva, and buccal mucosa have a local control rate of as much as 80%. In the absence of clinical evidence of spread to cervical lymph nodes, moderately advanced lesions of the floor of the mouth and anterior tongue are generally curable, with survival rates of as much as 70% and 65%, respectively.

Oropharynx

Introduction

Oropharyngeal cancers usually affect patients in their fifth through to their seventh decades of life, with a male preponderance (3–5:1).

The majority of tumours are SCC (85%). The high concentration of lymphoid tissue results in a higher incidence of lymphomas compared to other sites within the upper aerodigestive tract. These usually affect the palatine or lingual tonsils (10%) and are typically of the non-Hodgkin type. The remainder of tumours usually originate from minor salivary glands affecting the glands of the soft palate and tongue base. These are usually adenoid cystic carcinomas.

The commonest sites for malignancies within the oropharynx are the tonsil and tongue base; the remainder usually affect the faucial arch and pharyngeal wall.

Anatomy

The oropharynx extends from the soft palate superiorly down to the hyoid inferiorly. It communicates with the oral cavity anteriorly, with the nasopharynx superiorly, and the larynx and hypopharynx inferiorly. The lateral wall is comprised primarily of the tonsils and tonsillar fossa, the anterior and posterior tonsillar pillars, and the lateral pharyngeal wall. Posteriorly, it is bound by the pharyngeal wall mucosa, which extends from the superior to the inferior limits described previously. Subdivisions of the oropharynx include the tongue base (including the pharyngoepiglottic and glossoepiglottic folds and the vallecula), the faucial arch (including the soft palate, uvula, and anterior tonsillar pillar), the tonsil and tonsillar fossa, and the pharyngeal wall (including the posterior tonsillar pillar, the lateral and posterior pharyngeal walls).

Pathology

As with other head and neck squamous cancers, the most significant risk factors are smoking and alcohol consumption. Other risk factors include poor diet, low in fruits and vegetables, the chewing of betel quid, commonly used in various parts of Asia and infection with HPV, in particular subtype 16. HPV infection is an aetiological factor for a subset of tumours that arise predominantly from the lingual and palatine tonsils. Analogously, oral HPV infection has been associated with sexual behaviour, in particular with number of oral sex partners.

Clinical features and natural history

Initial presenting symptoms of oropharyngeal cancers are often vague and non-specific; consequently the majority of patients who present often have locally advanced disease at the time of diagnosis.

Presenting symptoms may include sore throat, odynophagia, muffled speech, and referred otalgia mediated though the glossopharyngeal nerve. Twenty per cent of patients may present with a neck lump as the only symptom. Whilst most neck metastases present as firm solid masses in the expected designated levels, there are certain cancers including those of the oropharynx that may present with a cystic neck mass. These are often erroneously misdiagnosed and treated as a branchial cyst, emphasizing the importance of an adequate diagnostic work-up prior to deciding on appropriate management.

Investigations

All patients should have a thorough history taken, eliciting potential risk factors and symptoms, as well as a careful examination of the upper aerodigestive tract and neck. This should also include a flexible nasal endoscopic examination.

An MRI scan will aid in delineating the extent of the disease both locally and regionally in the neck, allowing staging to be performed. Additionally the chest should be imaged, to check for second primaries.

In the case of a clinically palpable neck lump, an FNAC should be undertaken. Where there is less obvious neck disease, this may be performed under imaging guidance such as ultrasound or CT.

Assessment of the primary, under general anaesthesia, should be performed to stage the extent of the primary disease, with a biopsy being performed to confirm the diagnosis.

Management

As with all head and neck tumours, management decisions should be made in a multidisciplinary forum, with all the information required to hand, allowing the most appropriate treatment to be offered to the patient.

Early stage disease is generally treated with radiotherapy, although equivalent rates of local control may be achieved with either surgery or radiotherapy. The functional effects of either treatment modality should be considered in this situation. Surgery may be the preferred modality where the functional deficit is minimal avoiding the potential complications of radiotherapy such as xerostomia. Severe xerostomia is usually avoided by utilizing conformal or IMRT approaches. For node positive cases, it is often appropriate to attempt to spare some or all of the ipsilateral parotid.

In patients with advanced stage disease, the general trend has been to adopt a multimodality approach. Neck dissection followed by chemoradiotherapy is often used for bilateral base of tongue cancer; more lateralized lesions may be suitable for radical excision with free-flap reconstruction.

In these patients, access to the tumour is usually not possible via a conventional peroral approach; approaches to the oropharynx include the use of a stepped paramedian mandibulotomy, allowing preservation of the inferior dental nerve.

Prognosis

Prognosis of oropharyngeal tumours depends on site and stage. For early stage tonsillar tumours (T1–2), the local control rates exceed 80% with primary radiotherapy. Long-term follow-up is the same as for any HNSCC, to exclude locoregional recurrence, distant metastases, and second primaries. The morbidity to the patient in terms of function can be very significant, especially in patients undergoing radical surgery, where the effect on speech and swallow can be profound, warranting significant rehabilitation postoperatively.

Stratification of treatment by HPV status should be considered and oral HPV tests are becoming available. Overall survival is improved and risk of second cancers reduced in HPV-16 positive patients.

Further reading

Agrawal Y, Koch WM, Xiao W, et al. Oral human papillomavirus infection before and after treatment for human papillomavirus 16 positive and human papilloma virus 16 negative head and neck squamous cell carcinoma. *Clin Cancer Res* 2008; **14**:7143–50.

Hypopharynx

Epidemiology

More than 95% of hypopharyngeal cancers are epithelial in origin, predominantly SCCs. Other types and variants include basaloid squamous carcinomas, spindle cell carcinomas, small cell carcinomas, undifferentiated carcinomas, and carcinomas of the minor salivary glands, which comprise <5%. It is a rare disease with a prevalence of <1 per 100,000 of the population, with approximately 2500 new cases annually in the US. Peak incidences usually occur in the fifth and sixth decade, with a greater incidence in men (3:1) than women.

Anatomy

The hypopharynx extends from the inferior limit of the oropharynx at the level of the hyoid bone down to the level of the cricoid cartilage. The UICC recognizes three anatomical sites for purposes of tumour classification:

- *Piriform fossa*: this extends from the pharyngoepiglottic folds to the upper end of the oesophagus.
- *Posterior pharyngeal wall*: this extends from the floor of the vallecula down to the inferior border of the cricoid cartilage.
- *Postcricoid*: this extends from the arytenoid cartilage and connecting folds to the inferior border of the cricoid cartilage, therefore forming the anterior wall of the hypopharynx.

Aetiology

Whilst smoking has been implicated in the development of hypopharyngeal cancer, the association as in other head and neck sites is not as clear. Alcohol has been shown to be a significant cofactor, and it is likely that it promotes the mutagenic effects of tobacco.

Other predisposing factors include nutritional deficiencies in iron and vitamin C. In the past, links between Plummer–Vinson syndrome and postcricoid tumours in women have been suggested although this is more likely to be associated with excessive use of alcohol and cigarette smoking.

Natural history and patterns of spread

Hypopharyngeal cancers tend to be aggressive and demonstrate a natural history that is characterized by diffuse local spread, early metastasis, and a relatively high rate of distant spread. The majority of patients have advanced disease at presentation, with 60% having locoregional disease, reflecting the regional lymphatics and the anatomy of the region. The piriform fossa is the most common site of origin (60%) followed by the postcricoid (30%) and the posterior pharyngeal wall (10%); however, advanced presentation may make it difficult to identify the site of origin. The tumours demonstrate multisite involvement within the hypopharynx, often extending into adjacent mucosal areas. Dissemination in the submucosal lymphatics can also lead to a high incidence of 'skip' lesions, with >10% of patients having a second primary in the oesophagus.

Superiorly the tumour can extend into the posterior pharyngeal wall and tongue base. Anteriorly tumour spread can occur into the larynx, breaching the paraglottic space and entering the larynx via the pre-epiglottic space. Vocal cord fixation may occur from involvement of the cricoarytenoid joint and invasion of the posterior cricothyroid

muscle, paraglottic space, or the recurrent laryngeal nerve. The thyroid gland can be involved by its proximity to the lateral wall of the hypopharynx, although this is clearly a poor prognostic factor.

The presence of nodal metastasis is also a poor prognostic factor of significant importance, occurring more commonly in hypopharyngeal cancer than in other head and neck subsites. The hypopharynx has the highest incidence of distant metastases at presentation (17–24%) compared to other subsites within the head and neck (10%). The most common site of metastases is the lung (80%) followed by liver and bone. In the presence of distant metastases, survival is dramatically decreased, usually to <1 year.

Clinical features

The principal signs and symptoms include dysphagia, initially for solids then liquids, hoarseness as a result of laryngeal invasion, odynophagia, neck mass, and the sensation of a lump in the throat.

Patients may also complain of referred otalgia, mediated via the auricular branch of the vagus nerve. The hypopharynx may be the site of an occult primary in patients presenting with a metastatic neck node from an unknown primary, and should always be considered in the work-up of such patients.

Management

As with all patients, decisions must be made in a multidisciplinary forum. This is often complicated by the considerable comorbidity these patients have as well as the poor social support. The nature of the disease and the various treatment options available along with their associated morbidities can complicate management decisions.

In the majority of patients who present with large volume, advanced stage disease, surgery is the preferred option with postoperative radiotherapy. Surgery is radical, and often comprises a total pharyngolaryngectomy with reconstruction of any residual defects, using myocutaneous pectoralis major flaps, radial forearm flaps, or visceral interposition grafts using stomach or small bowel.

Early stage disease though rare can be treated with radiotherapy with salvage surgery used for recurrent disease. The use of neo-adjuvant chemotherapy in combination with radiotherapy has been shown to confer comparable survival rates to surgical treatment in patients with advanced hypopharyngeal cancers, offering the patients the option of laryngeal preservation. This also potentially gives the patient the option of salvage surgery in the case of recurrent disease. The use of radiotherapy versus surgery in this group has to be weighed up against the risks of radionecrosis resulting in an incompetent larynx, as well as the possibility of a tracheostomy and gastrostomy tube feeding.

Prognosis

The main prognostic factors affecting outcome are clinical stage, age of the patient, and PS. Generally hypopharyngeal cancers have a poor prognosis compared to other head and neck subsites, although figures vary between different series, ranging from 18–65% for 5-year disease-free survival rates. In addition to the risk of developing locoregional recurrence the risk of second primaries is also high. Poor prognosis may also be related to the poor comorbid health of the patient group.

Larynx

Epidemiology

Cancer of the larynx represents the most common malignancy within the head and neck; 90% are SCCs of varying degrees of differentiation. There are approximately 12,500 new cases each year in the US with 2200 in the UK. The incidence within the UK is 4 per 100,000 per year. It is more common in men than women (5:1). Epidemiology is complicated by the difficulty in clinically distinguishing between the various anatomical subsites within the larynx as well as the close relationship to the hypopharynx.

Aetiology

Smoking is strongly associated with the development of laryngeal cancer. The carcinogenic effects of tobacco are due to an interplay between carcinogen-DNA adduct formation, tumour-specific mutations, and cancer risk. It is significantly associated with an increased risk of TP53 mutations. Tobacco initiates a linear dose-response carcinogenic effect in which the duration is more important than the intensity of exposure. Other factors increasing the carcinogenic potential include hand-rolled versus commercially available cigarettes, the use of black versus blond tobacco, and the age of the patient when they start smoking. The carcinogenic potential has also been shown to be dependent on gender, where females with identical smoking histories are more susceptible to developing laryngeal cancer than males.

The risk of laryngeal cancer is increased (1.9–3.3-fold) with alcohol intake; however, alcohol potentiates the effect of tobacco acting synergistically to dramatically increase the risks.

There is a subset of patients in whom infection with HPV may be responsible, in particular types 16 and 18. The association between HPV and laryngeal cancer is weakest compared to other sites within the head and neck. Biologically, HPV positive tumours appear to have a better prognosis than HPV negative, by virtue of a lower rate of TP53 mutations. Various studies have suggested the association of gastro-oesophageal reflux disease with the development of laryngeal cancer; however, there are often several confounding factors which cloud the issue, including the role of smoking and alcohol.

Natural history and patterns of spread

There is a wide variation in outcome between different subsites of the larynx (locoregional control: glottis >supraglottis >subglottis). This may reflect in part differences in the regional lymphatics resulting in different rates of metastases as well as the T stage at diagnosis with glottic cancers often presenting with T1 disease.

Clinical features

The clinical features are related to the primary tumour, secondary spread, or the general effects of the cancer.

Hoarseness is the most common symptom, particularly in glottic cancers where it may be an early symptom, due to vocal cord involvement.

Supraglottic tumours generally present later with symptoms of pain, which may be perceived as a sore throat, or may be referred otalgia. Dysphagia or odynophagia may occur due to involvement of the pharynx.

Airway compromise in the form of stridor is usually a late sign, which necessitates urgent referral to an ENT team for further assessment and management (see box).

The patient may occasionally present with metastatic neck disease, with no obvious symptoms of the primary.

Emergency management of stridor
- Multidisciplinary team approach:
  - Involve ENT/anaesthetist
- Treatment depends on underlying cause
- Measures that may buy time include:
  - Nebulized adrenaline (5mL of 1:1000)
  - Heliox (helium and oxygen)
  - Dexamethasone IV
- Needs early recognition!

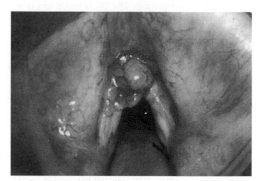

Fig. 4.1.5 Endoscopic view of laryngeal carcinoma involving anterior commissure.

Management

The most important factor used to determine management of laryngeal cancer is stage. Early stage disease (Stage I–II) is generally managed with single-modality therapy. The choice of surgery or radiotherapy is determined by the location of the tumour and the likely morbidity, particularly voice quality. The popularization of conservation techniques including transoral laser surgery allows the chance of organ-preserving conservation surgery to be offered. In carefully selected patients with early stage disease, or small volume disease, these conservation procedures may be considered and include partial laryngectomy, supracricoid/supraglottic, and various similar procedures. Although broadly categorized, the final procedure is tailored to the individual patient with the goal of achieving control of the cancer, and obtaining a functional outcome of speech and swallowing avoiding a permanent tracheostomy.

Irradiation for early stage tumours is delivered using small portals of 5–6cm. The determinants of choice between surgery and radiotherapy are complex and multifactorial.

Until recently, patients with advanced disease (Stage III–IV) tended to receive radical surgery and postoperative radiotherapy. However, the landmark Veterans Administrational Laryngeal Cancer Study in the 1980s demonstrated that induction chemotherapy followed by radiotherapy resulted in comparable survival rates to surgery with postoperative radiotherapy, demonstrating that organ preservation was possible with potentially curative therapy (The Department of Veterans Affairs Laryngeal Cancer Study Group 1991). The simultaneous administration of chemotherapy and radiotherapy (concurrent chemoradiotherapy) has been shown to be superior to radiotherapy alone (Pignon et al. 2000) and indeed to induction chemotherapy. In patients with advanced stage laryngeal cancer, surgical treatment is in the form of a total laryngectomy, resulting in the formation of a permanent tracheostomy.

Decision making for these patients needs to occur in a multidisciplinary forum, taking into consideration both patient-related factors as well as those related to the primary tumour itself. The team should fully discuss with the patient the advantages and disadvantages of larynx-preservation options compared with treatments that include total laryngectomy.

In patients who present acutely with stridor, endoscopic debulking should be carried out prior to planning of definitive management, although if this is not feasible then a tracheostomy may be required initially.

Radiotherapy

T1/T2 glottic cancers do not warrant elective nodal irradiation. Most T1 glottic cancers are in the anterior glottis and are well encompassed by an anterior oblique pair of beams; T2b glottic cancer should be treated with a lateral parallel pair of beams; local control with conventional fractionation is <70% such that modified fractionation should be considered. For larger volume tumours, elective nodal irradiation should be performed; if level IIA is clinically and radiologically negative then level II2B is unlikely to be involved.

Prognosis

Following radiotherapy glottis cancers have an initial local control of 90% for T1, 75% for T2, and 60% for selected T3 tumours. In supraglottic tumours the control rates are lower stage for stage, due to the larger tumour volumes. With surgical salvage, 5-year cancer specific survival is 95–100% for T1 and 85–90% for T2 glottic tumours. An important point to reiterate to patients is that smoking during radiotherapy has been shown to decrease the chance of locoregional control.

Rehabilitation

The psychosocial consequences of a total laryngectomy are well recognized and are related not just to the loss of voice, but also the presence of a permanent tracheostomy.

Social isolation, job loss, and depression are common sequelae.

Voice rehabilitation

Patients undergoing a laryngectomy should be seen preoperatively by the speech therapist for counselling, education and support.

There are three main options available for voice rehabilitation.

1. The use of voice prosthesis with a one-way valve inserted either primarily at the time of the surgery or secondarily after the surgery, uses a fistula created between the trachea and oesophagus to create a voice. When the stoma is occluded pulmonary air passes through the one-way valve in the tracheoesophageal wall, and causes the pharyngo-oesophageal segment to vibrate. Undoubtedly the best results are obtained with use of a voice prosthesis; however, the patient is dependent on the hospital for maintenance of the prosthesis and management of any associated problems. This clearly needs to be factored into making the appropriate choice of voice rehabilitation for the patient. Appropriate training in the maintenance and use of the valve is required and patients must be advised about the possible aspiration of food, fluids and secretions.

2. Oesophageal speech uses the swallowing of air to create an artificial voice, with the patient having to learn to separate respiration from phonation. The production of a functional voice may take months to acquire, with success dependent on patient motivation.

3. In those patients where these methods are not successful, then an electrolarynx allows a method of communication albeit less realistic. This battery powered source is held against the neck to produce sound. The advantages are that little effort is required; however, the voice created is artificial and robot like.

Further reading

Pignon JP, Bourhis J, et al. Chemotherapy added to locoregional treatment of head and neck squamous cell carcinoma: three meta-analyses of updated individual data. *Lancet* 2000; **355**(9208):949–55.

The Department of Veterans Affairs Laryngeal Cancer Study Group. Induction chemotherapy plus radiation compared with surgery plus radiation in patients with advanced laryngeal cancer. *N Engl J Med* 1991; **324**(24):1685–90.

Uncommon tumours of head and neck

Adenoid Cystic Carcinomas (ACCs)

ACCs arises from mucous secreting intercalated ducts in salivary gland tissue derived embryonically from small gut. They arise in minor salivary glands in 60% of cases (predominantly oral) and major salivary glands in 40%. ACCs account for approximately 1% of all head and neck malignancies, and are characterized by an indolent yet persistent growth with a tendency for local recurrence and distant metastases several years after initial presentation. Patients are generally younger and fitter than those with SCC of the head and neck. There is a female preponderance with peak incidence in the fourth to sixth decades. Tumours typically have a predilection for perineural infiltration. Unlike squamous cell head and neck cancer, ACC often spreads systemically, the commonest metastatic site being the lung. Other sites affected include bone. The primary treatment modality of choice is usually surgical resection followed by adjuvant radiotherapy; however there is significant work being undertaken examining the use of systemic therapies and biomarkers that may predict clinical outcome.

Mucosal melanoma

Primary mucosal melanoma of the head and neck is undoubtedly a rare disease associated with a very poor prognosis (mean survival of 17% at 5 years). The commonest sites affected include the nasal cavity, oral cavity, and paranasal sinuses. In contrast to cutaneous melanoma, mucosal disease generally occurs in an older age group typically affecting patients in their sixth to ninth decades. Common presentations include nasal obstruction and epistaxis. The primary treatment modality has been surgical wide en bloc excision. The role of radiotherapy has generally been shown to be of some benefit when given in the adjuvant setting, improving likelihood of local tumour control. Definitive radiotherapy may be used in patients with unresectable tumours or in those where the functional/cosmetic deficits would be too severe and may result in comparable survival rates to surgically treated patients. The role of chemotherapy and immunotherapy at present remains speculative.

Sarcomas

Sarcomas of the head and neck are rare, accounting for approximately 10% of all soft tissue sarcomas and approximately 1% of all head and neck tumours. There is typically a male preponderance with presentation usually in the sixth decade with a painless mass. Common sites include the scalp, face, and neck. The majority are high grade tumours. The risk of distant metastases is related to histological grade and tumour size, the commonest site being the lungs. Treatment modality of choice is surgical resection, with adjuvant radiotherapy in patients with high grade tumours, or close/positive margins. Radical radiotherapy is usually reserved for large unresectable tumours. The role of adjuvant chemotherapy is unclear, although studies suggest improvements in local control and distant metastases.

Plasmacytomas

Extramedullary plasmacytoma is a relatively uncommon malignancy that can present in the head and neck. The most common sites include the nasal cavity, paranasal sinuses, and nasopharynx, typically affecting the submucosa. There is a male predilection with patients typically presenting in their sixth to eight decades. Clinical presentation is usually with localized disease. The treatment of choice is radiotherapy. Surgery may be employed in patients with small localized lesions, where complete resection is possible with minimal functional deficit. The incidence of a monoclonal gammopathy is nearly 50%. The chance of local control is high (80–90%). The commonest cause of poor outcome is progression to systemic disease, with survival closely related to the chance of developing this.

Paragangliomas

Chemodectomas or paragangliomas are rare, comprising 0.6% of all head and neck tumours. They have a female preponderance, with a slow indolent history. They originate from neuroectodermal tissue, thought to play a role in monitoring changes in CO_2, pH, and O_2 levels. Ten per cent of these patients will have an inherited familial form, warranting appropriate genetic counselling and screening. Tumours can be multicentric in 20% of sporadic cases and 80% of familial cases. Patients therefore require further screening in the form of 24-hour urine collection for catecholamines as well as abdominal scanning to pick up an additional tumour. The definition of malignant disease is variable but is generally thought to be the presence of metastatic disease in tissue other than neuroendocrine tissue. Common presentations may include a neck mass with associated dysphonia (vagal paraganglioma). Carotid body tumours occur at the bifurcation of the carotid artery. The jugulotympanic paragangliomas (glomus jugulare) can present as a temporal bone mass involving the middle/external ear or the jugular bulb. Surgical removal remains the treatment of choice. Radiotherapy is effective at halting progression of these tumours though complete radiological resolution is unlikely.

Neuroendocrine tumours

Neuroendocrine tumours encompass a broad spectrum of neoplasms. They are of two types, depending on whether they have a neural or an epithelial origin. Paragangliomas represent those of neural origin, whilst neuroendocrine carcinomas represent those of epithelial origin. The actual cell of origin in cases of neuroendocrine carcinomas is not clearly known. It is thought they are derived from endocrine cells of the dispersed neuroendocrine system, although some believe they arise from pluripotential stem cells that are capable of dual epithelial and endocrine differentiation. They are further classified into three subtypes: typical carcinoid tumour (well-differentiated neuroendocrine carcinoma), atypical carcinoid tumour (moderately differentiated neuroendocrine carcinoma), and small cell carcinoma (poorly differentiated neuroendocrine carcinoma). These are rare tumours; tending to occur more commonly in the larynx, where they represent 0.5–1% of epithelial cancers. The laryngeal neuroendocrine tumours have an overall male predilection and the same seems to be true of non-laryngeal neuroendocrine carcinomas of the head and neck. Outside the larynx common sites include the paranasal sinuses. Clinically neuroendocrine tumours of the head and neck are usually locally advanced at the time of presentation. Symptoms at presentation are not diagnostic, and differ according to site and extent of disease. Diagnosis requires recognition of typical neuroendocrine architecture, morphology, and the immunohistochemical confirmation of neuroendocrine differentiation. Differentiation of these tumours from SCCs is essential both for purposes of management and prognosis. The treatment of choice is radical surgery with postoperative radiotherapy

Further reading

Bradley PJ. Adenoid cystic carcinoma of the head and neck: a review. *Current Opin Otolaryngol Head Neck Surg* 2004; **12**(2):127–32.

Dodd RL, Slevin NJ. Salivary gland adenoid cystic carcinoma : A review of chemotherapy and molecular therapies. *Oral Oncol* 2006; **42**:759–69.

Mendenhall WM, Mendenhall CM, Mendenhall NP. Solitary plasmacytoma of bone and soft tissues. *Am J Otolaryngol* 2003; **24**(6):395–9.

Mendenhall WM, Mendenhall CM, Werning JW, *et al.* Adult head and neck soft tissue sarcomas. *Head Neck* 2005; **27**(10):916–22.

Susnerwala SS, Shanks JH, Banerjee SS, *et al.* Extramedullary plasmacytoma of the head and neck region: clinicopathological correlation in 25 cases. *Br J Cancer* 1997; **75**(6):921–7.

Wagner M, Morris CG, Werning JW, *et al.* Mucosal melanoma of the head and neck. *Am J Clin Oncol* 2008; **31**(1):43–8.

Management of neck nodes

Anatomy of neck nodes (Fig. 4.1.6)

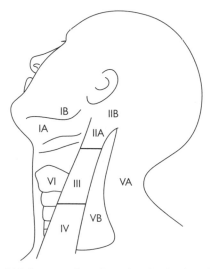

Fig. 4.1.6 One nomenclature (surgical) used to describe neck nodes is based on an anatomical basis, developed at the Memorial Sloan Kettering Centre, classifying nodes from levels I–VI (Table 4.1.1).

Table 4.1.1 The Memorial Sloan Kettering Centre node classification

IA	Submental
IB	Submandibular
IIA	Anteroinferior to the accessory nerve
IIB	Posterosuperior to the accessory nerve
III	Middle jugular nodes
IV	Lower jugular
VA	Posterior triangle (above cricoid level)
VB	Posterior triangle (below cricoid level)
VI	Central compartment—located between both carotid arteries

This can be adapted to cross sectional imaging taking into account specific radiological landmarks easily identifiable on CT or MRI slices (Gregoire et al. 2003). Cross sectional imaging is essential in the work-up of head and neck cancer patients allowing assessment of both the primary tumour site as well as the extent of any nodal disease. MR scanning tends to be the primary imaging modality of choice for tumours above the hyoid bone, whilst CT and MRI are equivalent below this level. In many sites (e.g. paranasal sinuses) CT and MRI are complementary.

Advances in the use of functional imaging techniques such as PET-FDG (fludeoxyglucose (^{18}F); Fig. 4.1.7) or CT-PET may provide greater information in specific situations such as patients with unknown primary disease, or in patients with suspected recurrence.

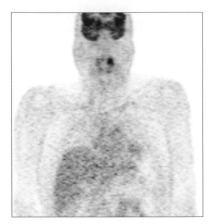

Fig. 4.1.7 Coronal FDG-PET showing increased uptake in the tongue base.

Management of neck nodes in known primary tumour

The N0 neck

The presence of neck disease is a significant prognostic marker of outcome, with a reduction in cure rate by up to 50%. There is some contention as to whether elective neck treatment for potential microscopic disease (clinical stage N0) improves survival among patients with T1–4 lesions with no clinically apparent nodal metastases. Radiation therapy and neck dissection are seemingly equally effective at eradicating subclinical disease. Therefore, management of the neck depends on the management of the primary tumour. If treatment is surgical, an elective neck dissection is frequently performed, resulting in control of subclinical disease in >90% of cases. If the primary treatment is radiotherapy, then radiation therapy can be used. In general, elective neck treatment is advocated for patients with a risk of subclinical disease of greater than 15%, i.e. it is not usually done for T1N0 cases.

The N positive neck

The management of clinically positive cervical lymph nodes (stage N1–3) is also related to the management of the primary tumour. Small nodes may be treated with radiation therapy alone. When the primary treatment is surgical, a neck dissection represents sufficient treatment for small volume nodal metastasis (stage N1). In this situation, treatment of the neck with a selective neck dissection may be appropriate, the choice of levels being made according to the site of the primary. In patients with advanced nodal disease, treatment of the neck is usually in the form of a modified radical neck dissection, with preservation of various non-lymphatic structures. The use of modified radical neck dissection is not associated with an increased risk of locoregional failure if the non-lymphatic structures are not affected by disease. Postoperative radiation therapy is added for advanced nodal disease (stage N2 or N3), increasing local control in the neck postoperatively as well as control of subclinical disease on the opposite side of the neck. In cases with extracapsular nodal disease, synchronous chemotherapy is added to postoperative radiotherapy. There is a view that adding chemotherapy to definitive radiotherapy for N2 disease with a neck dissection in reserve does not prejudice outcome compared with performing a neck dissection *ab initio* along with radiological follow-up. In those patients where tumours infiltrate the accessory/ internal jugular vein (IJV) or sternocleidomastoid (SCM), preservation may not be possible, and conversion to a radical neck dissection may be necessary.

Surgery

In 1991, the American Academy of Otolaryngology—Head and Neck Surgery (AAO-HNS) developed a system of classification of neck dissections, which is universally accepted.

Radical neck dissection

This is the standard procedure originally described by Crile in 1906, from which other procedures represent a modification. It is defined as an en bloc removal of all the neck nodes from levels I–V, along with the IJV, the SCM, and the accessory nerve.

Modified radical neck dissection

The significant morbidity caused by radical neck dissection has resulted in various modifications, with an attempt to preserve the non-lymphatic structures, namely the accessory, IJV, and SCM, whilst excising the nodal tissue from levels I–V. Conversion to a radical neck dissection may be required in tumours which infiltrate or involve these non-lymphatic structures.

Selective neck dissection

The rationale behind the use of a selective neck dissection is to surgically remove those levels of nodes likely to be affected by metastases, whilst also preserving non-lymphatic structures. The decision on which levels to remove is based on the study of the patterns of lymphatic spread from a particular primary site. Tumours of the oral cavity tend to metastasize to levels I–III, whilst tumours of the oropharynx tend to spread to levels II–IV.

1. *Supraomohyoid neck dissection (SOHND)*: removal of levels (I–III)—commonly performed in patients with oral cavity tumours, particularly in those with N0 necks. It includes the resection of soft tissue in the submental triangle, along with the submandibular triangle contents, including the submandibular gland and the fibrofatty tissue along the IJV from the skull base to the omohyoid muscle. The dissected contents include the fascia that covers the medial aspect of the sternocleidomastoid muscle; the muscle itself is laterally retracted and preserved. These neck contents are peeled off from the IJV and from around the accessory nerve, sparing these structures.
2. *Lateral neck dissection*: removal of levels (II–IV)—for oropharyngeal, laryngeal, and hypopharyngeal tumours. The lymph nodes are removed from the skull base superiorly down to the clavicle, and from the cutaneous branches of the cervical plexus at the posterior border of the sternocleidomastoid muscle posteriorly to the sternothyroid muscle anteriorly.
3. *Posterolateral neck dissection*: removal of levels (II–V)—often used in patients with cutaneous malignancies, consists of an en bloc removal of the lymph nodes in the suboccipital, postauricular, and upper, middle, and lower jugular nodes, along with posterior triangle nodes situated superior to the accessory nerve.
4. *Anterior compartment neck dissection*: removal of nodal tissue from (level VI)—usually performed in thyroid

cancers, with dissection to the level of the hyoid bone superiorly, the suprasternal notch inferiorly, and the carotid sheaths on both sides.

Extended radical neck dissection

In certain patients with very advanced neck disease, other structures not routinely removed in a radical neck dissection may have to be removed to ensure oncological clearance. Such structures may include the prevertebral muscles, the hypoglossal nerve, and the carotid artery.

Radiotherapy

The use of primary radiotherapy in early stage neck disease can have comparable regional control rates to a selective neck dissection alone. Radiotherapy used postoperatively has been shown to confer improved locoregional control rates. Various histopathological factors can be used and include margins of resection, number of nodes involved, and extracapsular spread.

In selected patients, the use of chemoradiotherapy with surgery to salvage any residual neck disease has the benefit of offering the patient a chance of organ preservation, in terms of speech or swallow. This does however need to be offset against the technical difficulties and increased risks in operating in a field which has previously been irradiated. Elective irradiation utilizes a dose of 50Gy in 25 fractions over 5 weeks or its biological equivalent. Treatment can be delivered to levels III/IV using a single anterior field below the hyoid level, with midline shielding of larynx, pharynx, and spinal cord with a 2-cm wide strip, a so called anterior-split approach. Using IMRT this sparing of midline structures is enhanced through stipulating constraint doses to contoured volumes in the midline such as the larynx.

For macroscopic disease 70Gy (2Gy/fraction) is conventionally used; for postoperative extracapsular spread 60–66Gy with synchronous chemotherapy. Lymph node disease in the lower neck from a head and neck primary is unusual; definitive treatment of this area with radiotherapy requires a consideration of the proximity/tolerance of the brachial plexus.

Management of neck nodes in unknown primary

Neck nodes from an unknown primary account for 1–2 % of head and neck cancer cases where despite thorough clinical, endoscopic, and conventional radiological evaluation, no primary site will be detected. Functional techniques such as PET-FDG may be useful. Treatment of such patients remains controversial.

SCC in upper neck nodes usually arises secondary to a (presumed) head and neck primary, whilst nodes in the supraclavicular fossa tend to be associated with a primary malignancy below the clavicles. In the majority of patients with metastatic cervical lymphadenopathy, a careful assessment will identify the primary site of the cancer. The diagnostic work-up of such a patient includes a comprehensive history and thorough physical examination concentrating on areas most likely to harbour an occult primary such as the tonsil, base of tongue, piriform fossa, and postnasal space. The use of cross-sectional imaging including PET should be performed prior to any surgical interventional (following nodal FNAC).

Management is often a combination of surgery and/or radiotherapy; however, this is dependent on the centre. Most centres adopt a wait and watch policy following neck dissection for N1 disease with no extracapsular spread. However for the majority of cases, postoperative radiotherapy is advisable and this is given either as wide-field mucosal irradiation or to the ipsilateral neck only. There is no evidence that either of these strategies is superior to the other in terms of impact on overall survival. Wide-field irradiation includes the oropharynx, hypopharynx, larynx, and possibly nasopharynx as well as the neck and is associated with significant morbidity, particularly xerostomia, although the advent of parotid sparing IMRT has made the effects of wide-field irradiation less morbid. Additionally wide-field irradiation poses the difficulty of re-irradiation in the case of a subsequent primary emergence.

Further reading

Gregoire V, Levendag P, Ang KK, et al. CT based delineation of lymph node levels and related CTVs in the node negative neck. Radiother Oncol 2003; 69(3):227–36.

Primary brain tumours: introduction

Tumours of the CNS are characterized by a remarkable diversity of pathological type and behaviour. Although rare, they affect people of all ages and hence have a disproportionate influence on the number of years of life lost to cancer. With few exceptions there is a marked consistency of incidence worldwide. Some types of brain tumour are increasing in incidence and, after many years of therapeutic stagnation, there have recently been some important improvements in treatment and outcome. For both of these reasons the subdiscipline of neuro-oncology is of increasing relevance in cancer medicine.

Classification and grading of CNS tumours

Unlike tumours of many other body systems there is, in general, no satisfactory staging system for CNS tumours. The brain does not have a lymphatic system. Tumours rarely spread systemically and tumour size is a weak prognostic factor. Hence systems, such as TNM, that work well in other parts of the body are of little or no value for CNS tumours.

The outcome from treatment of CNS neoplasms is determined principally by the underlying pathology and, to some extent, the tumour site.:

* Management is determined far more by the tumour grading than by any staging system.
* The most widely accepted grading system is the WHO classification of tumours of the CNS, currently in its fourth edition (Louis 2007). In this system tumours are allocated a grade I–IV based on their pathology.
* Within this grading system it is becoming clear that molecular features can provide additional highly relevant prognostic information even within one tumour type and grade. For example, the presence or absence of loss of heterozygosity on chromosomes 1p and 19q can have a profound effect on outcome, particularly in oligodendroglioma.

Benign or malignant?

The terms 'benign' and 'malignant' may be confusing when applied to CNS tumours. Low grade glial tumours almost never metastasize and show little cellular pleomorphism or mitosis. They are frequently called 'benign'. Usually, however, even these low grade tumours infiltrate widely into brain parenchyma, which is a cardinal feature of malignancy. It is better that they are labelled by their WHO grade, which is a reliable guide to behaviour, rather than the terms benign or malignant.

Truly benign tumours do exist (meningioma, choroid plexus papilloma); however even these can also appear in intermediate (atypical) and truly malignant forms. Again the WHO grading system is most useful.

Finally there is a tendency for many 'low grade' brain tumours to transform to a more malignant phenotype over time as they acquire additional genetic damage. At this point in their evolution, mixtures of grade can appear in the same tumour specimen. They are labelled by the highest grade identified in the biopsy sample.

Incidence

* The overall incidence of primary CNS tumours in the UK and the USA is around 16 per 100,000 per year. Slightly less than half of these are primary malignant tumours (NICE 2006; Bondy et al. 2008).
* The incidence of malignant tumours is higher in more developed countries, (around 5 per 100,000) than is the global incidence (3 per 100,000). There are around 4000 new malignant brain tumours diagnosed per year in the UK.
* Men have a nearly 50% higher risk of CNS tumour than women, particularly of malignant tumours, whereas women have higher rates of non-malignant tumours, particularly meningiomas.
* Mortality rates for malignant tumours are only slightly less (by 20%) than incidence rates, indicating the high lethality of these tumours.
* There is evidence of an increasing incidence of the most malignant type of brain tumour (glioblastoma). Whilst this may be partly due to improved diagnostic capability there is a strong suggestion that the overall incidence is increasing (Lynch et al. 2006).
* Whilst brain tumours may occur at any age, the age-specific incidence shows a small peak in early childhood and a rapidly increasing rate in middle age, with a second major peak in the eighth decade.
* The tumour pathology spectrum varies with age. Low grade glial tumours and medulloblastomas are the most common tumours of childhood whilst the rapidly increasing incidence in middle-aged adults is largely due to malignant tumours particularly glioblastoma (Rampling et al. 2008).

Aetiology

The great majority of brain tumours are sporadic, and have no known cause. However, an important minority are associated with a variety of genetic syndromes and a few tumours have environmental or occupational links.

Genetic syndromes associated with brain tumour

* *Neurofibromatosis I* (autosomal dominant [AD] NF1 on 17q11)—neurofibromas, gliomas, sarcomas
* *Neurofibromatosis II* (AD NF2 on 22q12)—schwannomas (acoustic neuromas), meningiomas, gliomas
* *Von Hippel–Lindau syndrome* (AD VHL on 3p25–26)—haemangioblastoma
* *Cowden's syndrome* (AD PTEN/MMAC1 on 10q23)—dysplastic gangliocytoma of cerebellum
* *Turcot's syndrome* (AD 5q21)—glioblastomas, medulloblastomas
* *Tuberose sclerosis* (TSC1 on 9q34 TSC2 on16p13)—subependymal giant cell astrocytoma, hamartomas
* *Li–Fraumeni syndrome* (AD TP53 on 17p13)—gliomas, PNETs
* *Basal naevus syndrome* (AD PTCH on 9q22)—medulloblastomas (Rampling et al. 2008)

Other aetiological factors

* There is very strong evidence that ionizing radiation is a potent cause of brain tumour, particularly meningioma and gliomas with a relative risk of approximately 4.6 per Gy for benign meningiomas and 2 per Gy for malignant brain tumours (Bondy et al. 2008). The latent period is typically 10 years but may be as long as 30 years.
* In contradistinction, non-ionizing radiation, particularly exposures in the RF range including those used by cellular phones, have no proven association with brain tumours.

- There is an increased risk of glioma in higher social class.
- There is no established association between viral infection of any type and CNS tumours.
- Although certain compounds, particularly polycyclic aromatic hydrocarbons, can induce brain tumours in animal models no neurocarcinogens have been identified in humans, hence there is no proven link between brain tumours and occupational exposure of any kind (other than radiation).
- Primary CNS lymphoma is associated with immune suppression either naturally occurring (HIV) or iatrogenic (organ transplants).
- There is an association between breast cancer and meningioma.
- There is an inverse association between atopic disease and glioma.

Referral pathways

Most patients currently who present with symptoms suspicious of tumour will be referred for an early brain scan. The discovery of a tumour is then normally an indication for a secondary referral to a neuro-oncology MDT either directly or via a neurosurgical unit. The case should be discussed at the meeting (MDT) or tumour board. Comprehensive guidelines for the constitution and functioning of such a Board must be drawn up. An example is given by the NICE document *Improving Outcomes for People with Brain and other CNS tumours* (NICE 2006).

Key 'NICE' recommendations

- All patient care should be coordinated through a designated MDT.
- All patients should have face-to-face contact with healthcare professionals to discuss their care at critical points in their care pathway, and be provided with high quality written information to support this
- All patients should have a clearly defined key worker.
- Patients should have ready access to specialist care services as appropriate.

- Palliative care specialists should be core members of the neuroscience MDT.
- Cancer networks should ensure that clinical trials on brain tumours carried out by the National Cancer Research Institute (NCRI) are supported.

Where possible, patients with a new diagnosis of brain tumour should be evaluated in the preoperative setting so that a management plan can be formulated by the MDT prior to surgical intervention. Sometimes this will not be possible and surgical intervention needs to be undertaken urgently. In this case protocols agreed by the MDT should be available.

Core membership of the Brain Tumour MDT should comprise: Neurosurgeon(s), Neuroradiologist(s), Neuropathologist(s), Neurologist(s), Oncologist(s), Clinical nurse specialist(s), Palliative care physician(s), Neuropsychologist(s), Specialist AHP(s), Coordinator(s)

The patient care plan will frequently begin in the neurosurgical unit but may pass to oncology, neurology, palliative care, and other disciplines. At all times a 'key worker' should be allocated who, for the period of allocation, is the main management reference professional for the patient. This will often be the clinical nurse specialist

Further reading

Bondy M, Scheurer M, Malmer B, *et al.* Brain tumor epidemiology: consensus from the Brain Tumor Epidemiology Consortium. *Cancer* 2008; **113**(7 suppl):1953–68.

Louis DN, Ohgaki H, Wiestler OD, *et al. WHO Classification of Tumours of the Central Nervous System.* Lyon: International Agency for Research on Cancer, 2007.

Lynch D, Sibernaller Z, Ryken T. Trends in brian cancer incidence and survival in the United States: Surveillance, Epidemiology and End Results Program, 1973 to 2001. *Neurosurg Focus* 2006; **20**(4):E1.

NICE, B.o.C.G.D.G. *Improving Outcomes for People with Brain and other CNS tumours.* London: National Institute for Health and Clinical Excellence, 2006.

Rampling R. Central nervous system tumours. In: Price P, Sikora K, Illige T (eds) *Treatment of Cancer*, pp.287–319. London: Hodder Arnold, 2008.

Brain tumours: clinicopathology

Understanding CNS tumour pathology and grading is key to their management. There is virtually uniform international acceptance of the WHO classification system (Louis et al. 2007), shown in abbreviated form here.

Classification is based on the presumed tissue of origin.

Grading is based on the predicted biological and clinical behaviour of the tumour.
- Grade 1 tumours have low proliferative potential and afford the possibility of cure with surgery alone.
- Grade 2 lesions have low proliferative potential but are infiltrative and some tumours progress to higher grade lesions.
- Grade 3 implies cytological evidence of malignancy (nuclear atypia, mitotic activity). These lesions are rarely curable.
- Grade 4 lesions are histologically highly malignant, often incorporating necrosis and associated with rapid disease progression and often fatal outcome.

WHO Classification System 2007
Tumours of neuroepithelial tissue
Astrocytic tumours
- Grade 1: pilocytic astrocytoma, subependymal giant cell astrocytoma, pleomorphic xanthoastrocytoma
- Grade 2: diffuse astrocytoma (variants: fibrillary, protoplasmic, gemistocytic, mixed)
- Grade 3: anaplastic (malignant) astrocytoma
- Grade 4: glioblastoma (variants: giant cell, gliosarcoma)
- (various grades) gliomatosis cerebri

Oligodendroglial tumours
- Grade 2: oligodendroglioma
- Grade 3: anaplastic oligodendroglioma

Oligoastrocytic tumours
- Grade 2: oligoastrocytoma
- Grade 3: anaplastic oligoastrocytoma

Ependymal tumours
- Grade 1: subependymoma, myxopapillary ependymoma
- Grade 2 (cellular): ependymoma
- Grade 3: anaplastic ependymoma

Choroid plexus tumours
- Grade 1: choroid plexus papilloma
- Grade 2: atypical choroid plexus papilloma
- Grade 3: choroid plexus carcinoma

Neuronal and mixed neuronal-glial tumours
- Grade 1: gangliocytoma, ganglioglioma, dysembryoplastic neuroepithelial tumour (of childhood)
- Grade 2: central neurocytoma
- Grade 3: anaplastic ganglioglioma

Pineal tumours
- Grade 1: pineocytoma
- Grade 4: pineoblastoma

Embryonal tumours
Grade 4: medulloblastoma. atypical teratoid/rhabdoid tumour, primitive neuroectodermal tumours (PNET including neuroblastoma)

Tumours of cranial and paraspinal nerves
- Grade 1: schwannoma (neurilemmoma, neurinoma), neurofibroma
- Grade 2, 3, or 4: malignant peripheral nerve sheath tumour

Tumours of the meninges
Meningiomas
- Grade 1: meningioma (and variants)
- Grade 2: atypical meningioma
- Grade 3: anaplastic (malignant) meningioma

Mesenchymal (non-meningothelial) tumours
- Grade 1: haemangioblastoma, solitary fibrous tumour
- Grade 2: haemangiopericytoma
- Grade 3: anaplastic haemangiopericytoma

Haematopoietic neoplasms (not graded)
- Primary malignant lymphomas (PCNSL)

Germ cell tumours
- Germinoma
- Teratoma (Immature, mature)
- Choriocarcinoma
- Mixed

Tumours of the sellar region
- Craniopharyngioma, pituicytoma

Metastatic tumours

Clinical pathological behaviour
In children and young adults there is a marked tendency for tumours to arise in the infratentorial compartment (pilocytic astrocytoma, medulloblastoma) whilst in adults the great majority arise supratentorially.

WHO grade I tumours
- Grow by expansion. Infiltration into brain parenchymal tissue is an unusual feature.
- In general, therefore, grade I tumours are surgically curable.
- Some grade I tumours (e.g. craniopharyngioma) grow into invaginations and tend to recur even after apparent surgical excision. This, however, does not represent true invasion.

WHO grade II gliomas
- These (and all higher grades) demonstrate infiltration as a major feature. Tumour cells tend to migrate along white matter tracks from early in their growth and widespread dissemination is common.
- Migrating tumour cells are clonogenic. Hence surgical cure of these tumours is rare.
- Cerebrospinal fluid (CSF) dissemination of glial tumours is unusual and spread beyond the CNS is very rare. When systemic dissemination occurs, sites of predilection are lung and bone.
- A cardinal feature of gliomas is their transformation from lower grade to higher grade through the acquisition of increasing numbers of genetic mutations.

WHO grades 3 and 4 glioma
- Demonstrate rapid expansive and infiltrative growth.

- Are never curable but relapse locally even after aggressive treatment.
- Glioblastomas are highly angiogenic tumours and enhance avidly on scan.
- Glioblastomas are characterized by the formation of regions of necrosis.
- Oligodendrogliomas and some 'mixed tumours' have considerably better prognosis.

Central neurocytoma
- Is an intraventricular tumour predominantly of young adults.
- Is slow growing and may reach a large size before presentation, often with CSF obstruction.

Gliomatosis cerebri
- Is defined as a diffuse glial tumour involving two or more lobes, often bilaterally.
- Is usually low grade but may transform to higher grade.
- Is easily confused with other diffuse pathological brain processes and diagnosis may be difficult.

Medulloblastomas
- Are highly malignant tumours that arise in the posterior fossa of children and young adults.
- Metastasize readily throughout the CNS and treatments directed towards the whole neuraxis are appropriate.
- May metastasize outside the CNS particularly if ventricular peritoneal shunts are used to decompress hydrocephalus.

Mesenchymal tumours
- Meningiomas are slow growing benign tumours that arise at any site bearing a meningeal surface.
- High grade (atypical and malignant) forms occur but are rare.
- Haemangioblastoma, solitary fibrous tumours and haemangiopericytoma are slow growing tumours that can sometimes be associated with troublesome recurrence and occasional metastasis.

Primary CNS lymphomas
- The great majority of PCNSL is high grade diffuse B cell lymphoma. T cell lymphoma can occur but is rare.
- They are often multifocal and periventricular and may disseminate through the CSF.
- PCNSL that is not related to immunosuppression has maximal incidence in late middle age. HIV (and other immune suppressed) related PCNSL is more common in younger patients.

Germ cell tumours
- Arise predominantly in the pineal region but also in suprasellar and other midline sites.
- May secrete markers (β-hCG, AFP). Measurement of tumour markers in the blood and CSF may be of use in diagnosis and monitoring disease response.

- Germ cell tumours may disseminate through the CSF.

Molecular biology of brain tumours
Astrocytoma
Low grade astrocytoma
Commonly show loss of heterozygosity on chromosome 17p that is associated with mutations of p53. PDGFR (platelet-derived growth factor receptor) amplification commonly occurs.

Anaplastic astrocytoma
Show p53 mutations and loss of heterozygosity on chromosome 17p with a similar frequency to low grade astrocytomas. Loss of heterozygosity on 10q is also reported and PTEN mutations are also quite frequent.

Glioblastoma
Glioblastomas are recognized to arise in two distinct patterns (The Cancer Genome Atlas Research Network 2008).
- Primary glioblastoma occurs in older patients with no prior history of tumour. They are characterized by loss of heterozygosity on chromosome 10q, EGFR (epithelial growth factor receptor) amplification and PTEN mutations.
- Secondary glioblastoma appears to arise from a pre-existing low grade tumour and, as well as carrying loss of heterogeneity (LOH) of chromosome 10q, there are persisting p53 mutations. On the other hand EGFR and PTEN mutations are much less common.
- In both tumour types the methyl guanine-DNA methyl transferase (MGMT) gene has a promoter methylation in approximately 40% of patients. This has prognostic significance.

Oligodendrogliomas
Oligodendrogliomas exhibit loss of heterozygosity on chromosomes 1p and 19q in up to 80% of patients. This is highly significant with respect to prognosis (Cairncross et al. 1998).

Medulloblastoma
The commonest abnormality occurs on chromosome 17q; the significance of this is not clear.

Meningioma
Deletions on chromosome 22 are common and mutations in the NF2 (neurofibromatosis 2) gene are detected in the majority of NF2 associated tumours and in 60% of sporadic meningiomas.

Further reading
Cairncross JG, Ueki K, Zlatescu M, et al. 1998. Specific genetic predictors of chemotherapeutic response and survival in patients with anaplastic oligodendrogliomas. *J Natl Cancer Inst* **90**:1473–9.

Louis D, Ohgaki H, Wiestler O, et al. *WHO Classification of Tumours of the Central Nervous System.* Lyon: International Agency for Research on Cancer, 2007.

The Cancer Genome Atlas Research Network. Comprehensive genomic characterization defines human glioblastoma genes and core pathways. *Nature* 2008; **455**(23):1061–8.

Brain tumours: presentation and general management

Presentation

Brain tumours affect the entire age spectrum. They occur in any part of the brain. Symptoms are caused by excitation, infiltration, or compression of normal CNS tissues. Hence, brain tumours present in a bewildering variety of ways although certain recognizable patterns emerge.

Headache

- Is the most common symptom recorded in patients with brain tumours, though it is the main presenting symptom in far fewer.
- Brain tumours are a rare cause of headache in the general population.
- Various schemes are available to facilitate the referral of a patient with headache and a possible brain tumour (Scottish-Executive 2002). In particular these look for evidence of raised intracranial pressure, an association with neurological deficit, or personality change in addition to headache.

Seizures

- Occur in approximately half of patients with brain tumours over the duration of their disease.
- Seizure is the most common presenting symptom in low grade glial tumours. Typically these begin as focal seizures but may become generalized.
- Tumour should be considered in all adults newly presenting with seizure that has no other obvious explanation.
- Tumour is more likely in patients with:
  1. Focal seizures
  2. Significant postictal focal deficit (excluding confusion)
  3. Epilepsy presenting as status epilepticus
  4. Associated interictal focal deficit
  5. Associated preceding persistent headache of recent onset
  6. Seizure frequency accelerating over weeks or months

Progressive neurological deficit

- Suspicion of tumour should be high in a patient presenting with progressive neurological deficit (e.g. progressive weakness, sensory loss, dysphasia, ataxia) developing over days to weeks.
- Some symptoms may be grouped into specific neurological syndromes associated with tumours in particular regions of the brain. Obvious examples are motor or speech dysfunction due to parietal tumours. Less obvious are complex syndromes such as Parinaud's (abnormalities of eye movement and pupil dysfunction) occurring in patients with pineal tumours.

Personality or cognitive change

- Patients frequently present with subtle changes in personality or cognition or a deterioration of performance. A high index of suspicion must be maintained in a person presenting with such features especially if associated with headache.
- Tumours in the elderly may be missed or put down to vascular disturbance. Again progressive neurological deterioration in an older person may be an indication for evaluation through imaging.

General medical management

Steroids

The use of steroids is ubiquitous in the care of patients with brain tumours. Their value in reducing intracranial pressure and reversing symptoms is undoubted. However, the side-effect profile is severe and many patients are probably left overtreated for long periods.

- Introduce steroid at the maximum dose likely to be useful in a situation and then rapidly titrate the dose downward against the patient's symptoms. The optimal dose is just above that at which deterioration occurs.
- Patients should always be assessed for response. If symptoms do not improve, the steroid should be stopped.
- The most commonly used steroid is dexamethasone in doses between 2mg and 16mg daily. The plasma half-life is long and at low doses dexamethasone can be given once daily. At higher doses it is best divided into 2–4 equally spaced doses.
- Betamethasone can be substituted for dexamethasone as a mg for mg (x1) replacement. Prednisolone (x7.5) and hydrocortisone (x30) can also be used but are less satisfactory due to their even greater glucocorticoid side effects.
- It is standard to cover brain surgery with steroid but protocols should be in place to reduce or eliminate the drug as quickly as safely possible after the operation. Even if steroids need to be re-introduced later, say during radiotherapy, a short period off the drugs can be beneficial.
- It is tempting to treat seizures with steroid but this should be resisted except as a very short-term expedient. It should quickly be replaced by modification of the anticonvulsant programme.
- It is normal practice to combine these steroid doses with an antacid (ranitidine 150mg bd or omeprazole 20mg daily). The evidence for the effectiveness of this in protecting against the GI complications of steroid use is lacking.

Antiepileptic drugs (AEDs)

- Over half of all patients diagnosed with malignant brain tumours will suffer a seizure at some time.
- Almost any patient with a brain tumour who suffers a seizure should be treated with an AED. However, prophylactic use of AED before a seizure has occurred is not recommended.
- Epilepsy in patients with brain tumours can be difficult to control. All such patients should be managed by a specialist in this area.
- Some brain tumour treatments such as chemotherapy and antidepressants impair the effectiveness of AEDs.
- First-line AEDs are successful in suppressing seizure in less than half of patients. Of those that fail less than half of these will be controlled with either second-line monotherapy treatments or polypharmacy.
- Many AEDs modify the cytochrome p450 enzyme system of the liver which is responsible for the metabolism of many other drugs including some antcancer agents (Vecht and van Breemen 2006). Many of the classic AEDs, (e.g. phenobarbitone, phenytoin, and carbamazepine) are enzyme-inducing AED drugs (EIAEDs), as are, to a lesser extent, lamotrigine and topiramate.
- Non-(or weak) enzyme-inducing drugs are preferred for patients with brain tumours in whom treatment with chemotherapy or some biological therapies is considered. It has been shown that substantially larger doses of some agents (e.g. irinotecan, erlotinib®) are required for the same effect when EIAEDs are being used (Vecht and van Breemen 2006).

- No EIAED is ideal. Lamotrigine (a weak inducer) has good activity but must be introduced slowly. Keppra® (levetiracetam) can be introduced rapidly at therapeutic dose but can produce unwanted mood disturbance in some patients. Valproate is an older but still excellent drug for all types of seizures (particularly if generalized). It may act to alter drug metabolism by suppressing liver activity.
- Of the older enzyme-inducing drugs, both phenytoin and carbamazepine have excellent antiseizure activity and are frequently used perioperatively. However, their side-effect profiles as well as their effects on liver make them less suitable for patients with brain tumours.

Anticoagulants

The incidence of thromboembolic disease in patients with a brain tumour is dramatic with a 45% reported incidence of deep vein thrombosis (DVT). The prevalence of pulmonary embolus (PE) at autopsy is 8.4%. This is due to coagulins released by the tumour itself, and loss of mobility in the patients (Hamilton et al. 1994). There is always anxiety with respect to anticoagulation because of the risk of intratumoural bleed.

- For patients with no prior history of tumour bleed, the balance of risk is in favour of anticoagulation.
- Low-molecular-weight heparins can be used in standard doses. Alternatively warfarin can be used in which case it may be prudent to manage the patient slightly less aggressively with an international normalized ratio (INR) 20% lower than for non-tumour cases.
- For patients with a prior history of bleeding or who are in generally poor health, simple measures such as antithrombotic stockings and analgesia may be more appropriate.

Analgesics

Pain is a relatively minor problem (numerically) in the brain tumour population. However, raised intracranial pressure and meningeal and blood vessel involvement can be a potent source of pain in a minority of cases. Appropriate analgesics should not be withheld from these patients.

- Use of the conventional WHO cancer analgesic 'ladder' is recommended for pain in patients with brain tumour.
- Paracetamol, (dihydrocodeine, and morphine and its newer analogues all have their place.
- Non-steroidal anti-inflammatory drugs (NSAIDs) and anticonvulsants (gabapentin) have a lesser role but can be used if there is an inflammatory or neuropathic component respectively.
- The value of steroids for relieving pain from raised pressure should not be forgotten.

Antidepressants

True clinical depression is common in patients with brain tumours. Once recognized, treatment with antidepressants and psychotherapy should be considered (Arnold et al. 2008).

- There is a concern that some antidepressants, particularly tricyclic compounds, might exacerbate seizure. Whilst this is also true to a lesser extent for selective serotonin antagonists (SSIs), these drugs are probably safe if seizures are absent or well controlled. SSIs probably represent the drugs of choice in such patients.
- There is a high incidence of stress and anxiety in this patient group which does not reach the level of true depression. The value of psychological and counselling

support should not be underestimated in this and the depressed population.

Other agents

- *Osmotic diuretics* (mannitol) have little place in the management of patients with brain tumour. They can be used in the acute situation to relieve pressure before the introduction of a more definitive management strategy. However more than one or two infusions can have detrimental systemic side effects.
- *Ulcer healing drugs* such as H2 antagonists (ranitidine) or proton pump inhibitors (omeprazole) can be used either to prevent or treat dyspeptic symptoms associated with steroid use. Their value as prophylaxis is not proven but conventionally they are used in the majority of patients.

Prognostic factors in brain tumours

The outcome for patients with brain tumours depends on a variety of prognostic factors.

Detailed pathology

The importance of a precise pathological diagnosis has already been emphasized (see p.84). Patients with grade II astrocytomas live on average three times as long as patients with grade III tumours. Grade for grade oligodendroglial tumours are associated with at least 50% better survival than that achieved for patients with astrocytic tumours.

Age

In adults there is a direct correlation between increasing age and poorer outcome for almost all brain tumours but particularly for those derived from the neuroepithelium.

Performance status

As with age, PS is a strong determinant of survival in patients with brain tumours. The PS should be estimated according to a suitable scale (Karnofsky, WHO) as a guide to treatment, before and after optimal general medical treatments have been given (including steroids)

Surgery

There is no satisfactory comparative study that has examined the impact of the extent of surgical excision on survival in any primary brain tumour (see p.89). However, there is extensive observational evidence that patients who have less residual disease after surgery have a better prognosis.

It is possible to combine the discussed features into a prognostic index which can be valuable in determining the management of patients (Scott et al. 1998).

Molecular factors are being discovered that correlate well with outcome in certain tumour types (see p.97).

Further reading

Arnold, S., Forman, L. Brigidi, B. *et al*. Evaluation and characterization of generalized anxiety and depression in patients with primary brain tumors. *Neuro-Oncology* 2008; **10**(2):171–81.

Hamilton M, Hull R, Pineo G. Venous thromboembolism in neurosurgery and neurology patients: a review. *Neurosurgery* 1994; **34**(2):280–96.

Scott C, Scarantino C, Urtasun R, *et al*. Validation and predictive power of Radiation Therapy Oncology Group (RTOG) recursive partitioning analysis classes for malignant glioma patients: a report using RTOG 90–06. *Int J Radiat Oncol Biol Phys* 1998; **40**(1):51–5.

Scottish-Executive. Scottish Referral Guidelines for suspected Cancer. Edinburgh: Scottish Office, 2002.

Vecht C, van Breemen M. Optimizing therapy of seizures in patients with brain tumors. *Neurology* 2006; **67**(Suppl 4):S10–S13.

Brain tumours: surgical management

Surgery has three major roles in brain tumour management:

- *Diagnosis*: a pathological diagnosis is required in virtually all patients in whom subsequent antitumour treatment is contemplated. The brain stem is the only site where risk of harm may still prevent biopsy.
- *Symptom control*: relief of pressure symptoms is the most common aim; however, sometimes surgery may be performed for seizure or other symptom.
- *Cure*: surgery is capable of curing most grade 1 tumours and may contribute to prolongation of survival in others.

Preparation for surgery

- Where possible, the patient should be operated electively after stabilization of any general medical problems. Drugs affecting coagulation (e.g. NSAIDs) should be eliminated prior to surgery.
- Steroids are routinely used to improve tolerance to the operative procedure. Daily dexamethasone doses around 16mg are used. This should be phased out as soon as possible after the operation and protocols for doing this should be in place and communicated to the next principal carer.
- Anticonvulsants need not be given routinely to patients undergoing surgery for brain tumour. However, they should be used in selected patients considered to be at risk of seizure (e.g. low grade and cortical location). If seizures were not present preoperatively, anticonvulsants can be phased out in the postoperative period. For patients already on anticonvulsants, the dose should be optimized to maximize the chance of control in the perioperative period.

Surgical technique

Biopsy

- *Closed biopsy* is now nearly always done using image guided (stereotactic) localization.
- Fusion of functional images with structural MRI or CT improves localization to the part of the tumour most likely to yield a diagnosis.
- Multiple biopsies taken along a single tract or multiple tracts can be used to maximize diagnostic accuracy.
- Intraoperative diagnosis (frozen section, smear) is essential to ensure adequate tissue has been sampled and to guide subsequent procedures.
- Diagnostic rates of >90% with <6% complications and <2% mortality should be achievable (Krieger et al. 1997).
- *Open biopsy* under direct vision may be needed for some lesions where there is surgical risk (bleeding, pressure) or where large quantities of tissue are needed.
- In many units snap frozen tissue is collected and stored to enhance the range of diagnostic tests available.

Surgical resection

General principles

- Access is gained by craniotomy. A scalp incision is made and a flap of skin and pericranial tissue turned. The siting of the craniotomy will depend on the position of the tumour.
- Usually a free bone flap is created first by making burrholes, freeing the dura and then cutting the flap using a high-speed craniotome. The dura is opened only by an amount that will give adequate exposure of the tumour-bearing brain. The operating microscope is routinely used to give good visualization.
- Minimal retraction of the brain is performed to permit access to the tumour.
- It is common practice to confirm the diagnosis with an intraoperative frozen section or cytological smear, prior to performing the full resection. The resection itself is typically performed by internal decompression using a mixture of bipolar coagulation, sharp dissection, cautery, ultrasonic aspiration and, if appropriate, laser vaporization. The aim is always to remove as much of the tumour as is safely possible.
- The operation is completed with dural closure, replacement of the bone flap and skin closure.
- The devitalized free bone flap is a potential site for infection that will be resistant to antibiotics. Infection in the flap following surgery will necessitate its removal.

Image-guided stereotactic resection

Obtaining three-dimensional image data and referencing it to a stereotactic frame allows the surgeon to plan an operative approach to minimize injury to neighbouring critical structures. This technique is particularly valuable in technically challenging locations, e.g. perithalamic.

Neuronavigation

- Normal brain anatomy is often distorted by the presence of tumour and its associated oedema making it difficult for the surgeon to resect according to conventional landmarks.
- Neuronavigation systems allow the registration of stored imaging data with 'real time' physical space. There is interaction with a localization device so that the surgeon can use the recent imaging information to guide the resection. Registration is done by either using natural landmarks or external fiducial markers. The system may be 'frame based' or more usually is 'frameless' which gives the surgeon much more freedom of access.
- A problem for the surgeon is the shift of structures during the operation which makes stored images obsolete. This can be addressed by incorporating real time, intraoperative imaging into the neuronavigation system.
- Real time intraoperative imaging may be based on ultrasound or more powerfully on MRI.
- Intraoperative MRI may be achieved either by moving the patient into the magnet during the surgical procedure or more conveniently by bringing the MR scanner into the operating suite. This introduces many complexities. The operating room must be shielded against the strong magnetic fields and all equipment in the operating room must be non-magnetizable.
- The particular advantage of intraoperative MRI is likely to be in the resection of low grade tumours where differentiation from normal brain is otherwise difficult.
- Intraoperative MRI is still only available in relatively few centres.

Cortical mapping 'awake craniotomy'
- Resection of tumours inside or adjacent to functional brain areas may not be safe even if the surgeon remains within obvious tumour boundaries.
- Intraoperative stimulation of cortical and subcortical sites and related tracts allows active areas to be identified and marked. This functional information facilitates avoidance of these areas during resection and allows the surgeon to perform a safer and more extensive tumour removal.
- In 'awake craniotomy' the initial craniotomy and preliminary stimulation is performed with the patient asleep. After arousal, sedative/hypnotic anaesthesia allows the patient to respond to motor and language commands but still provides subsequent amnesia.
- Core temperature and oxygen saturation must be carefully maintained and meningeal anaesthesia provided.
- Seizure is a risk during stimulation.

Fluorescence guided surgery
- 5-aminolevulinic acid (ALA) is the lead compound in fluorescence directed surgery. It is a prodrug that leads to intracellular accumulation of fluorescent porphyrins in malignant gliomas (Stummer et al. 2006). It is given preoperatively by mouth.
- The surgeon operates using violet–blue excitation light and appropriate light filters to identify the tumour bearing fluorescent regions against the dark, normal tissue, background.
- In a study comparing this technique with conventional microsurgery, it was shown that rates of complete resection, and progression free survival were both significantly improved using the fluorescence system. There was no increase in morbidity (Stummer et al. 2006). Whether this technique is adopted as standard remains to be seen.

Surgery and individual tumours
The scope and role of surgery varies according to tumour type

WHO grade 1 tumours
Surgery alone is frequently curative and maximal safe removal should be attempted. However, even if this is incomplete, tumours may fail to progress subsequently and the patients remain well without further intervention. In those where regrowth does occur, second surgery is usually indicated, possibly followed by non-surgical treatment.

WHO grade 2 gliomas
- The role of surgery is unclear.
- If the lesion is amenable to complete (or near complete) macroscopic excision then this group of patients can do well in the longer term without other intervention (Duffau et al. 2005).
- The value of resection when only a small proportion can be removed is unproven. In these cases, a biopsy followed by surveillance or non surgical anti tumour treatment may be more appropriate.
- If the patient has relevant symptoms, (pressure, seizure), and the appropriate region of tumour can be safely removed then surgery directed at improving the patient's condition should always be considered.

- Low grade ependymomas, although technically grade 2, should always be considered for resection, which if 'complete' may give long-term control.

WHO grade 3 and 4 gliomas
- There is no satisfactory randomized study that demonstrates a survival advantage for surgical resection as opposed to biopsy alone.
- There are numerous studies that show an association between extent of surgical resection and longevity (Proescholdt et al. 2005) and time to progression (Stummer et al. 2006) and it is a matter of common experience that patients undergoing resection have lower steroid requirement and tolerate radiotherapy better than those undergoing biopsy only.
- It is recommended that patients with high grade glioma undergo maximal safe resection prior to subsequent non-surgical therapy.
- Patients should not be put at unreasonable risk to achieve resection however. Where necessary, safety enhancing techniques such as ALA assisted resection and functional imaging can be considered to improve outcome.
- The brain stem is a surgically challenging region where even biopsy can be associated with high levels of morbidity and mortality. Whilst some exophytic tumours can be biopsied, most cannot and a clinicoradiological diagnosis must suffice.

Medulloblastoma
- There is an association between extent of resection and outcome in medulloblastoma. Maximal safe surgical resection should be attempted for all localized disease.
- The patient is often operated lying prone to avoid air embolus and subdural haematoma. A ventriculostomy is often performed to assist in postoperative management.

Lymphoma
There is no evidence that surgery improves outcome in PCNSL. Biopsy sufficient to allow complete pathological typing is all that is required.

Germ cell tumours
These typically arise in the pineal region—a site where biopsy can be problematic due to access problems and tumour vascularity. Biopsy is necessary however except in those cases where tumour marker positivity and imaging make a diagnosis unequivocal even without tissue. Surgical resection may be necessary when troublesome masses remain after non surgical treatment.

Intraoperative, non-resective approaches
Local chemotherapy
- Gliadel is the lead product. It comprises BCNU impregnated biodegradable polymer wafers. Up to eight are used to line the cavity following surgical excision. BCNU then diffuses into the adjacent tumour bearing tissue.
- Randomized studies have shown a modest improvement in median survival (approximately 8 weeks) in both newly diagnosed and recurrent high grade gliomas (Westphal et al. 2003).
- Disadvantages are that it is only applicable to tumours where a complete resection can be achieved and which do not communicate with the ventricles.

- Treatment is associated with increased postoperative complications such as seizures, brain oedema, problems with wound healing, and intracranial infection.
- Other chemotherapeutic approaches using free intracavitary drugs have not been useful.

Convection enhanced delivery

Using fine interstitial catheters connected to a constant intermediate pressure pump, it is possible to convect large molecules and even viruses through tumours and along white matter tracts following migrating tumour cells. Whilst this technique has been the subject of randomized trials using toxins and antibodies, it has yet to find a place in routine management.

Local radiotherapy

Various systems are commercially available for irradiating the surgical bed following tumour removal. These may use externally generated X-rays distributed through the surface of a sphere, or a system based on a radioactive solution confined within a balloon (Glia Site).

Further reading

Duffau H. Lessons from brain mapping in surgery for low-grade glioma: insights into associations between tumour and brain plasticity. *Lancet Neurol* 2005; **4**:476–86.

Krieger M, Chandrasoma P, Zee C-S, *et al.* Role of stereotactic biopsy in the diagnosis and management of brain tumors. *Semin Surg Oncol* 1997; **14**(1):13–25.

Proescholdt M, Macher C, Woertgen C, *et al.* Level of evidence in the literature concerning brain tumor resection *Clin Neurol Neurosurg* 2005; **107**:95–8.

Stummer W, Pichlmeier U, Meinel T, *et al.* Fluorescence-guided surgery with 5-aminolevulinic acid for resection of malignant glioma: a randomised controlled multicentre phase III trial. *Lancet Oncol* 2006; **7**(5):392–401.

Westphal M, Hilt DC, Bortey E, *et al.* A phase 3 trial of local chemotherapy with biodegradable carmustine (BCNU) wafers (Gliadel wafers) in patients with primary malignant glioma. *Neuro Oncol* 2003; **5**(2):79–88.

Brain tumours: radiotherapy

Radiotherapy is the major life-prolonging treatment for patients with brain tumours. In recent years it has been refined to a high level of sophistication.

Indications for radiotherapy

Grade 1 tumours Radiotherapy has a limited role in these lesions. Although routinely used in a few tumours (craniopharyngioma), it is usually confined to the setting of recurrent disease that defies complete surgical resection (e.g. pilocytic astrocytoma, meningioma).

Grade 2 tumours Radiotherapy can undoubtedly produce tumour shrinkage and symptomatic improvement in diffuse gliomas. However, its role in prolonging life is unproven and delayed radiotherapy seems as effective as immediate treatment (Karim et al. 2002). Observation for some small, slow growing asymptomatic tumours is acceptable though surveillance in a specialist clinic is required so that timing of intervention can be optimized.

Grade 3 and 4 tumours All patients with high grade tumours should be considered for radiation after surgery. Younger, fitter patients will receive radical treatments, older patients may receive short course palliative regimens, and those with very poor performance status may receive supportive care only. Virtually all patients with PNETs will receive craniospinal irradiation.

Radiotherapy process

Immobilization

- Since modern brain irradiation requires highly accurate localization, firm immobilization is required.
- Solid beam direction shells have largely been replaced by masks made of perforated, lightweight materials such as 'Orfit' that can be created in a single visit.
- Shells may be cast in either the supine or prone position to facilitate beam placement for anterior or posterior tumours respectively. Lateral casts give poor fixation and are not recommended.

Imaging

- Radiotherapy planning for brain tumour is based on the CT planning scan.
- This is acquired with the patient immobilized in the treatment position.
- Intravenous contrast should be given where this is likely to enhance tumour delineation.
- Cross-sectional images at 2.5mm spacing (approx) should be acquired from vertex to second cervical spine
- Other images should be available for the planning process. These might include preoperative images (CT, MRI) or postoperative images acquired specifically for the planning process.

Volume delineation

Many brain tumours are highly infiltrative so that very large volumes are at risk of harbouring microscopic disease. Further, many brain tumours are incurable even with doses at tolerance limits to normal brain. For these reasons the concept of GTV/CTV/PTV needs to be modified for brain tumour radiotherapy (see p.43).

- PTV should be drawn on every slice of the planning scan to create the three-dimensional planning target.

- Sensitive organs should also be drawn (eyes, brain stem, chiasm, etc.) to facilitate the limiting of dose to these structures in subsequent planning.
- Bone and meninges form natural barriers against the progress of tumour cells and reduced margins can be used at these borders (say, 5–7mm beyond the GTV).

Radiotherapy planning

- Treatments are planned for a 4–8MV linear accelerator.
- Most treatment plans will require three (or more) fields though wedged, paired fields can be used for small, peripheral tumours.
- A typical arrangement will comprise two wedged lateral fields and an unopposed plain antero/superior field.
- Rarely a parallel pair will be needed for large tumours.
- All fields should be conformed to the PTV.
- Dose uniformity should be maintained according to ICRU reports 50 and 62 (ICRU 1999)
- Replanning may be necessary part way through to keep sensitive structures within tolerance.
- Digital reconstructed radiographs (DRRs) should be produced to allow field checks.
- Dose volume histograms (DVH) of target and sensitive structures should be calculated to facilitate plan assessment.
- The field arrangement is either checked on a simulator or preverified on the treatment machine.

Dose prescription

- The dose is prescribed to the isocentre.
- The normal daily dose (for radical treatments) is 2Gy per fraction for high grade tumours and 1.8Gy or less for low grade (or benign) lesions
- An exception is whole neuraxis treatment where radiation delivery is always delivered at <2Gy per fraction.

Timing of radiotherapy

- For high grade tumours, delays in starting radiotherapy are associated with reduced survival.
- For patients undergoing biopsy only, radiotherapy should begin as soon as possible.
- Following craniotomy there is a need to allow wound healing and restoration of physiognomy. Planning here optimally begins at 10–14 days and radiotherapy a week later.
- For low grade tumours, timing is less critical and longer delays to allow complete healing and to accommodate patient preference are possible.

Radiotherapy delivery and patient assessment

- Patients are normally treated once daily, 5 days per week.
- Admission to hospital is generally not required.
- Steroid cover may be needed if the tumour has not been resected or large volumes are treated. Doses of dexamethasone vary from 2mg in low-risk situations to 16mg where raised pressure already exists. Attempts should be made to reduce the steroid dose during the course of treatment.
- Patients should be seen at least weekly to monitor treatment, assess symptoms, and modify medication.

Palliative treatments

- Simple planning is possible for patients requiring a purely palliative approach.
- An immobilization mask is still required.
- Rectangular radiation fields are 'screened on' either using a conventional simulator or using a CT simulator. Simple shielding can be added as necessary.
- Opposed beam arrangements are used.

Stereotaxy

Stereotactic radiotherapy localizes intracranial structures to an external reference frame for enhanced accuracy.

- For stereotactic treatments immobilization is enhanced by the use of an invasively attached frame (for stereotactic radiosurgery, SRS) or a re-locatable frame, frequently based on a mouth bite.
- The CT planning scan is done at 1-mm slice spacing
- Fusion with other imaging modalities (MRI, angiography) is the rule.
- Delivery is by means of a modified linear accelerator using non-coplanar dynamic arcs, or multiple fixed conformal beams or alternatively by a multicobalt source 'gamma knife'.
- Stereotactic radiotherapy (SRT) is multifraction stereo tactically guided radiotherapy and is performed almost exclusively on a linear accelerator.
- Stereotactic radiosurgery (SRS) is single fraction high dose treatment and can be performed on either system.

Individual tumour types

- For low grade gliomas the GTV is the high signal region on T2 or FLAIR MR images. The PTV is created by 'growing' the GTV by 1–2cm. Doses in the range 45–54Gy are prescribed in 1.8-Gy fractions.
- For high grade gliomas, the GTV is taken as the enhancing tumour margin and/or resection bed. The PTV is created by growing the GTV by 2–3cm. (This may be reduced in the vicinity of sensitive structures or natural barriers). The prescribed dose is 60Gy in 30 fractions. Alternatively a two-phase technique can be used, covering the entire oedematous area in phase 1 with a phase 2 boost to 2cm around the GTV. However, this has not been shown to be superior to the single-phase treatment and may be more toxic.

  A palliative treatment for high grade glioma comprises a screened pair of opposed fields to cover the tumour bed plus 2–3cm, prescribed to a dose of 30Gy in 6 fractions over 2 weeks (or similar).

  A regimen of particular use in the elderly population comprises a three-dimensional planned volume treated to 40Gy in 15 fractions. This has compared favourably to standard radiotherapy in this population with GBM.
- Planning in medulloblastomas may be performed according to anatomical landmarks rather than visualized tumour. Phase 1 (craniospinal) requires careful inclusion of the entire meningeal surface. The primary site boost usually comprises the posterior fossa and brain stem.
- Meningiomas rarely invade brain parenchyma so the margin at the brain interface can be small (1–2cm). They may, however, spread along the meninges and these margins should be more generous.
- The PTV for pituitary (and some other benign) tumours is often the GTV plus 5–10mm if conventionally planned

since spread beyond the enhancing margin is infrequent. If stereotactic localization is used then margins can be reduced still further (1–3mm).

- Radiotherapy for PCNSL is given as a salvage treatment or as consolidation after chemotherapy in younger patients. It is generally given to the whole brain to a dose of 35–40Gy.

Normal tissue reactions to radiotherapy

Sparing normal tissue

- Radiation will damage normal tissue in a dose dependant fashion.
- The concept of 'radiation tolerance' concerns the acceptable level of radiation damage to a tissue in a particular clinical circumstance. Thus a higher tolerance dose is acceptable when treating a high risk, highly malignant tumour than a lower risk tumour with a good prospect of survival.

Radiation tolerance limits in different risk situations

- Optic chiasm: 45Gy (low risk) to 55Gy (high risk).
- Brainstem 40–45Gy (low risk, e.g. meningioma) to 55Gy for high risk (e.g. medulloblastoma).
- Retina: 55Gy.
- Lens: 7–10Gy.
- In general the CNS is a 'late responding tissue' although both early and intermediate effects can also occur.
- Radiation injury in the CNS depends on treatment parameters (total dose, dose per fraction, volume irradiated) and patient related factors (age, vasculopathy, infection).

Acute effects

- Symptoms are generally those of acute raised intracranial pressure or a worsening of neurological symptoms caused by the lesion itself.
- Symptoms begin within days or even hours.
- Using conventional dosing, acute effects are rarely troublesome if steroids are appropriately given.

Early delayed (intermediate) effects

- Begin within weeks of completing radiation therapy and may continue for 6–10 weeks thereafter.
- The syndrome comprises somnolence, lethargy, and frequently recurrence of the original presenting symptoms and signs.
- Symptoms are usually self-limiting but will respond to steroids. Recovery is the rule.
- The pathogenesis is believed to relate to interruption of myelin synthesis secondary to damage to the oligodendroglial cells.
- A corresponding condition occurs after spinal irradiation and presents with Lhermitte's sign.

Delayed radiation damage

- This is the most sinister form of radiation damage and is uniformly irreversible.
- The onset may be from around 3–4 months up to many years after the exposure.
- Injury is predominantly to the white matter and is dose- and volume-dependent. Radiation necrosis is the most severe form of damage.
- The generally accepted tolerance dose for late damage (for malignant tumour) is 60Gy in 30 fractions. In less

demanding situations, 50–54Gy in 2-Gy fractions is considered the upper limit.

- To minimize late damage, fraction sizes for radical brain treatments should not exceed 2Gy.
- Other late consequences of brain irradiation include hormone (pituitary/hypothalamic) failure, damage to optic tracts, and second malignancy.

Further reading

ICRU. *Prescribing, Recording and Reporting Photon Beam Therapy (Supplement to ICRU Report 50), ICRU Report 62*. Bethesda, MD: ICRU, 1999.

Karim A., Afra D, Cornu P, *et al.* Randomized trial on the efficacy of radiotherapy for cerebral low grade glioma in the adult: EORTC study 22845 with the MRC study BRO4: an interim analysis. *Int J Radiat Oncol, Biol Phys* 2002; **52**(2): 316–24.

Brain tumours: chemotherapy and new agents

Cytotoxic chemotherapy of brain tumours is hampered by the intrinsic resistance of many tumours and the poor penetration caused by the blood–brain barrier (BBB). BBB resistance may not exist to the same extent in the vicinity of tumours. Chemotherapy has found an increasing role in recent years. Agents with best penetration are either small molecules (e.g. temozolomide) or lipid soluble (e.g. nitrosoureas). Chemotherapy can be given in a neo-adjuvant, adjuvant, concomitant, consolidation, or palliative setting.

Active agents

Nitrosoureas

- The chloroethyl nitrosoureas are highly lipid soluble, non-ionized drugs that rapidly cross the BBB.
- Carmustine (BCNU intravenous), and lomustine (CCNU oral) are the most commonly used drugs in Europe and the USA.
- Different nitrosoureas have different pharmacokinetic properties whilst retaining the same basic chemical activity and toxicity problems. None has proved more effective than any other.
- Major adverse effects include delayed and cumulative myelosuppression and lung fibrosis.

Procarbazine

- Procarbazine is an oral agent which is activated in the liver to become an alkylating agent.
- Adverse effects include nausea, vomiting, and myelosuppression.
- It interacts adversely with alcohol and some smoked and preserved foods. Dietary restriction is necessary.

Temozolomide

- Temozolomide is a small molecule that acts as an alkylating agent by adding methyl groups to the O^6 position of guanine in DNA.
- It has high oral bioavailability and is converted spontaneously into the active compound at physiological pH on entering the bloodstream.
- It penetrates readily into brain tumours.
- Methylation by temozolomide is opposed by methyl guanine methyl transferase (MGMT), a ubiquitous enzyme.
- Protracted, fractionated delivery of temozolomide is more effective than short courses of drug.
- Toxicity includes general myelosuppression, moderate emesis, skin rashes, and selective lymphopenia when given continuously.
- Temozolomide can be used as concomitant treatment with radiotherapy in patients with newly diagnosed glioblastoma.

Gliadel®

- Gliadel® is system comprising a biodegradable polymer in wafer form that is impregnated with BCNU.
- A number of these wafers are used to line the cavity left after resecting a brain tumour.
- After wound closure, the polymer slowly breaks down, delivering the BCNU in a more concentrated and protracted fashion than is possible to achieve by systemic delivery (see p.89).

Epipodophyllotoxins and platinum compounds

Drugs such as VP-16, cisplatin and carboplatin, are valuable for treating non-glial brain tumours such as medulloblastoma and germ cell tumours. They have only minor activity against gliomas and are typically used as third line agents.

Topoisomerase inhibitors

Topoisomerase inhibitors such as irinotecan have shown activity against glial tumours including glioblastoma both as single agents and in combination (Gruber et al. 2004). However, whether they have a role in routine management has yet to be determined.

Vinca alkaloids

Vinca alkaloids are highly polar molecules with very limited access to the brain. In spite of this vincristine appears regularly in the treatment of brain tumours. Its value is not clear.

Combination chemotherapy

Few drugs are effective as single agents in glioma therapy and hence the potential for combinations is limited. Few have been studied. The combination procarbazine, CCNU, and vincristine (PCV) was considered to be a standard first-line treatment in glioma treatment. However, the evidence that it is superior to single agent nitrosourea is very sparse.

Chemotherapy for individual tumours

Gliomas

WHO grade 1

- There is no clear role for chemotherapy in WHO grade 1 tumours in adults.

WHO grade 2

- Nitrosoureas and temozolomide can each produce clear symptomatic and radiological response in low grade gliomas at first diagnosis and relapse.
- (1p,19q) Co-deleted oligodendrogliomas are particularly responsive.
- A pan-European study is examining the relative effectiveness of radiotherapy and chemotherapy in newly diagnosed disease.

WHO grades 3 and 4

- PCV and temozolomide appear to be equi-effective in patients with relapsed astrocytoma.
- The objective response rate is around 10% with disease stabilization and symptomatic improvement in around 20–30%.
- Response is better in patients with grade 3 tumours.
- Temozolomide ($75mg/m^2$) given concurrently with radiation followed by adjuvant monthly treatment ($200mg/m^2$ days 1–5) for patients with newly diagnosed glioblastoma produces a survival advantage at 2 years of 16% sustained at 4 years when compared to radiation alone (10%–26%). Hence this is the treatment of choice for high grade gliomas (Stupp et al. 2005).
- Patients with methylation of the MGMT gene promoter have better prognosis with this regimen than those with unmethylated promoter.
- The value of concomitant treatment in grade 3 astrocytoma and oligodendroglioma is not proven.

- Gliadel has been shown in randomized study to prolong survival modestly in patients with newly diagnosed and relapsed disease who are able to undergo macroscopic tumour removal.
- Patients with oligodendroglioma demonstrating LOH on 1p,19q have very high response rates when treated with alkylating chemotherapy. Prolonged remissions are common. Previously untreated patients should receive chemotherapy at relapse following radiation treatment. A study comparing radiotherapy and chemotherapy as primary treatment is in preparation.
- Ependymomas are highly chemoresistant. The most effective agents are probably platinum compounds.

Medulloblastoma
- Adjuvant chemotherapy with cisplatin, CCNU and vincristine has become standard treatment for children with medulloblastomas following (reduced dose) radiotherapy.
- This regimen is too toxic for use in most adults and radiotherapy alone is used.
- Effective agents at relapse include carboplatin, epipodophyllotoxins, cyclophosphamide, and temozolomide.
- High-dose alkylating treatment with stem cell rescue has been used in attempts to prolong remission but the results are poor.

Primary CNS lymphoma
- The principal agent used in the treatment of PCNSL is high dose methotrexate ($>3Gm/m^2$), which may be used singly or combined with other BBB penetrating agents (e.g. Ara-C, BCNU, procarbazine).
- At relapse a variety of agents may be effective particularly alkylating agents (temozolomide, nitrosoureas).
- High dose therapies have been tried but with little success and high toxicity.

Germ cell tumours
- Agents similar to those used for systemic disease (cisplatin, carboplatin, epipodophyllotoxins, ifosfamide) are used.
- In the primary treatment of germinomas, chemotherapy can be used to reduce the extent of radiotherapy.
- Chemotherapy is an integral part of the treatment for nearly all patients with teratoma.
- Chemotherapy alone (without radiation) is not adequate for the curative management of these diseases.

Meningiomas
Chemotherapy has little part to play in the management of meningioma.
   Hydroxyurea has a low level of activity and can be useful to stabilize disease in some patients at relapse.

New agents
The greater understanding of the aberrant cellular pathways identified in brain tumours has lead to an explosion of interest in novel biological agents directed at correcting them. Few have gained acceptance as single agents but many are in clinical trials as combinations with other similar agents and conventional treatments. Most trials are in gliomas.

Antiangiogenesis inhibitors
- Marked neovascularization is a hallmark of glioma.
- Vascular endothelial growth factor (VEGF) has been identified as a potent mediator of angiogenesis, vascular permeability, and tumour growth (Pietsch et al. 1997).

- VEGF expression is particularly upregulated in glioblastoma and its expression may be a prognostic factor for survival. The expression of VEGF is related to prognosis.
- Protein kinase C (PKC) supports glioma cell proliferation, suppresses apoptosis, and imparts chemo- and radio-resistance (da Rocha et al. 2002).
- The VEGF receptor and regulators such as PKC are targets for the inhibition of angiogenesis. Lead compounds are bevacizumab, a monoclonal anti-VEGF antibody, and enzastaurin, a PKC inhibitor.
- Bevacizumab alone or in combination with conventional chemotherapy is used by some for the treatment of recurrent glioblastoma multiforme (GBM).
- The role of these agents in newly diagnosed disease is being explored.

Growth factor signalling pathways
- Growth factor signalling pathways are often upregulated in brain tumours and contribute to oncogenesis through autocrine and paracrine mechanisms.
- Excessive growth factor receptor stimulation can also lead to overactivity of the downstream Ras signalling pathway.
- The EGFR is frequently amplified and overexpressed in GBM and is usually accompanied by gene-rearrangements and deletions.
- The most common mutant in GB is the truncated EGFRvIII which does not recognize EGF but it is constitutively (ligand independent) activated and escapes normal regulation.
- EGFRvIII enhances cell proliferation through the P13-K/AKT pathway (Smith et al. 2001).
- The presence of EGFR amplification by itself does not seem to be of prognostic significance.
- EGFR antagonists may work by blocking the receptor itself (e.g. the monoclonal antibody cetuximab) or by inhibiting transmission at the intracellular portion of the receptor (e.g. the TK inhibitor erlotinib (Tarceva®).
- Although responses to these agents are seen in recurrent gliomas, they have not reached a level to make their routine use worthwhile.
- Trials are ongoing to explore their use in combination with other biological treatments and conventional therapy in newly diagnosed disease

Other cell signalling agents
- Platelet-derived growth factor (PDGF) and its receptors are commonly coexpressed in high grade gliomas, suggesting that autocrine PDGF receptor stimulation may contribute to their growth. Experiments using the PDGF antagonist imatinib Glivec® have been done with and without conventional cytotoxic agents (e.g. hydroxyurea). In spite of occasional responses, there has been no convincing evidence of worthwhile efficacy though research is ongoing.
- Other internal signal transduction pathways that may become dysregulated during transformation include Raf, MEK, PI3K, Akt (protein kinase B), and mTOR (mammalian target of rapamycin). Specific small molecules against these targets have been developed which include sorafenib against Raf; LY294002 against PI13 and temsirolimus against mTOR. All are currently in clinical trial.
- Farnesyltransferase has been considered a target in glioma and the FTase inhibitor tipifarnib is a candidate for study.

Further reading

Gruber MLMD, Buster WPDO. Temozolomide in combination with irinotecan for treatment of recurrent malignant glioma. *Am J Clin Oncol* 2004; **27**(1)33–8.

Pietsch T, Valter M, Wolf H, *et al.* Expression and distribution of vascular endothelial growth factor protein in human brain tumors. *Acta Neuropathol* 1997; **93**(2):109–17.

da Rocha A., Mans D, Regner A, *et al.* Targeting protein kinase C: new therapeutic opportunities against high-grade malignant gliomas? *Oncologist* 2002; **7**(1):17–33.

Smith J, Tachibana I, Passe S, *et al.* PTEN mutations, EGFR amplification, and outcome in patients with anaplastioc astrocytoma and glioblastoma multiforme. *J Natl Canc Inst* 2001; **93**:1246–56.

Stupp R, Mason W, van den Bent M, *et al.* Radiotherapy plus concomitant and adjuvant temozolomide for glioblastoma. *N Engl J Med* 2005; **352**(10):987–96.

Outcome and management of recurrence

Outcome

WHO grade 1 tumours

- By definition, the outcome in this group of tumours is good with long-term control or cure in 80–90% and low morbidity.
- Even if a complete resection is not achieved at primary surgery, regrowth may not occur.
- Outcome correlates with the volume of residual tumour.
- When recurrence occurs it is nearly always local.

WHO grade 2 gliomas

- Since the management of these tumours is so variable and prognostic factors so influential, the value of averaged outcome measures is limited. Important positive prognostic variables are:
  - Smaller tumour size (<6cm)
  - Non-encroachment of the midline
  - Oligodendroglioma rather than astrocytoma
  - Lack of neurological deficit
  - Young age (<40)
- Median survival is around 5–10 years.
- Median time to recurrence is 3–8 years.
- Most (75%) of patients will die of their disease, the majority following malignant transformation.

WHO grades 3 and 4 glioma

- More than 80% of high grade glioma recur within 2cm of the original tumour or its resection margin.
- Spinal spread can occur but is rare and systemic spread is very rare.

Anaplastic astrocytoma

- The median survival of patients with anaplastic astrocytomas is 2–5 years.
- The same prognostic factors operate as for glioblastoma.
- Recurrence is often accompanied by transformation to glioblastoma.

Glioblastoma

- Overall median survival remains <1 year for all patients.
- For patients treated with combined chemo-radiotherapy median survival is 14.6 months (Stupp et al. 2005)
- The major prognostic factors are age, PS, and extent of surgery.
- For patients in the best prognostic category, median survival is >2 years.
- Patients whose tumours have methylated MGMT promoter and are treated with chemoradiotherapy may have a median survival as high as 26 months (Hegi et al. 2005)

Anaplastic oligodendroglioma

- Median survival for this group of patients is 3–6 years; however, outcome is strongly influenced by the presence of LOH1p,19q.
- For tumours with no LOH, the behaviour is as for glioblastoma. With LOH of (at least) 1p the median time to progression following radiotherapy or chemotherapy is several years.

- Retreatment can produce a remission of similar duration.

Medulloblastoma

- Medulloblastoma in adults is a rare disease and survival figures are unreliable. A typical figure is around 70% 5-year survival for patients over 18.
- Patients continue to relapse many years after treatment and 5-year survival is not synonymous with cure.
- Good prognostic factors are the absence of metastatic disease, complete resection of primary tumour and timely completion of craniospinal irradiation.
- Relapse may be local, disseminated through the neuraxis or systemic.
- Lung and bone are sites of preference for systemic spread.

Meningioma

- The prospect of local control depends on:
  - The extent of resection (Simpson grade, see Table 4.2.1; Simpson 1957) and hence the site of tumour and the growth pattern
  - The histological grade
- Not all meningiomas regrow even after incomplete removal.
- Recurrence is nearly always local although grade 3 tumours may metastasize.
- Recurrence following Simpson grade 1 resection is rare.
- Grade 3 tumours frequently recur even after surgical excision and radiotherapy.

Lymphoma

- Approximately 50% of patients completing treatment with chemotherapy and radiation will live 5 years.
- Median survival for patients receiving chemotherapy alone is around 30 months.
- Patients not achieving complete remission following chemoradiotherapy have very poor survival.
- Deteriorating cognitive function is very common in patients surviving combined chemoradiotherapy.

Table 4.2.1 Simpson grading according to extent of resection

Grade	Extent of surgery	Risk of recurrence (%)
I	Gross total resection of tumour, dural attachments, and abnormal bone	9
II	Gross total resection of tumour, coagulation of dural attachments	19
III	Gross total resection of tumour without resection or coagulation of dural attachments or extradural extensions	29
IV	Partial resection of tumour	44
V	Simple decompression (biopsy)	

Treatment of relapse

WHO grade 1 tumours

- Treatment of relapse is surgical where possible.
- Treatment with radiotherapy of any residuum following surgery may be justified.

WHO grade 2 gliomas

- Many patients will have received radiotherapy as part of their initial treatment and many patients will have evidence of malignant transformation at relapse.
- Surgery should be considered particularly if there are pressure symptoms or there is the opportunity to insert Gliadel® wafers to a transformed tumour.
- Repeat radiotherapy is unlikely to be an option.
- The main treatment is likely to be with chemotherapy.
- Chemotherapy regimens will be as for high grade glioma.

High grade glioma

- Most patients will have received radiotherapy, and many temozolomide chemotherapy, as initial treatment.
- Further surgery should be considered for patients with pressure symptoms or those who might benefit from Gliadel® insertion.
- Chemotherapy should be considered for patients who relapse and who have a reasonable performance status (WHO 0–2).
- A recent MRC study has shown no difference in outcome between PCV and 5-day temozolomide in chemo-naive patients at relapse.
- For previously (temozolomide) treated patients the options are re-challenge with temozolomide (if initial treatment was beneficial) or PCV.
- Third-line chemotherapy, typically with etoposide and/or carboplatin is rarely of value.
- Chemotherapy should always be considered for patients with anaplastic oligodendroglioma. PCV and temozolomide are equi-effective and have response rates up to 90% in co-deleted patients.
- The antiangiogenesis agent bevacizumab has demonstrated unequivocal activity against recurrent glioblastoma both as a single agent and in combination with conventional chemotherapy (irinotecan) (Cloughesy et al. 2008). Whilst it undoubtedly produces radiological responses and symptomatic improvement in some patients, its value in prolonging life is unproven.

Medulloblastoma

- Medulloblastoma recurrence is a sinister event, rarely compatible with survival. Further remission can often be obtained however.
- Surgical resection of 'solitary' recurrences should be considered.
- Recurrences will remain sensitive to a variety of agents including platinum compounds, epipodophyllotoxins and alkylating agents. Appropriate chemotherapy is the treatment of choice.
- High-dose therapy with stem cell rescue has been tried but its benefit in adults is not established.
- Radiotherapy to isolated metastases can be repeated in some circumstances, particularly to regions not previously irradiated to high dose. Stereotactic localization should be considered.

Meningioma

- The principal treatment for relapsed meningioma is repeat surgery, where possible.
- Radiotherapy can be given for incompletely excised tumours or those where resection is not possible.
- Radiosurgery (SRS) is useful for small recurrences.
- Chemotherapy has little value for relapsed meningioma. Continuous oral hydroxyurea has been used to stabilize disease.
- In selected patients, somatostatin analogues can cause temporary tumour regression (Chamberlain et al. 2007).

Lymphoma

- The majority of tumours will relapse.
- Those not previously irradiated can receive radiotherapy (typically whole brain).
- Palliative treatment with salvage chemotherapy (temozolomide) should be considered.
- High-dose therapy and stem cell rescue has been advocated but is not generally accepted.

Palliative care input

Patients with progressive, incurable brain tumours have a number of particular needs that should be addressed by specialists working with this type of patient. Representative specialists should form part of the MDT.

- CNS symptoms such as seizure, headache, nausea, and movement disorder may need input from a specialist neurologist or palliative care physician.
- Appropriate support after loss of motor function or speech should be offered from physiotherapy, occupational therapy, and speech and language therapy.
- Cognitive dysfunction and depression are common in patients with brain tumours. Access to specialist psychological and psychiatric help should be available.
- Loss of function and life expectancy create profound social problems such as loss of employment. Social care specialists should be available to provide support.

New approaches

New generation radiosensitizers

- PARP-1 is a DNA-binding enzyme that is activated by DNA breaks and facilitates their repair.
- PARP inhibitors should enhance the action of antitumour agents that act through causing DNA damage (radiotherapy and some alkylating agents).
- Combination studies of PARP-1 and conventional cytotoxic agents in patients with brain tumours are ongoing.

Vaccines

- Cancer vaccines represent a promising new approach to the treatment of GBM.
- Various strategies can be taken including vaccination with cytokine-transfected tumour cells, adoptive transfer of tumour-activated T cells, administration of antigen-pulsed dendritic cells (DC), or direct vaccination with GBM tumour associated peptides.
- Most approaches have been clinically tested and show enhanced immunity, some with favourable clinical outcomes (Wheeler et al. 2006).

Gene therapy

- Gene therapy in brain tumours is most commonly delivered by modified viruses though approaches with liposomes and naked DNA have been attempted.
- The major killing strategies have been 'suicide' therapy where a gene is selectively inserted into the cancer cells whose product will transform an otherwise innocuous drug into a cellular poison (e.g. the HSV-tk gene sensitizes cells to gancyclovir) and oncolytic viruses that have been disabled such that they are harmless to normal cells but lethal to malignant tissue (e.g. the herpes simplex virus HSV1716).
- The first generation of gene therapy agents did not lead to therapeutic advance but second-generation strategies are looking more promising (Tyler et al. 2008).

Further reading

Chamberlain M, Glantz M, Fadul C. Recurrent meningioma: Salvage therapy with long-acting somatostatin analogue. *Neurology* 2007; **69**(10):969–73.

Cloughesy T, Prados M, Wen P, *et al.* Bevacizumab in recurrent glioblastoma. *J Clin Oncol* 2008; **26**(Suppl.): 2010b.

Hegi M, Diserens A, Gorlia T, *et al.* MGMT Gene silencing and benefit from temozolomide in glioblastoma. *N Engl J Med* 2005; **352**(10):997–1003.

Simpson D. The recurrence of intracranial meningiomas after surgical treatment. *J Neurochem* 1957; **20**:22–39.

Stupp R, Mason W, van den Bent M, *et al.* Radiotherapy plus concomitant and adjuvant temozolomide for glioblastoma. *N Engl J Med* **352**(10):987–96.

Tyler M, Sonabend A, Ulasov I, *et al.* Vector therapies for malignant glioma: shifting the clinical paradigm. *Expert Opin Drug Deliv* 2008; **5**(4):445–58.

Wheeler C, Black K, Liu G, *et al.* Vaccination elicits correlated immune and clinical responses in glioblastoma multiforme patients. *Cancer Res* 2008; **68**(14):5955–64.

Brain tumours: summary of management

WHO grade I tumours

- The principal treatment is surgical excision where possible.
- The ambition is total (microscopic) removal.
- Some asymptomatic tumours may be observed.
- Adjunctive treatments are rarely appropriate as part of primary treatment even if excision is incomplete.

WHO grade 2 gliomas

- The majority of patients present with seizures that should be managed with anticonvulsants.
- Small tumours whose symptoms are controlled can be managed with a policy of imaging and close follow-up.
- Alternatively a macroscopic removal can be attempted.
- Tumours with, or developing, adverse risk factors (tumour of >6cm, encroaching the midline, oligodendroglioma, with neurological deficit or age >40 years) should be offered maximal safe tumour removal and postoperative radiotherapy.
- Chemotherapy may be an alternative to radiation (subject currently of an international randomized trial EORTC 22033)
- All tumours with an oligodendroglial component should be tested for LOH 1p and 19q.

WHO grades 3 and 4 glioma

Anaplastic astrocytoma

- Patients should be offered maximal safe debulking surgery.
- Postoperative radical radiotherapy is required for nearly all patients.
- The value of concomitant/adjuvant chemotherapy is not proven and is the subject of a randomized clinical trial (the CATNON study [EORTC, RTOG, MRC])

Glioblastoma

- The patient's condition should be optimized (steroids, anticonvulsants, etc.) prior to a management decision. The steroid dose should be optimized throughout the perioperative period through clear protocol guidelines.
- Treatment decisions should be made on the basis of the known major prognostic factors of performance status, age, and tumour operability.
- Most patients should be offered maximal safe debulking surgery.
- In some patients biopsy only is possible. Multiple biopsies are desirable with acquisition of sufficient tissue for adequate pathological testing (including molecular) and deep freezing.
- Gliadel® insertion can be used in cases where near macroscopic removal has been obtained.
- Where possible an MRI should be done within 48 hours of surgery to assess the extent of resection and to assist radiotherapy planning.
- A decision on subsequent therapy should be made in the postoperative setting.
- The methylation status of the promoter of the MGMT gene should be estimated. However, at the time of writing this should not be used for clinical decision making but for audit and trial eligibility.
- Patients <70 years with performance status WHO 0–1 should be considered for radical radiotherapy (see p.92) and concomitant/adjuvant chemotherapy (see p.96).

- The outcome from combined Gliadel® and concomitant/adjuvant temozolomide has not been adequately explored and the combination is not recommended.
- For older patients (>70 years) or those with a poor performance status (WHO >1) shorter course palliative radiotherapy alone is indicated (see p.93)
- The value of concomitant/adjuvant temozolomide in the older population not clear. It is currently being explored in a NCIC/EORTC trial using a regimen of 40Gy in 15 fractions with daily temozolomide.
- In some patients only supportive/symptomatic care is indicated. Patients >80 years or with PS >3 rarely benefit.
- In such cases, where the radiological diagnosis is secure, even a biopsy may be withheld.

Anaplastic oligodendroglioma

- The same general principles apply as for anaplastic astrocytoma.
- LOH1p,19q should be performed in every case as a guide to prognosis and chemosensitivity.
- There is no clear evidence whether radiotherapy or chemotherapy is the better postoperative treatment.

Gliomatosis cerebri

- Surgery is restricted to obtaining a diagnosis.
- Wide-field radiotherapy (possibly to whole brain) can be helpful. Typically 45–50Gy in 1.8-Gy fractions are given.
- Chemotherapy with the usual agents (PCV or temozolamide) can produce responses that are sometimes durable.

Medulloblastoma

- Patients with medulloblastoma may present as an emergency with hydrocephalus. In these cases the patients should, where possible, be stabilized prior to definitive surgery.
- If surgical drainage is required, a non-dominant ventriculostomy is preferable to a shunt.
- In all cases where medulloblastoma is suspected, preoperative whole neuraxis imaging (MRI) is mandatory.
- Surgery is performed with the aim of obtaining as complete a resection as possible consistent with good neurological function.
- CSF should be sampled at the time of surgery (or earlier if a drain is placed) to aid staging.
- Postoperative staging according to the Chang system (which took account of metastasis, age, pathology and extent of resection) has been modified to define high or average risk (Chang et al. 1969) (see Table 4.2.2).
- All patients should be offered whole neuraxis radiotherapy (35Gy) with boosts to primary site and sites of residual bulk disease (20Gy).
- There is no evidence that adjuvant chemotherapy is valuable in adults (as it is in children).
- Delays in starting radiotherapy are accompanied by inferior outcomes.
- Neoadjuvant chemotherapy might be of value in high-risk patients (e.g. residual bulk disease) awaiting radiotherapy.

Table 4.2.2 Modified Chang staging

T1	1.5cm residual tumour
T2	≥1.5cm residual tumour
M0	No tumour
M1	Tumour in CSF
M2	Gross tumour nodules in the intracranial, subarachnoid or ventricular space
M3	Gross tumour in the spinal subarachnoid space
M4	Systemic metatasis
Average risk	M0 disease arising in the posterior fossa, age >3 years and <1.5cm residual tumour
High risk	All others

Mesenchymal tumours

• Patients with small asymptomatic meningiomas can be kept under imaging surveillance.
• Patients requiring treatment should be considered for surgery with a view to a maximal removal consistent with good neurological function.
• The outcome of surgery should be recorded in terms of an appropriate reporting system (e.g. Simpson grading) to aid surveillance and management decisions.
• Postoperative treatment should be withheld in the great majority of cases for grade 1 tumours.
• Incompletely excised grade 2 tumours should be considered for radiotherapy treatment or followed closely if radiotherapy is not given.
• All grade 3 tumours should be considered for radiation treatment. If given, the dose and fractionation is as for high grade glioma.
• Haemangioblastoma and solitary fibrous tumour can usually be managed with surgery alone.
• Haemangiopericytoma should be considered for postoperative radiotherapy.

Primary CNS lymphoma

• The role of surgery is confined to obtaining sufficient material for adequate tissue diagnosis.
• All patients should have whole neuraxis (MRI) imaging, slit lamp ophthalmological examination of the eye for tumour deposits, CSF examination for lymphoma cells, and immune status evaluation, including HIV.
• The value of full lymphoma staging is debated as the pick-up of systemic disease is low. However, it is still performed in many units.
• All patients should be considered for high-dose methotrexate-based chemotherapy as first-line treatment (see p.97).
• Patients <60 years should be considered for consolidation radiotherapy after discussion of the likely effect on cognitive function.
• Radiation should be withheld in patients >60 achieving remission with chemotherapy.
• Patients not going into remission with first-line chemotherapy should be considered for radiotherapy.

Gangliocytoma (and variants)

These are predominantly low grade tumours, managed by surgical excision.

Central neurocytoma

• An intraventricular tumour predominantly of young adults.
• Although designated WHO grade 2, the primary treatment is usually with surgery alone.
• Radiation (and even chemotherapy) can be helpful in tumours appearing particularly aggressive on histology or that relapse following surgery.

Choroid plexus tumours

• Surgery is the mainstay of treatment for choroid plexus papillomas (CPP) and carcinoma (CPC).
• Complete resection usually achieves cure in CPP. Incompletely removed tumours should be reoperated or observed.
• The value of adjuvant treatment in CPC is unclear though metastatic or locally advancing tumour can be managed palliatively with chemotherapy or radiation.

Pineocytoma/pineoblastoma

• Form a spectrum of tumours arising from the pineal parenchyma.
• Pathology and behaviour varies from the benign pineocytoma (WHO grade 1) to the highly malignant pineoblastoma (WHO grade 4).
• Low grade tumours are treated with surgery alone.
• High grade tumours are treated as medulloblastoma.

Germ cell tumours

• A tissue diagnosis may not be necessary if the tumour markers (AFP, hCG) are raised and the history and imaging are indicative.
• Non-secreting germinomas can be managed with whole brain radiotherapy and a pineoventricular boost or chemotherapy plus pineoventicular irradiation.
• Secreting germinomas and all teratomas require combined (germ cell) chemotherapy and radiotherapy, often to the entire neuraxis.
• Residual masses after treatment are often benign and may be followed.

Craniopharyngioma

• Primary treatment is with surgical excision.
• Postoperative radiotherapy should be considered if excision is incomplete.

Chordoma

• Chordomas arise mainly in the region of the clivus though they can be found at other midline sites.
• Surgical excision is the first treatment of choice but complete excision is rarely possible.
• High-dose highly localized radiotherapy (protons, stereotactically delivered photons) should be considered for residual/unresectable disease.

Further reading

Chang C, Housepain E, Herbert, C. An operative staging system and a megavoltage radiotherapeutic technique for cerebellar medulloblastomas. *Radiology* 1969; **93**:1351–59.

Simpson D. The recurrence of intracranial meningiomas after surgical treatment. *J Neurochem* 1957; **20**:22–39.

Brain metastases: introduction

- Brain metastasis is an extremely common complication of malignancy occurring in around 25% of all systemic cancers. They are approximately four times as common as primary brain tumours.
- The incidence of brain metastases may be increasing because of improved systemic control of those cancers which typically spread to the brain.
- In adults, the commonest sources of brain metastases are lung, breast, and GI cancers, some genitourinary cancers, especially kidney and malignant melanoma.
- A few tumour types, most notably prostate, almost never give rise to brain metastases.
- The great majority of patients who develop brain metastases are considered 'incurable'. However, some with solitary metastases may enjoy extended survival following appropriate management.
- Metastases from some rare tumours (particularly germ cell) may form exceptions to the general rules in that they have a better prognosis even with apparently advanced disease.

Single or solitary?
- Strictly, the term 'single brain metastasis' refers to one isolated lesion within the brain without regard to systemic disease. The term 'solitary brain metastasis' describes a single brain lesion that is the only known metastatic site in the body. These terms are often, erroneously, used interchangeably, even in peer reviewed literature.
- Between 20–50% of brain metastases are single at first presentation. Some cancers are more likely to produce single metastases (breast >small-cell lung cancer).
- The term 'oligometastasis' is used to describe a solitary metastasis, or a small number of metastases, that might be aggressively treated.

Incidence
- The approximate percentage of patients developing brain metastases over the duration of their disease is:
  - Small-cell lung cancer (overall) 30–50%
  - Small-cell lung cancer (without prophylaxis) 50–80%
  - Non-small-cell lung cancer 33%
  - Breast cancer 18–30%
  - Renal cancer 5–10%
  - Melanoma 10–20%
  - Prostate 0% (almost)
- The prevalence at postmortem in patients dying from their cancer may be more than double that found clinically.
- It is noticed that women with HER2-positive breast cancer have a high incidence of brain metastases. Possible reasons are a predisposition in these patients and the failure of Herceptin® to pass the BBB.

Presentation
- 80% of brain metastases will be diagnosed later than the primary cancer (metachronous); the remaining 20% are synchronous or precede the primary diagnosis.
- Headache is the most common symptom, especially in patients with multiple brain metastases or posterior fossa lesions.
- 10–20% of patients will have focal or generalized seizures.
- Other symptoms and signs include focal weakness, gait ataxia, speech disturbance, mental change, sensory disturbance, visual impairment, and papilloedema.
- 5–10% may present with an acute neurological syndrome caused by haemorrhage into a metastasis or cerebral infarction due to embolic or compressive occlusion of a vessel. Haemorrhage into a metastasis is particularly common with cholangiocarcinoma and melanoma.
- A high index of suspicion is required in any patient with a known 'metastasizing' cancer and a change in their neurological symptoms.

Clinicopathology
Metastasis to the brain is the result of haematogenous spread, mostly via the arterial circulation, but also via the vertebral venous system—Batson's plexus. In the cerebrum, metastases are most commonly found at the junction between the cortex and the white matter where the decreased size of blood vessels acts as a trap for tumour emboli. They are also common at terminal watershed areas of arterial circulation. Eighty per cent are found in the cerebral hemispheres, 15% in the cerebellum, and 5% in the brainstem. On CT scanning, more than half of patients have multiple metastases. With MRI, this figure is higher. Due to improved MRI, contrast agents and resolution, the proportion of patients found to have multiple brain metastases is likely to increase. Melanoma and lung cancer are most likely to produce multiple brain metastases.

Histopathology
Where a metastasis has been resected or biopsied, detailed histopathology is required either to confirm the site of origin, if the primary is known, or to help establish the site if it is not.
- Routine light microscopy will establish malignancy and usually allow classification into a broad histological type.
- Positive immunoperoxidase staining may identify subgroups of tumour e.g.
  - Carcinoma: cytokeratin, EMA (breast cancer: ER, PR, CK-7; lung cancer: CK-7, TTF-1, Colon cancer: CK-20)
  - Melanoma: HMB-45, s-100, vimentin, NSE
  - Germ cell tumour: hCG, AFP
  - Lymphoma: CLA
  - Sarcoma: vimentin
- Electron microscopy, and cytogenetic analysis may add further diagnostic accuracy.

Natural history
- The natural history for patients with untreated symptomatic cerebral metastases is extremely gloomy. The median survival is 4–8 weeks.
- Death is due to progressive loss of neurological function or raised intracranial pressure.
- Treatment with optimal dose steroids relieves symptoms by reducing peritumoural oedema but has little cytotoxic effect. Steroids improve median survival only to 8–12 weeks
- The great majority of patients with brain metastases will die an early neurological death. Hence the focus of

disease management and symptom control centres on the management of the brain metastases even in the presence of systemic disease.

Evaluation of the patient with brain metastasis

The management and outcome of the patient with metastatic disease to the brain is critically dependent on a number of prognostic and predictive factors. Careful evaluation is mandatory in every case.

Brain imaging
- Brain metastases usually show as discrete iso- or hyperdense lesions on CT; or T1 bright lesions on MRI. They arise typically in the junction of grey and white matter of the brain and enhance strongly following the injection of contrast. They may have necrotic regions and are frequently multiple.
- Where a management decision depends on the confirmation of brain metastasis, axial scanning (CT or MRI) with and without contrast is mandatory.
- MRI is more sensitive than CT (up to 30%) in detecting brain metastases (Suzuki et al. 2004). It is the preferred investigation where the diagnosis is in doubt following CT or where radical treatment is considered for the patient with oligometastases.
- Double dose contrast, multiplanar imaging, and fine slice thickness can all enhance diagnostic accuracy.
- Gadolinium-enhanced MRI is the appropriate investigation for the detection of meningeal spread.
- Other pathological processes (abscess, inflammation, primary tumour) may mimic metastasis in the patient with known malignancy. Biopsy may be necessary in some cases.

Clinical evaluation
- The outcome in patients treated for brain metastases is strongly dependent on their clinical condition and PS.
- A careful clinical evaluation (history and examination) is required to establish:
  - The presence or absence of active systemic malignancy
  - The performance status (e.g. WHO, Karnofsky performance score KPS)

Laboratory and imaging investigations
If a patient is being considered for aggressive treatment to their brain metastasis then a vigorous search for active systemic disease should be made. This might include disease in the following organs.
- Bone marrow (FBC, possible aspirate/trephine)
- Bone (bone profile, isotope bone scan, MRI)
- Liver and kidneys (hepatic and renal function tests)
- Chest imaging (CXR or CT)
- Abdomen (ultrasound specific organs, CT)
- Tumour markers where appropriate (CEA, CA-125, AFP, hCG)

Classification of the patient with brain metastases

- The principal adverse prognostic factors operating for patients with brain metastases are: poor PS, age, multiple brain metastases, and the presence of active systemic disease.

- Integration of these to form a prognostic classification has enhanced clinical decision making. A widely accepted and prospectively validated scheme is the RTOG classification into three groups based on recursive partitioning analysis (RPA) of prognostic factors (Gaspar et al. 2000).
  - Class 1: Patients with KPS at least 70, under 65 years of age, with controlled primary disease and no extracranial metastases
  - Class 2: all patients not in class 1 or 3.
  - Class 3: patients with (KPS) <70
- Exceptions to this scheme are patients with certain chemosensitive tumour types (e.g. germ cell tumours).
- The median survivals for RPA Classes 1, 2 and 3 are approximately 7.1 months, 4.2 months, and 2.3 months respectively.

Diagnostic evaluation for brain metastasis from unknown primary

Brain metastasis from an unknown primary is diagnosed when a metastatic lesion is discovered and after adequate investigation no primary site can be identified. A biopsy and full pathological examination of the presenting lesion is required in all cases. The pathology may give a clue as to the site of origin and direct further investigation. A thorough work-up (as listed) is required either before or after the biopsy has been done and evaluated.

All cases
- Thorough clinical history
- Physical examination (may include skin, rectum, breasts, testes and the oral cavity and nose)
- Full blood count, routine biochemistry.
- CXR

Selected cases
- Tumour markers CEA, CA-125, AFP, hCG
- CT chest abdomen and pelvis
- More detailed radiographic or invasive tests should be restricted to those with organ specific complaints, radiographic abnormalities or as directed from the pathology. These might include investigation of the:
  - *GI tract* (contrast studies, endoscopy)
  - *Abdomen and pelvis* (ultrasound and biopsy of specific organs)
  - *Chest* (bronchoscopy)
  - *Head and neck* (head imaging, endoscopy)
  - *Bone* (nuclear medicine scans)
  - *Lymph nodes* (biopsy, fine needle aspirate)
  - *Skin* (biopsy)
- FDG-PET may be useful in some cases but its value in routine management is not established.

Further reading

Gaspar, L.E., L. Scott, C. Murray, K. *et al.* 2000. Validation of the RTOG recursive partitioning analysis (RPA) classification for brain metastases. *Int J Radiat Oncol, Biol Phys* 2000; **47**:1001–6.

Suzuki, K., Yamamoto, M. Hasegawa, Y. *et al.* 2004. Magnetic resonance imaging and computed tomography in the diagnoses of brain metastases of lung cancer. *Lung Cancer (Netherlands)* **46**(3):357–60.

Brain metastases: treatment options for brain metastases

Initial management of the patient with brain metastases

- The great majority of patients with brain metastases will be symptomatic at the time of diagnosis.
- The commonest symptoms are pain, seizure, and neurological dysfunction.
- The mainstay of early management is the administration of steroids, usually dexamethasone.
- The rules for management of steroids are the same as for patients with primary brain tumours (see p.86)
- Whilst steroids will frequently reverse many of the symptoms, this is often incomplete and short lived. Other specific treatments (anticonvulsants, antiemetics, analgesics) should be administered as required (see p.86, 7)

Whole brain radiotherapy (WBRT)

- WBRT for cerebral metastases is established to be of value in improving survival and quality of life (Borgelt et al. 1980).
- WBRT is the treatment of choice for the majority of patients discovered to have multiple brain metastases.
- Not all patients benefit and those in the poorest group (RTOG RPA 3) still have a median survival of <3 months (Gaspar et al. 2000). Most of these patients should probably not receive WBRT.
- WBRT is normally delivered on a linear accelerator with appropriate immobilization using a pair of unmodified parallel opposed fields.
- Planning is usually by field placement either at the simulator or using a CT-simulator. Dose prescription is either to midplane or to the isocentre.
- A series of randomized studies in the 1980s (Borgelt et al. 1980) established a dose of 30Gy in 10 daily fractions as the 'international standard'.
- In poorer prognosis patients (RTOG RPA 2, 3) a dose of 20Gy in 5 daily fractions appears to produce similar survival and quality-of-life benefits (Borgelt et al. 1980).
- Shorter dose fractionation schemes are not internationally accepted for general use though ultrashort schemes such as 8Gy in 1 fraction and 12Gy in 2 fractions have been advocated.
- Steroid cover is usually given for patients receiving WBRT. Dexamethasone in doses of 4–16 mg is prescribed depending on symptoms. This should be reduced to optimal levels after the radiation is complete.
- Acute side effects of WBRT include transient worsening of neurological symptoms, nausea, vomiting, headache, fever, and hair loss. These will normally resolve or are abrogated by increase in steroid dose.
- Late effects from the radiation develop 12 months or more after irradiation. Hence long-term effects have not been an issue numerically because of short survival. However, >10% of patients who survive for >12 months will develop symptoms such as cognitive loss, ataxia, and urinary incontinence some of which are severe (De Angelis et al. 1989).
- WBRT may be given as an adjuvant to radical treatment of a single metastasis. Here survival prospects may be better and more protracted and more 'brain sparing' dosing schemes may be appropriate.

Other treatment modalities in patients with multiple brain metastases

Chemotherapy

- The BBB is known to be incomplete in the vicinity of brain metastases. A variety of chemotherapy agents effect good and moderate penetration and have the potential to be effective in patients with brain metastases.
- Patients with chemosensitive disease (e.g. small cell lung cancer and breast cancer) who develop brain metastases do respond to conventional chemotherapy.
- Non-conventional agents (temozolomide, nitrosoureas) may also be useful in these patients.

Neurosurgery

Neurosurgery is little used in patients with multiple brain metastasis other than to establish a diagnosis (where necessary) or for the relief of symptoms due to pressure or obstruction. However, surgery may be particularly useful to relieve symptoms due to disease in the posterior fossa especially if there is obstruction. In these conditions radiotherapy alone may worsen pressure problems.

Radiosurgery

Radiosurgery may be used in patients with multiple brain metastases but there is no evidence that it prolongs survival.

Best supportive care

Some patients with poor clinical condition and brain metastases should not have them actively treated. Also the majority of patients who are treated will progress with intracranial disease, often within months. The need for supportive care cannot be over emphasized. Early involvement of the palliative care services, home support and social care is vital in order to manage the resulting progressive disability and deteriorating symptoms.

Management of the patient with oligometastasis

Patients with a single brain metastasis have a better prognosis than those with multiple metastases provided other factors are similar. There is evidence that aggressively treating the index lesion with either surgery or radiation improves outcome.

Role of surgery

- Surgery should be considered for patients with a single brain metastasis in an accessible location. Multiple studies have shown improved survival when a single brain metastasis was excised prior to WBRT compared to treatment with WBRT alone (Patchell et al. 1990).
- Patients showing most benefit were younger (age <65 years) with a KPS score of at least 70, and no evidence of extracranial progression over the previous 3 months.
- In addition surgery may provide immediate relief of symptoms due to pressure of mass effect or from obstructive hydrocephalus.
- Surgery delivers tissue for pathological assessment.
- The major disadvantages of surgery are the need for an inpatient stay, limitation to accessible intracranial sites and clinical conditions which may preclude surgery in some patients.
- Surgical resection for more than one metastasis has been advocated by some but there are no studies to demonstrate convincingly a survival benefit.

Whole brain radiotherapy in addition to surgery
• There is evidence that WBRT following extirpation of a single brain metastasis reduces both intracranial relapse and neurological death in the irradiated patients. However, there is no evidence that overall survival is improved. This may be due to patients dying early from systemic disease.
• Following resection of a single metastasis in a patient with good prognosis either close clinical and imaging follow-up or WBRT should be offered.

Role of radiosurgery
• Radiosurgery is the delivery of a single high dose of radiation to a precisely localized target (metastasis) with the view of tissue sterilization. Single doses are typically in the range 14–21Gy depending on tumour size.
• This is normally delivered using stereotactic localizing techniques (SRS) (see p.93).
• The outcome following treatment for a single metastasis is similar to outcome following surgery but with lower overall cost.
• Use of either linac based systems or gamma knife yields equal results

Advantages of SRS compared to microsurgery.
• SRS can be delivered to 'brain eloquent' and surgically inaccessible sites.
• SRS does not require inpatient stay.
• SRS allows the simultaneous treatment of multiple metastases in different brain regions and multiple sequential treatments for metachronous metastases.
• SRS may be less expensive.

Disadvantages compared to microsurgery
• Only metastases smaller than about 3cm can be treated effectively.
• Pressure symptoms are not relieved and may even be exacerbated by the radiation. Particular caution is needed in patients with cerebellar metastases.
• SRS does not provide a tissue diagnosis.
  • For patients treated with radiosurgery, RPA classification predicts prognosis; but an alternative system (Score index for Radiosurgery, SIR) may prove to be more accurate (Weltman et al. 2005) (see Table 4.2.3)
• The strongest evidence for the value of SRS is a large randomized study which compared WBRT with or without SRS in patients with 1–3 metastases (Andrews et al. 2005). Patients receiving SRS had a significantly longer median survival (6.5 vs. 4.5 months) and improved PS (43% vs. 27%). However, subgroup analysis showed that the survival advantage was confined to patients with a single metastasis.
• Numerous other non-randomized studies indicate a survival advantage for SRS as an alternative as well as in addition to WBRT in patients with single metastases.
• In patients with oligometastases, SRS may represent an alternative to WBRT with less toxicity but without improving survival.
• Whether WBRT in addition to SRS adds further benefit remains an open question. It appears to have a similar role to surgery (see p.108).

Prophylactic cranial irradiation
• Some cancers have a very high rate of intracranial metastasis during their clinical course in spite of systemic treatment. Small-cell lung cancer has a 50–80% cumulative risk of intracranial relapse at 2 years.
• It has been common practice to offer prophylactic irradiation to the brain (prophylactic cranial irradiation, PCI) to try to prevent their occurrence.
• Meta-analysis data show an overall survival advantage with a relative risk of death of 0.82–0.84, and a reduction in rate of brain metastases (relative risk 0.46–0.48) when PCI is given.
• The benefits of PCI appear limited to patients achieving a complete response following induction chemotherapy.
• PCI may be associated with later cognitive impairment and it is recommended that dose fractions of 3Gy or less are used. A typical regimen is 30Gy in 10 fractions.
• PCI may have a role in other diseases with an improving prognosis and a high incidence of brain metastasis (e.g. HER2-positive breast cancer)

Management of special cases of brain metastases
• Special management is required for CNS involvement in highly chemosensitive malignancies which offer the prospect of cure even in the case of advanced disease (e.g. germ cell tumours, haematological malignancy).
• Initial treatment will often be with chemotherapy (and sometimes surgery) with subsequent radiation treatment for consolidation in some cases.
• High-dose protocols with bone marrow/stem cell rescue have been explored in this situation.
• WBRT can be given for palliation in the case of incurable disease.

Re-irradiation
• Virtually all patients irradiated for multiple brain metastases will relapse intracranially provided they survive long enough.

Table 4.2.3 Score index for radiosurgery in brain metastases

	0	1	2
Age	≥60	51–59	≤50
KPS	≤50	60–70	>70
Systemic disease status	Progressive disease	Partial remission/ stable	Complete remission/no evidence of disease
Largest lesion volume (cm 3)	>13	5–13	<5
Number of lesions	≥3	2	1

Score	Median survival (months)
1–3	2.91
4–7	7
8–10	31.4

- There is evidence that patients who have benefited from WBRT for at least 4 months may also benefit from re-irradiation (Cooper et al. 1990). The initial dose used in these studies was usually 30Gy in 10 fractions. The retreatment doses were 20–30Gy, usually given in 10 fractions.
- The studies reported little evidence of toxicity.

Further reading

Andrews D, Scott C, Sperduto P, et al. Whole brain radiation therapy with or without stereotactic radiosurgery boost for patients with one to three brain metastases: Phase III results of the RTOG 9508 randomised trial. Lancet 2005; 363(9422):1665–72.

Borgelt B, Gelber G, Kramer S, et al. The palliation of brain metastases: final results of the first two studies by the Radiation Therapy Oncology group. Int J Radiat Oncol, Biol Phys 1980; 6:1–9.

Cooper J, Steinfeld A, Lerch I. Cerebral metastases: value of reirradiation in selected patients. Radiology 1990; 174:883.

De Angelis L., Delattre J, Posner JB, et al. Radiation induced dementia in patients cured of brain metastases. Neurology 1989; 39:789–96.

Gaspar L, Scott C, Murray K, et al. Validation of the RTOG recursive partitioning analysis (RPA) classification for brain metastases. Int J Radiat Oncol, Biol Phys 2000; 47:1001–6

Patchell R, Tibbs P, Walsh J, et al. A randomised trial of surgery in the treatment of single metastases to brain. N Eng J Med 1990; 322:494–500.

Weltman E, Salvajoli J, Brandt R, et al. Radiosurgery for brain metastases: A score index for predicting prognosis. Int J Radiat Oncol Biol Phys 2000; 46:1155–161.

Brain metastases: outcome and summary

Outcome
Multiple metastases
- In general, patients with multiple metastases from most common cancers have very poor survival prospects, even after treatment, usually with WBRT. Overall survivals of approximately 7, 4, and 2 months for patients in RPA classes 1, 2, and 3 are typical.

Solitary metastases
- Patients with single brain metastases who are treated aggressively with either surgery or radiotherapy have a median survival of 6–12 months.
- The addition of WBRT does not appear to improve survival though it does reduce intracranial relapse and neurological death. It is likely therefore that death from systemic disease explains the failure to prolong median survival.
- It is also known that some patients treated with surgery or SRS and WBRT will maintain control of their brain metastases and survive long term (2+ years) provided their systemic disease is controlled. Reducing intracranial relapse in these patients is clearly of great importance as it may enhance survival.
- An appropriate study in patients with a single metastasis and no systemic disease to assess the impact of treatment on survival has not been done.

Summary of management
Patients with multiple brain metastases and unknown primary
- These patients require appropriate staging and evaluation (see p.564).
- If a tissue diagnosis is not obtained in this process then a biopsy from the brain metastasis is required.
- Once a full diagnosis and staging is established, the patient is treated as having a 'known primary'.

Patients with multiple brain metastases and known primary
- Should undergo systemic staging and general medical work-up appropriate to the overall clinical picture.
- They should then be classified according to an appropriate system (e.g. RTOG RPA system).
- RPA class 1 should be considered for WBRT (30Gy in 10 fractions or 20Gy in 5 fractions).

- RPA class 2 should be considered for WBRT (30Gy in 10 fractions or 20Gy in 5 fractions). Some will require best supportive care only.
- RPA class 3 should generally be considered for best supportive care only. Some may merit WBRT. Generally this will be restricted to 20Gy in 5 fractions.

Single brain metastases
- All patients <70 years of age with an apparently single metastasis who are in good clinical condition (Karnofsky >70) should have a high-quality gadolinium enhanced MRI to confirm the diagnosis.
- All patients should have appropriate staging and be classified according to an appropriate prognostic scoring system.
- Patients without systemic disease and with good prognosis should be considered for aggressive treatment to the index lesion (surgery or SRS) (see p.108).
- These patients should then be considered for WBRT (40Gy in 20 fractions or 30Gy in 10 fractions) or close imaging follow-up.
- Patients with systemic disease and otherwise good prognostic scores should still be considered for aggressive treatment with SRS. WBRT may be given or withheld until needed.
- Patients with poor prognostic scores should be treated with WBRT and/or best supportive care.

Oligometastasis
Patients with more than one aggressively treatable brain metastasis can be treated with SRS with or without WBRT. It may be justified to use just WBRT if the patient's outlook is poor.

PCI
PCI should be offered to patients with small-cell lung cancer who achieve remission after induction chemotherapy.

Patients with further intracranial relapse following treatment
- If relapse has occurred soon after initial treatment then best supportive care only is appropriate.
- If there has been benefit from the initial treatment and a period of months or more have elapsed then retreatment with WBRT maybe justified.
- SRS may be performed for new oligometastases appearing after initial treatment with either SRS, surgery or WBRT provided the patient's condition merits it.

Spinal cord tumours: introduction

Primary spinal cord tumours account for 2–4% of all primary CNS tumours. They occur within or adjacent to the spinal cord, i.e. they are intra-axial in location. Metastatic lesions can also occur, particularly from lung and breast primaries.

Tumour sites
- *Intramedullary tumours* arise within the spinal cord. The majority are glial tumours, either ependymomas or astrocytomas. Oligodendrogliomas occur but are rare. Metastases also occur.
- *Intradural-extramedullary* tumours arise within the dura, but outside the spinal cord itself. These are typically meningiomas or nerve sheath tumours.
- *Extradural tumours* are usually metastatic or primary tumours of bone and cartilage. They most often arise in or adjacent to the vertebral bodies. They are not the subject of this chapter.

Clinicopathology
A similar spectrum of tumours arises in the spine as in the brain, though the frequency of occurrence is markedly different and some types are absent. The great majority are low grade. High grade tumours do occur but are rare (see below).
- Gender prevalence is roughly equal though meningiomas are more common in females and ependymomas in males.
- Incidence is greatest in young and middle-aged adults and less common at the extremes of the age spectrum. Astrocytomas occur earlier in life than ependymomas.

Low grade tumours
Astrocytomas
- Spinal astrocytomas are rare (brain: spine 10:1).
- They arise most commonly in the cervical and cervico-thoracic parts of the cord.
- Histologically they divide broadly into pilocytic (WHO grade 1) and non-pilocytic (fibrillary, WHO grade 2) types, though mixed forms occur.

Ependymomas
- Ependymomas account for >60% of spinal gliomas.
- They are not encapsulated tumours but they are usually well circumscribed and tend not to invade adjacent brain.
- They may occur anywhere along the spinal cord but 50% arise in the conus or filum terminale. They may be intra or extramedullary. There are two main types:
  - Myxopapillary variant (WHO grade 1) has a predilection for the distal spine. It is characterized by perivascular and intracellular mucin. It is slow growing and does not transform to a more malignant phenotype.
  - Cellular variant (WHO grade 2) resembles its cerebral counterpart and arises usually in the proximal spine.

Haemangioblastoma
Haemangioblastomas are rare intramedullary tumours that are well circumscribed but not encapsulated. A quarter of patients will have VHL.

Meningioma (WHO grade 1)
- Spinal meningiomas occur mainly in women, the majority in the thoracic spine.
- Most meningiomas are entirely intradural, though a few may be all or partly extradural.
- They tend to be found near the nerve root without involving it directly, hence they often present with myelopathy without radiculopathy.
- They are usually solitary though multiple meningiomas can occur, particularly in association with NF.
- Most spinal meningiomas occur in the thoracic region. Lumbar tumours are rare.

Peripheral nerve sheath tumour (WHO grade 1)
- These are categorized as either schwannoma or neurofibroma and constitute 25% of intradural tumours. Schwannomas are the more common and occur maximally in the fourth to sixth decades.
- They more commonly affect the dorsal root and may extend through the dural root sleeve to form a 'dumbbell tumour'.
- Histologically neurofibromas comprise an abundance of fibrous tissue and there is a conspicuous presence of nerve fibres in the stroma. There is fusiform enlargement of the involved nerve and it can be very difficult to separate normal and neoplastic tissue.
- Schwannomas produce masses of elongated cells with dark fusiform nuclei which do not produce enlargement of the nerve but tend to hang from it.

Other low grade lesions
- There is a plethora of additional uncommon benign tumours which include dermoids, epidermoids, lipomas, teratomas, and neurenteric cysts that are managed with surgery and have an excellent outcome.

High grade tumours
- WHO grades 3 and 4 astrocytomas account for about 10% of intramedullary astrocytomas. Histologically they appear similar to their brain counterparts. Their clinical course is rapid and CSF dissemination is common.
- Anaplastic ependymomas are rarely found in the spinal cord. When they are they have the usual anaplastic features of necrosis, mitosis, vascular proliferation, cellular pleomorphism, and overlapping of nuclei.
- A very small minority (2.5%) of nerve sheath tumours are or become malignant.

Genetic associations
- As in brain disease, NF1 and NF2 are associated with excess tumours in the cord. NF1 is particularly (but not exclusively) associated with astrocytoma and NF2 with ependymoma and meningioma.
- In VHL syndrome there is an excess of spinal haemangioblastoma.

Presentation
Tumours of the spine cause symptoms through disruption of normal neural elements and pathways, producing both local and distant effects.
- *Pain* is the commonest presenting symptom. It usually occurs at the level of the lesion, in the spine itself or in the appropriate root distribution (radicular pain). It typically causes nocturnal wakening.
- The pain may be exacerbated by straining or coughing.

- Functional loss is caused by direct pressure from the tumour itself and associated oedema. Deficit may also occur through spinal infarction and through invasion into spinal tissue and growth along nerve roots.
- Functional loss is at and below the level of the lesion. For tumours of the thoracic or cervical spine, typical sequelae are spasticity, muscle weakness, loss of balance, sensory loss (pain, light touch, vibration), and difficulties with ambulation. Difficulties with bowel and bladder function may be reported due to loss of sphincter control.
- Tumours of the conus/filum region typically present with low back pain, lower motor neuron leg weakness, and sphincter disturbance.
- A Brown–Séquard syndrome, reflecting effective hemisection of the spinal cord, may occur particularly with slow growing nerve sheath tumours.

Examination
- A full neurological examination is required with particular attention to the extent and distribution of any neurological or muscular abnormalities found.
- A general examination is also needed. The majority of tumours in or near the spine are metastatic. Therefore a thorough assessment for evidence of other malignant disease is necessary.
- Assessment of ambulatory status must be done as this has prognostic significance.
- In general, expect upper motor neuron signs below the level of the spinal lesion with a combination of upper and lower motor neuron signs at the level of any tumour.
- Presentations can be complex and do not necessarily conform to expectation.
- In the adult, the spinal cord segmental level is approximately two above the bony vertebral level.
- The cord ends in the conus at the level of L1–2. Lesions below this level can only produce lower motor neuron signs.
- Clinical localization of the upper vertebral limit of the symptoms and signs (sensory level) is notoriously difficult and can be unreliable. If done with care, it can be a useful guide to identifying the position of the tumour within the spine. However, it should always be confirmed with imaging.

Differential diagnosis
- The symptoms caused by a spinal tumour may be mimicked by a wide variety of conditions. A list of differential

diagnoses following clinical examination might include, multiple sclerosis, syringomyelia, transverse myelitis, amyotrophic lateral sclerosis, spinal bony disease, Guillain–Barré syndrome, syphilis, nutritional deficiencies, malignant meningitis, ruptured disc, and others.

Investigation
The investigation of spinal cord tumours is almost entirely confined to imaging.

Plain X-ray
- Plain X-ray is of almost no value in the evaluation of spinal cord tumours.

Magnetic resonance imaging
Overwhelmingly MRI is the imaging modality of choice in spinal disease, including tumours. T1 (with and without gadolinium enhancement), and T2 sequences are needed in transverse and sagittal presentation.
It is possible to evaluate the internal structure of the cord including oedema, atrophy, haemorrhage, infarct, cyst, and syringomyelia.
- *Intramedullary tumours* will nearly always show as expansions of the cord and many enhance in spite of low grade. Individual features may help differentiate different tumour types.
- *Astrocytomas* are hypo- or isointense on T1 and hyperintense in T2. They may be centrally or eccentrically located. They are infiltrative and have an indistinct margin. They tend to enhance more strongly than ependymomas (particularly the pilocytic subtype). High protein cyst inclusions are frequent.
- *Ependymomas* tend to enhance intensely on MRI, and occur centrally within the cord, expanding it symmetrically as they grow. The spinal cord may be expanded along several segments, and a tumour-associated cyst (i.e. syrinx) is commonly seen.
- *Meningiomas* tend to be isointense on both T1 and T2 but enhance avidly with gadolinium.
- *Nerve sheath tumours* and haemangioblastomas are isointense on T1 and hyperintense on T2 imaging. Both enhance avidly on Gd-T1 MRI.

CT scan
CT scan is reserved primarily for patients in whom MRI is contraindicated. The investigation of CT with myelography is then performed. Information from CT on intramedullary tumours is indirect and relies mainly on evidence of architectural change or flow obstruction.

Spinal cord tumours: management

Management

General management

Spinal cord tumours often present insidiously. At presentation patients may have a combination of pain and disability that needs immediate attention. Appropriate analgesia should be offered (see p.87). As well as the usual drugs used in neuro-oncology, gabapentin and other nerve stabilizing anticonvulsants may be helpful for neurogenic pain. Steroids may benefit both pain and neurological deficit but their side effects make them inappropriate for long-term use. Early institution of rehabilitation (physiotherapy and functional aids) can help prevent further deterioration and improve the patient's quality of life. As soon as possible definitive treatment should be considered.

Surgery

• Surgery is by far the most important modality in the management of spinal tumours. Although in some cases some may argue for a watch policy until symptoms demand action, this can be a dangerous policy as it might render a previously operable tumour inoperable or allow a deficit to develop that cannot be reversed. In general, therefore, early surgery is advocated if it can be performed safely.

• Most spinal surgery, particularly if intramedullary, is performed through a posterior laminectomy with a midline durotomy. More ventrally positioned lesions (e.g. meningiomas) may need a posterolateral approach. When complete resection of an intramedullary tumour, particularly ependymoma is considered, the myelotomy should extend over the entire rostrocaudal extent of the tumour.

• Unless the intention is simply to obtain a biopsy, a maximal safe removal is usually the intention. This is always undertaken using the operating microscope and often tools such as intraoperative ultrasound and the cavitating ultrasonic aspirator (CUSA).

• In many benign and low grade tumours it is possible to find a plane of cleavage. For meningiomas it is often necessary to complete the operation with electrocautery of the involved dural base.

• Surgery is covered by the use of corticosteroids to reduce spinal oedema.

• Somatosensory- or motor-evoked potential during surgery can be used to evaluate intraoperative spinal function.

• If there has been extensive bony removal a spinal arthrodesis may be necessary.

• Immediately following surgery, neurological deterioration from the preoperative baseline is common. This usually improves back to baseline or better in the following weeks with sensory improvement usually occurring before motor improvement.

• Early specialized rehabilitation following surgery will improve outcome. Antithrombotic prophylaxis should be undertaken. Care must be taken to recognize and manage orthostatic hypotension which can occur following upper thoracic/cervical spinal surgery. Enthusiastic physio- and occupational therapy is helpful in optimizing rehabilitation.

Radiotherapy

• Radiotherapy is usually given with 'radical' intent. (For general principles see p.92–94.)

• Patients often require stabilization in a mouldable immobilization device. Stereotactic localization can improve accuracy.

• Patients are scanned with CT in the treatment position (frequently prone) to provide information to the planning computer. The tumour and planning outlines are drawn from these images and knowledge of the tumour and its pattern of spread.

• Planning usually involves using an oblique pair of wedged fields, or variant, taking into account normal organs that might be exposed to radiation from the exit beams.

• For treatments to low grade tumours, doses of 45–50Gy in 1.8Gy fractions are usual but for highly malignant tumours, doses up to 56Gy may be appropriate. Whilst the risk to the spinal cord from the radiation is increased at these doses, it may be less than previously thought, provided megavoltage X-rays are used and the dose per fraction is kept below 2Gy (Rampling and Symonds 1998). This risk must be balanced against the risk of under-treating the tumour and the consequences of early re-growth.

Chemotherapy

Chemotherapy has little established role in spinal cord tumours. The same agents used for brain tumours (see p.692) can be tried but responses are few and short-lived.

Management strategies

Low grade astrocytoma

• Surgery is the initial management of choice with the intention to effect as complete a removal as possible without causing neurological deficit.

• This may be difficult, particularly in the diffuse (fibrillary) tumours as there is not usually a clear plane of cleavage.

• Patients with some degree of deficit may still benefit from surgery but those with complete transection of cord function or who have extensive tumours are not surgical candidates.

• *WHO grade 1 (pilocytic) tumours*: surgery is the treatment of choice. Radiotherapy is not needed whether resection is complete or incomplete.

• *WHO grade 2 tumours*: for completely excised lesions radiotherapy can be withheld. For incompletely excised tumours postoperative radiotherapy should be considered.

Ependymoma

• Surgery is the initial treatment of choice. This is often more successful than for astrocytomas because of the presence of a recognizable plane of cleavage. Most patients are cured following gross total resection.

• *Myxopapillary ependymoma*: for the myxopapillary variant even when excision is subtotal, remission may be prolonged and there is no indication for further treatment (with irradiation).

• *Cellular ependymomas*: optimal management consists of gross total resection. Although these are infiltrative tumours, a total or near-total resection can often be achieved. The value of postoperative radiotherapy is controversial though the balance is in favour of offering it only if a total resection has not been achieved. Typical doses are 45–50Gy in 1.8Gy fractions.

Meningioma
- The essential treatment is complete surgical removal.
- Radiotherapy has a limited role but might be considered for patients with more malignant phenotypes (atypical, anaplastic) particularly if resection has been incomplete.
- Patients with multiple meningiomas should be investigated for neurofibromatosis.
- Although the great majority of meningiomas are benign, recurrence rates are relatively high, particularly for en plaque lesions. Regular follow-up with interval imaging is recommended.

Haemangioblastoma
- Patients with spinal haemangioblastoma should be investigated for VHL.
- For sporadic haemangioblastoma and for a first lesion in a patient with VHL, early removal is recommended for both diagnostic and therapeutic purposes.
- For patients with multiple lesions (usually VHL) it is reasonable to observe asymptomatic patients and operate once symptoms occur. If surgery is not indicated or otherwise not possible, radiotherapy can produce symptomatic improvement, particularly for small lesions. Stereotactic localization has been used in some units.

Nerve sheath tumours
The aim of treatment is complete surgical excision which is achievable in the majority of patients.

Other benign tumours
Tumours mentioned in p.84, 85 are managed either by watchful waiting or surgery.

High grade tumours
- The value of surgery, beyond biopsy, in patients with high grade glial tumours is not established.

- Radiotherapy can be offered. This usually comprises localized high dose treatment to the tumour and a generous margin. Some advocate whole neuraxis radiotherapy in high grade ependymoma but the value of this is not clear.
- Chemotherapy may be worth considering in rare patients whose tumours carry a majority oligodendroglial component.

Prognostic factors
- *Histological type*: low grade tumours, particularly WHO grade 1, have a significantly better prognosis than grade 2 tumours. Ependymomas, grade for grade, have a better prognosis than astrocytomas. High grade tumours (WHO grade 3 and 4) have a very poor prognosis.
- *Age*: youth is associated with better outcome but this may be due to variations in the distribution of tumour types in different age groups.
- *Functional status*: there is an association between outcome and functional status before surgery (usually indicated by mobility). Functional deficits present preoperatively are often not reversible.
- *Size*: tumour size is an important factor, probably because it is associated with operability and functional status. Also tumour location can dictate the ease with which a surgeon can remove a tumour. Anterior tumours are more difficult to remove.
- *Extent of resection*: there is clear evidence that if a complete removal of a tumour is able to be done the outcome is much improved (Abdel-Wahab et al. 2006).

Further reading
Abdel-Wahab M, Blessing E, Palermo J, et al. Spinal cord gliomas: a multi-institutional retrospective analysis. *Int J Radiat Oncol Biol Phys* 2006; **64**(4):1060–71.

Rampling RP, Symonds RP. Radiation myelopathy. *Current Opin Neurol* 1998; **11**:627–32.

Spinal cord tumours: outcome

Outcome in spinal tumours

Astrocytoma

- Overall, the 5-year survival figures for patients with spinal astrocytomas are reported as 50–90%. However, the outcome depends critically on the histology. In a large series treated with surgery alone, patients with grade 1 tumours had a 5-year survival of >90% whilst for those with grade 2 tumours it was <60% and all the patients with high grade tumours were dead (Raco et al. 2005).
- Treatment failure is predominantly through local relapse.
- Irrespective of radiotherapy, patients with complete resection and patients with grade 1 (pilocytic) tumours with or without complete resection have excellent control prospects.

Ependymoma

- Spinal ependymomas are associated with a better prognosis than cerebral lesions, particularly when complete resection is possible.
- In a large series, the 5-year progression free survival rate for patients with completely resected spinal ependymomas was >90% compared to <60% for incompletely resected tumours. The 10-year overall survivals were 98% and 70% respectively (Abdel-Wahab et al. 2006).
- Outcome relates to histological type. Patients with myxopapillary and cellular tumours have regrowth rates of approximately 10% at 10 years if completely resected, but the rates are approximately 20% for cellular tumours and this rises to >50% if a cellular ependymoma is incompletely resected.
- Tumours may recur up to 20 years after initial surgery.

Haemangioblastoma

Ninety per cent of patients are either clinically stable or improved after removal of a solitary haemangioblastoma.

Meningioma

- Surgical removal of a spinal meningioma is associated with clinical improvement in >50% of cases. Outcome is worse in patients with en plaque tumours, those in an anterior location and those which are entirely extradural. Older patients do less well.
- The overall recurrence rate is around 10% but rises to 40% for en plaque lesions.

Nerve sheath tumours

Although the majority of patients operated for nerve sheath tumours will be cured, recurrence rates of 20% are reported. This is especially common in patients with NF2 associated tumours.

Recurrence

- Many patients with truly benign tumours who have done well after surgery can be discharged after a year of follow-up. Patients with meningiomas and those whose tumours were not completely removed should be followed longer.
- Patients with spinal astrocytomas and incompletely excised ependymomas require long-term follow-up.

- Recurrence in all these tumours can occur after many years.
- If a tumour recurs and remains low grade, surgery should again be considered although reoperation is often more difficult than initial surgery
- Radiotherapy can be considered for some conditions if second surgery is not possible but the value in most cases is not clearly proven. There is a stronger case for radiotherapy following partial removal of a recurrence, particularly in astrocytoma, ependymoma, and meningioma.
- The value of chemotherapy in recurrent disease is very limited. For high grade lesions, response can sometimes be obtained with nitrosoureas or platinum-based regimens. However, if it occurs, it is generally short lived.
- Radiotherapy can be considered for patients following surgery for an early recurrence of meningioma.

Late sequelae of treatment

Surgery

- The spinal cord may be damaged during the operation itself either directly or by interruption of the blood supply. This can lead to neurological deficit. Some contusive injury and peripheral nerve damage is expected in many operations but recovery of function over many months is common. With good technique serious damage to the cord is rare.
- Following surgery, adhesions, gliosis, and fibrosis can develop, sometimes leading to pain and functional deficit.

Radiation

- Late radiation damage in the cord may be sudden or insidious in onset with sensory and motor abnormalities (paraplegia or quadriplegia), bowel and bladder sphincter disturbance, and diaphragm dysfunction in high lesions.
- The most serious consequence is complete transection of the cord at the irradiated level.
- The pathology—a combination of vascular lesions with demyelination and malacia—is characteristic of radiation myelopathy. The pathogenesis is obscure with both the vasculature and oligodendrocytes identified as principal targets (Schultheiss et al. 1995).
- Imaging may aid diagnosis. MRI performed within eight months of the onset of symptoms shows low signal intensity on the T1-weighted image and high signal intensity on T2-weighted images often with cord swelling. Gadolinium enhancement is common. Late scans show an atrophic cord with normal signal intensity.
- Accepted wisdom has been that spinal cord tolerance at conventional fractionation is 45–50Gy, depending on the clinical situation.
- A dose of 57–60Gy carries a 5% risk of myelitis (Schultheiss et al. 1995). There is evidence that re-irradiation of CNS tissue is possible. Some tolerance develops with increasing time from the initial radiation and is virtually complete (50–70%) by 2 years. However, full tolerance is never regained.

• Some chemotherapeutic drugs can enhance radiation damage in CNS tissue. These include methotrexate, cytosine arabinoside, and the nitrosoureas.

Further reading

Abdel-Wahab M, Blessing E, Palermo J, et al. Spinal cord gliomas: a multi-institutional retrospective analysis. Int J Radiat Oncol Biol Phys 2006; **64**(4):1060–71.

Raco A, Esposito V, Lenzi J, et al. Long-term follow-up of intramedullary spinal cord tumors: a series of 202 cases. Neurosurgery 2005; **56**(5):972–81.

Schultheiss TE, Kun LE, Ang KK, et al. Radiation response of the central nervous system. Int J Radiat Oncol Biol Phys 1995; **31**(5):1093–112.

Primary tracheal tumours

Primary tracheal tumours represent <1% of all respiratory malignancies and can arise from the respiratory epithelium, salivary glands, and mesenchymal structures of the trachea. Most tumours in adults are benign while this is the case in only 30% of tumours in children. Primary tumours in adults are predominantly of adenoid cystic or squamous cell histology (Gaissert et al. 2006).

Squamous cell carcinoma (SCC) is linked to cigarette smoking and more than a third of patients will have either mediastinal or pulmonary metastases at diagnosis. Metachronous or synchronous lesions are common. Up to 40% of tracheal tumours can develop before, concurrently, or after carcinoma of the oropharynx, larynx, or lung. In contrast, adenoid cystic carcinomas (ACC) are not associated with cigarette smoking, tend to spread along both submucosal and perineural planes, and only 10% of patients have regional lymph node or remote metastases at presentation. ACC also progresses slowly, often over several years, which is characteristic even of untreated cases.

Symptoms

Tracheal tumours present with symptoms and signs of upper-airway obstruction, cough, and haemoptysis, or symptoms arising from direct invasion and involvement of continuous structures such as the recurrent laryngeal nerve. Patients with ACCs are more likely to present with long-standing symptoms of wheezing or stridor for months before a definitive diagnosis is made.

Treatment

Evaluation in a specialist centre by a MDT is of particularly importance for these uncommon tumours. Resection should be considered, as a complete surgical resection ensures the best local control and greatest likelihood of cure in almost all patients with tumours of intermediate aggressiveness or/and malignant tumours. Absolute contraindications to surgery that have been cited in the literature include the presence of multiple lymph node metastases, involvement of >50% of tracheal length in adults and 30% in children, mediastinal invasion of unresectable organs, and distant metastases in SCC.

The primary treatment of a non-resectable or node-positive SCC is concurrent chemoradiotherapy with a cisplatin-based scheme and the maximum tolerated dose of radiotherapy. Data are sparse in terms of the optimal radiotherapy dose. For gross residual tumour, >60Gy in 2Gy per fraction is recommended, aiming to give 70Gy if feasible. For postoperative residual disease, 60Gy in 30 fractions is used. Chemotherapy is cisplatin based though there are no prospective studies.

The primary management of tracheal ACC is surgical resection, and patients treated with resection show a 52% 5-year OS. The role of postoperative radiotherapy is unclear although it is often administered if the operation failed to achieve a clear resection margins in the trachea. In unresectable ACC, radiotherapy (either alone or after debulking) is reported to achieve an OS of 30%. There are limited data suggesting that concurrent chemoradiotherapy may achieve good short-term responses. The majority of patients treated without surgery develop local recurrences.

Further reading

Gaissert HA, Mark EJ. Tracheobronchial gland tumours. *Cancer Control* 2006; **13**(4):286–94.

Licht PB, Friis S, Pettersson G. Tracheal cancer in Denmark: a nationwide study. *Eur J Cardiothorac Surg* 2001; **19**:339–45.

Macchiarini P. Primary tracheal tumours. *Lancet Oncol* 2006; **7**(1):83–91.

Lung cancer: introduction, screening and smoking cessation

Introduction

Lung cancer is the most commonly diagnosed cancer worldwide. In the USA, an estimated 213,380 new cases will be diagnosed each year, with 160,390 deaths in 2007 (Jemal et al. 2007). For women in the USA, lung cancer surpassed breast cancer as the leading cause of cancer death in 1987 and is expected to account for 26% of all female cancer deaths in 2008. In Europe, lung cancer is the third most common form of cancer with 386,300 new cases (12.1% of all cancers), but it was the commonest cause of death as indicated by the estimated 334,800 deaths (19.7% of total). The incidence across countries varies widely. Tobacco use is the most important aetiological factor (Doll et al. 2004), with the risk of dying of lung cancer <1% in people who have never smoked. Of all smokers, 16% will die from lung cancer by age 75, if they do not die earlier from other smoking-related causes.

Screening

The dismal survival of patients with lung cancer, as well as the fact that only 16% of all new lung cancers are localized (i.e. stages I–II) at diagnosis, has led to interest in screening programmes. The best cure rates are achieved in stage I NSCLC, and untreated lung cancer is a fatal disease in most patients with stage I disease. Screening for lung cancer remains a controversial issue. Some investigators have suggested that a longer survival in patients who participated in non-randomized, observational studies of low-dose spiral CT demonstrate the effectiveness of screening. Others have pointed out the shortcomings in coming to the above conclusion without evidence derived from randomized clinical trials. Points of concern about screening include the expense of CT screening, the large number of false positive studies, which in turn results in high-risk interventions for benign disease, and radiation exposure that may in turn increase the risk for malignancy.

The outcomes of two randomized clinical trials of screening are awaited. The first, a multicentre National Lung Screening Trial in the US has randomized >53,000 high-risk participants in the period from 2002–2004 to either low-dose CT screening or chest radiography. Participants received a prevalence and two annual incidence rounds of screening, followed by annual questionnaires after the screening rounds. The trial was designed to detect a 20% decrease in cumulative lung cancer mortality and results are expected in 2010. A second study, the NELSON trial, has also completed accrual and 20,000 high-risk participants were randomized to either low-dose CT screening or no screening of any type. CT scans were performed at baseline, year 1, and year 3, and the study will have an 80% power to detect a mortality reduction of 25%.

At present, no authoritative medical organization recommends screening for lung cancer in asymptomatic individuals, even if they are at high risk. As efforts at early detection have not yet demonstrated any reductions in mortality of lung cancer, and given the considerable risks associated with lung biopsy and surgery, both the American Cancer Society and American College of Chest Physicians (ACCP) do not recommend the routine use of low dose CT for screening for lung cancer.

Smoking cessation

Smoking is common in patients who present with lung cancer. As continuation of smoking is associated with poorer survival, patients who have undergone a curative treatment should be strongly encouraged to stop smoking, and offered pharmacotherapeutic and behavioural therapy. Smoking abstinence of at least 4 weeks prior to surgery is associated with reduced perioperative respiratory complications. Short-term benefits of cessation include a rapid decline in risk of acute myocardial infarction and stroke. In addition, continued cigarette smoking results in a significantly worse disease-free and OS in patients who have undergone a curative resection for stage I NSCLC. A poorer survival is also seen in patients who continued to smoke after treatment for limited-stage SCLC. Smoking cessation at the time of diagnosis of lung cancer may also reduce the rate of development of second tumours of the lung and aero-digestive tract. Continuing smoking increases the risk of second lung cancers even more in some groups of patients. For example, the risk of a second lung cancer is increased 13-fold among survivors with SCLC who received chest irradiation, and is higher in patients who continue smoking.

Smoking cessation remains a formidable challenge for many patients, and ACCP guidelines recommend offering intensive tobacco cessation programmes, including counselling, behavioural therapy, the use of sustained-release bupropion and nicotine replacement, and telephone follow-up, all of which have been shown to increase successful abstinence significantly. On a population basis, efforts to decrease smoking work remarkably well, and achieving a major decrease in tobacco deaths in the first half of the 21st century does require many current smokers to stop. In contrast, a big decrease over the next decade or two in the number who start smoking in the population as a whole, will only produce a big decrease in deaths around the middle and the second half of the present century

Further reading

Doll R, Peto R, Boreham J, et al. Mortality in relation to smoking: 50 years' observations on male British doctors. *BMJ* 2004; **328**:1519–28.

Ferlay J, Autier P, Boniol M, et al. Estimates of the cancer incidence and mortality in Europe in 2006. *Ann Oncol* 2007; **18**:581–92.

Jemal A, Siegel R, Ward E, et al. Cancer statistics, 2008. *CA Cancer J Clin* 2008; **58**:71–96.

Rubins J, Unger M, Colice GL; American College of Chest Physicians. Follow-up and surveillance of the lung cancer patient following curative intent therapy: ACCP evidence-based clinical practice guideline (2nd edition). *Chest* 2007; **132**(3 Suppl): 355S–367S.

Internet resource

http://www.deathsfromsmoking.net

Lung cancer: diagnosis and staging

Clinical features

Symptoms of lung cancer are often non-specific and difficult to distinguish from symptoms related to chronic obstructive airway disease, which commonly coexists in such patients. Consequently, most patients present with late stage disease, and only a minority present with early stage disease. General symptoms related to advanced stage of the tumour include fatigue, weight loss, and anaemia. Common thoracic symptoms at presentation include persistent cough, shortness of breath, chest pain, and haemoptysis. Other symptoms may relate to sites of metastases, with the commonest sites being the lung, liver, adrenals, bone, and brain.

Staging

All patients with newly diagnosed lung cancer should have a clinical history taken and physical examination performed. Particular note should be made of the performance status of the patient (Table 4.3.1). Simple blood investigations including haemoglobin, alkaline phosphatase, transaminases, and LDH may suggest the presence of distant metastases.

A correct diagnosis and appropriate staging are essential for determining the treatment plan and for providing prognostic information. All staging should be according to the TNM system (Table 4.3.2). The goals of staging are to obtain a precise pathological diagnosis, determine the extent of disease, to assess comorbidity and determine fitness of patients with non-metastatic disease to undergo either a resection or curative radiotherapy after evaluation of comorbidity and pulmonary function. Staging investigations should be performed in a logical fashion in order to minimize unnecessary, expensive, or invasive tests. In a patient with a histological diagnosis, extensive staging is inappropriate if initial investigations have already identified metastatic disease. For small cell lung cancer (SCLC), the tumour is further grouped into limited or extensive stage, with the former including tumours that can be encompassed within one radiation port.

Table 4.3.1 ECOG performance status scale (Oken et al. 1982)

Grade	ECOG
0	Fully active, able to carry on all pre-disease performance without restriction
1	Restricted in physically strenuous activity but ambulatory and able to carry out work of a light or sedentary nature, e.g. light house work, office work
2	Ambulatory and capable of all self-care but unable to carry out any work activities. Up and about >50% of waking hours
3	Capable of only limited self-care, confined to bed or chair >50% of waking hours
4	Completely disabled. Cannot carry on any self-care. Totally confined to bed or chair
5	Dead

Clinical imaging

Patients should undergo a CT scan of the chest and upper abdomen, which should include the liver, upper abdomen, and adrenal glands. Intravenous contrast should be administered unless contraindicated. A CT scan provides good anatomical detail which allows the T-stage to be established, and may provide information on the resectability of the tumour, although a definitive decision on resectability should be made only after discussion within a multidisciplinary team that includes a thoracic surgeon. A short-axis nodal diameter of ≥10mm is considered to be suspicious for metastases, and a contrast-enhanced CT can accurately detect such nodes. However, staging in this manner is of limited value as small nodes may contain metastasis and large nodes may be benign. Studies correlating nodal size with pathology reveal low sensitivity (57%) and a positive predictive value of only 56%. CT scans can assist in selecting the best procedure for sampling suspect LN regions.

FDG-PET is superior to CT in estimating T, N, and M disease. The routine use of PET is now recommended by the American College of Chest Physicians as a standard staging investigation for stages IB-IIIB prior to a curative treatment. Interpretation of PET images is improved by using fusion PET-CT scanners that allow for better anatomical localization of PET abnormalities. The latter can in turn further improve the accuracy of T, N, and M staging. PET is clearly superior for staging mediastinal nodal disease, and an overview of published studies showed the sensitivity of PET versus CT was 85% versus 61%, with a specificity of 90 versus 79% (Gould et al. 2003). However, PET is more sensitive but less specific when the CT scan shows enlarged mediastinal lymph nodes than when it does not (Ung et al. 2008). Therefore, positive findings on PET should be confirmed by biopsy before curative surgery is excluded as a treatment option, and negative PET findings should be interpreted in the light of a patient's pre-test probability of mediastinal metastases and whether CT reveals enlarged mediastinal nodes. The negative predictive value of PET is decreased in the case of patients with central tumours, hilar N1-disease on PET scan, bronchoalveolar cell carcinoma, and PET-negative mediastinal nodes measuring ≥16 mm.

A major role of PET is in excluding patients with distant metastasis from local treatment, and extrathoracic metastases are detected in 4–17% of patients in whom conventional staging showed no evidence of metastases (Ung 2008). Specifically, staging PET scans reduce the number of unnecessary thoracotomies in patients diagnosed with lung cancer, and shorten the median time to establishing a diagnosis of lung cancer when compared to a traditional staging workup. Up to 30% of conventionally-staged stage III patients referred for radical radiotherapy are excluded after a PET scan, mainly due to the detection of occult metastatic disease.

For solitary pulmonary nodules, PET has high sensitivity and intermediate specificity for identifying malignant pulmonary nodules but data for nodules measuring 1cm in diameter is limited. Additional studies of PET are required in populations with low prevalence of NSCLC. In some regions and countries, a higher percentage of false negative FDG-PET scans for both parenchymal lesions and nodes

Table 4.3.2 TNM staging system

T:	**primary tumour**
T1:	tumour ≤3cm diameter, surrounded by lung or visceral pleura, without invasion more proximal than lobar bronchus
• **T1a:**	tumour ≤2cm in diameter
• **T1b:**	tumour >2cm but ≤3cm in diameter
T2:	tumour >3 cm but ≤7cm, or tumor with any of the following features**:**
• Involves main bronchus, ≥2cm distal to carina	
• Invades visceral pleura	
• Associated with atelectasis or obstructive pneumonitis that extends to the hilar region but does not involve the entire lung	
• **T2a:**	tumour >3cm but ≤5cm
• **T2b:**	tumour >5cm but ≤7cm
T3:	tumour >7cm or any of the following**:**
• Directly invades any of the following: chest wall, diaphragm, phrenic nerve, mediastinal pleura, parietal pericardium, main bronchus <2cm from carina (without involvement of carina)	
• Atelectasis or obstructive pneumonitis of the entire lung	
• Separate tumour nodules in the same lobe	
T4:	tumour of any size that invades the mediastinum, heart, great vessels, trachea, recurrent laryngeal nerve, oesophagus, vertebral body, carina, or with separate tumour nodules in a different ipsilateral lobe
N:	**regional lymph nodes**
NX:	regional lymph nodes cannot be assessed
N0:	no regional lymph node metastasis
N1:	metastasis in ipsilateral peribronchial and/or ipsilateral hilar lymph nodes and intrapulmonary nodes, including involvement by direct extension
N2:	metastasis in ipsilateral mediastinal and/or subcarinal lymph nodes
N3:	metastasis in contralateral mediastinal, contralateral hilar, ipsilateral or contralateral scalene, or supraclavicular lymph nodes
M: distant metastasis	
MX:	distant metastasis cannot be assessed
M0:	no distant metastasis
M1:	distant metastasis
M1a:	separate tumour nodule(s) in a contralateral lobe; tumour with pleural nodules or malignant pleural or pericardial effusion
M1b:	distant metastasis
Composite staging	
Stage 0:	TisN0M0
Stage Ia:	T1N0M0
Stage Ib:	T2aN0M0
Stage IIa:	T1–2aN1M0, T2bN0M0
Stage IIb:	T2bN1M0; T3N0M0
Stage IIIa:	T1–2N2 M0; T3N1–2 M0, T4N0–1M0
Stage IIIb:	T4N2M0; any TN3M0
Stage IV:	any T, any NM1

are seen due to granulomatous or other inflammatory diseases.

MRI is of limited value except in special circumstances, such as assessing the relationship of tumour with large blood vessels, soft tissues, or vertebral body in patients with tumours of the superior sulcus. MRI is also superior to CT scan in detecting brain metastases.

Invasive staging: preoperative

In patients who do not have distant metastases, the presence and extent of mediastinal nodal disease is essential for determining treatment strategy (Robinson et al. 2003). Invasive nodal staging procedures can be omitted in patients with peripheral tumours and negative mediastinal PET images. As stated earlier, however, invasive staging is recommended for central tumours, hilar N1 disease on PET, low FDG uptake in the primary tumour and nodes with a short axis diameter of ≥16mm on CT scan. PET-positive mediastinal findings should always be confirmed by means of cytology or histology. Mediastinoscopy has long been considered as the gold standard in mediastinal staging, since the era preceding high quality CT scans and PET scans. There is growing evidence for the efficacy of endobronchial ultrasound (EBUS) and oesophageal ultrasound fine needle aspiration (EUS-FNA) approaches to mediastinal staging in NSCLC. Routine use of EUS-FNA in diagnosis and staging of lung cancer in 242 consecutive patients prevented 70% of the scheduled surgical procedures (mediastinoscopy or exploratory thoracotomy), and accuracy of EUS-FNA in mediastinal staging was 93% (Annema et al. 2005).

Intraoperative staging

Clear definitions for the use of procedures such as nodal sampling, systematic nodal sampling, systematic nodal dissection, and lobe-specific systematic nodal dissection have been published by the European Society of Thoracic Surgery (De Leyn et al. 2007). Systematic sampling or nodal dissection improves intraoperative nodal staging in contrast to selective lymph node sampling, especially regarding the detection of multilevel N2 disease. It is unclear if more extensive LN dissection influences survival or recurrence rate of the disease and the results of completed clinical trials are awaited. A removal of at least six lymph nodes from hilar and mediastinal stations is recommended in order to stage nodal disease accurately. It has been recommended that lymph node assessment be performed before performing any lung resection. Data on the compliance with these guidelines in routine practice is awaited.

Further reading

Annema JT, Versteegh MI, Veselic M, et al. Endoscopic ultrasound-guided fine-needle aspiration in the diagnosis and staging of lung cancer and its impact on surgical staging. *J Clin Oncol* 2005; **23**:8357–61.

De Leyn P, Lardinois D, Van Schil P, et al. European trends in preoperative and intraoperative nodal staging: ESTS guidelines. *J Thorac Oncol* 2007; **2**:357–61.

Gould MK, Kuschner WG, Rydzak CE, et al. Test performance of positron emission tomography and computed tomography for mediastinal staging in patients with non-small-cell lung cancer: a meta-analysis. *Ann Intern Med* 2003; **139**:879–92.

Oken MM, Creech RH, Tormey DC, et al. Toxicity And Response Criteria Of The Eastern Cooperative Oncology Group. *Am J Clin Oncol* 1982; **5**:649–55.

Robinson LA, Ruckdeschel JC, Wagner H Jr, et al.; American College of Chest Physicians. Treatment of non-small cell lung cancer-stage IIIA: ACCP evidence-based clinical practice guidelines (2nd edition). *Chest* 2007 Sep; **132**(3 Suppl):243S–265S

Toloza EM, Harpole L, McCrory DC. Noninvasive staging of non-small cell lung cancer: a review of the current evidence. *Chest* 2003; **123**:137S–146S.

Ung YC, Maziak DE, Vanderveen JA, et al. 18Fluorodeoxyglucose positron emission tomography in the diagnosis and staging of lung cancer: a systematic review. *J Natl Cancer Inst* 2007; **99**:1753–67.

Internet resource

National Comprehensive Cancer Network: http://www.nccn.org

Lung cancer: pathology and therapeutic implications

Histological types

The WHO classification system is based upon morphological features of diagnosis and the molecular biology of the various lung malignancies (Travis et al. 2004). A practical, treatment-based approach broadly divides lung tumours into NSCLC and SCLC.

NSCLC include SCC, adenocarcinoma, and large-cell carcinoma (LCC), but broadly includes any epithelial tumour that lacks a small cell component. SCC typically presents as a central mass but approximately 25% are located peripherally. In the past, this was the predominant histological subtype of lung cancer. However, adenocarcinoma is the predominant histological subtype of lung carcinoma in many countries, and the incidence in Europe has increased in the last three decades. Adenocarcinoma consists of five subtypes, namely acinar, papillary, bronchioloalveolar, adenocarcinoma with mixed subtypes, and solid carcinoma with mucus formation. The mixed subtype is the commonest histological type of adenocarcinoma as most tumours are histologically heterogeneous and consist of more than one subtype. Adenocarcinoma is the most prevalent form of lung cancer in younger males and in women of all ages, in never smokers (smoked <100 cigarettes in lifetime), and in former smokers. Differences in tobacco smoking habits (e.g. use of filters, light tobacco cigarettes, deep inhalation) have been postulated as the reason for favouring the development of distal bronchiolar and alveolar carcinogenesis at the expense of proximal SCC.

Bronchioloalveolar carcinoma (BAC) is a subtype of lung adenocarcinoma with unique pathological, clinical, and molecular characteristics. The definition of BAC requires that the tumour be comprised entirely of a lepidic pattern of growth without evidence of stromal, vascular, or pleural invasion. Three types of BAC are recognized, including non-mucinous, mucinous, and mixed mucinous and non-mucinous. The initial radiographic presentation varies considerably, from single ground glass opacities (GGOs) or nodules of mixed ground glass and solid attenuation to diffuse consolidative or bilateral multinodular disease. Classically, BAC demonstrates a relatively slow growth pattern and indolent clinical course. However, rapid growth and death from bilateral diffuse consolidative disease occurs within months of diagnosis or recurrence in a subset of patients.

A final diagnosis of BAC requires examination of the entire tumour to rule out areas of invasion, and should not be made on a small biopsy or cytological specimen. BAC represents <5% of adenocarcinomas, but as many as 20% of adenocarcinomas have some features of BAC and these tumours are more likely to have mutations in the EGFR gene and to be sensitive to EGFR tyrosine kinase inhibitors. The rising incidence of BAC is also reflected in recent lung cancer screening studies employing helical CT.

LCC accounts for approximately 10% of all lung cancers, and is defined as an undifferentiated non-SCC that lacks cytological features of SCC and glandular or squamous differentiation. LCC includes five variants: the subtypes of large-cell neuroendocrine carcinoma (LCNEC), basaloid carcinoma, lymphoepithelial-like carcinoma, clear cell carcinoma, and LCC with rhabdoid phenotype.

Tumours with neuroendocrine morphology

Neuroendocrine tumours of the lung are a distinctive subset which share morphological, immunohistochemical, and ultrastructural features (Beasley 2005). The main sub-types include low-grade typical carcinoid (TC), the intermediate grade atypical carcinoid (AC), and the two high-grade tumours, LCNEC and SCLC.

TC is defined as a neuroendocrine tumour with <2 mitoses per $2mm^2$ and lacking necrosis, while AC is defined as a neuroendocrine tumour with either 2–10 mitoses per $2mm^2$ or necrosis. Most AC will meet both criteria but occasional AC will have necrosis and <2 mitoses per 2mm.

LCNEC is defined as a neuroendocrine tumour with >10 mitoses/$2mm^2$ and cytological features of LCC. Evidence of neuroendocrine differentiation must be demonstrated by ancillary methods such as immunohistochemistry using a specific marker such as chromogranin or synaptophysin. Only tumours showing *both* neuroendocrine morphology and positive staining should be classified as LCNEC as up to 20% of conventional adenocarcinoma, SCC, or LCC, will stain with neuroendocrine markers. Such tumours have been designated as non-small cell lung carcinoma with neuroendocrine differentiation (NSCLC-ND). It is presently unclear if NSCLC-ND has a worse prognosis or responds differently to chemotherapy than conventional NSCLC, as reports have been conflicting.

SCLC is defined as a neuroendocrine tumour with >10 mitoses/$2mm^2$ and small cell cytological features. Cells are typically oval to slightly spindled in shape and have scant cytoplasm. Nuclei are hyperchromatic and have absent to very small nucleoli. SCLC comprises approximately 20% of all lung cancers and most present as central tumours with extensive mediastinal adenopathy. Only 5% of SCLC present as a peripheral coin lesions.

Therapeutic implications

An accurate histological diagnosis of the subtype of lung cancer is essential in order to formulate the treatment plan and it is no longer sufficient to simply separate NSCLC from small cell lung cancer. Subtypes of NSCLC can differ in their response to chemotherapeutic agents such as pemetrexed and gemcitabine, and some molecular targeted agents show more activity in adenocarcinoma, while others are more active in SCC. Consequently, the role of pathology is playing a greater role in choice of local and systemic therapy.

Key points

Main sub-types of lung cancer are
- NSCLC, including SCC, adenocarcinoma, and LCC
- SCLC

Subtypes of NSCLC are increasingly important in determining therapeutic strategies with new targeted therapies and systemic chemotherapy regimens.

Further reading

Travis WD, Garg K, Franklin WA, *et al.* Bronchioloalveolar carcinoma and lung adenocarcinoma: the clinical importance and research relevance of the 2004 World Health Organization pathologic criteria. *J Thorac Oncol* 2006; **1**(9 Suppl):S13–9.

Travis WD, Muller-Hermelink H-K, Harris CC, *et al.* *Pathology and Genetics of Tumours of the Lung, Pleura, Thymus and Heart.* Lyon: IARC Press, 2004.

Treatment of stage I non-small-cell lung cancer

Background

Only 20% of patients with lung cancer present with stage I NSCLC (T1–2N0M0). Even after a complete surgical excision, the 5-year survival is <70% due to tumour recurrence, non-cancer related mortality, and second malignancies (Rami-Porta et al. 2007). Long-term follow-up reveals that survival rates decrease further between 5 and 10-years, from 62% to 49%, respectively (Pasini et al. 2003). Extrapulmonary malignancies other than lung cancer occur in 11.2%, within a median time of 52 months. The presence of a previous tumour is an independent prognostic factor in a resected case of pathological stage I NSCLC, with the probability of death increasing by 1.5 times at 5 years (Lopez-Encuentra et al. 2007).

A wait-and-see policy is inappropriate as the 5-year OS in untreated stage I NSCLC is 6–14%, and the median survival ranges from 9–14 months (Haasbeek et al. 2008). It is therefore recommended that surgical resection or other ablative therapies should not be delayed for even small lung tumours.

In addition to the standard staging procedures discussed for a case of suspected lung cancer, addition of a PET scan correctly shows more advanced disease stages IIIA–IV in approximately 7.4% of patients with a clinical stage IA NSCLC (Kozower et al. 2008). However, due to a high false positive rate, the positive predictive value for advanced disease was only 33.3% and the negative predictive value of PET to predict benign lesions was only 57%. A total of 43% of patients with a PET-negative primary lung lesion in this analysis actually had cancer, and all of these had resectable disease (stages IA–IIB). The role of PET is more useful in this setting for the detection of distant metastases that it is for confirming the primary diagnosis of malignancy.

Surgery

The belief that surgery offers the best hope of a cure is based on retrospective data from the literature, and surgery is the present standard of care. All patients with early stage NSCLC should be seen and evaluated in a MDT, which includes a thoracic surgeon, in order to determine whether they are a candidate for surgical exploration and resection. Other local therapies such as stereotactic radiation or RF ablation may be appropriate for patients who are medically unfit for surgery. The use of these techniques in patients who are surgical candidates should not occur outside the context of a clinical research study.

A lobectomy is the recommended procedure but 8–10% of patients undergo a pneumonectomy for a stage I NSCLC, a finding which is of concern as pneumonectomy adversely influences survival. Previous trials had suggested that sublobar resections (e.g. wedge resection or segmentectomy) were associated with an increase in local recurrence, although a meta-analysis of reported studies to compare survival of stage I patients undergoing limited resection and standard lobectomy revealed no impact on survival.

It has been recommended that the surgical mortality risk for lobectomy should be expected to be <4%, and for a pneumonectomy <9%. Mortality rates after surgery for lung cancer are lower in patients whose operation was performed by specialist thoracic surgeons as opposed to general surgeons. Another study revealed that patients who undergo resection for lung cancer at hospitals that perform large numbers of such procedures are likely to survive longer, and also develop fewer postoperative complications with lower 30-day mortality, than patients who have such surgery at hospitals with a low volume of lung-resection procedures (Bach et al. 2001). The increased mortality in elderly patients is of concern as population-based studies reveal a mortality after lobectomy of 2.4% in patients aged 60–65 years, compared with a mortality of 4.9% in patients aged ≥70 years. This finding is of concern as nearly 50% of new patients are aged ≥70, with 14% aged ≥80 years.

The extent of lymph node evaluation at the time of surgical resection of stage I tumours continues to be a matter of debate. Current guidelines of the European Society of Thoracic Surgeons recommend a systematic nodal dissection in all cases, but lobe-specific systematic nodal dissections were considered acceptable for peripheral squamous T1 tumours and if hilar and interlobar nodes were negative on frozen section studies (Lardinois et al. 2006). Lobe-specific nodal dissections imply removal of at least three hilar and interlobar nodes and three mediastinal nodes from three stations, which always includes the subcarinal nodes.

Serious postoperative complications occur in up to 38% of patients operated for a stage I NSCLC, including air-leaks exceeding 7 days, chest drain placement for >7 days, atrial arrhythmia, and respiratory complications (Allen et al. 2006). In patients with stage I–II NSCLC, surgery has a substantial impact on health-related quality of life, and at 2 years after surgery, 31–33% of patients with disease recurrence reported the same or worse chest pain and arm or shoulder pain compared with before surgery (Kenny et al. 2008).

Postsurgical adjuvant treatment

Large differences in outcome are observed within stage I after surgery, with 5-year OS ranging from 77% for small T1 tumours to 35% for large T2 tumours. Approximately 20% of patients staged with both conventional imaging and PET will develop recurrent NSCLC, and the sites of recurrence with the addition of PET are similar to those reported with staging by conventional imaging alone. The most common site of first recurrence is the thorax, followed by the brain, bone, and adrenal glands. Neither postoperative radiotherapy nor adjuvant systemic chemotherapy have been shown to improve survival in resected stage I NSCLC. Recent work identifying gene expression profiles that predict for poor outcome indicates that this may be an approach to identify patients with stage I NSCLC prospectively who are most likely to benefit from adjuvant therapy. However, these prognostic factors will first have to be tested in prospective randomized clinical trials in order to determine their usefulness as predictive factors for adjuvant chemotherapy.

Primary radiotherapy

The results of conventional radiotherapy for stage I NSCLC have been poor, with SEER data showing lung cancer-specific survival rates ranging from 69% at 1 year, 29% at 3 years and 15% at 5 years. The poor local control after conventional radiotherapy has been explained partly by errors in target definition for radiotherapy due to tumour motion, and to low biological tumour doses.

Conventional radiotherapy fractionations used are 60–66Gy in 30–33 fractions and 55Gy in 20 fractions. A randomized study of continuous hyperfractionated accelerated radiotherapy (CHART) delivering 54Gy in 36 fractions over 12 consecutive days (3 fractions per day, 6 hours apart) produced a 10% improvement in survival.

A major development in the last decade has been stereotactic radiotherapy, which is a non-invasive technique characterized by accurate patient repositioning during treatment simulation and delivery, and by use of ablative doses that are typically delivered in 3–5 fractions. Stereotactic radiotherapy can achieve 2-year local control rates in excess of 90% (Lagerwaard et al. 2008). High-grade toxicity is limited to approximately 5% of patients despite the use of very high doses of radiation. In non-randomized studies, the reported local control achieved using this approach is far higher than that achieved using 6–7 weeks of conventional radiotherapy or even with accelerated schemes such as CHART. Departments within Europe have been quick to implement SRT and tailored treatment planning is generally performed using respiration-correlated (or four-dimensional) CT scans.

Despite the high local control rates, the late CT appearance after stereotactic radiotherapy may require careful

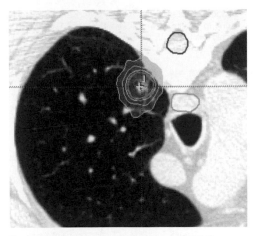

Fig. 4.3.1 Stereotactic radiotherapy for stage I NSCLC. Dose distributions achieved in high-dose stereotactic radiotherapy for a paravertebral tumour. Using nine non-coplanar beams, a dose of 12Gy was prescribed per fraction to the 80% isodose (light green). Rapid dose-fall off results in <20% of the prescribed dose to the contoured oesophagus and spinal cord. The biological effective dose achieved is 180Gy, which contrasts to the 66–7Gy typically delivered using conventional radiotherapy (see also colour plate section).

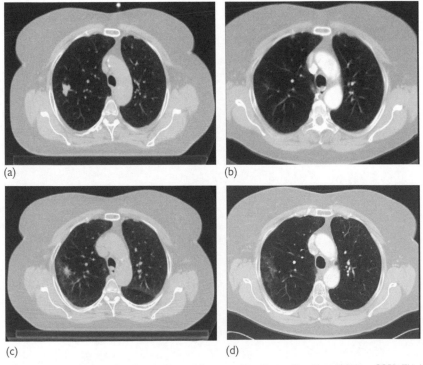

(a) (b)

(c) (d)

Fig. 4.3.2 Radiological changes after stereotactic radiotherapy in lung cancer in a 60-year-old patient with severe COPD. This lesion (A) was treated to a dose of 60Gy in 3 fractions in 2003, 2 years after the patient first presented with a growing lesion in the right upper lobe which showed intense FDG-PET uptake. Attempts at obtaining histology were unsuccessful. Serial post-treatment CT scans revealed residual ground glass changes at 12 months (B), but the parenchymal changes became more extensive at 26 (C) and 46 months (D). Repeat FDG-PET scans at 26 and 52 months revealed no uptake in the treated region.

evaluation as radiation fibrosis may give rise to a mass-like pattern in nearly 20% of cases (Figs. 4.3.1 and 4.3.2). Watchful waiting, with serial CT scans and, where indicated PET scans, is useful in distinguishing fibrosis from residual tumour.

Prospective study of quality of life and pulmonary function reveals that these are generally well preserved in patients treated using stereotactic radiotherapy. Randomized clinical trials of primary surgery versus stereotactic radiotherapy in patients with operable stage IA NSCLC are currently in progress.

Further reading

Allen MS, Darling GE, Pechet TT, et al. Morbidity and mortality of major pulmonary resections in patients with early-stage lung cancer: initial results of the randomized, prospective ACOSOG Z0030 trial. Ann Thorac Surg 2006; 81:1013–9.

Bach PB, Cramer LD, Schrag D, et al. The influence of hospital volume on survival after resection for lung cancer. N Engl J Med 2001; 345:181–8.

Haasbeek CJ, Senan S, Smit EF, et al. Critical review of nonsurgical treatment options for stage I non-small cell lung cancer. Oncologist 2008; 13:309–19.

Kenny PM, King MT, Viney RC, et al. Quality of life and survival in the 2 years after surgery for non small-cell lung cancer. J Clin Oncol 2008; 26:233–41.

Kozower BD, Meyers BF, Reed CE, et al. Does positron emission tomography prevent nontherapeutic pulmonary resections for clinical stage IA lung cancer? Ann Thorac Surg 2008; 85:1166–9.

Lagerwaard FJ, Haasbeek CJ, Smit EF, et al. Outcomes of risk-adapted fractionated stereotactic radiotherapy for stage I non-small-cell lung cancer. Int J Radiat Oncol Biol Phys 2008; 70:685–92.

Lardinois D, De Leyn P, Van Schil P, et al. ESTS guidelines for intra-operative lymph node staging in non-small cell lung cancer. Eur J Cardiothorac Surg 2006; 30:787–92.

López-Encuentra A, Gómez de la Cámara A, Rami-Porta R, et al. Previous tumour as a prognostic factor in stage I non-small cell lung cancer. Thorax 2007; 62:386–90.

Pasini F, Pelosi G, Valduga F, et al. Late events and clinical prognostic factors in stage I non small cell lung cancer. Lung Cancer 2002; 37:171–7

Rami-Porta R, Ball D, Crowley J, et al. The IASLC Lung Cancer Staging Project: proposals for the revision of the T descriptors in the forthcoming (seventh) edition of the TNM classification for lung cancer. J Thorac Oncol 2007; 2:593–602.

Lung cancer: treatment of stages II and III non-small-cell lung cancer

The approach to treatment of stages II and III NSCLC has been the subject of reviews by the American College of Chest Physicians and National Comprehensive Cancer Network, as well as a meta-analysis of trials evaluating adjuvant chemotherapy.

Assessing patient fitness to undergo surgery

Fitness to undergo an anatomical resection requires assessment of both comorbidity and pulmonary function tests (Colice et al. 2007). In patients who have impaired lung function, as evidenced by either an FEV_1 or DLCO value of <80% of predicted, the likely postoperative pulmonary reserve should be estimated. An estimated postoperative FEV_1 or DLCO <40% predicted indicates an increased risk for perioperative complications following a standard resection. In case of the latter, cardiopulmonary exercise testing to measure maximal oxygen consumption (VO_2max) should be performed to further define the perioperative risk of surgery. It has been recommended that the surgical mortality risk for lobectomy should be expected to be ≤ 4%, and for a pneumonectomy ≤9%.

Stage II

A complete surgical resection is the treatment of choice in patients with stage II NSCLC (N1 node metastases), and parenchyma-sparing excisions such as a sleeve lobectomy are preferred to a pneumonectomy. In spite of a complete resection, the 5-year disease-specific survival in such patients is only around 44%, with corresponding 5-year OS being around 34%. Following a resection in patients with a good PS, the use of platinum-based adjuvant chemotherapy leads to a significantly better survival (Pignon et al. 2008). The effect of chemotherapy did not vary significantly with the associated drugs, including vinorelbine, etoposide, or vinca alkaloids. The benefits of chemotherapy were higher in patients with better PS.

Medically-inoperable stage II NSCLC

For patients with stage II NSCLC who are not candidates for surgery ('medically inoperable') or who refuse surgery, curative concurrent chemoradiotherapy should be considered in patients who are fit to receive both treatments. If any form of chemotherapy is contraindicated, accelerated fractionated radiotherapy is recommended in order to minimize the amount of accelerated tumour-cell repopulation observed once therapy is initiated. Some groups perform accelerated radiotherapy by delivering two or three treatments per day, with time allowed between each dose to minimize late radiation toxicity. Another approach that was used in a recent European phase III trial was to use once-daily fractions of 2.75Gy to deliver a dose of 66Gy in 5 weeks, and this scheme is feasible in patients with small volume disease who have received prior induction chemotherapy.

Stage III

Approximately 30% of new NSCLC cases present with stage III disease, of which 12.1% have stage IIIA and 17.6% stage IIIB disease. The 5-year OS figures for clinically staged IIIA and IIIB disease are only 18% and 8% respectively, and corresponding figures for pathologically staged IIIA and IIIB disease 25% and 19%, respectively. The poor outcomes observed are due to locoregional failure rates of approximately 30%, with distant failure rates in the range of 40–60%. Two randomized phase III trials in patients with stage IIIA NSCLC have compared chemoradiotherapy only with combined modality treatments that included surgery, and they showed no survival benefit for surgery in patients with stage III N2 disease. In a study where responders to induction chemotherapy were randomized to receive either surgical resection or radiotherapy, the median and 5-year OS were 16.4 versus 17.5 months and 15.7% versus 14%, respectively (van Meerbeeck et al. 2007). Rates of PFS were also similar in both groups.

ACCP guidelines state that in NSCLC patients with N2 disease identified preoperatively, induction therapy followed by surgery is not recommended except as part of a clinical trial. In particular, surgery should be avoided in patients with 'bulky nodal disease' which was defined as lymph nodes ≥2cm in short-axis diameter measured on chest CT scan, especially with extranodal involvement, multiple station nodal disease, and/or groupings of multiple positive smaller lymph nodes. In addition, there is strong evidence to indicate that surgical resection should be avoided after induction therapy in patients who have definite biopsy-proven residual tumour in the mediastinal nodes.

In stage IIIB NSCLC, surgery appears indicated for carefully selected patients with T4N0–1M0 such as tumours of the superior sulcus, a potentially unique subgroup of patients for whom surgery may contribute to long-term survival and cure. When technically operable, these relatively uncommon superior sulcus tumours are widely treated with cisplatin-based concurrent chemoradiotherapy to around 46Gy, followed by surgical resection. All other patients with stage IIIB NSCLC with a good performance score and minimal weight loss, are treated with combined chemoradiotherapy.

Chemoradiotherapy delivered concurrently is the preferred treatment for prospectively recognized stage IIIA lung cancer with all degrees of mediastinal lymph node involvement (Robinson et al. 2007). A meta-analysis of trials comparing sequential chemoradiation with concomitant chemoradiation found no difference in pulmonary toxicity between the sequential and concomitant treatments, but the relative risk of grade 3 or 4 oesophagitis was higher in the group treated with concomitant therapy (Auperin et al. 2007). There was improved survival in the group receiving concomitant treatment, translating to an absolute improvement in survival of 5.7% at 3 years. Compared to the sequential group which had a survival of 10.6% at 5 years, the survival of 15.1% at 5 years in the concomitant group represented an absolute increase of 4.5%. These benefits seem primarily attributable to a decrease in locoregional progression in the concomitant therapy group, albeit at the expense of increased oesophageal toxicity. Although most clinicians use a combination of a platinum-containing regimen and radiotherapy, no reference regimen for inoperable stage III NSCLC has yet been established by randomized trials.

Choice of chemotherapy schemes

The greatest body of data from phase III trials has been reported using full-dose cisplatin–etoposide. The optimal chemotherapy agents and the number of cycles of treatment to combine with radiotherapy are uncertain. The addition of full-dose chemotherapy before or after concomitant therapy, with the aim of reducing the burden of systemic micro-metastases, may theoretically improve these results. There are few randomized trials that have addressed the question of whether additional chemotherapy given outside the setting of the concomitant phase of therapy enhances the overall efficacy of the treatment.

Choice of radiotherapy schemes

Total doses ranging from 60–66Gy, delivered in once-daily fractions of 1.8–2Gy have been the commonest scheme used with full dose chemotherapy. Recommendations for minimal standards of radiotherapy planning and delivery have been published by EORTC (Senan et al. 2004). Although higher radiation doses are feasible, there is little evidence to support the routine use of a dose >60Gy when systemic doses of chemotherapy are administered concurrently with radiation. Involved-field radiotherapy is the current standard of care in all stages of NSCLC. Recent advances in radiotherapy imaging, such as four-dimensional CT scans and cone-beam CT scans, allow for individualized treatment planning margins to account for motion, and also ensure improved patient set-up during daily treatments. The benefits of the traditional approach of using radiotherapy fields which encompassed the uninvolved mediastinal nodal stations, and occasionally the ipsilateral supraclavicular region, in order to treat potential subclinical disease have not been clearly demonstrated. Multiple daily fractions of radiotherapy when combined with chemotherapy have not been shown to result in improved survival compared with standard once-daily radiotherapy combined with chemotherapy. Accelerated radiotherapy schemes, using either multiple daily fractions or larger once-daily doses, are commonly applied in patients who are unfit to undergo optimal concurrent chemoradiotherapy.

Adjuvant management of completely resected stages II and III NSCLC

The adjuvant management of stage III disease consists of cisplatin-based chemotherapy which improves survival with a HR of 0.83 (95% CI, 0.72–0.94). However the locoregional failure rate remains 20–40% in this setting, and data from non-randomized trials suggest higher survival in patients with N2 disease who had postoperative radiotherapy than in those with observation only. This finding has renewed interest in adjuvant radiotherapy after resection and a large phase III European trial will shortly address this question.

Options for patients with a poor performance status

A significant proportion of stage III patients cannot tolerate optimal chemoradiotherapy due to significant comorbidities. In patients who are at risk of toxicity, sequential CT-RT remains a viable option as radiation oncologists can tailor treatment to a reduced dose and/or volume in patients who are deemed too frail. Postplanning assessment of a proposed treatment includes a calculation of the V_{20} (percentage volume of normal lung minus PTV which receives doses of 20Gy or more). Patients with a V_{20} in excess of 35% not only have an increased risk of high-grade radiation pneumonitis, but also a significantly poorer survival. Presentations such as extensive N2 involvement, bilateral hilar node disease and a peripheral tumour in the lower lobe with contralateral upper mediastinal nodes are examples of cases where clinicians can assume a large V_{20} will result from any radiotherapy plan, and thus make alternative decisions regarding treatment up front.

Further reading

Auperin A, Rolland E, Curran WJ, et al. Concomitant radio-chemotherapy (RT-CT) versus sequential RT-CT in locally advanced non-small cell lung cancer (NSCLC): A meta-analysis using individual patient data (IPD) from randomised clinical trials (RCTs). J Thorac Oncol 2007; 2:S310.

Colice GL, Shafazand S, Griffin JP, et al. Physiologic evaluation of the patient with lung cancer being considered for resectional surgery: ACCP evidenced-based clinical practice guidelines (2nd edition). Chest 2007; 132(3 Suppl):161S–77S.

Goldstraw PF. The IASLC Lung Cancer Staging Project: Proposals for the revision of the TNM stage groupings in the forthcoming (Seventh) edition of the TNM Classification of Malignant Tumours. J Thorac Oncol 2007; 2:706–14.

Pignon JP, Tribodet H, Scagliotti GV, et al. Lung adjuvant cisplatin evaluation: A pooled analysis by the LACE Collaborative Group. J Clin Oncol 2008; 26:3552–9.

Robinson LA, Ruckdeschel JC, Wagner H, Jr, et al. Treatment of non-small cell lung cancer-stage IIIA: ACCP evidence-based clinical practice guidelines (2nd edition). Chest 2007; 132:243S–65S.

Scott WJ, Howington J, Feigenberg S, et al.; American College of Chest Physicians. Treatment of non-small cell lung cancer stage I and stage II: ACCP evidence-based clinical practice guidelines (2nd edition). Chest 2007; 132(3 Suppl):234S–242S.

Senan S, De Ruysscher D, Giraud P, et al. Literature-based recommendations for treatment planning and execution in high-dose radiotherapy for lung cancer. Radiother Oncol 2004; 71:139–46

van Meerbeeck JP, Kramer GWPM, Van Schil PEY, et al. Randomized controlled trial of resection versus radiotherapy after induction chemotherapy in stage IIIA-N2 non-small-cell lung cancer. J National Cancer Inst 2007; 99:442–50.

Wisnivesky JP, Yankelevitz D, Henschke CI. Stage of lung cancer in relation to its size: Part 2. Evidence. Chest 2005; 127:1136–9.

Chemotherapy in stage IV non-small-cell lung cancer

The benefits of chemotherapy for stage IV NSCLC have become more clearly defined during the last decade. This review is based upon guidelines from National Comprehensive Cancer Network (2009) and American Society of Clinical Oncology (2009), as well as UK guidelines from NICE (2005), SIGN (2005), and COIN (2001).

First-line therapy

When is chemotherapy appropriate?

Patients with stage IV NSCLC and stage IIIB NSCLC with malignant pleural effusion are generally considered incurable. There is consensus that palliative chemotherapy should be offered to selected patients with incurable NSCLC in order to improve survival, symptom control and quality of life (NSCLC Meta-Analyses Collaborative Group 2008).

Those who receive chemotherapy in addition to best supportive care (BSC) have a significant increase in both 1 year survival from 20% to 29%, and median survival from 4.5 months to 6 months with chemotherapy treatment. Quality of life (QoL) in patients receiving chemotherapy was either no worse, or improved, and disease symptoms improved by approximately 60%, a larger proportion of patients than those demonstrating a radiological response.

The most significant factor used in selecting patients for chemotherapy treatment is WHO performance status (PS). Overall, patients with a PS ≤2 receive benefit from chemotherapy; however, the degree of benefit is less in patients with PS 2, in comparison to those with PS 0–1. In addition PS 2 patients are more susceptible to the adverse effects of chemotherapy. Therefore in PS 2, the benefit:risk ratio becomes more equal. As a result, PS 2 patients are often treated with less toxic agents, to increase the benefit:risk ratio, and there is often a lower threshold for withholding or withdrawing chemotherapy. There is no evidence to support the use of chemotherapy in patients with PS 3–4.

Patients of PS 0–1

In patients who are PS 0–1, in general first-line therapy is a combination of a platinum cytotoxic (carboplatin or cisplatin), with a third-generation cytotoxic (paclitaxel, docetaxol, gemcitabine, pemetrexed, or vinorelbine).

When compared with single-agent regimens, doublet regimens improved both radiological response and OS (Delbaldo et al. 2004). All trials of triplet regimens versus doublet regimens have failed to demonstrate a survival benefit and have consistently showed an increase in toxic adverse effects. Therefore the use of two cytotoxic agents in combination is the accepted standard.

Platinum doublets have demonstrated statistically significant improved survival compared with non-platinum doublets (D'Addario et al. 2005). However, there is no consensus on whether carboplatin or cisplatin is preferable. Although there is evidence from some meta-analysis that cisplatin is superior to carboplatin in terms of response rates and in some cases may be superior in terms of survival, it is generally felt to be more toxic, specifically with more nausea, hearing loss, and peripheral neuropathy. It is also time-consuming to administer cisplatin with the required hydration. In the absence of firm evidence that cisplatin improves OS, it is difficult to recommend cisplatin as the platinum of choice and, therefore, it is an individual decision for the clinician and patient whether the possible benefits outweigh the known risks.

Chemotherapy is stopped at disease progression or after four cycles. The recommended number of first-line chemotherapy cycles is 3 or 4. Three different trials have studied the optimal number of chemotherapy courses. The numbers of cycles compared have included: 4 versus 6, 3 versus 6, and 3 versus continuous therapy until progression. Although there is some evidence to suggest time-to-progression (TTP) and PFS can be increased by delivering 6 cycles of chemotherapy compared with 3 or 4, there is no OS advantage with >4 cycles of first-line chemotherapy (Park et al. 2007).

Individualized therapy

Until recently, there were no real tailored chemotherapy regimens based on patient or tumour characteristics as numerous trials comparing one platinum-based regimen with another failed to identify a superior regimen (Scagliotti et al. 2002). More recent trials have addressed how chemotherapy could be individualized, and this is the subject of much ongoing research. Although these are single trial findings and therefore should not be the sole deciding factor in selecting a chemotherapy regimen, they can be used in combination with a number of patient factors to direct therapy:

Selection by histology

It may be appropriate to select cisplatin/pemetrexed for patients with adenocarcinoma or LCCs, while opting for cisplatin/gemcitabine in SCCs. A preplanned subset analysis of a trial comparing cisplatin/pemetrexed to cisplatin/gemcitabine showed that those with adenocarcinoma (12.6 vs. 10.9 months) and LCC (10.4 vs. 6.7 months) had an increased OS with cisplatin/pemetrexed whilst those with SCC had a statistically significant increase in OS with cisplatin/gemcitabine (10.8 vs. 9.4 months) (Scagliotti et al. 2008).

Selection by EGFR mutation status

In patients with an EGFR mutation, first-line gefitinib, an EGFR inhibitor, can be used. Patients with a mutation have a statistically significantly improved PFS if they receive gefitinib as opposed to carboplatin/paclitaxel. If the patient does not have an EGFR mutation, they have an improved PFS with the platinum doublet and hence, in unselected patients, EGFR inhibitors should not be used as first-line treatment (Mok et al. 2009).

Selection by performance status

In those with PS 0–1, cisplatin/docetaxel doublet may be more appropriate than cisplatin/vinorelbine as the median survival has been shown to increase from 10.1 to 11.3 months with the use of cisplatin/docetaxel. However there is increased toxicity with cisplatin/docetaxel, so to maintain the benefit:risk ratio at an acceptable level, only very fit patients should be considered for this regimen (Fossella et al. 2006).

The addition of biological agents to a platinum doublet

There have been two trials published advocating the addition of different biological agents to a standard platinum doublet in selected patients:

The addition of bevacizumab to platinum doublet

In patients with PS 0–1, with non-squamous histology, no risk factors for bleeding and no hypertension, the addition of bevacizumab, a VEGF inhibitor, to carboplatin/paclitaxel improved OS from 10.3 to 12.3 months. If this platinum doublet is selected for a patient who fulfils the study inclusion criteria, it may be appropriate to add bevacizumab (Sandler et al. 2006).

The addition of cetuximab to platinum doublet
In patients who have had immunohistochemical confirmation of EGFR expression, the addition of cetuximab, a monoclonal antibody to EGFR, to cisplatin/vinorelbine increased OS to 11.3 months in the cetuximab arm versus 10.1 months in the placebo arm in a phase III trial (Pirker et al. 2009).

Survival and toxicity data for both of these biological agents have only been reported for one specific platinum doublet. The use of these agents with alternative regimens may result in different results and have different toxicity profiles and therefore should not be advocated.

Patients of PS 2
The meta-analysis advocating chemotherapy in incurable patients included patients of PS 2 and suggested there is a survival advantage in chemotherapy for PS 2 patients.

Patients who are PS 2 are known to gain less benefit with chemotherapy than those with PS 0–1, have greater toxicity, and shorter survival whether or not they have systemic therapy. As a result, the benefits of chemotherapy in this group must be reviewed carefully and separately from those with PS 0–1.

As a result of the discussed factors, clinicians will often opt for single-agent regimens as they are less toxic. There is certainly evidence that a number of single-agent regimens, such as vinorelbine or gemcitabine, increase survival. There have been a number of phase II and III trials looking at doublets versus single agent in PS 2 patients; however because of the large heterogeneity among patients classified as PS 2, it is difficult to interpret these studies with confidence.

The heterogeneity in PS 2 patients is due to a number of factors: firstly, the scales of PS are such that they are open to subjective interpretation, resulting in a broad range of patients being labelled as PS 2; it is often difficult to know whether patients are PS 2 as a result of comorbidities, or as a result of the physiological effects of cancer which may dictate whether chemotherapy will offer a benefit; patients labelled PS 2 in a clinical trial differ from those assigned this PS in routine clinical practice as many trials are not open to PS 3 patients which may sway interpretation; in addition, patients who are PS 2 are often considered with elderly patients, further diversifying the study group.

In summary, single-agent regimens have been demonstrated to offer a survival advantage. There is currently no convincing evidence that doublets offer any additional advantage in this group. In addition, there may be a subset of patients of PS 2 in which best supportive care (BSC) is the most appropriate course of action.

Second-line therapy
There are two agents that have been compared to BSC in second-line and have shown both an OS benefit and an improvement in QoL.

Docetaxol and erlotinib
In a seminal publication, docetaxol was reported to improve the OS to 7.5 versus 4.6 months, and the 1-year survival to 37% versus 11%, when compared to BSC (Shepherd 2000). In a similar trial evaluating the use of erlotinib, the EGFR inhibitor, versus BSC, erlotinib increased the OS to 6.7 versus 4.7 months when compared to BSC (Shepherd et al. 2005).

As a result of these trials, it was no longer considered ethical to randomize patients to BSC in the second-line setting; therefore the following drugs have shown their efficacy in second-line treatment by demonstrating non-inferiority to docetaxel.

Pemetrexed and gefitinib
Pemetrexed has been demonstrated to be non-inferior to docetaxel with OS of 8.3 versus 7.9 months in each arm respectively. A retrospective subset analysis showed that pemetrexed was comparable with docetaxel in adenocarcinomas, whereas patients with squamous carcinoma did better with docetaxol. Consequently, the use of pemetrexed in second-line is perhaps best reserved for non-squamous carcinomas (Hanna et al. 2004). Gefitinib also has demonstrated non-inferiority to docetaxol in this setting, and it has been shown to have fewer serious adverse events (Kim et al. 2008).

The optimal duration of second-line treatment has not been studied. In the earlier mentioned trials, the agents were given until progression; however the median number of cycles given in most of these trials was 4 cycles and therefore it would seem appropriate to stop, or have a low threshold for stopping after 4 cycles.

Third-line therapy
The trial that confirmed the role of erlotinib in second-line treatment included patients with both one and two previous chemotherapy regimens. Hence there were a group of patients who received it as third-line therapy. A subgroup analysis was undertaken in this group and it was reported that neither response rates, nor survival differed in this group in comparison with those receiving erlotinib second-line. This would indicate that receiving erlotinib third-line continues to offer a survival advantage (Shephard et al. 2005).

No other large trials have specifically addressed treatment in a third-line setting; therefore there is no conclusion as to whether chemotherapy in these patients is appropriate. Patients who receive more lines of therapy show decreasing response rates, disease control rates, and survival. Therefore, the benefit of systemic therapy becomes more questionable, and fit patients who have undergone treatment using two previous regimens should preferably be treated within clinical trials or receive experimental therapies.

Maintenance chemotherapy
There are two types of maintenance therapy. 'Continuous maintenance therapy' prolongs the use of one or both of the agents used in the first-line combination, after the standard 4 cycles of combination chemotherapy. 'Switch maintenance therapy' is when the patient completes 4 cycles of standard combination chemotherapy and immediately switches to an alternative chemotherapy despite demonstrating no progressive disease.

Continuous maintenance chemotherapy
Continuing platinum doublet regimen for >4 cycles has been discussed earlier. A further trial considered whether continuing one of the agents within a doublet may offer a survival advantage. A study investigated this possibility with a group that had completed 4 cycles of cisplatin/gemcitabine following which they were randomized to receive either continuous gemcitabine or BSC. Although time to progression was longer in the continuous gemcitabine arm,

there was no statistical survival advantage (Brodowicz et al. 2006).

Switch maintenance chemotherapy

A number of trials of switch maintenance chemotherapy have recently been published using pemetrexed, erlotinib, and docetaxel. Some have shown increased OS, and some have demonstrated increased time to progression or PFS. However, a problem with all of these trials is that only a small proportion of the patients in the BSC arm received the drug, therefore it is difficult to ascertain whether the improvement in OS is due to the timing of the agent or the fact that it is given at all. Certainly if the patients in the BSC arm who received the agent, are compared with those in the maintenance arm, OS, TTP, and PFS are very similar. This indicates that the timing of the second-line therapy is not as important as whether or not the patient receives the therapy and perhaps we should be monitoring patients after first-line therapy more closely so that the window of opportunity for second-line therapy is not missed.

Further reading

Brodowicz T, Krzakowski M, Zwitter M, et al. Cisplatin and gemcitabine first-line chemotherapy followed by maintenance gemcitabine or best supportive care in advanced non-small cell lung cancer: a phase III trial. *Lung Cancer* 2006; 52:155–63.

D'Addario G, Pintilie M, Leighl NB, et al. Platinum-based versus non-platinum-based chemotherapy in advanced non-small-cell lung cancer: A meta-analysis of the published literature. *J Clin Oncol* 2005; 23:2926–36.

Delbaldo C, Michiels S, Syz N, et al. Benefits of adding a drug to a single-agent or a 2-agent chemotherapy regimen in advanced non-small-cell lung cancer: A meta-analysis. *JAMA* 2006; 292:4405–11.

Fossella F, Pereira JR, von Pawel J, et al. Randomized, multinational, phase III study of docetaxol plus platinum combinations versus vinorelbine plus cisplatin for advanced non-small-cell lung cancer: The TAX 326 study group. *J Clin Oncol* 2006; 21:3016–24.

Hanna N, Shepherd FA, Fossella FV, et al. Randomized phase III trial of pemetrexed versus docetaxel in patients with non-small-cell lung cancer previously treated with chemotherapy. *J Clin Oncol* 2004; 22:1589–97.

Kim ES, Hirsh V, Mok T, et al. Gefitinib versus docetaxel in previously treated non-small-cell lung cancer (INTEREST): A randomised phase III trial. *Lancet* 2008; 372:1809–18.

Mok TS, Wu Y-L, Thongprasert S, et al. Gefitinib or Carboplatin-paclitaxel in pulmonary adenocarcinoma. *NEJM* 2009; 361:947–57.

NSCLC Meta-Analysis Collaborative Group: Chemotherapy in addition to supportive care improves survival in advanced non-small cell lung cancer: A systematic review and meta-analysis of individual patient data from 16 randomized controlled trials. *J Clin Oncol* 2008; 26:4617–25.

Park JO, Kim S-W, Ahn JS, et al. Phase III trial of two versus four additional cycles in patients who are non-progressive after two cycles of platinum-based chemotherapy in non-small-cell lung cancer. *J Clin Oncol* 2007; 25: 5233–9.

Pirker R, Pereira JR, Szczesna A, et al. Cetuximab plus chemotherapy in patients with advanced non-small-cell lung cancer (FLEX): An open-label randomised phase III trial. *Lancet* 2009; 373:1525–31.

Sandler A, Gray R, Perry MC, et al. Paclitaxel-carboplatin alone or with bevacizumab for non-small-cell lung cancer. *NEJM* 2006; 355: 2542–50.

Scagliotti GV, De Marinis F, Rinaldi M, et al. Phase III randomised trial comparing three platinum-based doublets in advanced non-small-cell lung cancer. *J Clin Oncol* 2002; 20:4285–91.

Scagliotti GV, Parikh P, von Pawel J, et al. Phase III study comparing cisplatin plus gemcitabine with cisplatin plus pemetrexed in chemotherapy-naïve patients with advanced-stage non-small-cell lung cancer. *J Clin Oncol* 2008; 26:3543–51.

Shepherd FA, Dancey J, Ramlau R, et al. Prospective randomized trial of docetaxel versus best supportive care in patients whith non-small-cell lung cancer previously treated with platinum-based chemotherapy. *J Clin Oncol* 2000; 18:2095–103.

Shepherd FA, Rodrigues Pereira J, Ciuleanu T, et al. Erlotinib in previously treated non-small-cell lung cancer. *NEJM* 2005; 353:123–32.

Small-cell lung cancer

Background

The incidence of SCLC is strongly linked with tobacco use. SCLC is a rapidly fatal disease without treatment. The SEER database reported a decrease in incidence of SCLC as a percentage of all types of lung cancer, from 17% in 1986, to 13% in 2002 (Govindan et al. 2006), but the proportion of women with SCLC increased from 28% in 1973 to 50% in 2002.

The WHO and International Association for the Study of Lung Cancer pathology committees developed a revised classification of lung and pleural tumours which was published in 1999 (Travis et al. 1999). In this classification, LCNEC is no longer considered as a variant of SCLC but included as a variant of LCC.

Patients can be staged as having either limited (LS-SCLC) or extensive disease (ES-SCLC), based upon a simplified two-stage system developed by the Veteran's Administration. LS-SCLC was defined as disease 'that can be encompassed by one port of radiotherapy', and ES-SCLC as tumour extension beyond the chest or that cannot be encompassed by one radiotherapy port. A recent International Association for the Study of Lung Cancer (IASLC) analysis of an international database suggests that TNM staging may be important as survival rates for clinical stages I and II are significantly different than those for stage III with N2 or N3 involvement (Shepherd 2007). Patients with malignant pleural effusion are not candidates for thoracic radiotherapy, but the IASLC analysis found that such patients without extrathoracic metastases had a better survival than those with stage IV disease.

At initial diagnosis, up to two-thirds of patients will have evidence of haematogenous metastases (M1). Of the remaining one-third, most patients have clinical evidence of extensive nodal involvement in the hilar, mediastinal, and supraclavicular nodal regions. In treated patients, the median survival ranges for LS-SCLC and ES-SCLC are 15–20 months and 8–13 months, respectively (Lally 2007). Approximately 20–40% of LSSCLC and 5% of ES-SCLC patients survive 2 years.

SCLC: diagnosis and staging investigation

A diagnosis can be obtained by biopsy using flexible bronchoscopy, mediastinoscopy, EUS, transthoracic needle aspiration, or thoracoscopy, depending on the localization of the tumour. Biopsy of a metastatic lesion can substitute for a biopsy from the primary tumour. Staging includes a full blood count and biochemistry, CT scan of chest and upper abdomen, an MRI scan or brain CT scan, and bone scan. Other investigations should be performed to exclude distant metastases when indicated by symptoms. Some small studies have shown that FDG-PET scans add to conventional staging by improving sensitivity in detecting extracranial disease. Sensitivity for staging extensive- versus limited-stage disease ranges from 89–100% and specificity from 78–95% (Ung et al. 2008). However, the frequency of changes in stage attributable to PET as a staging procedure are unknown and prospective randomized studies are awaited before PET scans can be recommended for routine use in staging SCLC.

SCLC: treatment of limited disease

The treatment of patients with LS-SCLC and a good performance score (WHO 0–1) is concurrent chemoradiotherapy with cisplatin–etoposide, followed by prophylactic cranial irradiation (Auperin et al. 1999). The addition of thoracic radiotherapy to chemotherapy improves survival, and cisplatin-containing schemes are preferred (Pujol et al. 2000). Furthermore, the toxicity of cisplatin-etoposide combined with concurrent thoracic radiotherapy is predictable and generally reversible (Turrisi 1999). Issues of optimal timing, dose, and fractionation of radiotherapy are not fully resolved, although recent reviews support the early start of concurrent chemoradiotherapy.

The Intergroup 0096 trial randomized patients to receive 45Gy of concurrent thoracic radiotherapy given either twice daily over 3 weeks or once daily over 5 weeks (Turrisi 1999). All patients received four 21-day cycles of cisplatin–etoposide, and radiation commenced with the start of chemotherapy. The 5-year OS favoured twice-daily radiation, 26% versus 16%, and the rate of local failure was lower with twice-daily radiation 52% versus 36%. The most important toxicity observed with twice-daily radiation was grade 3 or higher oesophagitis, which was seen in 27% of patients receiving twice-daily radiotherapy versus 11% with once-daily radiotherapy. However, twice-daily fractionation has not been adopted widely in the community for reasons which include logistics. Studies to compare this scheme with once-daily fractionation to a dose of 66Gy or higher are currently in progress. Another unresolved issue is the question of omission of elective irradiation of mediastinal nodes, and involved-field radiotherapy is increasingly being used, both within clinical trials and in routine practice.

Prophylactic cranial irradiation (PCI) is part of the standard of care for patients with LS-SCLC as the magnitude of survival benefit with PCI is similar to that achieved using thoracic radiotherapy in limited disease SCLC. For patients who achieve a complete response to chemotherapy, PCI decreases the cumulative incidence of brain metastases from 58.6% (controls) to 33.3%, which in turn is accompanied by an improved 3-year OS from 15.3% vs 20.7% (Auperin 1999). Currently, the standard dose used for prophylactic cranial radiotherapy is 25Gy, in 10 once-daily fractions of 2.5Gy (Fig. 4.3.3).

SCLC: treatment of very limited disease

There is no good evidence to support use of surgery in patients who present with stage I and II SCLC (Sorensen 2006). However, the diagnosis is occasionally made after a radical surgical excision for a patient presenting with a peripheral lung tumour without a preoperative histological diagnosis. In cases where adequate lymph node sampling reveals no evidence of metastases, a reasonable approach would be to administer 4 cycles of postoperative cisplatin–etoposide followed by prophylactic cranial radiotherapy (10 once-daily fractions of 2.5Gy).

Treatment of extensive stage SCLC

The standard treatment for patients with ES-SCLC and a good performance score (WHO 0–1) is sequential chemotherapy with a platinum-based scheme, followed by prophylactic cranial irradiation in all patients who show a response. Since the 1980s, the standard chemotherapy scheme used in North America has been the combination of cisplatin and etoposide. Subsequently, a meta-analysis revealed that cisplatin-containing regimens yield a higher

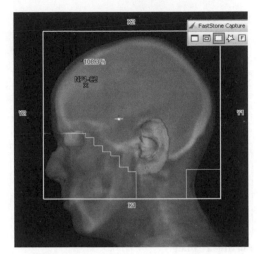

Fig. 4.3.3 Standard radiotherapy portals fields used for delivery of prophylactic cranial radiotherapy. The lens and oral cavity are shielded to reduce toxicity (see also colour plate section).

response rate and probability of survival than does chemotherapy containing other alkylating agents, without a perceptible increase in risk of toxic-death (Pujol et al. 2000). The corresponding increase in the probability of survival was 2.6% and 4.4%, respectively, at 6 months and 1 year. Carboplatin can be an appropriate substitute for cisplatin in older patients or those with renal insufficiency. The response rates to first-line chemotherapy range from 70–85%, with complete response rates of 20–30%. A recent study randomized ES-SCLC patients who showed any response to chemotherapy to either PCI or no PCI. The PCI scheme used in the majority of patients was 20Gy, in once-daily fractions of 4Gy. The risk of symptomatic brain metastasis was significantly reduced, and the 1-year OS rate was 27.1% for PCI and 13.3% for the control arm (Slotman et al. 2007).

SCLC: recurrence and new agents

Despite response rates to first-line chemotherapy which range from 70–85%, with complete response rates of 20–30%, virtually all patients relapse. Patients with good PS relapsing after response to first-line chemotherapy should be considered for second-line chemotherapy as second-line chemotherapy increases survival.

Several new systemic agents and therapeutic strategies have been tested during the last three decades in ES-SCLC. A Japanese trial found cisplatin plus irinotecan to be superior to cisplatin–etoposide (Noda et al. 2002). However, a similar US study failed to confirm this finding (Hanna et al. 2006). The addition of a third cytotoxic agent produces a higher response rate but at the cost of greater toxicity, and without improving the median survival duration over that seen with cisplatin plus etoposide alone (Lally et al. 2007). Similarly, raising the dose intensity of chemotherapy with ifosfamide, carboplatin, and etoposide by 3-fold did not improve the long-term outcome of SCLC (Leyvraz et al. 2008). In elderly patients with poor performance status, a greater benefit is seen from two-drug regimens than when single-agent regimens are used. After four cycles of standard cisplatin plus etoposide, treatment with either maintenance therapy or 4 cycles of topotecan has failed to improve survival (Sculier et al. 1998; Schiller et al. 2001).

Follow-up

In patients who have completed treatment, ESMO guidelines found no evidence to support routine follow-up assessment in asymptomatic patients. Monitoring of long-term survivors with LS-SCLC for the development of a second primary tumour should be considered.

Further reading

Auperin A, Arriagada R, Pignon JP, et al. Prophylactic cranial irradiation for patients with small-cell lung cancer in complete remission. Prophylactic Cranial Irradiation Overview Collaborative Group. N Engl J Med 1999; **341**:476–84.

Govindan R, Page N, Morgenstern D, et al. Changing epidemiology of small cell lung cancer in the United States over the past three decades: Analysis of the Surveillance, Epidemiologic and End Results Database. J Clin Oncol 2006; **24**:4539–44.

Hanna N, Bunn PA Jr, Langer C, et al. Randomized phase III trial comparing irinotecan/cisplatin with etoposide/cisplatin in patients with previously untreated extensive-stage disease small-cell lung cancer. J Clin Oncol 2006; **24**:2038–43.

Leyvraz C, Pampalloma S, Martinelli G, et al. A threefold dose intensity treatment with ifosfamide, carboplatin, and etoposide for patients with small cell lung cancer: a randomized trial. J Natl Cancer Inst 2008; **100**: 533–41.

Noda K, Nishiwaki Y, Kawahara M, et al. Irinotecan plus cisplatin compared with etoposide plus cisplatin for extensive small-cell lung cancer. N Engl J Med 2002; **346**:85–91.

Okamoto H, Watanabe K, Kunikane H, et al. Randomised phase III trial of carboplatin plus etoposide vs split doses of cisplatin plus etoposide in elderly or poor-risk patients with extensive disease small-cell lung cancer: JCOG 9702. Br J Cancer. 2007; **97**(2):162–9.

Pignon JP, Arriagada R, Ihde DC, et al. A meta-analysis of thoracic radiotherapy for small-cell lung cancer. N Engl J Med 1992; **327**:1618–24.

Pujol JL, Carestia L, Daurès JP. Is there a case for cisplatin in the treatment of small-cell lung cancer? A meta-analysis of randomized trials of a cisplatin-containing regimen versus a regimen without this alkylating agent. Br J Cancer 2000; **83**(1):8–15

Schiller JH, Adak S, Cella D, et al. Topotecan versus observation after cisplatin plus etoposide in extensive-stage small-cell lung cancer: E7593–a phase III trial of the Eastern Cooperative Oncology Group. J Clin Oncol 2001; **19**:2114–22.

Sculier JP, Berghmans T, Castaigne C, et al. Maintenance chemotherapy for small cell lung cancer: A critical review of the literature. Lung Cancer 1998; **19**:141–51.

Simon GR, Turrisi A. Management of small-cell lung cancer. ACCP Evidence-Based Clinical Practice Guidelines (2nd Edition) 2007; Chest **132**;324–39.

Small-cell lung cancer: ESMO Clinical Recommendations for diagnosis, treatment and follow-up. Ann Oncol 2007; **18**(Suppl 2): ii32–ii33.

Slotman B, Faivre-Finn C, Kramer G et al. Prophylactic cranial irradiation in extensive small-cell lung cancer. N Eng J Med 2007; **357**:644–72.

Sorensen M. Primary surgery revisited in very limited small cell lung cancer: does it have a role? A commentary. Lung Cancer 2006; **52**:263–4.

Travis WD, Colby TV, Corrin B, et al. World Health Organization International Histological Classification of Tumours: Histological Typing of Lung and Pleural Tumours, 3rd edition. Berlin: Springer Verlag, 1999

Ung YC, Maziak DE, Vanderveen JA, et al. 18Fluorodeoxyglucose positron emission tomography in the diagnosis and staging of lung cancer: a systematic review. J Natl Cancer Inst 2007; **99**:1753–67.

Warde P, Payne D. Does thoracic irradiation improve survival and local control in limited-stage small-cell carcinoma of the lung? A meta-analysis. J Clin Oncol 1992; **10**:890–5.

Lung cancer: follow-up

Guidelines of the ACCP recommend follow-up lasting 3–6 months by the specialists responsible for the curative intent therapy, in order to manage treatment-related complications (Rubins et al. 2007). Following surgery, a significant percentage of patients may experience post-thoracotomy pain syndromes and other adverse effects which can impair their QoL (Kenny et al. 2008). Similarly, patients who have undergone chemoradiotherapy can develop symptomatic radiation pneumonitis in the first 6–12 months. Appropriate diagnosis and adequate management of treatment-related complications are important for the QoL and functioning of patients.

The risk of disease recurrence is greatest in the first 3 years after curative treatment. The majority of patients who have undergone surgery for early stage disease will present with extrathoracic disease as the first site of recurrence. Although palliative treatment is often the only available option for patients with distant metastases, patients with solitary metastases may achieve long remission after appropriate treatment. Following curative therapy, new primary lung cancer can develop at a rate of 1–2% per patient per year, and a 13-fold increase in risk for second lung cancer has been reported in patients undergoing chemoradiotherapy for LS-SCLC.

Patients who have been treated for lung cancer are also at increased risk for other cancers of the aerodigestive system, particularly head and neck and oesophageal cancer. ACCP guidelines recommend that those patients having adequate performance and pulmonary function undergo surveillance with a history, physical examination, and imaging study (either CXR or CT) every 6 months for 2 years and then annually (Rubins et al. 2007). It is unclear if there are benefits in counselling patients to recognize important symptoms, but advice to contact their physician in the event of new and persistent symptoms appears reasonable.

Key points

Aims of post-treatment follow-up

- Manage treatment-related complications
- Detect second primary lung cancers
- Detect and manage other cancers of the aero-digestive systems

---

Further reading

Kenny PM, King MT, Viney RC, et al. Quality of life and survival in the 2 years after surgery for non small-cell lung cancer. *J Clin Oncol* 2008; **26**:233–41.

Rubins J, Unger M, Colice GL; American College of Chest Physicians. Follow-up and surveillance of the lung cancer patient following curative intent therapy: ACCP evidence-based clinical practice guideline (2nd edition). *Chest* 2007; **132**(3 Suppl):355S–367S.

Pleural mesothelioma

Epidemiology and clinical features

Malignant pleural mesothelioma (MPM) is an aggressive, locally invasive tumour which is most strongly associated with occupational asbestos exposure to crocidolite or amosite forms of the fibre. Its incidence has increased over last 20 years, with the number of cases expected to peak between 2011 and 2015 in Britain (Hodgson et al. 2005). Mesothelioma arises primarily from the surface serosal cells of the pleural, peritoneal, and pericardial cavities, with about 85% arising in the pleura. The mean time from first exposure to asbestos to symptoms is 30–40 years, and MPM is usually diagnosed in the fifth to seventh decades of life. A strong male predominance is seen where occupational exposure to asbestos is involved, and the burden of this disease in the developing world is likely to increase due to continued exposure in these populations to asbestos in recent decades.

Pathology and staging

Histological diagnosis can be established by thoracocentesis and closed pleural biopsy, biopsy under thoracoscopy, and occasionally by open pleural biopsy. Histologically, MPM can show an epithelial morphology (epithelial type), a fibrous morphology (fibrous type, also called sarcomatoid type), or a combination of both. Nearly 50–60% of cases of MPM are of the epithelial type, approximately 10% are sarcomatoid, and the rest are biphasic malignant mesotheliomas.

The commonest staging system used is the AJCC system, which was adopted from that of the International Mesothelioma Interest Group in 1995 (Table 4.3.3).

Clinical features

Shortness of breath and chest pain are the commonest presenting symptoms, but patients may also be asymptomatic, with evidence of a pleural effusion noted incidentally on a chest radiograph. Metastatic disease is uncommon at presentation and patients with MPM die principally from pulmonary insufficiency. Nearly all patients will have pleural thickening on CT scans, with pleural effusions present in 87% (Seely et al. 2008). Pleural thickening is nodular in 86% of patients, and ipsilateral volume loss is seen in 46%.

The pattern of nodal metastases differs from that typically observed for lung cancer, with internal mammary lymphadenopathy observed in 52% of patients and cardiophrenic lymphadenopathy in 46%. The role of FDG-PET scans in staging remains to be established although early reports suggest a role in identifying lymph nodal disease and otherwise occult metastatic disease. Preliminary data suggest that high FDG uptakes before treatment may predict for response to chemotherapy and correlate with poorer survival.

Management

Approximately 85–90% of patients with MPM present with unresectable disease at diagnosis and such patients are candidates for palliative treatment. Survival outcomes reported for interventions in non-randomized studies of MPM must be interpreted with caution as factors such as gender, PS, white-blood-cell count, histological subtype, and probability of histological diagnosis identify prognostic groups that can discriminate between patients receiving the same systemic treatment (Curran et al. 1998). For example, the median survival of the low-risk group (i.e. patients with two or fewer poor prognostic factors) was 10.8 months, compared with 5.5 months in the high-risk group.

Palliation: pleurodesis

Pleural effusion can be a difficult problem in MPM. A Cochrane systematic review of randomized trials concluded that the use of talc pleurodesis is superior to placebo or use of any other sclerosant, and that video-assisted thoracoscopic surgery (VATS) resulted in better control of effusion than bedside pleurodesis (Shaw and Agarwal 2004). In addition, representative tissue for a diagnosis can be obtained at VATS.

Palliation: chemotherapy

The majority of patients with MPM are eligible only for palliative treatments. MPM is relatively unresponsive to chemotherapy, and reviews found cisplatin to be the most active agent. The median age at diagnosis of malignant mesothelioma is increasing, and baseline PS and survival appears worse than in the selected literature. Only 37% of

Table 4.3.3 New international TNM staging system for diffuse MPM according to the IMIG*

T1	
T1a	Tumour limited to the ipsilateral parietal pleura, including mediastinal and diaphragmatic pleura
	No involvement of the visceral pleura
T1b	Tumour involving the ipsilateral parietal pleura, including mediastinal and diaphragmatic pleura; scattered foci of tumour also involving the visceral pleura
T2	Tumour involving each of the ipsilateral pleural surfaces (parietal, mediastinal, diaphragmatic, and visceral pleura) with at least one of the following features:
	• Involvement of diaphragmatic muscle
	• Confluent visceral pleural tumour (including the fissures) or extension of tumour from visceral pleura in the underlying pulmonary parenchyma
T3	Describes locally advanced but potentially resectable tumour

Table 4.3.3 (Cont'd)

	Tumour involving all of the ipsilateral pleural surfaces (parietal, mediastinal, diaphragmatic, and visceral pleura) with at least one of the following features:
	• Involvement of the endothoracic fascia
	• Extension into the mediastinal fat
	• Solitary, completely resectable focus of tumour extending into the soft tissues of the chest wall
	• Non-transmural involvement of the pericardium
T4	Describes locally advanced technically unresectable tumour
	Tumour involving all of the ipsilateral pleural surfaces (parietal, mediastinal, diaphragmatic, and visceral) with at least one of the following features:
	Diffuse extension or multifocal masses of tumour in the chest wall, with or without associated rib destruction
	Direct transdiaphragmatic extension of tumour to the peritoneum
	Direct extension of tumour to the contralateral pleura
	Direct extension of tumour to one or more mediastinal organs
	Direct extension of tumour into the spine
	Tumour extending through to the internal surface of the pericardium with or without a pericardial effusion, or tumour involving the myocardium
N, lymph nodes	
NX	Regional lymph nodes cannot be assessed
N0	No regional lymph node metastases
N1	Metastases in the ipsilateral bronchopulmonary or hilar lymph nodes
N2	Metastases in the subcarinal or the ipsilateral mediastinal lymph nodes, including the ipsilateral internal mammary nodes
N3	Metastases in the contralateral mediastinal, contralateral internal mammary, ipsilateral, or contralateral supraclavicular lymph nodes
M, metastases	
MX	Presence of distant metastases cannot be assessed
M0	No distant metastasis
M1	Distant metastasis present
Stage I	
Ia	T1aN0M0
IB	T1bN0M0
Stage II	T2N0M0
Stage III	Any T3M0
	Any N1M0
	Any N2M0
Stage IV	Any T4
	Any N3
	Any M1

patients in a British population-based study were considered candidates for palliative chemotherapy, and <20% accepted this treatment option (Chapman et al. 2008). Chemotherapy has been compared with active symptom control (ASC) alone in one randomized trial (Muers ASCO 2007). The two chemotherapy regimens chosen for investigation had shown good symptom palliation in phase II studies, and patients with MPM were randomized to either ASC alone (regular follow-up in a specialist clinic, and treatment could include steroids, analgesics, bronchodilators, palliative radiotherapy, etc), ASC + MVP (4 × 3-weekly cycles of mitomycin $6g/m^2$, vinblastine $6mg/m^2$, and cisplatin $50mg/m^2$), or ASC + N (12 weekly injections of vinorelbine $30mg/m^2$). Good symptom palliation, which was defined as prevention, control or improvement, was achieved in all 3 groups, and no between-group differences were observed in 4 predefined QL subscales (physical functioning, dyspnoea, pain and global QL). A small, non-significant survival benefit was seen for ASC + CT (HR 0.89, 95% CI 0.72–1.12, p = 0.32)

When patients with a good performance and stable symptoms were randomized between immediate chemotherapy, consisting of mitomycin $6g/m^2$, vinblastine $6mg/m^2$, and cisplatin $50mg/m^2$ (MVP), or the same chemotherapy at symptomatic progression (O'Brien et al. 2006), chemotherapy in the second arm was delayed with a median of 4 months, and some patients never received any. In patients who received chemotherapy, immediate treatment was associated with a significantly longer time to symptomatic progression, but the increase in OS was not significant, and delayed patients had a poorer quality of life.

Two phase III studies have evaluated the combination of cisplatin combined with a third-generation antifolate. Pemetrexed and cisplatin in medically fit patients provided 3–4 months of survival benefit over cisplatin administered as a single agent (Vogelzang et al. 2003). Another randomized study combining cisplatin with raltitrexed reported significant improvements in efficacy and disease-related symptoms (pain and dyspnoea) with the combination versus cisplatin only (van Meerbeeck et al. 2005). These two pivotal randomized trials concluded that contemporary chemotherapy improved symptoms and had no deleterious effect on quality of life, despite the associated toxicity. PFS was improved with the raltitrexed–cisplatin regimen compared with cisplatin alone (5.3 months PFS for the combination vs. 4 months for cisplatin; p = 0.058). By contrast the pemetrexed–cisplatin regimen produced significantly better PFS than cisplatin alone (3.7 vs. 5.7 months; p = 0.001). Survival in the cisplatin-only arm of both of these phase III trials was similar.

Radiotherapy: prophylactic and palliative
Malignant seeding in surgical scars and biopsy tracks in the chest wall, has been reported in 19–40% of patients. Subcutaneous nodules from MPM are painful and often refractory to radiotherapy or respond only transiently to this treatment. An earlier randomized trial had suggested that prophylactic radiation to these sites significantly reduces scar recurrences. However, two recent studies evaluating prophylactic radiation reported no benefit for this procedure (Bydder et al. 2004; O'Rouke et al. 2007).

Palliative external radiotherapy can palliate chest pain associated with mesothelioma in 50–68% of patients but all patients experience a recurrence of their symptoms several months after such radiation (de Graaf-Strukowska et al. 1999). Daily doses of 4Gy appear to be more efficacious than fractions of <4Gy in providing symptom relief.

Surgery as a component of bi- or trimodality treatment
A number of institutions in the USA and Europe have explored radical surgery in patients with MPM in recent decades. A large single-institution analysis concluded that surgical procedures such as extrapleural pneumonectomy, which was performed in 22% of all patients, or pleurectomy/decortication (in 19%) could be performed with low operative mortality rates (4%) (Flores et al. 2007). However, the assertion that use of multimodality therapy including surgery was superior due to a median survival of 20.1 months, must be viewed with caution due to possible confounding variables in such an analysis (Treasure et al. 2007).

Single modality treatment with surgical resection such as pleurectomy/decortication, or extrapleural pneumonectomy (EPP) has produced poor results. EPP is defined as an en bloc resection of the entire pleura, lung, and diaphragm, with or without resection of the pericardium (Rusch et al. 2001), and the local recurrence rate after surgical resection, either alone or in combination with low-dose postoperative RT, ranges from 35–78%. (Pass et al. 1997; Rusch et al. 1991). Similar recurrence rates were observed when EPP was followed by low-dose hemithorax irradiation to 30Gy, and a boost dose of radiation to sites of previous bulk disease. However, disease control was far superior with locoregional recurrences reported in only 13% of patients after high dose radiotherapy (54Gy) to the entire hemithorax (Rusch et al. 2001). Delivery of high-dose radiotherapy after EPP is technically challenging due to the proximity of dose-limiting adjacent organs such as the spinal cord, the heart, and the liver. Although initial reports using intensity-modulated radiotherapy (IMRT) suggested that this technique could reduce treatment-related toxicity, later reports indicated that toxicity was of real concern. An analysis of 63 consecutive patients who underwent extrapleural pneumonectomy and IMRT reported that 23 patients (37%) had died within 6 months of IMRT. The volume of contralateral lung receiving a dose of 20Gy or higher (i.e. the V_{20}) was the only independent determinant for risk of death related to pulmonary causes and to non-cancer-related deaths in the first 6 months (Rice et al. 2007). The importance of radiation doses to the contralateral lung was emphasized in another report where six of 13 patients developed fatal pneumonitis after IMRT following EPP (Allen et al. 2006).

The role of combined modality treatments incorporating surgery should be established within controlled clinical trials. The Mesothelioma and Radical Surgery (MARS) trial is an ongoing pilot study in Great Britain that aims to evaluate EPP within trimodality therapy with a control arm of any other treatment (Treasure 2006).

Key points

- Malignant pleural mesothelioma is associated with exposure to asbestos
- Pleural mesothelioma is a disease of mainly elderly patients
- Palliative therapy is the only option for many patients
- Systemic chemotherapy can palliative symptoms
- The role of surgery remains investigational

Further reading

Allen AM, Czerminska M, Jänne PA, et al. Fatal pneumonitis associated with intensity-modulated radiation therapy for mesothelioma. Int J Radiat Oncol Biol Phys 2006; **65**:640–5.

Bydder S, Phillips M, Joseph DJ, et al. A randomised trial of single-dose radiotherapy to prevent procedure tract metastasis by malignant mesothelioma. Br J Cancer 2004; **91**:9–10.

Chapman A, Mulrennan S, Ladd B, Muers MF. Population based epidemiology and prognosis of mesothelioma in Leeds, UK. Thorax 2008; **63**:435–9.

Curran D, Sahmoud T, Therasse P et al. Prognostic factors in patients with pleural mesothelioma: the European Organization for Research and Treatment of Cancer experience. J Clin Oncol 1998; **16**:145–52.

de Graaf-Strukowska L, van der Zee J, van Putten W, et al. Factors influencing the outcome of radiotherapy in malignant mesothelioma of the pleura–a single-institution experience with 189 patients. Int J Radiat Oncol Biol Phys 1999; **43**:511–16.

Flores RM, Zakowski M, Venkatraman E, et al. Prognostic factors in the treatment of malignant pleural mesothelioma at a large tertiary referral center. J Thorac Oncol 2007; **2**:957–65.

Hodgson JT, McElvenny DM, Darnton AJ, et al. The expected burden of mesothelioma mortality in Great Britain from 2002 to 2050. Br J Cancer 2005; **92**:587–93.

O'Brien ME, Watkins D, Ryan C, et al. A randomised trial in malignant mesothelioma (M) of early (E) versus delayed (D) chemotherapy in symptomatically stable patients: the MED trial. Ann Oncol 2006; **17**:270–5.

O'Rourke N, Garcia JC, Paul J, et al. A randomised controlled trial of intervention site radiotherapy in malignant pleural mesothelioma. Radiother Oncol 2007; **84**:18–22.

Pass HI, Kranda K, Temeck BK, et al. Surgically debulked malignant pleural mesothelioma: results and prognostic factors. Ann Surg Oncol 1997; **4**:215–22.

Rice DC, Smythe WR, Liao Z, et al. Dose-dependent pulmonary toxicity after postoperative intensity-modulated radiotherapy for malignant pleural mesothelioma. Int J Radiat Oncol Biol Phys 2007; **69**:350–7.

Rusch VW, Piantadosi S, Holmes EC. The role of extrapleural pneumonectomy in malignant pleural mesothelioma. A Lung Cancer Study Group trial. J Thorac Cardiovasc Surg 1991; **102**:1–9.

Rusch VW, Rosenzweig K, Venkatraman E, et al. A phase II trial of surgical resection and adjuvant high-dose hemithoracic radiation for malignant pleural mesothelioma. J Thorac Cardiovasc Surg 2001; **122**:788–95.

Seely JM, Nguyen ET, Churg AM, et al. Malignant pleural mesothelioma: Computed tomography and correlation with histology. Eur J Radiol 2008; **246**:288–97.

Shaw P, Agarwal R. Pleurodesis for malignant pleural effusions. Cochrane Database Syst Rev 2004; **1**:CD002916.

Treasure T, Tan C, Lang-Lazdunski L, et al. The MARS trial: mesothelioma and radical surgery. Interact Cardiovasc Thorac Surg 2006; **5**:58–9.

Treasure T, Utley M. Mesothelioma: benefit from surgical resection is questionable. J Thorac Oncol 2007; **2**:885–6.

van Meerbeeck JP, Gaafar R, Manegold C, et al. Randomized phase III study of cisplatin with or without raltitrexed in patients with malignant pleural mesothelioma: an intergroup study of the European Organisation for Research and Treatment of Cancer Lung Cancer Group and the National Cancer Institute of Canada. J Clin Oncol 2005; **23**:6881–9.

Vogelzang NJ, Rusthoven JJ, Symanowski J, et al. (2003) Phase III study of pemetrexed in combination with cisplatin versus cisplatin alone in patients with malignant pleural mesothelioma. J Clin Oncol **21**:2636–44.

Thymic tumours

Pathology and clinical features

Thymic tumours are uncommon, with the incidence of all thymic epithelial tumours in the Dutch population reported to be 3.2 per 1,000,000 (de Jong et al. 2008). Analysis in the USA revealed an incidence of 1.5 per 1,000,000 for 'malignant thymomas' (Engels et al. 2003). Up to 90% of all mediastinal tumours occur in the anterior mediastinum, and common causes of a mass at this location include thymoma, teratoma, thyroid disease, and lymphoma. Masses of the middle mediastinum are typically congenital cysts, including foregut and pericardial cysts, while tumours arising in the posterior mediastinum are often neurogenic tumours. The differential diagnosis of mediastinal tumours can be derived from the location, CT findings, and possible paraneoplastic syndromes.

Thymomas and thymic carcinomas constitute the most common neoplasm arising in the anterior mediastinum. Although epithelial cells in thymomas typically show no atypical features, thymomas may behave as locally invasive tumours and can therefore be considered as potentially malignant. In contrast, thymic carcinomas which also arise from thymic epithelial cells have both a malignant cellular appearance and behaviour.

Diagnosis

Up to half of all patients are asymptomatic, with the diagnosis made on routine examination or investigations. Of the patients presenting with symptoms, up to 50% have symptoms of paraneoplastic syndromes, a further 40% present with symptoms related to intrathoracic mass, for example, compression of neighbouring structures, and the remainder may have generalized systemic symptoms such as weight loss or tiredness. Myasthenia gravis (MG) occurs in approximately 10% of thymoma cases, and is the commonest paraneoplastic syndrome. MG occurs in approximately 33% of patients with thymoma, but the presence of MG does not adversely influence survival in thymoma.

The modified Masaoka's classification is used for the clinical staging of patients with thymoma (Table 4.3.4). The Masaoka staging system distinguishes between thymomas that are completely encapsulated, and those with invasion of the mediastinal fat, direct extension into adjacent structures or with tumour nodules separate from the main mass or lymph node/ distant metastases (Figs. 4.3.4 and 4.3.5).

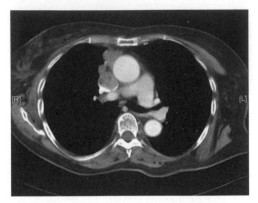

Fig. 4.3.5 CT image showing a thymoma invading the superior vena cava (Masaoka stage III).

Table 4.3.4 Masaoka staging system

Stage	Description
Stage 1	Macroscopically completely encapsulated and microscopically no capsular invasion
Stage II	Macroscopic or microscopic invasion into surrounding fatty tissue or mediastinal pleura
Stage III	Macroscopic invasion into neighbouring organ, i.e. pericardium, great vessels, or lung
Stage IVa	Pleural or pericardial dissemination
Stage IVb	Lymphatic or haematogeneous metastases

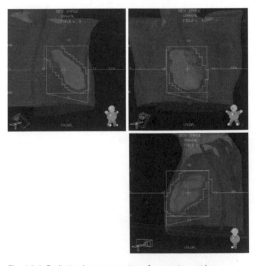

Fig. 4.3.6 Radiation beams-eye-views for a patient with a resected stage III thymoma. CT planning is used to ensure coverage of the planning target volume, and beams shaped to allow for shielding of lung and spinal tissue.

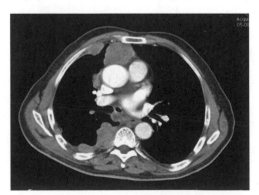

Fig. 4.3.4 CT image showing a thymoma with diffuse pleural metastases (Masaoka stage IV).

Table 4.3.5 WHO classification system for thymoma
(Rosai 1999)

Type	Histological description
A	Medullary thymoma
AB	Mixed thymoma
B1	Predominantly cortical thymoma
B2	Cortical thymoma
B3	Well-differentiated thymic carcinoma
C	Thymic carcinoma

The histological subtypes of thymoma are defined according to the WHO classification (Table 4.3.5), with subtypes AB and B2 the most frequent, and type C (or thymic carcinoma) representing about 5–15% of cases (Kim et al. 2005)

A population-based study revealed that the first definitive diagnostic approach performed in 56% of all patients was a primary resection (De Jong et al. 2008), and this was particularly the case in younger patients and in those with smaller tumours. The percentage of primary resection as the initial diagnostic procedure decreased with increasing Masaoka stage (76%, 75%, 46%, and 23% from stages I to IV, respectively). A preoperative pathological diagnosis was available in 24% of all cases undergoing a resection, and transthoracic needle biopsy was used to obtain the preoperative diagnosis in 64% of cases. Some authors have argued against preoperative needle biopsy due to the presumed risk of dissemination of disease following the procedure, and have argued in favour of immediate thoracic surgery in patients in whom a curative resection is possible. However, the reported risk of recurrences in the needle-track is very low. Another drawback is the limited accuracy of cytology in diagnosing thymomas as this depends on the acquisition of both epithelial and lymphoid elements in one sample.

Thymic tumours: prognosis and management

WHO classification, Masaoka disease stage, resection, and age are significant prognostic factors of overall and relative 5-year survival (De Jong et al. 2008). Stage I thymomas are encapsulated and non-invasive, and can often be resected completely. Treatment results from a surgical resection alone are excellent; 5–10-year survival rates are 95–100% and the local recurrence rate is <5%. Late recurrences that are limited to the mediastinum or thorax can be treated by repeated re-excision. Adjuvant radiotherapy does not appear to be required in a completely resected stage II thymoma (Mangi et al. 2002; Singhal et al. 2003; Rena et al. 2007). However, factors such as an unfavourable histological subgroup (e.g. subtype B3 or worse) and gross fibrous adhesion to the pleura have been linked to an increased risk of postoperative recurrence. Recent publications continue to support the use of postoperative radiotherapy in completely resected stage III thymic tumours (Ogawa et al. 2002; Strobel et al. 2004). A retrospective analysis found that radiotherapy for patients with completely resected type B2 and B3 thymomas prevented tumour recurrence, while a 33% local recurrence rate was seen in patients with stage III disease who did not receive adjuvant radiotherapy (Ogawa et al. 2002). However, disease-specific survival at 10 years in patients with stage III thymomas who did not receive radiation can be as high as 75% (Mangi et al. 2005).

Postoperative radiotherapy is also indicated in patients with stage IV disease in whom the disease can be encompassed in a radiotherapy volume that is likely to be associated with acceptable toxicity. Adjuvant radiotherapy is not indicated in patients with large volume disease (e.g. pleural metastases) as salvage surgery may be used for late recurrences (Blumberg et al. 1995), as opposed to the immediate risk of radiation-induced morbidity.

Treatment of incompletely excised thymoma or gross tumour

For patients with incompletely resected or unresectable thymomas, a combined multimodality approach using initial chemotherapy, followed by ± surgery and/or radiotherapy is recommended. Patients with an incomplete resection do not necessarily have a poorer prognosis than those with completely resected tumours (de Jong et al. 2008). A phase II multicentre study performed using 4 cycles of cisplatin–doxorubicin–cyclophosphamide chemotherapy and local radiotherapy to 54Gy achieved 5-year progression-free and OS rates of 54% and 52%, respectively (Loehrer et al. 1997). A prospective phase II study in which 22 patients with unresectable malignant thymomas were treated using induction chemotherapy followed by surgical resection, postoperative radiotherapy, and consolidation chemotherapy reported a 5-year OS of 95% (Kim et al. 2004). Similar results were described using such an approach in an Italian study (Bretti et al. 2004).

Recommendations for chemotherapy scheme and dose

In the metastatic or recurrent setting, thymoma exhibits sensitivity to a number of single agents including cisplatin, ifosfamide, doxorubicin, cyclophosphamide, and corticosteroids. Most reported studies have been are small but combination schemes have shown an ability to produce prolonged durable responses. A prospective intergroup trial showed activity with a cisplatin–doxorubicin–cyclophosphamide regimen in patients with metastatic or locally progressive recurrent disease. Other schemes showing activity include etoposide–ifosfamide–cisplatin and cisplatin–etoposide.

Radiation treatment: dose and techniques

Radiotherapy planning for thymoma should always be based upon CT scans in order to define the tumour volume (involved fields) which is based upon reconstructing the tumour bed and/or gross residual tumour (Fig. 4.3.6). Due to the lack of prospective trials in this uncommon tumour, there is limited evidence on dose–response relationship. In the preoperative setting, a dose of 40–45Gy is typically administered in once-daily fractions of 1.8–2.0Gy. The dose used for postoperative radiation is generally 50Gy, while doses of up to 60Gy are used for patients with incompletely excised tumours and those with inoperable tumours. There is little good evidence to support irradiation of uninvolved mediastinal or supraclavicular nodal regions, nor for hemithorax radiotherapy to prevent pleural metastases.

Further reading

Bretti S, Berruti A, Loddo C, et al: Multimodal management of stages III-IVa malignant thymoma. Lung Cancer 2004: **44**:69–77.

de Jong WK, Blaauwgeers JL, Schaapveld M, et al. Thymic epithelial tumours: a population-based study of the incidence, diagnostic procedures and therapy. Eur J Cancer. 2008; **44**:123–30.

Engels EA, Pfeiffer RM. Malignant thymoma in the United States: demographic patterns in incidence and associations with subsequent malignancies. *Int J Cancer* 2003;**105**:546–51.

Kim DJ, Yang WI, Choi SS, *et al.* Prognostic and clinical relevance of the World Health Organization schema for the classification of thymic epithelial tumours: a clinicopathologic study of 108 patients and literature review. *Chest* 2005; **127**:755–61.

Kim ES, Putnam JB, Komakl R, *et al.* Phase II study of a multidisciplinary approach with induction chemotherapy, followed by surgical resection, radiation therapy, and consolidation chemotherapy for unresectable malignant thymomas: final report. *Lung Cancer* 2004; **44**:369–79

Loehrer PJ Sr, Chen M, Kim K, *et al.* Cisplatin, doxorubicin, and cyclophosphamide plus thoracic radiation therapy for limited-stage unresectable thymoma: an intergroup trial. *J Clin Oncol* 1997; **15**:3093–9

Mangi AA, Wright CD, Allan JS, *et al.* Adjuvant radiation therapy for stage II thymoma. *Ann Thorac Surg* 2002; **74**:1033–7

Mangi AA, Wain JC, Donahue DM, *et al.* Adjuvant radiation of stage III thymoma: is it necessary? *Ann Thorac Surg* 2005; **79**:1834–9.

Ogawa K, Uno T, Toita T, *et al:* Postoperative radiotherapy for patients with completely resected thymoma: a multi-institutional, retrospective review of 103 patients. *Cancer* 2002; **94**:1405–13.

Rena O, Papalia E, Oliaro A, *et al.* Does adjuvant radiation therapy improve disease-free survival in completely resected Masaoka stage II thymoma? *Eur J Cardiothorac Surg* 2007; **31**:109–13.

Rosai J. Histological typing of tumours of the thymus. World Health Organization International Histological Classification of Tumours. 2nd ed. New York, Berlin: Springer-Verlag; 1999.

Singhal S, Shrager JB, Rosenthal DI, *et al.* Comparison of stages I-II thymoma treated by complete resection with or without adjuvant radiation. *Ann Thorac Surg* 2003; **76**:1635–41.

Strobel P, Bauer A, Puppe B, *et al:* Tumour recurrence and survival in patients treated for thymomas and thymic squamous cell carcinomas: a retrospective analysis. *J Clin Oncol* 2004; **22**:1501–9.

Carcinoid

Carcinoids are uncommon neuroendocrine tumours which account for only 2–3% of all primary lung neoplasms (Davila et al. 1998). More than 80% of thoracic carcinoid tumours arise in the bronchial tree and 20% of cases present as solitary pulmonary nodules in asymptomatic individuals. Endobronchial carcinoids are frequently symptomatic, presenting with unilateral wheezing, cough, haemoptysis or recurrent obstructive pneumonias. Bronchopulmonary carcinoid is more prevalent in patients with multiple endocrine neoplasia type 1 (MEN1) (Sachithanandan et al. 2005), although the majority occur as non-familial isolated tumours. MEN1 is an autosomal-dominant syndrome associated with neoplasia of pituitary, pancreas, parathyroid, and foregut lineage neuroendocrine tissue.

Bronchial carcinoids can manifest a spectrum of histopathological features and clinical behaviour, and the distinction between 'typical' and 'atypical carcinoids' is clinically important. It is based on both the number of mitoses (which is the best predictor of prognosis) and the presence of necrosis. 'Typical' carcinoid is defined as <2 mitoses per $2mm^2$ with no necrosis, whereas 'atypical' carcinoid is defined as having 2–10 mitoses per 2 mm^2 or coagulative necrosis, or both (Travis et al. 2004). In 10–15% of cases the tumour can present with regional lymph nodal metastases, and may be classified as malignant neoplasms, even if with a low malignant potential. Distant metastases occur in 15% of cases, and are typically located in the liver, bone, adrenal gland, and brain.

Radiological findings are typically related to bronchial obstruction, with central bronchial carcinoids manifesting as an endobronchial nodule or hilar or perihilar mass with a close anatomical relationship to the bronchus. Associated atelectasis, air trapping, obstructing pneumonitis, and mucoid impaction are also seen. Peripheral bronchial carcinoids appear as solitary nodules, with calcification often visualized at CT. In lung cancer presenting as peripheral nodules, PET scanning has a sensitivity of 96% (Ung et al. 2007). However, carcinoids presenting as peripheral nodules show a lower overall PET sensitivity, with a recent publication citing a 75% sensitivity (Daniels et al. 2007). Reasons for the reduced sensitivity of FDG-PET for diagnosis of primary pulmonary carcinoids are believed to be due to lower metabolic activity and slow growth of these tumours.

Treatment

Typical carcinoids are low-grade malignancies which are usually treated by excision, with parenchyma-sparing sleeve or bronchoplastic resections indicated whenever possible. Atypical carcinoids are aggressive malignancies, and radical surgical resection is indicated. Endobronchial treatment can be useful, both to treat airway obstruction before surgery and to look behind the tumour to estimate the extent of bronchoplastic surgery. Endobronchial treatment is inappropriate without careful imaging using high-resolution CT scans to detect the 10% or more of patients who may have nodal metastases, and for the early detection of local recurrences for salvage therapy. Locoregional failure rates of 8.4% have been reported for typical carcinoids and 22.7% for atypical carcinoids (Kaplan et al. 2003) Up to 64% of patients with atypical carcinoid can develop systemic metastases at a median time of 17 months after diagnosis (Thomas et al. 2001). Local relapse can be treated successfully with surgery, whereas distant metastases have a poor prognosis even after chemotherapy.

Further reading

Davila, DG, Dunn, WF, Tazelaar, HD, et al. Bronchial carcinoid tumours. Mayo Clin Proc 1993; **68**:795–803.

Jeung MY, Gasser B, Gangi A, et al. Bronchial carcinoid tumours of the thorax: spectrum of 303 radiologic findings. RadioGraphics 2002; **22**:351–65.

Kaplan B, Stevens C, Allen P, et al. Outcomes and patterns of failure in bronchial carcinoid tumours. Int J Radiat Oncol Biol Phys 2003; **22**(1):125–31.

Sachithanandan N, Harle RA, Burgess JR. Bronchopulmonary carcinoid in multiple endocrine neoplasia type 1. Cancer 2005; **103**(3):509–15.

Thomas CF Jr, Tazelaar HD, Jett JR. Typical and atypical pulmonary carcinoids: outcome in patients presenting with regional lymph node involvement. Chest 2001; **119**(4):1143–50.

Travis WD, Muller-Hermelink H-K, Harris CC, et al. Pathology and Genetics of Tumours of the Lung, Pleura, Thymus and Heart. Lyon, IARC Press, 2004.

Ung YC, Maziak DE, Vanderveen JA, et al. 18 Fluorodeoxyglucose positron emission tomography in the diagnosis and staging of lung cancer: a systematic review. J Natl Cancer Inst 2007; **99**: 1753–67.

Solitary fibrous tumour of the pleura

Solitary fibrous tumours (SFTs) of the pleura are uncommon slow-growing neoplasms arising from mesenchymal cells on serosal surfaces such as the visceral pleura, although an origin from the parietal or the diaphragmatic pleura has been reported in about 20% of cases. SFT are estimated to constitute <5% of all neoplasms involving the pleura.

Although they are considered to be benign tumours, SFTs of the pleura can occasionally express malignant behaviour. Criteria of malignancy include abundant cellularity, pleomorphism with cytonuclear atypia, >4 mitoses per 10 high-power field, large necrotic or hemorrhagic areas, associated pleural effusion, atypical location, and invasion of adjacent structures (England et al. 1989). Using these criteria, up to 33% of SFTs can be considered malignant (Rena et al. 2001). Immunohistochemistry can differentiate SFTs from other pleural tumours (mesothelioma, sarcoma, and other tumours).

Small tumours are typically sharply delineated, pedunculated neoplasms originating from the visceral pleura and present as incidental findings. Larger tumours most commonly present with chest pain and dyspnoea, but cough, haemoptysis, weight loss, and fatigue are other symptoms. Associated paraneoplastic syndromes include hypertrophic pulmonary osteoarthropathy and hypoglycaemia. CT scan of the thorax typically reveals an intrathoracic homogeneous sharply delineated round or lobulated mass sometimes associated with ipsilateral pleural effusion. Pulmonary atelectasis with opacification of the complete hemithorax has also been described. Complete surgical resection is the treatment of choice. A margin of 1–2cm of healthy tissue is recommended. The most important prognostic factor is complete excision with microscopically free margins. Paraneoplastic syndromes usually disappear after complete resection. Late local recurrences have been reported and long-term follow-up is necessary.

Further reading

Cardillo G, Facciolo F, Cavazzana AO, et al. Localized solitary fibrous tumours of the pleura: an analysis of 55 patients. Ann Thorac Surg 2000; 70:1808–12.

England DM, Hochholtzer L, McCarthy MJ. Localized primary tumours of the pleura. Am J Surg Pathol 1989; 13:640–58.

Rena O, Filosso PL, Papalia E, et al. Solitary fibrous tumour of the pleura: surgical treatment. Eur J Cardiothorac Surg 2001; 19:185–9.

Suter M, Gebhard S, Boumghar M, et al. Localised fibrous tumours of the pleura: 15 cases and review of literature. Eur J Cardiothorac Surg 1998; 14:453–9

Breast cancer: introduction

Epidemiology

It is estimated that more than one million women are diagnosed with breast cancer every year and more than 410,000 women die from breast cancer representing 14% of female cancer deaths.

Breast cancer is the most common female malignancy in the UK and USA. In the UK, 30,000 new cases and 15,000 deaths occur each year due to breast cancer. In the USA, there are 192,000 new cases and 43,300 breast cancer deaths every year. The lifetime risk of developing breast cancer for a woman is 1 in 12 in the UK and 1 in 8 in the USA.

There is considerable variability in the incidence of breast cancer based on ethnicity and geography. Studies show that the incidence of breast cancer is increasing in Japan, China, and India. Approximately 70% of breast cancers diagnosed in Western countries tend to be early stage whereas in developing countries 75% of breast cancers are diagnosed with clinical stages III and IV.

Aetiology and risk factors

The reported risk factors include hormonal, genetic, dietetic, and radiation. Table 4.4.1 shows risk factors and protective factors for breast cancer.

Hormonal and reproductive factors

The effect of hormones, notably oestrogen, is the most significant aetiological factor in breast cancer. Long menstrual history (early menarche and late menopause) increases the risk of breast cancer. Conversely, surgical menopause decreases the risk of breast cancer.

The risk of breast cancer due to exogenous hormone supplementation is controversial. A meta-analysis showed that breast cancer is increased by a factor of 1.3 in current and recent users of hormone replacement therapy (HRT). It has also been estimated that in postmenopausal women, HRT increases the annual risk of breast cancer by 2.3% for each year of hormone intake. Short-term use of HRT may be not associated with a high risk of breast cancer.

Young age at first childbirth is associated with reduction in breast cancer. It has been estimated that age at first birth of 20–25 gives a 50% relative reduction in breast cancer and those who are >35 years at first childbirth have a higher risk of breast cancer than those who are nulliparous. Breastfeeding reduces the relative risk of cancer by 4.3% for each year of breastfeeding.

Genetic risk factors (p.24)

Less than 5% of breast cancer is associated with genetic factors. The most common are high-penetrance mutations of BRCA1 and BRCA2 genes. Though a significant proportion of familial breast cancer may be due to these mutations, some of the familial aggregation of breast cancer is associated with unknown genetic changes.

BRCA1 mutation- associated cancers tend to occur at an early age, are highly aggressive and are typically negative for oestrogen (ER), progesterone (PgR) and human epithelial growth factor receptor 2 (HER2/neu) ('triple negative'). Breast cancers with BRCA2 mutation, which accounts for 1% of breast cancers, are often ER and PgR positive.

Dietetic factors

• Alcohol intake: alcohol intake increases the risk of breast cancer. Women who consume 4 or more alcoholic drinks daily have a 50% increase in risk of breast cancer. It has been estimated that the relative risk (RR) of breast cancer is increased by 7.1% (95% confidence interval [CI], 5.5–8.7, p <0.00001) for each drink of alcohol consumed on a daily basis.

• Obesity: increases the risk of breast cancer. Women with a body mass index (BMI) of >31kg/m² have a 30% higher risk of breast cancer than those with a BMI of 20. In obesity there is an increased production of oestradiol from fatty tissue.

• Physical activity: there is some suggestion that physical activity is protective.

Radiation

Prior radiation to the breast or part of the breast increases the risk of cancer (RR 3) (e.g. mantle radiotherapy for Hodgkin disease). The risk of breast cancer is related to the dose of radiotherapy to the chest wall. Women who have chest wall radiotherapy at or before the age of 25 years to a dose of 40Gy have a cumulative absolute risk of breast cancer of 1.4% at 35 years, 11.1% at 45 years, and 29% at 55 years.

Other risk factors include:

• Previous breast cancer: increases the risk of a contralateral breast cancer (0.5–1% per year).

• Some benign conditions of the breast (e.g. atypical hyperplasia RR 4–5, lobular carcinoma in situ RR 8–10, proliferative lesion without atypia RR 2).

Table 4.4.1 Risk factors in breast cancer

	Relative risk
Factors which increase the risk of breast cancer	
Early menarche (before 11 years)	3
Late menopause (after 54 years)	2
First pregnancy after 40 years	3
Nulliparity	3
HRT	1.7
Oral contraceptive	1.2
1 maternal first-degree relative	1.5–2
2 first-degree relatives	3–5
First-degree relative diagnosed before 40 years	3
Alcohol	4
Protective factors	
Artificial menopause before 35 years	0.5
Increased parity	
Age at first pregnancy <30 years	
Breastfeeding	0.8

Breast cancer: pathogenesis and pathology

Pathogenesis

Breast cancer arises from the epithelial cells lining the terminal duct lobular unit. Development of invasive breast cancer is thought to be due to a multistep process. The WHO classification of breast cancer is shown in the box.

Modified WHO classification of breast cancer

Precursor lesions
- Lobular carcinoma *in situ*
- Intraduct proliferative lesions
  - Atypical ductal hyperplasia
  - Ductal carcinoma *in situ* (DCIS)
- Microinvasive carcinoma

Malignant lesions
- Invasive ductal carcinoma (NST) and subtypes
- Invasive lobular carcinoma
- Tubular carcinoma
- Invasive cribriform carcinoma
- Medullary carcinoma
- Mucinous carcinoma
- Neuroendocrine tumours (small cell carcinoma)
- Metaplastic carcinoma
- Sarcoma

Precursor lesions

- Lobular carcinoma *in situ* is considered as a precursor of invasive cancer, but in most cases it does not progress to the invasive stage. It is regarded as a marker for either lobular or ductal carcinoma. It represents <15% of all non-invasive breast cancer and the usual age at diagnosis is 45 years.
- Atypical ductal hyperplasia is characterized by intraductal epithelial proliferation with some of the features of DCIS. These increase the risk of invasive cancer 4–5 times.
- In DCIS, malignant epithelial proliferation is confined to a duct with no stromal invasion. It accounts for 3–5% of palpable breast cancer and 15–20% of screen-detected cancer. It exhibits a spectrum of histological characteristics from non-comedo, low-grade DCIS to comedo, high-grade DCIS. It is graded according to the appearance of cell nuclei. Low-grade micropapillary DCIS can occur as a multicentric tumour whereas high-grade comedo carcinoma DCIS can be associated with invasive tumour in the same quadrant. Broadly there are five subtypes of DCIS: comedo, solid, cribriform, micropapillary, and papillary. Comedo type is characterized by large cells with poorly differentiated nuclei and central necrosis. Solid DCIS is characterized by ductal spaces filled with neoplastic cells. Cribriform DCIS is characterized by microlumens and fenestrations. Micropapillary DCIS is characterized by intraluminal projections with no fibrovascular core whereas, papillary DCIS has a fibrovascular core.
- Microinvasive carcinoma is a focus of invasive cancer of <1mm in maximum extent. When there are multiple microinvasive cancers, the size of the largest focus is used to classify the microinvasion.

Malignant breast lesions

- Invasive ductal carcinoma: 70–80% of all invasive carcinomas are classified as invasive ductal carcinomas, which are thought to arise from DCIS. Histologically they appear as solid cords of groups of ductal cancer cells of varying size, cytoplasmic content, and differentiation. They occur most commonly as 'ductal no special type' (ductal NST). Ductal NST is a diagnosis of exclusion. Other special subtypes of ductal carcinomas include:
  - Tubular carcinoma: constitutes 1–2% of breast cancer. These have an indolent growth pattern and an excellent prognosis. Histologically they are composed of tubular structures lined by a single layer of well differentiated epithelium. Axillary nodal metastasis occurs in <15% of cases of tubular carcinoma. After conservative treatment, local recurrence occurs in <5% and death from metastatic disease is extremely rare.
  - Medullary carcinoma: constitutes 4–9% of breast cancer. They are composed of cords and masses of large cells with pleomorphic nuclei and prominent nucleoli. These tumours have a good prognosis and are commonly associated with younger women and BRCA1 mutations.
  - Mucinous carcinoma: constitutes 2% of breast cancer. They are slow growing tumours seen generally in older women. Axillary lymph node involvement occurs in <5% of cases.
  - Micropapillary carcinoma: constitutes 1–2% of breast cancers. More than 75% of patients have nodal involvement at diagnosis. The prognosis is poor.
- Invasive lobular carcinoma: constitutes 10–15% of invasive cancers. These tumours infiltrate diffusely leading to a discrepancy between imaging findings and histological tumour size. Histologically these are characterized by cells appearing as single or small clusters in a targetoid or single-file (Indian file) pattern. These tumours are generally ER positive and can present as late diffuse recurrences on pleural or peritoneal surfaces.
- Rare histological subtypes include:
  - Adenocystic carcinoma: this resembles its counterpart in the salivary gland. These tumours have less risk of axillary recurrence and have a good prognosis
  - Small cell carcinoma: this resembles small cell carcinoma of lung. It should be differentiated from a metastasis from elsewhere. Treatment should be aggressive with surgery, chemotherapy, and radiotherapy
  - Metaplastic carcinoma: rare. These tumours have a high risk of axillary metastasis, and are generally hormone receptor negative. Some studies suggest that these, especially those with a sarcomatoid component, respond poorly to chemotherapy and have a poor outcome
  - Other cancers: include lymphoma, sarcoma, melanoma and metastasis.

Therapeutic pathology

Pathology plays an important role in deciding postoperative management. The postoperative pathology report should include: number of tumours, maximum diameter of largest tumour, histological type and grade (see Table 4.4.2), circumferential excision margin and minimal margin, vascular invasion, number of nodes retrieved, number of nodes involved, and extent of involvement (e.g. micrometastasis or metastasis), presence of DCIS and immunohistochemical status of oestrogen (ER) and progesterone (PgR) (see box) and HER2. Patients with an ambiguous

Table 4.4.2 Nottingham grading of breast cancer

Characteristics	Score 1	Score 2	Score 3
Degree of tubule formation	>75%	10–75%	<10%
Nuclear pleomorphism	Mild	Moderate	Severe
Mitoses/10 HPF		Score of 1–3 based on the diameter of high power field and mitotic frequency	

Grade I: score 3–5

Grade II: score 6–7

Grade III: score 8–9

HER2 (2+) status on immunohistochemistry require fluorescent *in situ* hybridization (FISH) to look for gene amplification (see box).

Molecular profiling has identified five subtypes of breast cancer: luminal A, luminal B, HER2+, normal breast-like, and basal-like. The luminal tumours are ER+ whereas others are ER−. The outcome for these types is different.

The role of molecular profiling in routine clinical practice is evolving but it is possible in the future that these subtypes will be treated differently (see p.171).

ER and PgR scoring systems

McCarty's semiquantitative H scoring (total score 0–300) (percentage of stained cells multiplied by a number, 0–3, reflecting the intensity of staining)

- Negative: Score ≤50 (−)
- Weakly positive: 51–100 (+)
- Moderately positive: 101–200 (++)
- Strongly positive: 201–300 (+++)

Her-2/neu scoring

Immunohistochemical scoring

- Score 0–1+: negative
- 2+: borderline—needs further testing
- 3+: positive

FISH score

- <2.0, not amplified: negative
- >2.0, amplified: positive

Breast cancer: clinical features, diagnosis, staging, and prognostic factors

Clinical features

Many early breast cancers are detected during screening by mammography.

The usual presentations are painless lump (65–75%), distortion of the breast (5%), and nipple discharge (2%). A small proportion of patients present with isolated axillary lymphadenopathy. Some patients present with metastatic manifestations such as bone pain, respiratory symptoms, and features of liver metastases and brain disease. Up to 30–40% of women with a clinically negative axilla may have microscopic involvement of axillary nodes.

Breast examination may reveal a non-tender, well- or ill-defined lump with or without fixity to the skin or chest wall. The skin may be dimpled, invaded, reddened, indurated or with nodular irregularity.

Axillary and supraclavicular lymph nodes may be enlarged. Hepatomegaly, pleural effusion and spinal tenderness (usually thoracic and lumbar) can occur in metastatic disease.

Diagnosis

Patients can present with early stage disease or with features of metastatic disease. In patients with early stage disease, the initial investigation involves triple assessment in a one-stop clinic. Indications for urgent evaluation of patients with suspected breast cancer are given on p.5.

Triple assessment

'Triple' assessment of patients with suspected breast cancer includes a combination of clinical examination, breast imaging (mammography and/or ultrasound), and pathological evaluation (core biopsy). With this approach, a definite diagnosis of breast cancer can be made in 99% of cases.

Clinical examination

Patients should be examined both sitting up and lying down. Both breasts should be examined and physical examination findings such as the location, size and consistency, mobility, and fixity of the tumour should be well documented. Physical examination should also include evaluation of the axilla and supraclavicular fossa. If there are any palpable nodes, the number, consistency, tenderness, fixity, and size should be documented. Examination of the chest and abdomen (for liver enlargement) and evaluation of bone for tenderness are essential. Clinical examination contributes to tumour and nodal staging.

Breast imaging

- *Mammography*: mammography is the most important component of breast imaging. The commonest mammographic abnormality of DCIS is microcalcification (in 50% cases). Other features include asymmetric density and mass. High-grade DCIS is associated with linear and branching calcification, whereas low-grade DCIS is associated with fine and granular calcification. Invasive cancer appears as a spiculated mass. Although calcification can occur in various conditions, a linear small (<1mm in diameter), irregular, and clustered calcification is suggestive of malignancy. In general, mammography has a sensitivity of 90% and specificity of 94%. However, it has a low sensitivity in breasts with considerable fibroglandular tissue, particularly in young women and those

on HRT. The evolving digital mammography has the advantages of better imaging of dense breast tissue and computer-assisted detection.

- *Ultrasound*: ultrasound examination complements physical examination and mammography. It is also helpful to distinguish between solid and cystic lesions of >1cm in size. Malignancy appears as a hypoechoic lesion with associated distortion of the surrounding tissues and an acoustic shadow on the breast tissue below it. It is also useful to assess axillary nodal status as well as to guide FNA and core biopsy. Ultrasound is less sensitive than mammography for early detection and hence is not used for screening.

- *MRI scan*: the role of MRI in breast cancer is rapidly increasing. MRI can more accurately define the size of the tumour compared with mammography and is better in delineating intraductal disease and multifocal disease. MRI has a high sensitivity in detecting cancers (almost 100%) and lower sensitivity in detecting DCIS (80%), but has a higher false positivity. MRI is more useful for young women who have dense breast tissue. MRI is particularly useful in screening women <40 years with a high risk of breast cancer, to rule out multifocal disease prior to conservation, for imaging breasts with implants, and to distinguish scars from tumour recurrence. MRI also has a clear role in evaluating patients presenting with axillary metastasis but without evidence of a breast lump on physical examination and mammography. Some recent studies suggest that MRI is also useful in detecting a contralateral breast cancer.

Pathological diagnosis

Pathological diagnosis may be obtained by core biopsy or open surgical biopsy. Core biopsy can be obtained by conventional or vacuum-assisted means such as a mammotome. Vacuum-assisted core biopsy yields a larger sample and may in some cases allow complete removal of the target abnormality in the breast. Clinically impalpable lesions may necessitate image localization using mammography or ultrasound and hook wire placement before open biopsy.

Investigations after triple assessment

Most patients with early stage disease without clinical evidence of metastatic disease will proceed to surgery after preoperative assessment. Patients who require neoadjuvant systemic treatment prior to definitive surgical management need staging investigations including:

- Full blood count, liver and renal function tests, and serum alkaline phosphatase
- CXR and CT scan of chest and abdomen to rule out distant metastasis
- Bone scan

There is no established role for routine CT scan staging in patients with early stage breast cancer. Since the yield of positive findings on CT scan is low in patients with node-negative and intermediate-risk node-positive disease, routine CT scan is advised only for patients with ≥4 positive lymph nodes and T4 disease postoperatively. In those with <4 positive nodes, normal biochemistry, and no symptoms suggestive of metastasis, the incidence of metastasis is 2–4% and hence routine staging is not advised.

There is no established role for PET scan. It may be useful for patients who present with isolated axillary nodal disease without a primary breast tumour, to decide further management.

Staging

TNM staging of breast cancer is given in the box on p.154.

Prognostic factors and survival

Breast cancer has a considerable spectrum of prognosis depending on a variety of clinical, biological, and genetic characteristics. The American College of Pathologists has categorized the prognostic factors in breast cancer into three categories as follows:

- Category I: factors associated with proven prognostic importance and useful in clinical management. These include tumour size, nodal status, grade, hormonal receptor status, lymphovascular invasion, and HER2 status
- Category II: factors which have been studied but whose importance is not known. These factors include p53 mutations, and DNA ploidy.
- Category III: factors are those not studied sufficiently. These factors include BCL2, cathepsin D expression etc.

Tumour size

Tumour size is correlated with survival and risk of lymph node involvement and distant metastasis. In patients with node-negative disease, tumour size remains the strongest prognostic factor.

Axillary nodal status

Lymph node status is the strongest predictor of disease-free survival (DFS) and overall survival (OS). The number of lymph nodes involved has prognostic implications. The current prognostic grouping for breast cancer patients is based on number of nodal sites of involvement (negative, 1–3 node involved, 4–10 nodes involved, and >10 nodes involved) which has implications for postoperative management (see p.160 and p.162).

Tumour grade

There are a number of grading systems of which one of the commonly used is that of the Nottingham group. Studies have shown that grade has strong correlation with prognosis.

Hormonal receptor status

Several studies have shown that patients with ER and PgR positive tumours have significantly higher survival. One study has shown that the 1-year survival for ER positive tumours was 65.9% compared with 56% for ER negative tumours.

Recently molecular profiling has further refined prognostication of ER positive tumours based on HER2 status. However, its therapeutic implications are still evolving.

HER2/neu status

The HER2/neu proto-oncogene, located on chromosome 17, is amplified or overexpressed in 25–30% of breast cancer. The overexpression is associated with aggressiveness of the cancer as well as decreased DFS. Currently HER2 status is an important factor in deciding whether to recommend adjuvant systemic treatment with trastuzumab (see p.163) as well as in selection of hormonal treatment in some patients.

Other prognostic factors

- Age has proven recently to be an important prognostic factor. Studies show that women aged <35 years have twice the risk of local recurrence and 1.6 times higher risk of distant metastasis compared with those >35 years. This has important implications in deciding the primary surgery (age <35 years is increasingly being considered as a relative contraindication for conservative surgery) and adjuvant systemic treatment.
- Lymphatic/vascular invasion has been shown to be an important independent prognostic factor in a number of studies. It has been associated with an increase in both local and systemic recurrence. Hence it is an important factor in deciding adjuvant treatment.

Composite stage continues be an important prognostic factor. The estimated 5-year survival of stage I breast cancer is 85%, stage II 70%, stage III 50% and stage IV 20%.

Estimation of prognosis

A number of predictive models can be used to estimate the long term prognosis thereby guiding the choice of appropriate systemic treatment. The most commonly used methods are the Nottingham prognostic index (Table 4.4.3) and an online tool called adjuvant online.

Table 4.4.3 Nottingham prognostic index and 10-year survival. (Index applicable only to patients aged ≤70 years and tumour size ≤5cm) Nottingham prognostic index score = N stage + grade + (maximum T size in cm x 0.2) (N0: no nodal disease; N1: 0–3 positive nodes; N2: 4–10 nodes; and N3: >10 nodes)

Prognostic group	Score	% 10-year survival
Excellent	2.08–2.4	96
Good	2.42–≤3.4	93
Moderate I	3.42–≤4.4	81
Moderate II	4.42–≤5.4	74
Poor	5.42–≤6.4	50
Very poor	6.5–6.8	38

Internet resource

Adjuvant! Online: http://www.adjuvantonline.com

Staging of breast cancer

Stage 0
- Tx: primary tumour cannot be assessed.
- T0: no evidence of primary tumour.
- Tis: carcinoma in situ and Paget's disease with no tumour

Stage I (T1N0M0)
- T1: tumour ≤2cm in its greatest dimension.
- N0: no regional lymph node metastasis
- M0: no distant metastases

Stage II

IIA (TxN1M0, T1N1M0, T2N0M0)
- T2: tumour >2 cm but not >5cm
- N1: ipsilateral non-fixed lymph node metastasis

IIB (T2N1M0, T3N0M0)
- T3: tumour >5cm

Stage III

IIIA (Tx–2N2M0, T2–3N1–2M0)
- N2: ipsilateral fixed axillary node or ipsilateral internal mammary lymph nodes

IIIB T4N0–2M0
- T4 : tumour of any size with:
  - T4a: extension to chest wall
  - T4b: oedema (including peau d'orange) or ulceration of the breast skin, or satellite skin nodules confined to the same breast
  - T4c: both T4a and T4b
  - T4d: inflammatory breast cancer

IIIC (any T, N3M0)

N3: metastasis to ipsilateral supraclavicular lymph nodes or infraclavicular lymph nodes or metastasis to the internal mammary lymph nodes with metastasis to the axillary lymph nodes

Stage IV (any T, any N, M1)
- M1: distant metastasis

Breast cancer: management of carcinoma *in situ*

Ductal carcinoma *in situ*

Introduction

DCIS is a heterogeneous clonal proliferation of epithelial malignant cells confined to the lumen of the mammary ducts without evidence of basement membrane invasion. DCIS constitutes 20–45% of screen-detected cancers and 10% of all breast cancers. It is a highly curable disease with 10-year survival exceeding 95%. The most common mammographic feature of DCIS is microcalcification (up to 90%), which is typically clustered, pleomorphic, variable in size and density, and often arranged in a linear or segmental fashion. Ten per cent of mammographic lesions may not have calcification. MRI scan of DCIS may show non-specific features and its role is still evolving.

Diagnosis

Preoperative diagnosis of DCIS is established by open surgical biopsy, wire-localization, or mammotome biopsy (stereotactic vacuum-assisted biopsy).

Treatment

Surgery

The treatment of DCIS is aimed at preventing local recurrence, particularly of invasive cancer. After biopsy alone, 40% will progress to invasive cancer. Treatment options include surgery alone, or surgery followed by radiotherapy and hormones.

Surgery of unicentric DCIS includes conservative surgery and simple or skin-sparing mastectomy. Conservative surgical options include wide excision, segmental resection, or quadrantectomy. Those who undergo mastectomy may be considered for immediate reconstruction. These choices should be discussed with patients.

Most patients can be treated with conservative surgery with good survival and cosmetic result. The optimal margin for wide excision is not well defined; a margin of >10mm is adequate and <1mm is inadequate (NICE recommends 2mm).

Patients with a persistent positive margin after repeat (two or more) surgical excision, widespread DCIS (involving two or more quadrants), suspicious microcalcification throughout the breast, and those likely to have an unacceptable cosmetic result with conservative surgery are considered for simple mastectomy. Young patients with a strong family history of breast cancer may also be considered for mastectomy. The local recurrence rate following skin-sparing mastectomy is similar to that after simple mastectomy. Skin-sparing mastectomy with immediate autologous myocutaneous flap reconstruction achieves a better cosmetic result than simple mastectomy with reconstruction. This is because skin preservation provides skin coverage of identical colour and texture to the opposite breast.

Axillary staging and dissection are unnecessary for patients with pure DCIS. However, the breast cancer-specific mortality rate in DCIS is 1–2% suggesting the presence of occult invasive disease. Some series report up to 2% incidence of axillary node metastasis due to an unrecognized invasive cancer. In clinical practice, axillary lymph node status is assessed in patients undergoing mastectomy and may be considered in situations where there is a high chance of invasive disease such as mammographic tumour of >4cm, age <55 years, high-grade DCIS, and diagnosis made with core biopsy. There is no proven role for sentinel node biopsy (SNB).

Postoperative radiotherapy

After conservative surgery, there is a 15% risk of local recurrence at 5 years. This risk depends on a number of factors such as size of the tumour, grade, margin, etc. Randomized studies show that postoperative radiotherapy (45–50Gy in 1.8–2Gy per fraction) reduces breast recurrence (both *in situ* and invasive) to approximately 8% with no impact on OS and the benefit is independent of prognostic factors. A recent systemic review of 3925 patients (from four randomized studies) showed that addition of radiotherapy reduced ipsilateral breast events (HR = 0.49; 95% CI 0.41–0.58, p <0.00001) in all subgroups of patients (Goodwin 2009). The NNT to prevent one ipsilateral breast recurrence was 9 and there was no evidence of excess radiotherapy late toxicities.

There is ongoing debate on whether radiotherapy can be omitted in patients with a low risk of recurrence such as the subgroup characterized by a tumour of <10–15mm, low/intermediate grade DCIS, and a clear margin of >1cm in all directions (<10% local recurrence at 10 years). Given the potential benefit of 50% reduction in local recurrence rate with radiotherapy, it is important to assess the potential risks, benefits, and cost implications when recommending radiotherapy for all patients with DCIS. On balance it would be advisable to consider radiotherapy based on an individual risk–benefit assessment.

The role of boost radiotherapy in DCIS is not known. The ongoing TROG 07.01 study is evaluating the role of dose escalation in non-low-risk DCIS. For practical purposes, boost radiotherapy may be considered if there is a close or positive margin and further excision to obtain a wider margin is likely to compromise cosmetic results, and in young patients (<45 years).

Adjuvant systemic treatment

Two studies compared the benefits of tamoxifen in DCIS. NSABP B-24 showed that tamoxifen reduced local recurrence of DCIS and invasive cancer (11% vs. 7.7% p = 0.02) whereas UKCCCR trial showed that tamoxifen had no beneficial effect in reducing local recurrence when combined with whole breast radiotherapy (15 vs. 13% p = 0.42). In the absence of radiotherapy, tamoxifen reduced the risk of DCIS recurrence (10 vs. 6% p = 0.03) but not invasive recurrence. There is no universally accepted recommendation for adjuvant hormones. Current studies are evaluating various other hormonal agents (e.g. IBIS II comparing anastrozole with tamoxifen).

Prognosis and outcome

With mammographic follow-up, breast cancer DFS in DCIS approaches 100%. Women with DCIS in one breast are at risk of a contralateral tumour occurring at a rate of 0.5–1% per annum.

DCIS has a variable potential for development into an invasive disease. A number of factors have been evaluated to predict the invasive potential including nuclear grade, architectural pattern, and presence of necrosis. However, these factors are more useful in predicting the risk of recurrence than the risk of malignant transformation. Grade of DCIS is the most important predictor of recurrence. High-grade tumours have 32% recurrence rate, intermediate grade 10%, and low grade 0%.

Summary of recommendations

Surgery is the definitive treatment of DCIS. In all patients, except those with low-risk disease, postoperative radiotherapy is indicated after conservative surgery. Boost radiotherapy is considered in those with close/positive margin if further surgery is not contemplated. There is no role for recommending adjuvant hormones routinely.

Lobular Carcinoma *In Situ* (LCIS)

Introduction

LCIS is an incidental histological finding. LCIS comprises 30–50% of carcinoma *in situ*, and is often multifocal (50%) and frequently bilateral (35–60%). It is associated with invasive cancer in 10%. However, it is not clear whether LCIS is a direct precursor of invasive lobular carcinoma. Many consider it as a marker of increased risk of subsequent breast cancer (7–18 times higher risk than general population) rather than a malignant lesion. There is an increased risk of cancer in both breasts and the risk is probably lifelong. Most of the invasive cancers are ductal in type. A recently identified variant, pleomorphic LCIS, has high-grade features and may have biological behaviour similar to DCIS.

It is usually undetectable clinically and cannot be seen on mammogram due to the lack of central necrosis. The mean age at diagnosis is 44–46 years. One-third of people develop invasive cancer in the same or contralateral breast over 20 years.

Treatment

Isolated LCIS following biopsy is managed with close observation. There is no evidence that a re-excision to obtain clear margins is likely to reduce risk significantly. The rate of progression to cancer after biopsy alone is approximately 1% per annum. Mastectomy is generally reserved for patients with the highest risk of invasive recurrence such as young age, diffuse high-grade lesions, and significant family history.

There is no evidence that radiotherapy has a role in the management of LCIS.

A subset analysis of patients with LCIS in the NSABP P-1 study has shown that tamoxifen reduces the risk of invasive cancer recurrence by 56%. Similar benefit has been confirmed with raloxifene in the NSABP P-2 study. In the absence of long-term data, patients are encouraged to participate in clinical trials.

LCIS associated with DCIS or invasive cancer is managed according to the dominant malignant histology. There is no need to pursue additional surgery to obtain a clear margin for LCIS.

There is no evidence that follow-up mammography will improve the outcome in LCIS.

Further reading

Afonso N and Bouwman D. Lobular carcinoma in situ. *Eur J Cancer Prev* 2008; **17**:312.

Goodwin A, Parker S, Ghersi D, *et al*. Post-operative radiotherapy for ductal carcinoma in situ of the breast – A systematic review of the randomised trials. *Breast* 2009; **18**:143–49.

Lakhani SR, Audretsch W, Cleton-Jensen A, *et al*. The management of lobular carcinoma in situ (LCIS). Is LCIS the same as ductal carcinoma in situ (DCIS)? *Eur J Cancer* 2006; **42**:2205–11.

Sakorafas G, Farley D, Peros G. Recent advances and current controversies in the management of DCIS of the breast. *Cancer Treat Rev* 2008; **34**:483–97.

Internet resource

American College of Radiologists: Practice Guideline for management of ductal carcinoma in-situ of breast—available at http:// www.acr.org

Management of breast cancer: surgery

After triple assessment, initial treatment options for early stage (non-inflammatory T1–2N0–1M0) include:
* Conservative surgery with axillary surgery
* Mastectomy with axillary surgery
* Neoadjuvant chemotherapy followed by conservative surgery (when primary surgery is likely to result in unacceptable cosmesis)

Surgery

Surgical management of early stage breast cancer involves surgery of the primary tumour and assessment and treatment of the axilla whenever indicated. Primary surgery of the tumour can be either conservative surgery or a mastectomy. The choice between conservative surgery and mastectomy is an important step in the management of early breast cancer. Randomized studies have shown that in carefully selected patients both approaches result in equal long-term survival. Conservative surgery followed by postoperative radiotherapy offers a better cosmetic outcome than mastectomy. However, not all patients are suitable for breast conservation (see box).

Nodal management can be nodal biopsy, node dissection or biopsy followed by dissection for node positive disease.

Breast surgery

Breast conservation surgery involves removal of the primary tumour with a circumferential margin of normal tissue. It can be wide local excision (WLE), segmental mastectomy, or quadrantectomy. WLE aims to remove the cancer with a macroscopic margin of 1cm which should achieve at least a >1mm circumferential microscopic disease-free margin. There is no consensus on the minimal safe circumferential microscopic margin. Worldwide values range from 1mm to 1cm. A number of clinicopathological factors increase the risk of local recurrence after WLE. These include:
* Close (<1mm) or positive margin. The risk of recurrence is 16–21% with a positive margin compared with 2–5% with a negative margin. Hence all patients with a close or positive margin should be considered for a re-excision if technically feasible.
* Age ≤35 years (2–3 times increased risk of local recurrence). Recently these patients are being increasing treated with a mastectomy.
* Extensive intraductal component (defined as an infiltrating ductal cancer where >25% of the tumour volume is DCIS and DCIS extends beyond the invasive cancer into the surrounding normal breast parenchyma).
* Lymphovascular invasion—increases the risk of recurrence by 1.5 times.
* Grade (grade I tumours have 1.5 times less risk of recurrence than grade II–III)

Mastectomy involves complete removal of the breast from the pectoral fascia. There are a number of variations of this procedure, namely radical mastectomy, extended radical mastectomy, modified radical mastectomy, simple mastectomy (total mastectomy), skin-sparing mastectomy, and nipple-sparing mastectomy based on the extent of the surgery. Details of these procedures are listed here:
* Radical mastectomy: removal of breast tissue with pectoralis major muscle with level I/II axillary dissection.
* Extended radical mastectomy: radical mastectomy with internal mammary node dissection with or without level III axillary node dissection.
* Modified radical mastectomy: removal of breast tissue with level I/II axillary node dissection.
* Simple mastectomy: removal of breast tissue alone.
* Skin-sparing mastectomy: simple or modified radical mastectomy with preservation of a significant proportion of skin of the breast to facilitate immediate reconstruction. This is usually done in patients who are unlikely to have postoperative radiotherapy.
* Nipple-sparing mastectomy: preservation of nipple and/or nipple areola complex. This procedure is not advised routinely.

The clinicopathological factors that increase the risk of chest wall recurrence after mastectomy include tumour of >5cm, more than four axillary nodes involved, margin <1mm. Grade 3 and vascular invasion are not independent risk factors for recurrence.

Breast reconstruction after mastectomy
Reconstruction can be done at the same time as mastectomy (immediate) or at a later date (delayed). Immediate reconstruction can be offered to patients with diffuse DCIS and early breast cancer who may not require postoperative radiotherapy (radiotherapy to a reconstructed breast can result in poor cosmetic outcome). Delayed reconstruction is appropriate when postoperative radiotherapy is planned and there is concern about tumour clearance.
Methods of reconstruction include:
* Tissue expanders: initially the expander is placed in the pocket deep to pectoralis muscle, which is later replaced with a permanent implant containing silicone gel or saline after a few months. Complications include infections, failure of expansion, and capsular contracture (particularly after radiotherapy).
* Autologous tissue: using either a pediculated flap (e.g. latissimus dorsi flap) or a free flap (free transverse rectus abdominis myocutaneous—TRAM flap).

Contraindications to breast conservation surgery

* Prior radiotherapy to the breast or chest wall
* Breast cancer during pregnancy
* Diffuse suspicious or malignant appearing microcalcification
* Widespread or multifocal disease that cannot be completely excised with satisfactory cosmesis through a single incision
* Persistent positive pathological margin
* Active connective tissue disease involving skin (scleroderma and lupus)
* Tumours of >5cm
* Women ≤35 years or premenopausal with BRCA1/2 mutation
* Inflammatory breast cancer
* No response or progression to neoadjuvant chemotherapy (see Chapter 4.4, Locally advanced breast cancer: concepts in management, p.166)

Axillary surgery

Standard axillary procedures include SNB, SNB followed by axillary dissection, or axillary dissection alone.

SNB is increasingly being used in patients with clinically node-negative breast cancer. The sentinel node is localized by preoperative intradermal injection of technetium-labelled colloid and lymphoscintiscan, or by intraoperative injection of blue due, or using both techniques. SNB has >95% detection rate. However, SNB is not recommended in cases of high risk of axillary node involvement (e.g. palpable axillary node, >3cm or T3 or T4 tumours, multicentric tumours), previous history of surgery to breast or axilla, during pregnancy or lactation (contraindication of dye and radioisotope) and after neoadjuvant systemic treatment outside clinical trials (role not defined), where dissection is the norm.

The current standard for patients with positive SNB is completion axillary dissection. However, the benefit of this approach is being questioned. The prospective randomized trial of Adjuvant Management of the Axilla, Radiotherapy or Surgery (AMAROS) compares postoperative radiotherapy with axillary dissection in sentinel node-positive patients.

Many patients with clinically positive nodes will undergo axillary dissection during primary breast surgery. The extent of dissection is based on the level of axillary contents. Level I contains tissue lateral to pectoralis minor muscle and between the axillary vein and latissimus dorsi. Level II is behind the pectoralis minor muscle whereas level III is between the medial border of pectoralis minor muscle and the apex of axilla. A complete axillary dissection (level I–III) is associated with a high incidence of lymphoedema but is without proven survival advantage. Before the advent of SNB, the traditional treatment of a clinically node-negative patient was level I/II dissection. A meta-analysis of six randomized studies has shown that this approach resulted in an average overall survival benefit of 5.4%. However, a meta-analysis of three randomized trials published after 2000, showed no overall survival advantage.

Further reading

Orr RK. The impact of prophylactic axillary node dissection on breast cancer survival: a Bayesian meta-analysis. *Ann Surg Oncol* 1999; **6**:109–16

Sanghani M, Balk EM, Cady B. Impact of axillary node dissection on breast cancer outcome in clinically node negative patients: a systematic review and meta-analysis. *Cancer* 2009; **115**:1613–20.

Breast cancer: role of adjuvant radiotherapy

Benefit of adjuvant radiotherapy

A meta-analysis suggests that adjuvant radiotherapy in breast cancer results in a reduction of local recurrence by two-thirds and improves 15-year survival by 5%. It also suggests that at 15 years one breast cancer death is avoided for every four local recurrences prevented.

Radiotherapy after conservative surgery

Randomized studies have shown that conservative breast surgery followed by postoperative radiotherapy results in equal long-term survival to that of mastectomy in stage I and II patients. A meta-analysis suggests that radiotherapy reduces the risk of local recurrence after breast conservation (5-year local recurrence of 7% with radiotherapy and 26% without radiotherapy) and is the current standard after WLE.

Young age appears to be a significant risk factor for local recurrence after conservative surgery. In the EORTC 22881/10882 study, the addition of boost radiotherapy resulted in the reduction of 5-year local recurrence from 26% to 8.5% in patients aged ≤35 years compared with a reduction from 3.9% to 2.1% in those aged ≥60 years. Because of this increase in the risk of local recurrence, some centres consider young age as a relative contraindication for breast conservation.

The role of routine radiotherapy after breast conservation in elderly patients is debatable. One study showed that in patients >70 years with good prognostic factors (<2cm tumour, grade 1 or 2, ER positive, node negative, and no lymphovascular invasion) omission of radiotherapy may not compromise survival. The ongoing PRIME study investigates the role of routine radiotherapy in women aged >65 years with hormone receptor-positive tumour of <3cm.

Role of boost radiotherapy

Two randomized studies have evaluated the role of tumour bed boost radiotherapy. It has been shown that the addition of radiotherapy to the tumour bed after whole breast radiotherapy reduces local recurrence (10-year local recurrence rate of 6.2% with boost and 10.2% without boost p <0.001). On multivariate analysis, age was the only significant predictor of local recurrence and the greatest benefit was seen in those aged <40 years. Boost radiotherapy did not improve 10-year OS. Many centres now follow a risk adapted policy for boost.

Postmastectomy chest wall radiotherapy

There is ongoing debate on the role of radiotherapy after mastectomy. Chest wall recurrence is thought to arise from tumour that has involved dermal lymphatics. Patients with a tumour of ≥5cm size and ≥4 positive lymph nodes are at high risk of chest wall recurrence (20–30%) and routine postoperative chest wall radiotherapy is advised. This results in less local recurrence (6% vs. 23%) and improvement of 15-year survival by 5%.

The role of post-mastectomy radiotherapy in patients with tumour <5cm with 0–3 positive nodes are less clear.

There is some evidence that radiotherapy improves local control and survival irrespective of number of involved lymph nodes. Hence postmastectomy radiotherapy and supraclavicular irradiation may be considered in women with T1 tumour with 1–3 positive nodes until further clinical trial results are available. A number of randomized trials are assessing the role of postmastectomy radiotherapy in patients with intermediate risk breast cancer (EORTC 22922/10925, NCIC MA20, and SFRO CM1). The Selective Use of Postoperative Radiotherapy after Mastectomy (SUPREMO) study randomizes patients with 1–3 positive axillary nodes and pT2pN0 tumours with grade 3 tumours and/or lymphovascular invasion between chest wall radiotherapy and follow-up.

The role of radiotherapy in patients with pT2N0 tumours with features of biological aggressiveness (ER−, HER2+, grade 3, and high proliferative index) is not known and postoperative radiotherapy may be considered, especially in young people.

Regional nodal radiotherapy

Axillary nodal radiotherapy

Current indications for axillary nodal radiotherapy include:

- Incomplete axillary surgery in a node-positive patient.
- Positive sentinel node where further axillary dissection is not intended.
- Patients with high risk of axillary nodal disease but no axillary surgery is intended (e.g. primary of >10mm and/or grade 3 tumour, neoadjuvant chemotherapy followed by consolidation radiotherapy).

Axillary radiotherapy is not recommended after axillary dissection as there is 30–40% risk of significant lymphoedema and the risk of isolated axillary recurrence without radiotherapy is only 1–4%. However, it may be considered in rare instances of residual macroscopic disease in the axilla or a positive dissection margin.

The role of axillary radiotherapy after SNB is being evaluated in the ongoing AMAROS trial.

Supraclavicular nodal radiotherapy

Patients with ≥4 involved nodes after axillary dissection are at risk of supraclavicular recurrence (>15%) and hence supraclavicular radiotherapy is advised.

Internal mammary node radiotherapy

The incidence of internal mammary node metastasis varies from 3–65% depending on the tumour stage and location of the primary tumour. There is no proven role for routine internal mammary chain radiotherapy. The early results of the EORTC 22922/10925 trial, evaluating the role of internal mammary chain and medial supraclavicular nodal radiotherapy in stage I–III breast cancer are expected in 2012. A 3-year toxicity analysis of this trial did not show any increased risk of toxicity in patients who received radiotherapy.

Role of radiotherapy after neoadjuvant chemotherapy and surgery

There are no prospective studies evaluating the role of radiotherapy in patients treated with preoperative chemotherapy. Retrospective studies show that initial clinical stage and postoperative pathological extent are independent risk factors for locoregional recurrence irrespective of an excellent response to systemic treatment.

In clinical practice, all patients who undergo conservative surgery after systemic treatment need postoperative radiotherapy to the breast. Patients with cT3–T4 disease and histologically positive nodes after chemotherapy are recommended to have chest wall and regional nodal radiotherapy.

The role of radiotherapy in stage II patients with negative nodes after chemotherapy is not known.

Further reading

Huang EH, Tucker SL, Strom EA, *et al.* Statement of the science concerning locoregional treatments after preoperative chemotherapy for breast cancer: A National Cancer Institute Conference. *J Clin Oncol* 2008; **26**:791–7.

Poortmans P. Evidence based radiation oncology: Breast cancer. Radiotherapy *Oncol* 2007; **84**:84–101.

Rowell N. Radiotherapy to the chest wall following mastectomy for node-negative breast cancer: A systematic review. *Radiotherapy Oncol* 2009; **91**:23–32.

Early stage breast cancer: adjuvant systemic treatment

Adjuvant systemic therapy has lead to significant reductions in cause-related mortality of breast cancer, particularly over the past decade. Adjuvant systemic therapies include chemotherapy, hormonal therapy, and trastuzumab. However, not all women with early stage disease will require adjuvant treatment and some may benefit from one or more modalities. The decision to administer adjuvant systemic treatments depends on a multitude of factors including patient age and comorbidities, tumour size, nodal status, hormone receptor status, and HER2 positivity.

Adjuvant chemotherapy

Results from the Early Breast Cancer Trialists' Collaborative Group's (EBCTCG) most recent review in 2000 showed that the addition of adjuvant chemotherapy provided a risk reduction in disease recurrence and death in patients <70 years of age. Patients >70 years could not be adequately assessed as only few numbers of these patients were included in the studies. However, most guidelines recommend individualizing decision making and considering chemotherapy in this patient population as well, depending on the balance of risks and benefits.

The magnitude of benefit from chemotherapy appears to favour patients younger than 50 more than those aged 50–69. For women younger than 50, the 15-year risk of recurrence was decreased from 54% to 41% and death from 42% to 32%. In the population aged 50–69, these reductions were from 58% to 53% and from 50% to 47%, respectively.

Node-positive and node-negative patients have similar proportional reductions from chemotherapy although the node-positive younger patients derive a greater magnitude of benefit. Node-positive patients <50 years of age have a 15% reduction in recurrence versus 10% in node-negative patients of similar age. The reduction is 6% versus 5% in women 50–69 years of age. However, among node-negative patients, most guidelines do not advise the use of chemotherapy in tumours that are <0.5cm in size, due to the low likelihood of benefit. Lastly, tumours that are hormone receptor negative are more likely to respond than hormone positive tumours.

Algorithms, such as Adjuvant! Online, have been developed to take into account these factors and assist clinicians and patients in making decisions about chemotherapy. Another available tool for risk assessment, Oncotype DX™, is a 21-gene assay using reverse transcriptase polymerase chain reaction (RT-PCR) of tumour tissue. This analysis provides a risk recurrence score that is most useful in node-negative, hormone receptor positive patients.

CMF and anthracyclines

CMF-type regimens (cyclophosphamide, methotrexate, fluorouracil) and anthracycline-based chemotherapies were some of the earlier widely used regimens for adjuvant therapy. Examples of anthracycline regimens include AC (doxorubicin and cyclophosphamide), FAC/CAF (fluorouracil, doxorubicin, and cyclophosphamide), FEC/CEF (fluorouracil, epirubicin, and cyclophosphamide), and EC (epirubicin and cyclophosphamide).

An overview by the EBCTCG comparing CMF-based chemotherapy with anthracycline regimens showed a modest but significant additional reduction in annual risk of recurrence (12%) and annual risk of death (11%); the absolute benefit was about 3% at 5 years. However, there has been much debate by investigators over these results. The exclusion of HER2 status in the analysis is a primary reason for the debate. Most of the advantage of anthracyclines may be derived from HER2-positive patients. Based on these results, current recommendations generally advise the use of anthracycline-containing regimens rather than CMF and especially so in HER2-positive tumours.

AC chemotherapy given as 3-week cycles over 12 weeks produces equivalent results for risk of relapse and death as compared with 6 months of CMF. Due to the decreased time in administration and results of the data mentioned earlier, AC is favoured over CMF. A randomized trial investigating AC (with sequential paclitaxel) given in a dose-dense fashion every 2 weeks demonstrated a significant reduction in risk of recurrence and death when compared to the 3-weekly schedule. Dose-intensification of doxorubicin and cyclophosphamide does not appear to provide any advantage to standard dosing.

FEC/CEF, FAC/CAF, and EC have been investigated in several randomized prospective trials with results overall showing improvements in reducing risk of recurrence and death compared with CMF. In addition to AC, these regimens are also recommended as appropriate to use.

Cardiac-related toxicity can be a limitation to using anthracyclines, particularly in patients with underlying heart disease. More recently, a small but increased risk of future development of leukaemia has been recognized. One analysis showed a 1.5% 10-year rate of treatment-induced leukaemia. In general this risk does not outweigh the benefits of adjuvant chemotherapy but a discussion with patients of this risk is advised.

Taxanes

The addition of taxanes, namely paclitaxel and docetaxel, has provided additional benefits to adjuvant treatment regimens.

Two randomized trials investigated AC chemotherapy with or without sequential paclitaxel therapy in node-positive patients. Both trials showed an increase in DFS and one showed an increase in OS. One caveat is that retrospective analysis appears to show most of this advantage being derived from ER-negative tumours. A separate series favours weekly paclitaxel versus an every 3-week schedule.

Results from a trial comparing TAC (docetaxel, doxorubicin, and cyclophosphamide) with CAF showed superiority of TAC over CAF. Although the 5-year survival was not significantly increased (87% versus 81%), the DFS was significantly improved (75% versus 68%). The patients had node-positive disease and results were equal for hormone status.

Another regimen, TC (docetaxel and cyclophosphamide), demonstrated significant improvements in OS and DFS compared with four cycles of AC. The acceptance of TC has been limited by its comparison with AC followed by a taxane, which is considered a superior regimen for high-risk patients.

Timing with radiotherapy and systemic therapy

The concurrent use of chemotherapy with radiotherapy is generally not recommended due to toxicity issues. There does not appear to be an advantage in timing of radiotherapy either before or after administration of chemotherapy in terms of risk of death or disease recurrence. However, the general recommendation is to deliver adjuvant radiotherapy after chemotherapy is completed.

For hormonal therapy, current recommendations suggest sequential chemotherapy followed by hormonal therapy. This recommendation is primarily based on the data from the EBCTCG that showed a non-significant improvement in OS and DFS for a sequential strategy versus a concurrent one. The underlying belief is that tamoxifen places cancer cells in a resting state, thus not allowing cytotoxic chemotherapy to adequately exert its effect. This suggestion has also been made about concurrent hormonal treatment with radiotherapy, but currently the data are lacking to provide a recommendation for a sequential approach in this setting.

Adjuvant hormonal therapy

Patients with hormone receptor-positive tumours should be considered for adjuvant hormonal therapy. The rationale is to block the oestrogen stimulus to breast cancer cells. Ovarian ablation was the method of choice in the 1950s. However this method has been replaced by pharmacological methods.

Tamoxifen

The efficacy of tamoxifen has been well established. The EBCTCG showed a reduction in 15-year disease recurrence (from 45% to 33%) and improved survival (35% from 26%) in patients receiving 5 years of tamoxifen versus no adjuvant tamoxifen. This finding was irrespective of menopausal status.

Tamoxifen is a selective oestrogen receptor modulator (SERM). It inhibits breast cancer cells by acting as a competitive antagonist at the oestrogen receptor. However, it also acts as a partial agonist at locations such as the uterus and bones. Thus it can have a positive impact on bone health but increase the risk of uterine cancer (approximately 3-fold) and thromboembolic events (approximately 2–3-fold).

Tamoxifen is metabolized by the CYP2D6 enzymatic system to the active metabolite, endoxifen. There is an increasing movement to test patients for their CYP2D6 metabolism status as it appears that poor metabolizers may not benefit from tamoxifen therapy.

Aromatase inhibitors (AI)

AIs block the conversion of androgens to oestrogen. The three most common medications are anastrozole, letrozole, and exemestane. Current evidence does not suggest a meaningful difference in efficacy or toxicity between the three drugs. AIs should not be used in women with functioning ovaries.

AIs have been investigated in a number of trials of postmenopausal patients looking at AIs alone, tamoxifen for 2–3 years followed by AIs, extended therapy with AIs after 4.5–6 years of tamoxifen, or tamoxifen alone. Differences in patient populations and study designs have made it difficult to provide strong recommendations. In general, if hormonal therapy is to be utilized in the care of postmenopausal patients, current guidelines support the use of AIs either as initial treatment, sequential after 2–3 years of tamoxifen, or as extended therapy after 4.5–6 years of tamoxifen.

Both tamoxifen and the AIs have similar common side effects including hot flushes, vaginal dryness, and night sweats. However, AIs have increased rates of osteoporosis, fractures, and musculoskeletal complaints. They do not have increased rates of thromboembolic events or uterine cancer though, as seen with tamoxifen.

Trastuzumab

Trastuzumab (also known by the trade name Herceptin®) is a humanized monoclonal antibody directed towards the HER2 receptor (EGFR2, also HER2/neu). Approximately 20% of tumours will show overexpression of HER2.

Several prospective randomized trials have demonstrated the efficacy of trastuzumab in the adjuvant setting. Two of the larger studies, the NSABP (National Surgical Adjuvant Breast and Bowel Project) B-31 and NCCTG (North Central Cancer Treatment Group) N9831, were reported in a joint analysis that included 3968 patients. The patients were randomized to either four cycles of AC every 3 weeks followed by four cycles of paclitaxel every 3 weeks versus the same regimen plus trastuzumab started with paclitaxel and given for 52 weeks. Median follow-up was 4 years. The risk of disease recurrence was reduced by 52% and risk of death by 35%. The results appear to be independent of ER hormonal status. Cardiac toxicity associated with trastuzumab is the most concerning side effect associated with the medication. Of the current studies evaluating cardiotoxicity, Grade III/IV congestive heart failure and cardiac-related death was as high as 4.1% (from the NSABP B-31 trial).

The HERA trial investigated trastuzumab given for 1 or 2 years versus none in patients with tumours >1cm. At 1 year of follow-up, risk of recurrence was improved 46% when trastuzumab was given for 1 year versus none. Analysis of the same groups at 2 years showed an OS advantage in favour of trastuzumab (HR of 0.66, p = 0.0115). Cardiac toxicity was considered acceptable at the 1-year point. Currently, a European trial is underway investigating 6 months of trastuzumab versus the current standard of 12 months.

The regimen TCH (docetaxel, carboplatin, and trastuzumab) is also an acceptable regimen for HER2 patients and can be considered in those patients with concern for cardiac toxicity.

Summary and recommendations

The recommendations for adjuvant systemic treatment for early breast cancer are constantly evolving. An important step in determining the need for adjuvant systemic treatment and the choice of systemic treatment is the assessment of risk of recurrence (Table 4.4.4). There is no consensus on the definition of various risk groups. In Europe, the St Galen consensus meeting incorporates new advances in the management of breast cancer whereas in the USA, the National Comprehensive Cancer Network updates the advances and changing philosophies of breast cancer management. Many clinicians also use Adjuvant Online! as a rough guide to make clinical recommendations for adjuvant systemic treatment.

All patients with tumours with any detectable ER are recommended to have hormonal therapy. In premenopausal women, tamoxifen with or without ovarian suppression is the standard choice. In postmenopausal women, AI is included as part of the standard treatment. A subset of patients with low-risk disease may be treated with tamoxifen.

Patients with ≥1cm tumours which are HER2 positive on either IHC (3+ defined as uniform intense membrane staining of >30% of invasive tumour cells) or FISH test (HER2 gene amplification ratio ≥2.0) are considered for

Table 4.4.4 Risk categories of early breast cancer (Goldhirsch et al 2009)

Risk group	Features	Treatment recommendations
Low risk	All of the following: • Tumour of ≤2cm • Grade 1 • No lymphovascular invasion • Node negative • ER+/PgR+ • HER2− • Low proliferation index (Ki 67 ≤15%) (if available) • Gene assay—low score (if available)	Adjuvant endocrine treatment is the mainstay of treatment. Consideration for adjuvant chemotherapy is individualized and should take into consideration of all the risk factors. Patient should be encouraged to participate in the ongoing clinical trials
Intermediate risk	Any of the following: • Tumours of 2.1–5cm • Grade 2 • 1–3 nodes positive • Intermediate proliferation index (Ki 67 16–30%) (if available) • Gene assay—intermediate score (if available)	Decision on adjuvant treatment is individualized taking into consideration all patient and tumour related prognostic factors. Patients with ER− tumours are treated with chemotherapy and those with HER2+ tumours receive trastuzumab. Patients receiving trastuzumab will also receive chemotherapy. The role of chemotherapy in ER+ and HER− tumours is not well defined. Patients should be encouraged to participate in on-going clinical trials to assess the benefit of chemotherapy.
High risk	Any of the following: • Tumour of >5cm • Grade 3 • Extensive lymphovascular invasion≥4 lymph nodes positive • ER−/PgR− or low level • High proliferation index (Ki 67 >60%) (if available) • Gene assay—high score (if available)	These patients are generally considered for an appropriate combination of systemic treatments. Patients with ER+/PgR+ tumours are considered for chemotherapy with the addition of hormones. All patients with HER2+ tumours will also receive trastuzumab.

trastuzumab therapy for 1 year. The role of trastuzumab for HER2+ tumours of <1cm size with no nodal involvement or high-risk features is not known and hence not recommended.

Patients with high-risk disease (see Table 4.4.4), and triple-negative tumours are generally considered for chemotherapy along with other appropriate systemic treatments. In other situations the role of chemotherapy is less clearly defined. Chemotherapy is given to patients with HER2-positive disease as the evidence for the use of trastuzumab is limited to its use with chemotherapy. Anthracycline-containing combinations are the commonly used chemotherapy regimens. There is an increasing trend to incorporate taxanes in the adjuvant regimens for patients with high-risk disease. Some histological subtypes such as medullary carcinoma and adenoid cystic carcinoma do not need chemotherapy despite being triple negative due to low risk of recurrence provided there is no nodal involvement or high-risk features.

Recent trials to define the role of chemotherapy in low- to intermediate-risk patients with breast cancer are incorporating molecular prognostic factors. The ongoing TAILORx trial is evaluating the role of chemotherapy in patients with node-negative breast cancer and with an Oncotype Dx recurrence score of 11–25. The European study of MINDACT is comparing 70-gene expression signature with Adjuvant! Online in selecting patients with negative or 1–3 positive nodes for adjuvant chemotherapy.

Further reading

Berry C, Cirrincione C, Henderson I, et al. Estrogen-receptor status and outcomes of modern chemotherapy for patients with node-positive breast cancer. *JAMA* 2006; **295**:1658–67.

Diamandidou E, Buzdar A, Smith T, et al. Treatment-related leukemia in breast cancer patients treated with fluorouracil-doxorubicin-cyclophosphamide combination adjuvant chemotherapy: the University of Texas M.D. Anderson Cancer Center Experience. *J Clin Oncol* 1996; **14**:2722–30.

Early Breast Cancer Trialists' Collaborative Group (EBCTCG). Effects of chemotherapy and hormonal therapy for early breast cancer on recurrence and 15-year survival: an overview of the randomised trials. *Lancet* 2005; **365**:1687–717.

Early Breast Cancer Trialists' Collaborative Group (EBCTCG). Polychemotherapy for early breast cancer: an overview of the randomised trials. *Lancet* 1998; **352**:930–942.

Gennari A, Sormani M, Pronzato P, et al. HER2 status and efficacy of adjuvant anthracyclines in early breast cancer: a pooled analysis of randomized trials. *J Natl Cancer Inst* 2008; **100**:14–20.

Goldhirsch A, Ingle JN, Gelber RD, et al. Thresholds for therapies:highlights of the St Gallen International Expert Consensus on the primary therapy of early breast cancer 2009. *Ann Oncol* 2009; **20**:1319–29.

Piccart-Gebhart M, Procter M, Leyland-Jones B, et al. Trastuzumab after adjuvant chemotherapy in HER2-positive breast cancer. *N Engl J Med* 2005; **353**:1659–72.

Smith I, Procter M, Gelber R, et al. 2-year follow-up of trastuzumab after adjuvant chemotherapy in HER2-positive breast: a randomized controlled trial. *Lancet* 2007; **369**:29–36.

Internet resources

National Comprehensive Cancer Network (NCCN) Clinical Practice Guidelines in Oncology™—available at http://www.nccn.org

UpToDate Inc.: http://www.uptodate.com

Locally advanced breast cancer: concepts in management

Locally advanced breast cancer (LABC) in general refers to patients with stage IIIA, IIIB, and IIIC disease. Inflammatory breast cancer is also frequently included in this group and will be discussed separately at the end of this section. Patients with LABC have one or more of the following characteristics.
• Large primary tumours (>5cm)
• Extensive lymph node involvement (usually N2 nodes)
• Inoperable tumours without distant metastases
• Tumours involving the chest wall or skin

Work-up for these patients is the same as for earlier stage patients (stage I and II). The routine use of MRI, chest/abdomen/pelvis CT, PET/CT scan, or bone scan is generally not recommended in the initial evaluation unless symptoms or abnormalities in other studies (ultrasound for example) dictate their use.

Most of these patients are considered inoperable at presentation, meaning a low likelihood of achieving negative margins from resection. One exception is noted among stage IIIA patients, specifically T3N1M0. These patients are frequently operable and can be managed in a similar fashion to early stage disease (see prior sections).

However, the majority of LABC patients require a multimodality approach to their treatment. The general approach involves induction, or neoadjuvant, chemotherapy followed by surgery and/or radiation. There are several reasons for providing neoadjuvant chemotherapy:
• Shrinkage of the tumour to allow for adequate surgical resection or breast conservation surgery.
• Early treatment for possible unseen distant disease and to the tumour through intact vasculature.
• The tumour can be assessed clinically for response during treatment.

About three quarters of patients will have a major clinical response and one half a complete clinical response.

Neoadjuvant (induction) chemotherapy
Guidelines generally recommend the use of anthracycline-based regimens in neoadjuvant chemotherapy. Although there is no clearly superior regimen, the most commonly studied ones include FAC/CAF, FEC/CAF, AC, CMF, and CMFVP (CMF with vincristine and prednisone). Taxanes can also be added. They appear to increase the probability of achieving a pathological clinical response at time of resection versus not including them, but demonstration of an OS advantage has been conflicting among studies. Current guidelines do not clearly delineate indications for their addition although they are commonly used. For tumours which overexpress HER2, trastuzumab should be added to the neoadjuvant regimen as well. The number of cycles and treatment schedules for neoadjuvant chemotherapy in general follows the approach of the adjuvant regimens.

Neoadjuvant hormonal therapy does show some clinical response in shrinking tumours but lacks the data to be recommended as standard of care in neoadjuvant treatment. However, older women and women with comorbidities or organ dysfunction may be candidates for neoadjuvant hormonal treatment.

Response to induction chemotherapy is an important prognostic feature. Several studies have determined a correlation between residual tumour in the breast and axilla, and subsequent DFS and OS.

Surgical management
If the patient has a clinical response to induction chemotherapy, then they proceed to locoregional treatment, which is typically surgery. The two primary options include:
• Mastectomy with level I/II lymph node dissection, with or without subsequent delayed breast reconstruction
• Lumpectomy with level I/II lymph node dissection

Results from several studies show a 50–90% rate of success in proceeding to breast conservation therapy (BCT) after neoadjuvant chemotherapy. However, not all women are indicated for having BCT (see box in Chapter 4.4, Management of breast cancer: surgery, p.158).

Role of radiotherapy
Patients with LABC are at a sufficiently high risk for local recurrence that all should undergo postsurgical radiation to the chest wall and supraclavicular lymph nodes. Radiation treatment to the internal mammary nodes should also be included if these nodes were involved as well. Some consideration can be given to irradiating the internal mammary nodes even if they were not involved, depending on the clinical situation. Capecitabine may be administered concurrently with radiation as a sensitizer.

Adjuvant systemic management for LABC
Following locoregional treatment, patients should complete the planned course of chemotherapy if not finished previously. ER-positive or PgR-positive tumours should be treated with adjuvant hormonal therapy with either tamoxifen or AIs (subsequently after chemotherapy). Trastuzumab should be completed for a total of up to 52 weeks in HER2-positive patients. Trastuzumab can be given concurrently with radiation therapy, hormonal therapy, and capecitabine (if used as a radiation sensitizer).

Non-responders
Typically, patients should not be considered non-responders until at least four cycles of chemotherapy are completed. As mentioned earlier, a lack of response or progression on treatment is a poor prognostic feature.

Several options can be employed to elicit a response and proceed to subsequent locoregional therapy:
• Change chemotherapy to an alternative regimen that does not include the initial drugs (i.e. taxanes for anthracycline failure).
• Add or change to endocrine therapy if hormone-receptor positive.
• Provide pre-operative radiotherapy.
• Trastuzumab, if not used previously, should be used in HER2-positive tumours.

Inflammatory breast cancer (IBC)
IBC is an aggressive form of LABC that comprises about 1–6% of all breast cancers. Prognosis tends to be much worse than in non-inflammatory LABC. Data from the NCI Surveillance, Epidemiology and End Results (SEER) program from 1998–2000 showed a median survival of 2.9 years for IBC versus 6.4 years for non-inflammatory LABC. In addition to poorer prognosis, IBC patients tend

to be younger and have tumours that are HER2-positive and hormone-receptor negative.

Diagnosis, staging, and work-up

The diagnosis of IBC is made on a clinical basis. The characteristic features are induration and oedema of the skin (referred to as peau d'orange), involving a third or more of the breast, and having a raised edge. Other similarly appearing diseases, such as mastitis or abscess, need to be ruled out. Histology frequently shows dermal lymphatic invasion by tumour emboli, but this finding is not necessary for diagnosis. The primary tumour is, by definition, T4d, despite the presence or lack of a definable breast mass. IBC is thus either stage IIIB, IIIC, or IV, depending on the absence or presence of distant metastases.

Unlike the pretreatment evaluation for early stage breast cancer and LABC, IBC warrants routine staging with a bone scan and CT of the chest, abdomen, and pelvis. Breast MRI is optional and other testing is derived from patient symptoms.

Treatment management for IBC

The approach to treatment for IBC is actually nearly the same as for LABC (see earlier). Anthracycline-based neo-adjuvant chemotherapy regimens with or without taxanes are generally recommended. One study from MD Anderson demonstrated a 28% DFS at 15 years using anthracycline-based chemotherapy. A randomized trial of an epirubicin-based regimen showed a 44% 5-year survival rate.

Surgical management is the same for IBC as for LABC with the caveat being that BCT is contraindicated in IBC. Postsurgical radiotherapy and adjuvant systemic therapy follow similar guidelines to those for LABC. Stage IV disease should be treated using the metastatic management guidelines discussed later in the chapter.

Further reading

Hortobagyi G, Ames F, Buzdar A, et al. Management of stage III primary breast cancer with primary chemotherapy, surgery, and radiation therapy. Cancer 1988; **62**:2507–176

Hortobagyi G, Singletary S, Strom E. Locally advanced breast cancer. In: Harris J, Lippman M, Morrow M, et al. (eds) Diseases of the Breast, 3rd edition. Philadelphia, PA: Lippincott Williams & Wilkins, 2004.

Internet resources

National Cancer Institute (NCI) Surveillance, Epidemiology and End Results (SEER) data; 1998, 2000—available at: http://seer.cancer.gov/

National Comprehensive Cancer Network (NCCN) Clinical Practice Guidelines in Oncology™—available at http://www.nccn.org

UpToDate Inc.: http://www.uptodate.com

Management of recurrent and metastatic breast cancer

Recurrence of breast cancer can be either local (ipsilateral preserved breast tissue or chest wall), regional (lymph nodes), or distant. The work-up for recurrent and metastatic disease entails the following tests:

- Complete blood count (CBC) and liver function tests
- Bone scan
- Chest radiograph
- Radiographs of symptomatic bones
- Biopsy if first recurrence
- Determination of ER/PR and HER2 status if not completed previously
- CT of the chest, abdomen, and/or pelvis is optional, depending on clinical situation

Local recurrence management

Local recurrence will occur in about 5–20% of patients 10 years after BCT and in 10–15% after mastectomy. Patients with local recurrence can be divided into those who had BCT, mastectomy with radiation, and those without radiation.

For prior BCT, patients should have a total mastectomy and axillary lymph node dissection. Systemic chemotherapy should also be given and guidelines generally suggest using regimens and schedules for adjuvant treatment discussed previously.

For patients with prior mastectomy, the goal of management is surgical excision of the recurrence, as long as negative margins can be expected. If no radiation was administered previously, patients should also receive involved-field radiotherapy to the chest wall and internal mammary lymph nodes. Chemotherapy is considered in the same manner as for BCT patients.

Metastatic disease

Less than 10% of patients initially present with metastatic disease. However, when breast cancer does recur, it tends to be with distant metastases rather than local recurrence. The most common sites of distant disease include bones, liver, brain, lungs, and subcutaneous tissues. The approach to treating metastatic disease is generally considered non-curative in nature and is aimed at palliation, improving quality of life, and prolonging survival.

Endocrine therapy

As the main goal of treatment for metastatic disease is palliation, agents with the most activity and least toxicity are employed first if possible. Thus, hormonal therapy is usually attempted before cytotoxic chemotherapy in ER-positive or PgR-positive patients. Some general guidelines are listed below:

- In postmenopausal patients with prior antioestrogen exposure within 1 year, therapy should be with selective AIs (such as letrozole, anastrozole, or exemestane).
- In postmenopausal patients without prior antioestrogen exposure or without exposure for >1 year, AIs may have a slight advantage over tamoxifen but either can be used.
- In premenopausal patients with prior antioestrogen exposure within 1 year, therapy should be oophorectomy (either surgical or radioablative), or by suppression with LHRH analogues combined with antioestrogens (preferred approach)
- In premenopausal patients without prior antioestrogen exposure or without exposure for >1 year, initial treatment is with antioestrogens or ovarian ablation/suppression.

If patients have disease response or stabilization with initial antioestrogen therapy, then subsequent endocrine treatments should be given at time of progression. Antioestrogens can also be tried in patients whose tumours are ER negative/PgR negative as some metastases may express different hormone receptors from the primary tumour.

Several other hormonal options exist for postmenopausal patients including the antioestrogen fulvestrant, the progesterone derivative megestrol acetate, the androgen fluoxymesterone, and high-dose oestrogen. For premenopausal patients, options include the LHRH agonists luprolide and goserelin, fluoxymesterone, and high-dose oestrogen.

Cytotoxic chemotherapy

Chemotherapy in the metastatic setting is usually reserved for hormone-refractory patients, ER-negative/PgR-negative, rapidly progressive disease, or symptomatic visceral metastases. Both single agent and combination regimens are available options. Combination therapy will lead to higher response rates and increased time to progression, but not necessarily survival benefits. Toxicities of combination regimens also need to be weighed against the benefits. Thus either combination or single-agent therapy is reasonable. In general, therapy is continued until progression.

A multitude of agents are used in the metastatic setting. In general, many are either the combination regimens used in the adjuvant setting (i.e. AC, FAC/CAF, FEC/CEF, CMF) or the individual drugs themselves (i.e. taxanes, anthracyclines). Other examples include antimetabolites (capecitabine and gemcitabine), non-taxane microtubule inhibitors (vinorelbine), and platinum agents (cisplatin). Taxanes tend to be favoured frequently in initial management although there is no clear consensus.

One of the newer agents, ixabepilone, an epitholine B analogue that acts as a microtubule stabilizer, has been investigated as a single agent and in combination with capecitabine for tumours refractory to anthracyclines and taxanes. A phase III study did show a progression-free survival (PFS) advantage when combined with capecitabine versus capecitabine alone (5.8 months vs. 4.2 months) but OS was not assessed and neutropenia was significantly more in the combination arm.

Bevacizumab, a humanized monoclonal antibody against VEGF, was investigated in a study in combination with paclitaxel versus paclitaxel alone. The PFS was statistically improved from 5.9 months to 11.8 months, but no difference was noted in OS between the groups.

HER2-positive disease

Assessing HER2 status of the tumour is important in determining if agents directed against this receptor can be used. As in early stage breast cancer and LABC, trastuzumab is very effective in HER2-overexpressing tumours. Trastuzumab can be used either as a single agent or in combination with chemotherapy in hormone-receptor negative patients. It has also been combined with capecitabine and shown benefit in the first-line setting as well. The optimal duration of treatment for patients responding to trastuzumab-containing regimens or with stable disease is unknown in the metastatic setting.

Lapatinib, an oral tyrosine kinase inhibitor of both HER2 and EGFR, has also developed a niche in HER2-positive metastatic disease. It is approved in the USA for use with capecitabine in patients who have failed an anthracycline, taxane, and trastuzumab. Lapatinib combined with letrozole endocrine therapy appears to improve PFS and it also shows some promise in treatment of brain metastases. Preliminary results of a phase III trial looking at lapatinib combined with trastuzumab show an increase in OS from 41.4 weeks to 60.7 weeks. Completion of the study and further analysis will be needed to determine the place of this combination in treatment.

Bone metastases and bisphosphonates

For patients with bony metastases, especially lytic lesions, bisphosphonate therapy in conjunction with adequate calcium and vitamin D supplementation is helpful in reducing fractures and other skeletal-related events. Bisphosphonates are for palliative treatment with no evidence at this time of a survival advantage. Serum creatinine monitoring is important when dosing these medications due to renal toxicity issues.

Patients should have a dental exam and complete any needed interventions before starting therapy because of the increased risk of osteonecrosis of the jaw (ONJ). ONJ is a recently recognized complication of bisphosphonates, occurring in 5.48 out of 100 patients in one study, and increases in risk with cumulative dosing.

Surgery and radiotherapy

Currently, the role for surgery and radiotherapy in metastatic disease is generally for palliative purposes. Patients with painful bony metastases, for example, may benefit from palliative radiotherapy to the lesion.

Surgical excision of the intact primary tumour may be helpful in a subset of patients who require palliation of symptoms such as pain, ulceration, and infection. Several retrospective analyses suggest a survival benefit in surgical resection of the primary tumour, but much caution is advised due to the potential for selection bias of these studies. Surgical excision of metastases also may have benefit but currently does not have a clear role.

Further reading

Perez E, Josse R, Pritchard K, et al. Effect of letrozole versus placebo on bone mineral density in women with primary breast cancer completing 5 or more years of adjuvant tamoxifen: a companion study to NCIC CTG MA.17. *J Clinc Oncol* 2006; **24**:3629–35.

Internet resources

National Comprehensive Cancer Network (NCCN) Clinical Practice Guidelines in Oncology™—available at http://www.nccn.org

UpToDate Inc.: http://www.uptodate.com

Breast cancer: new agents and future perspectives

Many questions about breast cancer remain despite the relative abundance of breast cancer data that is currently available.

Hormonal therapy

An area of interest in tamoxifen therapy involves the metabolism of the drug to its active metabolite endoxifen by the liver enzyme CYP2D6. A currently held belief is that patients who are poor metabolizers of tamoxifen will not convert enough of the prodrug to its active component, endoxifen, and thus will not benefit from this therapy. Recommendations do not currently include routine testing for CYP2D6 metabolizer status although studies are ongoing to further elucidate this issue. Additionally, certain antidepressants are inhibitors of CYP2D6 and their role in tamoxifen therapy is being further investigated as well.

Chemotherapy and targeted therapy

Targeted therapies are a fast growing field in nearly all areas of cancer treatment. Several agents are being investigated in breast cancer.

PARP inhibitors

PARP-1, or poly (ADP-ribose) polymerase-1, is a protein that binds to DNA and is involved in the repair of strand breaks. PARP-1 inhibitors appear to exert their effect mostly on BRCA-deficient cells. A phase II study investigating gemcitabine and carboplatin with or without the PARP-1 inhibitor, BSI-201, in metastatic triple-negative breast cancer shows encouraging efficacy with minimal to no increased toxicity. Triple-negative breast cancer shares features similar to BRCA1-related tumours.

VEGF inhibitors

As well as bevacizumab, other established VEGF inhibitors, such as sorafenib and sunitinib, may show some promise as single agents or in combination with chemotherapy. Novel agents targeting more than one of the VEGF receptors are also being developed in phase I and II trials.

HER2 agents

Labatinib continues to be investigated in conjunction with other chemotherapies and endocrine treatments. It is also being investigated in other settings than metastatic disease such as being used adjuvantly with trastuzumab. Other agents similar to lapatinib, such as neratinib, are also being developed and investigated.

Other agents

Many other cellular targets are the source of ongoing research. The insulin-like growth factor-1 receptor (IGF-1R) has been implicated in tumourigenesis through activation of the AKT signalling pathway and inhibition of apoptosis. Antagonists to IGF-1R are being studied in early trials.

TKI258 is a novel, multitargeted tyrosine kinase inhibitor that was presented at the 2009 ASCO meeting. TKI258 targets several growth factor receptors and intracellular pathways. It demonstrated potent antitumour effects in breast cancer cell lines.

Internet resources

National Comprehensive Cancer Network (NCCN) Clinical Practice Guidelines in Oncology™—available at http://www.nccn.org

UpToDate Inc.: http://www.uptodate.com

Triple-negative breast cancer

Triple-negative breast cancer lacks the expression of oestrogen, progesterone, and HER2 receptors. Up to 15% of breast cancer falls into this category which is associated with a high rate of local and systemic recurrence. These tumours are similar to BRCA1-associated breast cancers. Histologically these are characterized by poor differentiation, presence of central necrosis, and immunohistochemical staining for cytokeratin 5/6.

Currently, these tumours are treated as other breast cancers and there is no special recommended chemotherapy regimen. Data shows that these tumours are sensitive to platinum-based chemotherapy and hence a number of studies are underway to evaluate various platinum regimens. Recent understanding of the role of BRCA1 gene pathway dysfunction in these tumours has lead to ongoing research on the role of platinum chemotherapy and PARP inhibitors as potential therapeutic strategies.

Further reading

Cleator S, Heller W, Coombes R. Triple negative breast cancer: therapeutic options. *Lancet Oncol* 2007; **8**:235–44.

Gluz O, Liedtke C, Gottschalk N, *et al*. Triple-negative breast cancer-current status and future directions. *Ann Oncol* 2009; **20**:1913–27.

Tan A, Swain S. Therapeutic strategies for triple-negative breast cancer. *Cancer J* 2008; **14**:343–51.

Bilateral breast cancer

Bilateral breast cancer can be either synchronous (tumours occur simultaneously or within 6 months of initial diagnosis) which occurs in <2% of patients, or metachronous (tumours diagnosed 6 months or more after initial diagnosis) with an incidence of 1–2% per year after the first cancer diagnosis. Bilateral breast cancer commonly occurs in those with a strong family history of breast cancer and those who had breast cancer at early age.

The general principle in managing bilateral breast cancer is to treat as for two separate primary tumours. Surgical management depends on the characteristics of each individual tumour. Breast conservation is advisable if surgically feasible and the patient prefers this. Adjuvant systemic treatment is based on the cancer with the worst prognosis. If tumours have discrepant ER status, both chemotherapy and hormones may be considered.

It is believed that prognosis is dictated by the worse prognosis cancer. There is no clear evidence that bilateral breast cancer has a different survival compared with matched unilateral breast cancer. Some studies report the same prognosis as unilateral breast cancer but others a worse one. Part of the problem is attributed to the method of calculating survival. It has been suggested that survival should be calculated from the time of development of the second breast cancer whereas many authors calculate it from the time of diagnosis of the first breast cancer.

Further reading

Heron D, Komarnicky L, Hyslop T, *et al.* Bilateral breast carcinoma: risk factors and outcomes for patients with synchronous and metachronous disease. *Cancer* 2000; **88**:2739–50.

Irvine T, Allen D, Hamed G, *et al.* Prognosis of synchronous bilateral breast cancer. *Br J Surg* 2009; **96**:376–80.

Paget's disease

Paget's disease is a premalignant condition of the nipple and areola occurring in the 5th or 6th decade (mean age 54 years) and its incidence is approximately 0.5–5%. Clinically there is erythema, dryness, and fissuring of the nipple.

Microscopically it is characterized by Paget's cells located throughout the epidermis. More than 95% of patients with Paget's disease have an associated ductal carcinoma. Fifty per cent of patients with Paget's disease have a lump which in >90% cases is an invasive carcinoma. Of the patients without a lump, 30% will have invasive carcinoma and 70% have DCIS.

A typical clinical presentation is with an eczematoid reaction with raised, irregular, and sharply demarcated edges. There may be associated nipple retraction or deformity. It is often associated with discharge or staining of clothes. The lesion most often appears in the breast and spreads to the areola.

In patients with previous conservative treatment for breast cancer, the appearance of Paget's disease may suggest tumour recurrence and hence early biopsy is indicated.

Investigations include breast examination, mammography and full thickness skin biopsy. Prognosis is dependent on the characteristics of the associated malignancy.

Conservative surgery followed by radiotherapy is the treatment of choice. The local recurrence rate with surgery alone is 25–40% from various small series. An EORTC study of complete excision with the nipple-areolar complex followed by postoperative radiotherapy showed a local recurrence of 5.2%. Mastectomy is offered based on patient choice and for multifocal disease. Management of regional nodes and recommendations for systemic treatment are based on the features of the underlying malignancy.

Further reading

Sakorafas G, Blanchard K, Sarr M, *et al.* Paget's disease of the breast. *Cancer Treat Rev* 2001; **27**:9–18.

Male breast cancer

Introduction

Male breast cancer (MBC) accounts for 1% of all breast cancers and 0.1% of male cancer deaths. There is a worldwide variation in incidence with the highest rate in Uganda and Zambia and the lowest in Japan.

Risk factors for MBC include the following:

- Genetic/familial factors: it has been estimated that 15% of MBC is familial. A family history of breast cancer increases the risk of male breast cancer by 2.5 times. MBC is associated with BRCA1 and BRCA2 mutation and is more common in those with BRCA2 mutation. Other genetic mutations associated with MBC include androgen gene mutation, PTEN mutation (Cowden syndrome), CHEK 2 mutation (Li–Fraumeni syndrome), and the Lynch syndrome.
- Hormonal factors: imbalance in testosterone and oestrogen levels as occurs in men with undescended testis, or after orchiectomy, and lifestyle factors. Klinefelter's syndrome is associated with a 50-fold increase in breast cancer. Obesity, a common cause for hyperoestrogenism in men, doubles the risk of MBC.
- Lifestyle factors: these include alcoholism, and exogenous oestrogen intake by transsexuals.
- Prior radiotherapy for unilateral gynaecomastia and thymic enlargement also increases the risk of MBC (1.6–1.9-fold).
- A history of MBC increases the contralateral breast cancer risk by 30-fold.
- Occupational exposure to high temperatures (e.g. steel works, blast furnaces) is thought to increase the risk of MBC.

Clinical presentation

The average age at diagnosis (63 years) is 10 years later than women. The usual presentation is with a painless mass (85%) and other features include nipple retraction, ulceration, discharge, and pain. Rarely breast cancer can present as axillary nodal metastasis. More than 40% of men with breast cancer present with stage III/IV disease.

Investigations

Investigations include ultrasound, mammography, and histological confirmation. All patients with locally advanced or clinically node-positive disease need staging to rule out distant metastasis. On ultrasound the tumours appears as solid lesions. Mammography has a sensitivity and specificity of >90%. Mammographic appearance is often of a mass with well-defined or speculated margins with or without microcalcifications.

Ninety per cent of tumours are invasive, of which 80% are infiltrating ductal carcinoma, 5% papillary, and 1% lobular. Ten per cent of tumours are DCIS. Eighty to ninety per cent of tumours are ER positive and 75–96% are PR positive.

Treatment

Surgery is the definitive treatment of choice in localized disease. It involves total mastectomy with an axillary procedure as in female breast cancer. There are data that show SNB is useful in clinically node-negative patients.

Many centres advise adjuvant radiotherapy after conservative surgery and for tumours of >1cm, grade III tumours, tumours with vascular invasion, and for node positive disease. The radiotherapy target volume includes the mastectomy scar, skin, and underlying muscle. Care should be taken to avoid unnecessary irradiation of the heart when irradiating the left chest wall. Axillary radiotherapy is not recommended after a dissection. Supraclavicular fossa and internal mammary chain radiotherapy may be indicated depending on the tumour characteristics.

Since the majority of MBC are ER positive, tamoxifen is the standard of care, though there is no prospective randomized data to confirm the benefit. The role of gonadal ablation and AIs are not known.

There is some evidence that adjuvant chemotherapy may improve the OS and hence may be considered for high-risk patients, especially those with hormone negative, node positive tumours. The role of trastuzumab has not been studied; it may be considered for high-risk HER2-positive MBC.

Patients with locally advanced cancer are treated with preoperative hormone- or chemotherapy to facilitate future definitive surgery.

Metastatic breast cancer can be treated with hormonal manipulation or chemotherapy. Eighty per cent of oestrogen in men is produced peripherally and 20% from the testis. Hence, AIs may not be effective as first-line therapy. However, the circulating level of oestrogen is found to be high in patients who develop tamoxifen resistance and hence AIs may be useful as second-line treatment. Other methods of hormonal manipulation include orchiectomy, antiandrogens, and aminoglutethimide.

Prognosis and survival

Stage and nodal status are the most important prognostic factors. The reported 5-year survival is 40–65%. Stage-wise 5-year survivals are: 75–100% for stage I, 50–80% stage II, and 30–60% for stage III. Node-positive patients have a worse prognosis compared with node-negative patients (10-year survival 84% vs. 44%). With >4 positive nodes the 10-year survival falls to 14%.

Further reading

Fentiman I, Fourquet A, Hartobagyi G. Male breast cancer. *Lancet* 2006; **367**:595–604.

Kamila C, Jenny B, Per H, *et al*. How to treat male breast cancer. *Breast* 2007; **16**:S147–S154.

Oesophageal cancer: epidemiology and clinical features

Epidemiology

Oesophageal cancer is a common cancer in the UK with an annual incidence of 16.5 for men and 8.5 for women per 100,000 and >7000 new cases per year (ONS 2004). The incidence has risen steadily over the last 20 years mainly due to an increase in adenocarcinomas, whereas SCCs have decreased slightly. Despite advances in the treatment OS rates remain poor at <15% (ONS 2004).

Worldwide it is the eighth commonest cancer and has the fifth highest mortality rate (Parkin et al. 2005). There is a large geographical variation in the incidence and histological types, being less common in the Western world although rates of adenocarcinoma are increasing exponentially. The incidence in countries such as China and in the Eastern Mediterranean is extremely high, consisting mainly of SCC. There is a male to female ratio of 2.5:1 although the incidence of cervical oesophageal cancer is higher in women. Incidence increases with age for both sexes.

Aetiology and pathology

The majority of oesophageal malignancies are adenocarcinomas, SCCs, or undifferentiated carcinomas. Worldwide, 85% are squamous carcinomas. The increase in adenocarcinomas in the Western world over the last 20 years is thought to be associated with GORD as a consequence of increasing obesity.

The majority of tumours arise within the middle and lower third of the oesophagus with 15% in the upper third. Most adenocarcinomas occur at or immediately above the gastro-oesophageal junction (GOJ). It is often difficult to determine whether an adenocarcinoma extending through the GOJ originated in the oesophagus or in the stomach.

Oesophageal reflux is a recognized causative factor in and is thought to account for the increased risk seen in conditions such as achalasia and hiatus hernias. This risk is also significantly increased in the presence of Barrett's oesophagus, a dysplastic condition resulting in columnar epithelium containing mucous glands. Barrett's itself is related to oesophageal reflux. Most adenocarcinomas arise in Barrett's epithelium although a small number arise in glands within the oesophageal wall.

Multiple environmental factors are known to play a role in the aetiology of SCC although their role in adenocarcinoma is less clear. High salt intake, alcohol, smoking, and excessive starchy food such as rice and maize are all associated with an increased risk. A diet rich in fruit and vegetables has been shown to reduce the relative risk (Nakachi et al. 1988; Franceschi 1993).

The role of genetic alterations in oesophageal cancer is yet to be fully established. However, studies have indicated the potential role of a number of tumour-related genes including p53, pRb, and bcl-2 (Parenti et al. 1997; Mathew et al. 2002).

Other uncommon malignant histological types include sarcoma variants, GISTs, SCCs, neuroendocrine tumours, adenocystic type tumours, and NHL.

Clinical features

Most patients present with dysphagia from mechanical obstruction, often describing difficulty with specific food types and the need to employ techniques such as liquidizing food. Difficulty in swallowing liquids is indicative of the progression to an advanced stage.

Other symptoms related to local disease include odynophagia, reflux, regurgitation, and vomiting following eating. Generally patients will have rapid weight loss assumed to be due to poor calorific intake.

Locally advanced disease can cause pain due to invasion of neighbouring structures to the oesophagus such as the mediastinum and vertebral bodies. Other signs can include Horner's syndrome, recurrent laryngeal nerve palsy, and a raised hemidiaphragm.

Advanced metastatic disease can result in liver capsule discomfort, painful bony metastases, ascites, or peritoneal deposits. Other sites of blood-borne spread include the lungs and brain. Patients may be jaundiced and by this stage most will have significant cachexia.

Further reading

Franceschi S. Role of nutrition in the aetiology of oesophageal cancer in developing countries. *Endoscopy* 1993; **25**:613–16.

Mathew R, Arora S, Khanna R, *et al.* Alterations in p53 and pRB pathways and their prognostic significance in oesophageal cancer. *Eur J Cancer* 2002; **28**:832–41.

Nakachi K, Imai K, Hoshiyama Y, *et al.* The joint effects of two factors in the aetiology of oesophageal cancer in Japan. *J Epidemol Community Health* 1988; **42**:355–64.

Office for National Statistics. *Cancer Statistics Registrations in England and Wales*. London: HMSO, 2004.

Parenti AR, Rugge M, Shiao YH, *et al.* Bcl-2 and p53 immunophenotypes in pre-invasive, early and advanced oesophageal squamous cancer. *Histopathology* 1997; **31**:430–5.

Parkin DM, Bray F, Ferlay J, *et al.* Global cancer statistics 2002. *AC Cancer J Clin* 2005; **55**:74–108.

Oesophageal cancer: screening, diagnosis, and staging

Screening and surveillance

Oesophageal cancer has a poor prognosis. Even if detected early enough for radical treatment the chance of cure remains no more than 30%.

When screening for any condition the benefit in terms of improved outcome must be weighed up against the costs in terms of resource usage and risk to the patient. The screening test used to detect oesophageal cancer is upper GI endoscopy. As oesophageal cancer is not particularly common in the Western world, screening on this basis is unlikely to be beneficial. In countries where SCC of the oesophagus is endemic, screening may be beneficial.

In the UK a more pragmatic approach is adopted for the screening of high-risk groups. No firm guidelines exist although high-risk patients with conditions such as tylosis and Plummer–Vinson syndrome are regularly screened with endoscopy. Guidelines published by the British Society of Gastroenterology (2005) state that surveillance in patients with chronic reflux is not justified as the absolute risk to individual patients is <1 in 1000 per annum. In patients with non-dysplastic Barrett's oesophagus this risk is increased 10-fold to 1% per annum. Whether this represents a justifiable benefit compared to the morbidity associated with endoscopy is a matter for discussion between the patient and their doctor. If the decision is to screen, it should be done every 2 years. There is currently insufficient evidence to reject screening in such cases on economic grounds alone (British Society of Gastroenterology 2005).

In patients with Barrett's oesophagus diagnosed with mild dysplasia, a more intensive course of action is recommended with acid suppression therapy followed by a repeat endoscopy and multiple biopsies at 8–12 weeks. If this remains stable, repeat biopsy is recommended every 6 months. Patients with high-grade dysplasia on endoscopic biopsy have a 30–40% risk of having invasive adenocarcinoma found in the resection specimen. Therefore, the recommendation is to consider full staging with a view to oesophagectomy.

Diagnosis

Clinical assessment of the patient is the key starting point. History of dysphagia and upper GI symptoms can point towards the potential diagnosis and may be associated with weight loss. Examination may reveal findings in keeping with metastatic spread such as hepatomegaly, lymphadenopathy, cachexia, bone pain, or Horner's syndrome.

Barium swallow

This will identify any region of obstruction due to tumour or compression. Strictures can often be distinguished between benign and malignant. Most abnormal lesions seen on barium swallow need further assessment with endoscopy to allow for direct tumour visualization and biopsy.

Endoscopy and endoscopic ultrasound

This is the cornerstone for diagnosis and subsequent follow up of oesophageal cancer. It enables the operator to visualize and record the position and extent of the tumour and also to obtain tissue for a histological diagnosis. The main limitation of endoscopy is that only the mucosal surface of the oesophagus can be seen and biopsied.

EUS combines a conventional endoscope with a high-frequency (resolution) ultrasound probe attached to the tip. This allows the operator to see the depth of tumour invasion through the five layers of the oesophageal wall and extension of tumour into adjacent structures such as the pleura. Assessment of lymph nodes is based on size as well as signal characteristics. EUS-guided FNA of any suspicious lesions, particularly lymph nodes, can improve the diagnostic accuracy. For locoregional staging, EUS is the most accurate means of predicting local tumour (T) stage and lymph node involvement (N stage) (Pfau et al. 2007).

Computer tomography and magnetic resonance imaging

A staging CT scan of the thorax, abdomen, and pelvis is recommended routinely in all patients to demonstrate the size of the primary tumour and its relationship with adjacent organs as well as any enlarged mediastinal, supraclavicular fossa, or perigastric/coeliac lymph nodes. However, the layers of the oesophageal wall are not sufficiently defined on CT to provide accurate local (T) or nodal (N) staging information. CT is good for assessing direct invasion into the bronchial tree and detecting distant metastases. The use of CT and EUS improve the accuracy of staging (Maerz et al. 1993).

Whilst MRI avoids ionizing radiation, it offers no benefit beyond a combination of CT and EUS in staging oesophageal cancers. New developments in MRI technology may allow for better staging in the future.

Positron emission tomography

The use of ^{18}FDG-PET scanning is becoming more widespread in oesophageal cancer. Its main role is to detect sites of distant metastases not easily identified on CT, as well as second primary cancers (such as lung, head and neck, colon, and breast) (Bruzzi et al. 2007). The use of PET for locoregional staging is limited by low specificity and resolution.

Laparoscopy

Laparoscopy allows the visualization and biopsy of small peritoneal metastases which may not have been detected on CT or PET. Up to 20% of patients would avoid major surgery as a result of a diagnostic laparoscopy (de Graaf et al. 2007). This is particularly useful in lower-third oesophageal and GOJ tumours rather than upper- and middle-third cancers where the risk of intra-abdominal dissemination is low.

Bronchoscopy

Many upper- or middle-third oesophageal cancers impinge on the bronchial tree causing compression or direct invasion. This is often visible on CT but bronchoscopy may be required to determine whether or not the tumour is potentially operable.

Staging

Accurate staging of oesophageal cancer is essential to determine prognosis and management options. It will also allow for meaningful comparison of outcomes between different centres and different countries. The UICC TNM classification (Tumour, Nodes, Metastases) (Sobin and Wittekind 2002) is used to define extent of local, nodal and metastatic disease:

T: tumour

- T0: no evidence of tumour
- Tx: primary tumour cannot be assessed
- Tis: *in situ* changes only
- T1: invasion of lamina propria or submucosa

- T2: invasion of the muscularis mucosa
- T3: invasion of the adventitia
- T4: invasion of adjacent structures

N: nodal
- Nx: regional nodal involvement cannot be assessed
- N0: no nodal disease
- N1: regional nodal involvement

M: metastasis
- Mx: metastatic disease cannot be assessed
- M0: no metastasis
- M1: metastatic disease

Tumours of lower thoracic oesophagus
- M1a: metastasis in coeliac lymph nodes
- M1b: other distant metastasis

Tumours of upper thoracic oesophagus
- M1a: metastasis in cervical lymph nodes
- M1b: other distant metastasis

Tumours of mid-thoracic oesophagus
- M1a: not applicable
- M1b: non-regional lymph node or other distant metastasis

Stage grouping
- Stage I: T1N0/xM0
- Stage IIa: T2/3N0/xM0
- Stage IIb: T1/2N1M0
- Stage III: T3N1M0 or T4N0/1M0
- Stage IV: any T any N M1
- Stage IVa: any T any N M1a
- Stage IVb: any T any N M1b

Stage I disease on both clinical staging and subsequent pathological review is uncommon with the majority of patients with localized disease being stage II or III.

Siewert classification

It is often difficult to distinguish whether adenocarcinomas arising in the vicinity of the oesophagogastric junction have originated at the junction, the stomach, or the lower oesophagus. The Siewert classification aims to standardize how these tumours are described and treated (Siewert and Stein 1998).
- Type I: adenocarcinoma of the distal oesophagus which may infiltrate the oesophagogastric junction from above.
- Type II: true carcinoma of the cardia often referred to as 'junctional carcinoma'.
- Type III: subcardial gastric carcinoma which infiltrates the oesophagogastric junction and distal oesophagus from below.

References

British Society of Gastroenterology. *Guidelines for the diagnosis and management of Barrett's columnar-lined oesophagus.* London: British Society of Gastroenterology, 2005.

Bruzzi JF, Munden RF, Truong MT, *et al.* PET/CT of esophageal cancer: its role in clinical management. *Radiographics* 2007; **27**:1635–52.

de Graaf GW, Avantunde AA, Parsons SL, *et al.* The role of staging laproscopy in oesophagogastric cancers. *Eur J Surg Oncol* 2007; **33**:988–92.

Maerz LL, Deveney CW, Lopez RR, *et al.* Role of computed tomographic scans in the staging of esophageal and proximal gastric malignancies. *Am J Surg* 1993; **165**:558–60.

Pfau PR, Perlman SB, Stanko P, *et al.* The role and clinical value of EUS in a multimodality esophageal carcinoma staging program with CT and positron emission tomography. *Gastrointest Endosc* 2007; **65**:377–84.

Sobin LH, Wittekind C (eds). *TNM Classification of Malignant Tumours Sixth Edition.* UICC International Union Against Cancer. New York: Wiley-Liss, 2002.

Siewert JR, Stein HJ. Classification of adenocarcinoma of the oesophagogastric junction. *Brit J Surg* 1998; **85**:1457–9.

Oesophageal cancer: treatment of localized disease

Principles of management

Less than half of newly diagnosed patients with oesophageal cancer are curable. All curative treatment options are associated with significant short- and long-term morbidity. Therefore accurate staging is essential to deliver appropriate treatment. Patient selection for stage, physical fitness, and mental attitude are important considerations.

The two main curative options are surgical resection or radiation therapy. Cure rates from single modality therapies are poor and attempts to improve survival using multimodality approaches, such as combining surgery with chemotherapy or radiotherapy or all three have been made. However, any benefit from multimodality therapy must be weighed up against the increased toxicity, particularly in a generally frail and elderly population of patients.

There have been two small trials comparing surgery alone with radiotherapy alone. Both trials showed a survival advantage in favour of surgery (Fok et al. 1994; Badwe et al. 1999). A third trial by the MRC failed to accrue.

Surgery

The overall 5-year survival of patients with oesophageal cancer referred for surgery is <10% (Muller et al. 1990). Major surgery should be avoided in patients who are unlikely to be surgically curable. The best results are achieved in specialist centres with established MDTs. These centres can achieve 5-year survival rates of 35% and postoperative mortality <5% (Lerut et al. 2005) and patients with very early cancers can expect a 5-year survival of 80% (Holscher et al. 1997).

The specific surgical approach is dependent on site of the tumour, histology, and the extent of lymphadenectomy intended. The most common procedure for middle- and lower-third cancers is the two-stage Ivor Lewis approach. The first stage consists of laparotomy and mobilization of the stomach, followed by right thoracotomy to remove the tumour and to form an oesophagogastric anastomosis.

Tumours in the upper third of the oesophagus are often resected using a three-phase approach to achieve adequate longitudinal margins. This will also allow more extensive lymph node removal, particularly in the mediastinum and supraclavicular fossa. However, this operation is associated with significant morbidity and in less fit patients it may be more appropriate to offer a non-surgical treatment such as radiotherapy with or without concurrent chemotherapy.

Radiotherapy

Radical radiotherapy for oesophageal cancers can cause significant acute and late morbidity and patients need to have a minimum level of fitness to tolerate treatment. Patients selected for radiotherapy tend to be less fit and have a more advanced disease than those having surgery. This different 'case mix' between surgical and radiotherapy series makes comparison of results difficult. In a literature review of 49 published series the combined 5-year survival was 6% (Earlam and Cunha-Melo 1980).

Definitive chemoradiotherapy

The main reason for adding chemotherapy to radiotherapy concurrently is to exploit the radio-sensitizing interaction in order to improve local control. Randomized trials comparing CRT with radiotherapy alone in oesophageal cancer have shown improved outcome for CRT.

The Radiation Therapy Oncology Group trial (RTOG 85-01) randomized 123 patients to definitive radiotherapy (64Gy) or CRT (50Gy) with 2 cycles of concurrent cisplatin and 5FU followed by a further 2 cycles. Interim analysis showed significant survival improvement with CRT resulting in early termination of the trial. A further 69 patients were treated using the CRT regimen. The 3-year OS in the randomized and non-randomized CRT arms was 30% and 26% respectively compared to 0% in the radiotherapy alone arm (Al-Sarraf et al. 1997).

A second trial by the Eastern Cooperative Oncology Group (EST-1282) also showed a significant improvement in survival for CRT compared with radiotherapy alone (Smith et al. 1998). Subsequent publications have shown that 3-year survival of around 30% can be consistently achieved with definitive CRT (Minsky et al. 2002). Despite improved outcomes with CRT, locoregional failure remains a major problem at around 50%. In an attempt to improve local control, the Intergroup trial (INT 0123) explored radiation dose escalation by randomizing 236 patients to high-dose (64.8Gy) versus standard-dose (50.4Gy) CRT. There was no improvement in locoregional control or OS (Minsky et al. 2002). More treatment-related deaths occurred in the high-dose arm (10% vs 2%), but most of the events occurred prior to receiving dose escalation.

No randomized trials have compared definitive CRT with surgery in resectable oesophageal cancer. Most of the data on CRT are for SCCs, which usually arise in the mid to upper oesophagus and are more likely to be surgically unresectable. Two trials have compared definitive CRT against a trimodality approach (CRT followed by surgery).

The EORTC trial (FFCD 9102) treated 444 patients (90% SCC) with induction CRT (using cisplatin and 5-FU) (Bedenne et al. 2007). A total of 259 patients who had made a clinical response were then randomized to surgery or further CRT. OS was similar (median 17.7 vs. 19.3 months and 2-years 34% vs. 40% respectively). However, treatment-related mortality was higher in the surgery arm (9% vs. 1%; p = 0.002).

The German Oesophageal Cancer Study Group Trial compared induction chemotherapy followed by CRT (40Gy) and surgery with induction chemotherapy followed by CRT alone (65Gy) (Stahl et al. 2005). A total of 172 patients with locally advanced SCC were randomized. The data showed that although local PFS was better in the surgery group (64% vs 41%; p = 0.003), it did not improve OS (median 16.4 vs 14.9 months and 2 years 40% vs. 35% respectively). Again, treatment-related mortality was higher in the surgery arm (13% v 3%; p = 0.03).

Most trials of definitive CRT use cisplatin and 5-FU. To improve the effectiveness of CRT, new chemotherapy regimens and drugs are being tested. One example is the UK SCOPE 1 trial, which is testing the addition of cetuximab (an EGFR inhibitor) to standard CRT (SCOPE).

Preoperative chemotherapy

There have been numerous randomized trials comparing preoperative chemotherapy followed by surgery versus surgery alone. Only one major trial has shown a statistically significant benefit in survival (Medical Research Council Oesophageal Cancer Working Party 2002). Most of the other trials were underpowered to detect a difference. A meta-analysis of 10 trials has shown improvement in survival with preoperative chemotherapy (7% difference at 2 years; p = 0.05) (Gebski et al. 2007). The largest trial was the Medical Research Council (MRC) OEO2. A total of 802 patients were randomized to either surgery alone or two cycles of preoperative cisplatin and 5FU followed by surgery. The use of chemotherapy improved OS from 34% to 43% at 2 years (p = 0.004). This strategy is now the standard of care in most UK centres. In an attempt to improve outcomes further, the current UK OEO5 trial is comparing 2 cycles of cisplatin and 5-FU with 4 cycles of epirubicin, cisplatin, and capecitabine (ECX) (OEO5).

Preoperative chemoradiotherapy

The role of preoperative CRT has also been investigated in numerous randomized trials. A large number of different preoperative CRT schedules using varying radiation doses and fractionations and varying chemotherapy regimens have been published. Pathological complete response (pCR) rates range from 7–56% (Geh et al. 2001). Most randomized trials showed no survival improvement, partly due to small patient numbers. However, meta-analyses show a statically significant improvement in OS (p = 0.016) (Urschel and Vasen 2003; Gebski et al. 2007) with preoperative CRT followed by surgery compared with surgery alone. This benefit was only seen when chemotherapy was given concurrently with radiotherapy (p = 0.005) rather than sequentially (p = 0.36). However, treatment-related mortality was increased with preoperative CRT (p = 0.053).

In an attempt to find the optimal CRT regimen, a systematic analysis of 26 trials showed that there is a dose–response relationship between radiotherapy and chemotherapy dose and pCR rate (Geh et al. 2006). One gram/m^2 of 5FU was calculated to be equivalent to 1.9Gy of radiation and 100gm/m^2 was equivalent to 7.2Gy.

Further reading

Al-Sarraf M, Martz K, Hesskovic MA, et al. Progress report of combined chemoradiotherapy versus radiotherapy alone in patients with esophageal cancer: An Intergroup study. J Clin Oncol 1997; 15:277–84.

Badwe RA, Sharma, Bhansali MS, et al. The quality of swallowing for patients with operable esophageal carcinoma. A randomized trial comparing surgery with radiotherapy. Cancer 1999; 85:763–8.

Bedenne L, Michel P, Bouche O, et al. Chemoradiation followed by surgery compared with chemoradiation alone in squamous cancer of the oesophagus: FFCD 9102. J Clin Oncol 2007; 25:1160–8.

Earlam R, Cunha-Melo JR. Oesophageal squamous cell carcinoma: I. A critical review of radiotherapy. Br J Surg 1980; 67:457–61.

Fok M, McShane J, Law SYK, et al. Prospective randomized study on radiotherapy and surgery in the treatment of oesophageal cancer. Asian J Surg 1994; 17:223–9.

Gebski V, Burmeister B, Smithers BM, et al. Survival benefits from neoadjuvant chemoradiotherapy or chemotherapy in oesophageal cancer: a meta-analysis. Lancet Oncol 2007; 8:226–34.

Geh JI, Crellin AM, Glynne-Jones R. Preoperative (neoadjuvant) chemoradiotherapy in oesophageal cancer. Br J Surg 2001; 88:338–56.

Geh JI, Bond SJ, Bentzen SM, et al. Systematic overview of preoperative (neoadjuvant) chemoradiotherapy trials in oesophageal cancer: Evidence of a radiation and chemotherapy dose response. Radiat Oncol 2006; 78:236–44.

Holscher AH, Bollschweiler, Schneider PM, et al. Early adenocarcinoma in Barrett's oesophagus. Br J Surg 1997; 84:1470–3.

Lerut T, Nafteux PH, Moons J, et al. Quality in the surgical treatment of cancer of the esophagus and gastroesophageal junction. Eur J Surg Oncol 2005; 31:587–94.

Medical Research Council Oesophageal Cancer Working Party. Surgical resection with or without pre-operative chemotherapy in oesophageal cancer: a randomised controlled trial. Lancet 2002; 359:1727–33.

Minsky BD, Pajak TF, Ginsberg RJ, et al. INT 0123(Radiation Therapy Oncology Group 94-05) phase III trial of combined modality therapy for esophageal cancer: high-dose versus standard dose-dose radiation therapy. J Clin Oncol 2002; 20:1167–74.

Muller JM, Erasmi H, Stelzner M, et al. Surgical therapy of oesophageal carcinoma. Br J Surg 1990; 77:845–57.

OEO5. A randomised controlled trial comparing standard chemotherapy followed by resection versus ECX chemotherapy followed by resection in patients with resectable adenocarcinoma of the oesophagus. MRC/CRUK clinical trial.

SCOPE 1 Trial: Study of chemoradiotherapy in oesophageal cancer plus or minus Erbitux. 2007. NCRI Upper GI Clinical Studies Group.

Smith TJ, Ryan LM, Douglass HO, et al. Combined chemoradiotherapy vs radiotherapy alone for early stage squamous cell carcinoma of the esophagus: a study of the Eastern Cooperative Oncology Group. Int J Radiat Oncol Biol Phys 1998; 42:269–76.

Stahl M, Stuschke M, Lehmann N, et al. Chemoradiation with and without surgery in patients with locally advanced squamous cell carcinoma of the oesophagus. J Clin Oncol 2005; 23:2310–17.

Urschel JD, Vasan H. A meta-analysis of randomized controlled trials that compared neoadjuvant chemoradiation and surgery to surgery alone for respectable esophageal cancer. Am J Surg 2003; 185:538–43.

Oesophageal cancer: treatment of advanced disease, symptom control, and palliation

Principles of management

Over two-thirds of oesophageal cancer patients present with advanced, incurable disease. In addition, a significant number of patients who initially undergo radical treatment will relapse and enter this group.

In this situation, palliative treatment aims to improve symptoms and quality of life. It has to be weighed against potential toxicity before a decision to proceed, particularly in a population whose PS is often poor and toxic treatments such as chemotherapy may not be appropriate.

A multidisciplinary approach is essential. This should include not only medical and nursing teams in the hospital but also those in the community including hospice services.

The main symptom encountered in advanced oesophageal cancer is dysphagia and palliation is aimed at improving swallowing. The most appropriate option is dependent on local tumour extent as well as the individual patient.

Localized treatments for dysphagia

Dilatation

This is performed using a number of different graded oesophageal dilators. It results in immediate improvement of dysphagia but is generally short lived, usually 2–4 weeks. It is associated with a complication risk of 10–15% (including perforation and haemorrhage), even in the most experienced hands.

Stenting/intubation

Early stenting techniques involved intubating the oesophagus with a rigid plastic tube but were associated with perforation, bolus obstruction, and stent migration. The use of self-expandable plastic stents has improved palliation and reduced complication rates. These are deployed once they are in the correct position. Uncovered stents imbed into the surrounding tissue becoming fixed and immoveable over time. Covered stents reduce the likelihood of imbedding allowing potential removal and/or repositioning but, however, are associated with an increase risk of migration. Covered stents are particularly useful for occluding a tracheo-oesophageal fistula.

Stenting may be combined with other local therapies for dysphagia. However it may be associated with a higher rate of morbidity if used following chemoradiotherapy (Lecleire et al. 2006).

Injection/thermal ablation

Alcohol injection or thermal ablation with YAG laser or photodynamic therapy can improve dysphagia. The benefit is often short lived and may need to be repeated regularly. All techniques are also associated with potential morbidity including haemorrhage and perforation in 10–15%.

Radiotherapy

This can be delivered either by EBRT or by brachytherapy (insertion of iridium-192 radioactive source into the oesophagus). Improvement in swallowing will not occur immediately and sometimes could initially deteriorate before improving. EBRT is often given as 30Gy in 10 fractions over 2 weeks or 20Gy in 5 fractions. Brachytherapy has been shown to be effective using a high-dose rate machine to give 16Gy in 2 fractions or 18Gy in 3 fractions over 5 days. Both techniques can be utilized with other local therapies in order to try and maximize symptom control.

Chemotherapy

Chemotherapy for advanced oesophageal and gastric cancer has been shown to improve survival when compared with best supportive care alone. A recent meta-analysis showed that the benefit was greatest when using a three-drug regimen including 5-FU, an anthracycline, and cisplatin (Wagner et al. 2006). In the UK the combination of epirubicin, cisplatin, and 5-FU (ECF) has been used as randomized trials have established this regimen to be superior to other combinations (Webb et al. 1997; Ross et al. 2002). The main disadvantage of ECF is the need for permanent central venous access to deliver the 5-FU as a continuous infusion and this is associated with significant toxicity.

The recently published REAL-2 trial evaluated oral capecitabine and oxaliplatin as an alternative to infusional 5-FU and cisplatin in a 2x2 trial design (Cunningham et al. 2008). A total of 1002 patients with advanced oesophagogastric cancer were randomized. The data showed that capecitabine and oxaliplatin were as effective as infusional 5-FU and cisplatin in terms of response rate and PFS. Although toxicity of 5-FU and capecitabine were similar, oxaliplatin resulted in increased neuropathy and diarrhoea but reduced renal toxicity, thromboembolism, alopecia, and neutropenia when compared with cisplatin. Patients receiving EOX survived longer than with ECF (38% vs 47% at 1 year; p = 0.02).

Before proceeding with chemotherapy, it is vital that the patient has been fully assessed in terms of staging and fitness to tolerate treatment. The patient must be closely monitored and treatment promptly stopped if symptoms are not improving or indeed deteriorating.

General palliation

Patients should be managed on an individual basis with interventions only being used when it is likely to improve symptoms and QoL. This often involves analgesia and steroids for the improvement of pain and appetite/general well-being. Painful bone metastases may benefit from a single 8-Gy fraction of EBRT.

References

Cunningham D, Starling N, Rao S, et al. Capecitabine and oxaliplatin for advanced esophagogastic cancer. N Eng J Med 2008; **358**:36–46.

Lecleire S, Di Fiore F, Ben-Soussan E, et al. Prior chemoradiotherapy is associated with a higher life-threatening complication rate after palliative insertion of metal stents in patients with oesophageal cancer. Aliment Pharmacol Ther 2006; **23**:1693–702.

Ross P, Nicholson M, Cunningham D, et al. Prospective randomized trial comparing mitomycin, cisplatin and protracted venous-infusion flurouracil (PVI 5-FU) with epirubicin, cisplatin and PVI 5-FU in advanced esophagogastric cancer. J Clin Oncol 2002; **20**:1996–2004.

Wagner AD, Grothe W, Haerting J, et al. Chemotherapy in advanced gastric cancer: a systematic review and meta-analysis based on aggregate data. J Clin Onc 2006; **24**:2903–9.

Webb A, Cunningham D, Scarffe JH, et al. Randomized trial comparing epirubicin, cisplatin and fluorouracil versus fluorouracil, doxorubicin and methotrexate in advanced esophagogastric cancer. J Clin Oncol 1997; 15:261–67.

Gastric cancer: introduction and clinical features

Epidemiology

There are significant differences in the geographical, ethnic, and socioeconomic distribution of gastric cancer in the world. It is the eighth commonest cancer in the UK with an incidence of 17.2 for men and 8.7 for women per 100,000 (ONS 2008) and approximately 8200 new cases per year (Cancer Research UK website). There has been a significant change in the pattern of disease over the past 30 years in the Western world. Although the overall incidence has decreased significantly (Dolan et al. 1999), there has been an exponential rise in tumours involving the proximal stomach and cardia (Cancer Research UK website). During this period, incidence of lower oesophageal adenocarcinomas has also increased at the same rate. The overall 5-year survival remains low at around 15% (Cancer Research UK website).

Gastric cancer remains the fourth commonest cancer and the second commonest cause of cancer death in the world (Stewart and Kleihus 2003). Prevalent areas include Japan, China, South America, and Eastern Europe, whilst the lowest rates are observed in North America, Northern Europe, and most countries in Africa and South Eastern Asia. It is more common in men than women and incidence increases with age. The rapid decline of incidence is likely to be due to improved living conditions and increased consumption of fresh fruit, vegetables, and vitamins (Hohenberger and Gretschel 2003).

Pathology

The term gastric cancer is generally applied to adenocarcinomas which account for approximately 95% of all gastric neoplasms. The Laurén classification divides gastric adenocarcinomas into two different histological variants, intestinal and diffuse (Laurén 1965). In the intestinal subtype, tumour cells adhere to each other in a tubular or glandular formation, similar to adenocarcinomas arising in other parts of the intestinal tract. In the diffuse subtype, tumour cells lack adhesion molecules and have a more infiltrative appearance with little in the way of tubule or gland formation. The intestinal subtype tends to affect older patients and arise in the distal stomach, whereas the diffuse subtype is more common in younger patients. A variant of the diffuse subtype which extensively infiltrates the stomach wall is known as linitis plastica.

Other malignant tumours which arise in the stomach include lymphomas, GISTs and carcinoid tumours. The stomach is the most common site for GISTs and extra-nodal lymphomas.

Aetiology

The aetiology of gastric cancer is multifactorial. The causes of proximal/ cardia tumours are thought to be similar to lower oesophageal adenocarcinomas and are distinct from distal gastric cancers, accounting for the dramatic change of disease pattern over recent years (Stewart and Kleihus 2003). Increasing population weight and high calorific intake are associated with GORD and proximal cancers. Chronic reflux disease causes Barrett's oesophagus, which is a premalignant step to developing lower oesophageal adenocarcinoma. Higher socioeconomic status is associated with proximal cancers, whereas distal cancers are associated with poorer socioeconomic status. Migrant studies indicate an important role of environmental factors in the aetiology of gastric cancer. Diets rich in nitrates and salt are associated with an increased risk of developing gastric cancer, whereas fruits and vegetables high in vitamin C and E, and antioxidants are considered to have a protective effect. Smoking is also associated with an increased risk. The association with high alcohol intake is less robust. Radiation exposure is an associated risk factor.

Helicobacter pylori (*H. pylori*) is recognized as a group I carcinogen (carcinogenic to humans) for gastric cancer (IARC 1994). Its role as a risk factor for gastric cancer has been investigated in prospective epidemiological studies (Uemura et al. 2001). *H. pylori* infection is associated with both intestinal and diffuse subtypes of gastric cancer, as well as gastric MALToma. The role of *H. pylori* eradication in reducing the risk of gastric cancer remains controversial (Wong et al. 2004; Takenaka et al. 2007). *H. pylori* eradication is indicated in patients with gastric MALToma.

Germline mutations in the E-cadherin (CDH1) gene have been found in families with hereditary diffuse gastric cancer. This disorder is inherited in an AD fashion. Gastric cancer is associated with certain other cancer syndromes including hereditary non-polyposis colorectal cancer, familial adenomatous polyposis, and Peutz–Jeghers syndrome. Blood group A is associated with a 20% increased risk of developing gastric cancer.

Other risk factors include chronic atrophic gastritis and hypochlorhydria, pernicious anaemia, gastric surgery, Epstein–Barr virus infection, hypertrophic gastropathy, and various immunodeficiency syndromes. Regular use of aspirin and other NSAIDs is associated with a reduced risk of non-cardia gastric adenocarcinomas.

Clinical features

Weight loss and persistent abdominal pain are the most common symptoms. Nausea, anorexia, and early satiety are common features. Dysphagia occurs with tumours involving the proximal stomach or GOJ. Patients may describe preceding symptoms of indigestion. Distal tumours can present with symptoms of gastric outlet obstruction. Iron deficiency anaemia due to occult GI bleeding is not uncommon, whilst approximately 20% present with haematemesis or melaena. In countries such as Japan where gastric screening is routine, up to 60% have asymptomatic early gastric cancers.

Up to 50% of patients in the Western world present with symptoms of metastatic disease. Clinical signs indicating advanced disease include a palpable epigastric mass, an enlarged stomach with succussion splash, hepatomegaly, obstructive jaundice, and cachexia. Presence of ascites usually indicates peritoneal carcinomatosis. Virchow's node (left supraclavicular adenopathy) occurs with distant lymphatic spread. Peritoneal spread can result in a Sister Mary Joseph nodule (periumbilical metastasis), Krukenberg tumour (ovarian metastasis), and Blumer's shelf (mass in the anterior rectal wall on rectal examination). Associated paraneoplastic syndromes include dermatomyositis, acanthosis nigricans, sudden appearance of diffuse seborrhoeic keratoses (sign of Leser–Trelat), circinate erythemas, and microangiopathic haemolytic anaemia. Patients can also present with symptoms and clinical features suggestive of bone, lung, and CNS metastases.

Further reading

Dolan K, Sutton R, Walker SJ, *et al.* New classification of oesophageal and gastric carcinomas derived from changing patterns in epidemiology. *Br J Cancer* 1999; **80**:834–42.

Hohenberger P, Gretschel S. Gastric Cancer. *Lancet* 2003; **362**:305–15.

IRAC. Schistosomes, liver flukes and Helicobacter pylori. *IARC Monogr Eval Carcinog Risks Hum* 1994; **61**:177–240.

Laurén P. The two histological main types of gastric carcinoma: Diffuse and so-called intestinal-type carcinoma. *Acta Path Microbiol Imunol Scand* 1965; **64**:31–49.

ONS. Cancer Statistics Registrations 2005. London, HMSO 2008.

Stewart BW, Kleihus P (eds): *World Cancer Report* Lyon: IARC Press, 2003.

Takenaka R, Okada H, Kato J, *et al. Helicobacter pylori* eradication reduced the incidence of gastric cancer, especially of the intestinal type. *Aliment Pharmacol Ther* 2007; **25**:805–12.

Uemura N, Okamoto S, Yamamoto S, et al. Helicobacter pylori infection and the development of gastric cancer. *N Eng J Med* 2001; **345**:784–9.

Wong BC, Lam SK, Wong WM et al. Helicobacter pylori eradication to prevent gastric cancer in a high-risk region of China. *JAMA* 2004; **291**:187–94.

Internet resource

Cancer Research UK: http://info.cancerresearchuk.org

Gastric cancer: screening, diagnosis, staging and prognosis

Screening

The role of screening asymptomatic individuals for gastric cancer is not entirely proven. Such programmes have been implemented in countries with a high incidence such as Japan, Korea, and Chile (Leung et al. 2008). In Japan, initial screening is with barium studies and any suspicious lesions are investigated endoscopically (Leung et al. 2008). Uptake in the eligible population is approximately 20%, and there is a paucity of data on the cost-effectiveness of mass screening, even in a population with such a high incidence of gastric cancer. Although retrospective studies have shown a reduction in incidence and mortality, data from prospective studies remain inconsistent, with very little evidence from randomized trials (Leung et al. 2008).

Although endoscopy increases the rate of detection of gastric cancer compared to barium studies (Tashiro et al. 2006), as a tool for mass population screening it is limited by cost and availability of experienced operators. More recently, interest has been focused on the use of serological markers to identify patients at risk of developing gastric cancer.

A low serum pepsinogen (PG) I concentration and a low ratio of PGI/PGII are both recognized as serological markers of atrophic gastritis. The sensitivity and specificity of PG screening for gastric cancer in a Japanese population has been shown to be 84.6% and 73.5% respectively (Kitahara et al. 1999). A separate Japanese prospective study analysed the usefulness of a combination of serum PG and H. pylori antibody concentration as a marker of gastric cancer (Watabe et al. 2005). Individuals with features consistent with severe atrophic gastritis were found to have the highest risk of developing gastric cancer (Watabe et al. 2005). The authors concluded that H. pylori antibody and serum PG are good markers for the development of gastric cancer. Whether these findings are applicable to populations with a low incidence of gastric cancer would need investigating.

In the UK, the national screening committee has not recommended routine screening for gastric cancer or H. pylori on the basis of insufficient evidence to support such a policy (UK Screening Portal website). A more pragmatic approach has been recommended, for example, following-up patients with gastric ulcers with repeated biopsies until complete healing (Allum et al. 2002). For patients with hereditary diffuse gastric cancer, annual chromoendoscopic surveillance may have a role (Shaw et al. 2005). No guidelines are available for routine surveillance of other high-risk groups, e.g. pernicious anaemia.

Diagnosis and staging

Clinical assessment is an important starting point. The Department of Health in the UK has issued guidance specifying the 'at risk' symptoms including dysphagia, dyspepsia with high-risk factors, jaundice, and upper abdominal mass which should initiate specialist referral to aid earlier diagnosis of upper GI cancers (Allum et al. 2002). Patients with early gastric cancer are often asymptomatic or present with non-specific symptoms such as uncomplicated dyspepsia. A high index of suspicion is required to identify correctly the 'at risk' group of patients in such cases.

The presence of clinical signs such as an enlarged Virchow's (left supraclavicular fossa) lymph node or a palpable epigastric mass usually indicates advanced disease.

Routine blood tests may reveal anaemia or deranged liver function. Tumour markers, including CEA, CA 19-9, and CA 125 may be elevated, but are neither sensitive nor specific enough to be diagnostic in gastric cancer.

Endoscopy

Flexible OGD is the diagnostic procedure of choice. It permits direct visualization and biopsy of any suspicious lesions. The sensitivity of OGD is about 95% when multiple (≥7) biopsies are taken from any suspicious lesion. Newer techniques, such as chromoendoscopy, may enhance the detection of subtle lesions or dysplasia. However, the diagnosis of the diffuse-type gastric cancer can be difficult endoscopically as the overlying mucosa may appear normal.

Barium studies

Double-contrast barium studies have a continuing but limited role in detecting malignant lesions and some early gastric cancers when endoscopy is not feasible. It is particularly useful in the diagnosis of diffuse-type gastric cancer (linitis plastica). In this situation, the endoscopic appearance may be normal as the infiltration is submucosal and the rigid appearance on barium studies, commonly described as 'leather bottle', may be the only radiological indication of disease.

Computed tomography and magnetic resonance imaging

Contrast enhanced multislice CT scan following gastric distension with 600–800mL of water should be performed routinely in the staging of gastric cancer. The thorax, abdomen, and pelvis should be included to detect distant metastases and to provide an indication of the local tumour and lymph node stage. However, there are limitations of CT. Up to 30% of peritoneal metastases will not be detectable. Although CT is accurate for staging locally advanced (T3 and T4) tumours, its accuracy for staging early cancers is poor.

MRI has similar accuracy to CT but is not routinely used in the staging of gastric cancer because of the greater availability of CT.

Endoscopic ultrasound

EUS combines high-frequency ultrasonography with OGD and provides a more accurate prediction of depth of tumour invasion, particularly in early cancers. The accuracy for lymph node staging is similar to CT; however EUS-guided FNA of suspicious lymph nodes can improve the accuracy of EUS.

Positron emission tomography

Limited data are available regarding the use of FDG-PET for the evaluation of gastric cancer. Results from relatively small retrospective studies indicate comparatively low sensitivity of 70% and specificity of 69% (Chin and Wahl 2003). PET scanning is not routinely used in the staging of gastric cancer.

Laparoscopy and peritoneal cytology

Laparoscopy allows direct visualization of the liver surface, peritoneum, and local lymph nodes. Up to 20–30% of gastric cancer patients will have peritoneal metastases which are not detected on CT. Positive identification of such lesions will prevent the patient undergoing a futile laparotomy and resection. Laparoscopy is recommended in all patients with gastric cancer and gastro-oesophageal cancer where there appears to be a gastric component (Allum et al. 2006). There is inconsistent data regarding the additional benefit of peritoneal cytology in the staging of gastric cancer (SIGN 2006).

Staging systems

Accurate staging is essential to determine prognosis and appropriate treatment. A standardized staging system allows for meaningful comparison of treatment outcomes within clinical trials, and between centres in the same country as well as between countries.

Two major classification systems are currently used for the staging of gastric cancer. The Japanese system is more detailed and requires a more rigorous pathological assessment of the nodal stage compared to its counterpart, the AJCC/UICC system. The AJCC/UICC system is mainly used in the western world although it is increasingly used in other Asian countries. A comparison of the Japanese and AJCC/UICC staging system found that the AJCC/UICC system was more accurate in estimating prognosis (Ichikura et al. 1999). It is summarized below (Sobin and Wittekind 2002).

T: primary tumour
- TX: primary tumour cannot be assessed
- T0: no evidence of primary tumour
- Tis: carcinoma *in situ*: intraepithelial tumour without invasion of the lamina propria
- T1: tumour invades lamina propria or submucosa
- T2: tumour invades muscularis propria or subserosa
- T2a: tumour invades muscularis propria
- T2b: tumour invades subserosa
- T3: tumour penetrates serosa (visceral peritoneum) without invasion of adjacent structures
- T4: tumour invades adjacent structures

N regional lymph nodes
- NX: regional lymph nodes cannot be assessed
- N0: no regional lymph node metastasis
- N1: metastasis in 1–6 regional lymph nodes
- N2: metastasis in 7–15 regional lymph nodes
- N3: metastasis in >15 regional lymph nodes

M: distant metastasis
- MX: distant metastasis cannot be assessed
- M0: no distant metastasis
- M1: distant metastasis

Stage grouping
- Stage 0: TisN0M0
- Stage IA: T1N0M0
- Stage IB:
  T1N1M0
  T2a/bN0M0
- Stage II:
  T1N2M0
  T2a/bN1M0
  T3 N0M0
- Stage IIIA:
  T2a/bN2M0
  T3N1M0
  T4N0M0
- Stage IIIB: T3N2M0

- Stage IV:
  T4 N1,N2,N3M0
  T1,T2,T3 N3M0
  Any T, Any N, M1

Two other classification systems have been established to unify nomenclature relating to gastric cancers. The Vienna classification system of GI epithelial neoplasia (Schlemper et al. 2000) aimed to resolve differences between Western and Japanese pathologists in the description of such lesions. The Siewert classification system standardizes nomenclature used to describe adenocarcinomas arising at the GOJ (Siewert and Stein 1998). Siewert type 3 cancers are treated as gastric cancers.

Prognosis

Important prognostic factors in resectable gastric cancer include depth of invasion, number of lymph nodes involved, and positive resection margins. In the UK 5-year survivals rates remain low at approximately 15%. Estimated 5-year survival by stage is:
- Stage 1: 70%
- Stage 2: 40%
- Stage 3: 20%
- Stage 4: <5%

Further reading

Allum WH, Griffin SM, Watson A, *et al.* Guidelines for the management of oesophageal and gastric cancer. *Gut* 2002; **50**(supplement V):v1–v23.

Chin BB, Wahl RL. 18F-Fluoro-2-deoxyglucose positron emission tomography in the evaluation of gastrointestinal malignancies. *Gut* 2003; **52**(suppl 4):iv23–iv29.

Ichikura T, Tomimatsu S, Uefuji K, *et al.* Evaluation of the new American Joint Committee on Cancer/ International Union against Cancer Classification of lymph node metastasis from gastric carcinoma in comparison with the Japanese Classification. *Cancer* 1999; **86**:553–8.

Kitahara F, Koboyashi K, Sato T, *et al.* Accuracy of screening for gastric cancer using serum pepsinogen concentrations. *Gut* 1999; **44**:693–7.

Leung WK, Wu M, Kakugawa Y, *et al.* Screening for gastric cancer in Asia: current evidence and practice. *Lancet Oncol* 2008; **9**:279–9–87.

Schlemper RJ, Riddell RH, Kato Y, *et al.* The Vienna classification of gastrointestinal epithelial neoplasia. *Gut* 2000; **47**:251-5.

Scottish Intercollegiate Guidelines Network. Management of oesophageal and gastric cancer: A national clinical guideline. Edinburgh: SIGN, 2006.

Shaw D, Blair V, Framp A, et al. Chromoendoscopic surveillance in hereditary diffuse gastric cancer: an alternative to prophylactic gastrectomy? Gut 2005; 54:461–8.

Siewert JR, Stein HJ. Classification of adenocarcinoma of the oesophagogastric junction. *Br J Surg* 1998; **85**: :1457-9.

Sobin LH, Wittekind Ch (eds). *TNM Classification of Malignant Tumours, 6th edition* New York: Wiley-Liss, 2002.

Tashiro A, Sano M, Kinameri k, Fujita K, *et al.* Comparing mass screening techniques for gastric cancer in Japan. *World J Gastroenterol* 2006; **12**:4873–4.

Watabe H, Mitsushima T, Yamaji Y, *et al.* Predicting the development of gastric cancer from combining *Helicobacter pylori* antibodies and serum pepsinogen status: a prospective endoscopic cohort study. *Gut* 2005; **54**:764–8.

Internet resource

UK Screening Portal: http://www.nsc.nhs.uk

Gastric cancer: treatment of localized disease

Principles of treatment

Surgical resection offers the only curative treatment option for gastric cancer but is only appropriate in <50% of newly diagnosed patients in the West, as the majority present with locally unresectable or metastatic disease. Patients being considered for curative surgery should be accurately staged and assessed for physical fitness to avoid subjecting patients to unnecessary risk of morbidity and mortality (McCulloch et al. 2003), particularly if they are subsequently found to have incurable disease.

Cure rates from surgical resection as a single modality treatment range from 13–50% in Western series (Wanebo et al. 1993). Multimodality treatment results in a modest survival benefit but at the cost of increased toxicity. The standard of care varies from country to country and current issues of controversy include extent of resection and lymphadenectomy and the role of neoadjuvant and adjuvant chemotherapy and radiotherapy.

Early gastric cancer (EGC)

EGC is tumour that is limited to the gastric mucosa or submucosa (T1) irrespective of nodal involvement. It is associated with a favourable prognosis compared to cancers that invade beyond the submucosa (≥T2). Following resection, 5-year survival rates of >90% have been reported (Everett and Axon 1997).

The risk of lymph node metastasis in EGC is 10–15% and depends on the size of tumour, histological subtype, and presence of submucosal invasion (Folli et al. 2001). If untreated, up to two-thirds of patients with EGC can progress to advanced cancer over 5 years (Tsukuma et al. 2000). Patients with a low risk of nodal involvement may be considered for less radical treatment options such as endoscopic mucosal resection (EMR). Five-year survival rates of 84% have been reported with EMR (Uedo et al. 2006). Limitations of EMR include risk of incomplete tumour resection and tumour/lymph node understaging despite optimal work-up.

H. pylori is classified as a group I carcinogen for gastric cancer. The evidence for *H. pylori* eradication in reducing the incidence of gastric cancer remains controversial. In a Japanese randomized trial, 554 patients with EGC treated endoscopically received *H. pylori* eradication or no eradication. At 3-years follow-up, the OR for development of metachronous gastric cancer was 0.353 (95% CI 0.161-0.775) in favour of eradication (Fukase et al. 2008). Further studies are required to confirm these findings.

Surgery

The aim of surgical resection is to achieve complete removal of the tumour and involved lymph nodes. Guidelines from ESMO recommend recovery of a minimum of 14 lymph nodes (Cunningham et al. 2007).

The size and location of the primary tumour determine the extent of gastric resection. Three randomized trials compared distal versus total gastrectomy for distal gastric cancer. The largest involved 648 patients and showed no difference in 5-year survival (Bozzetti et al. 1999). Distal gastrectomy reduces morbidity, results in better function, and is the preferred surgical option when the primary tumour can be completely resected. Tumours involving the proximal stomach or the GOJ (Siewert types I and III) require total gastrectomy.

Lymphatic drainage of the stomach is extensive and multidirectional. D1 lymphadenectomy involves dissection of the perigastric lymph nodes within 5cm of the primary tumour. D2 lymphadenectomy involves dissection of lymph nodes along the major vessels (coeliac axis, hepatic artery, and splenic artery) and in the splenic hilum in addition to D1 lymphadenectomy. D3 lymphadenectomy includes the porta hepatis and para-aortic lymph nodes in addition to D2 lymphadenectomy. The recommended extent of lymph node dissection remains controversial.

Although results of prospective surgical series suggested significant survival advantage of D2 lymphadenectomy over D1 (Hohenberger and Gretschel 2003), the MRC (Cuschieri et al. 1999) and Dutch Gastric Cancer Group (Bonenkamp et al. 1999, Hartgrinket al. 2004) randomized trials showed no difference in overall survival. Patients undergoing D2 resection had higher surgical morbidity and mortality. This was attributed to the pancreatico-splenectomy component of the D2 arm. A subset analysis of patients undergoing D2 lymphadenectomy without pancreaticosplenectomy suggested improved survival compared to D1 (Cuschieri et al. 1999). However, the quality assurance of both trials has been questioned. The Japanese Clinical Oncology Group trial compared D2 with D3 lymphadenectomy (Sasako et al. 2008). There was no difference in 5-year survival (69% vs. 70%) or recurrence-free survival. Surgical complications were more common in the D3 arm (Sasako et al. 2008).

The UK recommendation is to perform D2 lymphadenectomy without pancreatico-splenectomy in patients considered to be sufficiently fit to tolerate this procedure (Allum et al. 2002; SIGN 2006).

Gastric cancer surgery is associated with significant morbidity and mortality. Patients should be treated in high- volume regional specialist centres to improve outcomes (SIGN 2006). Patients need intensive support to minimize the physical and psychosocial morbidity associated with gastrectomy to enhance recovery.

Chemotherapy

Most patients who have undergone surgical resection for gastric cancer remain at high risk of recurrence. Multiple trials have investigated the role of adjuvant chemotherapy and meta-analyses suggest some survival improvement although individual trials have failed to demonstrate benefit. A recent Japanese randomized trial using S-1 (an oral fluoropyrimidine pro-drug combined with a DPD antagonist and potassium oxonate which reduces GI toxicity) showed survival improvement compared to surgery alone (Sakuramoto et al. 2007).

An alternative approach is to use preoperative (neo-adjuvant) therapies. The potential advantages include improving curative resection rates, earlier treatment of micro-metastases, and better treatment compliance. The UK MRC MAGIC trial compared 3 cycles of preoperative ECF (epirubicin, cisplatin, and continuous infusional 5-FU) followed by a further 3 cycles postoperatoperatively against surgery alone for resectable gastric and lower oesophageal cancers (Cunningham et al. 2006). Five-year survival was significantly better in patients receiving chemotherapy (36% vs 23%; HR for death 0.75 p = 0.009).

Results of the MAGIC trial are supported by a French trial randomizing to perioperative cisplatin and 5-FU chemotherapy versus surgery alone. Results from the trial appear to show improved 5-year survival rates for perioperative chemo-therapy (24% vs 38%; p = 0.02), but full publication of the trial is awaited (Boige et al. 2007).

Adjuvant chemoradiotherapy
The role of post-operative radiotherapy was explored following high rates of loco-regional failure in American patients (van de Velde and Peeters 2003). The Intergroup trial 0116 randomized 556 patients to post-operative chemotherapy, and chemoradiation versus surgery alone (Macdonald et al. 2001). Patients received 5-FU and leucovorin before, during, and after radiotherapy, which consisted of 45Gy in 25 fractions. The 3-year survival rate was better in the chemoradiation arm (50% vs 41%; p = 0.005). However, this trial has been criticized in a number of areas. Firstly over 50% of patients entered had sub-optimal lymph node removal (Estes et al. 1998). The role of adjuvant chemoradiation following adequate surgical resection remains in question. Secondly the acute toxicity of this treatment was significant.

Adjuvant chemoradiotherapy is not accepted as standard treatment in the UK and Europe.

Targeted therapies
Targeted therapies include monoclonal antibodies and small molecules targeting intracellular signalling cascades which promote cancer cell proliferation. Data on targeted therapies for gastric cancer are limited to phase I trials. The role of bevacizumab (a monoclonal antibody against the VEGFR receptor) in addition to conventional chemotherapy is being investigated by the current UK NCRN ST03 trial (see 'Internet resource').

Further reading
Allum WH, Griffin SM, Watson A, et al. Guidelines for the management of oesophageal and gastric cancer. Gut 2002; 50:1–23.

Boige V, Pignon B. Saint-Aubert P, et al. Final results of a randomized trial comparing pre-operative 5-fluorouracil (F)/cisplatin (P) to surgery alone in adenocarcinoma of the stomach and lower oesophagus (ASLE): FNLCC ACCORD07-FFCD 9703 trial. J Clin Oncol 2007; 25(18S):4510.

Bonenkamp JJ, Hermans J, Sasako M, et al. Extended lymph node dissection for gastric cancer. N Eng J Med 1999; 340:908–14.

Bozzetti F, Marubini E, Bonfati G, et al. Subtotal versus total gastrectomy for gastric cancer: Five-year survival rates in a multicentre randomized Italian trial. Ann Surg 1999; 230:170–8.

Cunningham D, Oliveira J. Gastric cancer: ESMO clinical recommendations for diagnosis, treatment and follow-up. Ann Oncol 2007; 18(suppl 2):ii17–ii18.

Cunningham D, Allum WH, Stenning SP, et al. Perioperative chemotherapy versus surgery alone for resectable gastroesophageal cancer. N Eng J Med 2006; 355:11–22.

Cuschieri A, Weeden S, Fielding J, et al. Patient survival after D1 and D2 resections for gastric cancer: long-term results of the MRC randomized surgical trial. Br J Cancer 1999; 79:1522–30.

Estes NC, MacDonald JS, Touijer K, et al. Inadequate documentation and resection for gastric cancer in the United States: a preliminary report. Am Surg 1998; 64:680–5.

Everett SM, Axon ATR. Early gastric cancer in Europe. Gut 1997; 41:142–50.

Folli S, Morgagni P, Roviello F, et al. Risk factors for lymph node metastasis and their prognostic significance in early gastric cancer (EGC) for the Italian Research Group for Gastric Cancer (IRGGC). Jpn J Clin Oncol 2001; 31:495–9.

Fukase K, Kato M, Kikuchi S, et al. Effect of eradication of Helicobacter pylori on incidence of metachronous gastric cancer after endoscopic resection of early gastric cancer: an open-label, randomised controlled trial. Lancet 2008; 372:392–7.

Hartgrink HH, van de Velde CJH, Putter H, et al. Extended lymph node dissection for gastric cancer: who may benefit? Final results of the randomized Dutch Gastric Cancer Group trial. J Clin Oncol 2004; 22: 2069–77.

Hohenberger P, Gretschel S. Gastric cancer. Lancet 2003; 362: 305–15.

Macdonald JS, Smalley SR, Benedetti J, et al. Chemoradiotherapy after surgery compared with surgery alone for adenocarcinoma of the stomach or gastroesophageal junction. N Eng J Med 2001; 345:725–30.

McCulloch P, Ward J, Tekkis PP. Mortality and morbidity in gastro-oesophageal cancer surgery: initial results of the ASCOT multicentre prospective cohort study. BMJ 2003; 327:1192–7.

Sakuramoto S, Sasako M, Yamaguchi T, et al. Adjuvant chemotherapy for gastric cancer with S-1, an oral fluoropyrimidine. N Eng J Med 2007; 357:1810–20.

Scottish Intercollegiate Guidelines Network. Management of oesophageal and gastric cancer: A national clinical guideline. Edinburgh: SIGN, 2006.

Sasako M, Sano T, Yamamoto S, et al. D2 lymphadenectomy alone or with para-aortic nodal dissection for gastric cancer. N Eng J Med 2008; 359:453–62.

Tsukuma H, Oshima A. Narahara H, et al.Natural history of early gastric cancer: a non-concurrent, long term, follow up study. Gut 2000; 47:618–21.

Uedo N, Iishi H, Tatsuta M, et al. Longterm outcomes after endoscopic mucosal resection for early gastric cancer. Gastric Cancer 2006; 9:88–92.

van de Velde CJ, Peeters KC. The gastric cancer treatment controversy. J Clin Oncol 2003; 21:2234–6.

Wanebo HJ, Kennedy BJ, Chmiel J, et al. Cancer of the stomach. A patient care study by the American College of Surgeons. Ann Surg 1993; 218:583–92.

Internet resource
National Cancer Research Network: http://www.ncrn.org.uk

Gastric cancer: treatment of advanced disease, symptom control, and palliative care

Principles of management

The majority of patients with gastric cancer either present with metastatic disease or will develop recurrent disease following resection. Management of advanced disease is a significant challenge in the treatment of gastric cancer.

In this situation, palliation of distressing symptoms to improve QoL is the priority. A holistic approach is paramount and all patients should be managed by a MDT including the community palliative care team. Oncological treatment may be offered to increase life expectancy but this should be balanced by the potential negative impact from toxicity on the patient's quality of life.

Endoscopic treatment

Tumours at the cardia and GOJ often cause dysphagia and regurgitation, whilst distal tumours can cause gastric outlet obstruction. Endoscopic stent placement can be effective in relieving symptoms and improving QoL. In tumours causing gastric outlet obstruction, endoscopic stent placement appears as effective as gastric bypass in relieving symptoms (Maetani et al. 2005; Mehta et al. 2006). However, 15–40% may require further intervention due to recurrent symptoms.

Up to 20% of patients will develop frank GI bleeding. Endoscopic laser photocoagulation or argon plasma coagulation can be effective in palliating tumour-related haemorrhage.

Surgery

Indications for surgical intervention include gastric outlet obstruction and occasionally uncontrollable haemorrhage. Options include bypass surgery (gastrojejunostomy) or palliative gastrectomy. Palliative gastrectomy is rarely performed in clinical practice as most patients can be adequately palliated using other modalities. Laparoscopic approaches can results in lower morbidity and more rapid recovery.

Radiotherapy

EBRT can be useful in palliating local symptoms such as haemorrhage, dysphagia, and pain. It is also useful in treating painful metastatic disease. There is no evidence of a dose–response relationship (Tey et al. 2007), and doses of 8Gy in a single fraction, 20Gy in 5 fractions, or 30Gy in 10 fractions have been used.

Chemotherapy and targeted therapies

Prior to a decision to embark on palliative chemotherapy treatment, the patient's ability to tolerate treatment must be assessed. Patients should be monitored closely and treatment ceased where there is disease progression or where toxicity from treatment outweighs any potential benefit. A significant proportion will not be sufficiently fit for chemotherapy.

The use of chemotherapy has been shown to improve OS as well as QoL when compared with BSC in multiple randomized trials. A recently published systematic review demonstrated the superiority of combination chemotherapy when compared with monotherapy and chemotherapy when compared with BSC; the survival benefit of combination chemotherapy was estimated to be around 6 months (Wagner et al. 2006).

In the UK the combination of epirubicin, cisplatin, and continuous 5-FU (ECF) has been the reference regimen following results of two randomized trials (Webb et al. 1997; Ross et al. 2002). The main disadvantage of this regimen is that an indwelling venous catheter is required to deliver the 5-FU and this is associated with infection and thromboembolic risk. Capecitabine (X), an oral pro-drug of 5-FU, has been successfully integrated into the ECX regimen as a direct substitute for infusional 5-FU. The REAL-2 trial demonstrated equivalence of capecitabine to 5-FU when combined with either cisplatin or oxaliplatin (O) in terms of efficacy and toxicity. In a subset analysis there was suggestion of prolonged survival with EOX when compared to ECF (Cunningham et al. 2008).

Other chemotherapy agents have been shown to be active in gastric cancer including the taxanes and irinotecan. A US/European randomized trial showed that the addition of docetaxel to cisplatin and 5-FU (DCF) was superior to cisplatin and 5-FU in terms of OS and response rate; however this was at the expense of greater grade 3/4 toxicity (Van Cutsem et al. 2006). A randomized trial compared the combination of S-1 with cisplatin versus S-1 alone and showed improved survival and response rates in Japanese patients using the combination, but again this was more toxic (Koizumi et al. 2008).

There is a relative lack of randomized trials addressing the management of patients who progress following first-line palliative chemotherapy. Options include further chemotherapy using regimens containing a taxane or irinotecan. Patients responding to second-line chemotherapy experience symptomatic benefit and may survive longer compared to non-responders (Wilson et al. 2005).

Targeted therapies have demonstrated only modest benefit in advanced gastric cancer (Field et al. 2008). A phase II trial reported response rates of 65% for a combination of bevacizumab with irinotecan and cisplatin (Shah et al. 2006).

A recent phase III international study of trastuzumab in patients with HER2- positive gastric cancer showed a 26% reduction in risk of death in comparison with those who received chemotherapy alone. Overall survival was increased by 2.7 months. There was no increase in cardiac morbidity (Van Cutsem et al. 2009)

Best supportive care

Simple measures including adequate analgesia and steroids can improve a patient's quality of life. Access to hospice care and other relevant specialists, where appropriate, should be made easily accessible in accordance with National Service Framework guidelines (see 'Internet resources').

Further reading

Cunningham D, Starling N, Rao S, et al. Capecitabine and oxaliplatin for advanced esophagogastric cancer. N Eng J Med 2008; **258**:36–46.

Field K, Michael M, Leong T. Locally advanced and metastatic gastric cancer: current management and new treatment developments. Drugs 2008; **68**:299–317.

Koizumi W, Narahara H, Hara T, et al. S-1 plus cisplatin versus S-1 alone for first-line treatment of advanced gastric cancer (SPIRITS trial): a phase III trial. Lancet Oncol 2008; **9**:215–21.

Maetani I, Akatsuka S, Ikeda M, et al. Self-expandable metallic stent placement for palliation in gastric outlet obstructions caused by gastric cancer: a comparison with surgical gastrojejunostomy. J Gastroenterol 2005; **40**:932–7.

Mehta S, Hindmarsh A, Cheong E, et al. Prospective randomized trial of laparoscopic gastrojejunostomy versus duodenal stenting for malignant gastric outflow obstruction. Surg Endosc 2006; **20**: 239–42.

Ross P, Nicolson M, Cunningham D, et al. Prospective randomized trial comparing mitomycin, cisplatin, and protracted venous-infusion fluorouracil (PVI 5-FU) with epirubicin, cisplatin, and PVI 5-FU in advanced esophagogastric cancer. J Clin Oncol 2002; **20**:1996–2004.

Shah MA, Ramanathan RK, Ilson DH, et al. Multicentre phase II study of irinotecan, cisplatin, and bevacizumab in patients with metastatic gastric or gastroesophageal junction adenocarcinoma. J Clin Oncol 2006; **24**:5201–6.

Tey J, Back MF, Shakespeare TP, et al. The role of palliative radiation therapy in locally advanced gastric cancer. Int J Radiat Oncol Biol Phys 2007; **67**:385–8.

Van Cutsem E, Moisenyenko VM, Tjulandin S, et al. Phase III study of docetaxel and cisplatin plus fluorouracil compared with cisplatin and fluorouracil as first-line therapy for advanced gastric cancer: a report of the V325 study. J Clin Oncol 2006; **24**:4991–7.

Van Cutsem E, Kang Y, Chung H, et al. Efficacy results from the ToGa trial: a phase III study of trastuzumab added to standard chemotherapy in first-line human epidermal growth factor receptor 2 (HER2) positive advanced gastric cancer. J Clin Oncol 2009; **27**:18s.

Wagner AD, Grothe W, Haerting J, Kleber G, Grothey A, Fleig WE. Chemotherapy in advanced gastric cancer: a systematic review based on aggregate data. J Clin Oncol 2006; **24**: 2903–9.

Webb A, Cunningham D, Scarffe JH et al. Randomized trial comparing epirubicin, cisplatin and fluorouracil versus fluorouracil, doxorubicin and methotrexate in advanced esophagogastric cancer. J Clin Oncol 1997; **15**:261–7.

Wilson D, Hiller L, Geh I. Review of second-line chemotherapy for advanced gastric adenocarcinoma. Clin Oncol 2005; **17**:81–90.

Internet resources

Department of Health: http://www.dh.gov.uk

NHS: National Service frameworks and strategies—available at: http://www.nhs.uk/nhsengland/NSF/pages/Cancer.aspx

Hepatocellular cancer: introduction

Epidemiology

Hepatocellular cancer (HCC) accounts for 90% of all primary liver cancers. It is the fifth most common neoplasm in the world and accounts for as many as 500,000 deaths annually (Bosch et al. 2004).

Geographical variation in HCC incidence (per 100,000):

- Asia: 20
- Mediterranean countries: 11–20
- UK and Germany: 5–10
- USA and Canada: 5

In Western countries the incidence and mortality rate from HCC are increasing. This is attributed to chronic HCV infection, ageing of the population, increased detection rates, the obesity epidemic, and associated non-alcoholic fatty liver disease (NAFLD) (Fattovich et al. 2004)

Aetiology

Chronic liver disease is the most important risk factor for the development of HCC with 80–90% of cases arising in patients with cirrhosis or hepatic fibrosis.

Population at risk of HCC:

- HBV infection
- HCV infection
- High alcohol consumption
- NAFLD
- Genetic haemochromatosis

HBV and HCV account for three-quarters of all cases of HCC. The annual incidence of HCC among cirrhotic patients ranges from 2–9% (Fattovich et al. 2004).

Hepatitis B virus infection

The carcinogenic potential of HBV infection has been established from both epidemiological observation and biological studies. The HBV-related oncogenesis is related to genomic integration (Lok and McMahon 2007). The risk of HBV-associated HCC is increased by a young age at infection, active viral replication, prolonged duration of infection, and advanced cirrhosis. HBV infection acquired early in life or during pregnancy is more likely to be associated with HCC than infection acquired at a later stage through sexual or parenteral routes. The annual incidence of HCC is 0.5% in chronic hepatitis and 2% in cirrhotic patients. Vaccination against HBV has resulted in a decrease in the incidence of HCC. Spontaneous reductions or reducing HBV DNA levels with antiviral drugs can decrease the future cancer risk (Fattovich et al. 2004; Lok and McMahon 2007).

Hepatitis C virus infection

This accounts for the increased incidence of HCC observed over the last 10 years. Case–control studies have shown the risk of HCC is increased 17-fold in HCV infected patients. HCV related HCC is rare before 40 years of age and the incidence subsequently increases linearly with age. The risk of HCC correlates with the severity of hepatitis, age, male gender, and the duration of disease (Degos et al. 2000). A synergistic role of high BMI, alcohol, HBV, and HIV coinfection in the development of HCV-related HCC has also been demonstrated. The mechanism of HCV-related HCC is not very clear. Replicating HCV-RNA and virus-specific protein expression has been detected in infected livers but no genomic integration has been documented. As no anti-HCV vaccination is available, the prevention of HCV infection developing to cirrhosis and HCC is only through anti-viral treatment (Degos et al. 2000; Fattovich et al. 2004).

Alcohol

Heavy and prolonged alcohol intake is a risk factor. It accounts for 10% (Asia) and 20% (Europe and North America) of HCC. Alcohol is also an important cofactor in the development of HCV- or HBV- related HCC (Bosch et al. 2004; Fattovich et al. 2004).

Non- alcoholic fatty liver disease

This has recently been recognized as one of the most common causes of liver disease in Western countries. It is frequently associated with type 2 diabetes and morbid obesity. It progresses to liver cirrhosis in 5% of cases and predisposes to HCC development. It is also a cofactor for HCV-related HCC (Bugianesi et al. 2002; Bosch et al. 2004; Fattovich et al. 2004).

Aflatoxin

Ingested in food as a result of contamination of imperfectly stored crops with *Aspergillus flavus*. It is thought to induce HCC through mutation of the tumour suppressor gene p53. HCC in this setting frequently develops in a non-cirrhotic liver. Some studies suggest it could be a co-carcinogen in patients infected with HBV (Bosch et al. 2004; Fattovich et al. 2004)

Metabolic disease

The relative risk of HCC development in haemochromatosis with cirrhosis in comparison to the normal population is >200 and rises with age (Bosch et al. 2004; Fattovich et al. 2004). An increased risk of HCC is also recognized with other metabolic disorders including alpha-1-antitrypsin deficiency, porphyrias, cutanea tarda tyrosinaemia and hypercitrullinaemia, glycogenosis type 4, hereditary fructose intolerance, and Wilson's disease.

Adenoma, contraceptive, androgenes

The risk of transformation of adenoma to HCC secondary to contraceptive use is real but probably <10%. The risk of malignant transformation with multiple hepatic adenomas surprisingly is less (Fattovich et al. 2004).

Risk factors for HCC development in cirrhosis:

- Male gender
- Age
- Disease severity
- High liver cell proliferation activity (Degos et al. 2000; Bosch et al. 2004)

The risk of tumour development varies with the type of cirrhosis with the highest risk for chronic viral hepatitis and a low risk with primary biliary cirrhosis.

Screening

HCC fulfils most of the required criteria for surveillance and screening to be justified. It is common in endemic areas and is associated with high mortality. Tests with low morbidity and high efficacy exist that allow the tumour to be recognized at an early stage when effective treatment is available. The two most common tests used for screening are serum AFP and ultrasonography.

AFP levels greater > 500ng/mL indicates HCC with 95% confidence but the test lacks both sensitivity and specificity. AFP is normal in 40% of patients with HCC and 30% of chronic active hepatitis patients have moderately high levels.

Tumours other than HCC can also produce high AFP levels.

Ultrasonography identifies 85–95% of HCCs >3–5cm and 60–80% of lesions of 1cm. The main difficulty is differentiating regenerative and dysplastic nodules from HCC. It is highly operator dependent. CT and MRI are most useful for confirming the diagnosis. Surveillance for HCC should be performed using ultrasonography (Bruix et al. 2005).

Patients who should be screened for HCC

Hepatitis B carriers
• Asian males >40 years
• Asian females >50 years
• Africans >20 years
• Family history of HCC
• All cirrhotic hepatitis B carriers
• Non-cirrhotic hepatitis B carriers with high HBV DNA concentrations and those with ongoing hepatic inflammatory activity

Non-hepatitis B cirrhosis
• Hepatitis C
• Alcoholic cirrhosis
• Genetic haemochromatosis
• Primary biliary cirrhosis

Patients who may benefit from screening
• Alpha-1 antitrypsin deficiency
• Non-alcoholic steatohepatitis (NASH)
• NAFLD
• Autoimmune hepatitis

Patients on the liver transplant waiting list should be screened for HCC because the development of HCC gives increased priority for liver transplantation.

Surveillance interval
Screening is usually performed every 6 months because available data suggest that the time taken for an undetectable lesion to grow to 2cm is 4–12 months. It takes 5 months for most rapidly growing HCC to reach the size of 3cm. The impact of screening programme for HCC on survival remains controversial although data indicate that screening improves the chance of successful treatment and improves survival (Bruix et al. 2005).

Pathology
Macroscopically HCC are classified into three types:
• Unifocal expansive
• Infiltrating
• Multifocal diffuse

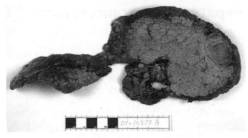

Fig. 4.5.1 Multifocal HCC on the background of cirrhotic liver.

Tumours are multiple in >50% of cases and have a distinct fibrous capsule in 80% of cases. The frequency of microscopic invasion into the surrounding parenchyma is influenced by tumour size.

HCC have a tendency to spread locally and invade blood vessels, particularly the portal vein. The presence of portal vein invasion is an important factor associated with recurrence after treatment. The tumour thrombus has its own arterial supply and can block the main portal vein leading to varices, liver decompensation, and encephalopathy. In addition tumour fragments can embolize and spread via the portal vein. Rarely HCC invades the biliary tract leading to obstructive jaundice and haemobilia.

Metastases are most frequently found in the lungs. Other locations with decreasing frequency are the adrenal glands, bones, lymph nodes, meninges, pancreas, brain, and kidney.

Further reading
Bosch FX, Ribes J, Diaz M, *et al.* Primary liver cancer: worldwide incidence and trends. *Gastroenterology* 2004; **127**(5 Suppl 1): S5–S16.

Bruix J, Sherman M. AASLD practice guideline: management of hepatocellular carcinoma. *Hepatology* 2005; **42**:1208–36.

Bugianesi E, Leone N, Carucci P, et al. Expanding the natural history of nonalcoholic steatohepatitis: From cryptogenic cirrhosis to hepatocellular carcinoma. *Gastroenterology* 2002; **123**:134–40.

Degos F, Christidis C, Ganne-Carrie N, et al. Hepatitis C virus related cirrhosis: time to occurrence of hepatocellular carcinoma and death. *Gut* 2000; **47**:131–6.

Fattovich G, Stroffolini T, Zagni I, et al. Hepatocellular carcinoma in cirrhosis: incidence and risk factors. *Gastroenterology* 2004; **127**(Suppl 1):S35–S50.

Lok ASF, McMahon BJ. AASLD practice guideline on chronic hepatitis B. *Hepatology.* 2007; **45**:507–39.

Hepatocellular cancer: clinical features and staging

Clinical features

The clinical findings depend on the stage of the tumour and the function of the liver. HCC is increasingly being detected early as a result of screening programmes at which stage there may be no signs or symptoms related to the cancer.

Large HCC may present with abdominal pain associated with malaise, weight loss, asthenia, anorexia, and fever. Spontaneous haemorrhage and rupture of HCC occurs in 5–15% of patients. A small bleed may manifest as abdominal pain or haemorrhagic ascites. A large bleed can result in hypovolaemic shock. Portal vein invasion by HCC may present with upper GI bleeding from varices or the acute development of ascites due to portal hypertension. Invasion of the hepatic veins or IVC may result in sudden death from a PE. A small number of patients may present with obstructive jaundice due to infiltration of the bile duct or haematobilia producing haematemesis or melaena. Only large and superficial tumours are palpable.

Patients may have clinical signs of chronic liver disease such as jaundice, parotid enlargement, spider naevi or cutaneous bruising, palmar erythema, clubbing, ascites, splenomegaly, caput medusa, pedal oedema, or testicular atrophy. Paraneoplastic syndromes may occur and include hypercalcaemia and hypoglycaemia.

HCC on the background of a normal liver often presents with a large cancer mass but this does not preclude curative treatment.

Diagnosis

The tests used to diagnose HCC include radiology, biopsy, and AFP serology. Diagnosis of HCC can usually be established by non-invasive means. In the setting of a patient with known chronic liver disease a mass found incidentally or on screening ultrasound has a high likelihood of being HCC. The sequence of tests used to diagnose HCC depends on the size of the lesion (Bruix and Sherman 2005; Aljabiri et al. 2007) Fig 4.5.2.

In cirrhotic patients, nodules found on ultrasound surveillance that are <1cm should be followed with ultrasound at intervals of 3–6 months. If there has been no growth over a period of up to 2 years, one can revert to routine surveillance.

Nodule 1–2cm found on ultrasound screening of a cirrhotic liver should be evaluated with two dynamic studies, either CT scan, contrast enhanced ultrasound (CEUS), or MRI with contrast. If the appearances are typical of HCC (arterial phase hypervascularity with washout in the portal venous phase Fig 4.5.3) in two techniques the lesion should be treated as HCC. This double imaging confirmation avoids a false positive diagnosis. However, almost half of the HCC of 1–2cm will not exhibit this specific contrast enhancement pattern on CT or MRI. For these a biopsy may be required if a precise diagnosis would change the therapeutic option.

A biopsy could be delayed or avoided depending on the timing of potential therapy. If the patient is being

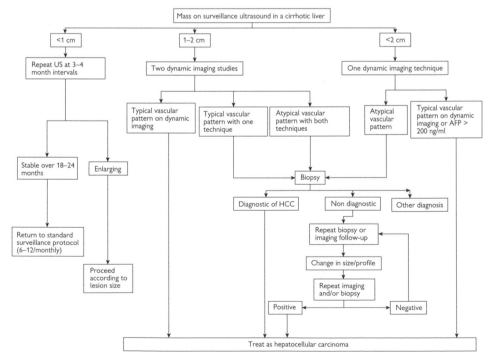

Fig. 4.5.2 Algorithm for evaluation of a liver mass in a cirrhotic patient detected during HCC surveillance according to AASLD guidelines (Bruix and Sherman 2005).

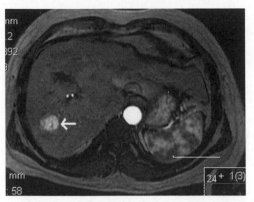

Fig. 4.5.3 Hepatocellular carcinoma characterized by hypervascular lesion in arterial phase. Arterial phase.

Staging systems

Historically HCC has been classified by the TNM or Okuda staging systems (Mazzaferro et al. 1996; Marrero et al. 2005). The TNM system is based on pathological findings and does not have prognostic accuracy. The Okuda classification is based on tumour size and liver function but is unable adequately to stratify patients with early or intermediate stage disease. Several scoring systems have been developed in the last few years, attempting to stratify patients according to expected survival.

A treatment algorithm for HCC should include

• Tumour stage

• Liver function

• Physical status

These are incorporated in the Barcelona Clinic Liver Cancer (BCLC) staging system (Fig. 4.5.4) which was developed based on data from several independent studies (Bruix and Sherman 2005). It identifies those with early HCC who may benefit from curative therapies and those at intermediate or advanced disease stage who may benefit from palliative therapy.

Prognosis

Considerable progress has been made in the diagnosis and treatment of HCC over the last decade. Prognosis depends on two variables, the cirrhosis and the cancer. In patients with HCC. 50–60% of deaths are due to cancer, while hepatic failure and GI bleeding account for 30% and 10% respectively (Bruix and Sherman 2005; Aljabiri et al. 2007; Llovet 2007

The BCLC staging system is the best prognostic model at the present time as it takes into account all three important variables of the disease process as mentioned previously. Patients with BCLC stage 0 with very early HCC (tumours <2 cm and Childs–Pugh A) and patients with stage A with

considered for liver transplantation on the basis of background liver cirrhosis ultrasound or CT, scanning could be repeated at 3–6-monthly intervals until the nodule either disappears, enlarges, or displays diagnostic radiological characteristics of HCC. Another option is to treat as HCC with ablative therapy in the absence of a histological diagnosis because the risk of seeding is not increased by ablative therapy (Aljabiri et al. 2007).

Nodule >2cm with typical features of HCC on one dynamic imaging: a biopsy is not necessary to confirm the diagnosis. However, if the vascular profile on imaging is not characteristic biopsy should be performed.

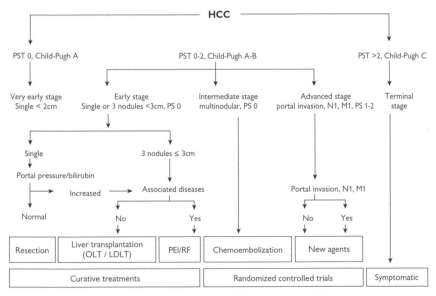

Fig. 4.5.4 Strategy for staging and treatment in patients diagnosed with HCC according to the BCLC protocol (Bruix and Sherman 2005). RF, radiofrequency ablation; LDLT, living donor liver transplantation; OLT, orthotopic liver transplantation; PS, performance status.

early HCC (single or 3 nodules <3cm, Child–Pugh A–B) are candidates for radical therapies (resection, transplantation, or percutaneous treatment) and have 5-year survival of 50–70%. Untreated patients at an intermediate stage (BCLC stage B, multinodular asymptomatic tumours without an invasive pattern) have a median survival of approximately 16 months. Untreated patients with advanced stage disease (BCLC class C, PS 1–2, vascular invasion, extrahepatic disease) have a median survival of approximately 6 months.

Further reading

Aljabiri RM, Lodato F, Burroughs AK. Surveillance and diagnosis of HCC. *Liver Transplant* 2007; **13**(11 Suppl 2):S2–S12.

Bruix J, Sherman M. AASLD practice guideline: management of hepatocellular carcinoma. *Hepatology* 2005; **42**:1208–36.

Knight SR, Friend PJ, Morris PJ. Role of transplantation in the management of hepatic malignancy. *Br J Surg* 2007; **94**:1319–30.

Llovet JM, Clinical and molecular classification of hepatocellular carcinoma.; *Liver Transplant* 2007; **13**(11 Suppl 2):S13–S16.

Marrero JA, Fontna RJ, Barrat A, et al. Prognosis of hepatocellular carcinoma: comparison of 7 staging systems in an American cohort. *Hepatology* 2005; **41**:707–16.

Mazzaferro V, Regalia E, Bozzetti F, et al. Liver transplantation for the treatment of small hepatocellular carcinomas in patients with cirrhosis. *N Engl J Med* 1996; **334**:693–9.

Hepatocellular cancer: management

Principles of management

Historically, HCC was usually diagnosed at an advanced stage when patients were symptomatic with impaired liver function. Today with screening and improved imaging many patients are diagnosed at an early stage when liver function is preserved and there are no cancer-related symptoms. There are several treatments available that have a positive impact on survival. To achieve the best outcome requires the careful selection of candidates for each treatment option and the expert application of these treatments. This requires the skills of MDTs. Therapies that are known to offer a high rate of complete responses and thus a potential for cure are:
• Liver resection
• Liver transplantation
• Percutaneous tumour ablation

Among non-curative therapies transarterial chemoembolization (TACE) and the tyrosine kinase inhibitor sorafenib have been shown to improve survival. Other options such as arterial embolization without chemotherapy or internal radiation, systemic chemotherapy with several other agents have marginal activity, frequent toxicity, and no survival benefit. Finally, agents such as tamoxifen, antiandrogens or octreotide are completely ineffective.

Surgical resection

Non- cirrhotic liver

This is the treatment of choice for HCC in non-cirrhotic patients. HCC are usually large and solitary in this setting. They occur in relatively young patients and the liver has a good regenerating capacity. The 5-year survival is >50% with a morbidity of 15% and mortality of 1% in large series. No other treatment equals these results (Llovet et al. 2005). Percutaneous ablation is not usually feasible in this group due to the large size of the cancers. Liver transplantation does not improve the outcome for this group and is associated with a higher early mortality and the risks of lifelong immunosuppression.

Cirrhotic liver

Criteria for liver resection for HCC in cirrhosis:
• Single tumour
• No jaundice
• No portal hypertension
• No extra-hepatic disease.

The size of the tumour dictates the extent of resection and hence the risk of postoperative liver failure. Vascular invasion and dissemination also increase with the size of the HCC (Bruix et al. 2005; Llovet et al. 2005) although some tumours attain a large size without vascular invasion and their resection is associated with a good outcome. Patients with HCC on the background of cirrhosis should be carefully selected for resection to diminish the risk of postoperative liver failure and mortality. A normal preoperative level of bilirubin and portal pressure are the best predictors of excellent outcomes after surgery and an overall 5-year survival of 70% can be achieved with this approach in early stage HCC (Llovet et al. 2007). Surgical techniques and patient selection have improved and surgery-related mortality is currently <5% (Llovet et al. 2005). Pre-operative techniques such as transarterial and portal venous embolization may render some patients with large or centrally placed tumours suitable for resection.

Risk of recurrence

Tumour recurrence rate exceeds 70% at 5 years and the risk factors are (Todo et al. 2007):
• Large HCC
• Poorly differentiated
• Microvascular invasion
• Multifocal HCC
• Resection margin positive
• Blood transfusion

There is no proven adjuvant therapy that can reduce recurrence rates. Recurrence is usually multifocal. A solitary recurrence may be considered for repeat liver resection. Salvage transplantation has been used for recurrence following resection but most recurrences appear early, are due to tumour dissemination and have an aggressive biological pattern (Llovet et al. 2005). An alternative strategy is to transplant patients whose resected HCC has histological criteria suggesting a high risk of recurrence (Bruix et al. 2005).

Liver Transplantation

This removes the HCC and replaces the cirrhotic liver. The shortage of donor organs has prompted the application of strict selection criteria (Mazzaferro et al. 1996). Indications for liver transplantation for HCC *(Milan criteria)* are: –
• Solitary HCC <5cm
• Up to three HCC all <3cm

The 5-year survival of these patients following transplantation exceeds 70%. As only 10% of HCC patients meet these strict criteria there is considerable interest in extending the criteria to include selected patients with larger tumours. Most groups have reported a 5-year survival of around 50% in patients transplanted for extended criteria (Bruix et al. 2005).The lack of sufficient organ donors is the major limitation and waiting for a suitable organ allows the tumours to grow beyond criteria for transplantation. The waiting list drop out rate may be as high as 25% if the waiting list is >12 months (Duffy et al. 2007). Considering patients with more advanced tumours for LT will increase the waiting list dropout rate and will translate into poorer post- transplant survival unless selection criteria are improved and effective methods of preventing disease progression are established (Llovet et al. 2005).

Loco regional therapy as a bridge to transplantation for HCC

Data is available on RF ablation and TACE. Locoregional therapies are known to improve survival in patients with HCC (Chen et al. 2006). RF ablation is safe and decreases the drop out from the transplant waiting list and may increase the long- term survival after transplantation (Llovet and Bruix 2003). TACE before transplantation is of unproven benefit.

Priority listing for transplantation for HCC

In the USA patients with HCC are prioritized for organ allocation to prevent tumour progression during the waiting period for transplantation. The most effective approach to reduce the dropout rate on the OLT waiting list is to expand the number of available donor livers.

Strategies to increase donor organ availability for patients with HCC include:
• Domino transplants (e.g. amyloidosis)
• Livers from viral carriers
• Split liver transplantation
• Non-heart beating donors
• Live donor transplants

Live donor liver transplant for HCC
The outcome after live donor liver transplantation is similar to that of cadaveric donation. However, this is a complex intervention and in the best hands has a donor complication rate of 20–40% and mortality risk of 0.3–0.5%. Since live donor transplantation can be done without the delays of cadaveric transplantation, living donation might be a good option for patients with more locally advanced HCC. This remains a controversial issue (Todo et al. 2003).

Post-transplant management
Effective therapy is available for HBV to prevent or treat viral graft re-infection using lamivudine and HBIG. Treatment of HCV with interferon and ribavirin is less satisfactory. Immunosuppression may increase the risk of HCC recurrence as a result of decreased immune surveillance. Calcineurin inhibitors have been associated with an increase in tumour recurrence. However, sirolimus inhibits tumour growth and angiogenesis and trials are currently evaluating whether its use reduces recurrence of HCC post transplant.

> **Author tips**
> • Liver transplantation is an effective option for patients with HCC corresponding to the Milan criteria: solitary tumour <5cm or up to three nodules <3cm. Expanding these criteria results in significantly poorer outcomes.
> • Locoregional tumour therapy should be considered while patients await transplantation.
> • Living donor transplantation should be considered if the transplant waiting time is long.

Percutaneous ablation
This is considered the best treatment option for patients with early stage HCC who are not suitable for resection or transplantation. Destruction of tumour cells can be achieved by:
• Injection of chemical substances (ethanol, acetic acid, boiling saline)
• Thermal ablation (RF, microwave, laser, cryotherapy).

Ethanol injection has been used extensively, is highly effective, inexpensive, and is most effective in tumours <2cm. RF ablation provides better local disease control that may result in an improved survival. The main drawback of RF is its higher cost, higher rate (up to 10%) of adverse events (pleural effusion, peritoneal bleeding), and recurrence rate. Procedure-related mortality is low at <0.5%. Subcapsular location and poor tumour differentiation have been associated with increased risk of peritoneal seeding following local ablation (Mazzaferro et al. 2004). Recurrences are mainly due to microscopic satellites not included in the ablation zone. In Child–Pugh A patients with successful tumour necrosis, a 50% survival at

5 years can be achieved. This compares favourably with the results of surgical resection for early stage HCC (Chen et al. 2006).

> **Authors tip**
> • Local ablation is a safe and effective therapy for patients who cannot undergo liver resection or as a bridge to transplantation.
> • Alcohol injection and radiofrequency are equally effective for tumours <2 cm. Radiofrequency is more effective for larger tumours.

Non-curative treatment
Transarterial embolization (TAE) and TACE are considered for patients with HCC who are not candidates for liver resection or transplantation and whose tumours are beyond an effective size for local ablation (3cm) (Llovet and Bruix 2003). Patients with lobar or segmental portal vein occlusion from thrombosis or tumour infiltration and advanced stage liver disease (Child–Pugh class B or C) are poor candidates as they have a risk of developing liver failure postembolization. The side effects include nausea, vomiting, bone marrow depression, alopecia, renal failure, and postembolization syndrome. The latter occurs in >50% of patients and consists of fever, abdominal pain, and ileus which is usually self-limiting.

TAE and TACE induce extensive tumour necrosis in >50% of patients. Fewer than 2% of treated patients achieve a complete response (Llovet and Bruix 2003). Tumour re-growth is common and repeat TAE is often required. Response to treatment is associated with improvement in survival ranging from 20–60% at 2 years (Llovet and Bruix 2003). Meta-analysis of published randomized controlled trials suggest that patient survival is improved following TACE. TAE alone remains unproven.

Systemic chemotherapy
Systemic chemotherapy has had a limited role because of low response rates and no clear impact on survival. However, sorafenib, a multi-kinase inhibitor, has recently been shown to prolong survival in patients with advanced HCC with good liver function. Overall survival was 10.7 months for treated patients vs 7.9 months in controls (Llovet et al. 2007). Benefit has not been reproduced in patients with more advanced tumours and poor liver function (Pinter et al. 2007). Selective radiation through intra-arterial injection of 131I-lipiodol or yttrium-90 labelled microspheres and multiple other treatment modalities have been trialled including octreotide, interferon, external radiation, tamoxifen, or antiandrogenic therapy, but none have been shown to improve survival.

> **Author tips**
> • TACE is recommended for cirrhotic patients with large or multi-focal HCC in the absence of extra-hepatic disease
> • Systemic chemotherapy has shown little evidence of improving the length or quality of life, although early results of tyrosine kinase inhibitors seem promising.
> • Radio-labelled Yttrium microspheres, radio-labelled Lipiodol or immunotherapy cannot be recommended outside trials

Further reading

Bruix J, Sherman M. AASLD practice guideline: management of hepatocellular carcinoma. *Hepatology*. 2005; **42**:1208–36.

Chen MS, Li JQ, Zheng Y, Guo RP, *et al*. A prospective randomised trial comparing percutaneous local ablative therapy and partial hepatectomy for small hepatocellular carcinoma. *Ann Surg* 2006; **243**:321–8.

Duffy JP, Vardanian A, Benjamin E, *et al*. Liver transplantation criteria for hepatocellular carcinoma should be expanded: a 22-year experience with 467 patients at UCLA. *Ann Surg* 2007; **246**(3):502–11.

Llovet JM, Bruix J. Systematic review of randomized trials for unresectable hepatocellular carcinoma: Chemoembolization improves survival. *Hepatology* 2003; **37**:429–42.

Llovet JM, Schwartz M, Mazzaferro V. Resection and liver transplantation for hepatocellular carcinoma. *Semin Liver Dis* 2005; **25**(2):181–200.

Llovet J, Ricci S, Mazzaferro V, *et al*., for the SHARP Investigators Study Group. Sorafenib improves survival in advanced hepatocellular carcinoma (HCC): results of a phase III randomized placebo-controlled trial (SHARP trial). Posters and abstracts from the 43rd annual meeting of the American Society of Clinical Oncology; June 1–5, 2007; Chicago, IL.

Mazzaferro V, Regalia E, Bozzetti F, *et al*. Liver transplantation for the treatment of small hepatocellular carcinomas in patients with cirrhosis. *N Engl J Med* 1996; **334**:6939.

Mazzaferro V, Battiston C, Romito R, *et al*. Radiofrequency ablation of small hepatocellular carcinoma in cirrhotic patients awaiting liver transplantation: a prospective study. *Ann Surg* 2004; **240**:900–9.

Pinter MW, Sieghart W, Graziader I, *et al*. Sorafenib in multifocal hepatocellular carcinoma and advanced liver dysfunction. *Hepatology* 2007; **46**:410A.

Todo S, Furukawa H, Tada M. Extending Indication: Role of living related liver transplantation for hepatocellular carcinoma. *Liver Transl* 2007; **13**:S48–S54.

Biliary tract tumours: introduction

Epidemiology

Cholangiocarcinoma (CCA) accounts for approximately 3% of all GI cancers and is the second most common hepatobiliary cancer. Our ability to diagnose this cancer has improved over the last decade which may partly explain a worldwide increasing incidence. There is a slight male preponderance. Peak incidence occurs around 65–70 years (Ben-Menachem 2007).

On the basis of anatomical distribution, CCA has been classified as either intrahepatic (IHCCA) or extrahepatic EHCCA). Justification for this classification is supported by differences in the epidemiology, pathogenesis, clinical presentation, and therapeutic approach to IHCC versus EHCC (Khan et al. 2003; Ben-Menachem 2007). EHCC is defined as a neoplasm arising from the extrahepatic common bile duct, gallbladder, or ampulla of Vater. Studies from several countries have reported an increase in the incidence and mortality rates of IHCC, but a decrease in the incidence and mortality of EHCC (Khan et al. 2003; Shaib and El-Sarag 2004). The cause of the rising incidence of IHCC is not clear but could be related to the increasing prevalence of chronic hepatitis B and C (Khan et al. 2003; Ahrens et al. 2007; Ben-Menachem 2007).

A common site for the development of CCA is at the confluence of the bile ducts as they arise from the liver and these are termed Klatskin tumours. Their position may lead to confusion in classification as Klatskin tumours were previously classified as IHCC (Bergquist et al. 1998; Khan et al. 2003; Ahrens et al. 2007).

There is a wide geographical variation in the incidence of CCA largely related to the distribution of risk factors. For example Thailand and China, which report the highest rates of IHCC, are also regions with high rates of liver fluke infestation (Watanapa and Watanapa 2002).

Aetiology

Risk factors for cholangiocarcinoma include:
* Primary sclerosing cholangitis
* Liver fluke infestation
* Hepatolithiasis
* Congenital biliary cysts
* Toxic damage, e.g. thorotrast

Primary sclerosing cholangitis (PSC)

PSC is one of the most common risk factors for CCA. The lifetime risk of CCA for patients with PSC is 8–20% (Bergquist et al. 1998; Shaib and El-Sarag 2004; Ben-Menachem 2007). The median age of diagnosis is earlier for patients with PSC than for sporadic cases of CCA Surprisingly the risk of CCA appears to be unrelated to the duration of PSC (Bergquist et al. 1998; Shaib and El-Sarag 2004). Although the majority of patients with PSC have inflammatory bowel disease, there is no proven association between the risk of CCA and the presence, severity, and extent of inflammatory bowel disease (Watanapa and Watanapa 2002). Surgical or medical treatment of ulcerative colitis does not decrease the risk of developing CCA. CCA in the presence of PSC tends to be diffuse and multi-centeric.

Parasitic biliary infections (liver flukes)

This is the most important risk factor for CCA in East Asia. Both epidemiological and experimental data strongly support the role of *Opisthorchis viverrini* in the pathogenesis of CCA (Watanapa and Watanapa 2002; Ben-Menachem 2007). Several potential carcinogenic mechanisms have been described including hyperplasia and dysplasia caused by chronic inflammation, nitric oxide formation, intrinsic nitrosation, and activation of cytochrome P450 isoenzymes.

Hepatolithiasis (recurrent pyogenic cholangiohepatitis or Oriental cholangiohepatitis)

This is more common in Asia and represents a risk factor for CCA, primarily IHCCA. It is thought to result from chronic portal bacteraemia and gives rise to intrahepatic duct stones. This leads to recurrent episodes of cholangitis and ductal stricture and carries a 10% risk of developing CCA. (Khan et al. 2003; Ahrens et al. 2007; Ben-Menachem 2007).

Congenital cystic dilation of the bile ducts

Choledochal cysts are associated with an increased risk of EHCCA. The lifetime risk of developing CCA secondary to a choledochal cyst is 3–15% (Shaib and El-Sarag 2004; Ahrens et al. 2007; Ben-Menachem 2007). The average age for development of CCA is 34 years. The risk is highest after the age of 20 years and in those treated with drainage rather than excision. Malignant transformation is more frequent in choledochal cysts associated with an anomalous pancreatico-biliary ductal junction and more recently mutations of tumour suppressor genes p53 and Smad-4 as well oncogene K-ras have been identified in patients with choledochal cysts. There is no increased risk of cancer with simple biliary cysts.

Chronic exposure to DNA-damaging chemical agents

The best documented association is with thorium dioxide (thorotrast), a radiological contrast agent that has been removed from sale (Shaib and El-Sarag 2004; Ahrens et al. 2007; Ben-Menachem 2007).

Risk factors with a weaker association or conflicting reports include (Shaib and El-Sarag 2004; Welzel et al. 2006; Ahrens et al. 2007; Ben-Menachem 2007).
* Liver fluke Clonorchis sinensis
* Excess alcohol consumption
* Tobacco use
* Chronic viral hepatitis without cirrhosis
* Surgical biliary-enteric bypass procedures
* Obesity
* Asbestos, aflatoxins, methylene chloride, vinyl chloride monomer, and nitrosamines

Although a clear genetic predisposition has not been established, polymorphism of the CYP1A2 and glutathione-S-transferase omega 1 and 2 genes have been shown to be associated with CCA. These may influence the metabolism of toxic environmental agents such as asbestos or dioxin that are risk factors for cholangiocarcinoma (Ben-Menachem 2007). Only 10% of CCA are associated with a recognized risk factor (Ben-Menachem 2007).

Pathology

The vast majority of cancers (90%) of the bile duct are adenocarcinomas. Malignancies associated with cystic anomalies of the bile duct or bile duct stones may be adenosquamous or squamous carcinomas. Carcinoid tumours may rarely arise from the biliary tree. Kaposi's sarcoma and

lymphomas of the biliary tree have been described in patients with AIDS. Intrahepatic CCA may present with a liver mass and needs to be differentiated from a metastasis by immunohistochemical analysis. Based on tumour morphology and growth pattern they are described in three different categories:
• Sclerosing—infiltrating
• Nodular—mass forming
• Papillary—intraductal

The sclerosing variant accounts for 70% of tumours and is commoner in the hilar area. The duct wall appears thickened and is difficult to differentiate from inflammatory stricture. Sclerosing CCA grows along the bile duct to produce a concentric thickening that eventually produces complete obliteration of the duct lumen (see Fig. 4.5.5). Sclerosing tumours often do not form an easily identifiable mass, but rather manifest radiologically and clinically as a poorly defined stricture. These tumours are also associated

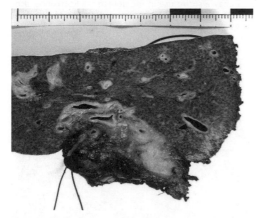

Fig. 4.5.5 Resected specimen of sclerosing type cholangiocarcinoma showing thick walled bile duct with infiltration into surrounding tissue.

with a dense desmoplastic reaction and have a propensity for vascular invasion.

Nodular tumours usually affect the upper and mid bile duct and account for 20% of CCA. Nodular cholangiocarcinomas arise in the mucosa, grow within the lumen, and then penetrate the bile duct wall. This growth and the accompanying desmoplastic reaction result in a hard white mass with well-defined margins.

Papillary tumours are usually found in the mid and distal part of the common bile duct and account for 10% of CCA. Papillary tumours contain numerous papillary infoldings formed by proliferations of columnar cells supported by fibrovascular stalks. They do not tend to invade the bile duct wall but grow intraluminally, and are therefore associated with a better prognosis. The papillary projections of this tumour are long and friable; tumour debris or mucin produced by these lesions can cause intermittent bile duct obstruction that may be mistaken clinically for stone disease. Papillary tumours grow along the mucosal surface and produce multiple metastatic deposits along the adjacent bile ducts.

Further reading

Ahrens W, Timmer A, Vyberg M, et al. Risk factors for extrahepatic biliary tract carcinoma in men: medical conditions and lifestyle. Eur J Gastroenterol Hepatol 2007; **19**:623–30.

Ben-Menachem Risk factors for cholangiocarcinoma. Eur J Gastroenterol Hepatol. 2007; **19**(8):615–17.

Bergquist A, Glaumann H, Persson B, et al. Risk factors and clinical presentation of hepatobiliary carcinoma in patients with primary sclerosing cholangitis: a case-control study. Hepatology 1998; **27**:311–16.

Khan SA, Taylor-Robinson SD, Toledano MB, et al. Changing international trends in mortality rates from liver, biliary and pancreatic tumours. J Hepatol 2003; **37**:806–13.

Shaib Y, El-Sarag HB. The epidemiology of cholangiocarcinoma. Semin Liver Dis 2004; **24**:115–125.

Watanapa P, Watanapa WB. Liver fluke-associated cholangiocarcinoma. Br J Surg 2002; **89**:962–70.

Welzel TM, Mellemkjaer L, Gloria, et al.(2006) Risk factors for intrahepatic cholangiocarcinoma in a low-risk population: a nationwide case-control study. Int J Cancer 2006; **120**:638–41.

Biliary tract tumours: clinical features, staging, and prognosis

Clinical features

The presentation of CCA depends on the anatomical location and can be divided into three categories
- Intrahepatic:5– 10%
- Hilar:60–70% (Klatskin)
- Distal :20–30%

Intrahepatic CCA typically presents as a mass lesion detected by abdominal imaging or with non-specific symptoms. In contrast, hilar or extrahepatic lesions usually present with jaundice, pruritus, weight loss, and abdominal pain.

Patients with PSC are at a high risk for developing CCA. The diagnosis of malignancy in these patients is clinically challenging as the presentation and cholangiographic findings of biliary tract strictures in PSC are similar to those of CCA. The new development of jaundice and a dominant bile duct stricture in an individual with previously stable PSC should raise the suspicion of malignancy.

Diagnosis and staging

Serum tumour markers

Serum CEA and CA-19.9 may be increased, but are not diagnostic of CCA. They may be elevated with other causes of jaundice and several other GI malignancies. They can be useful in follow-up of treatment response and to detect recurrence.

Imaging

Often several imaging modalities are required for the full evaluation of patients with suspected CCA.

Ultrasonography

This is used as a first- line test in patients presenting with abnormal liver function tests, jaundice, or abdominal pain. Ultrasonography can differentiate obstructive from non-obstructive jaundice, detect a mass lesion in intra-hepatic CCA, and confirm ascites in patients with advanced disease. Further imaging is always needed to evaluate and stage the disease.

Computed tomography

CT is commonly used to evaluate patients with suspected CCA. The location of the lesion, extent of local spread, vascular involvement, atrophy of liver, and metastases may be determined. Combining chest and pelvic CT with abdominal CT can help in determining distant metastases. CT cholangiography is a promising technique that may expand the value of CT scanning in assessing CCA.

Magnetic resonance imaging

MRI is a valuable alternative to CT for further evaluation of a patient suspected of having CCA on the basis of ultrasound assessment. It can determine the local extent of tumour, relationship to blood vessels, and extent of hepatic atrophy, lymph node involvement, and intrahepatic or distant metastases. MR cholangiography (MRCP) can identify the upper extent of luminal involvement, which is essential for accurate surgical staging. MRCP is comparable to endoscopic retrograde cholangiopancreatography (ERCP) and has a similar sensitivity and specificity for the detection of malignancy. It has the advantage of being non-invasive with minimal procedure-related risk and avoids introducing enteric organisms to the biliary tract. MRI is the single most useful modality for the further evaluation

of CCA (see Fig. 4.5.6), particularly hilar CCA (Malhi and Gores 2006; Singh and Patel 2006).

Endoscopic retrograde cholangiography (ERC) and percutaneous transhepatic cholangiography (PTC)

These are methods of obtaining access to the biliary tract to determine the extent of bile duct involvement by cancer, to allow drain insertion for resolution of jaundice and to obtain samples for culture, biliary cytology, or histology. Staging and an assessment of a patient's suitability for resection should be completed before considering biliary tract drainage. ERC is usually favoured in patients with distal bile duct strictures and PTC for proximal lesions.

Positron emission tomography (PET)

PET is more sensitive than CT in the diagnosis of CCA but provides limited information on local disease spread. FDG-PET may also be useful for detecting recurrence after resection. Patients with biliary tract infections or inflammatory cholangiopathies such as PSC may have false positive scans, and acellular mucinous cancers may not be visualized (Malhi and Gores 2006; Singh and Patel 2006).

Cytology and biopsy

Obtaining a tissue diagnosis in suspected CCA is vital if staging suggests unresectable or metastatic disease.

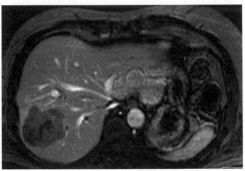

(a)

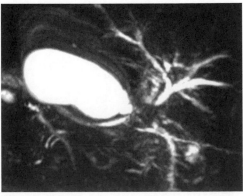

(b)

Fig. 4.5.6 MRI Showing intrahepatic CCA (A) and MRCP showing type 3 CCA (B).

For patients with resectable disease there is no indication for a pre-operative biopsy. Recent advances in biliary cytology diagnostic methods include the use of digital image analysis (DIA) or the use of fluorescence *in-situ* hybridization (FISH). DIA involves the use of DNA stains to quantitate aneuploidy, whereas FISH analysis uses a commercial probe set to assess polysomy of chromosomes 3, 7, 17, and 9p21. The sensitivity of brush cytology has also been shown to be increased by the use of RT-PCR for the detection of human aspartyl (asparaginyl) beta-hydroxylase and homeobox B7 mRNA (Malhi and Gores 2006; Singh and Patel 2006).

Endoscopic ultrasound with fine needle aspiration
This is as good as CT-guided FNA for hepatic lesions in anatomically accessible regions, namely the hilum, left lobe of liver, and proximal biliary tract. EUS-FNA may allow a tissue diagnosis in distal biliary strictures. However, the negative predictive value is low and a negative biopsy does not therefore exclude malignancy.

Laparoscopy ± laparoscopic ultrasound
This is useful in identifying patients with superficial liver or peritoneal metastases in whom an unnecessary laparotomy could be avoided.

Emerging technologies
Advances in endoscopic technologies hold promise for the diagnosis and evaluation of cholangiocarcinoma. Examples of such technologies include optical coherence tomography (OCT), peroral cholangioscopy, or duodenoscope-assisted cholangioscopy. OCT uses infrared light to evaluate duct wall structure which is disrupted by cancer. Cholangioscopy is useful to directly visualize the biliary tract lumen and obtain tissue samples for analysis. Cholangioscopy is likely to be of most use with mucin producing tumours in which the upper limit of the lesion is indeterminate on MRI (fMalhi and Gores 2006; Singh and Patel 2006).

Author tips

- All patients should have an initial ultrasound scan followed by combined MRI and MRCP (where MRI/MRCP is not available, patients should have contrast enhanced spiral/helical CT).
- Invasive cholangiography should be reserved for tissue diagnosis or therapeutic decompression where there is cholangitis, or stent insertion in irresectable cases.
- The techniques are complementary and sometimes several are necessary as part of a surgical assessment.

Staging
Bismuth and Corlette classification (Fig. 4.5.7)
Bismuth and Corlette classification of proximal bile duct cancers (1975) stratifies patients based on the location and the extent of involvement of the biliary tree by cancer (Malhi and Gores 2006).

- Type 1:bile duct cancers proximal to the bifurcation.
- Type 2:cancer involves the hepatic duct confluence but neither the right nor left hepatic ducts.
- Type 3:cancer occluding the hepatic duct confluence and extending into the right (type 3A) or left (type 3B) hepatic ducts.
- Type 4:cancers of the hepatic duct confluence which extend into both the right and left hepatic ducts or with multi-focal duct involvement.

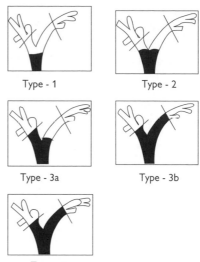

Type - 1   Type - 2

Type - 3a   Type - 3b

Type - 4

Fig. 4.5.7 Bismuth–Corlette staging system.

The Bismuth–Corlette staging system is a simple and helpful way of describing tumours and the extent of bile duct involvement. The BC stage also indicates the extent of bile duct and liver resection required for curative surgery.

American Joint Committee on Cancer staging system
The AJCC staging system describes the extent of local invasion as well as the presence of lymph node or distant metastases (Green et al. 2005).

T stage
- T0: n - no evidence of primary tumour
- Tis: c - carcinoma *in situ*
- T1: t - tumour confined to the bile duct
- T2: t - tumour invades beyond the bile duct wall
- T3: t - tumour invades the liver, gallbladder, pancreas, and/or unilateral branches of the portal vein or hepatic artery
- T4: t - tumour invades any of the following: main portal vein or its branches bilaterally, common hepatic artery, or adjacent structures (colon, stomach, duodenum, abdominal wall)

N stage
- N0: no regional lymph node metastases
- N1: regional lymph node metastases

M stage
- M0: no distant metastases
- M1: distant metastases

Stage
- Stage 0:TisN0M0
- Stage I:T1 N0M0
- Stage II:T2 N0M0
- Stage III:T1 or T2N1 or N2M0
- Stage IVa:T3 Any NM0
- Stage IVb:Any T Any NM1

Prognosis

A complete surgical resection with histologically negative resection margins (R0 resection) is the only way to
cure patients. Five- year survival following resection of
hilar cholangiocarcinoma ranges from 20–40%. The best
predictor of survival is an R0 resection. For intrahepatic
tumours, 5 year survival ranges from 20–43% and good
prognostic factors are R0 resection, absence of vascular
invasion and N0 status.

Survival data according to therapy (Malhi and Gores 2006)

Surgery and 5-year survival

- R0 resection: 20– 40%
- R1 resection: 5– 10%
- R2 resection: 0%

Liver transplantation

For localized unresectable disease with no lymph node and
vascular involvement after chemoradiation 5- year survival
is 82%.

Palliative therapy and median survival

- Stenting: 4–6 months
- PDT and stenting: 12 months
- Chemotherapy: 4–16 months

Further reading

Greene FL, Page DL, Fleming ID. *AJCC Cancer Staging Manual*, 6th
edition. New York: Springer, 2005.

Malhi H, Gores GJ. Cholangiocarcinoma: modern advances in
understanding a deadly old disease. *J Hepatol* 2006; **45**:856–67.

Singh P, Patel T. Advances in the diagnosis, evaluation and management
of cholangiocarcinoma. *Curr Opin Gastroenterol* 2006; **22**:294–9.

Biliary tract tumours: management

Principles of management (see Fig. 4.5.8)

Role of surgery and resectability

The aim of treatment for patients with cholangiocarcinoma is to perform a complete resection of the cancer with histologically negative resection margins (R0 resection). This offers the only hope of cure. The emerging trend in the surgical approach to cholangiocarcinoma is to combine an extended liver resection and lymphadenectomy with excision of the bile duct cancer (Khan and Davidson 2002,; Halazun et al. 2007). This radical approach has been shown to decrease recurrence and improve survival in hilar lesions without a significant increase in postoperative morbidity and mortality (Sano et al. 2006). Achieving clear resection margins is technically demanding in hilar tumours as the bile duct bifurcation is close to the vascular inflow of the liver. Portal vein and hepatic artery resection and reconstruction in selected cases allows negative margins to be achieved and may improve survival. Portal vein embolization is being increasingly used pre-operatively to ensure there is adequate functioning liver following resection.

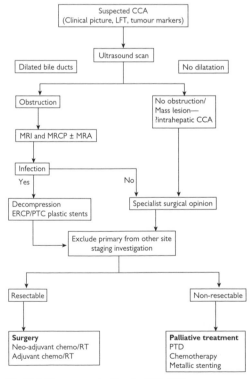

Fig. 4.5.8 Management algorithm for CCA. CCA, Cholangiocarcinoma; RT, radiotherapy; ERCP, endoscopic retrograde cholangiography; LFT, liver function test; MRA, magnetic resonance angiography; PTC, percutaneous cholangiography; PTD, photodynamic therapy.

Our own survival data which correlate with world literature is shown in Fig. 4.5.9.

> **Author tips**
>
> - Bismuth classification is a guide to the extent of surgery required:
>   - Types I and II: en bloc resection of the extrahepatic bile ducts and gall bladder, regional lymphadenectomy, and Roux-en-Y hepaticojejunostomy
>   - Type III: as above plus right or left hepatectomy;
>   - Type IV: as above plus extended right or left hepatectomy.
> - Microscopic seeding to the caudate lobe (segment 1) is well recognized justifying its resection with hilar cholangiocarcinoma (stages II–IV).
> - Distal cholangiocarcinomas are managed by pancreatoduodenectomy as with ampullary or pancreatic head cancers.
> - The intrahepatic variant of cholangiocarcinoma is treated by resection of the involved segments or lobe.

Criteria of unresectability
- Distant metastases
- Encasement of coeliac trunk
- Portal vein occlusion with collaterals
- Lymph node metastases (N2 nodes)
- Insufficient future liver remnant
- Poor clinical status and co-morbidities

Adjuvant treatment

There is no evidence for adjuvant treatment after potentially curative surgery (R0 resection) and patients should be encouraged to participate in ongoing clinical trials. Neoadjuvant treatment involving chemoradiation has been proposed as a method of improving outcome or for downstaging unresectable disease. Limited data are available and review at a specialist centre is vital to ensure that a resection option has been fully explored. Neoadjuvant therapy should be considered within a clinical trial.

Liver transplantation

The results of liver transplantation for cholangiocarcinoma have been disappointing with high recurrence rates and poor long-term survival. Recently transplantation has been combined with neoadjuvant chemoradiotherapy in highly selected patients with unresectable localized disease in the absence of lymph node and vascular involvement. The 5-year survival has been reported as 82% (Rosen et al. 2007). With CCA developing secondary to PSC, liver transplantation rather than resection is an attractive option as the liver function may be poor, the cancer may be multifocal, and recurrence after resection is common.

Management of unresectable tumours

Treatment of biliary obstruction

The aim of palliation is the relief of jaundice and related pruritis, prevention of cholangitis and hepatic dysfunction, and improvement of QoL. This can be achieved endoscopically or surgically.

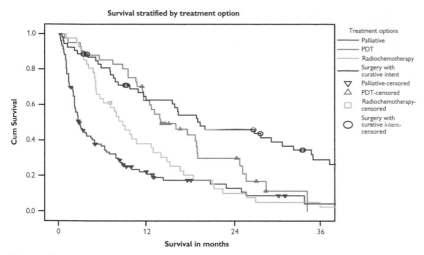

Fig. 4.5.9 Survival with various treatment options (Royal Free and University College Hospital London data).

These techniques are equally effective in resolving jaundice. However non-surgical procedures offer significantly lower morbidity, mortality, and cost (Smith et al. 1994). The optimal use of palliative stents depends on the life expectancy of the patient and location of the tumour in the biliary tree. In Bismuth type I and distal CCA, placement of a single biliary stent is adequate. With the peri-hilar tumours multiple stents may provide better drainage and improved survival.

Expanding metal and plastic stents have advantages and disadvantages. Once employed, metallic stents cannot be removed and therefore tissue confirmation of cancer is mandatory prior to placement. For distal tumours, metal stents provide a longer patency and are more cost-effective for patients surviving at least 3 months. Patency of hilar plastic stents is <4 weeks and they are at high risk of distal migration. To achieve adequate biliary drainage involves a combination of endoscopic and percutaneous approaches in one third of patients.

Photodynamic therapy (PDT)
The principle of PDT is to administer a photosensitizer agent which accumulates within the neoplastic tissue and becomes cytotoxic when the tumour is directly exposed to low-energy light of a specific wavelength. The only randomized trial (Ortner et al. 2003) comparing PDT using Photofrin® plus stenting vs stenting alone was stopped prematurely due to a significant survival advantage in the PDT group (493 vs 98 days, p < 0.0001). QoL was also significantly improved in this study.

The main side effect of PDT treatment is skin photosensitivity and patients need to temporarily avoid bright sunlight. The survival of patients treated with PDT and stenting may be similar to those who have undergone palliative surgery (R1 and R2 resections) with a median survival of 12 months. Combining PDT with stenting is an attractive palliative option to reduce tumour growth, improve biliary drainage, and decrease biliary sepsis, and is associated with low complication rates. Preliminary studies are now starting using high-intensity focused ultrasound (HIFU), RF ablation, and drug coated stents.

Palliative radiotherapy
Palliative radiotherapy has been proposed for patients with locally advanced unresectable tumours. In published trials EBRT has been used alone or in combination with brachytherapy. No survival benefit has been demonstrated. The use of conformal radiation combined with chemosensitizing agents provides opportunities for new trials.

Systemic chemotherapy and new targeted agents
Chemotherapy has had a limited impact on the overall survival of patients with CCA. 5-FU-based chemotherapy has a response rate of only 5–10% but has been shown to improve QoL for biliary cancer patients versus BSC. A recent phase III study showed that a combination of gemcitabine and cisplatin improved survival and reduced the risk of cancer progression compared with gemcitabine alone. Patients who received the combination of cisplatin and gemcitabine had a PFS of 8.5 months compared with 6.5 months with gemcitabine alone. Overall survival was also better with the combination (11.7 months vs. 8.2 months) (Valle et al. 2009).

Growth factor receptors HER-1 and HER-2 have been shown to be over expressed in biliary tract cancers and can be targeted by monoclonal antibodies or the small molecules erlotinib (HER1 tyrosine kinase inhibitor) or lapatinib (HER1/HER2 kinase dual inhibitor). A small phase II trial has reported promising activity with erlotinib in biliary tract cancer with a 50% response rate. These receptor targeting therapies may require patient selection on the basis of tumour receptor expression to optimize outcome.

Further reading

Khan SA, Davidson BR, Goldin R, et al. Guidelines for the diagnosis and treatment of cholangiocarcinoma: consensus document Gut 2002; **51**(Suppl VI):vi1–vi9.

Halazun KJ, Toogood TG, Lodge PA, et al. Right hepatic trisectionectomy for hepatobiliary diseases results and an appraisal of its current role. - Ann Surg 2007; **246**(6):1065–74.

Nagino M, Kamiya J, Nishio H, et al. Two hundred and forty consecutive portal vein embolizations before extended hepatectomy for biliary cancer: surgical outcome and long-term follow-up. Ann Surg 2006; 243:364–372.

Ortner MA, Caca K, Berr F, et al. Successful photodynamic therapy for nonresectable cholangiocarcinoma: a randomized prospective study. Gastroenterology 2003; 125(5):1355–63.

Rosen, CB, Heimbach, JK, Gores, GJ. Current status of liver transplantation for hilar cholangiocarcinoma. Curr Opin Organ Transplant. 2007; 12(3):215–19.

Sano T, Shimada K, Sakamoto Y, et al. One hundred and two consecutive hepatobiliary resections for perihilar cholangiocarcinoma with zero mortality. Ann Surg 2006; 244:240–7.

Smith AC, Dowsett JF, Russel RC, et al. Randomised trial of endoscopic stenting versus surgical bypass in malignant low bile duct obstruction. Lancet 1994; 344(8938):1655–60.

Valle JW, Wasan HS, Palmer DD, et al. Gemcitabine with or without cisplatin in paients with advanced or metastatic biliary tract cancer (ABC): Results of a mulcicentre, randomised phase III trial (the UK ABC-02 trial). J Clin Oncol 2009; 27(; 15s):, (abst 4503.)

Pancreatic cancer: introduction

Epidemiology

Pancreatic ductal adenocarcinoma is the commonest cancer affecting the exocrine pancreas. It is the sixth cause of cancer death in the UK. In 2002, there were 232, 306 new cases of pancreatic cancer and 227, 023 deaths worldwide (CANCERMondial website). In 2004 there were 7398 new cases in the UK, with similar numbers in men and women (Cancer Research UK website) In the USA in 2006 there were 33, 730 new cases and 32, 300 deaths.

The peak incidence is in the 65–75- year age group with 60% of patients being > 65 years of age.

Without active treatment, metastatic pancreatic cancer has a median survival of 3–6 months and 6–10 months for locally advanced disease, which increases to around 11–15 months with surgical resection (Alderson et al. 2005).

Due to late presentation only a minority (10–15%) of patients can undergo potentially curative surgery. Major advances have included improvements in operative mortality and morbidity through the development of specialist regional centres and improved survival using systemic chemotherapy.

Aetiology

Major risk factors include:
• Increasing age
• Tobacco smoking
• Chronic pancreatitis
• Late onset diabetes mellitus
• Hereditary pancreatitis
• Cancer family syndromes
• Increased BMI

Weaker associations include:
• Increased consumption of red meat and processed meat
• Reduced methionine intake from food
• Reduced folate intake from food
• Westernized society

Tobacco smoking is a major risk factor and the risk is approximately 2-fold and accounts for approximately 30% of all cases.

Chronic pancreatitis is now recognized as a risk factor, with approximately 15–25-fold risk. Patients may have chronic pancreatitis for at least 20 years before the development of pancreatic cancer. These patients tend to have severe disease, increased calcification of the gland, and a higher rate of complications.

Hereditary pancreatitis

An uncommon disorder inherited as an AD condition with an estimated 80% penetrance and an equal gender incidence, presenting in children and younger adults. The gene responsible was identified as the PRSS1 gene, and mutations have a causative role, resulting in a gain of function of the digestive enzyme trypsin. It is associated with a 70- fold increase in risk of developing pancreatic cancer (Howes et al. 2004).

Cancer family syndromes

A variety of familial cancer syndromes are associated with an increased risk of pancreatic cancer; these account for approximately 10% of cases (see Table 4.5.1.)

Table 4.5.1 Cancer family syndromes affecting the pancreas

Syndrome	Lifetime risk of pancreatic cancer
Familial pancreatic cancer	Up to 50%
Peutz–Jeghers	36%
Hereditary pancreatitis	35%
FAMMM	17%
Cystic fibrosis	~5%
Fanconi anaemia	?~5%
Li–Fraumeni syndrome	?~5%
Von Hippel–Lindau	?~5%
Ataxia telangiectasia	?
Familial breast ovarian	?
FAP	?
HNPCC	?

FAMMM, familial atypical multiple mole melanoma; FAP, familial adenomatous polyposis; HNPCC, hereditary non-polyposis colon cancer

Secondary screening

Familial pancreatic cancer itself is rare and the European Registry of Hereditary Pancreatitis and Familial Pancreatic Cancer (EUROPAC) has been established to provide a database of these families for long-term follow-up, with the aim of identifying people at risk and developing a screening programme in the future.

Diagnostic criteria are:
• Two or more first-degree relatives with pancreatic ductal adenocarcinoma
  or
• Two or more second-degree relatives with pancreatic cancer, one of whom has early-onset pancreatic cancer (age <50 years at diagnosis).

Overall, the observed to expected rate of pancreatic cancer is significantly raised by 9-fold, rising specifically from 4-fold in families with one first-degree relative, to 6.4-fold where there are two affected relatives to 32.0-fold with three relatives with pancreatic cancer.

Screening in Pancreatic Cancer

• Primary screening for pancreatic cancer in the general population is not feasible at present.
• All patients with an increased inherited risk of pancreatic cancer should be referred to a specialist centre.
• They should be offered clinical advice and genetic counselling and, where appropriate, genetic testing.
• Secondary screening for pancreatic cancer in high-risk cases should only be part of an investigational programme.

Pathology

Ductal adenocarcinoma is the most common malignant tumour of the pancreas. The variants are:
- Undifferentiated (anaplastic)
- Adenosquamous
- Adenosquamous carcinoma
- Signet ring cell carcinoma
- Mixed ductal endocrine carcinoma
- Mucinous non-cystic
- Mucinous non-cystic carcinoma
- Osteoclast-like giant cell tumour

Characteristically, there is an intense desmoplastic reaction in the stroma surrounding these tumours. In about 20% of cases it is not possible to distinguish the tissue of origin and the term 'peri-ampullary cancer' is often applied.

Ductal adenocarcinoma develops through an adenoma–carcinoma sequence of epithelial preneoplastic lesions called pancreatic intra-epithelial neoplasia (PanIN).

Intraductal pancreatic mucinous neoplasms (IPMNs) are pre-malignant with main branch IPMNs having the greater risk of progression compared to side-branch IPMNs.

Mucinous cysts are highly pre-malignant.

Sixty-five per cent are located within the head of the pancreas, 15% in the body, 10% in the tail, and 10% are multifocal.

The TNM classification for pancreatic cancer (Sobin and Wittekind 2002):

T: primary tumour
- TX: primary tumour cannot be assessed.
- T0: no evidence of primary tumour.
- Tis: carcinoma *in situ*.
- T1: tumour limited to the pancreas, ≤2cm or less in greatest dimension.
- T2: tumour limited to the pancreas, >more than 2cm in greatest dimension.
- T3: tumour extends beyond pancreas, but without involvement of coeliac axis or superior mesenteric artery.
- T4: tumour involves coeliac axis or superior mesenteric artery.

N: regional lymph nodes
- NX regional lymph nodes cannot be assessed.
- N0 no regional lymph node metastasis.
- N1 regional lymph node metastasis.

M: distant metastasis
- MX distant metastasis cannot be assessed.
- M0 no distant metastasis.
- M1 distant metastasis.

Clinical features

Tumours of the head of the pancreas tend to present with obstructive jaundice or acute pancreatitis, but the onset is usually insidious. Tumours of the body and tail tend to present even later and are associated with a worse prognosis.

Symptoms
- Painless jaundice
- Pruritis secondary to jaundice
- Fatigue
- Weight loss
- Back pain
- Vague dyspepsia or abdominal discomfort
- Anorexia
- Constipation (reduced food intake)
- Steatorrhoea (fatty stools)
- Late- onset diabetes mellitus without risk factors for diabetes
- Acute pancreatitis of unknown cause
- Chronic pancreatitis
- Acute cholangitis
- Vomiting from duodenal obstruction
- DVT

Signs
- Jaundice
- Scratch marks secondary to jaundice
- Multiple bruises (ecchymoses) secondary to impaired clotting
- Hepatomegaly
- Palpable gallbladder: Courvoisier's sign
- Cachexia
- Troisier's sign: left supraclavicular node enlargement (Virchow's node)
- Anaemia
- Abdominal mass
- Metastasis at the umbilicus: Sister Joseph's sign
- Ascites
- Venous gangrene of the lower limbs
- Migratory thrombophlebitis

Further reading

Alderson D, Johnson CD, Neoptolemos JP, *et al.* Guidelines for the management of patients with pancreatic cancer periampullary and ampullary carcinomas. *Gut* 2005; **54**(Suppl 5):v1–16.

Howes N, Lerch MM, Greenhalf W, *et al.* Clinical and genetic characteristics of hereditary pancreatitis in Europe. *Clin Gastroenterol Hepatol* 2004; **2**:252–61.

Sobin KL, Wittekind C, (eds). *TNM Classification of Malignant Tumours.* 6th edition. New York: Wiley-Liss, 2002.

Internet resources

CANCER *Mondial*: http://www-dep.iarc.fr/
Cancer Research UK: http://info.cancerresearchuk.org/cancerstats/
EUROPAC: http://www.europac-org.eu/

Pancreatic cancer: diagnosis, staging, and prognosis

Diagnosis

Blood tests
Look for anaemia, check clotting profile, liver function tests, and serum proteins.

Tumour markers
- Serum CA19.9 most commonly used marker.
- Sensitivity 70–90% and specificity of 90%. Better than CA-50, DU-PAN-2, and CEA.
- False positives with obstructive jaundice, chronic pancreatitis, and ascites.
- Useful to assess response and identify tumour recurrence.

Non-invasive diagnostic imaging
Transabdominal ultrasound (TAUS)
May be the initial investigation and can detect dilated biliary and pancreatic ducts (double duct sign), tumours >2cm in size, and liver metastases. Not useful in early disease and obese patients.

Contrast-enhanced computed tomography (CE-CT)
Multislice CT is the gold standard for diagnosis and staging (see Fig. 4.5.10). Diagnosis rates of 97% for pancreatic cancer. Accuracy for unresectable lesion is 90% but accuracy for a resectable lesion is 80–85%. False negatives due to small liver metastases and peritoneal deposits.

Magnetic resonance imaging
Similar diagnostic accuracy as CT, better for the diagnosis of liver lesions. Useful for patients who are allergic to intravenous contrast.

Magnetic resonance cholangio-pancreatography
MRCP may enhance diagnosis by revealing a double duct sign and is important for diagnosing and assessing cystic tumours.

Positron emission tomography and PET-CT
Difficult to differentiate inflammatory conditions from tumours accurately; sensitivity is 71–87% with specificity of around 64–80%. The use of PET-CT adds little to the use of CT alone. Further evaluation is needed (Doran et al. 2004).

Invasive diagnostic imaging
Endoluminal ultrasonography (EUS)
Highly sensitive in the detection of small tumours (see Fig. 4.5.11) and small lesions can be biopsied for increased accuracy in diagnosing malignant lesions (not seen on CT). Poor for distant metastases and distant nodal involvement.

Endoscopic retrograde cholangiopancreatography
The sensitivity and specificity of ERCP alone are 70–82% and 88–94%, respectively for pancreatic cancer. With EUS and MRCP now available, ERCP should only be used for the insertion of stents to relieve jaundice and to obtain biopsy or brush cytology.

Percutaneous transhepatic cholangiography (PTHC)
Used for the relief of jaundice when ERCP has failed or is not possible. Can also obtain brushings or biopsy for diagnosis.

Percutaneous fine needle aspiration biopsy
Percutaneous FNA cytology has a sensitivity and specificity of 69% and 100%, respectively, for tissue diagnosis, but a risk of intraperitoneal seeding up to 16%. The diagnostic accuracy of EUS with FNA carries a sensitivity and specificity of >90% and approximately 100%, respectively.

Staging

Diagnostic imaging
Most centres will use multi-slice CE-CT scan as the main modality to stage pancreatic cancer and determine resectability in combination with EUS and ERCP/MRCP. As part of the staging process, laparoscopy plus laparoscopic ultrasound are used on a selective basis.

Laparoscopy and laparoscopic staging
Laparoscopy with laparoscopic ultrasound enables intraoperative scanning of the liver and pancreas to be performed and is highly predictive of resectability, altering the management of 15% of patients already assessed as resectable by dual-phase multislice CT (Ghaneh et al. 2007). Selective laparoscopy based on the serum level of CA19-9 is a more efficient strategy, reducing the proportion of

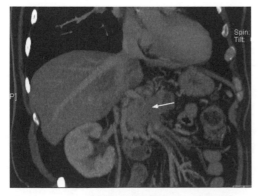

Fig. 4.5.10 Coronal section of multidetector CT scan demonstrating pancreatic tumour encasing the portal vein (white arrow). This patient has unresectable disease.

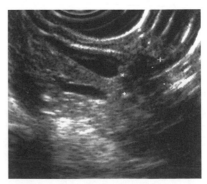

Fig. 4.5.11 Endoluminal ultrasound demonstrating a small pancreatic cancer (between two crosses).

patients undergoing laparoscopic ultrasound from 100% to around 45% while increasing the yield from 15% to 25% (Connor et al. 2005).

Peritoneal cytology

Malignant cells can be identified in 7–30% of peritoneal washing samples from patients with pancreatic cancer. The relationship between positive cytology and survival is not entirely clear and requires further study.

Stage grouping for pancreatic cancer— UICC (Sobin and Wittekind 2002)

Stage grouping
- Stage 0: TisN0M0
- Stage IA: T1N0M0
- Stage IB: T2N0M0
- Stage IIA: T3N0M0
- Stage IIB: T1, T2, T3N1M0
- Stage III: T4, Any NM0
- Stage IV: Any T, Any NM1

Tis=carcinoma in situ; T1= limited to the pancreas ≤2cm; T2= limited to the pancreas >2cm; T3= beyond pancreas; T4=coeliac axis or superior mesenteric artery involved; N1= regional lymph node metastasis; M1= distant metastasis.

Prognosis

The most important determinants of survival in pancreatic cancer are (Ghaneh et al. 2006):
- Surgical resectability
- PS.

Median survival following surgical resection ranges from 11–20 months. Five- year survival ranges from 7–25%.

The other prognostic factors can be categorized into tumour- related, patient- related, and treatment- related groups.

Tumour- related factors

- Stage of tumour: patients with locally advanced disease have a better prognosis than those with metastatic disease.
- Histological type: undifferentiated (anaplastic) carcinoma has a worse prognosis than ductal adenocarcinoma.
- Grade of tumour differentiation: well-differentiated tumours have a better prognosis.
- Lymph node involvement–and lymph node 8a (antero-superior group of the lymph nodes along the common hepatic artery) involvement indicates poor prognosis.

- Location (head lesions better than body and tail).
- Presence of perineural invasion associated with decreased survival.
- Resection margins involvement is associated with decreased survival (positive resection margin is defined as at least one cancer cell within 1mm of any surface).
- CA19.9 ≥100 U/mL is a marker for poor prognosis in advanced disease before treatment.
- Molecular markers, e.g. K-ras mutation, TGF beta, VEGF, Bax, PD-ECGF, DPC4, S100A6, MUC4, MMPs (Chaneh et al. 2007)

Patient- related factors

- Leucocytosis:–elevated white cell count is associated with poor survival (Engelken et al. 2006).
- Elevated gamma glutamine transferase is a biomarker of cholestasis and has a poor prognosis.
- Elevated C-reactive protein level is an independent prognostic marker in advanced disease.
- Presence of severe pain is a poor prognostic factor in advanced disease.
- High platelet/lymphocyte ratio indicates poor outcome.

Treatment- related factors

- Treatment centre with expertise and high case load.
- Relief of jaundice and gastric outlet obstruction in advanced disease.
- Systemic chemotherapy.

Further reading

Connor S, Bosonnet L, Alexakis N, et al. Serum CA19-9 measurement increases the effectiveness of staging laparoscopy in patients with suspected pancreatic malignancy. Dig Surg 2005; 22:80–5.

Doran HE, Bosonnet L, Connor S, et al.. Laparoscopy and laparoscopic ultrasound in the evaluation of pancreatic and periampullary tumours. Dig Surg 2004; 21:305–13.

Engelken FJ, Bettschart V, Rahman MQ, et al. (2003). Prognostic factors in the palliation of pancreatic cancer. Eur J Surg Oncol, 29:368–73.

Ghaneh P, Neoptolemos JP. Pancreas Cancer. In: Gaspodarowicz M, O'Sullivan B, Sobin L (eds). Prognostic Factors in Cancer, pp.153–156. Hoboken, NJ: John Wiley and Sons, 2006.

Ghaneh P, Costello E, Neoptolemos JP (2007). Biology and management of pancreatic cancer. Gut 2007; 56:1134–52.

Sobin KL, Wittekind C (eds). TNM Classification of Malignant Tumours, 6th edition. New York: Wiley-Liss, 2002.

Pancreatic cancer: treatment of resectable cancer

Definition of resectability

Once a diagnosis of pancreatic cancer has been made, the patient will be assessed for fitness to undergo resection and the tumour will be staged. Resectable disease is defined as:

- No coeliac, hepatic, or superior mesenteric artery involvement.
- A patent superior mesenteric-portal venous confluence.
- Portal venous involvement of not >2cm in length or > 50% circumference.
- No liver, peritoneal, or other distant metastases.
- Absence of portal hypertension and cirrhosis.
- No severe co-morbidity to exclude surgery.

Principles of management

These are, broadly:

- To treat patients in a centre of expertise with a high case load.
- To consider pre-operative biliary drainage in jaundiced patients.
- To resect all tumour to achieve R0 resection.
- Reduce/manage post-operative complications.
- Consider adjuvant chemotherapy for all patients.

Preoperative biliary drainage

There is no evidence from meta-analysis that preoperative biliary stenting is harmful or beneficial to surgical outcome (Sewnath et al. 2002). Stents are used mainly to facilitate logistical planning of staging and treatment.

- Plastic stents should be used and placed endoscopically if possible.
- Metal stents should be avoided as surgery can be more difficult, though still technically possible.

Surgical management

- The aim of surgery is to achieve an R0 resection (clear microscopic resection margins).
- Nevertheless, 30–60% of resections are R1 positive: complete clearance of macroscopic tumour with positive microscopic resection margins.
- Patients who have R2 resections (incomplete clearance of macroscopic tumour) should be treated as for locally advanced disease.

Tumours of the head of pancreas

The standard operation for tumours of the head of pancreas is the Kausch–Whipple partial pancreato-duodenectomy. The most commonly used approach at the present time is the pylorus-preserving partial pancreatoduodenectomy. There is no difference in long term outcome between these two approaches (Diener et al. 2002). Pancreato-jejunostomy, hepatico-jejunostomy and duodeno-jejunostomy are performed for the reconstruction. The benefit from a pancreato-gastrostomy rather than a pancreato-jejunostomy is still unclear, and there may be no advantage for the routine use of pancreatic stents.

- There is no survival advantage for extended radical lymphadenectomy in pancreatic cancer (Michalski et al. 2007).
- There is no survival advantage to be gained by performing a total pancreatectomy for a tumour of the pancreatic head, unless it is to achieve R0 resection.

- Resection of the portal or superior mesenteric vein may be necessary to achieve an R0 resection and can be done with an acceptable morbidity.

Tumours of the body and tail of pancreas

A left pancreatectomy is performed, which includes splenectomy and en bloc removal of the hilar lymph nodes.

Morbidity and mortality

- The overall mortality for major pancreatic resections is <5% in major centres.
- Post-operative morbidity is around 40%, so patients require high dependency care for at least the first 24 hours after surgery.

Management of complications

Intra-abdominal abscess

Occurs in 1–12% of patients. Usual cause is anastomotic leak at the pancreato-jejunostomy, hepato-jejunostomy, duodeno-jejunostomy, gastro-jejunostomy, or the jejuno-jejunostomy. CE-CT is indicated. Preferred management is CT-guided percutaneous drainage.

Haemorrhage

Postoperative haemorrhage occurs in 2–5% of patients. Bleeding within 24 hours is due to insufficient intra-operative haemostasis or bleeding from an anastomosis. Free intraperitoneal haemorrhage requires immediate reoperation. Management of anastomotic bleeding is initially conservative. Stress ulceration can be managed medically and/or endoscopically. Secondary haemorrhage (1–3 weeks after surgery) is commonly related to an anastomotic leak and secondary erosion of the retroperitoneal vasculature, or a pseudoaneurysm with a mortality rate of 15–58%. Investigations—CE-CT scan, endoscopy, selective angiography with embolization. Bleeding from a pancreato-jejunostomy may require completion total pancreatectomy or refashioning of the anastomosis.

Fistula after pancreatoduodenectomy

Incidence ranges from 2–24%. The mortality risk from a major pancreatic fistula may be as high as 28%; the cause of death is retroperitoneal sepsis and haemorrhage. Most leaks however can be managed conservatively with little upset to the patient.

Delayed gastric emptying

Incidence ranges from 14–70%. Resolves with conservative treatment and may require intravenous pro-kinetic therapy with erythromycin. Operative correction is rarely required.

Role of octreotide

Postoperative complications may be reduced by the prophylactic use of octreotide given just before the start of the operation for 7 days.

Role of neo-adjuvant and adjuvant treatment

Radical resection alone will result in 5-year survival rate of around 10%. Nearly all patients develop metastatic disease, most commonly of the liver and peritoneum but also the lungs, and this may occur with or without local recurrence.

Neoadjuvant therapy

Indications are:

- To convert tumours to resectability from being locally unresectable.

- To be used with adjuvant therapy to improve overall survival.

Results from small trials are useful to identify particular regimens and toxicity. A comparison of adjuvant and neo-adjuvant therapy did not demonstrate a significant difference in survival between the two groups. There is a suggestion that the proportion of R0 resections may be increased by neo-adjuvant therapy but this does not appear to translate into improved OS.
- To date there are no completed phase III studies of neo-adjuvant studies using either chemotherapy or chemoradiation.
- Neo-adjuvant therapy should only be assessed as part of a clinical trial.

Adjuvant therapy

Adjuvant chemotherapy
- The results from two large randomized trials (ESPAC-1 and CONKO-1) show that adjuvant systemic chemotherapy will increase the 5-year survival from 9–12% with resection alone to 21–29% and 23% with either 5FU and folinic acid (FA) or gemcitabine, respectively (Neoptolemos et al. 2004; Oettle et al. 2007)
- The survival benefit is maintained irrespective of the type of operation used and whether or not patients develop postoperative complications.
- The ESPAC-3(v2) trial comparing adjuvant gemcitabine and 5-FU/FA did not show any significant difference in treatment between the two treatments. Median survival from resection of patients treated with 5-FU/FA was 23.0 (95% CI 21.1–25.0) months and for patients treated with gemcitabine this was 23.6 (95%CI 21.4–26.4) months.

Adjuvant chemoradiotherapy
- Improved survival seen in small randomized and non-randomized series of patients. Not been confirmed in large randomizsed trials (Smeenk et al. 2006; Oettle et al. 2007).

Chemoradiotherapy and follow-on chemotherapy
- The RTOG 9704 trial (Regine et al. 2008) used background 5-FU-based chemoradiotherapy together with pre- and post-chemoradiation (systemic chemotherapy comprising either 5-FU or gemcitabine). The results showed no difference between the two groups in terms of median survival or 3-year survival in all patients.

Meta-analysis
- The results of meta-analysis using individual patient data reject the use of chemoradiation and provide powerful evidence for systemic chemotherapy (Stocken et al. 2005).

Key points
- Adjuvant 5FU-based chemotherapy significantly improves survival.
- Adjuvant gemcitabine chemotherapy improves disease free survival.
- Adjuvant chemoradiation has not been shown to improve survival in the absence of maintenance chemotherapy.
- Adjuvant chemoradiotherapy and follow-on chemotherapy may not offer improved survival compared with chemotherapy alone.
- Neo-adjuvant treatments should only be administered as part of a controlled clinical trial.

Further reading

Diener MK, Knaebel HP, Heukaufer C, et al. A systematic review and meta-analysis of pylorus-preserving versus classical pancreaticoduodenectomy for surgical treatment of periampullary and pancreatic carcinoma. Ann Surg 2007; **245**:187–200.

Michalski CW, Kleeff J, Wente MN, et al. Systematic review and meta-analysis of standard and extended lymphadenectomy in pancreaticoduodenectomy for pancreatic cancer. Br J Surg 2007; **94**:265–73.

Neoptolemos JP, Stocken DD, Friess H, et al. European Study Group for Pancreatic Cancer. A randomized trial of chemoradiotherapy and chemotherapy after resection of pancreatic cancer. N Engl J Med, 2004; **350**:1200–10.

Oettle H, Post S, Neuhaus P, et al. Adjuvant chemotherapy with gemcitabine vs observation in patients undergoing curative-intent resection of pancreatic cancer: a randomized controlled trial JAMA, (2007); **297**:267–77.

Regine WF, Winter KA, Abrams RA, et al. Fluorouracil vs gemcitabine chemotherapy before and after fluorouracil-based chemoradiation following resection of pancreatic adenocarcinoma: a randomized controlled trial. JAMA 2008; **299**:1019–26.

Sewnath ME, Karsten TM, Prins MH, et al. A meta-analysis on the efficacy of preoperative biliary drainage for tumors causing obstructive jaundice. Ann Surg 2002; **236**:17–27.

Smeenk HG, van Eijck CH, Hop WC, et al. Long-term survival and metastatic pattern of pancreatic and periampullary cancer after adjuvant chemoradiation or observation: long-term results of EORTC trial 40891. Ann Surg 2007; **246**:734–40.

Stocken DD, Büchler MW, Dervenis C, et al. Pancreatic Cancer Meta-analysis Group. Meta-analysis of randomised adjuvant therapy trials for pancreatic cancer. Br J Cancer 2005; **92**:1372–81.

Pancreatic cancer: treatment of unresectable and metastatic cancer

Unresectable cancer
Approximately 70% of patients will present with unresectable disease. The treatment of patients who have unresectable pancreatic cancer due to localized advanced disease, and/or metastases consists of symptom control and palliative therapy.

Principles of management
Pain relief
- Intractable pain is a major problem.
- Necessitates use of high- dose opiates.
- Additional approaches include intraoperative, percutaneous CT-guided or EUS neurolytic coeliac plexus block and bilateral or unilateral thoracoscopic splanchnicectomy.
- Pain control with coeliac plexus block was improved in a randomized study compared with systemic analgesia, but this was not reflected in the QoL or survival (Wong et al. 2004).

Jaundice and duodenal obstruction
- Jaundice best relieved using ERCP and biliary stent.
- PTC-endoscopy approach employed only if ERCP not technically possible.
- Main complications are acute cholangitis, bleeding, and peritonitis.
- Self-expanding metal (and covered) stents should be used for patients with a good PS and favourable prognosis (locally advanced primary tumour <3cm).
- Plastic stent for those patients with metastases and tumours >3cm in diameter.
- Endoscopically- placed expandable metal stents deployed for duodenal obstruction (occurs in approximately 15%).
- Success rate of around 85%. Complications include: perforation, fistula, bleeding, and recurrent obstruction due to stent migration or fracture.
- Surgical bypass (open and laparoscopic) can be used to relieve jaundice using a Roux-en-Y loop hepatojejunostomy, and duodenal obstruction by gastrojejunostomy, especially in younger patients. Both can be achieved laparoscopically.

Weight loss
- Initially is due to pancreatic exocrine insufficiency owing to obstruction of the main pancreatic duct as well as exclusion of bile acids from obstruction of the main bile duct.
- Fat maldigestion may also contribute to abdominal pain and bloating.
- Relief of biliary obstruction and pancreatic enzyme supplementation will alleviate these symptoms (Bruno et al. 1998).
- Cachexia can be a marked feature of the later stages of pancreatic cancer, with no good treatment.

Systemic chemotherapy
- See following section for metastatic disease treatment options.

Role of chemoradiotherapy
- External beam radiotherapy is used with 5-FU or gemcitabine as a radiosensitizing agent (chemoradiotherapy).

The main drawback is the limit on the dosage owing to the close proximity of adjacent radiosensitive organs.
- Newer techniques such as conformal radiotherapy are now being used, but these studies almost invariably employ follow-on chemotherapy once the chemoradiotherapy has been completed.
- Meta-analysis has demonstrated that chemoradiotherapy is better than radiotherapy alone but there is no survival difference between chemoradiotherapy plus follow-on chemotherapy and chemotherapy alone (Sultana et al. 2007a).
- Should only be evaluated as part of a clinical trial.

Metastatic disease
Principles of management
These include the relief of pain, jaundice, and reduction of weight loss outlined previously.

Treatment options
Systemic chemotherapy
Pancreatic ductal adenocarcinoma is highly resistant to conventional methods of cytotoxic treatment and radiotherapy. Few chemotherapeutic agents have been shown to have reproducible response rates of >10%.
- 5-FU is an inhibitor of thymidylate synthetase (essential for synthesis of DNA nucleotides) and has been the most widely used in advanced pancreatic cancer, with a median survival of around 5–6 months and is better than the BSC.
- The nucleoside analogue, gemcitabine, has replaced 5-FU as the preferred drug. Median survival increase in favour of gemcitabine compared with 5-FU (5.7 vs 4.4 months), the 1-year survival rate increase (18% vs 2%), toxicity relatively mild, and better clinical response (24% vs 5%, respectively) (Burris et al. 1997).
- A recent meta-analysis has confirmed that combination chemotherapy may improve the survival observed with gemcitabine alone (Sultana et al. 2007b). Two agents in combination with gemcitabine have improved survival compared to gemcitabine alone. Capecitabine (Xeloda) is a new oral, fluoropyrimidine carbamate that is sequentially converted to 5-FU by three enzymes located in the liver and in tumours, including pancreatic cancer and demonstrated significantly improved survival compared with gemcitabine alone. Platinum-based agents have also demonstrated improved survival.

Key points
- Chemotherapy improves survival and QoL in patients with advanced pancreatic cancer.
- Chemoradiotherapy and follow-on chemotherapy are no better than chemotherapy alone.
- The best chemotherapy combination available at the present time is gemcitabine with either capecitabine or a platinum agent.
- New agents will be expensive but will become increasingly targeted based on molecular profiling.

Table 4.5.2 Phase III trials of novel agents in pancreatic cancer

Trial	Regimen	Outcome
PA3 Canada/USA	Gem vs gem + erlotinib	MS 5.91 months, 1 year 17%
		MS 6.37 months, 1 year 24%
SWOG S0205 USA	Gem vs gem + cetuximab	Closed—no survival difference
CALGB 80303 USA	Gem vs gem + bevacizumab	Closed—no survival difference
Avita Europe	Gem + erlotinib vs gem + bev + erlotinib	Closed—no survival difference
Telovac UK	Gem + cap vs gem + cap then GV1001 vs Gem + Cap + GV1001	Active
RC-57 crossover Germany	Cap + erlot then gem vs gem + erlot then cap	Active
IPC-BAYPAN France	Gem + sorafenib vs gem	Active
Pfizer	Gem + axitinib vs gem	Active

gem=gemcitabine, bev=bevacizumab, cap=capecitabine, MS=median survival

Novel approaches

Recently there have been large phase III trials of novel agents in combination with gemcitabine in advanced pancreatic cancer. The results have been mixed with slightly improved survival (but nevertheless significant) seen only with the oral EGFR tyrosine kinase inhibitor erlotinib (Tarceva®).

Several phase III trials are now open and results are awaited (Table 4.5.2). Newer agents which rely on the molecular analysis of pancreatic cancer are at an early stage and may be incorporated into clinical trials in the near future (Ghaneh et al. 2007).

Further reading

Bruno MJ, Haverkort EB, Tijssen GP, et al. Placebo controlled trial of enteric coated pancreatin microsphere treatment in patients with unresectable cancer of the pancreatic head region. Gut 1998; **42**:92–6.

Burris HA 3rd, Moore MJ, Andersen J, et al. Improvements in survival and clinical benefit with gemcitabine as first-line therapy for patients with advanced pancreas cancer: a randomized trial. J Clin Oncol, 1997; **15**:2403–13.

Ghaneh P, Costello E, Neoptolemos JP, Biology and management of pancreatic cancer. Gut, 2007; **56**:1134–52.

Sultana A, Tudur Smith C, Cunningham D, et al. Meta-analyses on the management of locally advanced pancreatic cancer using radiation/combined modality therapy. Br J Cancer 2007a; **96**:1183–90.

Sultana A, Tudur-Smith C, Cunningham D, et al. Meta-analyses of chemotherapy for locally advanced and metastatic pancreatic cancer. J Clin Oncol 2007b; **25**:2607–15.

Wong GY, Schroeder DR, Carns PE, et al. Effect of neurolytic celiac plexus block on pain relief, quality of life, and survival in patients with unresectable pancreatic cancer: a randomized controlled trial. JAMA 2004; **291**:1092–9.

Internet resources

Useful sites for pancreatic cancer and clinical trials include:

http://www.cancer.gov/clinicaltrials

http://public.ukcrn.org.uk/Search/Portfolio.aspx?Level1=1&Level2=16&Level3=30&Status=All

http://www.lctu.org.uk/

http://www.pancreaticcancer.org.uk/

Uncommon pancreatic tumours

Carcinoid tumours

Epidemiology
Carcinoid tumours are neuroendocrine neoplasms arising from enterochromaffin cells. The tumours may be functioning or non-functioning (Modline et al. 2004; Soga 2005).
- Prevalence in the general population of 2–4 per 100,000.
- Pancreatic carcinoids represent 0.6–1.4% of all carcinoid tumours and 2.2% of GI carcinoid tumours.
- Male to female ratio is 1:1.5.
- Mean age (range) at presentation 49 years (22–78 years).
- Overall 5-year survival rate 30–37.5%.
- Median survival for patients with metastatic disease approximately 7 months.

Clinical presentation and diagnosis/staging
- May be non-specific. Abdominal pain, diarrhoea, flushing, and nausea are among the most frequently encountered symptoms in patients with pancreatic carcinoid tumours. Carcinoid syndrome occurs in around 25%.
- Main diagnostic modality is CE-CT scan. MRI with dynamic gadolinium enhancement and fat suppression may detect smaller pancreatic lesions. Tumours tend to be hypervascular on CT scan.
- Endoluminal ultrasound EUS will enable biopsy of suspect lesions.
- The role of PET scan is under evaluation.
- Further imaging includes ^{111}In-octreotide and ^{123}I-MIBG scans.
- Plasma chromogranin A.

Histology
Microscopy reveals trabecules of small- to medium-sized cells with argyrophilic, granular eosinophilic cytoplasm and monomorphic round nuclei. On immunohistochemical analysis, these lesions are positive for chromogranin A, synaptophysin, serotonin (93%), and NSE (neuron- specific enolase) (100%).

Treatment
Surgical
- If the tumour is resectable then pancreatectomy will be performed. Tumours of the head will require pancreatoduodenectomy; body and tail tumours will require left pancreatectomy.
- Liver metastases may be resected if superficial and small.
- Resection of the primary advised even in the presence of metastatic disease.

Non-surgical
Approximately 70–80% of patients will present with advanced disease. Treatment for advanced carcinoid disease is still to be standardized. Options for therapy include:
- Symptom control using octreotide long-acting repeatable (LAR).
- ^{131}I-MIBG or [III]In/90Y octreotide in patients with positive diagnostic scans. No randomized trials to date.
- Chemotherapy demonstrates only modest improvement in survival (streptozosin plus 5-FU/dacarbazine vs doxorubicin plus 5-FU).
- Disease limited to hepatic metastases only— hepatic arterial chemoembolization, RF ablation.
- Novel agents—angiogenesis inhibitors.

Pancreatic endocrine tumours

Epidemiology
Arise from the islet cells of the pancreas—main types are insulinoma, gastrinoma, glucagonoma, and VIPoma.
- Incidence of all pancreatic endocrine tumours 0.01–0.3 per 100,000.
- Mean age (range) 47 years (8–82years).
- WHO classification based on clinical, molecular, and histopathological features (Capella et al. 1995; Solcia et al. 2000).
- Metastases (i.e. malignancy) observed in 10% insulinomas, 60% gastrinomas, 60% glucagonomas, up to 70% VIPomas.
- Five- year survival following surgical resection 50–95%.

Aetiology
Poorly understood. There are four inherited diseases associated with pancreatic endocrine tumours (Table 4.5.3). These patients should undergo screening to identify early tumours which are treatable.

Clinical presentation and diagnosis/staging
Present with symptoms either from the tumour itself (non-functioning) or a defined syndrome from excessive peptide secretion.
- *Insulinoma*: typically there is faintness, fatigue, or even coma, associated with fasting or vigorous exercise and rapidly relieved by eating a snack or drinking a liquid rich in glucose. Diagnosis is based on a very low blood sugar (<2mmol/L) and a high level of insulin and C-peptide (indicative of endogenous insulin). Main differential diagnosis is self-administration of insulin.
- *Gastrinoma*: high gastric acid secretion resulting in refractory multiple peptic ulcers of a severe nature (Zollinger–Ellison syndrome) and sometimes diarrhoea.

Table 4.5.3 Inherited diseases associated with pancreatic endocrine tumours

Condition	Comment
Multiple endocrine neoplasia type 1 (MEN-1)	Pituitary, parathyroid, and pancreatic islet cell tumours (often multiple). Gastrinoma is the commonest Mutation MEN-1 gene 30–85% have clinical evidence of pancreatic endocrine tumour
Von Hippel– Lindau	AD Mutation VHL tumour suppressor gene
Type 1 neurofibromatosis (NF1)	Affects 1 in 4000, AD. Mutation of tumour suppressor gene NF1
Tuberous sclerosis	Rare. Mutation in TSC1 or TSC2 genes.

History of gastric or duodenal perforation or haemorrhage. Diagnosed by high gastrin levels (>100pg/mL, or > 200pgmL after secretin stimulation). Gastrin also elevated by H2-receptor blockers, proton pump inhibitors, or *Helicobacter pylori* infection.

- *Glucagonoma*: characteristic necrolytic migratory erythema of the skin, starting in the groin and perineum and may affect oral mucosa. Features include attacks of hyperglycaemia, stomatitis, vulvitis, anaemia, a rash, weight loss, diarrhoea, and psychiatric disturbances. High plasma glucagon levels are found.
- *Vasoactive intestinal polypeptide tumour*: a VIPoma causes watery diarrhoea and hypokalaemia (WDHA). Results in massive intestinal loss of sodium and bicarbonate, leading to hypovolaemia, hypokalaemia, and achlorhydria or metabolic acidosis. May be impaired glucose tolerance and hypercalcaemia. Diagnosis is by high plasma levels of vasoactive intestinal polypeptide.
- *Localization and staging investigations* may include CE-CT scan, MRI scan, EUS, ^{111}In-octreotide, and selective portal/splenic venous sampling and intra-operative ultrasound.

Treatment

Surgical
- Enucleation is the usual operation for benign insulinomas—small without metastases. Adult nesidioblastosis may require a left or total pancreatectomy.
- Radical resection. Gastrinomas are often multiple, may be found in the duodenal wall. Surgical resection is the only procedure that will provide cure with a normal life expectancy
- Hepatic resection. May be indicated for resectable disease.

Non-surgical
- Proton -pump inhibitor. Reduce gastric acid secretion from gastrinomas but will not prevent tumour growth and metastases.
- As for pancreatic carcinoid.

Uncommon histologies

Cystic tumours
Comprise at least 15% of all pancreatic cystic masses. The three most common primary pancreatic cystic neoplasms are:
- Serous cystic neoplasms predominantly affect women, are found mostly in the head of pancreas, and represent 30% of cystic neoplasms.

- Mucinous cystic neoplasms also are found more often in women, but mostly in the body and tail of the pancreas, and represent 40% of primary cystic neoplasms. The cyst does not communicate with the main pancreatic duct.
- Intraductal papillary mucinous neoplasms (IPMNs). Affect more men than women, can involve part or the whole of the pancreatic ductal system, affect older patients and represent 30% of pancreatic cysts. IPMNs are classified as arising either from the main duct or branch duct

Diagnosis
- CT/MRI scan, EUS, FNA cystic fluid, serum CA-19.9 tumour marker

Management
- Confirmed serous cystic neoplasm—a conservative approach with regular follow-up imaging is justified.
- Mucinous cystic neoplasms should be resected if the patient is fit for major surgery owing to the high malignant potential.
- All main duct IPMNs should be resected. Patients with relatively benign features of branch duct IPMN may be managed with regular follow-up imaging.

Pancreatic lymphoma
By definition, pancreatic lymphoma is restricted to the pancreas and draining lymph nodes. Resection should be undertaken if this is possible.

Metastases to the pancreas
The pancreas is a site for metastases from cancers arising in the abdomen, breast, bronchus or skin. Sometimes these metastases are isolated in which case radical resection is the treatment of choice.

Further reading
Capella C, Heitz PU, Hofler H, *et al.* Revised classification of neuroendocrine tumours of the lung, pancreas and gut. *Virchows Arch* 1995; **425**:547–560.

Modline I, Shapiro M, Kidd M (2004). An analysis of rare carcinoid tumours: clarifying these conundrums. *World J Surg*, **29**:92–101.

Soga J. Carcinoids of the pancreas. *Cancer* 2005; **104**:1180–7.

Solcia E, Kloeppel G, Sobin LH. World Health Organization: International Histological Classification of Tumours: Histological Typing of Endocrine Tumours. Berlin: Springer, 2000.

Internet resources
http://www.cancerbackup.org.uk/Cancertype/Endocrine/Overview
http://www.pancreaticcancer.org.uk/PCNeuroendocrine.htm

Tumours of small intestine

Epidemiology
The small intestine constitutes 75% of the length of the GI tract but is the site of only 2–3% of malignant GI cancers. In 2004 the incidence of small intestinal tumours was 0.6 per 100, 000 with a slight male preponderance. There has been a gradual increase in the age standardized rate since the mid 19-70s (Shack et al. 2006). This may be in part due to an increasing elderly population but may also reflect improved diagnostic techniques.

Pathology
There are four main types of small intestinal tumours:
• Adenocarcinomas (45%)
• Carcinoids or neuroendocrine tumours (NETs) (30%)
• Sarcomas (10%) (majority are GISTs, 20% occur in the small bowel)
• Lymphomas (15%)

The majority of small bowel adenocarcinomas (SBAs) occur in the duodenum or jejunum with a minority occurring in the ileum. NETs and lymphoma commonly arise in the terminal ileum. Sarcomas are more evenly distributed although more common in the ileum (Shack et al. 2006). Metastatic lesions are more common than primary tumours and may occur from direct invasion or by intraperitoneal seeding (colon, ovary, uterus, and stomach cancers), or by haematogenous spread (melanoma, breast and lung cancer).

The SBAs are mostly non-specific adenocarcinoma but mucinous adenocarcinoma and signet ring carcinoma are frequent findings; the latter are often grouped with poorly differentiated tumours. Other rarer epithelial cancers include papillary adenocarcinoma, villous adenocarcinoma, and small- cell carcinoma. NETs arise from neuroendocrine cells. The jejunum and ileum are the second most common sites in the body behind the rectum although there are racial variations (Yao et al. 2008).

Five distinct types of small bowel lymphoma have been described; adult-western type, paediatric type, immunoproliferative small intestinal disease or Mediterranean type, enteropathy-associated T-cell lymphoma, and HD. The western type is the most common and is a form of extranodal B-cell (NHL) that is normally high grade.

The most frequent malignant mesenchymal tumour (sarcoma) is the GIST. These are defined by the overexpression of the growth factors c-kit or PDGFR-A with a specific set of histological features including spindle cell, epithelioid, and rarely pleomorphic morphology. Leiomyosarcomas occur much less frequently in the small intestine. They form polypoid intraluminal masses and if excised have a better prognosis than GISTs.

Benign mesenchymal tumours that arise in or involve the GI tract include leiomyomas, uterine type leiomyomas, schwannomas, and desmoid tumours. Desmoids occur sporadically or in association with Gardner syndrome, a sub-type of familial adenomatous polyposis (FAP). These tumours are locally invasive and can cause bowel obstruction but do not metastasise.

Age
There is an increase in the age- specific incidence of tumours of the small intestine from the mid-40s, plateauing in the 80s. The median age at presentation for SBA is in the mid-60s; the age distribution for carcinoid tumours and sarcomas is similar although peaks slightly earlier. The peak incidence for lymphomas is in the mid to late 50s. Specific subtypes may present earlier, some in childhood.

Race
The incidence of tumours of the small intestine varies among populations. Higher rates are seen in the Maori people of New Zealand and among ethnic Hawaiians, with low rates in India, Romania, and other parts of Eastern Europe. Data from the SEER database from the USA shows a higher incidence of adenocarcinoma and malignant carcinoid tumours in the black population. Mediterranean-type lymphoma and enteropathy-associated T-cell lymphoma are seen in younger age groups in the Middle East and Africa, where they constitute the most common small bowel malignancy (Neugut et al. 1998).

Aetiology
The adenoma–carcinoma sequence of large bowel adenocarcinoma is generally accepted. Several findings suggest that SBA also arise as a result of a malignant transformation in adenomatous polyps. Invasive carcinoma is frequently seen within small bowel adenomas. Patients with SBA are on average several years older than those presenting with adenomas suggesting an appropriate temporal relationship and the majority of SBA shows adenomatous change in adjacent tissue. In accordance, conditions that give rise to adenomas such as FAP are associated with an increased risk of SBA. Indeed SBA is the major cause of death in such patients post colectomy. Other risk factors for SBA include:
• Crohn's disease
• Coeliac disease
• Neurofibromatosis
• Urinary diversions (i.e. ileal conduits)

Bile acid may be a causative carcinogen as tumours often cluster around the ampulla of Vater. Moreover cholecystectomy also increases the risk of SBA (Neugut et al. 1998).

The aetiology of carcinoid tumours is poorly understood. The majority are sporadic although there may be a familial component. First-degree relatives of affected patients have a 4-fold increased risk, which rises to 12- fold if a further first- degree relative is affected. Affected individuals may have a generalized increased cancer risk. From a series of > 13, 000 patients, 20% went on to have a further malignancy, one-third of which arose in the GI tract (Modlin et al. 2003).

Coeliac disease and tropical sprue have been associated with lymphoma and to a lesser extent with SBA. In a national survey, in 39% of small intestine lymphomas and 13% of SBA there was a diagnosis of carcinoid. Lymphoma associated with coeliac disease was largely enteropathy-associated T-cell as opposed to B-cell type, tended to be a more proximal than normal, and have a worse prognosis (Howdle et al. 2003). An increased incidence of small bowel lymphoma occurred during the 1980's related to the HIV/ AIDS epidemic (Neugut et al. 1998).

GISTs are believed to originate from interstitial cells of Cajal. These are intermediates between the GI autonomic nervous system cells and smooth muscle cells regulating GI motility. Mutually exclusive mutations in c-kit or PDGFR-A receptor tyrosine kinase proteins are seen in 80% of GISTs. These mutations are somatic. They cause functional change in c-kit and PDGFR-A proteins leading to ligand-independent activation and subsequent activation of downstream effectors. The end result is an increase in cellular proliferation and a reduction in apoptosis. Ninety-five per cent of GISTs are sporadic. A minority are associated with three tumour syndromes: neurofibromatosis type 1 (NF1), Carney triad, and familial GIST syndrome. GISTs that occur in NF1 have a high predilection for the small bowel and are normally clinically indolent. GISTs in Carney triad occur in the stomach together with paraganglioma, pulmonary chondroma, or both. These also have an indolent behaviour (Miettinen and Lasota 2006)

Clinical features

The presenting symptoms of SBA depend on site and size. These include:

- Non-specific symptoms: abdominal pain, anaemia, nausea, bleeding and weight loss, palpable mass
- Obstructive jaundice
- Surgical emergencies: intussusception, perforation

Tumours in the duodenum frequently present with pain related to partial duodenal obstruction. Tumours of the ampullary region often present with jaundice. More distal tumours may present with small bowel obstruction. Occult bleeding is common but frank haemorrhage rare. Adenocarcinoma of the small and large bowel have a similar pattern of spread; common sites include regional lymph nodes, liver, lung, and the abdominal cavity. Because of late presentation many patients have metastatic disease at diagnosis.

Primary carcinoid tumours are often silent but can present with vague abdominal pain or obstruction. Carcinoid syndrome is a manifestation of secretory metastases in the liver. Intermittent abdominal pain occurs in 70% of affected patients, diarrhoea in 50%, flushing in 30%, and less frequently wheezing. With time, right-sided heart disease may occur and is associated with high levels of circulating amines; likewise pellagra can develop in patients with late presentation. Surgical insult to the primary may trigger a massive release of serotonin (5-HT) and other vasoactive amines and cause a carcinoid crisis that consists of bronchospasm, severe flushing, tachycardia, and fluctuating blood pressure. In addition to the liver, other common metastatic sites include the abdominal cavity, lymph nodes, lung, and bones.

Lymphomas commonly present with acute and/or chronic abdominal pain relating to bowel obstruction or less often perforation. Patients often have a history of weight loss and fatigue. A mass may be palpable and blood tests may reveal anaemia. Rarer types of lymphoma frequently have characteristic presenting symptoms. Paediatric lymphoma often presents with right lower quadrant pain associated with intussusception. Mediterranean-type lymphoma presents with a triad of fatigue, malabsorption, and clubbing. Enteropathy-associated lymphoma is also associated with malabsorption.

The most common presentation of GISTs is GI bleeding that may be insidious or haemorrhagic. Patients may present with an acute abdomen due to tumour rupture, bowel obstruction, or appendicitis-like pain. Smaller GISTs are often incidental findings at surgery. Patients with advanced disease may present with symptoms arising from metastases in the abdominal cavity, liver, rarely in bones, skin, and soft tissues, and extremely rarely in the lungs.

Diagnosis

Patients normally present with symptoms related to the primary tumour or, if the disease is initially silent, secondary symptoms of anaemia or manifestations of metastatic disease. A careful examination should be performed looking for evidence of metastatic disease. Plethoric facies due to chronic flushing and evidence of right-sided heart failure may suggest carcinoid syndrome.

The initial investigations will often be dictated by the presenting symptoms. They may include:;

- Small bowel follow-through
- Plain X-rays
- Abdominal ultrasound
- CT scan
- Endoscopic ultrasound (EUS)
- Small bowel endoscopy

Cross sectional imaging of the chest, abdomen, and pelvis may help delineate the primary tumour and provide staging information. Different tumour types have characteristic appearances on CT. Larger carcinoid tumours may be seen with fixation, separation, and angulation of bowel loops, and often calcification at the centre of a desmoplastic reaction giving a 'starburst' appearance. Diffuse segmental thickening of a length of small intestine is suggestive of lymphoma. GISTs are often well-circumscribed masses. Carcinoid tumours often differentially express somatostatin receptors (SSTRs) compared to normal tissue. Scintigraphy with [111] In-octreotide, a somatostatin analogue, can be used to identify carcinoid primaries and stage metastatic disease, exhibiting sensitivities of 67–100% (Ramage et al. 2005).

A tissue diagnosis is necessary prior to planning non-surgical treatment. For proximal tumours this may be obtained by an upper GI endoscopy. Occasionally tumour masses may be amenable to CT-guided biopsies- otherwise a diagnostic laparoscopy or laparotomy is required. In one national prospective series from the UK, laparotomy was required for diagnosis in 30–66% of adenocarcinoma, 78% of lymphoma, and 93% of carcinoid cases (Howdle et al. 2003).

Staging

Adenocarcinomas are staged using the AJCC TNM system which is similar to cancers of the large intestine.

- Stage I: T1–2N0M0
- Stage II: T3–4N0M0
- Stage III: T1–4N1M0
- Stage IV: T1–4N0–1M1

WHO guidelines of 2000 describe four categories of carcinoid tumours.

- Well-differentiated endocrine tumour of probable low malignant potential.
- Well-differentiated endocrine tumour of unknown malignant potential.
- Well-differentiated endocrine carcinoma.
- Poorly-differentiated endocrine carcinoma.

There is no TNM staging system for these tumours.

Lymphomas are staged using the Ann Arbor staging system (see p.437).

The most powerful and widely applied criteria for evaluating the biological potential of GIST are tumour size and mitotic activity. Using these criteria, tumours can be classified as very low risk, low risk, intermediate risk, and high risk (Miettinen and Lasota 2006).

Principles of treatment

When disease is localized a radical surgical resection with removal of all visible disease and regional lymph nodes should be undertaken. When there is evidence of metastatic disease the aim of treatment is to minimize symptoms and prolong life expectancy. Clear communication with the patient and relatives is paramount so that the physician understands the patient's expectations and the patient understands the possible gains and potential treatment related toxicity and inconvenience.

Surgery

Surgery is performed to obtain a histological diagnosis, to palliate symptoms, and to attempt to cure. A potentially curative approach necessitates complete resection of the primary tumour, often en bloc with adjacent organs and a radical lymph node dissection. Anatomical constraints permit this more often in distal than in proximal small intestine tumours. As a result, curative surgery is performed more frequently for distal tumours, 52% versus 90% in one large series (Howe et al. 1999). Failure to achieve a complete resection results in median survival of 10–14 months, similar to patients with inoperable disease.

For carcinoid tumours, cytoreductive surgery may be considered to control symptoms of functional tumours and improve survival (>50% at 5 years for patients undergoing liver resection). Potential techniques include surgical resection of liver metastases, RF ablation, cryotherapy, and embolization. Octreotide should be administered prior to surgery for functional carcinoid tumours to avert a carcinoid crisis.

Systemic therapy

Small bowel adenocarcinoma

Chemotherapy is commonly used for metastatic SBA. The approach and choice of chemotherapy is largely extrapolated from the management of large intestinal cancer. There are a few reported phase II clinical trials but no randomized data. The largest trial of palliative chemotherapy used a combination of 5-FU, doxorubicin, and mitomycin C, and had a response rate of 18% but with an unacceptably high toxicity. Single institution experiences have reported similar response rates with less toxicity using single-agent 5-FU or a combination of 5-FU and platinum agents in the first line setting and irinotecan and 5-FU in the second line setting. More recently a small phase II study of oxaliplatin and capecitabine reported a higher response rate of 50% and median survival of 20.3 months.

Carcinoid tumours

Therapeutic avenues for carcinoid tumours centre on targeting somatostatin receptors (SSTRs). Native somatostatin plays an inhibitory role regulating several organ systems and tissues, i.e. GI motility, secretion of pancreatic and intestinal hormones. Somatostatin analogues, octreotide, and lanreotide have been developed that suppress release of amines/hormones by functional carcinoid tumours. Diarrhoea and flushing can be controlled in 45–60% and 54–68% of patients, respectively. The main toxicities relate to bowel disorders, biliary disorders, and injection site pain. Initially immediate- release subcutaneous two to four times daily octreotide is used to establish the effective dose followed by use of long- acting formulations. Indications include symptomatic patients with functional tumours or rapidly progressing non-functional tumours. Resistance may be due to loss of inhibitory control of secretion or tumour growth (Oberg et al. 2004).

Small bowel lymphoma

Ann Arbour stage I and II B-cell NHL are treated surgically with or without chemotherapy. Stage III and IV disease are treated with primary chemotherapy with or without surgical debulking. Chemotherapy regimens are similar to nodal NHL. Low- grade NHL may be managed conservatively in the absence of symptoms.

Sarcoma

GIST: Imatinib is a competitive inhibitor of multiple tyrosine kinase inhibitors including c-kit and PDGFR. Large clinical trials report response rates of 40%, stable disease in a further 25%, and median PFS and OS of 18–20 and 51–55 months, respectively (Blay et al. 2007; Blanke et al. 2008). The role of adjuvant imatinib post resection is being explored in randomized clinical trials. These survival figures are clearly superior to those achieved with doxorubicin chemotherapy.

Non-GIST sarcomas: doxorubicin and ifosfamide remains the chemotherapy of choice.

Prognosis

Prognosis relates primarily to the stage of disease at diagnosis and to the type of tumour.

SBA frequently present with advanced disease. Overall 5-year survival rates in the region of 30% are commonly reported. This is increased to 55% if node negative and 0% if distant metastases are present.

The prognosis of carcinoids is dictated by site, stage, and the degree of differentiation. Within the small bowel proximal carcinoids are more frequently localized than those in the jejunum and terminal ileum. The median survival for localized tumours is 107–111 months, for regional disease is 101–105 months, and in the presence of distant metastases is 56–57 months. The median survival of patients with any grade 1 and 2 NET tumours is 124 and 64 months, respectively compared to just 10 months for those with grade 3 and 4 tumours (Yao et al. 2008)

Most series of small intestinal lymphomas include lymphoma of the stomach. For early stage disease, 10- year survival rates range from 60–86% but are worse for advanced disease.

The prognosis of small bowel GISTs depends on their size and mitotic rate. From one large series overall tumour related mortality was 39%. Eight-six per cent of tumours >10cm with a high mitotic rate index metastasized in contrast to only 2–3% of <5cm tumours with a low mitotic rate. The metastatic rate of intermediate tumours ranged from 24–50% (Miettinen and Lasota 2006)

Further reading

Blanke CD, Rankin C, Demetri GD, et al. Phase III randomized, intergroup trial assessing imatinib mesylate at two dose levels in patients with unresectable or metastatic gastrointestinal stromal tumors expressing the kit receptor tyrosine kinase: S0033. J Clin Oncol 2008; 26:626–32.

Blay JY, Le Cesne A, Ray-Coquard I, et al. Prospective multicentric randomized phase III study of imatinib in patients with advanced gastrointestinal stromal tumors comparing interruption versus continuation of treatment beyond 1 year: the French Sarcoma Group. J Clin Oncol 2007; 25:1107–13.

Howdle PD, Jalal PK, Holmes GKT, et al. Primary small-bowel malignancy in the UK and its association with coeliac disease. QJM 2003; 96:345–53.

Howe JR, Karnell LH, Menck HR, et al. The American College of Surgeons Commission on Cancer and the American Cancer Society. Adenocarcinoma of the small bowel: review of the National Cancer Data Base, 1985–1995. Cancer 1999; 86: 2693–706.

Kaltsas GA, Papadogias D, Makras P, et al. Treatment of advanced neuroendocrine tumours with radiolabelled somatostatin analogues. Endocr Relat Cancer 2005; 12:683–99.

Miettinen M and Lasota J Gastrointestinal stromal tumors: review on morphology, molecular pathology, prognosis, and differential diagnosis. *Arch Pathol Lab Med* 2006; **130**:1466–78.

Modlin IM, Lye KD, Kidd M. A 5-decade analysis of 13,715 carcinoid tumors. *Cancer* 2003; **97**:934–59.

Neugut AI, Jacobson JS, Suh S, *et al*. The epidemiology of cancer of the small bowel. *Cancer Epidemiol Biomarkers Prev* 1998; **7**:243–51.

Oberg K, Kvols L, Caplin M, *et al*. Consensus report on the use of somatostatin analogs for the management of neuroendocrine tumors of the gastroenteropancreatic system. *Ann Oncol* 2004; **15**:966–73.

Ramage JK, Davies AHG, Ardill J, *et al*. Guidelines for the management of gastroenteropancreatic neuroendocrine (including carcinoid) tumours. *Gut* 2005; **54**(Suppl 4):iv1–16.

Shack LG, Wood HE, Kang JY, *et al*. Small intestinal cancer in England & Wales and Scotland: time trends in incidence, mortality and survival. *Aliment Pharmacol Ther* 2006; **23**:1297–306.

Yao JC, Hassan M, Phan A, *et al*. One hundred years after 'carcinoid': epidemiology of and prognostic factors for neuroendocrine tumors in 35,825 cases in the United States. *J Clin Oncol* 2008; **26**:3063–72.

Colorectal cancer: introduction

Colorectal cancer (CRC) is a common and lethal cancer, comprising 13% of all cancers diagnosed in UK. Around two-thirds of the cancers arise in the colon and one-third in the rectum. However, the sigmoid colon and rectum account for more than half of the cases.

The cancer registry data from 2004 revealed the following site-specific distributions: rectum (29%), sigmoid colon (19%), caecum (13%), rectosigmoid junction (7%), ascending colon (5%), transverse colon (4%), splenic or hepatic flexures (4%), descending colon (2%), and other non-specified sites (17%) (Toms 2004).

Epidemiology
In 2004, 36,109 new cases were registered in the UK. Furthermore, 16,092 deaths from CRCs were reported in 2005. It is the second most common cause of cancer-related deaths after lung cancer. Age is a major risk factor for sporadic CRC.

Geographical variation
There is a significant worldwide geographical variation in the incidence of CRC. Highest rates are observed in the western countries and the lowest in parts of Africa and Asia. These appear to be attributable to differences in dietary and environmental exposures that are imposed upon a background of genetically determined susceptibility.

UK and Europe
In contrast to the USA, where the rates have fallen in the last two decades, the incidence of CRC in Europe is gradually increasing. Furthermore, the survival rates in UK are less than other European countries such as Scandinavia, the Netherlands, France, Germany, Italy, and Switzerland (Gatta et al. 2004). This is most likely related to better opportunities for screening in these countries (NICE-2004).

Age and incidence
The incidence of CRC increases with age with 83% of cases arising in people who are > 60 years. The annual incidence is 25 per 100,000 between the ages of 45–55 years. In contrast, the incidence rises by >10-fold to > 300 per 100,000 in people older than 75 years.

Sex distribution
These cancers are observed more frequently in men compared to women (1.2:1). The lifetime risk of men developing CRC in England and Wales is approximately 1 in 18 compared to 1 in 20 in women.

Aetiology
Multiple factors (dietary, environmental, and familial) play an aetiological role in the development of CRC. The majority (approximately two-thirds) of the tumours arise sporadically without any obvious predisposing factor. The remaining develop on the background of an increased familial risk (positive family history and hereditary CRC syndromes), and on the background of inflammatory bowel disease.

Colorectal polyps
• In approximately 80% of cases invasive cancer arises on the background of adenomatous polyp formation.
• Colorectal polyps are classified histologically as non-neoplastic (hyperplastic, inflammatory, hamartomatous) or neoplastic (adenomatous).
• Adenomatous polyps may be tubular (85%), tubulo-villous (15%), or villous (5%).
• The mean age of adenoma diagnosis is 10 years earlier than with carcinoma.
• Malignant potential of adenomatous polyps increases with size (>1cm), higher degrees of dysplasia, and increasing percentage of villous tissue within polyps.
• The risk of cancer development is approximately 4% after 5 years and 14% after 10 years. Villous adenomas have significantly higher risk (15–25% overall, but higher with size >2 cm).
• Risk factors that increase the probability of future malignant progression include male gender, presence of multiple/metachronous polyps, and positive family history of CRC.
• The progression of the adenoma–carcinoma sequence is characterized by the development of functional abnormalities in several genes that regulate important cellular functions, including proliferation and apoptosis. These processes promote development of an invasive phenotype. See Chapter 4.5.7, Colorectal cancer: genetics, screening, and prevention, (p.228).

Dietary risk factors
Previous epidemiological and experimental studies have demonstrated the presence of a possible relationship between dietary habits and risk of bowel cancer. Studies in migrant populations have suggested an increased risk with the adoption of Western dietary habits.

Fat and red meat
Consumption of a diet rich in animal saturated fat has been shown to increase the risk of developing bowel cancer.
• The EPIC study of 1,300 bowel cancer cases showed a significant 55% increase in risk for a 100g/day increase in consumption of red and processed meat (Larsson et al. 2006). Two recent meta-analyses reported a similar relationship between consumption of animal fat and bowel cancer (Norat et al. 2002).
• Excretion of faecal bile acids combined with their degradation into potential carcinogens by bacterial flora (e.g. Clostridium paraputrificum, anaerobic flora) have been proposed as possible factors.

Dietary fibre intake
• Dennis Burkitt first proposed that dietary fibre reduced the risk of bowel cancer by reducing the intestinal transit time and exposure of gut mucosa to potential carcinogens (Burkitt. 1972).
• The EPIC study showed a reduced risk of CRC with an increase in dietary fibre and the association was strongest for left-sided colon cancers. Interestingly, no risk reduction was observed for rectal cancers.
• However, results from a meta-analysis of prospective cohort studies failed to support this above association (Park et al. 2005).

Other dietary factors
• Meta-analysis of 14 pooled cohort studies showed a reduction in risk of distal colon cancer with an increased intake of fruit and vegetables (Koushik et al. 1996).
• Previous studies have also shown a reduced risk with an increased intake of folate, selenium, vitamin B6, calcium, and vitamin D.

Obesity and lifestyle

- Obesity increases the risk of bowel cancer. A recent meta-analysis showed a 25–50% increase in risk of colon cancer in overweight and obese men. The association was weaker in women, possibly related due to higher circulating levels of oestrogen (Moghaadam et al. 2007). See Chapter 3.1, Cancer prevention, p.18.
- Alcohol consumption has been shown to increase CRC risk by >40% (Cho et al. 2004).
- Smoking increases the risk of adenoma formation (up to 4-fold), but the association with CRC remains unclear. (Larsen et al. 2006). It may take three to four decades for increased risk of CRC to become apparent.

Familial risk factors

Approximately one-third of CRC cases have an underlying familial component (De la Chapelle. 2004). These include patients with positive family history, but no specific identifiable genetic mutation (undefined familial CRC), or patients with hereditary CRC syndromes characterized by well-defined germline mutations in particular gene subsets.

Undefined familial colorectal cancer

- Approximately 15–20% of patients present with a positive family history of CRC in the absence of a well-defined genetic abnormality.
- Presence of one affected first-degree relative is associated with a 2-fold higher risk of CRC, which doubles with two or more relatives. Risk is further enhanced with an affected younger relative (<45 years) and a family history of colon, rather than rectal, cancer.
- Inherited susceptibility is most likely due to genetic instability from low-penetrance/recessive mutations in genes regulating DNA repair and other important cellular functions.
- Previous observational studies have suggested that increased risk may be due to combined effect of genetic susceptibility and environmental factors (Kampman 2007).

Hereditary colorectal cancer syndromes (HCS)

The risk of CRC in major HCS is discussed as follows:

1 Familial adenomatous polyposis (FAP). AD inheritance; constitutes 1% of CRC; hundreds to thousands of polyps at young age (<35 years); deletions/mutations in APC gene (Wnt/wingless signalling pathway); 100% lifetime risk of CRC in 'classical' FAP; 20% lifetime risk in 'attenuated' FAP (Ashkenazi Jews); other associated tumours include duodenal adenoma, cerebral and thyroid tumours, medulloblastoma, and desmoids.

2 Hereditary non-polyposis colorectal cancer (HNPCC): AD inheritance; responsible for 3-5% of CRC; defects in mismatch repair (MMR) pathway leading to microsatellite instability; CRC at young age (<40 years); normal rate of adenoma formation but rapid rate of progression to carcinoma; 80% lifetime risk of CRC and 60% risk of endometrial cancer; other associated cancers include stomach, ovarian, small bowel, biliary, and kidney cancers.

3 Peutz–Jeghers syndrome: AD inheritance; constitutes <1% of CRC; STK11/LKB1 mutations; GI hamartomatous polyps combined with mucosal pigmentation develop during the first two decades of life; 39% lifetime risk of CRC; increased risk of gastric and pancreatic cancer.

Inflammatory bowel disease

IBD is associated with an increased risk of CRC. The overall prevalence of CRC in patients with UC is approximately 3.7% (Eaden et al. 2001). Patients with Crohn's disease who have associated colitis also have a similar risk of developing CRC.

Risk factors for CRC in IBD patients

- Duration of colitis is the most important factor. The cumulative incidence of CRC in UC patients is 2.5% after 20 years, 7.6% after 30 years, and 10.8% after 40 years of follow-up (Rutter et al. 2006).
- Extent of colonic involvement. A study of > 3000 UC patients in Sweden demonstrated a standardized incidence ratio (SIR) of 1.7 in patients with proctitis compared to 2.8 in left-sided colitis, and 14.8 in patients with pancolitis (Ekbom et al. 1990).
- Family history of CRC.
- Primary sclerosing cholangitis.

Further reading

Burkitt DP, Walker AR, Painter NS. Effect of dietary fibre on stools and the transit-times, and its role in the causation of disease. *Lancet.* 1972; **2**(7792):1408–12.

Cho E, Smith-Warner SA, Ritz J, et al. Alcohol intake and colorectal cancer: a pooled analysis of 8 cohort studies. *Ann Intern Med,* 2004; **140**(8):603–13.

De la Chapelle A.: Genetic predisposition to colorectal cancer. *Nat Rev* 2004; 4: 769–80.

Eaden JA, Abrams KR, Mayberry JF. The risk of colorectal cancer in ulcerative colitis: a meta-analysis. *Gut* 2001; **48**:526–35.

Ekbom A, Helmick C, Zack M, et al. Ulcerative colitis and colorectal cancer. A population-based study. *N Engl J Med* 1990; **323**: 1228–33.

Koushik A, Hunter DJ, Spiegelman D, et al. Fruits vegetables and colon cancer risk in a pooled analysis of 14 cohort studies. *J Natl Cancer Inst* JNCI 1996; **99**(19):147:1–83.

Kampman E. A first-degree relative with colorectal cancer: what are we missing? *Cancer Epidemiol Biomarkers Prev.* 2007; **16**(1):1–3.

Larsen IK, Grotmol T, Almendingen K, et al. Lifestyle as a predictor for colonic neoplasia in asymptomatic individuals. *BMC Gastroenterol* 2006; **6**:5.

Larsson, S.C, . and Wolk, A. Meat consumption and risk of colorectal cancer: a meta-analysis of prospective studies. *I J Cancer* 2006; **119** (11):2657–64.

Moghaddam A, Woodward M, Huxley R, et al. Obesity and risk of colorectal cancer: A meta-analysis of 30 studies with 70,000 events. *Cancer Epidemiol Biomarkers Prev,* 2007; **16**(12):2533–47.

NICE. *Improving Outcomes in Colorectal Cancers.* Manual Update, pp.8–11. London: NICE, 2004.

Norat T, Lukanova A, Ferrari P, et al. Meat consumption and colorectal cancer : dose-response meta-analysis of epidemiologic studies. *Int J Cancer* 2002; **98**(2):241–56.

Park Y, Hunter DJ, Spiegelman D, et al. Dietary fiber intake and risk of colorectal cancer: a pooled analysis of prospective cohort studies. *JAMA,* 2005; **294**(22):2849–57.

Rutter MD, Saunders BP, Wilkinson K, et al. Thirty-year analysis of a colonoscopic surveillance program for neoplasia in ulcerative colitis. *Gastroenterology* 2006; **130**:1030–1038.

Toms JR (ed). *CancerStats Monograph 2004.* London: Cancer Research UK, London 2004.

Colorectal cancer: genetics, screening, and prevention

Genetics

- A wealth of information is available on the complex genetic mechanisms prevalent in a CRC tumour cell. The understanding of these molecular mechanisms has provided considerable insight into the genetic events that regulate the multi-step process of colorectal carcinogenesis.
- Development of malignant potential involves procurement of specific cancer hallmarks by the tumour cell, including autonomous proliferation, resistance to apoptotic and immune mechanisms, and generation of an invasive and angiogenic phenotype.

Genomic instability

- Genomic instability promotes the development of a malignant phenotype by creating an environment in which subsequent mutations develop at rapid rate and allow the cell to gain autonomy and escape from normal cell regulatory mechanisms including cell cycle check points and apoptosis.
- The discordant and autonomous microenvironment of CRC can occur on a background of generalized chromosomal instability (CIN) which facilitates the development of various abnormalities (aneuploidy, allelic losses, amplifications, translocations, and mutation) in genes with important regulatory function.
- In addition, some cancers may develop from genomic instability arising from mutation in genes regulating the MMR pathway, which leads to detectable abnormality in segments of repetitive (microsatellite) DNA.
- Finally, a small minority of cancers may arise from epigenetic changes—methylation of promoter sequences—leading to a silencing of gene function.

Genomic instability in CRC

Most CRCs are acquired and develop from mutations or epigenetic changes in one or more of the genes regulating the two distinct pathways—CIN and microsatellite instability (MSI)—of genomic instability (see later section). Germline mutations in these genes give rise to the hereditary CRC syndromes (FAP and HNPCC).

CIN microsatellite stable (MSS) CRC

CRC arising 'classically' on the background of CIN is characterized by the development of sequential functional abnormalities in several genes including mutation/deletion of 5q (APC), ki-RAS, 18q and 17p (p53).

CIN and adenoma–carcinoma sequence

- Most CRCs arise from adenomatous polyps. Approximately 75–85% of CRCs arise on the background of CIN-associated genetic alterations, which stimulate the 'traditional pathway' of adenoma-carcinoma progression.
- Vogelstein et al (1988) first published the molecular analysis from 172 CRCs and outlined the genetic basis of a coordinated adenoma–carcinoma sequential progression observed in most tumours. (Vogelstein et al. 1988).
- The adenoma–carcinoma sequence is characterized by CIN and development of mutations in several important regulatory genes (e.g. APC, ki-ras, and TP53).
- Aberrant crypt foci arising sporadically usually develop on a background of activating ki-ras mutations that confer a cellular survival advantage. However, progression into adenoma requires development of additional abnormalities usually in the form of inactivating mutations of the APC/Wnt pathway. An environment of CIN is reinforced by the allelic loss of 18q and inhibition of important apoptotic and growth regulating proteins, including DCC, SMAD2, and SMAD4. Finally mutation of the 'gatekeeper' p53 heralds the progression into invasive phenotype.
- The sequential pathogenic molecular profile of FAP-associated CRC often follows this pattern. However, the incidence of k-ras mutation is significantly lower in early FAP-associated lesions. (Takayama. et al. 2001).
- However, most sporadic cancers do not incorporate the full complement of genetic changes mentioned earlier. This suggests the presence of other, as yet, undefined and pro-carcinogenic genetic mechanisms that possibly allow the bypass of some of the steps involved in the classical mutational sequence.

Adenomatous polyposis coli (APC) (5q21)

- APC gene is located on the long arm of chromosome 5 (band 21). It is large gene comprising 15 exons and several functional domains.
- APC mutations are usually associated with the generation of a truncated protein which has a reduced capacity for the binding and subsequent degradation of the β-catenin protein, an important component of the Wnt signalling pathway. Ineffectual degradation of β-catenin leads to constitutive activation of the Wnt pathway that plays a crucial role in the development of CRC.
- APC is a kinetochore-associated microtubular protein with a possible role in the organization and coordinated progression of mitosis. Loss of functional APC may promote CIN from a failure to arrest mitotic progression even in the presence of chromosome abnormalities.
- Patients with FAP are characterized by a germline mutation/deletion of one APC allele and development of thousands of polyps at a young age. Subsequent inactivation of the second allele initiates the development of CRC in these patients. Interestingly, the incidence of mutations in other known pro-carcinogenic genetic targets such as ki-ras is much lower, indicating the powerful influence that even relatively isolated APC mutations may have on CRC development. (Takayama et al. 2001). See Chapter 4.5, Hereditary colorectal cancer syndromes, p.227.
- APC mutations are observed in 60% of colonic and approximately 80% of rectal tumours. However, some sporadic cancers may develop in the absence of mutations involving the APC/Wnt pathway, indicating the presence of other independent pro-carcinogenic genetic mechanisms

k-ras (12p12)

- k-ras is GTP binding protein. In normal conditions ras is activated following ligand-binding and dimerization of EGFR. Activated ras transmits signals to the downstream MAPK/ERK and P-I3K/AKT pathways. The end result of this sequence of events is uncontrolled proliferation from an increased transcription of specific cell cycle proteins that stimulate progression through the G1/S restriction check point and inhibition of apoptosis.
- Mutations involving k-ras are commonly associated with loss of intrinsic GTPase activity which leads to an increase in GTP-bound and constitutively active ras.

- Tumour cells affected by activating k-ras mutations acquire survival advantage compared to their normal cell counterparts. However, development of invasive neoplasia is dependent on development of other sequential genetic events. (see later)
- Activating k-ras mutations are observed in >60% of aberrant crypt foci which represent the pre-adenomatous stage of colorectal carcinogenesis. In contrast, the incidence of k-ras mutations in adenomas and CRCs is much lower at approximately 35–40%. Furthermore, these mutations are infrequent in FAP-associated familial CRC. (Leslie et al. 2002).
- More recently, it has been shown that tumour k-ras status has important therapeutic and prognostic significance since only tumours with wild-type (wt)-ras proteomic profile respond to EGFR-targeted therapies. This is not surprising since a constitutively activated ras may 'fire' downstream proliferative signals independent of EGFR pathway. (De Reyniès A et al. 2008).
- This represents the first clinical use of a predictive marker (where k-ras mutant status determines the ineffectiveness of anti- EGFR therapy).

DCC, SMAD2, and SMAD4 (18q21)
- DCC, SMAD2, and SMAD4 genes are associated with the same locus on long arm of chromosome 18.
- DCC encodes a transmembrane receptor that promotes apoptosis whereas SMAD2 and SMAD4 represent components of the tumour growth factor (TGF)-β signalling pathway that regulates growth and differentiation.
- Sixty per cent of CRCs harbour allelic deletion at the chromosomal site of these genes.
- Germline mutations of SMAD2 are associated with juvenile polyposis syndrome that increases the risk of CRC.

p53 (17p13)
- p53 is a tumour suppressor protein that is stabilized and activated following DNA damage, leading to cell cycle arrest and facilitation of DNA repair. p53 also leads to induction of pro-apoptotic proteins and promotes cell death in the event of incomplete DNA repair.
- Genetic alterations acquired from other cellular mechanisms are non-sustainable in presence of wt-p53 because of p53-induced activation of the DNA repair or, alternatively, apoptotic pathways. In other words, for CIN to thrive, inactivation of p53 function is essential.
- Previous studies have shown that loss of p53 function from mutation or loss of heterozygosity (LOH) at 17p is related to the pathological stage of the lesion. p53 abnormalities are observed in 4–26% of adenomas, 50% of adenomas with invasive foci, and 50–75% of CRCs.
- p53 mutation in CRC development is usually a late event and indicates the transition into invasive stage.

Microsatellite instability
- In 1993, a report on another phenotypically distinct group of CRC was published. These tumours progressed more rapidly without a definitive adenoma–carcinoma transitional pattern. Furthermore, they had peculiar genetic features characterized by MSI from inactivating mutations in genes regulating the MMR pathway.
- Approximately 15–20% of CRC cases arise on the background of MSI and can be classified into the MSI-high (MSI-H) and MSI-low (MSI-L) subgroups based on the proportion of microsatellite lesions. (Worthley et al. 2007).

- Cancers arising on the background of MSI are characterisized by abnormalities of the MMR system composed of at least seven different proteins. hMLH1 and hMSH2 represent the two most important proteins which associate with other molecules to form functional heterodimers.
- Defective MMR induces errors in DNA replication that primarily affect the short-repeat DNA sequences (microsatellites). MSI is characterized by detectable abnormalities with these microsatellite sequences.
- MSI is defined in relation to a standardized panel of short-repeat DNA sequences—five in total (two mono- and three di-nucleotides)—that was developed to achieve uniformity of research and clinical practice.
- MSI-H phenotype is characterized by presence of abnormalities within two or more (≥40%) of the five specified sites. In contrast, MSI-L phenotype is associated with presence of mutation within one specified site, and MSS phenotype with no detectable mutation at any of the specified sites. (Worthley et al. 2007).
- Most MSI-H cancers are sporadic in origin and are related to epigenetic silencing of the hMLH1 gene. However, such cancers may also arise following germline mutation of the critical MMR genes (hMSH2 and hMLH1) as is observed in the HNPCC (Lynch syndrome). See Chapter 4.5, Hereditary colorectal cancer syndromes, p.227.

Molecular staging and 'genetic signatures'
- Scientific research in the field of CRC has been recently dominated by attempts at identifying specific genetic 'fingerprints' that may provide useful prognostic and therapeutic information. Identification of typical predictive patterns of gene expression may aid in selecting patients for a particular treatment.
- Using cDNA microarray technology in 78 CRC tissue samples, Eschrich et al (2005) identified 43 core genes with a 90% accuracy of predicting long- term survival. Furthermore, molecular staging was more accurate in predicting prognosis compared to conventional Dukes staging, especially for stage B and C patients (Eschrich et al. 2005).

Screening
- Previous research has demonstrated that screening performed to a high standard in a large population can potentially reduce CRC mortality rates by 15%.
- The U.S. Preventive Services Task Force (USPSTF) first laid down recommendations for CRC screening in 1996. More recently, these guidelines were updated as a joint effort of the USPSTF, the American Cancer Society (ACS), and the American College of Radiology. (Levin et al. 2008).
- The Advisory Committee on Cancer Prevention in the European Union endorsed mass screening for CRC in 2001. (Micksche et al. 2001).
- Since 90% of sporadic CRCs occur in people >50 years, most current screening programmes target the specific population subgroup ranging from 50–69 years. Earlier age of screening is recommended for high-risk individuals with other associated factors (e.g. familial, IBD, etc.).

UK CRC screening initiative
- The implementation of a screening programme in the UK has lagged behind the rest of Western Europe which is reflected in the higher CRC-associated mortality in this country compared to Denmark, France, Finland, and Austria.

- Recognizing the importance of CRC screening for improving patient outcomes, the NHS Cancer Plan (2000) proposed a strategic development of CRC screening services for the provision of a robust community-based screening programme. It recommended the use of a pilot study to evaluate the feasibility of faecal occult blood (FOB) testing and subsequent colonoscopy in the 50–69- year old population subgroup (DOH 2000).
- This initiative led to the development of the NHS Bowel Cancer Screening Programme in 2006. The current and future planned provisions of this service are specified in the DOH document on the Cancer Reform Strategy (DOH 2007).
- Implementation of the first phase involved setting up 15 screening centres (2006–2007) and a further 20 centres are expected to roll out as part of the second phase.
- By the end of October 2007, approximately 575,000 FOB kits were dispatched from which >50% were returned. Approximately 5500 were positive requiring further assessment. Colonoscopy was performed in 3,500 individuals with over >1600 polypectomies and detection of cancer in 400 patients.
- The NHS Bowel Screening Programme (NBSP) is currently targeted at the population in the range of 60–69 years. It aims to include those from 70–75 years by the year 2010, followed by a service review to decide on extension to the 50–60 year subgroup.

Screening protocols
- Previous studies have investigated the diagnostic utility of various procedures, including digital rectal examination (DRE), FOB, endoscopic (sigmoidoscopy and colonoscopy), and radiological assessment (e.g. double-contrast barium enema) for the early detection and prevention of CRC.
- More recently, other modern technologies, including faecal immunochemical testing (FIT), stool DNA (sDNA), and CT colonography have undergone evaluation for their possible use in CRC screening.

Digital rectal examination
- The potential sensitivity of screening DRE is low with < 10% of cases of CRC within reach of the examining finger. This limits the usefulness of DRE as a potential screening tool for CRC.
- A US case–control study found no difference in the frequency of DRE—during the preceding year prior to diagnosis—in CRC patients who died of their disease and selected matched controls (Herrinton et al. 1995).

Faecal occult blood test (FOBT)
- Guaiac-based FOBT detects the pseudoperoxidase activity of the iron-containing prosthetic subgroup haem. Different commercial kits are available for home-based use (e.g. Haemoccult ®). Patients with a positive test require further assessment such as colonoscopy or barium enema.
- Commonly used protocols recommend testing on three different days to improve sensitivity and prevent sampling error. A single-office FOBT is less sensitive detecting only 58% of cancers compared to those detected after a 3-card test. Test sensitivity may also be improved by sample rehydration.
- Sensitivity of a single unrehydrated FOBT for cancer is approximately 40%; its specificity seems to range

from 96–98%. Rehydration increases sensitivity to 50–60% (Pignone et al. 2002).
- Three randomized studies have demonstrated a significant reduction in CRC-associated mortality rates following the use of FOBT in the general population. The Minnesota trial, that employed a 3-card rehydrated test, showed a 33% and 21% cumulative reduction in mortality at 18 years of follow-up after annual and biennial screening, respectively. Similarly, two European studies (UK and Denmark) have shown a 15–18% reduction in mortality following the use of a biennial 3-card unrehydrated FOBT screening protocol.
- Based on this evidence, the NBSP incorporates screening with FOBT at biennial intervals. In contrast, the US screening guidelines recommend FOBT to be performed at annual intervals.
- One of the important caveats of using FOBT as an initial screening tool is the presence of false-positives leading to the performance of unnecessary colonoscopies. Similarly, a false-negative result may be falsely assuring.

Sigmoidoscopy
- One small randomized Norwegian study (800 individuals aged 50–59 years) of flexible sigmoidoscopy (FS) as a one time screening procedure demonstrated >50% reduction in CRC-associated mortality compared to no intervention. Similarly, a retrospective case–control study reported a 56% reduction in mortality following FS. It has been reported that one-time screening with FS can detect up to 70–80% of advanced neoplastic polyps and cancer. (Pignone et al. 2002).
- Previous randomized studies have shown that addition of sigmoidoscopy to FOBT doubles the detection rate of significant adenomas and cancer.
- USPSTF screening guidelines endorse FS as an acceptable screening procedure. It is recommended that FS should be performed every 5 years.

Colonoscopy
- Colonoscopy has been reported to have sensitivity of >90% for cancer and large adenomas and 75% for smaller adenomas (<1cm). The role of colonoscopy as a screening procedure has not been addressed in a randomized trial.
- The US National Polyp Study reported that approximately 75–90% of cancers can be prevented by regular colono scopies. Müller and Sonnenberg et al. (1995) reported on a case–control study that showed an approximately 60% reduction in CRC-associated mortality in patients with a previous colonoscopy.
- Colonoscopy is widely accepted as the gold standard for the diagnosis of CRC. However, it does not merit a similar status for CRC screening—except in high-risk patients (see below)—due to lack of randomized evidence, invasive nature, associated complications (e.g. perforation), poor adherence, and limited availability.
- USPSTF guidelines recommend that colonoscopy should be performed every 10 years.

Double- contrast barium enema
- There are no studies that have assessed the role of DCBE in reducing the incidence and death from CRC cancer.
- The accuracy of DCBE in diagnosing colorectal lesions has been compared to colonoscopy. The sensitivity of

DCBE for polyps <0.5cm is 32%; 53% for polyps 0.6–1cm; and 48% for polyps >1cm.

- USPSTF guidelines recommend that patients undergoing DCBE as a screening procedure should have it repeated every 5 years.

Faecal immunochemical test (FIT)

- Standard guaiac-based FOBT has relatively poor sensitivity and specificity which is further disadvantaged by dietary modulation from ingestion of red meat and certain peroxidase-containing vegetables. In contrast, FIT is based on the detection of globin moiety which is more sensitive and not affected by dietary habits.
- Several observational studies have reported improved sensitivity with the use of FIT. In a comparison study, FIT identified 50% more cancers and 256% more high-risk adenomas than guaiac-based FOBT (Guittet et al. 2007). This has led to many organizations around the world endorsing the use of FIT for screening purposes, despite the lack of randomized evidence.
- At the currently employed analytical threshold, FIT is associated with lower specificity (significantly higher false- positives) that will limit its usefulness in public screening programmes. It has been previously reported that 47 false-positive results would be required to detect 1 extra case of invasive CRC, and 2.2 false-positive results would be required to detect 1 extra advanced adenoma.
- In an attempt to reduce the number of false-positives and improve the future applicability of FIT, the Scottish Bowel Screening Centre proposed a two-tier reflex screening algorithm in which positive FOBT is followed by FIT prior to colonoscopy. In an observational study of 1124 individuals following this algorithm approximately 40% with a positive FIT were found to have cancer or high-risk polyps compared to <5% with negative FIT (Fraser GC et al. 2007).

Other modern technologies

- A prospective, multicentre study of stool DNA analysis—using a multitarget DNA testing panel—in 4404 participants demonstrated a 52% sensitivity for cancer detection. (Imperiale et al. 2004). Other small observational studies have shown 62–91% sensitivity for cancer detection with rates independent of cancer stage and site.
- Analysis of stool DNA has been approved by the USPSTF as one of the options for CRC screening. However, the optimal screening interval for stool DNA testing remains undefined.
- CT colonography is now regarded as an acceptable non-invasive substitute for colonoscopy in the diagnosis of CRC. Recently, it gained USPSTF approval for CRC screening with recommended interval duration of 5 years.

Screening in high-risk individuals

- First- degree relatives of individuals diagnosed with CRC or adenomatous polyps at <50 years should have colonoscopy starting at 40 years or 10 years earlier than the age of previous diagnosis, whichever came first. Subsequent examinations should be repeated at 5 years.
- Patients suspected of hereditary CRC syndromes should have first colonoscopy around the second to third decade followed by every 1–3 years.

- First colonoscopy in patients with IBD is recommended at 8–10 years after diagnosis and should be repeated every 1–3 years.

Prevention

- NSAIDs—by virtue of their ability to inhibit COX-2 enzyme—have undergone extensive investigation for their possible role in preventing adenoma formation and subsequent CRC development.
- In a prospective cohort of 662,424 patients enrolled in the ACS Cancer Prevention Study II, risk of colon cancer death decreased about 40% with the use of aspirin. Similarly, two randomized trials confirmed that aspirin reduces risk of colorectal adenomas. (Burt et al. 2004).
- However, in the Physicians Health Study of 22,000 men aged 40–84 years, who were randomly assigned to receive placebo or aspirin (325mg every other day) for 5 years, no reduction in invasive cancer or adenoma development was observed at a median follow-up of 4.5 years (Gann et al. 1993). The relatively lower dose and shorter duration of aspirin used in the study may have contributed to the negative outcome. Furthermore, the risk of GI-associated complications has limited the widespread use of NSAIDs as chemopreventive agents.
- Use of HRT and oral contraceptives has also been shown to reduce the risk of CRC development. Previous meta-analyses have shown an approximately 20% reduction in risk of CRC with the use of these agents. (Burt et al. 2004).

Further reading

Burt RW, Winawer SJ, Bond JH, et al. *Preventing Colorectal Cancer: A Clinicians' guide.* The American Gastroenterology Association, 2004.

De Reyniès A, Boige V, et al. KRAS mutation signature in colorectal tumours significantly overlaps with the cetuximab response signature. *J Clin Oncol* 2008; **26**(13):2228–30.

DOH. *NHS Cancer Plan.* London: Department of Health, 2000.

DOH. *Cancer Reform Strategy.* London: Department of Health, 2007.

Eschrich S, Yang I, Bloom GC, et al. Molecular staging for survival prediction of colorectal cancer patients. *J Clin Oncol* 2005; **23**:3526–35.

Fraser GC, Mathew CM, Mowat NA,GC et al. Evaluation of a card collection-based faecal immunochemical test in screening for colorectal cancer using a two-tier reflex approach. *Gut* 2007 **56**: 1343–44.

Gann PH, Manson JE, Glynn RJ, et al. Low-dose aspirin and incidence of colorectal tumours in a randomised trial. *J Natl Cancer Inst.* 1993; **85**(15):1220–4.

Garassino MC, Farina G, Rossi A, et al. Should KRAS mutations be considered an independent prognostic factor in patients with advanced colorectal cancer treated with cetuximab? *J Clin Oncol* 2008 May 20; **26**(15):2600.

Guittet L, Bouvier V, Mariotte N, et al. Comparison of a guaiac based and an immunochemical faecal occult blood test in screening for colorectal cancer in a general average risk population. *Gut* 2007; **56**:210–14.

Herrinton LJ, Selby JV, Friedman GD, et al. Case control study of digital-rectal screening in relation to mortality from cancer of the distal rectum. *Am J Epidemiol.* 1995; **142**:961–4.

Imperiale TF, Ransohoff DF, Itzkowitz SH, et al. Faecal DNA versus faecal occult blood for colorectal-cancer screening in an average-risk population. *N Engl J Med* 2004 **351**(26):2704–14.

Levin B, Lieberman DA, McFarland B, et al. Screening and surveillance for the early detection of colorectal cancer and adenomatous polyps: joint guideline from the ACS, USPSTF and Task Force on Colorectal Cancer, and the American College of Radiology. *CA Cancer J Clin* 2008; **58**:130–60.

Micksche M, Lynge E, Diehl V, *et al.* Recommendations pour le dépistage du cancer dans l'Union Eurpéenne [Recommendations on cancer screening in the European Union]. *Bull Cancer.* 2001; **88**:687–92.

Müller AD, Sonnenberg A. Protection by endoscopy against death from colorectal cancer, A case-control study among veterans. *Arch Intern Med.* 1995; **155**(16):1741–8.

Pignone M, Rich M, Teutsch SM, *et al.* Screening for colorectal cancer in adults at average risk: A Summary of the Evidence for the U.S. Preventive Services Task Force. *Ann Intern Med.* 2002; **137**:132–41.

Takayama T, Katsuki S, Takahashi Y, *et al.* Analysis of K-ras, APC, and beta-catenin in aberrant crypt foci in sporadic adenoma, cancer, and familial adenomatous polyposis. *Gastroenterology* 2001; **121**:599–611.

Vogelstein B, Fearon ER, Hamilton SR, *et al.* Genetic alterations during colorectal-tumour development. *N Engl J Med* 1988; **319**: 525–32.

Worthley DL, Whitehall VL, Spring KJ, *et al.* Colorectal carcinogenesis: road maps to cancer. *World J Gastroenterol.* 2007; **13**(28):3784–91.

Colorectal cancer: clinical features, diagnosis, and staging

Clinical features

Approximately 5–20% of cancers are asymptomatic and diagnosed during the course of screening procedures. Cancers that present as an emergency, with symptoms of obstruction and perforation, carry a worse prognosis. The remaining cancers often present in the primary setting with symptoms that may be difficult to distinguish from benign causes.

Rectal bleeding

Rectal bleeding is an important presenting symptom (in 20–58% of patients). However, it is also observed in 14–33% of the general population and is mostly from benign causes (Hamilton et al. 2005). Patients with bleeding observed in the presence of one or more of the following features should be urgently referred for further investigations (Hamilton, et al. 2005):

• Increasing age (>50 years).
• Change in bowel habit and abdominal pain.
• Positive FOB test.
• Passage of dark blood mixed with stools.
• Isolated rectal bleeding without anal symptoms. Presence of anal symptoms (soreness, lump, pruritus) may indicate other benign causes (fissure, haemorrhoids). However, it is important to note that rectal tumours also present with local symptoms (pain, tenesmus, pruritus).

Change in bowel habit

Many patients (39–85%) with CRC will experience change in bowel habit. Prevalence of bowel irregularity (constipation or diarrhoea) ranges from 10–25% in the general UK population. The following clinical features increase the probability of underlying CRC:

• Recent change in bowel habit, especially in older patients.
• History of passage of blood or mucus should be urgently referred for specialist opinion.
• History of persistent new onset diarrhoea (increased frequency or looseness).

Abdominal pain

• Prevalence of CRC in patients presenting with unexplained abdominal pain is 1%.
• Abdominal pain in a patient with CRC may be a sign of impending obstruction.
• Colicky abdominal pain combined with other obstructive symptoms (abdominal distension, nausea and vomiting) should be urgently investigated.

Other symptoms

• Chronic blood loss: iron-deficiency anaemia, tiredness, lassitude; more frequently observed in right-sided tumours.
• Abdominal mass: sign of advanced disease; right iliac fossa lump classically observed in caecal carcinoma.
• Rectal mass: DRE may reveal a palpable mass in low/mid rectal tumours.
• Weight loss, loss of appetite: suggestive of advanced/metastatic disease.

Emergency presentation

• Up to 20% of tumours may present as an emergency with obstruction or perforation/peritonitis.

• Worse prognosis.
• Sixty per cent of these patients would have seen the GP previously with one or more symptoms suggestive of CRC.
• Abdominal pain, weight loss, diarrhoea and anaemia are more common in this group (Cleary et al. 2007).

Features of hereditary colorectal syndrome-associated CRC

Diagnosis of one of the HCS should be suspected in presence of one or more of the following:

• Early age of onset (<40 years).
• Presence of multiple (>10) polyps.
• Synchronous or metachronous cancers (CRC or other associated).
• Positive family history for one or more of these features.

Features of CRC in inflammatory bowel disease

• Younger patients.
• Higher proportion of invasive tumours arising from flat non-polypoidal lesions.
• Higher frequency of tumours with mucinous and signet ring histology.
• Multifocality with higher rate of two or more synchronous primaries.

Diagnosis

History and physical examination

• Detailed history of onset and duration of local and systemic symptoms.
• Identify patients at risk of obstruction.
• Family history to identify patients with familial predisposition and hereditary CRC syndromes. Clinical suspicion of genetic susceptibility may have important implications for other members of the family. See Chapter 4.5, Colorectal cancer: genetics, screening, and prevention, p.228.
• Complete physical examination including DRE.

Endoscopy

Flexible sigmoidoscopy (FS)

• First most appropriate investigation for most patients.
• Diagnostic reach of 60cm (assess lesions in rectum, sigmoid and descending colon).
• Patients with rectal bleeding or change in bowel habit have a 0.2% risk of possible bowel neoplasm after negative FS (Anwar et al. 2004).
• Diagnostic assessment of rectal lesions should include evaluation of the length, position (distance of AV), and mobility of the primary tumour.
• Low risk of complications and is relatively easy and quick to perform.

Colonoscopy

• Employed to assess the colon beyond the reach of the sigmoidoscope
• Performed following a negative FS in patients with persistent bowel symptoms, especially abdominal pain and weight loss.
• Initial investigation in patients with history suggestive of right-sided lesions (anaemia, tiredness, abdominal pain).

- Average risk of perforation is 0.1–0.2%. However, this may be as low as 0.02% with surgeons performing at least 3 procedures per week or 100–200 per annum. Furthermore, increasing experience is associated with higher completion rates (Dafnis G, et al 2000).

Barium enema
- Less risk of complications, but also reduced diagnostic sensitivity compared to colonoscopy.
- Least preferred choice of patients compared to FS, colonoscopy and CT colonography (Taylor S, 2003).
- Use of barium enema in the diagnosis of CRC has significantly declined following the optimization and widespread availability of endoscopic procedures.

CT colonography
CT colonography (virtual colonoscopy) has greater accuracy than barium enema and is possibly as sensitive as colonoscopy for detection of larger polyps. A meta-analysis of data from 14 studies with a total of 1324 patients demonstrated an overall specificity of 95% for the detection of polyps ≥10mm (Sosna J, et al. 2003).

Endoscopic-guided biopsy
Patients should have endoscopic-guided biopsy to establish a diagnosis of colon cancer. Most CRC are adenocarcinomas exhibiting CK20 and CK7 positivity. Other histological variants include mucinous, squamous, signet-ring-cell, and neuroendocrine carcinomas.

Staging
Laboratory tests
Full blood count, liver function tests and urea and electrolytes should all be performed. A variety of serum markers have been associated with CRC, particularly CEA, and CA 19-9. However, these markers have a low diagnostic ability to detect primary CRC due to overlap with benign disease and low sensitivity. Non-cancer-related causes of an elevated CEA include gastritis, diverticulitis, liver disease, diabetes, and any acute or chronic inflammatory state.

Local staging of rectal tumours
MRI scanning
- Patients with rectal tumours should undergo an MRI scan to define the local extent of primary tumour.
- MRI helps in defining the relationship of primary tumour with mesorectal fascia and also identifies the presence of pelvic lymphadenopathy.
- Distance of <2mm between the primary tumour and mesorectal fascia is predictive of potential involvement of circumferential resection margin (CRM) (<1mm) following surgery.
- A large multicentre study (MERCURY) prospectively evaluated the correlation between preoperative MRI-predicted resection margin and the pathological outcome. In patients proceeding to curative resection the correlation between MRI-predicted clear margins (>1mm from mesorectal fascia) and pathological outcome (R0) was 0.92, with an observed agreement of 84% (MERCURY study group. 2006).

Rectal endosonography (RE)
- Sensitive technique for diagnosis of early rectal lesions. Previous studies have reported diagnostic accuracy of 76–100%.

- RE may be employed to differentiate between various early rectal lesions (Tcis, T1, T2). The depth of submucosa involvement can predict early T1 lesions (superficial one-third of submucosa) which may be amenable to local excision.

Exclusion of metastatic disease
- CT of thorax, abdomen, and pelvis is the most commonly performed investigation to exclude metastatic spread.
- Ultrasonography (USG) may be employed to assess metastatic spread to the liver. USG has low sensitivity (50–76%) compared to CT scan (>90%) for assessment of liver disease.
- There is no definitive evidence to support the routine use of PET/CT in staging of CRC. There is however a role for PET scanning when initial imaging is inconclusive for excluding metastatic disease, and for evaluation of patients who are thought to be candidates for resection of isolated CRC liver metastases

Staging protocols (Table 4.5.4)
The two most commonly employed staging protocols include the Dukes and TNM (AJCC/UICC) systems which divide the tumour into prognostic categories based on the extent of primary tumour, locoregional nodal involvement and the presence of metastatic disease.

The failure to address the resection margin status and the presence of residual tumour is a major limitation of these staging systems. Therefore, additional descriptors are used in conjunction with the TNM classification. These include classification of tumours on the basis of residual tumour (R) and vascular invasion (V).

The Royal College of Pathologists has recently published a national minimum dataset and methodology (RCPath). This proforma-based method of reporting results in the most complete data capture. The document described the techniques for assessment of the CRM for rectal cancer resections which is considered involved if microscopic tumour is present ≤1mm from the radial resection margin.

Molecular assays such as the Oncotype-DX may be used in combination with other pathological criteria to predict risk of recurrence. There is some evidence that failure to

Table 4.5.4 Staging protocols

Tcis: carcinoma *in situ* T1: confined to submucosa T2: invades muscularis propria (MP)	Stage I	Dukes A
T3: penetrates through MP (subserosa, mesorectum) T4: serosal surface, invasion of other structures	Stage II	Dukes B
N0: no nodal involvement N1: 1–3 nodes involved N2: 4 or more nodes involved	Stage III	Dukes C*
M0: no metastatic disease M1: metastatic disease	Stage IV	Dukes D

* C1= no apical nodes involved, C2=apical nodes

respond to EGFR inhibitors such as cetuximab may be associated with mutations in the BRAF gene.

Further reading

Anwar R, Flashman K, O'Leary DP, et al. Probability of proximal cancers of the rectum and left colon to 60cm in patients presenting with rectal bleeding to a surgical outpatient clinic. *Colorectal Disease* 2002; **4**(Suppl.1):47.

Cleary J, Peters TJ, Sharp D, et al. Clinical features of colorectal cancer before emergency presentation: a population-based case-control study. *Fam Pract* 2007; **24**:3–6.

Dafnis G, Blomqvist P, Pahlman L, et al. The introduction and development of colonoscopy within a defined population in Sweden. *Scand J Gastroenterol* 2000; **7**:765–71.

Hamilton W, Round A, Sharp D, et al. Clinical features of colorectal cancer before diagnosis: a population-based case-control study. *Br J Cancer* . 2005; **93**(4):399–405.

MERCURY Study Group. Diagnostic accuracy of preoperative magnetic resonance imaging in predicting curative resection of rectal cancer: prospective observational study. *BMJ* 2006; **14**:779.

NICE. *Improving Outcomes in Colorectal Cancers. Manual Update,* pp.30–1. London: NICE, 2004.

Royal College of Pathologists. Standards and Datasets for Reporting Cancers: Dataset for colorectal cancer (2nd edition) September 2007—available at: http://www.rcpath.org/resources/pdf/G049ColorectalDataset-Sep07.pdf

Sosna J, Morrin MM, Kruskal JB, et al. CT colonography of colorectal polyps: a metaanalysis. *Am J Roentgenol* 2003; **181**:1593–8.

Taylor S, Halligan S, Saunders B, et al. Acceptance by patients of multidetector CT colonography compared with barium enema examinations, flexible sigmoidoscopy, and colonoscopy. *Am J Roentgenol* 2003; **181**:913–21.

Colorectal cancer: treatment of localized disease

Surgery is the mainstay of treatment for localized CRC. For optimal results this should be performed by specialist surgeons, working within a dedicated MDT. Outcomes (e.g. survival, local recurrence, and histopathological prognostic measures) should be audited regularly to ensure a high-quality service.

Preparation for surgery

Patients require staging investigations prior to surgery. These aim to assess the local extent of disease, to exclude distant metastases and to identify any synchronous primary lesions elsewhere in the large intestine. In colon cancer, CT scanning of the chest, abdomen, and pelvis is the standard means of assessing the primary and looking for metastases (PET-CT at present is not standard) and colonoscopy or CT virtual colonography can all be used to assess the remainder of the large intestine. For rectal cancer, CT is used to identify distant metastases but pelvic MRI is the current standard for assessing local disease extent, by showing the tumour's relationship to the expected plane of resection. Endoscopic ultrasound is of use in the selection of early rectal tumours for local treatment.

There is evidence that preoperative antibiotic prophylaxis (usually with a cephalosporin and metronidazole) reduces postoperative infection. Patients also require thromboembolism prophylaxis (usually with low- molecular- weight heparin and graded compression stockings), anaesthetic assessment, and blood cross-match. The use of mechanical bowel preparation is controversial but it is performed less commonly than in the past due to concerns over dehydration. Patients are usually catheterized in theatre before the operation begins.

There is some debate concerning perioperative blood transfusion, which some believe can increase cancer relapse rates. Current practice is to be cautious about transfusing unless absolutely necessary.

Technique

Radical excision of a colonic tumour, along with the appropriate vascular pedicle and accompanying lymph nodes, is the standard approach to gaining local control and acquiring important prognostic information about nodal spread. Occasionally, a more limited procedure may be required in an unfit patient, or one with incurable disease, where relief of obstruction is the main purpose of the procedure.

The arterial supply to the segment of bowel to be resected determines the length of bowel removed. Ideally 5cm of normal bowel will be taken proximal and distal to the tumour.

Colon cancer

Elective procedures:

Right hemicolectomy

Tumours of the caecum, ascending colon and proximal transverse colon are removed by a right hemicolectomy. This involves division of the ileo-colic artery, right colic artery, and right branches of the middle colic artery. If the main branch of the middle colic artery is also taken then the remainder of the transverse colon is removed (an 'extended right hemicolectomy'). Included in the specimen will be the distal 10cm of the ileum.

Left hemicolectomy

Tumours of the descending and upper sigmoid colon are removed using a left hemicolectomy. This involves resection of the inferior mesenteric artery near its origin on the aorta.

The ideal procedure for tumours at the splenic flexure is less certain, since this is at the boundary between vessels supplied from the superior mesenteric and inferior mesenteric arteries. There is also heterogeneity between individuals as to the predominant feeder blood vessel. Technique is therefore individualized based on anatomy and the need to have well- vascularized bowel ends for the anastomosis.

Rectal cancer

Sphincter preservation and surgical approaches

Tumours of the distal sigmoid and mid to upper rectum are usually removed by an anterior resection. Lower rectal tumours also require removal of the anal canal (known as an abdomino-perineal resection), which then necessitates a permanent stoma. To avoid this, there has been a trend for lower anastomoses, joining the colon ever closer to the anal canal. These procedures require considerable skill and can be limited by increased complication rates (such as anastomotic leakage) and relatively poor functional results unless performed by experienced surgeons. It is important that such procedures are oncologically sound and do not unnecessarily increase the risk of residual disease.

Development of total mesorectal excision (TME)

For many years the results of surgery alone were poor in rectal cancer. Local recurrence rates were >20%. With the growing realization that involvement of the circumferential resection margin was predictive for local recurrence, the concept of total mesorectal excision (TME) developed. This procedure removes not just the rectum but also the surrounding envelope of fatty tissue (mesorectum). Evidence that this improves surgical results comes directly from individual surgical series, population- based studies and within the context of recently published, randomized-controlled trials. Current rates of local recurrence for surgery alone are often <10%.

Temporary stomas

Many patients having surgery for rectal cancer will require a temporary stoma. This allows the new pelvic anastomosis to heal and reduces the sequelae of any anastomotic leak.

Role of radiotherapy

Radiotherapy has a long track record in rectal cancer, with clear evidence from meta-analyses and randomized trials that it reduces local recurrence rates when used in combination with surgery. This is discussed in more detail in Chapter 4.5, Colorectal cancer: adjuvant treatment., p.240.

Quality of life

There is an increasing appreciation that treatments for rectal cancer can adversely affect patients' QoL. Bowel function is frequently abnormal following rectal surgery and this dysfunction can be increased further by adjuvant radiotherapy. Sexual function can also be affected (with radiotherapy and/or surgery potentially causing erectile dysfunction, low sperm counts, early menopause), dyspareunia, vaginal stenosis, and vaginal dryness. Combined with the adverse effect of a stoma on body image, many patients are starting to ask if less aggressive approaches can be taken to avoid the morbidity of treatment. One approach is to adopt a non-surgical or less aggressive surgical approach to early rectal cancers. Using a combination of endoscopic resection, external beam (chemo) radiotherapy and contact radiotherapy (applied directly to the rectum per-anally) some patients are spared a stoma. However, no direct comparison to the 'gold-standard' surgical techniques has been made and clinical trials are required to determine the benefits and risks.

Surgery for early stage disease

As screening for CRC increases in the UK, an increasing number of tumours are being discovered at an earlier stage of their development. Frequently, pre-malignant polyps are also identified. Many of these lesions can now be removed endoscopically using a variety of dissection techniques.

Benign polyps or very early T1 lesions can be removed by endoscopic mucosal resection (EMR), where saline is infiltrated into the base of a lesion (to raise it away from underlying layers) and it is then resected with diathermy or a hot loop. This technique can be applied around the whole colon at colonoscopy.

Transanal endoscopic microsurgery (TEMS) is another way of removing lesions up to 20cm from the anal verge. It uses a specially designed 40-mm diameter operating rectoscope with a three-dimensional, magnified optical system. Unlike EMR, TEMS allows a full-thickness excision to be performed. Nevertheless, it is an insufficient treatment on its own for all but the earliest rectal cancers because it fails to remove local lymph nodes and local recurrence rates are higher than with classical approaches.

Anastomotic technique

Anastomoses can be formed using a variety of stapling devices or by hand-sewing. For a long-time surgeons had individual preferences, but recent evidence suggests that staples produce fewer leaks and are otherwise very similar. They are therefore used increasingly.

Laparoscopic surgery

Laparoscopic surgery has become standard for many indications such as cholecystectomy and Nissen fundoplication. There has therefore been considerable enthusiasm for using the same techniques in colorectal surgery. However, it requires considerable experience and training to do well, takes longer in theatre, and is probably more expensive overall. No significant differences in terms of DFS rate, local recurrence rate, mortality, morbidity, anastomotic leakage, resection margins, or recovered lymph nodes have been found. There are however some important short-term benefits, including less blood loss, quicker return to normal diet, less pain, less narcotic use, and slightly shorter average stays in hospital. In the longer term, incisional hernias and adhesions are also reduced. Given the equivalent oncological outcomes, this has encouraged wider adoption of this approach.

Emergency procedures

In the UK, about 20% of patients with colon cancer present as an emergency. Commonly, this is with an obstructed bowel, but bleeding and perforation can also be responsible.

Ideally such patients should be treated in a unit where they can be seen and operated on by a specialist colorectal surgeon. Following resuscitation and initial investigations to establish the cause of the problem (which may include plain films, CT, endoscopy, or water soluble enemas) different options exist for treatment.

Surgical

Obstruction

The bowel is initially decompressed before proceeding. Right- sided obstruction is then usually dealt with by a right hemicolectomy. However, several options are available for left-sided lesions. These include a two-stage procedure using Hartmann's operation to bring out an end proximal colostomy with closure of the distal segment. The stoma may then be closed later if appropriate. Alternatively, some surgeons attempt one-stage procedures with anastomosis following resection (mainly for colonic tumours).

Perforation

Caecal perforation, due to a distal tumour, is usually treated by right hemicolectomy. When the cancer itself perforates, the resection can be technically demanding. For left-sided lesions a Hartmann's procedure is usually required.

Stenting

Emergency surgery has a high perioperative mortality rate, often reflecting the advanced stage of disease, electrolyte disturbances, poor nutritional state, and unprepared bowel that can be present. Recently there has been considerable interest in the use of endoscopically-deployed stents as either primary treatment, for those unfit for surgery, or as a 'bridge to surgery,' for those whose condition could be improved if the obstruction was relieved. Subsequent elective resection can then more safely include primary anastomosis.

Stents are expensive, require expertise to be inserted, and can cause various problems such as perforation, pain, bleeding, re-obstruction, and distal migration. Their cost is offset, however, by avoidance of subsequent stoma formation and shorter hospital stays. They can also be invaluable for the management of patients who would have been at high risk with conventional emergency surgery.

Postoperative care

Following surgery, postoperative care has traditionally been similar to that of other patients undergoing abdominal surgery. Analgesia has usually been provided with opiates, in a patient-driven system, for the first few days. Intravenous fluids have been used initially but oral intake has been gradually increased as normal bowel function returns (audible bowel sounds and passage of flatus). Patients have slowly been mobilized when they feel able to.

However, there has been a trend in recent years to develop 'enhanced recovery programmes' to reduce hospital stays after surgery. These include optimizing a patient's status preoperatively (education, nutrition, control of risk factors); efficient discharge planning; avoidance of mechanical bowel preparation and complete fasting preoperatively (risk of dehydration); optimized anaesthesia (including postoperative epidural analgesia); early feeding and mobilization; and multidisciplinary involvement (e.g. physiotherapy, social worker, dietician). Such techniques can be challenging to implement but have been shown to work, without affecting outcome.

Colorectal cancer: adjuvant treatment

In CRC, the definitive treatment is surgery. Many of the patients who receive adjuvant therapy do not benefit; either because they are cured already or because the treatment fails. Nevertheless, even a small effect in a common disease translates into many hundreds or thousands of lives saved. When counselling individual patients it is therefore important to outline some of these uncertainties, and to carefully evaluate any co-morbid factors, which may increase the risks of treatment.

Chemotherapy in colorectal cancer

Chemotherapy, based on 5-FU, is widely used as an adjuvant treatment in stage III colon cancer, where it confers a 5–10% improvement in absolute survival. More recently, 5-FU has increasingly been combined with oxaliplatin, especially in good PS patients at higher than average risk of relapse.

Why 5-FU?

Despite some effect in metastatic disease, early trials of 5-FU failed to show any adjuvant benefit. However, in 1989 and 1990 two large randomized trials clearly showed a survival benefit for 12 months of 5-FU plus levamisole over observation alone. The American National Institute of Health therefore recommended this combination strategy in stage III colon cancer patients.

Subsequent trials assessed the value of combining 5-FU with folinic acid (FA) (which potentiates its effect on the target enzyme thymidylate synthase) and examined the importance of levamisole (an anti-helminthic with immunostimulatory properties that had been proposed to enhance the effect of 5-FU). Studies were also performed addressing the optimum duration of therapy. In summary, these trials concluded that 6 months of chemotherapy with 5-FU/FA was equivalent to 12 months of 5-FU/levamisole, and superior to 6 months of 5-FU/levamisole. Furthermore, combining 5-FU/FA with levamisole gave no extra benefit.

Particularly influential in the UK was the Quick and Simple and Reliable (QUASAR) study (QUASAR Collaborative Group 2000). In this large study, patients were given either weekly bolus chemotherapy or 5 consecutive days every 4 weeks (the so-called 'Mayo regimen'). Although not randomly allocated, the weekly schedule appeared much less toxic, with equivalent efficacy. This very large trial encouraged widespread adoption of the weekly regimen in the UK.

Recent developments

In the last few years a variety of trials have combined 5-FU/FA with other chemotherapy agents in an attempt to increase the impact of adjuvant chemotherapy. Despite enhanced responses in metastatic disease the combination of 5-FU and irinotecan has so far shown no benefit, but more importantly, two large randomized trials (MOSAIC and NSABP-C07) have now shown a benefit in combining oxaliplatin with different 5-FU/FA regimens in the adjuvant setting (Andre et al. 2004; Wolmark et al 2005). Both have shown improved disease free-survival rates for the combination, at the expense of increased toxicity (see next section). Furthermore, subgroup analysis of MOSAIC has also shown a small but statistically significant 4.6% (72.9% vs 68.3%) improvement in overall survival for stage III

(but not stage II) patients, after a median follow up of 6 years (de Gramont et al. 2007).

Intravenous 5-FU can be inconvenient and in-dwelling lines for infusional therapy are also vulnerable to complications such as infection or thrombosis. There has therefore been interest in using oral fluoropyrimidines (the group of drugs to which 5-FU belongs). Capecitabine is one such drug, which has now been approved as an alternative adjuvant treatment to 5-FU/FA in the UK. Currently, its use in combination regimens for adjuvant therapy remains unproven (although relevant trial data are awaited).

Toxicity

5-FU can cause several side effects such as fatigue, nausea, vomiting, diarrhoea, stomatitis, plantar-palmar erythema, epistaxis, and sore eyes. Alopecia and significant myelosuppression are uncommon. The severity and site-specific side effects are dependent on the regimen used. Capecitabine tends to mimic infusional 5-FU, with plantar-palmar erythema and diarrhoea being particularly common. A rare complication is angina, which may be related to coronary artery spasm and is commoner in those receiving continuous infusions of 5-FU or capecitabine. This does not necessarily occur in patients with known coronary artery disease, although there is some evidence that this slightly increases the risk.

A small proportion of people are deficient for the enzyme dihydropyrimidine dehydrogenase (DPD), which is important in metabolizing 5-FU. Such individuals will be otherwise healthy but have extremely severe and early toxicity with standard doses of 5-FU and often require emergency admission to the oncology centre. If these toxicities can be successfully managed, it is sometimes possible to recommence treatment with a 50% dose reduction after careful consideration of the balance of benefit and risk.

Oxaliplatin in combination with 5-FU/FA increases toxicity. In the MOSAIC trial, significant neutropenia was much commoner in the combined arm (41.1% vs 4.7%), but was complicated by infection/fever in only 1.8%. However, perhaps the biggest problem in the clinic is the increased incidence of sensory neuropathy with oxaliplatin, which can be clinically significant and long-lasting. This was sufficiently severe to interfere with function in 12.4% of patients receiving combined treatment in MOSAIC, although for the majority this resolved in the subsequent months (down to 0.7% after 4 years' median follow-up; (de Gramont A et al. 2005)).

Patient selection

Most oncologists would now give high-risk (e.g. heavily node-positive) stage III patients the choice of combination oxaliplatin/5-FU/FA if they are sufficiently fit and aware of the toxicities. For others, however, 6 months of 5FU5-FU/FA or capecitabine remains the mainstay of treatment (a position supported by NICE).

Controversy persists in some areas. For instance, elderly patients are generally under-represented in clinical trials and yet form the majority of patients in clinic. There is some evidence to suggest that the magnitude of benefit in the elderly is the same as in younger patients, but subgroup analyses from influential randomized trials have often shown little benefit in older patients (>65–70) (Andre et al. 2004; Quasar Collaborative Group 2007).

Another area of considerable debate is the role of chemotherapy in stage II colorectal cancer. Such patients already have a reasonable prognosis and their benefit from chemotherapy is likely to be small. Indeed, one large UK study of adjuvant 5-FU-based chemotherapy demonstrated only a modest absolute survival benefit at 5 years (3.6% assuming a recurrence rate of 20% without chemotherapy).

Although not directly addressed by this study, it is known that some stage II tumours have a worse prognosis, such as those presenting with perforation, obstruction, extramural vascular invasion, peritoneal involvement, or poorly differentiated histology. Many clinicians would target this group of patients for adjuvant chemotherapy, on the basis that their absolute risk of relapse is higher and therefore the likely benefit is greater. Nevertheless, careful discussion is required in each case.

After resection of a primary rectal cancer, many patients are referred for chemotherapy with a defunctioning stoma. Despite their obvious desire to have a reversal as soon as possible this is commonly deferred until after chemotherapy. This is to allow chemotherapy to commence as soon as possible after surgery, as most of the clinical trials have required chemotherapy to commence within 6–8 weeks. There is inadequate evidence to define the benefit from chemotherapy at later time points or for interrupting chemotherapy to allow reversal.

Can current treatments be improved?
Adjuvant chemotherapy could be improved if:
• It was better tolerated
• It was more effective
• It was targeted more closely to the patients who would benefit/respond

Increasing tolerability
The increasing use of capecitabine in adjuvant therapy is one approach to improving the acceptability of chemotherapy for patients (by avoiding the need for intravenous access and in-dwelling line complications) but it is not without toxicity. For some patients, diarrhoea and plantar-palmar erythema may be greater than that seen with weekly 5-FU/LV. Furthermore, agents such as oxaliplatin continue to require intravenous access, meaning that some of the convenience is lost when contemplating combination approaches.

Much of the toxicity with conventional 6-month regimens could be reduced by treating for a shorter period. An interesting approach would be to determine if less chemotherapy had equivalent efficacy. This forms the basis of a large, multicentre trial (SCOT), which opened in the UK in 2008, comparing 3 or 6 months of oxaliplatin/5-FU based chemotherapy.

Increasing effectiveness
In advanced CRC, a range of targeted biological agents have been shown to enhance the benefits of conventional chemotherapy. Of particular interest are antibodies specific to the epidermal growth factor receptor (EGFR) and vascular endothelial growth factor (VEGF), which are both important for the growth and spread of CRC. Cetuximab and panitumumab are licensed products (in metastatic disease) targeting EGFR, whilst bevacizumab targets VEGF. Despite relatively modest improvements in outcome in metastatic disease, on-going trials are evaluating the benefit of adding these agents to conventional

adjuvant chemotherapy. Theoretically, these agents may be particularly effective in the adjuvant setting, interfering with the processes that allow residual tumour cells to proliferate but clinical trial evidence is awaited.

The recently reported NSABP C-08 study found that addition of bevacizumab to standard adjuvant chemotherapy (FOLFOX- fluorouracil, leucovocin and oxaliplatin) did not improve disease-free-survival in stage II–III colon cancer (Wolmark et al. 2009).

Better targeting
Various different molecular markers have been examined as potential predictive factors for response to adjuvant treatment (e.g. thymidylate synthase, DCC, MSI) and sensitive assays for the detection of micrometastases have been used to try and identify high-risk individuals. However, none of these strategies is sufficiently accurate to use in clinical practice at the present time. On-going trials are evaluating targeted therapy for tumours with MSS and loss of heterozygosity at chromosome 18q.

Rectal cancer
The largest evidence base supporting the use of chemotherapy exists in patients with colon cancer and its applicability to patients with rectal cancer remains controversial. Nevertheless, in the UK, it is common to use the same criteria to select patients, irrespective of the primary site within the large bowel.

Radiotherapy
Radiotherapy is the use of ionizing radiation to eliminate cancer cells. It is used almost exclusively for the treatment of rectal cancer, rather than colon cancer, since small bowel toxicity and the mobility of much of the colon limits treatments outside the pelvis. Local pelvic recurrence is also a particularly unpleasant feature of rectal cancer which is ideally prevented if possible.

Indications
There are three main indications for adjuvant radiation in rectal cancer:
• Reducing the risk of local recurrence in patients with resectable rectal cancer.
• Shrinking locally advanced rectal cancer to facilitate successful resection.
• Using radiation to shrink or 'downsize' resectable disease to achieve sphincter-preserving surgery.

Reducing local recurrence in resectable disease
Many early trials tested the value of adding radiotherapy to surgery. Two meta-analyses of these early studies, published in 2000 and 2001, demonstrated unequivocal evidence that adjuvant radiation reduced the risk of local recurrence in resectable rectal cancer (Camma et al. 2000; Colorectal Cancer Collaborative Group 2001). This is also the conclusion of a recent Cochrane review.

As well as a dose–effect, analysis of these data also demonstrated that preoperative treatment seemed more effective than postoperative radiotherapy. Only one of these overviews (Camma et al. 2000) demonstrated an improvement in overall survival, although both reported improvements in cancer-specific mortality.

The development of the 25Gy in 5 fractions preoperative schedule
To avoid unnecessary delays before surgery, many early studies used large (5Gy) fraction sizes in short

duration treatments. It was clear that these were well-tolerated as long as the radiotherapy was carefully planned, to spare excessive doses to normal tissues. The Swedish Rectal Cancer Trial was particularly influential since it showed an improvement in overall survival when 25Gy in 5 fractions short-course, preoperative radiotherapy (SCPRT) was added to surgery (Swedish Rectal Cancer Trial 1997),

In recent years, TME surgery has dramatically improved the outcome of surgery alone. It could therefore be hypothesized that radiotherapy in these early studies was simply compensating for inadequate surgery. Therefore, to establish the role of SCPRT in the TME era, the Dutch Colorectal Cancer Study Group trial and the Medical Research Council (MRC) CR07 trial were both designed to compare SCPRT with selective postoperative approaches, based on CRM status (radiotherapy alone in the Dutch study, chemoradiotherapy in CR07).

Results from the Dutch trial (Kapiteijn et al. 2001; Peeters et al. 2007) and early data from the CR07 study (Sebag-Montefiore et al. 2006) (presented in abstract form) both showed a reduction in local recurrence with routine SCPRT. CR07 also demonstrated a 5% improvement in 3-year DFS. Absolute benefit was greatest in those patients at highest risk of relapse. Overall, the proportional reduction in local recurrence appeared very similar to the pre-TME era, but the absolute reduction was that much smaller due to the better surgical outcomes.

SCPRT does have some well-established, long-term complications, including permanent sterility for men and pre-menopausal women. There is also an increased incidence of erectile dysfunction and impaired bowel function, although rates of pelvic fractures and bowel obstruction do not appear to be increased. It is therefore important to weigh up the pros and cons of SCPRT in different groups of patients. Many clinicians would not treat patients with stage I disease but opinions vary on where the threshold should be set for more advanced tumours.

Conventionally fractionated radiation schedules

An alternative approach to SCPRT is to use a longer course of radiation with a lower (more conventional) dose per fraction. This is an approach favoured in much of mainland Europe and North America. Most current long course schedules use 45–50.4Gy over 5–5.5 weeks using 1.8–2Gy per fraction. As with SCPRT, there is evidence for improved local control using this strategy but no trial evidence for improved survival.

There has been an increasing interest in long-course radiotherapy combined with concurrent chemotherapy (CRT), an approach that maximizes response rates when used in locally advanced disease. Recent randomized trials (Bosset et al. 2006; Gerard et al. 2006) have shown that preoperative CRT is more effective than radiotherapy alone, when used in resectable disease. There were fewer local recurrences, but no difference in DFS.

As yet it is not clear what the advantage of operative CRT may be over SCPRT, although the former is clearly more expensive and resource intensive. Only one trial, from Poland, has been performed to compare these strategies (Bujko et al. 2006a) and this was powered to detect differences in sphincter-preservation rather than local recurrence or survival. Unsurprisingly, CRT followed by a 4–6 week wait, led to greater tumour down-staging, pathological complete response rates, and CRM negative resections, but was also associated with higher rates of acute toxicity. Nevertheless, there was no significant difference seen in the rate of sphincter-preserving surgery and, interestingly, no statistical difference in local recurrence or late toxicity.

Postoperative approaches

Giving radiotherapy after surgery enables targeting of higher-risk individuals on the basis of surgical pathology. However, treatment is more toxic because of adherent small bowel in the pelvis and hypoxia in the tumour bed can compromise effectiveness. Although early trials showed improved local control the results were less impressive when compared to preoperative techniques.

Particularly in North America there was interest in trying to improve these results with the addition of chemotherapy to postoperative radiotherapy. In 1990, the results of three such studies led to a consensus statement from the National Institute of Health, making postoperative chemoradiation (adjuvant chemotherapy + concurrent CRT) for patients with pT3/4 or N+ve disease (TNM stage II and III) the North American standard of care (NIH consensus conference et al. 1990). Despite increased selection, only patients with stage I disease were spared treatment and the acute toxicities were more severe, making its applicability to the general population less certain. There was particular concern about older patients.

Preoperative versus postoperative radiation in resectable disease

Both the CR07 and Dutch trials have compared routine SCPRT with selective postoperative treatments (as described earlier), and both have shown less local recurrence with the preoperative approach. Nevertheless, many oncologists around the world remain wary of SCPRT because of a perception that it increases long-term toxicity.

Of particular significance, however, are the results of the recent German CAO/ARO/AIO 94 trial (Sauer et al. 2006) comparing pre- and postoperative CRT. This influential study, using standardized TME surgery and postoperative chemotherapy in all patients, showed that the preoperative approach resulted in lower local recurrence rates (6% vs 12%) and reduced complications (both acute and late). OS was unaffected.

This study (combined with the pre-operative superiority of CRT over long-course radiotherapy alone, described above) appears to have decisively changed the treatment paradigm in rectal cancer to a preoperative approach and is already influencing practice in North America. Nevertheless, whether preoperative CRT in resectable disease is superior to SCPRT, or justifies the extra costs, remains to be proven. Furthermore, with TME surgery producing very low local recurrence rates, it is likely that the extra toxicities of treatment are not justified in many low-risk patients.

Radiotherapy for locally advanced rectal cancer

Locally advanced disease can be defined clinically or on the basis of imaging. Transrectal ultrasound is considered a gold-standard for assessing trans-mural tumour extent and MRI the best way of demonstrating the relationship of the tumour to the mesorectal fascia (the intended 'CRM' for a mesorectal excision).

Given the difficulty of surgery alone in this group of patients there is limited randomized evidence to support the use of radiotherapy. Nevertheless, in recent years, neoadjuvant concurrent chemoradiotherapy has become a standard treatment for locally advanced rectal cancer, because of increased response rates seen in the very large number of phase II studies that have been performed. Many have used either infusional 5-FU or bolus 5-FU/LV but no direct comparison has been performed and there remains considerable uncertainty as to how to derive the optimum regimen or the most useful endpoint.

Currently, there is considerable interest in the use of other drugs such as capecitabine, oxaliplatin, irinotecan, and the targeted biologicals in chemoradiation schedules. Many studies utilizing these agents are underway but no phase III data have yet been reported comparing them to standard 5-FU based regimens.

There is considerable uncertainty as to the benefit of adjuvant chemotherapy following prior neo-adjuvant CRT. If it is to be used, should it be given to those who have responded well to CRT (and therefore have chemosensitive disease) or should combination treatment be given to those that have not responded to CRT containing a single agent? On-going trials are addressing these issues.

Improving sphincter preservation

It remains controversial whether preoperative treatment (usually with CRT) can increase rates of sphincter-preserving surgery in low rectal cancer (i.e. converting a planned abdomino-perineal resection into a low anterior resection). Indeed, a systematic review (Bujko et al. 2006b) has found no evidence of increased sphincter-preservation following preoperative treatment. The authors argue that surgeons are reluctant to change their initial plan, even after a good response, because of understandable concern over residual microscopic disease at the original site of the tumour. There is also concern about the functional outcome following very low anterior resections. Nevertheless, some series have shown it to be possible, without excessive local recurrence, and the debate continues.

Summary

Deciding on the optimal adjuvant therapy for colo-rectal cancer may be straightforward, but can often be complex. Increasing options are available and patients vary in their risk factors for recurrence, preferences for treatment, co-morbidities, perception of risk/benefit, and acceptance of toxicity. Many questions also remain unanswered which will be addressed by future studies.

Further reading

Andre T, Boni C, Mounedji-Boudiaf L, et al. Oxaliplatin, fluorouracil, and leucovorin as adjuvant treatment for colon cancer. N Engl J Med. 2004; **350**(23):2343–51.

Bosset JF, Collette L, Calais G, et al. Chemotherapy with preoperative radiotherapy in rectal cancer. N Engl J Med 2006; **355**(11):1114–23.

Bujko K, Nowacki MP, Nasierowska-Guttmejer A, et al. Long-term results of a randomized trial comparing preoperative short-course radiotherapy with preoperative conventionally fractionated chemoradiation for rectal cancer. Br J Surg 2006a; **93**(10):1215–23.

Bujko K, Kepka L, Michalski W, et al. Does rectal cancer shrinkage induced by preoperative radio(chemo)therapy increase the likelihood of anterior resection? A systematic review of randomised trials. Radiother Oncol 2006b; **80**(1):4–12.

de Gramont A, Boni C, Navarro M, et al. Oxaliplatin/5FU/LV in adjuvant colon cancer: Updated efficacy results of the MOSAIC trial, including survival, with a median follow-up of six years. J Clin Oncol 2007; **25** (suppl)(18S): Abstract 4007.

de Gramont A, Boni C, Navarro M, et al. Oxaliplatin/5FU/LV in the adjuvant treatment of stage II and stage III colon cancer: Efficacy results with a median follow-up of 4 years J Clin Oncol 2005; **23**(16S): Abstract 3501.

Quasar Collaborative Group. McConkey C, Hills RK, Williams NS, et al. Adjuvant chemotherapy versus observation in patients with colorectal cancer: a randomised study. Lancet 2007; **370**(9604):2020–9.

Camma C, Giunta M, Fiorica F, et al. Preoperative radiotherapy for resectable rectal cancer: A meta-analysis. JAMA 2000; **284**(8):1008–15.

Colorectal Cancer Collaborative Group. Adjuvant radiotherapy for rectal cancer: a systematic overview of 8,507 patients from 22 randomised trials. Lancet 2001; **358**(9290):1291–304.

Gerard JP, Conroy T, Bonnetain F, et al. Preoperative radiotherapy with or without concurrent fluorouracil and leucovorin in T3-4 rectal cancers: results of FFCD 9203. J Clin Oncol 2006; **24**(28):4620–5.

Kapiteijn E, Marijnen CA, Nagtegaal ID, et al. Preoperative radiotherapy combined with total mesorectal excision for resectable rectal cancer. N Engl J Med 2001; **345**(9):638–46.

NIH consensus conference. Adjuvant therapy for patients with colon and rectal cancer. JAMA 1990; **264**(11):1444–50.

Peeters KC, Marijnen CA, Nagtegaal ID, et al. The TME trial after a median follow-up of 6 years: increased local control but no survival benefit in irradiated patients with resectable rectal carcinoma. Ann Surg 2007; **246**(5):693–701.

QUASAR Collaborative Group. Comparison of flourouracil with additional levamisole, higher-dose folinic acid, or both, as adjuvant chemotherapy for colorectal cancer: a randomised trial. Lancet 2000; **355**(9215):1588–96.

Sauer R, Becker H, Hohenberger W, et al. Preoperative versus postoperative chemoradiotherapy for rectal cancer. N Engl J Med 2004; **351**(17):1731–40.

Sebag-Montefiore D, Stevens RJ, Steele R et al. Pre-operative radiotherapy versus selective post-operative chemoradiotherapy in patients with rectal cancer (MRC CR07 and NCIC-CTG CO16): a multi-centre randomized trial. Lancet. 2009; **373**: 811–820.

Swedish Rectal Cancer Trial. Improved survival with preoperative radiotherapy in resectable rectal cancer. N Engl J Med 1997; **336**(14):980–7.

Wolmark N, Wieand HS, Keubler JP. A phase III trial comparing FULV to FULV + oxaliplatin in stage II or III carcinoma of the colon: results of the NSABP protocol C-07. J Clin Oncol 2005; **23**:16s (abstract 3500).

Wolmark N, Yohters G, O'Connell MJ, et al. A phase III trial comparing mFolfox6 to mFolfox6+bevacizumab in stage II or III carcinoma of the colon: Results of NSABP protocol C-08. J Clin Oncol 2009; **27**:18s, (abstract LBA4).

Colorectal cancer: treatment of advanced colorectal cancer

Introduction

Advanced CRC can be defined as disease presenting with distant metastatic spread (stage IV disease by the AJCC staging system or modified Dukes stage D) or recurrence following surgery. In the advanced setting, the broad principles of management of colon and rectal cancer are the same and have thus been treated as one topic.

Approximately 30% of patients with CRC present with stage IV disease and around 25% of patients originally treated for localized disease will go on to develop distant recurrence.

The median OS for patients with metastatic disease managed by best supportive care alone is around six months. The use of modern chemotherapy regimens has extended this to >20 months in clinical trials.

Chemotherapy

Fluoropyrimidines

5-FU has been the most commonly used fluoropyrimidine since it was introduced in 1957. Active metabolites inhibit thymidylate synthase (TS) and are incorporated into RNA and DNA thereby inhibiting DNA synthesis and function. Oral bioavailability is poor due to inactivation of 5-FU by the gut mucosa. Co-administration of folinic acid (FA, or leucovorin) can enhance 5-FU by stabilizing the interaction with thymidylate synthase leading to an improvement in response.

A meta-analysis of several small studies has shown that 5-FU regimens extend median survival to 12 months. 5-FU is delivered using either bolus or infusional regimens. Infusional regimens are favoured as they improve response rates and reduce toxicity with comparable survival (Malet-Martino et al. 2002).

Capecitabine is an oral fluoropyrimidine pro-drug that undergoes a three- step conversion to 5-FU. The final step is mediated by thymidine phosphorylase (TP) in the liver and in the tumour. TP expression is higher in tumour cells, thus providing a degree of tumour selectivity. Capecitabine has equal efficacy to different 5-FU regimens. It is better tolerated than bolus 5-FU but less well tolerated than infusional 5-FU due to increased hand foot syndrome (HFS) and diarrhoea (Malet-Martino et al. 2002; Seymour et al. 2007a).

UFT is composed of another oral pro-drug, tegafur and uracil that inhibits 5-FU catabolism. Two randomized studies have shown equivalent efficacy and reduced stomatitis and myelosuppression compared to bolus 5-FU regimens (Malet-Martino et al. 2002). No randomized controlled trials have compared UFT with capecitabine or infusional 5-FU. Cross trial comparisons suggest there is less HFS than with capecitabine but more diarrhoea than with infusional 5-FU.

Irinotecan and oxaliplatin

Irinotecan is a topoisomerase I (topo I) enzyme inhibitor. Inhibition of topo I results in DNA strand breaks that trigger apoptosis. The active metabolite SN-38 is glucuronidated to SN-38G, an inactive product in the liver and is excreted in bile. The gut flora can reverse the inactivation, causing enterohepatic circulation of SN-38 and direct gut exposure, leading to myelosuppression and diarrhoea. Early trials using irinotecan found an excess of deaths due to severe diarrhoea. Guidelines now stipulate early initiation of anti-diarrhoeal therapy. Single- agent irinotecan improves median survival by 2–3 months following progression on first-line treatment with 5-FU (Cunningham et al. 2001).

Oxaliplatin is a platinum derivative. The active moiety binds to DNA guanine residues and forms intra- and interstrand cross links. These adducts are recognized as damaged DNA and trigger apoptosis or DNA repair pathways. Oxaliplatin is eliminated via the kidneys. The dose- limiting toxicity is a cumulative sensory neuropathy. It is highly active in combination with 5-FU but has limited activity as a single agent (Kuebler et al. 2003).

Combining irinotecan with 5-FU in the first-line setting improves response rates and overall survival. Initially irinotecan was combined with bolus 5-FU but high rates of diarrhoea meant this combination was almost unfeasible. Combinations with infusional 5-FU are better tolerated and have achieved even better survival outcomes (Cunningham et al. 2001; Seymour et al. 2007b).

Combining oxaliplatin with infusional 5-FU in the first-line setting has also been shown to increase response rates and prolong progression free survival (PFS). Overall survival was improved but did not reach statistical significance. Although some toxicities were increased these did not significantly impact on quality of life (Kuebler et al. 2003).

Comparisons of first-line oxaliplatin/ /5-FU and irinotecan/ /5-FU have not shown any significant difference in efficacy or tolerability. Deciding between these regimens is dictated by patient choice and co-morbidity (Kuebler et al. 2003). Both oxaliplatin and irinotecan have been combined with capecitabine. The oxaliplatin/capecitabine combinations have generally equivalent efficacy and tolerability compared to those with 5-FU. The use of the irinotecan/ / capecitabine combination has been limited by excessive GI toxicity although this has not been a consistent finding in all studies.

Newer agents

Bevacizumab is a humanized monoclonal antibody targeted against VEGF, a potent angiogenic growth factor. Common toxicities include hypertension and proteinuria. Rarer toxicities include a doubling of the risk of arterial thrombotic events (ATE), perforation, fistula formation, and haemorrhage. The highest risk group for ATE are patients >65 years and those with a history of ATE. Recent surgery or the presence of peritoneal disease increases the risk of perforation.

Internationally, bevacizumab is widely used in combination with irinotecan/ 5-FU or oxaliplatin/ 5-FU. The licensing study compared irinotecan and bolus 5-FU with or without bevacizumab. The addition of bevacizumab resulted in significant improvements in response rates and OS (Hurwitz et al. 2004). However the addition of bevacizumab to oxaliplatin and infusional 5-FU in the first- and second- line setting has been less impressive. The differences in the results are likely to be related to the use of infusional as opposed to bolus 5-FU in the latter studies. NICE has not approved the use of bevacizumab in the UK.

Cetuximab is a chimeric monoclonal antibody that binds to and inhibits the (EGFR). Panitunumab is a fully humanized monoclonal antibody against EGFR. In the third- line setting, both have been shown to confer a small survival benefit over best supportive care. Following progression on irinotecan, the addition of cetuximab has been shown to restore tumour sensitivity to irinotecan and improve PFS. However in the first-line setting the addition of cetuximab to combination chemotherapy has not improved survival.

Planned translational studies performed in multiple randomized studies containing EGFR targeted monoclonal antibodies have highlighted the importance of mutations in the KRAS growth factor. Patients with mutated KRAS are insensitive to EGFR- directed monoclonal antibodies. Patients with wild type KRAS conversely derive a survival benefit. Further studies may enable better selection of more sensitive patients.

Role of surgery

Surgery may be performed with usual oncological considerations for cure in the presence of potentially resectable metastases or for palliation of symptoms.

The latter is often performed in the emergency situation when patients present with obstruction or bleeding. Surgical options include resection with a stoma, an anastomosis, colo-colonic/ileocolonic bypass, or a defunctioning stoma alone. A preoperative diagnosis allows patient wishes to be considered when planning whether to use a defunctioning stoma. This allows fastest recovery and earlier chemotherapy. An alternative to surgery for an obstructing cancer is stenting, which avoids the need for general anaesthesia and the recovery time also permits early chemotherapy. Strictures on the right side and those at or close to the colonic flexures are difficult to stent. Stenting low rectal cancer also has a high risk of tenesmus. Some studies have found unacceptable perforation rates. Further scrutiny will be possible by ongoing randomized clinical trials.

Similar approaches are used in the semi-elective setting. Impending obstruction requires intervention prior to palliative chemotherapy as outcomes are worse following acute obstruction during treatment. Persistent anaemia requiring blood transfusion may warrant a limited resection. Advanced rectal cancer can present with significant pelvic symptoms and, whilst palliative chemotherapy may lead to some transient improvement in symptoms, surgery may give better palliation. In addition to the options previously listed, improvement of pelvic symptoms such as bleeding, tenesmus and obstructed defecation may be achieved through trans-anal endoscopic methods such as laser activated plasma coagulation and partial endoscopic resection. In some cases the only option for unresectable pelvic disease is a defunctioning stoma.

Resection of liver metastasis

Surgical series report that complete surgical resection of metastases confined to the liver has resulted in a 30% 5-year survival (Fong et al. 1999). Even though the evidence base lacks randomized controlled trials, liver resection has been accepted as part of the routine management of these patients. Currently 10% of patients have liver disease that is technically resectable at diagnosis, and a further 10% become operable following response to 'downstaging' chemotherapy. Patients responding to 'downstaging' chemotherapy have a similar survival to those with initially resectable disease. However numbers of metastases >3, size >3cm, or a lack of response may herald a worse outcome (Adam et al. 2008). At the multidisciplinary meeting disease need to be categorized as resectable, potentially resectable, or unresectable.

The criteria for resectability are continuously expanding. Currently for liver-only metastases, the criteria include disease that can be completely resected providing that: at least two adjacent liver segments can be spared, vascular supply and biliary drainage can be preserved, and at least 20% of the total organ volume is left to maintain liver function. A variety of surgical techniques are used including anatomical and non-anatomical resections and wedge excisions.

Several prognostic scoring systems have been developed for patients undergoing hepatic resection. One large series of 1001 cases identified extra-hepatic disease as a contraindication to resection and developed a scoring system based on criteria that could be measured preoperatively. These include node positive primary tumour, disease- free interval <12 months, number of metastases >1, preoperative CEA >200ng/ml and largest metastasis more than >5cm diameter. No patients with a score of five 5 survived beyond 2 years (Fong et al. 1999).

The surgical management of lung metastases has largely been extrapolated from those of the liver and likewise lacks any randomized evidence.

Special situations

Who to treat and when to start?

The ECOG performance status (PS) scoring system is a useful and easy assessment of a patient's fitness for chemotherapy. Those who score 0–2 are generally suitable (see 'Internet resource'). Co-morbidities also need to be taken into account. A recent ischaemic cardiac event contraindicates fluoropyrimidines. IBD and liver dysfunction contraindicate irinotecan and severe renal impairment contraindicates oxaliplatin and capecitabine. Oxaliplatin is also contraindicated in the presence of a peripheral neuropathy.

The majority of patients commence chemotherapy when they present with metastatic disease even if they are asymptomatic. However, if patients have low volume disease it is reasonable to opt for careful surveillance initially, especially if there are co-morbidities present that increase the risk of chemotherapy.

Do we need to use combination treatment first-line?

Initial studies clearly showed first-line combination chemotherapy improved survival compared to single- agent chemotherapy. However, the single agent chemotherapy arms of these studies lacked a planned crossover to combination chemotherapy on progression. Following these studies the term 'staged combination chemotherapy' was coined to describe such an approach. There have now been three large randomized clinical trials that have compared staged combination chemotherapy with first-line combination chemotherapy. The largest of these was the FOCUS trial that randomized over 2000 patients (Seymour et al. 2007). These studies have shown no detrimental effect on survival with the use of staged combination chemotherapy.

A retrospective molecular analysis of 1313 tumour samples from the FOCUS trial identified topo I as a predictive marker of benefit. Patients with tumours expressing high levels of topo I experienced a major overall survival benefit with first-line combination chemotherapy as opposed to staged combination chemotherapy. Patients with tumours with medium or low expression of topo I experienced no survival benefit with first-line combination chemotherapy (Seymour et al. 2008). This interesting data requires confirmation in a prospective trial.

Intermittent or continuous chemotherapy?

There is no clear consensus on whether chemotherapy can be delivered intermittently or whether the aim should be to treat until progression. Introducing a chemotherapy-free interval after 3 months of treatment may be a sensible option in responding patients without bulky symptomatic disease.

This issue has been interrogated by three randomized clinical trials. The MRC conducted a study where patients responding or achieving disease stabilization after 3 months of single- agent chemotherapy were randomized to either a treatment break with rechallenge on progression or continuing chemotherapy until progression. Intermittent chemotherapy had no detrimental effect on survival However, the study was closed early due to slow accrual and predated combination chemotherapy. A French group conducted a similar study, the OPTIMOX 1 trial, using combination chemotherapy. Patients were randomized to either continuous oxaliplatin/ 5-FU or planned hiatus in oxaliplatin after three months with reintroduction after nine months. Patients on the study arm experienced less neurotoxicity with again no detrimental effect on survival (de Gramont et al. 2007). No true chemotherapy- free intervals were used in this study as patients were maintained on 5-FU. Interestingly oxaliplatin reintroduction achieved disease control in 50% of patients and was associated with a better outcome highlighting the importance of rechallenging patients on progression. In the second-line setting a small UK study randomized responding patients at 24 weeks to either stopping or continuing irinotecan chemotherapy. No survival benefit was observed in the extended chemotherapy arm.

This question has been further assessed by the COIN study that randomized patients to either continuous or intermittent combination chemotherapy. Until the results of the COIN study are available decisions about the duration of therapy should be made on an individual patient basis. If an intermittent approach is used, patients should be carefully monitored off treatment with regular clinical assessment and CT scanning so that treatment can be restarted promptly on progression.

Second- line treatment and beyond?

Following progression on combination chemotherapy, fit patients are commonly treated with further combination or single- agent chemotherapy. The choice of drug is dictated by what they did not have as first-line. The evidence supporting this approach is based on the observation that patients who receive all three active chemotherapy drugs (a fluoropyrimidine, oxaliplatin, and irinotecan) have longer survival times than those who do not. Response rates in these circumstances are low although disease stabilization is common lasting for a short number of months. Fitness, low serum LDH, female gender, and no previous adjuvant chemotherapy predict for longer PFS in these circumstances.

On further progression if a long period has elapsed since first-line chemotherapy, rechallenge with the initial regimen may temporarily achieve disease control. Patients with wild type KRAS may benefit from cetuximab and irinotecan or panitunumab alone. Otherwise entry into early phase clinical trials should be considered for selected fit patients.

Is there a role for chemotherapy with operable metastases?

In cases that are initially technically operable there is no definite survival benefit for the use of preoperative chemotherapy. One randomized study has reported a strong trend for a PFS benefit for perioperative chemotherapy but this did not reach statistical significance nor did it translate into a survival benefit. If patients are chemotherapy naive, offering adjuvant chemotherapy is appropriate. One randomized study has reported a PFS benefit; otherwise evidence is extrapolated from the use of adjuvant chemotherapy following resection of the primary disease.

Conclusion

A steady improvement in outcomes of advanced CRC has been achieved in recent years through a combination of multidisciplinary management and developments in chemotherapy. Staged combination chemotherapy has been developed as a general approach to combine and sequence patient selection for different therapeutic approaches including when to use biological agents, when to use staged combination therapy, and how to avoid toxicity.

Further reading

Adam R, Wicherts DA, de Haas RJ, et al. Patients with initially irresectable colorectal liver metastases: Is there a possibility of cure by an oncosurgical approach? *Proc Am Soc Clin Oncol* 2008; 26:abstract 4023.

Braun MS, Richman SD, Quirke P, et al. Predictive biomarkers of chemotherapy efficacy in colorectal cancer: results from the UK MRC FOCUS trial. *J Clin Oncol* 2008; **26**:2690–8.

Cunningham D, Maroun J, Vanhoefer U, et al. Optimizing the use of irinotecan in colorectal cancer. *Oncologist* 2001; **6**(Suppl 4):17–23.

de Gramont A, Buyse M, Abrahantes JC, et al. Reintroduction of oxaliplatin is associated with improved survival in advanced colorectal cancer. *J Clin Oncol* 2007; **25**:3224–9.

Fong Y, Fortner J, Sun RL. et al. Clinical score for predicting recurrence after hepatic resection for metastatic colorectal cancer: analysis of 1001 consecutive cases. *Ann Surg* 1999; **230**:309–18; discussion 318–21.

Hurwitz H, Fehrenbacher L, Novotny W, et al. Bevacizumab plus irinotecan, fluorouracil, and leucovorin for metastatic colorectal cancer. *N Engl J Med* 2004; **350**:2335–42.

Kuebler JP, de Gramont A. Recent experience with oxaliplatin or irinotecan combined with 5-fluorouracil and leucovorin in the treatment of colorectal cancer. *Semin Oncol* 2003; **30**:40–6.

Malet-Martino M, Martino R. Clinical studies of three oral prodrugs of 5-fluorouracil (capecitabine, UFT, S-1): a review. *Oncologist* 2002; **7**:288–323.

Seymour MT, Maughan TS, Wasan HS, et al. Capecitabine (Cap) and oxaliplatin (Ox) in elderly and/or frail patients with metastatic colorectal cancer: The FOCUS2 trial. *Proc Am Soc Clin Oncol* 2007a; **25**:abstract 9030.

Seymour MT, Maughan TS, Ledermann JA, et al. Different strategies of sequential and combination chemotherapy for patients with poor prognosis advanced colorectal cancer (MRC FOCUS): a randomised controlled trial *Lancet* 2007b; **370**:143–52.

Internet resource

ECOG performance status: http://ecog.dfci.harvard.edu/general/perf_stat.html

Colorectal cancer: prognosis, follow-up, and management of recurrence

Prognosis

Approximately one-third of patients undergoing curative surgery will relapse. Relapse most often presents within 3 years, but rarely can occur up to 10 years after resection. Patients can develop local recurrence or may relapse at distant sites with liver and lungs representing the most common sites. Although the majority of patients who relapse are incurable, approximately one-third of patients with isolated local or distant recurrences are alive at 5 years (Manfredi et al. 2006).

Prognosis after surgery for CRC is primarily determined by the following factors.

Key prognostic factors

1. TNM staging: 5-year survival rate for patients with CRC is largely dependent on TNM stage. Stage-specific survival is as follows: stage I—70%, stage II—50%, stage III—35%, stage IV—5%
2. Vascular invasion: presence of tumour cells beneath the endothelium of unmuscularized veins and small vessels influences the rates of local and distant relapse. Previous studies using multivariate analysis have demonstrated vascular invasion as an independent adverse prognostic factor (Wiggers et al. 1988).
3. Residual tumour: presence of residual microscopic (R1) or macroscopic (R2) disease is associated with high rates of local and distant relapse. Presence of tumour within 1mm of the CRM (R1) adversely affects the clinical outcome following surgery (TME) for rectal cancer (Quirke et al. 1986).
4. Serum CEA: high preoperative CEA levels are associated with increased rates of recurrence possibly related to the higher incidence of micrometastases in these patients (Compton, et al. 2000).

Other prognostic factors

Tumour grading

- Higher tumour grades (poor glandular differentiation, atypia, mitotic figures) are associated with worse prognosis.
- Use of tumour grading as an independent prognostic factor is confounded by the presence of inter-observer variability.
- The American College of pathologists has recommended a two-tiered grading system (high vs. low) based on glandular differentiation as the sole criterion (>50% or <50% gland formation).

Tumour border and 'budding'

- Presence of an irregular infiltrating border without any associated stromal reaction is a negative prognostic factor.
- Similarly, a concentrated presence of tumour cells in front of the advancing infiltrative edge ('budding') is associated with an adverse prognosis.
- Absence of tumour budding has been correlated with the presence of intratumoural (ITL) and peritumoural lymphocytes, indicating a possible immune-mediated destruction of 'buds' which may lead to an improved prognosis (Zlobec and Lugli. 2008).

Perineural invasion

- Perineural invasion is quantified by the depth and number of foci of malignant cells per field.
- Perineural invasion has been reported to carry important prognostic significance following neoadjuvant chemoradiotherapy (Ruo et al. 2002).

Nodal micrometastasis

- Tumour deposits of <0.2 mm detected by detailed histological assessment or immunohistochemistry (IHC).
- However, the prognostic significance of sole nodal micrometastasis remains unclear, unless associated with foci of neovascularization or attainment of a certain size (Bilchik et al. 2003).
- At present the TNM staging protocol does not recognize nodal micrometastasis of < 0.2mm to be an independent prognostic factor. It is recommended that tumour deposits of >0.2mm, but <2mm, should be used to classify nodal status but designated as pN (mi).

Tumour immunity

- Increased number of tumour-infiltrating lymphocytes (TIL) is associated with an improved overall and recurrence-free survival. In addition, there is a possible inverse correlation with tumour stage (Ropponen et al. 1997).
- Favourable response is primarily mediated by CD8+ TILs expressing cytotoxic proteins (granzyme B, perforin).
- Galon et al, (2006) investigated the role of adaptive immune response in a large cohort of patients. Maximum protective effect was observed in tumours with lymphocyte infiltrate at both the centre and invasive margin.

Microsatellite instability

- A recent meta-analysis of 7000 patients showed that tumours with MSI were associated with superior survival compared to MSS cancers (Popat et al. 2005). Subsequently, it was shown that this may be related to an increased number of ITL (Baker et al. 2007). See Chapter 4.5, Colorectal cancer: genetics, screening and prevention, p.228.
- However, MSS tumours may derive a higher survival benefit from 5-FU based adjuvant chemotherapy (Popat et al. 2005).

Loss of heterozygosity (18q deletions and TP53)

- Chromosomal loss at 18q is observed in up to 70% of CRCs.
- 18q deletion affects the function of DCC gene which plays a crucial role in the late phase of colorectal carcinogenesis.
- Previous studies have shown that stage II and III cancers with 18q deletions have a worse prognosis (Compton et al. 2000).
- TP53 is mutated in 50% of CRCs. However, the association with clinical outcome remains unclear. TP53-CRC collaborative study showed that patients with Dukes C disease and wt-TP53 status probably derive a higher survival benefit from adjuvant chemotherapy (Russo et al. 2005).

Protein marker profiling (EGFR, VEGF, and ki-RAS)
- Currently there is a huge interest in identifying molecular markers with prognostic implications. Discovery of a tumour proteomic profile associated with specific patterns of aggressive biological behaviour or resistance to conventional therapeutic modalities can potentially have a huge impact on patient selection and individualization of treatment protocols.
- Although several proteins (e.g. β-catenin, TGFβ, bcl-2, Bax) have been investigated, the most consistent prognostic correlation has been observed for VEGF and EGFR.
- EGFR and VEGF expression can be detected in up to 75% of tumours and has been linked to several poor prognostic features, including increased potential for metastatic spread, inferior DFS and OS, and poor response to radiotherapy (Zlobec et al.and Lugli 2008).
- ki-RAS mutations are observed in 20–50% of CRC and most frequently involve the codon 12 in exon 1. The RASCAL study of >3000 cases demonstrated a significant reduction in DFS and OS in Dukes' stage C tumours harbouring ki-RAS mutation (Russo et al 2005).
- More recently, it has emerged that only patients with wt-RAS status derive a useful benefit from anti-EGFR targeted therapies.

Follow-up
- Primary aim of follow-up schedule is to detect any recurrence (loco-regional or distant) and metachronous tumours at an early asymptomatic stage.
- Patients with isolated local or limited systemic (liver and lung) recurrence may be amenable to surgical resection.
- Patients with image-detected recurrences have higher frequency of limited disease that is amenable to curative resection compared to those with symptoms.
- Previous meta-analyses have demonstrated a superior outcome following intensive follow-up schedules with a survival benefit of 7–10% compared to minimal or no follow-up (Gan S et al. 2007). However, there is no optimal follow-up schedule that is universally accepted.
- In the UK, there is no specific recommendations, but NICE advocates the presence of network-specific guidelines for follow-up based on the risk profile of individual patients and available resources. Whilst awaiting more definitive evidence, NICE emphasizes the importance of patient recruitment in national trials.
- The results from the large NCRN trial of follow-up strategies (FACS) in >4000 CRC patients are awaited. The trial was designed to investigate the effects of monitoring CEA in primary care compared to more intensive hospital follow-up with imaging of the liver or abdomen.
- Currently used follow-up schedules for CRC patients commonly involve a combination of regular clinical reviews, CEA monitoring, interval imaging, and colonoscopy.

Clinic reviews
Significant geographical variation in review patterns; no evidence that more frequent reviews improve outcome; most commonly patients are reviewed at 3–6 month intervals for first 2 years followed by 6–12 monthly.

Carcinoembryonic antigen
Frequently elevated in recurrent disease (especially liver) and often earlier compared to image-detected recurrences;

false-negative rate of 40%; false-positive of 10%; isolated CEA monitoring has no survival benefit; combining liver imaging and CEA monitoring reduces mortality; usually performed at 6–12 monthly intervals.

Liver imaging
Previous meta-analyses have shown that regular CT scan increases the detection rate of asymptomatic liver metastases, but does not increase the number of curative resections; usually performed at annual intervals.

Colonoscopy
Patients without a previous colonoscopy should have one within 6 months of curative surgery; other patients should have it performed at 3–5 yearly intervals depending on underlying risk; patients with limited life-expectancy are unlikely to benefit from colonoscopy.

Recurrence and management
- Patients with loco-regional and isolated liver and lung recurrences should be appropriately staged to identify those that would benefit from further curative resection. One-third of such patients will be cured and alive at 5 years.
- PET/CT is useful and should be considered in selected cases. However, there is no evidence to support its routine use in this situation.
- Twenty to thirty percent of patients with liver relapse will proceed to surgery. In contrast, a relative minority of patients with lung metastases will have localized disease that is amenable to surgical resection.
- Patients with multiple liver lesions are sometimes referred for neoadjuvant combination chemotherapy with the aim of downstaging disease prior to future surgery. NICE recommends the use of oxaliplatin/5-FU regimens in these patients.
- The incidence of loco-regional recurrence following surgery for rectal cancer is 5–30% depending on disease extent and the plane of surgical resection specimen achieved. If radiotherapy naïve, all patients with isolated local recurrence of rectal cancer should be considered for preoperative RT or CRT prior to rectal cancer resection if the disease is considered resectable.
- Patients with non-resectable disease at recurrence are incurable and have MS of 6–9 months. Selected patients with good PS should be considered for palliative chemotherapy that is associated with a significant improvement in survival (median survival of 18–22 months) combined with an improvement in QOL.

Further reading
Baker K, Zlobec I, Tornillo L, et al. Differential significance of tumour infiltrating lymphocytes in sporadic mismatch repair deficient versus proficient colorectal cancers: a potential role for dysregulation of the transforming growth factor-beta pathway. *Eur J Cancer* 2007; **43**:624–31.

Bilchik AJ, Nora DT, Sobin LH, et al. Effect of lymphatic mapping on the new tumor-node-metastasis classification for colorectal cancer. *J Clin Oncol* 2003; **21**:668–72.

Compton C, Fenoglio-Preiser CM, Pettigrew N, Fielding LF. American Joint Committee on Cancer Prognostic Factors Consensus Conference: Colorectal Working Group. *Cancer* 2000; **88**:1739–57.

Galon J, Costes A, Sanchez-Cabo F, et al. Type, density, and location of immune cells within human colorectal tumors predict clinical outcome. *Science* 2006; **313**:1960–4.

Gan S, Wilson K, Hollington P. Surveillance of patients following surgery with curative intent for colorectal cancer. *World J Gastroent* 2007; **13**:3816–23.

Manfredi S, Bouvier AM, Lepage C, *et al.* Incidence and patterns of recurrence after resection for cure of colonic cancer in a well defined population. *Br J Surg* 2006; **93**:1115–22.

Popat S, Hubner R, Houlston RS. Systematic review of microsatellite instability and colorectal cancer prognosis. *J Clin Oncol* 2005; **23**:609–18.

Quirke P. *et al.* Local recurrence of rectal adenocarcinoma due to inadequate surgical resection. Histopathological study of lateral tumour spread and surgical excision. *Lancet* 1986; **2**:996–9.

Ropponen KM, Eskelinen MJ, Lipponen PK, *et al.* Prognostic value of tumour infiltrating lymphocytes (TILs) in colorectal cancer. *J Pathol* 1997; **182**:318–24.

Ruo L, Tickoo S, Klimstra DS, *et al.* Long-term prognostic significance of extent of rectal cancer response to preoperative radiation and chemotherapy. *Ann Surg* 2002; **236**:75–81.

Russo A, Bazan V, Agense V, *et al.* Prognostic and predictive factors in colorectal cancer: Kirsten Ras in CRC (RASCAL) and TP53CRC collaborative studies. *Ann Oncol* 2005; **16** (Supplement 4):iv44–iv49.

Wiggers T, Arends JW, Schutte B, *et al.* A multivariate analysis of pathologic prognostic indicators in large bowel cancer. *Cancer* 1998; **61**(2):386–95.

Zlobec I, Lugli A. Prognostic and predictive factors in colorectal cancer. *J Clin Pathol* 2008; **61**:561–9.

Anal cancer: introduction

Anal cancer is a rare cancer which can be treated with combination radiotherapy and chemotherapy resulting in high overall 5-year survival rates and preservation of normal sphincter function. Moreover, despite its rarity, large randomized phase III trials have been successfully performed allowing treatment to be refined.

Epidemiology

Anal cancer is a rare cancer representing only 4% of all lower GI cancers and 1.5% of all GI cancers. In the UK the annual incidence is approximately 1 per 100,000 resulting in 600 new cases per year. According to SEER data 4,660 men and women were diagnosed with anal cancer in the USA in 2006 and 660 died of the disease. There is a slight predominance in women (1.5–2), with rates increasing in women over the last 10 years. Data from the Nordic countries have also suggested that the incidence rates might have increased by 2.5–5 fold in the last 50 years.

Prior to the AIDS epidemic there was known to be a higher incidence of anal cancer in men who have receptive anal sex with men (MSM), estimated at 12–35 per 100,000. Interestingly there is only a weak association in women (relative risk, RR 1.8). However, the incidence in HIV positive MSM is much higher and some studies have suggested it could be as high as 70–75 per 100,000, although this high incidence has not been the experience of the authors. The relative risk of invasive squamous cancer in HIV positive women is 6.8 and a similar increase is seen in HIV positive heterosexual males.

The relative risk of the precursor lesions for invasive cancer (see later) is also higher in HIV positive MSM with a value of 60 compared to 7.8 for HIV positive women.

Other groups of immunosuppressed patients, in particular renal transplant patients, have an increased risk of developing anal cancer. The relative risk for all ano-genital malignancies for this group of patients has been estimated to be up to 20- fold.

Aetiology

It had been believed that benign lesions, in particular chronic irritation, progressed to invasive anal cancer. However, despite an association, benign lesions are not thought to progress to invasive cancer. Listed next are the most important risk factors for the development for anal cancer.

Human papilloma virus

HPV infection is a common sexually transmitted disease which is usually cleared by the immune system. However, in a process similar to that seen in cervical cancer, high- risk subtypes (including 16 and 18 amongst others) have been shown to be associated with the development of the premalignant condition, anal intraepithelial neoplasia (AIN) which can progress from low to high grade and in a proportion of patients to invasive cancer. Several population- based studies have examined the association between HPV infection and anal cancer and have detected HPV DNA in up to 90% of cancers. HPV subtype 16 is most commonly associated with anal cancer, being detected in up to 70% of cases in population- based studies. It is hoped that one of the 'side effects' of vaccination against cervical cancer in girls will be a reduction in the incidence of anal cancer.

Immunosuppression

As discussed earlier, patients who are immunosuppressed either as a result of HIV infection or iatrogenic (post-transplant or corticosteroids) have a higher risk of anal cancer.

The data on the association between HIV infection and anal cancer is difficult to interpret due to confounders including sexual practices and the likelihood that HIV positive patients are infected with multiple sub-types of HPV. However, a number of observations have been made. In the pre- highly active antiretroviral therapy (HAART) era although an increased incidence of pre-malignant lesions were diagnosed in HIV positive patients this did not appear to lead to an increased incidence of invasive cancer. However, in the post- HAART era the incidence of invasive anal cancer has increased. This has led to the suggestion that firstly HIV alone is probably not a causative factor in invasive cancer, as if it were, a decrease in incidence would have been expected as has been the case for other malignancies. Secondly, the increased incidence has been postulated to be due to the fact that individuals are living longer and therefore have more time for pre-invasive lesions to progress to invasive disease.

Knowing that certain groups of patients are at risk of developing invasive disease, a number of investigators have advocated screening using swabs similar to those used in cervical cancer. However, this area remains controversial and there are currently no screening programmes.

Smoking

Smoking increases the risk of anal cancer by approximately four, slightly higher for men than women. The risk has also been shown to decrease on smoking cessation.

Anatomy of anal canal

The anal canal extends from the perianal region known as the anal verge to the rectal mucosa. It is 3–4 cm long. The upper portion commences at the anorectal ring which is formed by the junction of the upper portion of the internal sphincter, the distal portion of the longitudinal muscles, the puborectalis, and the deep portion of the external sphincter. This can be felt on rectal examination. The anal canal finishes at the junction of squamous epithelium and the perianal skin. It is divided into two sections by the dentate line. Below the dentate line the mucosa is lined with squamous epithelium and above, by columnar epithelium. This is not an abrupt histological demarcation but rather a transition zone that is 6–12mm in length. The recognized consensus is that all tumours arising between the anorectal ring and the anal verge are classified as anal canal tumours and those arising distal to this as anal margin. Using this definition approximately 15% arise at the margin only and the remainder in the canal.

The external sphincter muscles are skeletal and voluntary, being innervated by the inferior rectal nerves from the pudendal nerve whereas the internal sphincters are smooth muscle, involuntary, and innervated by the parasympathetic nerves from S4. The action of both of these muscles is to constrict the anal canal. Below the dentate line the mucosa is sensitive to touch.

The anal canal has a rich supply of lymphatics. Lymphatic drainage relates to the dentate line. Below the line, drainage is to the inguinal and femoral nodes and subsequently to the external iliac and common iliac nodes. Above, the dentate line drainage is to perirectal and superior rectal nodes, inferior mesenteric, and eventually the para-aortic. However, there are extensive interconnections which explain why patients with distal cancers may have involvement of mesenteric nodes.

Pathology

The most common tumours are squamous, constituting 75% of all cancers. They arise from the whole length of the canal and margin. Those arising below the dentate line are keratinizing whereas those arising above the line are more likely to be non-keratinizing. Basaloid, also known as cloacogenic, are sub-types of non-keratinizing SCC which arise around the dentate line. Despite this distinction, stage rather than sub-type is more important in determining prognosis, as all behave in a similar manor.

Adenocarcinoma of the anal canal, probably arising from ducts or glands are rare and tend to behave like, and are treated in a similar way to low rectal cancers. Small cell cancers can also occur but are exceptionally rare. At the margin, as well as squamous all other skin tumours including basal carcinoma, Kaposi's sarcoma, and malignant melanomas may occur.

Anal cancer shows many similarities to cervical cancer, and a spectrum of precancerous changes has been described. These are referred to as anal intra-epithelial neoplasia (AIN). AIN can be classified in a similar way to cervical intra-epithelial neoplasia as AIN1, AIN2, and AIN3, the latter representing full thickness mucosa pre-cancerous changes.

A more recent Bethesda system has classified these changes as low- grade or high- grade squamous intra-epithelial lesions (LSIL or HSIL respectively). Although few data are available to determine progression rates it is thought that at least 5% progress to invasive cancer.

Clinical features

The most common presentation is with bleeding per rectum, often bright red blood. Diagnosis can be delayed as bleeding is often attributed to haemorrhoids. At least a third of patients present with pain and/or a rectal mass. One in five patients has no symptoms at all.

Patients presenting with large tumours might have symptoms of incontinence associated with anal sphincter disruption. Apparent incontinence might also be related to vaginal infiltration and fistulation. In both of these situations patients require formation of a defunctioning stoma in order to proceed with definitive treatment. Large tumours can also extend into the lower rectum, perineum, and less commonly the prostate and bony pelvis.

Gynaecological assessment should also include cervical smear history and assessment of the vulva and cervix (if no recent smear) in view of the association with HPV- related malignancies.

In most reported series inguinal nodes are found to be involved at presentation in about 15–20% of patients. Pelvic nodal involvement is less common but if present is usually associated with tumours arising above the dentate line.

Anal cancer: management

Diagnosis and staging

The diagnosis is by biopsy and examination under anaesthetic, documenting the extent of tumour including any involvement of the vagina and palpation of the inguinal nodal regions for the presence of lymphadenopathy.

Staging requires MRI of the pelvis to determine the extent of local disease and CT of the chest and abdomen to exclude distant metastases. FNA of suspicious lymph nodes is of limited exclusion value and not routinely used. Excision biopsy of suspicious nodes is not recommended as it leads to increased morbidity and delays definitive treatment. Recently the role of PET-CT has been investigated prospectively in small series of patients undergoing chemo-radiotherapy (CRT) treatment. These suggest an increase in the proportion of patients with involved nodes by about 15–20%. At present whether this information directly leads to improved outcome is not clear.

Staging is based on the AJCC and UICC 1997 system (Tables 4.5.5 and 4.5.6).

Principles of management

Over the last few decades the management of anal cancer has changed dramatically. For a long time, an abdominoperineal resection (APR) was the treatment of choice. However, as early as 1974, it was shown that CRT could be an effective alternative to surgery. A series of randomized clinical trials have subsequently evaluated CRT as definitive treatment for anal cancer and confirmed that CRT with mitomycin-C (MMC) and 5-FU combined with 45–60Gy in 1.8–2 Gy fractions to the pelvis is standard of care.

Table 4.5.5 AJCC anal cancer stage grouping

Stage			
Stage 0	Tis	N0	M0
Stage I	T1	N0	M0
Stage II	T2	N0	M0
	T3	N0	M0
Stage IIIA	T1	N1	M0
	T2	N1	M0
	T3	N1	M0
	T4	N1	M0
Stage IIIB	T4	N1	M0
	Any T	N2	M0
	Any T	N3	M0
Stage IV	Any T	Any N	M1

Surgery

Up until the mid 1980's the treatment of choice for anal cancer was APR with permanent colostomy. Local failure rates were 27–47% and OS 50–70% depending on stage and extent of the disease. Although there has never been a randomized trial comparing surgery with radiotherapy or CRT, clinical experience of high local control and cure rates coupled with reduced morbidity of CRT has led to this being the standard of care for patients with anal carcinomas. APR is now reserved for salvage treatment, but should also be considered in young women who wish to

Table 4.5.6 UICC anal cancer TNM staging system

Primary tumour (T)	
Tx	Primary tumour cannot be assessed
Tis	Carcinoma *in situ*
T0	No evidence of primary tumour
	Tumour ≤2cm or less in maximum dimension
	Tumour > 2cm but not > 5cm in maximum dimension
	Tumour > 5cm in maximum dimension
	Tumour of any size invading adjacent organs(s), e.g. vagina, urethra, bladder (involvement of sphincter muscle(s) alone is not classified as T4)
Lymph nodes (N)	
Nx	Regional nodes cannot be assessed
N0	No regional lymph nodes
N1	Metastasis in perirectal nodes
N2	Metastasis in unilateral internal iliac and/or inguinal lymph nodes (s)
N3	Metastasis in perirectal and inguinal nodes and / or bilateral internal iliac and / or inguinal nodes
Distant metastasis (M)	
Mx	Presence of distant metastasis cannot be assessed
M0	No distant metastasis
M1	Distant metastasis

preserve their fertility at the expense of a permanent stoma (an uncommon clinical scenario).

Local excision should be considered for small anal margin tumours < 2cm in diameter, where there is no evidence of disease in the anal canal, nodal spread and clear margins can be achieved without compromising function. Adenocarcinoma of the anal canal is rare and should be managed in the same way as adenocarcinoma of the low rectum. This might require adjuvant radiotherapy or CRT followed by surgery, usually an APR.

Radiotherapy

A number of studies have investigated the role of radiotherapy alone. Most of these are from the late 1980s and early 1990s before the establishment of CRT as the treatment of choice. Treatment is either with external beam alone or in combination with a brachytherapy boost.

Local control and survival rates comparable to those seen with CRT have been reported with external beam alone. However high doses of radiotherapy, 60Gy or more, are required, resulting in higher reported rates of toxicity, with around 10%, requiring surgery. Very high rates of local control have also been reported for patients treated with combination EBRT and a brachytherapy boost. A brachytherapy boost is attractive as it allows sparing of normal tissue and thus minimizing the possibility of late toxicity. Local control rates comparable to CRT have been reported in the region of 75–79% with 5 year OS rates of up to 64%. However, apart from one French study of 276 patients, the majority of whom had T1 and T2 disease where a necrosis rate of 3% was seen, most report anal necrosis rates of 10% or more.

In summary, radiotherapy alone might be considered in patients who are unable to tolerate chemotherapy; however, high doses are required leading to higher rates of significant toxicity. Brachytherapy should only be used by clinicians with sufficient training and who have experience in treating other disease sites.

Combined modality treatment

Norman Nigro was the first to describe in a case report complete response in three patients treated with mitomycin C (MMC) and 5-FU combined with 30Gy radiotherapy. A subsequent report described the outcome for 45 patients treated with the same regimen with a complete response rate of 84% on biopsy 6 weeks after completion of treatment. A number of investigators reported encouraging results of initial non-surgical treatment either using radiotherapy alone or concurrent CRT. This in turn led to three pivotal randomized control trials that investigated the role of CRT.

Radiotherapy versus chemotherapy

The United Kingdom Coordinating Committee on Cancer Research (UKCCCR) reported the results of a trial comparing radiotherapy alone to CRT. Five hundred and eighty-five patients were randomized to either radiotherapy alone, 45Gy over 5 weeks or the same dose with the addition of 5-FU (1000mg/m^2 per day for 4 days or 750mg/m^2 per day over 5 days) during the first and last week of radiotherapy and mitomycin (12 mg/m^2 on day 1 only). Response was assessed at 6 weeks. Good responders received a boost of 15Gy in 6 fractions using either photons or electrons or a brachytherapy boost of 25Gy at 10Gy per day. The primary endpoint was local failure and secondary, overall and cause-specific survival. Approximately 50% of patients in each arm had T3/4 disease and 20% were

node positive. The local failure was 59% in the radiotherapy alone arm and 36% in the CRT arm. There was no OS benefit (58% versus 65% for CRT) probably due to the effect of salvage surgery; however, the risk of death from anal cancer was reduced in the CRT arm. Of note, early morbidity was higher in the CRT arm; however, reported late morbidity was similar for both arms. Of note in the first part of the trial, six deaths related to chemotherapy were reported; this led to a protocol amendment limiting the dose of MMC in elderly patients to 8mg/m^2 with no further deaths due to septicaemia.

A second similar trial was reported by the European Organization for Research and Treatment of Cancer (EORTC). One hundred and ten patients were randomized to either radiotherapy alone (45Gy in 5 weeks) followed by a boost of 15Gy for complete responders and 20Gy for poor responders 6 weeks after completion of initial treatment. In the CRT arm, patients received chemotherapy similar to that in the UKCCCR trial. CRT improved local control by 18% with a 32% higher colostomy- free survival rate in the CRT arm. They found no difference in acute toxicity whilst event-free survival (including tumour progression and late toxicity) was better for the CRT arm.

Following publication of these trials, CRT with combination 5-FU and MMC is accepted as the standard treatment for anal cancer.

Which chemotherapy?

MMC was felt to add significant toxicity and for this reason Flam and colleagues investigated CRT with 5-FU and MMC or 5-FU alone. Radiotherapy and chemotherapy doses were similar to those in the UKCCCR and EORTC trials. Evaluation was at 4–6 weeks with a biopsy and patients with residual disease went on to have a further 9Gy. The addition of MMC resulted in a significantly higher colostomy- free survival rate at 4 years (71% versus 59%) and DFS rate (73% versus 51%). However, these results were balanced by a higher significant toxicity rate (23% versus 7%) with 4 versus 1 death in the MMC compared with the 5-FU arm. The authors concluded that MMC was an important component of the treatment and remained the standard of care.

More recently The Radiation Therapy Oncology Group (RTOG) has reported the results of the 98-11 trial evaluating the role of cisplatin given both adjuvantly and concurrently in place of MMC. Six hundred and eighty-two patients were randomized to either 5-FU (1000mg/m^2 days 1–4 and 29–32) and MMC 10mg/m^2 days 1 and 29) combined with 45–59Gy of radiotherapy or the same doses of radiotherapy preceded by two cycles of 5-FU and cisplatin (75mg/m^2) and two cycles with the radiotherapy. Based on 634 evaluable patients there was no significant difference in DFS (60% in MMC group and 54% in cisplatin arm) and OS (75% versus 70%). However, the colostomy rate was higher in the cisplatin arm: 19% versus 10%. The second UK study, ACTII is a four-arm study using a factorial 2x2 design comparing 1) concurrent cisplatin 5FU CRT with MMC 5FU CRT (50Gy in both arms) and 2) maintenance chemotherapy post- CRT (two cycles of 5-FU and cisplatin) versus no maintenance chemotherapy. Until this trial reports the standard of care remain 5-FU and MMC without neo- or adjuvant chemotherapy. The radiotherapy technique used in the ACT2 trial is in two phases with 30.6Gy in 17 fractions to the primary and all nodal structures at risk in both the pelvis and inguinal regions followed by 19.8 Gy in 11 fractions to all sites of gross tumour volume with a 3-cm margin.

Treatment of elderly and HIV positive patients

All three randomized trails included patients with good PS and a median age of 55–60 years. Although many elderly patients are able tolerate full dose CRT there remains a group of patients where a palliative approach is required. The approach may range from a single or short fractionated course of radiotherapy treating the tumour plus margin only in an attempt to control bleeding or pain. However, if significant tumour regression is to be achieved then a modified CRT regimen of 30Gy encompassing the tumour and involved nodes combined with 600mg/m^2 of 5 FU days 1–4 can achieve long- term control in up to 70% of patients.

Data from small series suggest that outcome is similar to HIV negative patients, especially in the era of HAART; however, there is an increased level of acute and late toxicity. Prior to the era of HAART, a small series suggested that treatment-related toxicity was higher for patients with CD4 counts <200. Subsequently two later series have not shown any relationship between CD4 count and toxicity.

In general, HIV positive patients should be treated with standard protocols although modification in radiation volume and chemotherapy dose, especially MMC (if haematological abnormalities are present or a previous history of significant opportunistic infection) may be necessary. It is important to commence HAART prior to CRT treatment and modification of chemotherapy doses.

Role of post-operative CRT

A small number of patients will be referred following excision of a lesion which turns out to be a cancer, or following excision of small cancers. This occurs most commonly in anal margin tumours. Local excision should be avoided in anal canal tumours as incomplete excision can compromise sphincter function especially when excision is followed by CRT.

If a small tumour (<2cm) has been excised locally with close or involved margins a number of approaches have been advocated, including brachytherapy, full dose CRT, radiotherapy alone, or modified CRT (30Gy to an involved field only combined with 5 FU days 1–4 and MMC day 1). Although there are no randomized trials to support any of these approaches the authors have reported local control rates of 95% and no significant late toxicity for this group of patients.

Toxicity

Acute skin toxicity ranging from erythema to moist desquamation is universal, although the grade is variable. In some cases the severity can lead to treatment gaps or early discontinuation of treatment. Other acute toxicities include diarrhoea, urinary symptoms, and those related to chemotherapy.

Late toxicity includes anal ulceration, stenosis, and necrosis necessitating a colostomy in up to 10% of patients who are otherwise disease free. More common, and poorly documented in the literature, is the level of functional toxicity including urgency, frequency, incontinence, and 'toilet dependency'. Vaginal stenosis and premature ovarian failure can occur, although in very young women contraception should be continued until failure is proven. Male patients should be offered sperm banking as temporary or permanent azoospermia might occur.

Management of metastatic and recurrent disease

Salvage therapy should be considered for patients with either persistent or recurrent disease, in general with an APR. The definition of persistent disease is controversial. Response is generally assessed at 6–8 weeks following completion of CRT. Some advocate biopsy at 6 weeks, even if there has been a complete response whilst others, recognizing that squamous tumours can take up to 12 weeks to regress, closely monitor patients only performing biopsy of residual abnormalities at 3 months.

For patients with suspected recurrent disease a small biopsy should be performed followed by restaging (approximately one-third will have synchronous distant failure). For those patients with isolated local failure only around 60% will be able to undergo salvage surgery (usually APR) and the long- term disease control is in the region of 30–40% with similar overall survival.

Distant metastases occur in approximately 10% of patients with the liver being the commonest site. Only combination cisplatin and 5-FU has been widely reported as active. Other agents where activity has been reported include carboplatin, doxorubicin, irinotecan, and irinotecan in combination with cetuximab.

Prognosis

The risk of local failure is substantially higher for patients with T4 or node- positive disease. The overall risk of local failure for T1/2N0 patients is 10–15%. The majority of local failures are identified within the first 6 months of completion of CRT with the remainder found within 2–3 years.

Follow-up

Follow-up is dictated by the pattern of recurrence and the recognition that a proportion of patients can be salvaged with surgery. Most recurrences will occur in the first 2 years. Therefore it is recommended that patients are seen every 3 months for the first 2 years and then 6-monthly for year 3, and annually to 5 years. Digital rectal examination and examination of groins should be performed at each visit and other investigations dictated by symptoms or findings.

The role of regular CT scanning to detect metastatic disease is controversial as detection is rarely curable. The current ACT II study, where regular imaging is part of the follow-up protocol will hopefully answer this question. Tumour markers have no role in follow-up.

Cancer of kidney: introduction

Epidemiology

Renal cell carcinoma (RCC) accounts for approximately 2% of cancer diagnosis worldwide. It has the highest mortality of any urological cancer. Clear-cell renal cell carcinoma (CC-RCC) is the commonest RCC. CC-RCC has the highest prevalence in Eastern Europe and is the fifth commonest solid tumour in the UK. Incidence of primary CC-RCC rises after the age of 40 years old and there is a 2:1 male to female ratio.

Renal tumours are classified using the WHO system which defines histopathological tumour subtypes with different clinical behaviours and underlying genetic mutations. More than 90% of tumours are one of the common subtypes: CC(conventional)-RCC (75%), papillary RCC (10–15%), chromophobe RCC (5–10%), and renal oncocytoma. Mesenchymal renal tumours are rarer. CC-RCC has the highest rate of metastasis and poorest survival. Papillary and chromophobe carcinomas are less aggressive but can metastasize or transform to high-grade, sarcomatoid tumours. Oncocytomas and angiomyolipomas behave relatively benignly.

Aetiology

Familial syndromes

Several different genetic mutations are associated with RCC.

Pseudohypoxic syndromes

In these syndromes there is alteration of levels of expression of hypoxia-inducible factors (HIF) which are regulators of oxygen homeostasis. Loss of VHL or FH (described later) results in a pseudohypoxic state so that cellular response pathways are inappropriately activated.

- Von Hippel–Lindau (VHL) syndrome is manifest by germline loss of VHL at chromosome 3p. Multifocal and/or bilateral CC-RCC tumours are well recognized. VHL syndrome is divided into two types: in type 1 there is a low risk of developing phaechromocytoma and in type 2 a higher risk Type 2 is subdivided into types a and b based on the risk of developing RCC and hemangioblastomas.
- Mitochondrial germline deletions of enzymes involved within the tricarboxylic acid cycle (TCA) cycle, such as fumarate hydratase (FH) and succinate dehydrogenase (SDH), also can lead to CC-RCC with cutaneous/uterine leiomyomata or paragangliomas/abdominal phaechromocytomas, respectively.

Non-pseudohypoxic syndromes

- Birt–Hogg–Dube (BHD) syndrome: 15–30% of BHD patients develop RCCs. It is caused by homozygous deletion of the folliculin (FLCN) gene, and leads to fibrofolliculomas and pleural blebs causing pneumothorax.
- Hereditary leiomyomatosis renal cell carcinoma (HLRCC) leads to type II papillary RCCs (distinguished histologically from the better prognosis type I) which show lymphovascular invasion and can be very aggressive and metastasize rapidly, although they often present as single primary tumours. Cutaneous leiomyomata as well as uterine fibroids are also recognized.
- Hereditary papillary renal cell carcinoma—Type 1: germline mutation in c-Met; presents with slow growing primary papillary tumours (with type 1 papillary histology).
- Xp11.2 translocation involving the TFE3 gene on chromosome X is a recognized cytogenetic abnormality

leading to the development of CC-RCCs in children and young adults.

Pathology

Benign renal lesions may progress to malignancy. The most notable of these are renal cysts and oncocytomas. RCC arises from the nephron tubular epithelium. There are four main histological subtypes, with marked differences in incidence: Clear-cell (85%), papillary (10%), chromophobe (<5%), and collecting duct tumours (<1%). CC-RCCs arise from the proximal tubule and are histologically graded using Fuhrman's criteria. These are based on nucleoli size and morphology at x10 magnification. Fuhrman's grading can only be used for CC-RCC.

Rare RCC histological subtypes include neuroendocrine (carcinoid) tumours, PNETs, and Ewing's osteosarcomas.

Genetics of sporadic CC-RCCs

More than 85% of CC-RCCs are deficient in the expression or function of the tumour suppressor, pVHL, which is found on chromosome 3p. Sporadic CC-RCCs also arise in patients with end-stage renal failure (ESRF) on long-term haemodialysis, but their carcinogenesis may be different, although loss of pVHL is also recognized.

Genetics of sporadic non-CC-RCC tumours

- Papillary RCCs are thought to arise mainly through acquired mutations in c-Met.
- Chromophobe tumours have better OS than papillary and collecting-duct tumours. Collecting-duct tumours usually present at an advanced stage and are of higher histological grade than CC-RCCs.

Clinical features

- 'Incidentalomas' detected at routine ultrasound or CT scanning are increasing.
- Haematuria is the most common symptom.
- Twenty-five per cent of patients present with metastatic disease and the thorax is the commonest site.
- Less than 10% of primary CC-RCC present with the 'classical triad' of flank pain, haematuria, and fever.
- Bone lesions occur in up to 30% of patients with metastases and are typically osteolytic and painful.
- Soft tissue metastasis may be hypervascular and have an audible bruit.
- Atypical metastatic sites of disease may include the ovaries and small intestine, with the latter causing problematic GI tract bleeding.
- Para-neoplastic manifestations (common): weight loss and fever (IL-6 mediated); hypercalcaemia (PTHrP); polycythaemia and hypertension (erythropoietin, EPO).

Diagnosis

Imaging

There are no specific radiological characteristics suggesting RCCs. However, cystic lesions and contrast-enhancement are typical of CC-RCCs, particularly using CT.

- The Bosniak classification (I–IV) of CT-detected renal cysts can be used to predict the likelihood of malignancy (Table 4.6.1). Bosniak IV lesions are typically multiseptated, rim-enhancing lesions that invariably correlate with the pathological findings of CC-RCC.

Table 4.6.1 Bosniak classification of renal cysts on CT

Bosniak category	Features
I	A simple benign cyst with a hairline thin wall that does not contain septa, calcification or solid components. It measures as water density and does not enhance with contrast material.
II	A benign cyst that might contain a few hairline thin septa. Fine calcification might be present in the wall or septa. Uniformly high-attenuation lesions of <3 cm that are sharply marginated and do not enhance.
IIF	These cysts might contain more hairline thin septa. Minimal enhancement of a hairline thin septum or wall can be seen and there might be minimal thickening of the septa or wall. The cyst might contain calcification that might be nodular and thick but there is no contrast enhancement. There are no enhancing soft-tissue elements. Totally intrarenal non-enhancing high-attenuation renal lesions of >3 cm are also included in this category. These lesions are generally well marginated.
III	These lesions are indeterminate cystic masses that have thickened irregular walls or septa in which enhancement can be seen.
IV	These lesions are clearly malignant cystic lesions that contain enhancing soft-tissue components.

- *Pitfall:* Bosniak III lesions may occasionally represent necrotic cancers.
- Oncocytomas on CT may have a typical low-attenuation 'naked-eye' appearance.
- MRI is particularly used in the assessment of the superior extension of tumour-thrombus pre-cavotomy/thrombus resection.
- Transoesphageal echocardiogram (TOE) may also be useful for Mayo level III/IV tumour-thrombus in pre-operative planning.
- ^{99}Tc-isotope bone scan is not sensitive in the detection of CC-RCC bone metastasis and MRI has a better sensitivity.
- ^{19}FDG-PET scan has an undefined role at present, but initial studies suggest that it may have a significant impact in the surgical management of disease.

Staging

AJCC 2002 TNM classification is currently used:

Primary tumour (T):
- TX: primary tumour cannot be assessed
- T0: no evidence of primary tumour
- T1: tumour ≤7cm, limited to kidney
- T2: tumour >7 cm, limited to kidney
- T3: tumour extends into major veins/adrenal/ perinephric tissue; not beyond Gerota's fascia
- T3a: tumour invades renal sinus and /or adrenal/perinephric fat
- T3b: tumour extends into renal vein(s) or vena cava below diaphragm
- T3c: tumour extends into vena cava above diaphragm
- T4: tumour invades beyond Gerota's fascia

Regional lymph nodes (N)
- NX: regional nodes cannot be assessed
- N0: no regional lymph node metastasis
- N1: metastasis in a single regional lymph node
- N2: metastasis in more than one regional lymph node

Distant metastasis (M)
- MX: distant metastasis cannot be assessed
- M0: no distant metastasis
- M1: distant metastasis

Staging notes
- T3a stage now includes renal sinus invasion, as well as perinephric fat and adrenal gland involvement.
- T3b disease is classified as involvement of either renal vein (30% cases) or IVC (5–10%) tumour ± thrombus. Tumour-thrombus is not a detrimental prognostic finding.
- T3c disease is evaluated according to the Mayo classification which anatomically divides IVC involvement into 4 levels (Levels I–IV: I = renal, II = infra-hepatic, III = intrahepatic/suprahepatic, IV = right atrial involvement). Patients with either level III suprahepatic or level IV tumour-thrombus need careful cardiothoracic surgical assessment.

Cancer of kidney: prognosis and surgical management

Clinical risk stratification

Non-metastatic disease

The Mayo and UISS (UCLA integrated staging system) nomograms are commonly used (Leibovich et al. 2003). The Mayo system (Table 4.6.2) classifies primary tumours into low-, intermediate-, and high-risk groups. The UISS system stratifies clinical risk into five categories (I–V) based on TNM staging (AJCC 1997), Fuhrman's grade and ECOG PS. Such nomograms are useful in the allocation of patients into *adjuvant* trials.

Metastatic disease

The cornerstone of prognostic models in metastatic CC-RCC is the Memorial Sloan–Kettering Cancer Center (MSKCC) prognostic system, which was later modified (Table 4.6.3) (Motzer et al. 1999).
* Good prognosis (no risk factor): median survival 29 months.
* Intermediate prognosis (1–2 risk factors): median survival 15 months.

Table 4.6.2 The Mayo primary CC-RCC classification system (Leibovich et al. 2003)—Mayo scoring algorithm to predict metastases after radical nephrectomy in patients with clear cell renal cell carcinoma

Feature	Score
Primary tumour status (pathologic T stage)	
pT1a	0
pT1b	2
pT2	3
pT3a	4
pT3b	4
pT3c	4
pT4	4
Regional lymph node status (N stage)	
pNx	0
pN0	0
pN1	2
pN2	2
Tumour size (cm)	
<10	0
>10	1
Nuclear grade	
1	0
2	0
3	1
Histological tumour necrosis	
No	0
Yes	1

* Poor prognosis (3 or more risk factors): median survival 4.5 months.

Table 4.6.3 The modified MSKCC prognostic system (Motzer et al. 1999)

Modified MSKCC prognostic markers	Risk factor
Karnofsky score (KS)	<80%
Corrected calcium	>10mg/dL
Haemoglobin	<lower limit of local reference range
Serum LDH	>1.5x upper limit of local reference range
Time to immunotherapy from initial diagnosis of metastasis	<12 months

The Cleveland Clinic Foundation (CCF) extended-MSKCC prognostic system is currently the best clinical prognostic model for first-line therapy in the era of tyrokinase inhibitors (TKIs) (Mikhail et al. 2005). This consists of 4 prognostic markers from modified MSKCC and 4 additional markers (Table 4.6.4). (KS is not included since all patients within the initial study were either performance status 0 or 1). Both the models permit subdivision into good, intermediate-, and high-risk categories (see Table 4.6.5, p.261).
* Good prognosis (0–1 risk factors): median survival 26 months.
* Intermediate prognosis (2 risk factors): median survival 14.4 months.
* Poor prognosis (>2 risk factors): median survival 7 months.

Surgical management

Curative surgery

Radical nephrectomy is the cornerstone of the management of primary RCCs. The roles of nephron-sparing surgery (NSS) and laparoscopic approaches are being very actively developed. NSS is particularly suited to small (<4cm) lesions at the poles or periphery of the kidney, and anatomically isolated from the hilum or collecting-duct system. There are no randomized studies to date comparing open versus laparoscopic radical nephrectomy. Laparoscopic surgery has a lower complication rate and operative blood loss than open surgery, but a large tumour is an indication for open surgery.

Table 4.6.4 CCF extended MSKCC prognostic system

CCF extended-MSKCC model	Risk factor
Additional prognostic markers	
Prior radiotherapy	+
Hepatic metastasis	+
Pulmonary metastasis	+
Retroperitoneal lymph node metastasis	+

Table 4.6.5 Treatment algorithm for metastatic CC-RCC in the era of small molecule inhibitors using extended-MSKCC prognostic criteria

	Good risk	Intermediate risk	Poor risk
First-line	IFN, IFN + bevacizumab, or sunitinib	Sunitinib or sorafenib	Temsirolimus (USA)
Second-line	Sorafenib	Some data for TKI switch	Few data

In T3b disease, radical nephrectomy with vena cavotomy and resection of the caval thrombus can provide long-term survival rates up to 68% at 5 years. Tumour-thrombus in the IVC is an indication for anticoagulation with low-molecular-weight heparin. If significant haematuria is present, radiological assessment for an IVC filter should be made.

Radiofrequency ablation (RFA), cryoablation or the developing technique of high-intensity frequency ultrasound (HIFU), are alternatives to surgery that are actively being developed. Concerns remain as to the most reliable means of detecting dead tumour tissue treated with either RFA or HIFU.

Role of surgery in metastatic disease

Surgery of primary tumour
The usual indications for radical nephrectomy in metastatic disease are a symptomatic primary tumour and possible optimization of response to immunotherapy. Subtotal nephrectomy may also be used to manage uncontrolled haematuria and/or primary tumour pain.

Nephrectomy produces a response on metastatic (mainly thoracic) disease of <0.5%. However, the response rate to cytokine therapies may be increased by pretreatment nephrectomy. The SWOG 8949 trial of IFNα alone versus radical nephrectomy followed by IFNα demonstrated an increased PFS and improvement in OS from 8.1 to 11.1 months (p= 0.05). Retrospective studies have demonstrated that post-nephrectomy IL-2 may possibly be superior to IFNα (Flanagan et al. 2001).

Surgery of loco-regional metastasis
Retroperitoneal lymph node (RPLN) is the commonest loco-regional site of metastasis. RPLN metastasis increases the risk of distant metastasis 3–4 fold. Studies show that an isolated RPLN metastasis is as detrimental to OS as a single-site distant metastasis. However, prophylactic retroperitoneal lymph node dissection (RPLND) does *not* improve OS compared with radical nephrectomy alone, whereas in patients with proven RPLN metastases, lymphadenectomy improves OS and possibly increases the response to postoperative IL-2.

Surgery of distant metastasis (metastatectomy)
Surgery of distant metastases may be performed with either palliative or potentially curative intent.
Patient selection is paramount when considering potentially curative surgery. Many specialists would observe a patient with an apparently solitary lesion for 3–6 months before restaging to confirm that no new metastasis had arisen. The role of ^{18}FDG-PET is being evaluated in diagnosing CT-occult disease. Early studies suggest that it may alter the initial surgical decision in up to 35% of all CC-RCC cases. Favourable features for a curative metastatectomy include good performance status and a PFS of at least 1 year. Clinical benefit from surgery declines very rapidly if multiple metastases are present.

Resection of pulmonary metastasis is the most common surgical procedure with curative intent. Complete pulmonary metastatectomy may give 5-year OS of about 50%. Stereotactic neuro- or γ-knife radiosurgery can be used in the treatment of isolated brain or spinal cord metastasis. For potentially operable bone metastasis, with curative intent, assessment by an experienced orthopaedic cancer surgeon is mandatory.

Orthopaedic surgery is the commonest palliative surgical intervention and is often used prophylactically to prevent pathological fracture.

Further reading

Flanagan RC, Salmon SE, Blumenstein BA, *et al.* Nephrectomy followed by interferon alfa-2b compared with interferon alfa-2b alone for metastatic renal-cell cancer. *N Engl J Med* 2001; **345**(23):1655–9.

Leibovich BC, Blute ML, Cheville JC, *et al.* Prediction of progression after radical nephrectomy for patients with clear cell renal cell carcinoma: a stratification tool for prospective clinical trials. *Cancer* 2003; **97**:1663–71.

Mikhail T, Abou-Jawde RM, BouMerhi G, *et al.* Validation and extension of the Memorial Sloan-Kettering prognostic factors model for survival in patients with previously untreated metastatic renal cell carcinoma. *J Clin Oncol* 2005; **23**(4):832–41.

Motzer RJ, Mazumdar M, Bacik J, *et al.* Survival and prognostic stratification of 670 patients with advanced renal cell carcinoma. *J Clin Oncol* 1999; **17**(8):2530–40.

Cancer of kidney: non-surgical management

Radiotherapy

RCC displays a variable sensitivity to radiation in the metastatic setting. Radiotherapy is indicated to palliate pain (e.g. bone/soft tissue), bleeding (e.g. lung/GI metastasis), spinal cord compression, and brain metastases. Radiotherapy is beneficial for local treatment of inoperable primary tumours causing uncontrolled pain or haematuria. Radiotherapy is also useful if tumour pain and/or bleeding persist after subtotal nephrectomy. Selective arterial embolization can also be used for the same indications.

Special situations

Thorax

- Radio-frequency ablation (RFA) can be used in the management of small volume pulmonary metastasis.
- Symptomatic endobronchial lesions may be treated with cryotherapy or photocoagulation.
- Selective arterial embolization can also be used for inoperable bleeding pulmonary lesions that are not suitable for or refractory to radiotherapy.

Bone

- Bisphosphonate infusions are used in either focal or diffuse bony pain.
- Osseous selective arterial embolization and RFA can also be used to treat refractory focal bony pain.
- Percutaneous vertebroplasty with methyl methacrylate can be used in cases of vertebral collapse.

Systemic therapy in CC-RCC

CC-RCC is a chemoresistant disease.

Adjuvant (postnephrectomy)

None of the following are established as standard adjuvant therapy: chemotherapy, cytokines, chemo-immunotherapy, vaccine-based approaches or postoperative radiation to the renal bed.

Advanced/metastatic CC-RCC

Spontaneous remissions in low-volume, mainly intrathoracic disease are well documented. Metastatic CC-RCC has a <5% response rate to medoxyprogesterone acetate, but this is mainly used for palliation of constitutional symptoms.

Cytokine therapy

Cytokine therapy mainly involves the use of interferon α (IFNα) or interleukin-2 (IL-2). However, IFNα and IL-2 have no proven beneficial role in metastatic non-CC-RCCs. IFNα, which also has an antiangiogenic effect, has been the standard therapy in Europe and gives a response rate of up to 15% in metastatic CC-RCC, with <2% having a complete response. It has little activity in liver, bone, or brain metastasis, and in brain metastasis may precipitate seizures and tumour-induced cerebral oedema. IFNα therapy is restricted to extended-MSKCC good risk category patients with predominantly pulmonary metastasis or nodal disease.

High-dose IL-2 can also be considered as a first-line therapy in advanced CC-RCC patients with purely clear-cell histology, high carbonic anhydrase IX (CAIX) expression (which may predict efficacy of IL-2 therapy), and with extended-MSKCC classified good prognosis. High-dose IV IL-2 can lead to durable complete responses in <5% patients, mainly with intrathoracic disease. However, clinical utility of high-dose IV IL-2 is limited due to its toxicity and the frequent requirement for inotropic support.

Antiangiogenic multitargeted tyrosine kinase inhibitors (TKIs)

Development of TKIs such as sunitinib and sorafenib represents a paradigm shift in treatment for metastatic CC-RCC. These agents share the following side effects:

- Commonly cause fatigue, diarrhoea, rash, stomatitis, and nausea.
- Hand–foot syndrome, diarrhoea, and myelosuppression may be treatment limiting.
- Each drug can induce both hepatic and thyroid dysfunction, isolated thrombocytopenia, hyponatraemia, alopecia, skin discoloration, and VTE.
- Both TKIs can also precipitate pericardial or pleural effusions in intrathoracic metastatic disease.
- Both TKIs can induce drug interactions as they inhibit hepatic CYP3A4.
- Careful monitoring of the INR is recommended with warfarin.

Cardiovascular complications are important during the use of TKIs. Both TKIs can cause hypertension and cardiotoxicity. Hence, echocardiography, to assess LV function, is advised in patients with known cardiovascular co-morbidities both before and during treatment. Sunitinib should be avoided in patients with ventricular tachyarrhythmias since it can elongate the QT interval; similarly, concomitant use of clarithromycin should be avoided in patients on sunitinib.

In general sunitinib produces more clinically significant fatigue, stomatitis, and cardiovascular effects than sorafenib. Sorafenib produces more alopecia and skin toxicity.

Sunitinib

Sunitinib is a TKI against VEGFR-1, -2, -3, PDGFR-1, -2, and c-kit. In a randomized phase III, interferon-controlled trial of sunitinib as first-line treatment in advanced renal cancer, PFS was doubled to 11 months compared with 5 months in the interferon group (HR 0.415; p <0.000001) (Motzer et al. 2007). Patients who received sunitinib had a response rate (CR+PR) of 31% compared with 6% for the IFNα group (Fig. 4.6.1). There was also a reduction in the risk of death with sunitinib (HR: 0.65; p= 0.0219). The benefit of sunitinib seems to be retained within all MSKCC metastatic prognostic groups. Since patients were allowed to crossover therapies, there has been no proven benefit in overall survival. The suggested treatment schedule consists of sunitinib 50mg once daily orally for 28 days and the cycle repeated every 42 days. Radiological disease evaluation is usually performed every 2 cycles.

A continuous dosing regimen of 37.5mg once daily orally, is equivalent to the standard dosing schedule in terms of PFS, but has a lower response rate. The continuous schedule may be helpful for patients with:

- Cumulative drug toxicities
- Uncontrolled haematuria/metastatic deposit haemorrhage (to control bleeding)

Sorafenib

Acts as a TKI against VEGFR-1, -2, -3, PDGFR-1, -2, c-kit, FLT-3, c-RET, CSF-1, and has anti-MAP kinase activity.

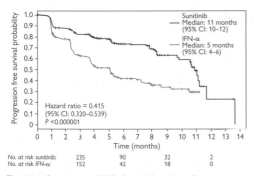

Fig. 4.6.1 Comparison of PFS of sunitinib and interferon-α. Reproduced from Motzer RJ, Hutson TE, Tomczak P, et al. Sunitinib versus interferon alfa in metastatic renal-cell carcinoma. *N Engl J Med* 2007; **356**(2):115–24.

First-line: it has no established clinical role, although response rates of 2–10% have been demonstrated. Addition of IFNα may increase response rates up to 19%.

Second-line: the TARGET trial demonstrated that in IFNα refractory patients, sorafenib has a response rate of 10% compared with 2% for placebo (2). There was an increase in PFS from 2.8 to 5.5 months in the sorafenib arm. Since patients were allowed to crossover trial arms, there has been no proven benefit in OS.

Dosing schedule: 400mg twice daily orally for 28 days (1 cycle).

Dose escalation of sorafenib (and sunitinib) may increase clinical activity of these agents, but level 1 evidence is currently lacking.

Non-CC-RCC
Immunotherapy is not effective in these histological sutypes of disease. TKIs may have efficacy in advanced non-CC-RCCs (Schrader et al. 2008). Novel VEGF targeting agents may have a role.

Chemotherapy generally has modest response in renal cell carcinoma (10–15%). In RCC with sarcomatoid features chemotherapy may have some benefit. In one study a combination of gemcitabine with adriamycin produced a response rate of 28% (David et al. 2006).

Alternative novel biological therapies
Antiangiogenic agents: bevacizumab is a recombinant humanized IgG1 monoclonal antibody against pan-VEGF isoforms. It has some role in second-line IL-2 refractory metastatic disease. Phase II trial evidence shows an increase in PFS from 2.5 months to 4.8 months compared with placebo (p <0.001) with 10mg/kg bimonthly, but only 3.0 months (p = 0.041) with 3mg/kg bimonthly. However, there was no effect on OS. Common side effects include hypertension, proteinuria, allergy, nausea, lethargy, venous thromboembolic disease and bleeding. It is used in a dose of 10mg/kg IV bimonthly.

AVOREN study demonstrates that addition of bevacizumab to IFNα improves PFS from 5.5 months to 10.4 months (HR 0.63, p <0.0001), with an increase in RR from 12.4% to 30.6% (p <0.0001). OS is increased from 21.3 to 23.3 months.

Growth factor pathway inhibitors: mTOR inhibition
In treatment-naïve patients within the high-risk MSKCC group, temsirolimus (CCI-779) improves PFS and OS when compared to IFNα alone (HR 0.73, p = 0.008), or the combination of the two drugs at lower doses (Hudes et al. 2007). The dose is 25mg IV weekly and radiological re-assessment is usually performed 8–12 weeks after commencement of therapy.

Side effects include anaphylaxis, diarrhoea, intestinal perforation, interstitial pneumonitis (acute and chronic), myelosuppression, hepatic/renal dysfunction, and drug interactions with steroids, non-steroidal anti-inflammatory agents, and macrolide antibiotics.

There is some evidence for effectiveness of everolimus used for progressive disease after sunitinib and/or sorafenib.

Experimental immunotherapies
Much effort in the last 20 years has been concentrated in various immunological trials in CC-RCC (e.g. dendritic cell vaccines). To date, no trial has provided a significant improvement in OS, although anecdotal cases of prolonged complete remissions are well documented.

Allograft stem-cell transplantation (allo-SCT or mini-allo-SCT) has also been used, and although disease control is known, treatment induced mortality can be as high as 30% in some studies. This should be considered strictly experimental.

Future prospects
The role of multitargeted antiangiogenic TKIs in the adjuvant setting is currently undefined. The ongoing SORCE (sorafenib vs. placebo), STAR (sunitinib vs. placebo) and ASSURE (sorafenib vs. placebo + sunitinib vs. placebo) trials will address these questions. The role of antiangiogenic TKIs in the neoadjuvant (prenephrectomy) setting will be investigated.

Better serum/tissue molecular prognostic profiles may enhance the current clinical nomograms used in both the postnephrectomy and metastatic disease settings. The development of robust biomarkers will also greatly assist the clinical usage of many novel biological therapies, and predict developing drug resistance/disease progression before any radiological progression becomes apparent.

Further reading
David KA, Milowsky MI, Nanus DM. Chemotherapy for non-clear-cell renal cell carcinoma. *Clin Genitourin Cancer* 2006; **4**(4):263–8.

Escudier B, Eisen T, Stadler WM. et al. Sorafenib in advanced clear-cell renal-cell carcinoma. *N Engl J Med* 2007; **356**:125–34.

Escudier B, Bellmunt J, Negier S, et al. Final results of the phase III randomized doiuble blind AVOREN trial of first line bevacizumab plus interferon alfa-2a in metastatic renal cell carcinoma. *J Clin Oncol* 2009; **18s**:(abstract 5020).

Hudes G, Carducci M, Tomczak P, et al. Temsirolimus, Interferon alfa, or both for advanced renal-cell carcinoma. *N Engl J Med* 2007; **356**:2271–81.

Motzer RJ, Hutson TE, Tomczak P, et al. Sunitinib versus interferon alfa in metastatic renal-cell carcinoma. *N Engl J Med* 2007; **356**(2):115–24.

Schrader AJ, Olbert PJ, Hegele A, et al. Metastatic non-clear cell renal cell carcinoma: current therapeutic options. *BJU Int* 2008; **101**(11):1343–5.

Urothelial and bladder cancer: introduction

Epidemiology
Bladder cancer is the seventh most common cancer worldwide, accounting for 3.2% of all cancers. There were an estimated 68,810 new cases and 14,100 deaths from bladder cancer in the USA in 2008. The highest incidence rates of bladder cancer in both sexes are observed in Europe, North America, and Australia. Most tumours occur rarely before age 40. In Europe, it is the seventh most common cancer in males and fourteenth in women. Each year approximately 36,500 deaths due to bladder cancer occur in males and nearly 13,000 in females.

Aetiology
Gene abnormalities resulting in disruption of cell-regulatory processes
- Proto-oncogenes involvement, e.g. Ras p21 proteins
- Tumour suppressor genes involvement, e.g. p53, p21, p27, retinoblastoma gene (pRB), thrombospondin-1
- EGFR 1–2
- VEGFR
- Loss of heterozygosity of chromosome 9

Chemical exposure
- Tobacco smoking
- Occupational exposures, i.e. aromatic amines, aniline dyes, nitrites, nitrates, plastics, tar, coal, asphalt

Chronic irritation
- Infection by Schistosoma hematobium (Egypt)
- Catheters
- Irradiation
- Diet
- Volume of liquid intake
- Analgesic abuse of phenacetin

Pathology
Anatomy of urinary bladder and natural spread
Primary site
The urinary bladder consists of three layers, the epithelium, the subepithelial connective tissue, the muscularis and the perivesical fat. In males, the, the bladder adjoins the rectum and seminal vesicles posteriorly, the prostate inferiorly, the pubis and the peritoneum anteriorly. In females, the vagina is located posteriorly and the uterus superiorly. The bladder is an extraperitoneal organ.

Regional lymph nodes
- Hypogastric
- Obturator
- Iliac (internal, external, NOS)
- Perivesical
- Pelvic (NOS)
- Sacral (lateral, sacral promontory [Gerota's])
- Presacral

Metastatic sites:
- Lymph nodes (common iliac nodes are considered M1)
- Lung
- Bone
- Liver

Anatomy of renal pelvis and ureter and natural spread
Primary site
The renal pelvis and ureter form a single unit that is continuous with the collecting ducts of the renal pyramids including calyces (major and minor) through the urinary bladder wall as the intramural ureter opening in the trigone of the bladder at the ureteral orifice. The renal pelvis and ureter are composed of three layers: epithelium, subepithelial connective tissue and muscularis, which is continuous with the connective tissue adventitial layer.

Regional lymph nodes
Regional lymph nodes of the renal pelvis:
- Renal hilar
- Paracaval
- Aortic
- Retroperitoneal, NOS
- Regional lymph nodes for the ureter
- Iliac (common, internal [hypogastric], external)
- Paracaval
- Periureteral
- Pelvic, NOS

Metastatic sites:
- Lung
- Bone
- Liver

Histology
Urothelial or transitional cell carcinoma (TCC)
This is cancer that begins in cells in the innermost tissue layer of the bladder. Approximately 90% of TCCs occur in the bladder and the remaining 10% develop from the renal pelvis, ureter, and urethra.

Squamous cell carcinoma
This tumour is characterized by keratinization which begins in squamous cells, which are thin, flat cells that may form in the bladder after long-term infection or chronic irritation. SCCs account for 5% of bladder tumours. This type of bladder cancer is frequent in countries where *Schistosoma hematobium* is endemic.

Adenocarcinoma
Adenocarcinoma is characterized by glandular (secretory) cells that may form in the bladder after long-term irritation and inflammation. Other less common bladder cancers include small cell carcinomas, giant cell carcinomas, and lymphoepitheliomas.

Histological grading
Classification of bladder tumours includes cellular characteristics such as grading into low- (G1) and high-grade (G2–3). This is most clinically significant in non-invasive tumours.
- Gx: grade can not be assessed
- G1: well differentiated

- G2: moderately differentiated
- G3/4: differentiated or undifferentated

Clinical features

Macroscopic haematuria may be painless in 75–95% of patients with ureteral, renal, pelvic, and bladder cancer and should always be followed by a sonogram and further clinical evaluation.

Further reading

American Cancer Society. Cancer Facts and Figures 2008. Atlanta, GA. American Cancer Society, 2008. Available online—http://www.cancer.org/Research/CancerFactsFigures/index

Greene GL, Page DL, Fleming ID, *et al. AJCC Cancer Staging Manual, Sixth Edition*, pp.329–31. New York: Springer-Verlag, 2002.

Urothelial and bladder cancer: diagnosis, staging, and prognosis

Diagnosis

Symptoms

Painless haematuria, urgency, dysuria, increased frequency, and pelvic pain. Pelvic pain and symptoms related to urinary tract obstruction may be found in more advanced tumours.

Physical examination

Includes rectal and vaginal bimanual palpation. A palpable pelvic mass may be found in patients with locally advanced tumours.

Imaging

Intravenous urography and CT scan

Tumours may be seen as filling defects in the bladder. Intravenous pyelography (IVP) is also used to detect filling defects in the calices, renal pelvis, and ureters, and hydronephrosis, which may indicate the presence of a ureteral tumour. In the majority of major centres, CT scans are used as an alternative to conventional IVP. CT scans give more information than IVP, especially in invasive tumours of the upper tract, and in terms of lymph nodes or other potential metastases.

Ultrasonography

Transabdominal ultrasonography permits characterization of renal masses, detection of hydronephrosis, and visualization of intraluminal filling defects in the bladder. Combined with plain abdominal films, it can be as accurate as IVP in diagnosing the cause of haematuria.

Urinary cytology and urinary markers

Examination of voided urine or bladder-washing specimen for exfoliated cancer cells has high sensitivity in high-grade tumours. It is, therefore, useful when high-grade malignancy or carcinoma *in situ* (CIS) is present. Positive urinary cytology may indicate urothelial tumour anywhere in the urinary tract including the calyces, ureters, bladder, and proximal urethra. Cytological interpretation is highly dependent upon the pathologist's experience; however, specificity usually exceeds 90%.

Cystoscopy

The diagnosis of bladder cancer ultimately depends on cystoscopic examination of the bladder and histological evaluation of the resected tissue. In general, cystoscopy is initially performed as an outpatient or in the office, using flexible instruments. A careful description should include the site, size, number, and appearance (papillary or solid) of the tumours as well as a description of mucosal abnormalities. Use of a bladder diagram is recommended.

Transurethral resection of invasive bladder tumours

The goal of transurethral resection of the bladder (TURB) is diagnostic, which means that bladder muscle must be included in the biopsies. Small tumours (<1cm) can be resected en bloc, where the specimen contains the complete tumour plus a part of the underlying bladder wall including the bladder muscle. Larger tumours should be resected separately in fractions, which include the exophytic part of the tumour, the underlying bladder wall with the detrusor muscle, and the edges of the resection area. The specimens from different fractions must be referred to the pathologist in separate containers to facilitate correct diagnosis.

Bladder and prostatic urethral biopsy

The involvement of the prostatic urethra and ducts in male patients with bladder tumours has been reported. Although the exact risk is not known, it seems to be higher if tumour is located on the trigone or bladder neck, in the presence of bladder CIS and when there are multiple tumours. In these cases and when cytology is positive or when abnormalities of the prostatic urethra are visible, biopsies of the prostatic urethra are recommended. Special care must be taken with tumours at the bladder neck and trigone in female patients where urethral preservation and an orthotopic neobladder is planned.

Fluorescence cystoscopy

Fluorescence cystoscopy is performed using filtered blue light after intravesical instillation of a photosensitizer, usually 5-aminolaevulinic acid (5-ALA) or hexaminolaevulinate (HAL). It has been confirmed that fluorescence-guided biopsy and resection are more sensitive than conventional procedures in detecting malignant tumours, particularly CIS. However, false-positive results can be induced by inflammation, recent TURB, or intravesical therapy.

Second resection

A second TURB should always be performed when the initial resection has been incomplete, e.g. when multiple and/or large tumours are present, and especially when the pathologist reports that the specimen doesn't contain muscle tissue. There is no clear consensus as to the timing of a second TURB. Most urologists recommend resection at 2–6 weeks after the initial TURB. The procedure should include resection of the primary tumour site.

Staging

The AJCC has designated staging by TNM classification to define bladder cancer as follows:

Primary tumour (T)

- TX: primary tumour cannot be assessed
- T0: no evidence of primary tumour
- Ta: non-invasive papillary carcinoma
- Tis: carcinoma *in situ* (i.e. flat tumour)
- T1: tumour invades subepithelial connective tissue
- T2: tumour invades muscle:
  - pT2a: tumour invades superficial muscle (inner half)
  - pT2b: tumour invades deep muscle (outer half)
- T3: tumour invades perivesical tissue:
  - pT3a: microscopically
  - pT3b: macroscopically (extravesical mass)
- T4: tumour invades any of the following: prostate, uterus, vagina, pelvic wall, or abdominal wall:
  - T4a: tumour invades the prostate, uterus, vagina
  - T4b: tumour invades the pelvic wall, abdominal wall

Regional lymph nodes (N)

- NX: regional lymph nodes cannot be assessed
- N0: no regional lymph node metastasis
- N1: metastasis in a single lymph node ≤2cm in largest dimension
- N2: metastasis in a single lymph node >2cm but ≤5cm in largest dimension; or multiple lymph nodes ≤5cm in largest dimension

- N3: metastasis in a lymph node >5cm in largest dimension

Distant metastasis (M)
- MX: distant metastasis cannot be assessed
- M0: no distant metastasis
- M1: distant metastasis

Additional descriptors
Lymphatic vessel invasion (L)
- LX: lymphatic vessel invasion cannot be assessed
- L0: no lymphatic vessel invasion
- L1: lymphatic vessel invasion

Venous invasion (V)
- VX: venous invasion cannot be assessed
- V0: no venous invasion
- V1: microscopic venous invasion
- V2: macroscopic venous invasion

AJCC stage groupings
Stage 0a:
- TaN0M0

Stage 0is;
- TisN0M0

Stage I:
- T1N0M0

Stage II:
- T2aN0M0
- T2bN0M0

Stage III:
- T3aN0M0
- T3bN0M0
- T4aN0M0

Stage IV:
- T4bN0M0
- Any T,N1M0
- Any T,N2M0
- Any T,N3M0
- Any T, any NM1

Prognosis
Prognostic factors of primary tumours
- Grading
- Stage
- Hydronephrosis
- Anaemia
- Size
- Expression of blood group substances
- Expression of EGFR
- Mutation of p53
- Upregulation of RB
- Other oncogene expression

Prognostic factors for metastatic disease
- Performance status poor (ECOG PS >2).
- Visceral metastasis.
- Abnormal liver function.
- Expression, upregulation or mutation of known onco-genes (e.g. p53; Rb; P21, etc.) is still under investigation, no consensus has been achieved and controversial results on p53 have been published.
- Loss of heterozygosity of chromosome 9 is associated with genesis of superficial bladder cancer.
- Loss of heterozygosity of chromosome 17 with mutation of the p53 suppressor gene seems to be associated with evolution of invasive disease and/or metastatic disease.
- Ploidy has been investigated in superficial disease. Aneuploid DNA content is associated with shorter DFS and higher chances of progression to higher stage.

Guidelines on assessment of tumour specimens after radical cystectomy
Mandatory evaluations
- Depth of invasion (categories pT2 vs. pT3a, pT3b or pT4).
- Margins, with special attention paid to the radial margin.
- Histological subtype.
- Extensive lymph node representation (>8).

Optional evaluations
- Bladder wall blood vessel invasion
- Pattern of muscle invasion

Comments
- The incidence of muscle invasive disease has not changed in the last 5 years.
- Active and passive tobacco smoking continues to be the major risk factor while occupational exposure-related incidence is decreasing.
- The estimated male to female ratio is 3.8:1.
- Currently, treatment decisions cannot be based on molecular markers.

Further reading
Aus G, Chapple C, Hanuz T, *et al*. The European Association of Urology (EAU) Guidelines Methodology: A critical evaluation. *Eur Urol* 2008; **56**: 859–64.

DeVita VH, Hellman S, Rosenberg, SA. Carcinoma of the bladder. In: DeVita VH, Hellman S, Rosenberg, SA (eds) *Principles and Practice of Oncology*, 8th edition, pp.1358–76 Lippincott, Williams and Wilkins, 2008.

Heidenreich A, Aus G, Bolla M. EAU Guidelines on Prostate Cancer. *Eur Urol* 2008; **53**:168–80.

Lerner SP, Schoenberg M, Sternberg C (eds). *Textbook of Bladder Cancer*. London: Taylor & Francis Group, 2006.

Smith, JA Jr, Labasky RF, Cockett AT, *et al*. Bladder cancer clinical guidelines panel summary report on the management of nonmuscle invasive bladder cancer (stages Ta, T1 and TIS). The American Urological Association. *J Urol* 1999; **162**(5):1697–701.

Internet resources
American Urological Association: http://www.auanet.org
European Association of Urology: http://www.uroweb.org
National Comprehensive Cancer Network: http://www.nccn.org

Bladder cancer: management of localized and muscle invasive disease

Surgery

Superficial bladder cancer

Transurethral resection of Ta and T1 bladder tumours

The goal of TURB in Ta and T1 bladder tumours is diagnostic and also has the scope of removing all visible lesions. The strategy of resection depends on the size of the lesion. Small tumours (<1 cm) can be resected en bloc, where the specimen contains the complete tumour plus a part of the underlying bladder wall. Larger tumours should be resected separately in fractions, which include the exophytic part of the tumour, the underlying bladder wall with the detrusor muscle, and the edges of the resection area. Specimens from different fractions must be referred to the pathologist in separate containers to permit correct diagnosis. Cauterization should be avoided during resection to prevent tissue destruction. A complete and correct TURB is essential for prognosis.

Cystectomy for non-muscle invasive bladder cancer

Many experts consider that it is reasonable to propose immediate cystectomy to patients with non-muscle invasive tumours who are at high risk of progression. According to the risk tables of the EORTC these are:
• Multiple recurrent high-grade tumours
• High-grade T1 tumours
• High-grade tumours with concomitant CIS.

Cystectomy is advocated in patients with non-muscle invasive disease who have failed BCG. Delaying cystectomy in these patients may lead to decreased disease-specific survival.

In all T1 tumours at high risk of progression (such as high-grade, multifocal, with CIS, and large tumour size, as outlined in the non-muscle-invasive bladder cancer EAU guidelines), immediate radical cystectomy is an option. In all T1 patients failing intravesical BCG therapy, cystectomy is the preferred option. A delay in cystectomy increases the risk of progression and cancer-specific death.

Invasive bladder cancer

Radical surgery

• *Aim*: removal of the tumour-bearing bladder.
• *Background*: radical cystectomy is the standard treatment for localized muscle invasive bladder cancer in most countries of the western hemisphere.
• *Timing*: delay in surgery beyond 90 days of primary diagnosis is associated with a significant increase in extravesical disease.
• *Indications*: radical cystectomy is recommended for patients with muscle-invasive bladder cancer T2–T4a, N0–Nx, M0. Other indications include high-risk and recurrent superficial tumours, BCG-resistant CIS, T1G3, as well as extensive papillary disease that cannot be controlled with TURB and intravesical therapy alone.
• *Technique and extent*: standard surgery for urothelial tumours infiltrating the muscularis propria, i.e. clinical stage T2 or greater, is a radical cystectomy with pelvic lymph node dissection. A radical cystectomy involves wide resection of the bladder with all of the perivesical fat and tissue in an attempt to achieve negative margins.

Men undergo prostatectomy and women require resection of the uterus, fallopian tubes, ovaries, anterior vaginal wall, and surrounding fascia. A conduit diversion or a continent reservoir is used to redirect urinary flow

Laparoscopic cystectomy

Laparoscopic cystectomy has been shown to be feasible both in males and females. Cystectomy and subsequent urinary diversion are most often performed by open surgery, but there is increasing use of hand-assisted or robot-assisted laparoscopic surgical techniques.

Urinary diversion after radical cystectomy

An increasing proportion of patients is given a continent reservoir which more often is an orthotopic neobladder which allows patients to void through the urethra. Although continent diversions are more technically demanding, postoperative complications are not, thereby improving QoL after cystectomy

Urinary diversion or bladder substitution after cystectomy can, however, be performed in several ways:
• Abdominal diversion such as uretero-cutaneostomy, ileal or colonic conduit, and various forms of cutaneous continent pouch.
• Urethral diversion which includes various forms of GI pouches attached to the urethra as a continent, orthotopic urinary diversion (neobladder, orthotopic bladder substitution.
• Rectosigmoid diversions, such as uretero(ileo-) rectostomy.

Conclusions

• Cystectomy is the preferred curative treatment for localized bladder neoplasms.
• Radical cystectomy includes removal of regional lymph nodes, although the extent of removal necessary has not been sufficiently defined.
• Radical cystectomy in both sexes must not necessarily include the removal of the entire urethra in all cases, which may serve as an outlet for an orthotopic bladder substitution.
• Terminal ileum and colon are the intestinal segments of choice for urinary diversions.
• The type of urinary diversion does not affect oncological outcome.

Role of radiotherapy

Primary radiotherapy

• Preoperative radiotherapy for operable muscle-invasive bladder cancer does not increase survival.
• Preoperative radiotherapy for operable muscle-invasive bladder cancer, using a dose of 45–50Gy in fractions of 1.8–2Gy may result in downstaging after 4–6 weeks, but is not standard treatment.

Radiotherapy

• EBRT alone should only be considered as a therapeutic option when the patient is unfit for cystectomy or as a multimodality bladder-preserving approach with radio-sensitizing chemotherapy.

- Radiotherapy can also be used to stop bleeding from the tumour when local control cannot be achieved by transurethral manipulation because of extensive local tumour growth.

Chemoradiotherapy

Multimodality treatment is an alternative in selected well-informed and compliant patients where cystectomy is not considered for clinical or personal reasons.

The algorithm of bladder preserving therapy for muscle-invasive cancer includes maximal TURBT of the bladder tumour, modern EBRT with radiosensitizing chemotherapy given concurrently, and a careful urology-based surveillance programme with prompt cystectomy for persistent or recurrent invasive tumours. Tumour presentations with the highest success rates include: solitary T2 or early T3 tumours <6cm, no tumour-associated hydronephrosis, tumours allowing a visibly complete TURBT, invasive tumours not associated with extensive carcinoma *in situ*, adequate renal function to allow cisplatin concurrent with radiation.

Agents which have been shown to be radiosensitizers include: cisplatin, paclitaxel, 5-FU, mitomycin C, and gemcitabine. Gemcitabine with RT is not standard, but if used the maximum tolerated dose (MTD) is $27mg/m^2$ twice weekly. Neoadjuvant cisplatin-based chemotherapy is not standard care before radiation or radiation concurrent with chemotherapy.

Role of chemotherapy

Neoadjuvant chemotherapy
Advantages include:
- Chemotherapy is delivered, when the burden of micro-metastatic disease is expected to be low.
- *In vivo* chemosensitivity is tested.
- The tolerability of chemotherapy is expected to be better before than after cystectomy.

Disadvantages of neoadjuvant chemotherapy include:
- Differences between clinical and pathological staging.
- Delayed cystectomy might compromise the outcome in patients not sensitive to chemotherapy.
- Side effects of chemotherapy might affect outcome of surgery and type of urinary diversion.
- In patients with muscle invasive disease, neoadjuvant cisplatin-containing combination chemotherapy improves OS by 5% at 5 years, based upon meta-analyses of randomized studies, particularly in cystectomy series.
- Neoadjuvant chemotherapy has its limitations regarding patient selection, and current chemotherapy combinations.

Adjuvant chemotherapy
The benefits of chemotherapy in the adjuvant setting include:
- Chemotherapy is administered after accurate pathological staging.
- Overtreatment in patients at low risk for micro-metastases is avoided.
- No delay in definitive surgical treatment, especially in patients not sensitive to chemotherapy.
The drawbacks of adjuvant chemotherapy are:
- Assessment of *in vivo* chemosensitivity of the tumour is not possible.
- Delay or intolerability of chemotherapy, due to postoperative morbidity.

There is insufficient evidence on which to reliably base adjuvant chemotherapy treatment decisions. Randomized trials have been underpowered and meta-analyses have not been conclusive. Failure to enrol patients into adjuvant chemotherapy trials after cystectomy has led to this dilemma. Further research and support of clinical trials is required.

Conclusions
Cisplatin-based combination neoadjuvant chemotherapy prior to cystectomy produces a 5% improval in survival according to meta-analysis of randomized trials.

There is not enough evidence of benefit for the routine use of adjuvant chemotherapy

Recommendations

Radical cystectomy
- Radical cystectomy is recommended for patients with T2–T4a, N0–NX, M0, and high-risk non-muscle invasive BC as outlined earlier.
- No preoperative radiotherapy is recommended.
- Lymph node dissection should be an integral part of cystectomy, optimal extent is not established.
- Preservation of the urethra is reasonable if margins are negative. If there is no bladder substitution, the urethra must be checked regularly.
- Laparoscopic and robot-assisted laparoscopic cystectomy may be an option. Current data, however, have not sufficiently proven its advantages or disadvantages.

Urinary diversion
- Treatment is recommended at centres experienced in major types of diversion techniques and postoperative care.
- Before cystectomy, the patient should be counselled adequately regarding possible alternatives, and the final decision should be based on a consensus between the patient and surgeon.
- An orthotopic bladder substitution should be offered to male and female patients without contraindications and who do not have tumour in the urethra and at the level of urethral dissection.

Intravesical therapy
- In patients at low risk of tumour recurrence and progression, one immediate instillation of chemotherapy is strongly recommended as adjuvant treatment.
- If chemotherapy is given, it is advised to use the drug at its optimal pH and to maintain the concentration of the drug during instillation by reducing fluid intake. The optimal schedule and the duration of the chemotherapy instillations remain unclear, but it should probably be given for 6–12 months.
- In patients at high risk of tumour progression, maintenance intravesical BCG is given for at least 1 year. Immediate radical cystectomy may be offered to the highest-risk patients.
- The absolute risks of recurrence and progression do not always indicate the risk at which a certain therapy is optimal. The choice of therapy may be considered differently according to what risk is acceptable for the individual patient and the urologist.

Neoadjuvant chemotherapy
- Neoadjuvant cisplatin-containing combination chemotherapy should be considered in muscle-invasive bladder cancer patients prior to cystectomy.

- Neoadjuvant chemotherapy is not recommended in patients with PS >2 and impaired renal function.

Adjuvant chemotherapy
The need for adjuvant chemotherapy for patients after radical cystectomy with pT3/4 and/or lymph node-positive (N+) disease without clinically detectable metastases (M0) has not been definitively proven in randomized studies.

Internet resources
American Urological Association: http://www.auanet.org
European Association of Urology: http://www.uroweb.org
National Comprehensive Cancer Network: http://www.nccn.org

Bladder cancer: management of advanced and metastatic disease

Principles of management

Metastatic disease

Approximately 30% of patients with urothelial cancer present with muscle-invasive disease. About half will relapse after radical cystectomy, depending on the pathological stage of the primary tumour and the nodal status. Local recurrence accounts for about 30% of relapses, whereas distant metastases are more common. About 10–15% of patients already have metastatic disease at the time of diagnosis. Before the development of effective chemotherapy, patients with metastatic urothelial cancer rarely had a median survival of >3–6 months.

Prognostic factors and treatment decisions

Bladder cancer is a chemosensitive tumour. Response rates differ with respect to patient-related factors and pretreatment disease. Prognostic factors for response and survival have been established. KPS of ≤80% and the presence of visceral metastases are independently prognostic of poor survival after treatment with M-VAC (methotrexate, vinblastine, adriamycin, and cisplatin). These prognostic factors have also been validated in other newer combination chemotherapy regimens. Additional data exist on the prognostic value of elevated alkaline phosphatase and the number of disease sites (>3 or <3). In elderly patients, an ECOG PS 2–3 and a haemoglobin level of <10mg/dL are independent predictors of poor survival. Age itself has no impact on response or toxic events. Besides these prognostic factors, treatment decisions should be based on whether a patient is 'fit' enough to receive a cisplatin-containing combination regimen; renal function (creatinine clearance >50mL/min, PS, comorbidities). So far, there is no generally accepted definition for 'fit' or 'unfit' patients.

Role of radiotherapy and multimodality treatment for muscle invasive disease

After a complete as possible TURB, radiation to the bladder and pelvic lymph nodes to 40Gy with a boost to bladder tumour to 64Gy is considered standard therapy. This is usually accompanied by cisplatin chemotherapy at weeks 1, 4, and 7. Close cystoscopic surveillance with salvage cystectomy for tumour persistence or for invasive recurrence is required

Tumour presentations with the highest success rates include: solitary T2 or early T3 tumours <6cm, no tumour-associated hydronephrosis, tumours allowing a visibly complete TURBT, invasive tumours not associated with extensive carcinoma *in situ* and adequate renal function to allow cisplatin concurrent with radiation.

Palliative radiotherapy

Radiotherapy can also be used to stop bleeding from the tumour when local control cannot be achieved by TURB because of extensive local tumour growth.

Role of chemotherapy

- Urothelial carcinoma is a chemosensitive tumour.
- PS and the presence or absence of visceral metastases are independent prognostic factors for survival. These factors are at least as important as the type of chemotherapy administered.
- Cisplatin-containing combination chemotherapy is able to achieve a median survival of up to 14 months, with long-term DFS reported in some 15% of patients with nodal disease and good PS.
- Single-agent chemotherapy provides low response rates usually of short duration.
- Carboplatin-combination chemotherapy is less effective than cisplatin-based chemotherapy in terms of CR and survival.
- Non-platinum combination chemotherapy has produced substantial responses in first- and second-line use, but has not been tested against standard chemotherapy in fit patients or in a purely unfit patient group.
- To date, there is no defined standard chemotherapy for 'unfit' patients with advanced or metastatic urothelial cancer.
- Small-sized phase II trials provide evidence of moderate response rates for single agents or non-platinum combinations for second-line use.
- Postchemotherapy surgery after a partial or complete response may contribute to long-term DFS.

Role of surgery

Palliative cystectomy for muscle-invasive bladder carcinoma

For patients with inoperable locally advanced tumours (T4b, invading the pelvic or abdominal wall), radical cystectomy usually is not a therapeutic option. Treatment of these patients remains a clinical challenge. These patients are candidates for palliative treatments, such as palliative radiotherapy or chemotherapy. Inoperable locally advanced tumours may be accompanied by debilitating symptoms, including bleeding, pain, dysuria, and urinary obstruction. There are several treatment options for patients with these symptoms. In advanced bladder cancer cases complicated by bleeding, cystectomy with urinary diversion is the most invasive treatment. It carries the greatest morbidity and should be considered only if there are no other options.

Low-volume disease and postchemotherapy surgery

With cisplatin-containing combination chemotherapy, patients with lymph node metastases only, good PS and adequate renal function may achieve excellent response rates, including a high degree of complete responses, with up to 20% of patients achieving long-term DFS. Stage migration may play a role in this positive prognosis.

Post-chemotherapy surgery may contribute to long-term DFS in selected patients.

Conclusions

- Primary radical cystectomy in T4b bladder cancer may be a palliative option in symptomatic patients where chemotherapy or radiation therapy is not indicated.
- Recent organ-preservation strategies combine TURB, chemotherapy, and radiation therapy (trimodality therapy). The rationale for performing TURB and radiation with radiosensitizing chemotherapy is to achieve bladder preservation. Neoadjuvant combination chemotherapy has not been shown to improve survival in patients who undergo radiation therapy and concomitant radio sensitizing chemotherapy.

• There are no randomized trials comparing radical cystectomy with or without chemotherapy to trimodality organ preservation chemoradiation therapy.

Palliative care

Palliative radiotherapy

Advanced carcinoma of the bladder with pelvic fixation carries a poor prognosis and no significant differences in results can be shown whether the patient is treated with radical or palliative intent. Patients should be carefully selected, as those in very poor condition or with grossly reduced bladder capacity can have their symptoms aggravated by radiation. Haematuria may be controlled by a short course of irradiation in about 50% of cases. Pelvic pain can be due to a bladder mass or to bone lesions, with or without nerve involvement. If the site of illness is well identified, pain control may be achieved in >50% of cases. Palliation is generally obtained with doses of about 30Gy in 2 weeks; shorter regimens are generally excluded in order to avoid toxicity. Single fraction treatments with 8Gy or 10Gy to a well circumscribed bladder volume are reported as safe and effective in controlling haematuria. Painful bone metastasis in other sites than the pelvis can be treated effectively with short course radiotherapy.

The evaluation of health-related quality of life (HRQoL)

Evaluation of QoL should consider physical, emotional, and social functioning. Several questionnaires, e.g. FACT (Functional Assessment of Cancer Therapy)-G, EORTC QLQ-C30, and SF (Short Form)-36, have been validated for assessing HRQoL in patients with bladder cancer. A psychometric test such as the FACT-BL should be used for recording bladder cancer morbidity.

Conclusions

• The overall HRQoL after cystectomy remains good in most patients, whichever type of urinary diversion is used. Some data suggests that continent diversions produce better HRQoL.
• Radiation oncologists also report excellent HRQoL as evidenced by urodynamic studies, QoL questionnaires and late pelvic toxicity analyses.

Recommendations

• For muscle invasive bladder cancer, there is evidence that radiotherapy alone is less effective than curative therapy (radical cystectomy or trimodality treatment).
• For patients with metastatic cancer first-line treatment for fit patients: cisplatin-containing combination chemotherapy with GC, M-VAC, preferably with G-CSF, or HD-MVAC with G-CSF.
• Carboplatin and non-platinum combination chemotherapy as first-line treatment in patients fit for cisplatin is not recommended.
• First-line treatment in patients unfit for cisplatin: carboplatin combination chemotherapy or single agents.
• Second-line treatment: consider single agents or paclitaxel/gemcitabine for patients with a good PS.
• Morbidity of surgery and QoL should be weighed against other options.
• TURB alone is not a curative treatment option for most patients with muscle invasive disease.
• Multimodality treatment is an alternative in selected, well-informed, and compliant patients where cystectomy is not considered for clinical or personal reasons.
• HRQoL in patients with muscle-invasive bladder cancer should be assessed using validated questionnaires.
• Continent urinary diversions should be considered when possible.

Further reading

Heidenreich A, Aus G, Bolla M. EAU Guidelines on Prostate Cancer. *Eur Urol* 2008; **53**:68–80.

Internet resources

American Urological Association: http://www.uroweb.org
European Association of Urology: http://www.uroweb.org
National Comprehensive Cancer Network: http://www.nccn.org

Non-transitional urothelial cancer: management

Introduction
- More than 90% of all bladder tumours are transitional cell carcinomas. Non urothelial bladder tumours are rare and account for <5% of all vesical tumours.
  1. Squamous cell carcinomas 3–5%
  2. Adenocarcinomas 0.5–2%
  3. Small cell carcinoma <0.5%
  4. Sarcomas < 0.1%

Other histological types such as melanomas and lymphomas may also be found in the bladder but are extremely rare and account for less than 0.5% of all bladder malignancies.

Squamous cell carcinomas
SCCs are the second most prevalent epithelial tumours of the bladder. They are usually aggressive tumours. The aetiology is chronic bladder inflammation, as for example from use of catheters with neurogenic bladders that rely on intermittent catheterization. A well recognized pathogenic factor is chronic infection with *Schistosoma hematobium*. SCC accounts for 30% of cancers and is the second most common malignancy in women in countries with endemic schistosomiasis. This is a poor prognosis disease, due to local invasion. Most patients have extravesical tumour extension at the time of diagnosis and death is usually related to locally recurrent disease. Treatment is therefore directed to local control of the disease with radical cystectomy and bilateral pelvic node dissection. Preoperative radiation for invasive (stages T2–3) SCC of the bladder can downstage the disease in up to 40% of the patients. Therefore, it may protect patients from pelvic recurrence which is usually the main cause of death. Two growth characteristics of carcinoma of the bilharzial bladder have been observed:
- High mitotic rate with a potential doubling time of 6 days
- Extensive cell loss factor

Tumours with such growth characteristics are expected to respond to radiation. Nevertheless, early experience with external beam radiation therapy for definitive control of these tumours was disappointing.

Adenocarcinomas
Pure adenocarcinomas of the bladder are the third most common type of epithelial tumour and represent 0.5–2% of all bladder tumours. The definition of vesical adenocarcinoma is still controversial. Pathological variations of tumours include: glandular structures resembling colonic adenocarcinomas (enteric type) and/or tumours that produce intra-(signet cell type) or extracellular mucin (mucinous type). Adenocarcinomas of the urinary bladder can be divided into 3 different subtypes depending on their origin.

Adenocarcinomas may arise from a urachal remnant (urachal adenocarcinoma, UA), from metaplasia of the bladder urothelium (non-urachal adenocarcinoma, NUA), or from a metastatic site from another primary tumour such as from the colon, rectum, prostate, stomach, breast, endometrium or ovary. NUAs arising from eutopic bladder urothelium account for 0.4–3.9% of all bladder tumours, whereas primary UAs account for only 0.17–1.18% of those tumours. Males are more frequently affected than females, with a ratio of approximately 7:3. Although there is no consensus regarding diagnostic criteria for UA, important clinical pathological features include location in the bladder dome, a sharp demarcation between the tumour and surface epithelium and exclusion of primary adenocarcinoma that may have metastasized to the bladder. Standard treatment for vesical adenocarcinomas is radical cystectomy and bilateral pelvic node dissection, followed by urinary diversion. In rare instances where patients have a well-differentiated UA localized to the bladder dome, partial cystectomy with removal of the urachus and umbilectomy may be considered. The largest series of UA reported 5 year survival rates ranging from 40% to 50% for patients with urachal adenocarcinomas. In the series from Siefker-Radtke et al., nodal status and surgical margins were significantly associated with survival. It is noteworthy that 13 of the 16 long-term survivors were treated with en bloc resections. In this largest published series, no patient had disease confined to the epithelium or urachal ligament at presentation, with most patients showing locally advanced disease. In addition, more than 29% of all cases presented with positive nodal or systemic disease. Local management usually required surgery and radiation therapy. For patients with NUA, radical cystectomy is usually the first choice treatment. Very few patients have been studied to make it possible to systematically recommend adjuvant treatment after cystectomy. The most effective regimens appear to contain 5-FU and CDDP, suggesting that a regimen for adenocarcinoma of the colon may be more beneficial for UA than the traditional urothelial cancer chemotherapy regimens. For patients with NUA, radical cystectomy is usually the first treatment choice. Surgery and radiation therapy are usually required for local management.

Web resources
American Urological Association: http://www.auanet.org
European Association of Urology: http://www.uroweb.org
National Comprehensive Cancer Network: http://www.nccn.org

Further reading
Siefker-Radtke AO, Gee J, Shen Y, *et al.* Multimodality management of urachal carcinoma: the MD Anderson Cancer Center experience. *J Urol* 2003; **169**:1295–8.

Prostate cancer: introduction

Epidemiology

• Prostate cancer accounts for 23% of cancers in European men.
• It is the second most common cancer in men worldwide.
• There has been a large increase in incidence over the past 20 years due to increased detection through prostate specific antigen (PSA) screening and surgery for benign prostatic disease. In 1985–1992, the age-adjusted incidence of prostate cancer in the USA more than doubled due to the introduction of PSA screening.
• In the UK there are 32,000 new diagnoses and 10,000 deaths from prostate cancer each year.
• There is significant geographical variation in incidence, with the highest rates in the USA (125/100,000 population). These rates are twice those in the UK, primarily due to wider availability of PSA screening in asymptomatic men. Black Americans have a particularly high incidence (274/100,000).
• Incidence rates are particularly low in China, India, and Japan.
• The majority of cases occur in the >70 age-group and the disease is rare in the <50s.
• As yet there is no evidence that PSA screening reduces mortality rates from prostate cancer.

Aetiology

• Age is the most important risk factor for prostate cancer
• Postmortem studies have shown that men >80 years of age have a 60–70% incidence of histological evidence of prostate cancer.
• Various environmental risk factors have been proposed, including a high fat diet, anabolic steroids, and oestrogen exposure.
• High circulating testosterone levels are associated with increased risk.
• Genetic risk factors have been identified, including a hereditary prostate cancer gene on chromosome 1p and genetic variation at the insulin-like growth factor-1 locus.
• Recent studies have concentrated on 8q24—single nuclear polymorphisms at multiple loci have been demonstrated to be independent risk factors for prostate cancer.
• Mutation of the vitamin D receptor gene may also lead to increased risk (vitamin D itself may be protective).
• Mutation of the androgen receptor domain may be associated with high-grade disease, extraprostatic extension, and distant metastases.
• Laboratory and observational studies have suggested that selenium, vitamin E, and beta-carotene may be protective. Evidence from prospective studies suggests that benefit is restricted only to those with particularly low dietary intakes or, in the case of vitamin E, to current smokers.

There is no strong support for population-wide use of antioxidant supplementation.
• Soy products may be protective, perhaps partly explaining the relatively low incidence of prostate cancer in Asian countries. This may be due to phyto-oestrogenic components of soy.

Pathology

• The majority (95%) of prostate tumours are adenocarcinoma.
• Cells tend to be uniform with relatively little anaplasia. Lymphatic, vascular, and perineural invasion differentiate from benign prostatic hypertrophy.
• Malignant areas are frequently multifocal and most often involve the posterolateral part of the gland.
• Seventy per cent arise in the peripheral zone of the prostate.
• Rare variations include mucinous, signet-ring, small cell, squamous cell, adenoid cystic, and endometrioid carcinoma. With the exception of mucinous and adenoid cystic carcinomas, prognosis tends to be poor. Squamous cell and endometrioid carcinomas are characterized by a normal PSA and lack of hormone response.
• Transitional cell carcinoma of the prostatic urethra may occur and there are rare reports of secondary spread from other tumours such as melanoma and lung cancer.

Gleason grade

The Gleason grading system, developed in the early 1970s, is used to describe the degree of differentiation and cytological atypia of the malignant cells (Gleason 1991). Each tumour is graded twice, each out of 5 to give a total score out of 10—the first grade relates to the most commonly observed pattern (primary pattern) and the second to the next most common pattern (see Table 4.6.6). This scoring system allows for the heterogeneity and multifocality of prostate cancer. The major pattern has prognostic significance—patients with Gleason 3+4 tend to do better than those with 4+3.

Table 4.6.6 Gleason grading

1	Well differentiated; uniform gland pattern
2	Well differentiated; glands variable
3	Moderately differentiated; papillary/cribriform features or well-spaced acini
4	Poorly differentiated; cords, sheets, fused cells
5	Very poorly differentiated; minimal gland formation and necrosis

Reference

Gleason DF. Histologic grading of prostate cancer: a perspective. *Hum Pathol* 1991; **23**:273

Prostate cancer: clinical features, diagnosis, and staging

Clinical features

- The majority of prostate cancers are initially detected following a raised serum PSA level, either as a result of investigations into non-specific lower urinary tract symptoms of bladder outflow obstruction such as hesitancy, frequency, nocturia, and terminal dribbling, or increasingly as part of a well-man screening programme.
- Approximately half of patients are completely asymptomatic.
- In symptomatic patients who require a transurethral resection of the prostate (TURP) for presumed benign prostatic hypertrophy, it is not uncommon to discover cancer cells in the prostatic chippings.

Locally advanced cancers can be detected on rectal examination, and occasionally patients may present with symptoms due to local extension such as pain, bleeding, or impotence. Metastases to bone are common and bone pain or pathological fracture can be presenting features, although this is becoming less frequent due to better availability of PSA testing. Occasionally patients will present with weakness or paraesthesia due to spinal cord or nerve root compression from vertebral metastases. Other areas of spread include obturator, perivesical, and para-aortic lymph nodes and rarely liver, lung, or brain metastases. It is unusual for patients to present with symptoms related to metastases in these areas.

Diagnosis

- Initial investigations should include a PSA blood test and DRE.
- Patients with raised PSA or suspicious examination may be offered transrectal ultrasound-guided biopsy (TRUS biopsy) of the prostate to obtain histological diagnosis.
- If clinical suspicion of advanced disease is high, with markedly raised PSA levels and evidence of metastases on imaging, then TRUS biopsy is not necessary to confirm the diagnosis.

Not all men with a raised PSA level require a biopsy. There has been a tendency to over-investigate modestly raised PSA levels, resulting in overdiagnosis of clinically insignificant prostate cancer. The large Prostate Cancer Prevention Trial (PCPT) showed that low-grade prostate cancers were also common in men with normal PSA levels. The aim of histological diagnosis of prostate cancer is to be able to offer treatment to those cancers which might impact on patients' life expectancy. Predictive models have been developed that define the need for biopsy. The PCPT identified variables predictive of prostate cancer including higher PSA level, positive family history of prostate cancer, and abnormal DRE result, whilst a previous negative prostate biopsy was associated with reduced risk. Age and PSA velocity did not appear to be predictive in this study. However other models have identified additional predictive factors such as prostate volume and PSA density (discussed later).

TRUS biopsy

TRUS biopsy is a short outpatient procedure performed under local anaesthetic. Typically 8–12 core biopsies are obtained, 4–6 from each lobe of the prostate, although current guidance supports a minimum of 10 cores for histological assessment.

If the biopsy is negative, then the risk factors should be reviewed, including PSA level, PSA density (see later), DRE findings, patient age, and prostate volume. If there is still concern, repeat biopsy is indicated. Various studies have revealed a 10–25% rate of detection of malignancy on second biopsy, although they differ in which of the PSA parameters are predictive of a positive repeat biopsy.

Prostate specific antigen

As well as the absolute PSA level, various other PSA parameters have been developed in an attempt to improve the predictive value of the test for diagnosis and monitoring:

- *PSA density* (PSA/volume of gland) allows for higher PSA levels in older men with large, hypertrophied glands. A value of 0.1ng/mL/cc is considered normal (e.g. a PSA of 5ng/mL with a 50cc prostate volume).
- *Percent-free PSA (fPSA)* is the ratio of how much PSA circulates free compared with the total PSA level, including that attached to blood proteins. The percentage of free PSA is lower in men who have prostate cancer than in men who do not and may be useful in determining which patients with intermediate PSA levels should have a prostate biopsy for diagnosis. There is some controversy over where the cut-off should lie, but fPSA levels of <10% are very suspicious.
- *PSA kinetics* give an indication of the rate of tumour growth, and include the PSA doubling time, expressed in months or years, and the PSA velocity, expressed as ng/mL/year (this is commonly utilized in patients on active surveillance—see later). To get an accurate indication of PSA velocity, at least 3 measurements should be taken over a period of 18 months.

Note that very poorly differentiated cancers may not secrete PSA and are therefore more difficult to diagnose, predict and monitor.

Staging (Table 4.6.7)

If cancer is confirmed, further staging investigations are determined by the grade, volume of disease and PSA level. These investigations are aimed at diagnosing advanced or metastatic disease, which would preclude radical local treatment options.

- Pelvic MRI to define extracapsular spread, seminal vesicle or lymph node involvement, or local extension of disease should be offered to patients in whom radical treatment is being considered with Gleason 4+3 disease or above, those with PSA levels >20ng/mL or those with clinical T3 or 4 disease on examination. For patients unable to tolerate MRI, CT scanning of the pelvis is a reasonable alternative.
- Bone scan is used to detect metastatic bone disease. Bone scans are sensitive but not specific, with a high rate of false positives. Any equivocal areas should be examined with plain radiographs and/or cross-sectional imaging. At PSA levels of <10ng/mL, the rate of true positive bone scans is <1%, so this investigation should only be requested in patients with PSA levels >10–15ng/mL.

If there is doubt over lymph node involvement on pelvic imaging, a laparoscopic retroperitoneal lymph node biopsy might be considered before proposed radical treatment.

Table 4.6.7 Staging of prostate cancer

Stage	Description		
I	T1a	Not palpable, confined to prostate	Diagnosed on TURP, <5% of chippings involved, Gleason grade 2–4 only
II	T1a		Diagnosed on TURP, <5% of chippings involved, Gleason grade ≥5
	T1b		Diagnosed on TURP, >5% of chippings involved
	T1c		Diagnosed by needle biopsy in response to a raised PSA
	T2a	Palpable, but confined to prostate	Confined to 1 lobe, <50% involved
	T2b		Confined to 1 lobe, >50% involved
	T2c		Both lobes palpably involved
III	T3a	Breaches prostate capsule	Extension through the prostate capsule
	T3b		Involvement of one or both seminal vesicles
IV	T4	Local invasion	Invasion of other nearby structures
	Any N1		Spread to regional lymph nodes
	Any M1		Distant metastases

Risk stratification (Table 4.6.8)
A commonly used risk stratification is into low, intermediate, and high risk based on PSA, Gleason score, and clinical stage:

Table 4.6.8 Risk stratification

Risk	PSA	Gleason score	Clinical stage
Low	<10ng/mL	<6	T1a–T2a
Intermediate	10–20ng/mL	7	T2b or T2c
High	>20mg/mL	8–10	T3 or T4

The strongest predictors of metastasis are a high PSA, high Gleason score (8–10), and age >70 years. The Partin tables, developed in 1997 by urologists at Johns Hopkins University and updated in 2001 (Partin et al. 2001), are commonly used in treatment algorithms to predict the risk of local extension and lymph node spread. The Roach formulae, based on the Partin tables, are simple equations that can be used to predict these risks (Roach 1993).

Roach formulae
- Percentage risk of lymph node involvement 2/3 PSA + 10(Gleason −6)
- Percentage risk of seminal vesicle involvement: PSA + 10(Gleason −6)
- Percentage risk of extracapsular extension: 3/2 PSA + 10(Gleason −3)

Further reading
Partin AW, Mangold LA, Lamm DM, et al. Contemporary update of prostate cancer staging nomograms (Partin Tables) for the new millennium. *Urology* 2001; **58**:843–8.
Roach M. Equations for predicting the pathologic stage of men with localized prostate cancer using the preoperative prostate specific antigen. *J Urol* 1993; **150**:1923–4.

Internet resources
Memorial Sloan–Kettering Cancer Centre Prostate cancer prediction nomograms: http://www.mskcc.org/applications/nomograms/prostate/index.aspx
Partin tables: www.http://urology.jhu.edu/prostate/partintables.php

Prostate cancer: natural history, screening, and prognosis

Natural history

- The natural history of prostate cancer is very variable and is poorly understood.
- Low-grade tumours tend to follow an indolent course, whilst higher-grade tumours present more risk of local extension and metastatic spread.
- For localized low-intermediate Gleason grade disease the first decision to be made is whether to treat radically or to initially plan a period of surveillance, with regular PSA monitoring and rectal examination. Many of these tumours might never progress to a point that they influence life expectancy, particularly in elderly patients.
- Cohort studies of untreated prostate cancer reveal that the majority of tumours follow an indolent course over the first 10 years with prostate cancer-specific survival rates of approximately 80%, but by 15–20 years deaths due to prostate cancer become more common (cancer specific survival of approximately 50%).
- For this reason if a patient has a life expectancy of <10 years due to age or comorbidity, then it is reasonable to defer radical treatment in the first instance.
- For tumours that do spread, local invasion is usually into the seminal vesicles, directly through the capsule of the prostate or, for transitional zone tumours, into the bladder neck. Metastases are most often to bone and pelvic lymph nodes.
- With the wider use of screening, there are more small, low-grade tumours being diagnosed in younger men and the natural history of these tumours in this group of patients is particularly poorly understood.

Screening

- Screening for prostate cancer principally employs PSA testing and/or DRE, with the aim of early detection of malignant disease.
- Various applications have been utilized to suggest the need for further investigation, including absolute PSA level (for example >4ng/mL), age-specific PSA, or per cent-free PSA.
- However, there is no convincing evidence that earlier detection and treatment of prostate cancer leads to improvements in mortality.
- There is potential harm associated with screening. False positive PSA tests have been shown to cause psychological harm for up to a year after the testing. Also many patients with low-risk cancer may end up having aggressive and debilitating treatment for limited or no benefit.
- A 2008 update of the US Preventive Services Task Force recommendation statement regarding screening for prostate cancer concludes that current evidence is insufficient to assess the balance of benefits and harms of screening for prostate cancer in men <75 years old. Screening for prostate cancer is not recommended in men aged ≥75 years.
- These statements are based on cross-sectional and cohort data only. Three large-scale randomized trials are underway or recently completed and the results are awaited:
- The European Randomised Study of Screening for Prostate Cancer (ERSPC) is the largest of these studies aiming to determine whether early detection and treatment of prostate cancer will lead to a reduction in mortality; 180,000 participants from 8 European countries are randomized between PSA screening (with or without DRE) or no screening. Results are expected in 2010.
- The large US screening trial is the PLCO study (prostate, lung, colorectal, and ovarian screening programme), which undertakes annual PSA screening and DRE for 5 years along with screening tests for the other tumour types. This study recruited 154,000 men and women in 1992–2001, half of whom were allocated screening tests and half received routine care as a control group.
- In the UK, the PROTECT study aims to evaluate the effectiveness, acceptability, and cost-effectiveness of treatments for men with localized prostate cancer and involves >100,000 men. Participants were recruited before diagnosis and underwent a screening programme, with the offer of randomization between active surveillance, radiotherapy, and surgery on detection of an abnormal PSA and diagnosis of prostate cancer. This study is unique in that it evaluates both the utility of screening and the relative benefits of different treatment approaches.

Prognosis

- Figures for survival from prostate cancer vary widely, depending on histology, stage, PSA level, and therapeutic intervention.
- The Partin tables, based on PSA level, Gleason score, and clinical stage, remain the best method of predicting spread and prognosis of prostate cancer.
- For well-differentiated tumours, the risk of developing metastases at 10 years is <20%.
- Patients with localized disease treated with either radiotherapy or radical surgery have 5-year bio-chemical control rates of 75–85% and 10-year OS rates of 60–70%.
- Patients with metastatic disease can survive for many years, particularly if the tumours are endocrine-responsive and if the metastatic spread is confined to the bones.
- There is some evidence that particular genetic polymorphisms influence prognosis. Polymorphisms affecting alleles of insulin-like growth factor 1 and cytochrome p450 may be associated with a worse outcome. Other polymorphisms (such as TGFB1) may be protective.

Internet resources

European Randomized Study of Screening for Prostate Cancer: http://www.erspc.org

National Cancer Institute—Prostate, Lung, Colorectal, and Ovarian Cancer Screening Trial: http://prevention.cancer.gov/programs-resources/groups/ed/programs/plco

ProtecT Study (Prostate testing for cancer and Treatment): http://www.epi.bris.ac.uk/protect/

Prostate cancer: treatment of localized disease

Principles of management

For localized low-intermediate Gleason grade disease the first decision to be made is whether to treat radically or to initially plan a period of surveillance. Patients with high-grade localized disease should be offered radical treatments if fit. Radical treatment options for prostate cancer include radical prostatectomy, EBRT, and brachytherapy (low-dose rate or high-dose rate). Each treatment has its own characteristics and may be suitable for certain types of patients, but reported success rates are similar if patients are chosen appropriately.

Active surveillance (Table 4.6.9)

Many patients will have slow-growing disease that might have little or no impact on their life expectancy, and they might therefore be spared the toxicities and inconvenience of radical treatment. Active surveillance implies close monitoring with early curative treatment offered to patients who show signs of progression.

There are no absolute criteria for considering active surveillance, but initial studies used the following parameters: T1–T2b disease, Gleason grade ≤7 and PSA ≤15 (with favourable kinetics). The approach is most suited, however, to those with the following characteristics:
- T1b/c disease
- Gleason 3+3
- PSA density of <0.15ng/mL
- Less than 50% of cores involved

A typical surveillance programme consists of 3-monthly visits for the first 2 years, followed by 6-monthly visits thereafter, with a DRE and PSA checked at each visit. Repeat transrectal biopsies should be performed at 18 months. Criteria for consideration of radical treatment would be PSA progression (doubling time <2 years), clinical progression or upgrading of the Gleason score on repeat biopsy.

The concept of active surveillance is relatively new, having been first reported by a group from Toronto in 2001 (Choo et al. 2001). After a median follow-up of 29 months, more than three-quarters of men remained under surveillance without progressing on to radical treatment. Similar results were confirmed from a UK series from the mid-1990s, where median PSA doubling time was found to be approximately 12 years, suggesting an indolent course of disease in many men. Prospective studies of active surveillance are underway, but preliminary results suggest that only around 20% of patients will require radical treatment. The PROTECT study randomizes suitable patients between active surveillance, primary surgery or radiotherapy.

Table 4.6.9 Active surveillance

Advantages	Disadvantages
Better quality of life	Risk of progression or metastases
Avoids treatment side effects	Anxiety of living with un-treated cancer
Cost savings if treatment expensive	Regular follow-up and re-biopsy
	Optimal schedule not established

Watchful waiting

The approach of watchful waiting is distinct from active surveillance. Patients deemed unsuitable for radical treatment are watched before being treated with endocrine therapy upon symptomatic progression. It is usually reserved for elderly or unfit patients who are thought unlikely to suffer significant cancer progression during their expected life-span.

Radical prostatectomy

- Radical prostatectomy is often considered the definitive treatment for localized prostate cancer.
- Perineal, retropubic, or laparoscopic approaches can be considered.
- Of the open techniques, the perineal approach gives better access to the urethra and less blood loss, whilst the retropubic approach allows lymph node staging and better nerve sparing. There have been suggestions that the perineal approach might result in positive surgical margins more commonly than the retropubic approach, but this has not been confirmed.
- Robotic-assisted laparoscopic surgery is now available. Short-term functional and PSA-related outcomes compare favourably with standard surgical approaches, but long-term data are not yet available.
- Surgical series of prostatectomies for organ confined disease report 5-year PSA-free survival rates of 69–84% with 10-year rates of 47–75%.
- Surgery is generally discouraged for T3 disease due to the risk of positive surgical margins and lymph node metastases, although there is a move to recommend surgery followed by immediate adjuvant radiotherapy in this group of patients. It should also be noted that there is a degree of overstaging, particularly with the prediction of seminal vesicle invasion on MRI—approximately 25% of patients thought to be T3 will in fact be T2 and therefore achieve good biochemical control from radical prostatectomy.
- There is a 5–15% risk of significant urinary dysfunction after surgery (stress incontinence, urine leak or fistulas).
- Nerve-sparing techniques have improved morbidity, with approximately 50% impotence rates, but these are very much surgeon-dependent and not appropriate for patients with high risk of extracapsular disease.

Radical radiotherapy

Radical radiotherapy is an alternative to surgery in localized prostate cancer. There are two small randomized trials comparing surgery and radiotherapy, but these suffer from methodological problems and relatively small numbers of participants. Historical series suggest similar success rates in terms of PSA control.

Radiotherapy techniques

Conformal CT planning is well established in prostate radiotherapy. Patients are scanned with an empty rectum (to minimize variation in prostate position) and target volumes are defined on CT. The clinical target volume (CTV) includes the whole prostate and any tumour extension. The seminal vesicles are generally included for intermediate/high risk patients (based on clinical stage, Gleason grade, and PSA). The CTV is expanded by 1cm in all directions to give the planning target volume (PTV). A second phase of treatment is planned with reduced margins of 0.5cm.

Conformal planning has enabled escalation of doses from 64–66Gy in 32–33 fractions to 74–78Gy in 37–39 fractions, whilst remaining within predefined tolerance doses to the rectum and bladder. Various studies have shown that improved local control is achieved with dose escalation. The Medical Research Council RT01 study randomized between 64Gy and 74Gy and found a hazard ratio for biochemical PFS of 0.67 in favour of the escalated group. However this was achieved at the expense of increased late bowel and bladder toxicity (Dearnley et al. 2007). Similarly an MD Anderson study found significantly better 5-year PSA control with 78Gy delivered conformally than with conventional 70Gy dose (Zelefsky et al. 1998). It is not yet known whether there will be any improvements in OS.

Typical rectal tolerance doses are 55.5Gy to no more than 50%, 70Gy to no more than 25%, and 74Gy to no more than 3% of the rectum. Less than 50% of the bladder should receive 67Gy.

Newer techniques such as intensity modulated radiotherapy (IMRT) might enable even further increases in the dose administered or further sparing of normal tissues.

Radiobiological studies have suggested a surprisingly low alpha-beta ratio for prostate cancer (1.2–1.5Gy), which implies that hypofractionated courses of radiotherapy with a high dose per fraction might result in improved cancer control for a similar level of side effects. For this reason, doses such as 57–60Gy in 19–20 fractions over 4 weeks are being investigated. These shortened schedules have the additional advantage of sparing resources and being more convenient for patients.

For patients with poor prognostic risk factors and a high risk of pelvic lymph node involvement (≥15% on Roach criteria, see p.277)), it is worth considering a larger first phase of treatment to include the pelvic nodes to a dose of 50Gy in 25 fractions, followed by a second phase of treatment to the prostate itself of 18–24Gy in 9–12 fractions, although any survival benefit from this approach remains to be demonstrated.

Acute side effects of radiotherapy include dysuria, frequency, diarrhoea, lethargy, and erythema. Late effects include proctitis (diarrhoea, rectal bleeding, tenesmus: 30% mild, 5% severe), impotence (30–40%), and urinary incontinence (1–5%). If radiation is given to large pelvic fields, there is a risk of small bowel damage.

Brachytherapy
Low-dose rate (LDR) brachytherapy:
Permanent radioactive seeds are implanted directly into the prostate via transperineal needles that are inserted with ultrasound guidance under general or spinal anaesthetic. Approximately 50–100 iodine-125 or palladium-103 seeds are implanted to achieve a prescribed dose of 145Gy. Patients are not suitable for LDR brachytherapy if the prostate is large (>50cc), if they have had a previous TURP or if they are at high risk of extracapsular extension or lymph node involvement. Generally this technique is restricted to Gleason ≤6, PSA≤15, T2 or less disease—a similar group to those suitable for active surveillance. Patients should have a TRUS volume study to assess suitability for brachytherapy.

Although there is good evidence to confirm the efficacy of brachytherapy in terms of PSA control and biopsy findings, there are as yet no long-term survival data. The procedure has not been directly compared with external beam radiotherapy or radical surgery in randomized studies, but comparative and cohort studies show similar 5-year biochemical recurrence-free and OS. The incidence of adverse events also appears to be similar to radiotherapy and prostatectomy.

High-dose rate (HDR) brachytherapy:
HDR brachytherapy is suitable for intermediate–high-risk patients—a similar group to those suitable for large-field pelvic radiotherapy with prostate second phase. It is typically given as a boost followed by a shortened course of EBRT but can also be used as monotherapy. Treatment is delivered via catheters implanted with ultrasound guidance into the prostate under general anaesthetic. The catheter positions are confirmed on CT scanning and target volumes are contoured, along with the urethra and rectum as organs at risk. Dwell positions for the radioactive source are defined and an individual treatment plan is produced. HDR boost patients are typically treated in two or three fractions, 6–12 hours apart, often necessitating overnight stay with the catheters and template *in situ*. Typical doses are 17Gy in 2 fractions of HDR followed by 46Gy in 23 fractions of EBRT to the pelvis, but there is considerable regional variation.

Cryotherapy
Cryotherapy is a minimally invasive technique in which the prostate is frozen to temperatures of −140°C with argon gas. Needles are inserted into the prostate through the perineum in a similar fashion to brachytherapy. A warming catheter is used throughout the procedure to protect the urethra, and particular attention should be paid to temperatures around the wall of the rectum. There is no long-term evidence of the success of cryotherapy as primary treatment of prostate cancer, with the literature restricted to short follow-up case series. However, reported biochemical control rates are good. Impotence rates are high at around 80% and there is a small (1–2%) risk of rectal perforation. Cryotherapy is not widely used as an initial treatment for localized prostate cancer, its use being mainly restricted to salvage therapy after previous radiotherapy.

High intensity frequency ultrasound (HIFU)
HIFU is administered via a transrectal probe, causing the prostate to heat to very high temperatures leading to cell death. As with cryotherapy, long-term outcome data is poor and reports are limited to relatively small case series. The most commonly reported side effects are urinary tract infection, impotence, and incontinence. Within the UK its use is mainly restricted to post-radiotherapy salvage treatment.

Role of endocrine therapy in localized disease
Neoadjuvant hormones
Patients undergoing radical radiotherapy are commonly treated with 3 months of neoadjuvant luteinising hormone releasing hormone (LHRH) analogues. This approach may enable a reduction in the volume of tissue irradiated due to shrinkage of the prostate gland.

An RTOG study by Pilepich et al. (2001) looked at the role of androgen deprivation for 2 months before and during radiotherapy. Interestingly the improvements in biochemical DFS and OS were confined to the better prognosis patients with low-grade disease (Gleason ≤6). Nevertheless, most institutions treat all radical radiotherapy patients with a period of neoadjuvant LHRH analogues.

The role of neoadjuvant endocrine therapy prior to radical prostatectomy is more controversial. A Cochrane review showed no overall or DFS advantage, but there were improvements in pathological variables such as organ-confined and clear margin rates.

Adjuvant hormones

There is good evidence of a benefit with prolonged endocrine manipulation in patients with locally advanced prostate cancer. An EORTC study (Bolla et al. 1997) compared radiotherapy alone versus radiotherapy with immediate androgen suppression started on the first day of radiotherapy and continued for 3 years. Five-year clinical DFS was 40% versus 74% and OS was 62% versus 78% in favour of the adjuvant endocrine group.

Prolonged adjuvant treatment for 2–3 years should be offered to all patients with high-risk disease (Gleason 8-10, clinical T3/4 tumours, or lymph node risk >30%). The role in low- and intermediate-risk patients is being assessed in randomized studies, but these patients are frequently treated with 3–6 months of LHRH analogues before and during radiotherapy.

It should be noted that LHRH analogues are not without side effects and can add considerably to the morbidity of patients undergoing radiotherapy.

There is no established role for adjuvant hormonal manipulation in patients undergoing radical prostatectomy, although the Cochrane review does suggest a benefit in DFS.

Postoperative adjuvant radiotherapy

There is increasing interest in the role of adjuvant radiotherapy to the prostatic bed following radical prostatectomy for patients with high-risk disease, particularly if there are positive surgical margins or if the PSA fails to suppress completely after surgery. Results from a randomized clinical trial have shown that adjuvant radiotherapy given after radical surgery for pathological T3N0M0 significant reduces risk of metastasis by 29%, improves survival by 28% and median survival by 1.9 years (Thompson et al. 2009).

Further reading

Bolla M, Gonzalez D, Warde P, et al. Improved survival in patients with locally advanced prostate cancer treated with radiotherapy and goserelin. N Engl J Med 1997; **337**(5):295–300.

Choo R, DeBoer, G., Klotz, L, et al. PSA Doubling time of prostate carcinoma managed with watchful observation alone. Int J Radiat Oncol Biol Phys 2001; **50**(3):615–20.

Dearnley DP, Sydes MR, Langley, et al. Escalated-dose versus standard-dose conformal radiotherapy in prostate cancer: first results from the MRC RT01 randomised controlled trial. Lancet Oncol 2007; **8**(6):475–87.

Pilepich MV, Winter K, Roach M, et al. Phase III radiation therapy oncology group (RTOG) trial 86-10 of androgen deprivation adjuvant to definitive radiotherapy in locally advanced carcinoma of the prostate. Int J Radiat Oncol Biol Phys 2001; **50**(5):1243–52.

Thompson IM, Tangen CM, Paradelo J, et al. Adjuvant radiotherapy for pT3N0M0 prostate cancer significantly reduces risk of metastases and improves survival: Long term follow-up of a randomized clinical trial. J Urol 2009; **181**:956–62.

Zelefsky MJ, Leibel SA, Graham JD, et al. Dose escalation with three-dimensional conformal radiation therapy affects the outcome in prostate cancer. Int J Radiat Oncol Biol Phys 1998; **41**(3):491–500.

Prostate cancer: treatment of advanced disease

Principles of management
- For patients with locally advanced disease and a high risk of micrometastases it is appropriate to offer primary endocrine therapy.
- Radical radiotherapy or surgery may add little or no additional benefit over hormone therapy alone in patients with T3b disease, a baseline PSA>50ng/mL, or those who are elderly or have significant co-morbidities.
- Treatment in the advanced or metastatic setting is aimed at controlling the disease, symptoms, and PSA levels. It is sensible therefore to work through the treatment options systematically with the aim of maximizing the benefit obtained from each step.

First-line treatment
- Treatment can be with surgical castration, LHRH analogues, or antiandrogens. Typically LHRH analogues such as goserelin, leuprolide, or triptorelin are used in the first instance.
- LHRH analogues effectively reduce testosterone levels by eliminating the hormonal signals for its production. There are various formulations available, given by subcutaneous implants or injections.
- When commencing LHRH analogues, there is an initial release of testosterone ('flare') and patients should therefore be given anti-androgens for 7–10 days before the first LHRH analogue injection and continued for 2 weeks afterwards.
- Prolonged treatment with LHRH analogues results in significant toxicity due to reduction of testosterone levels. Side effects include hot flushes, weakness/loss of muscle bulk, weight gain, fatigue, osteoporosis/fracture risk, loss of libido and erectile function, lipid abnormalities, mood changes, poor concentration/memory, and disordered glucose metabolism.
- Management of hot flushes is often difficult but the following approaches have been tried with varying degrees of success: cyproterone acetate, diethylstilboestrol, megestrol acetate, clonidine, homeopathic remedies, sage, and SSRIs.
- Androgen receptor inhibitors, such as bicalutamide, effectively reduce the delivery of testosterone to the prostate without reducing serum testosterone levels and therefore tend to have a better side effect profile, although they can cause significant gynaecomastia and mastalgia. Erectile function is often maintained. However, evidence suggests they are less effective than LHRH analogues in terms of OS in metastatic disease, and so bicalutamide monotherapy is currently only licensed for use in locally-advanced prostate cancer.
- Prophylactic radiotherapy to the breast buds or prophylactic tamoxifen 10–20mg/day can reduce and sometimes prevent the painful gynaecomastia. Typical radiotherapy doses are 8–10Gy in a single fraction or 15Gy in three fractions given on alternate days, using electron radiotherapy delivered to an 8–10 cm circle around each nipple.
- First-line hormonal therapy is generally continued until there is evidence of intolerance or progression of disease, either with the development of new symptoms or PSA progression. There is no consensus on the extent of rise in PSA which should trigger a change in treatment, but a doubling time of <6 months is a cause for concern.
- The typical duration of response to first-line endocrine therapy with LHRH analogues is 18–24 months.

Intermittent therapy
There is interest in intermittent endocrine therapy in patients established on treatment with good disease control. This has three possible benefits: patients are spared the side effects of treatment for a period of time, there is a cost saving and also the potential of extending the period of efficacy of first-line therapy. Trials are ongoing but a systematic review of five small randomized studies showed no difference in survival but an improved quality of life when compared with continuous therapy. Patients spent a median of 1 year off endocrine treatment. A typical approach is to discontinue the LHRH analogue once the PSA has stabilized at a nadir (<4ng/mL) and restart when it rises above 10ng/mL.

Second- and third-line treatments
- After failure of first-line LHRH analogue endocrine treatment (clinical or biochemical progression), the next step is combined or maximal androgen blockade (CAB or MAB) with the addition of antiandrogen therapy (e.g. 50mg of bicalutamide daily).
- Synthetic oestrogens such as diethylstilboestrol can result in a PSA response in patients failing CAB. There is a risk of thrombosis with oestrogen therapy—it is best avoided in men with a significant cardiovascular history, and in any case should be given with aspirin.

Hormone-refractory disease
- There is no universally agreed definition of hormone refractory prostate cancer (HRPC), which usually is designated when combined androgen blockade is failing to control the PSA or symptoms.
- Even when disease is classed as hormone refractory, the LHRH analogue is continued. There is often still some activity of the androgen receptor on the cancer cells and stopping the androgen deprivation is likely to speed up the progression of the disease.
- Chemotherapy is generally reserved for advanced metastatic prostate cancer that has become refractory to endocrine treatment, although it is moving forward in the treatment pathway.
- Docetaxel is now well established in this setting, with studies showing quality of life and OS benefits (in the region of 10–12 weeks) when compared with the previous standard regimen of mitoxantrone and prednisolone.
- Updated survival analysis of the TAX327 study, which randomized between 3-weekly docetaxel, weekly docetaxel and mitoxantrone (all given with prednisolone) showed OS figures of 19.2, 17.8, and 16.3 months respectively (Berthold et al. 2008).
- Doses of 75mg/m^2 of docetaxel are administered on a 3-weekly basis for up to 10 cycles.
- Low-dose oral steroids are typically given with the chemotherapy (prednisolone 5mg twice daily).

- Although low-grade neutropenia is fairly common, the rate of febrile neutropenic sepsis is surprisingly low (<3%) without need for granulocyte colony-stimulating factor support.
- Cytotoxic agents are now being investigated earlier, both in metastatic disease prior to the development of HRPC or as an adjunct to radical prostatectomy for localized disease.
- There is also interest in second-line chemotherapy after failure of taxanes. Current standard second-line chemotherapy is mitoxantrone + prednisolone. There is some evidence for PSA response with satraplatin, an orally active platinum-based drug, and other cytotoxic drugs are under investigation.
- In patients not suitable for chemotherapy, low-dose corticosteroids may be used. These can cause a fall in PSA

levels (due to reduction in adrenal androgen production) and also have symptomatic benefits due to their anti-inflammatory effect and appetite stimulation.
- Abiraterone, an orally active inhibitor of 17alpha-monooxygenase (a member of the cytochrome p450 family), effectively suppresses testosterone production by both the testes and the adrenals to castrate levels. Early studies have shown impressive PSA responses in heavily pre-treated patients and phase III trials are now underway.

Further reading

Berthold DR, Pond GR, Soban F, et al. Docetaxel plus prednisone or mitoxantrone plus prednisone for advanced prostate cancer: updated survival in the TAX 327 study. *J Clin Oncol* 2008; **26**(2):242–5

Prostate cancer: detection and treatment of recurrence

Significance of early detection of recurrence
- Following radical treatment with surgery, radiotherapy, or brachytherapy, disease will recur in a proportion of patients. This is often first detected with a rise in PSA levels following a post-treatment nadir.
- If the disease recurrence is localized to the prostate or prostate bed, there is potential for further curative interventions.
- Early detection of recurrence is therefore important to enable prompt salvage therapy in appropriate patients.

Postoperative recurrence
- A substantial proportion of patients who have undergone a radical prostatectomy (RP) for localized prostate cancer will have either persistently detectable PSA levels or a delayed rise in PSA. Approximately 25–40% of patients will experience recurrence after RP, manifested by a rising PSA, often without clinical or radiological evidence of disease.
- The optimum treatment for these situations is not known. The key question is whether the PSA is reflective of local or distant progression.
- For salvage radiotherapy to be most effective, treatment should be considered before the PSA is allowed to rise too high, when disease is more likely to be confined to the prostate bed. However, at low PSA levels, current imaging techniques are poor at detecting disease, making it difficult to differentiate local or distant recurrence and to target the radiotherapy appropriately.
- Theoretically any detectable level and/or rising PSA after RP should be considered as persistent or recurrent disease. The precise definition of biochemical failure varies from study to study. Though previous studies have suggested a threshold of ≥0.4ng/mL for biochemical failure, more recent work suggests that a PSA of >0.2ng/mL is an appropriate threshold to define PSA recurrence since these patients had a 3-year PSA progression of 100%.
- A European Consensus statement on the management of PSA relapse in patients with prostate cancer defined PSA relapse after RP as a value of 0.2ng/mL with one subsequent rise (Boccon-Gibod et al. 2004).
- Ultrasensitive PSA assays that detect serum PSA levels of <0.01ng/mL may detect relapse several months or even years earlier than conventional assays, but the clinical utility is limited by higher rates of false positive results.
- Although biochemical recurrence is accepted as a surrogate endpoint for defining treatment outcome and as an indication for salvage treatment, the clinical significance in terms of OS and clinical DFS remains unclear. Even in men who develop biochemical recurrence, clinical progression may take many years to manifest and hence the benefit of local treatment in terms of prostate cancer specific mortality is questionable. In one series of 1132 patients, those with rising serum PSA after RP had a 10-year survival rate of 88% compared to 93% of those without biochemical recurrence (Jhaveri et al. 1999).
- The European consensus suggested that secondary treatment after local failure of RP should be initiated when PSA levels reach 1.0–1.5ng/mL and salvage radiotherapy should be considered with or without hormonal therapy.
- Current practice is to treat with salvage radiotherapy for a rising PSA, without the need for imaging or biopsy evidence of local recurrence, accepting that current techniques may not be sensitive enough to detect small volume local disease. Imaging is primarily aimed at excluding metastatic disease and hence patients who would not benefit from salvage radiotherapy. Current evidence suggests that bone scan and pelvic nodal assessment with CT or MRI should not be performed prior to commencing radiotherapy unless the PSA velocity is rapid, although there is no well-defined cut-off value. Functional imaging techniques such as PET or antibody scintigraphy may prove useful in identifying patients with early metastatic disease not evident on current standard techniques and these warrant further investigation.

Treatment of persistent PSA elevation
- It is not clear whether selective adjuvant radiotherapy for high risk patients after RP is better than salvage radiotherapy for patients who develop biochemical relapse at a later date.
- This issue was addressed by a comparative study of postprostatectomy radiotherapy from two institutions, one adopting a prospective policy of adjuvant radiotherapy and the other salvage radiotherapy. The salvage group underwent radiotherapy after longer postoperative intervals (median, 40.3 vs. 2.9 months; p <0.0001) and had higher PSA values before starting radiotherapy (4.5 vs. 0.86ng/mL; p = 0.003), but radiotherapy was equally effective in either salvage or adjuvant setting when the pre- radiotherapy PSA level was <1ng/mL (Hagan et al. 2004).
- The UK RADICALS study addresses this issue further. It is open to patients following radical prostatectomy where there is uncertainty about the need for postoperative radiotherapy. Patients are randomized between immediate radiotherapy to the prostate bed and delayed radiotherapy on PSA relapse. A second randomisation amongst patients receiving radiotherapy is between no androgen deprivation therapy versus short-term (4 months) and long-term (2 years) endocrine treatment. Given the uncertainty around adjuvant and salvage treatment following prostatectomy, eligible patients should be encouraged to take part in this study.

Salvage radiotherapy technique
- A CT scan of the pelvis is obtained for treatment planning and a three-dimensional conformal radiotherapy technique is used. The preoperative CT scan and the location of surgical clips in the fossa of the prostate and seminal vesicles are used to help define the CTV.
- CTV includes the prostatic bed, periprostatic tissue, and any residual seminal vesicle. In the majority of series, pelvic lymph nodes are not included in the clinical target volume.
- The PTV for salvage radiotherapy includes 1–1.5 cm margin on the CTV. A lesser margin may be acceptable posteriorly for optimal sparing of rectum.

- After prostatectomy the bladder neck is pulled down into the prostatic fossa. Periprostatic bed surgical clips are typically located in the central lower aspect of the prostatic bed (from level with the top of pubic symphysis inferiorly) and in the upper region of the surgical bed (superior to the pubic symphysis and posterior to the bladder where the seminal vesicles are located).
- Radiotherapy dose is often limited by rectal tolerance, but the aim should be to treat to over 60Gy equivalent in 2Gy fractions. Studies have shown better biochemical control if doses of 66Gy and above are obtained.

Postirradiation recurrence

- The rate of biochemical failure following radiotherapy reported in the literature varies widely (from 20–66%).
- Local recurrence following radical radiotherapy is more problematic to salvage. Surgery is more difficult due to postradiation scarring, and many patients who underwent radiotherapy as the primary treatment may have been deemed unsuitable or unwilling for surgery in the first instance.
- There are various definitions of what constitutes a PSA relapse after radical radiotherapy, and for many years failure was defined as three consecutive rises in PSA. The 2005 ASTRO consensus group agreed the standard definition of biochemical failure after RT should be a rise in PSA by 2ng/mL or more above the post-treatment nadir.
- Patients are often offered a prostate biopsy following PSA-relapse. It is important that the pathologist is aware the gland has been previously irradiated.
- Prior to considering local salvage therapy, clinically apparent metastases should be excluded using bone scans and pelvic MRI.

- Current salvage options include cryotherapy and HIFU (see p.281). There are several published series with varying results.
- It is reasonable to consider a period of androgen deprivation prior to salvage therapy (3–6 months), to reduce the size of the gland and potentially decrease procedure-associated morbidity.

Distant recurrence

- In cases of patients with distant recurrence or the patient is not suitable for local salvage therapy, the mainstay of treatment is with endocrine therapy similar to advanced and metastatic disease (see p.281)).
- There is no clearly defined point at which endocrine treatment should be started. Although in practice many patients start endocrine therapy when they are diagnosed with metastatic recurrence, there is probably no detriment in waiting until the absolute PSA level climbs above 10ng/mL, the PSA velocity increases or the patient becomes symptomatic.
- For patients with recurrence that is well-controlled on endocrine treatment, it is reasonable to consider a long-term policy of intermittent therapy.

Further reading

Boccon-Gibod, L, Djavan WB, Hammerer P, et al. Management of prostate-specific antigen relapse in prostate cancer: a European Consensus. Int J Clin Pract 2004; **58**(4):382–90.

Hagan M, Zlotecki R, Medina C, et al. Comparison of adjuvant versus salvage radiotherapy policies for postprostatectomy radiotherapy. Int J Radiat Oncol Biol Phys 2004; **59**(2):329–40.

Jhaveri FM, Zippe CD, Klein EA, et al. Biochemical failure does not predict overall survival after radical prostatectomy for localized prostate cancer: 10-year results. Urology 1999; **54**(5):884–90.

Prostate cancer: palliative care and symptom control

The natural history of prostate cancer is such that palliative care may be needed for a long period of time, often over-lapping with active interventions as the disease progresses. It is important to involve palliative care services at an appropriate time and not to wait for the end of life setting.

Bone metastases

Radiotherapy

- EBRT is effective in controlling pain from bone metastases in approximately 80% of instances.
- Typical doses are 20Gy in 5 fractions or a single fraction of 8Gy. A trial comparing single and multiple fraction regimens found no difference in the speed of onset or duration of pain relief achieved.
- Re-irradiation to the same site at a later date is worth considering, particular if the first treatment gave significant benefit.
- Prophylactic antiemetics should be given when large-field radiotherapy is used.

Radioisotopes

- For patients with widespread metastases and diffuse or flitting pains, consider intravenous treatment with radio-isotopes that localize to the bone, such as strontium-89 or samarium-153.
- Radioisotopes provide effective pain control and improve quality of life indices but there is no evidence for any improvement in survival.
- Side effects include bone marrow suppression, so it is wise to restrict usage until after any envisaged courses of chemotherapy.
- Retreatment with radioisotopes is possible assuming adequate bone marrow function.

Bisphosphonates

- A systematic review of 10 randomized trials reveals that the benefit of bisphosphonates in metastatic prostate cancer is unclear. Many of the trials were small and the outcomes measured were different.
- Only one trial (using zoledronic acid) confirmed a modest reduction in skeletal events (an absolute reduction in events of 8% compared with placebo) (Saad et al. 2002). Pamidronate did not reduce the frequency of skeletal events in two trials.
- Of the 9 trials which evaluated pain, only 1 found a significant reduction, although the zoledronic acid trial did not specifically report on pain outcomes.
- It is reasonable to consider bisphosphonates for pain relief when other methods have failed.

Spinal cord compression

Spinal cord compression is a relatively common occurrence in late stage metastatic prostate cancer, and can occasionally be the presenting feature in previously undiagnosed individuals. Urgent MRI scan of the whole spine is indicated if patients present with neurological symptoms consistent with cord compression. Prompt treatment is essential to prevent permanent paralysis.

Decompressive surgery

For patients with previously good PS and relatively few metastases, consider decompressive spinal neurosurgery. If patients are correctly chosen, outcome in terms of function tends to be better following surgery and radiotherapy than following radiotherapy alone. In a randomized trial, significantly more patients were able to walk after the combined treatment (84% vs. 57%) (Patchell et al. 2005).

Radiotherapy

Aim to treat the involved vertebrae plus two vertebrae above and below if possible. Usual doses are 20Gy in 5 daily fractions. Patients should be commenced on high-dose steroids (e.g. dexamethasone 8mg twice daily) prior to commencing radiotherapy, and these can usually be tailed-off gradually on completion of treatment.

Obstructive uropathy

Patients may develop lower urinary tract symptoms due to prostatic enlargement or direct invasion into the base of the bladder or urethra. Flow studies and cystoscopy are appropriate, with a view to proceeding possibly to transurethral resection of the prostate for symptom relief. For men with significant prostatic enlargement and inadequately suppressed testosterone levels, 5-alpha reductase inhibitors may be beneficial. Some patients will require urinary catheters.

In severe cases, there may be significant back pressure, resulting in ureteric dilatation and hydronephrosis, necessitating ureteric stenting or nephrostomies.

Other symptoms

- Haematuria might be due to local invasion by the cancer and can be controlled with palliative doses of radiotherapy to the prostate/bladder. Patients should be examined cystoscopically to exclude other causes of haematuria such as radiation damage or unrelated bladder pathology. Sometimes bleeding points can be cauterized endoscopically.
- Bowel obstruction due to invasion of the prostate cancer is a rare but serious development. In the early stages it might be managed by diet, laxatives, and palliative radiotherapy. If the obstruction becomes more established, then defunctioning colostomy may be required.

Further reading

Saad F, Gleason DM, Murray R, et al. A randomized, placebo-controlled trial of zoledronic acid in patients with hormone-refractory metastatic prostate carcinoma. J Natl Cancer Inst 2002; 94:1458–68.

Patchell RA, Tibbs PA, Regine WF, et al. Direct decompressive surgical resection in the treatment of spinal cord compression caused by metastatic cancer: a randomised trial. Lancet 2005; 366(9486):643–8.

Testicular cancer: introduction

Epidemiology
In Western Europe, the incidence of malignant germ cell tumours (MGCTs) has been rising by an annual rate of 3% during the last 50 years, corresponding to a 2–4 fold increased incidence rate (Richiardi et al. 2004).

The incidence of MGCT shows large geographical variations. In general, the incidence is low in Asia and Africa and high in Caucasians, especially in the Northern part of Europe, and among North Americans of European origin. Denmark, Norway, and Sweden are among the countries with the highest rates of TC. Danish or Norwegian males have a 3–4 times higher risk of developing a MGCT compared with Finnish males. Testicular cancer (TC) is now the most frequent malignancy among Caucasian males aged between 15–40 years.

Aetiology
Causes for the development of MGCT and its rising incidence remain obscure. However, most authorities consider both genetic and environmental factors as important.

Genetic factors
Approximately 2% of TC patients have a first-degree family member who also is affected with this cancer. The relative risk (RR) is 8–10 between brothers and 4–6 between fathers and sons (Rapley 2007). These RRs exceed those commonly observed in other cancers (RR: 2–3) and indicate a genetic basis or an extremely potent, as yet unidentified, environmental risk factor.

However, a large international consortium has been unable to demonstrate distinct genes as risk factors for TC (Crockford et al. 2006).The authors concluded that no single gene could account for the substantial familial risk, and probably many genes contribute to the risk of MGCT.

Environmental factors
Despite numerous studies, a consensus on the importance of environmental factors for the risk of MGCT has not yet been reached.

However, substances with oestrogenic and antiandrogenic properties, so-called endocrine disrupters, are considered the most relevant type of substances (Aitken et al. 2004).

Maternal oestrogens and industrial chemicals such as pesticides, modified by polymorphic enzymes, might increase the risk of MGCT development.

Key points of this simplified process
- Endocrine disrupters and genetic susceptibility
- Decreased Leydig cell function → androgen insufficiency
- Disturbed Sertoli cell function → impaired germ cell differentiation
- Testicular dysgenesis syndrome

The Testicular Dysgenesis Syndrome comprises the following features (Skakkebaek et al. 2001):
- Poor semen quality
- Cryptorchidism
- Hypospadia
- Testicular cancer

The first three findings are clinically more subtle, probably more prevalent, and not as reliably registered as testicular cancer. Skakkebaek et al. (2006) consider the rising TC incidence as a 'whistle blower' for an increased prevalence of sub-infertility and genital malformations.

Individuals at high risk
Presence of one or more of the components of the Testicular Dysgenesis Syndrome indicates an increased risk for TC development.

Cryptorchidism, i.e. the incomplete descent of one or both testicles at birth, is associated with a 7–8 fold risk of developing TC. Furthermore, sons and brothers of men with TC are at increased risk of developing MGCT. The more pronounced increase in risk among brothers of TC patients compared to sons might be related to shared environmental risks.

Key points for individuals at risk:
- Cryptorchidism
- First-degree relative with TC
- Poor semen quality/subinfertility

Pathology
Histological examinations should be performed of the completely laminated testicle and spermatic cord.

In addition to staining with haematoxylin-eosin (HE), immunohistochemistry should be used:
- Mandatory:
  - AFP
  - β-hCG
- Recommended for detection of TIN:
  - Placental alkaline phosphatase (PLAP)
  - Oct 3/4

Histology differentiates mainly between:
- Seminoma
- Non-seminoma

Seminoma is composed of quite homogeneous cells and is found in approximately 50% of unselected series of TC patients (Horwich et al. 2006). Syncytiotrophoblastic cells may be found but do not impact on treatment or prognosis.

Non-seminoma can be quite heterogeneous and include one or several components. These components are usually classified according to the WHO and the British Tumour Panel schemes (Table 4.6.10) which refer to most components as malignant teratoma (MT).

Both seminomatous and non-seminomatous components are found in 10–20% of unselected patients (Horwich et al. 2006). Such combined tumours are treated as non-seminoma.

Teratoma is composed of slow growing somatic cell types of at least two germ layers (ectoderm, endoderm, and mesoderm). The variety of structures encountered, e.g. hair, teeth, cartilage, etc. probably explains its Greek name which means 'monster tumour'. In prepubertal children, this testicular tumour is benign and enucleation is adequate treatment. In adults however, this non-metastasizing tumour is considered malignant due to its potential to grow and to undergo malignant transformation into non-germ cell tumours, e.g. rhabdomyosarcoma, adenocarcinoma etc.

Table 4.6.10 WHO and the British Tumour Panel classification schemes

WHO	British Tumour Panel
Teratoma	MT* differentiated
Embryonal carcinoma	MT* undifferentiated
Choriocarcinoma	MT* trophoblastic
Teratocarcinoma	MT* intermediate
Yolk-sac tumour	Yolk-sac tumour

* MT: malignant teratoma

Teratoma is resistant to radio- and chemotherapy and is therefore treated surgically. Prognosis does not differ between mature (adult-type differentiation) and immature teratoma (foetal differentiation).

Key points
- Somatic cell types of at least two germ layers
- Slow growing
- May transform into non-germ cell tumours
- Resistant to radio- and chemotherapy

Embryonal carcinoma consists of undifferentiated somatic cells with high metastatic potential. These cells resemble counterparts of human embryonic stem cells with the potential to differentiate into teratoma, choriocarcinoma, or yolk sac tumours. Syncytiotrophoblastic cells may be found but have no impact on treatment or prognosis.

Yolk sac tumours, or endodermal sinus tumours usually produce AFP. Pure yolk sac tumours are rarely seen in adults but may be found in mediastinal extragonadal germ cell tumours.

Choriocarcinoma is composed of syncytiotrophoblasts and cytotrophoblasts which may invade blood vessels, leading to primary extralymphatic metastases, in, for example, liver or brain. Haemorrhage may occur with severe complications.

Testicular intraepithelial neoplasia (TIN) is considered the non-invasive precursor of all testicular MGCTs and is often found in the vicinity of these tumours. Spermatocytic seminoma is an exception from this rule.

Further reading

Aitken R J. Koopman P. Lewis SE. Seeds of concern, *Nature* 2004; **432**(7013):48–52.

Crockford GP. Linge R. Hockley S, *et al.* Genome-wide linkage screen for testicular germ cell tumour susceptibility loci. *Hum Mol Genet* 2006; **15**(3):443–51.

Horwich A. Shipley J. Huddart R. Testicular germ-cell cancer, *Lancet* 2006; **367**(9512):754–65.

Rapley E. Susceptibility alleles for testicular germ cell tumour: a review. *Int J Androl* 2007; **30**(4):242–50.

Richiardi L, Bellocco R, Adami HO, *et al.* Testicular cancer incidence in eight Northern European countries: Secular and recent trends. *Cancer Epidemiol Biomarkers Prev* 2004; **13**(12):2157–66.

Skakkebaek NE, Rajpert-De Meyts E, Main KM. Testicular dysgenesis syndrome: an increasingly common developmental disorder with environmental aspects, *Hum Reprod* 2001; **16**(5):972–8.

Skakkebaek NE, Rajpert-De ME, Jorgensen N, *et al.* Testicular cancer trends as 'whistle blowers' of testicular developmental problems in populations. *Int J Androl* 2007; **30**:198–204.

Testicular cancer: clinical features, diagnosis, TIN, staging, and prognosis

Clinical features

TC is the most common malignancy in 15–40-year old males. The cure rate is approximately 90% and treatment of TC is considered a success story of evidence-based medicine.

The majority of TCs are MGCT. For a discussion of the remaining rare histological types see p.305.

Typically, the diagnosis of MGCT is made in young men with painless enlargement of the testicle or a lump in an otherwise normal testicle (Bosl and Motzer 1997; Horwich et al. 2006). Pain may be caused by retroperitoneal lymph-node metastases, and persistent newly developed back pain in younger males should raise suspicion of TC, prompting palpation of the testes and CT examination. More rarely, dyspnoea, haemoptysis or seizures, caused by metastases in lungs and brain respectively, indicate this disease. Tumours of unknown primary in younger males should always raise suspicion of MGCT since these tumours are the most frequent solid malignancies in these patients.

> **Key points: clinical presentation of TC**
> - Enlarged painless testicle
> - A lump in an otherwise normal testicle
> - Persistent back pain
> - Gynaecomastia or tender breasts
> - Rarely: haemoptysis, supraclavicular mass or seizures
> - MGCT must be ruled out in younger males with tumours of unknown primary

MGCTs arising outside the testes, extragonadal germ cell tumours (EGGCTs), account for about 2–5% of male MGCT (Bokemeyer 2002). These tumours are located in the midline of the body in the retroperitoneal space, the anterior mediastinum, or in the brain in the pineal gland or the suprasellar region. Differentiation between metastases from burned-out testicular MGCT and EGGCT may be difficult. In particular, retroperitoneal tumours may represent metastatic TC rather than primary malignancies as one third of patients harbour testicular intraepithelial neoplasia (TIN) and another third have testicular scar tissue, indicative of a 'burned out' TC (EGCCCG 2008). Primary mediastinal EGGCTs have a poor prognosis (see p.296) and these tumours are over represented among men with Klinefelter's (47 XXY) and Down's syndromes. Haematological malignancies such as megakaryoblastic leukaemia may also be associated with these tumours (Bokemeyer 2002).

Initiation of treatment should not be delayed in critically ill patients if there unequivocal elevation of AFP or β-hCG. If the histological diagnosis is not straightforward, immunohistochemistry and examination of isochromosome 12p should be performed.

Diagnosis

Demonstration of a solid testicular mass by ultrasound must be followed by biopsy of the tumour, by retraction of

> **Key points: EGGCTs**
> - Located in the midline of the body (retroperitoneum, mediastinum, or brain)
> - Difficult to determine whether metastases are from TC or EGCCT
> - Associated with chromosomal alterations
> - If histology not available, AFP↑/hCG↑ strongly supports diagnosis

the affected testicle through an inguinal incision, and examination of a frozen section.

The histological diagnosis distinguishes mainly between seminoma and non-seminoma which are treated differently (for further details please refer to pathology section in Chapter 4, Testicular cancer: introduction, p.292).

The following tumour markers may be released by MGCT:
- β-HCG
- AFP
- LDH

AFP is strictly related to non-seminoma and a histologically pure seminoma must be considered to be and treated as non-seminoma if there is AFP elevation which is otherwise unexplained, for example, by liver disease or chemotherapy toxicity.

> **Key points: serum AFP**
> - Normal level: <10 µg/l or <14 kU/L or <10ng/mL
> - Raised level defines non-seminoma
> - ↑ in 40–60% of non-seminoma patients
> - ↑↑ levels → yolk sac tumour
> - (↑) levels → possibly unrelated to TC, e.g. liver disease
> - Half-life: 5–7 days

HCG may be elevated in both seminoma and non-seminoma. Moderately elevated levels may stem from cross-reaction of the test assay with the α-chain of other glycoprotein hormones, e.g. luteinizing hormone (LH) or follicle-stimulating hormone (FSH). High levels are found in choriocarcinoma, which may metastasize haematogenously to visceral organs like lungs, liver, or brain.

> **Key points: serum hCG**
> - Normal level: <5IU/L or < 5mUI/mL
> - ↑ in 25–60% of men with disseminated TC
> - ↑↑ levels → choriocarcinoma → MR brain
> - (↑) levels → possible cross-reaction with LH, FSH in sub-gonadal patients
> - Half-life: 1–2 days.

LDH is an enzyme which is elevated in most situations where there is high cellular turnover, e.g. infections, myocardial infarction, and is therefore the least specific marker for MGCT. However, LDH levels predict prognosis and help to identify relapses at follow-up.

AFP, HCG, and LDH may be released by treatment-induced tumour-lysis, and elevation during the first 10 days after initiation of treatment—a 'marker surge'—should not be interpreted as tumour progression. However, persistent elevation, rise, or slower decrease than calculated by respective serum half-lives may indicate insufficient treatment.

Pattern of metastases
TC spreads primarily through lymph vessels to the retroperitoneal lymph nodes. These are best assessed by CT of abdomen and pelvis. Metastases to visceral organs such as lung, liver, or brain are exceedingly rare if the abdominal CT is normal. Choriocarcinoma is the exception to this rule as it spreads primarily through blood vessels, leading to visceral metastases. High levels of HCG suggest this diagnosis and MR examination of the brain is essential.

Mandatory diagnostic work-up
- Palpation of both testicles
- Ultrasound of both testicles
- Serum tumour markers (HCG, AFP, LDH)
- CT abdomen/pelvis
- CXR
- Histological diagnosis

TIN (testicular intraepithelial neoplasia)
Up to 9% of TC patients have TIN in their remaining 'unaffected' testicle. This proportion increases to roughly one-third in case of testicular atrophy (<12mL volume) and age <40 years (EGCCCG 2008). The majority of patients with TIN will develop a TC within 10 years (Hoei-Hansen et al. 2005).

Prevalence of TIN:
- <1% general population
- 2–3% among sub-/infertile males
- 4–9% in the remaining testicle of TC patients
- Up to 33% of TC patients <40 years with atrophic testicle
- Up to 33% in patients with extragonadal germ cell tumour

Therefore, the possibility of a contralateral TC should be discussed with each patient. Self-examination after treatment is of particular importance for these patients (see p.304.).

In high-risk patients, TIN is diagnosed by a testicular biopsy, which may be performed during orchiectomy of the affected testicle.

Important: do *not* use formalin but Bouin's or Stieve's solution.

Treatment options of TIN in the contralateral testicle:
- Orchiectomy
- Radiotherapy
- Surveillance strategy

Orchiectomy and radiotherapy are effective treatments but either will render the patient infertile. Surveillance by annual testicular ultrasound examination and instruction in self-examination (see p.304.) is in our view a valid management option.

Staging
The Royal Marsden staging system is commonly used in Western Europe, see Table 4.6.11.

Table 4.6.11 The Royal Marsden staging system

Stage	
I	Testicular tumour only
IM	Elevated levels of AFP and/or HCG without visible metastases
II	Infradiaphragmatic lymphadenopathy
A: <2cm	
B: 2–5cm	
C: >5cm	
III	Supradiaphragmatic lymphadenopathy
A: <2cm	
B: 2–5cm	
C: >5cm	
IV	Extralymphatic metastases (lung, liver, bone, etc.)

Sensitivity to chemotherapy
The high curability of metastatic TC by cisplatin-based chemotherapy serves as a model for a curable neoplasm and is a remarkable clinical feature (Einhorn 2002). The reasons behind the 2–4 times higher sensitivity to cisplatin-based chemotherapy by TC compared to most other tumours are not yet fully understood, but the following findings are considered important (Masters et al. 2003):

MGCT cells lack or have only low activity of drug export pumps, cisplatin-inactivation enzymes, efficient DNA repair system, especially the nucleotide-excision-repair system. There are high intrinsic levels of pro-apoptotic proteins, e.g. wild-type p53 or BAX, and prompt cell death after chemotherapy. Furthermore, anti-apoptotic proteins such as BCL2 are either absent or present at only very low levels.

> *Key points: sensitivity to chemotherapy*
> - Lack of drug efficient export pumps
> - Inability to efficiently detoxify cisplatin
> - Inability to repair the respective DNA damage
> - Limited antiapoptotic factors
> - Intact apoptotic cascade

Some of these features might also explain the high radiosensitivity of seminoma.

Teratoma is slow-growing and resistant to chemo- and radiotherapy. These non-seminoma components are common findings in residual masses and complicate the management of residual post-chemotherapy masses.

Further reading
Bokemeyer C, Nichols CR, Droz JP, et al. Extragonadal germ cell tumors of the mediastinum and retroperitoneum: Results from an international analysis. *J Clin Oncol* 2002; **20**:1864–73.

Bosl GJ, Motzer RJ. Testicular germ-cell cancer. *N Engl J Med* 1997; **337**(4):242–53.

Einhorn LH. Curing metastatic testicular cancer, *Proc Natl Acad Sci USA* 2002; **99**(7):4592–5.

European Germ Cell Cancer Consensus group. 2008; European Consensus Conference on Diagnosis and Treatment of Germ Cell Cancer: A Report of the Second Meeting of the European

Germ Cell Cancer Consensus group (EGCCCG): Part I. *Eur.Urol* 2008; **53**(3):478–96.

Hoei-Hansen CE, Rajpert-De Meyts E, Daugaard G, *et al.* Carcinoma in situ testis, the progenitor of testicular germ cell tumours: a clinical review. *Ann Oncol* 2005; **16**(6):863–8.

Horwich A, Shipley J, Huddart R. Testicular germ-cell cancer, *Lancet* 2006; **367**(9512):754–65.

Masters JRW, Koberle B. Curing metastatic cancer: Lessons from testicular germ-cell tumours. *Nature Rev Cancer* 2003; **3**(7):517–25.

Testicular cancer: prognosis and management of advanced disease

Prognostic grouping (Table 4.6.12)

Several algorithms have been developed for prognosis prediction and treatment adjustments for patients with advanced MGCT. By far the most important one has been established by the International Germ Cell Consensus Classification Group (IGCCCG). International experts retrospectively analysed the outcome of a large number of patients with metastatic or extragonadal MGCT (non-seminoma n=5202, seminoma n=660) (IGCCCG 1997).

Usability in the clinical setting was a priority and three features were the basis for prognostication:

- Serum level of tumour markers (AFP, HCG, LDH)
- Localization of the primary tumour (i.e. mediastinal EGGCT vs. the remainder)
- Presence of visceral metastases outside the lungs

Three prognostic groups were established according to 5-year survival rate:

- Good (90%)
- Intermediate (80%)
- Poor (50%)

For seminoma only presence of non-pulmonary visceral metastases confers an intermediate prognosis (approximately 10%). The remaining 90% have a good prognosis. Due to good treatment results, no poor prognosis group could be established for patients with seminoma.

Cisplatin-based chemotherapy

Introduction of cisplatin in the treatment of metastatic TC during the late 1970s by Einhorn et al. transformed this disease into a model for a curable neoplasm (Einhorn et al. 1981).

The three-drug regimen of bleomycin, etoposide, and cisplatin (BEP) is today's gold-standard.

Dosage

- Bleomycin: (30,000 IU days 1 + 8 + 15
- Etoposide: $100mg/m^2$ days 1–5
- Cisplatin: $20mg/m^2$ days 1–5
- 3-weeks interval between cycles

Treatment intensity is important and dose reduction and prolonged intervals should be avoided. However, fever,

Table 4.6.12 Prognosis of metastatic germ cell tumors. International Germ Cell Cancer Collaborative Group. International Germ Cell Consensus Classification: A Prognostic Factor-Based Staging System for Metastatic Germ Cell Cancers. *J Clin Oncol* 1997; **15**:594–603, © 2008 American Society of Clinical Oncology. All rights reserved

Prognosis	Non-seminomatous MGCT	Seminomatous MGCT
Good	**56%** of patients fulfil all of the following: No non-pulmonary visceral metastases No mediastinal EGGCT AFP <1000 HCG <5000 LDG <1.5 x ULN	**90%** of patients are free from: non-pulmonary visceral metastases
5-year PFS(%)	89	82
5-year OS (%)	92	86
Intermediate	**28%** of patients fulfil the following: No non-pulmonary visceral metastases; No mediastinal EGGCT; And any of these: AFP 1000–10,000 HCG 5000–50,000 LDG 1.5–10 x ULN	**10%** of patients do have non-pulmonary visceral metastases
5-year PFS (%)	75	67
5-year OS (%)	80	72
Poor	**16%** of patients fulfil any of the following: Non-pulmonary visceral metastases Primary mediastinal MGCT AFP >10.000 HCG >50.000 LDG >10 x ULN	No patients with seminoma have poor risk
5-year PFS (%)	41	
5-yearOS (%)	48	

ULN, upper limit of normal

neutrophil counts $<0.5 \times 10^9$/L or platelets $<100 \times 10^9$/L at day 1 may necessitate some recovery time. Granulocyte colony-stimulating factor (G-CSF) should not be used routinely, but may shorten prolonged periods of neutropaenia and should be employed if there have been previous chemotherapy-induced serious infections or febrile neutropenia.

Carboplatin plays no role in treatment of patients with metastatic disease as it has been shown to be consistently inferior to cisplatin-based chemotherapy (Feldman et al. 2008).

Good risk

Conventional chemotherapy followed by adjunctive surgery cures approximately 90% of patients with a good risk according to IGCCCG (Kondagunta and Motzer 2006).

Patients with a good prognosis are primarily treated by 3 cycles of BEP.

If there are contradictions to using bleomycin, e.g. compromised lung function, 4 cycles of EP may be given.

Alternative regimens have not shown greater efficacy (equal or higher cure rates and equal or less toxicities). Other chemotherapy regimens should therefore only be employed in clinical trials (Kondagunta and Motzer 2006).

Intermediate or poor risk

Only 16% of all patients with MGCT have a poor prognosis according to IGCCCG and survival of these patients is best if treated in centres which have good experience in management of such patients (Collette et al. 1999). We recommend that patients with intermediate or poor prognosis disease are referred to hospitals especially dedicated to treatment of MGCT. The standard treatment is:

• 4 cycles of BEP

Most experts agree that improvement of the survival rate of patients with intermediate- or poor-risk MGCT is a priority. Consequently, many randomized trials have been undertaken with more intensified treatment approaches, e.g. high-dose chemotherapy with stem cell rescue. However, no alternative regimen has proved to be more effective; and most regimens caused higher toxicities (Feldman et al. 2008).

Management of residual tumour

Seminoma

Residual tumours, especially <3cm, consist usually of necrotic/fibrotic tissue (Heidenreich et al. 2008). Because of desmoplastic reactions of seminoma, surgical removal of such masses is more complicated than in non-seminoma and complete resection is sometimes impossible. Extensive biopsies should be taken and presence of viable seminoma should prompt salvage chemotherapy. PET may identify residual seminoma, particular in masses >3cm and salvage chemotherapy is the treatment of choice.

Key points for treating residual seminoma
• <3cm → usually fibrosis/necrosis, follow with CT, PET optional
• 3cm PET positive → salvage treatment (surgery, chemotherapy, or radiotherapy)
• 3cm PET negative → follow with CT

Non-seminoma

As a rule, residual tumour should always be removed (Heidenreich et al. 2008). Since the retroperitoneal lymph nodes represent the most frequent place of metastases, most residual tumours are located in the retroperitoneal space. Postchemotherapy (PC) retroperitoneal lymph node dissection is more challenging than primary RPLND and only experienced surgeons should perform this operation. The histological findings of PC-RPLND are:
• Necrosis (50%)
• Teratoma (35%)
• Viable non-teratomatous MGCT (15%)

Obviously only patients with either teratoma or viable MGCT can benefit from this operation, whereas 50% of patients with only necrosis will not.

This dilemma led to attempts to develop an algorithm to reliably predict the PC-histology. Unfortunately, no approach has been broadly accepted (EGCCCG 2008; Feldman et al. 2008).

Small lesions are less likely to contain viable MGCT than larger ones. This relationship led to the recommendation that residual masses should only be removed if they exceed 1–2cm in size. However, in lesions <2cm, teratoma and MGCT was present in 26% and 7% of retroperitoneal lymph nodes (Oldenburg et al. 2003). Five out of six patients with viable MGCT had residual lesions of <1 cm.

At our institution we therefore remove all visible lesions after chemotherapy irrespective of size.

Management of recurrence

More than 90% of patients who achieve a complete response to initial therapy are cured (EGCCCG 2008; Feldman et al. 2008). A single lesion without tumour marker elevation may be cured surgically without chemotherapy. In patients with recurrent seminoma, PET may help to differentiate viable MGCT from necrosis (De Santis et al. 2004). In non-seminoma patients, however, PET is of limited value since teratoma, a common histology of recurrent masses, is PET negative.

In patients with systemic relapse, i.e. tumour marker elevation and/or multiple metastases, second-line or even third-line chemotherapy may lead to cure.

Whether second-line chemotherapy should consist of standard dose three-drug regimens or high-dose chemotherapy with autologous stem-cell is controversial. Up to now, no randomized controlled trial has shown any survival benefit from intensified treatment compared with the standard chemotherapy.

Four cycles of TIP (Taxol, Ifosfamide, CisPlatin) have achieved >60% cure rate in patients relapsing after initial chemotherapy (Kondagunta et al. 2005) and this is our regimen of choice.

4 cycles of the following regimens are usually used:
• TIP (PacliTaxel, Ifosfamide, CisPlatin)
• VIP (Etoposide [VP-16], Ifosfamide, CisPlatin)
• VeIP (Vinblastine, Ifosfamide, CisPlatin)

High-dose chemotherapy with 2–3 cycles of etoposide and carboplatin (ifosfamide or cyclophosfamide may be added) may alternatively be used. This intensive chemotherapy has been better tolerated recently with the use of growth factor support (G-CSF) and mobilization of peripheral blood stem cells. Einhorn et al. (2007) achieved a

4-year complete remission in 110 of 184 (63%) patients with relapsing or initially cisplatin-resistant TC by high-dose chemotherapy.

Late relapses occur by definition after at least 2 years—but may be encountered decades after successful primary treatment. Such recurrences are, if initially treated by chemotherapy, usually resistant to cisplatin. However, a seminoma patient with a single retroperitoneal mass after surveillance will respond well to either radio- or chemotherapy.

In non-seminoma patients, surgery is an extremely important treatment strategy which cures many patients with single lesions (Oldenburg et al. 2006).

Achievement of a representative biopsy is important as almost all patients with teratoma only will survive whereas 50% or more of patients with viable MGCT will succumb to their relapse. Teratoma may differentiate by malignant transformation into for example rhabdomyosarcoma or adenocarcinoma and demonstration of isochromosome 12 proves MGCT clonality. Complete removal is the treatment of choice, but if not feasible, chemotherapy should be given as appropriate for the histological tumour type.

Treatment of late recurrences is complex and requires individual treatment which should be restricted to experienced centres only.

Brain metastases

Brain metastases occur in approximately 10% of patients with advanced MGCT. In patients with brain metastases at initial diagnosis survival is 30–40%, whereas those with systemic relapse or development of brain metastases during treatment have a dismal survival of 2–5% (EGCCCG 2008).

Treatment should comprise systemic chemotherapy and radiotherapy may be added. Neither the optimal sequence nor the role of surgery is defined yet.

Further reading

Collette L, Sylvester RJ, Stenning SP, et al. Impact of the treating institution on survival of patients with 'poor-prognosis' metastatic nonseminoma. European Organization for Research and Treatment of Cancer Genito-Urinary Tract Cancer Collaborative Group and the Medical Research Council Testicular Cancer Working Party. J Natl Cancer Inst 1999; 91:839–46.

De Santis M, Becherer A, Bokemeyer C, et al. 2-18fluoro-deoxy-D-glucose positron emission tomography is a reliable predictor for viable tumor in postchemotherapy seminoma: An update of the prospective multicentric SEMPET Trial. J Clin Oncol 2004; 22:1034–1039.

Einhorn, LH. Testicular cancer as a model for a curable neoplasm—the Richard and Hinda Rosenthal Foundation Award Lecture. Cancer Res 1981; 41:3275–80.

Einhorn L H, Williams SD, Chamness A, et al. High-dose chemotherapy and stem-cell rescue for metastatic germ-cell tumors. N Engl J Med 2007; 357:340–8.

European Germ Cell Cancer Consensus group. European Consensus Conference on Diagnosis and Treatment of Germ Cell Cancer: A Report of the Second Meeting of the European Germ Cell Cancer Consensus Group (EGCCCG): Part II. Eur Urol 2008; 53:497–513.

Feldman DR, Bosl GJ, Sheinfeld J, et al. Medical treatment of advanced testicular cancer. JAMA 2008; 299:672–84.

Heidenreich A. Thuer, D. Polyakov S. Postchemotherapy retroperitoneal lymph node dissection in advanced germ cell tumours of the testis. Eur Urol 2008; 53:260–74.

International Germ Cell Cancer Collaborative Group. International Germ Cell Consensus Classification: a prognostic factor-based staging system for metastatic germ cell cancers. International Germ Cell Cancer Collaborative Group. J Clin Oncol; 1997; 15:594–603.

Kondagunta GV, Motzer RJ. Chemotherapy for advanced germ cell tumors. J Clin Oncol 2006; 24:5493–502.

Kondagunta GV, Bacik J, Donadio A, et al. Combination of paclitaxel, ifosfamide, and cisplatin is an effective second-line therapy for patients with relapsed testicular germ cell tumors. J Clin Oncol 2005; 23:6549–55.

Oldenburg J, Alfsen GC, Lien H, et al. Postchemotherapy retroperitoneal surgery remains necessary in patients with nonseminomatous testicular cancer and minimal residual tumor masses. J Clin Oncol 2003; 21:3310–17.

Oldenburg J. Martin J M. Fossa SD. Late relapses of germ cell malignancies: Incidence, management, and prognosis. J Clin Oncol 2006; 24:5503–11.

Testicular cancer: management of low stage seminoma

Orchiectomy is usually the first step of treatment of TC and should be performed within 1 week after clinical diagnosis. However, in patients with advanced life-threatening TC, orchiectomy should not delay cisplatin-based chemotherapy (EGCCCG 2008).

Organ-sparing surgery may be considered in case of:
- Bilateral testicular cancer
- Small (<2cm) solitary tumour
- Sufficient endocrine function
- Benign tumour
- Treatment at experienced centre

Clinical stage I

Eighty per cent of seminoma patients present apparently without metastases, i.e. with clinical stage I disease. Approximately 20% of those harbour micrometastases in the retroperitoneal lymph nodes (Albers 2007). Disease-specific survival rate approaches 100%, independent of which of the following three management strategies are applied (de Wit and Fizazi 2006):
- Radiotherapy
- Surveillance and treatment in case of relapse
- Carboplatin

Radiotherapy

Radiotherapy to para-aortic and ipsilateral pelvic lymph nodes is one adjuvant treatment option. This approach exploits two features of seminoma:
- Extreme radiosensitivity
- Tumour spread through the lymphatic vessels

During the last 50–60 years it has been the standard treatment of stage I seminoma.

Approach: 20Gy in daily doses of 2.0Gy/ fraction, 5 days/ week

Target: para-aortic lymph nodes

Field borders:
- Upper: upper edge T11
- Lower: lower edge of L5
- Ipsilateral (to primary tumour): renal hilum
- Contralateral (to primary tumour): transverse process included

Before 1999, prophylactic radiation included ipsilateral iliac lymph nodes within a 'dog-leg field'. Due to similar relapse rates and less acute toxicity, para-aortic lymph node radiation became standard treatment (Fossa et al. 1999). Reduction of the radiation dose from 30 to 20Gy has further contributed to reduction in toxicity (Jones et al. 2005).

Chemotherapy or extension of the radiation field to ipsilateral iliac or inguinal nodes or the scrotal region may be considered if there is
- Inguinal violation, e.g. by prior hernia operation
- Scrotal violation, e.g. trans-scrotal biopsy
- Advanced primary tumour, i.e. pT3–4

The advantages and disadvantages of adjuvant radiotherapy are as follows:

Advantages
- Highly effective.
- Mostly well tolerated.
- Low relapse rate <5% (almost exclusively outside radiation field, removing need for abdominal CT scans during follow-up).
- Long observation data.

Disadvantages
- Unnecessary treatment to approximately 80% of unselected patients (those without retroperitoneal micrometastases).
- Disease outside the radiation field is left untreated.
- Risk of long-term toxicity, e.g. radiotherapy-induced malignancies.
- Risk of acute toxicity, e.g. nausea, fatigue, diarrhoea, peptic ulceration.

Surveillance

Surveillance, also called 'watchful waiting' or 'wait and see', is increasingly used, since metastases, developing mostly in retroperitoneal lymph nodes, can be cured by subsequent radio–or chemotherapy.

Approach

Frequent follow-up visits during the first 2–3 years with decreasing frequency later on (refer to follow-up chapter)

Salvage treatment by chemo- or radiotherapy if metastatic disease is found by radiological or clinical examination or by tumour marker elevation

Unfortunately, surveillance has not been investigated in randomized trials and the long-term risk/benefit ratio remains uncertain.

Advantages
- Avoidance of treatment and its toxicities for the majority of patients
- Salvage treatment highly effective

Disadvantages
- Late relapses may occur after 2, 5, and even 10 years
- Long follow-up, including CT examinations, is necessary
- Requires high degree of compliance
- May be psychologically demanding

Carboplatin

Carboplatin as adjuvant treatment of clinical stage I seminoma is considered to be as effective as adjuvant radiotherapy (Oliver et al. 2005).

Approach: one course of carboplatin as single agent intravenously

Dose: 7 x AUC (area under the curve), i.e. 7 x (glomerular filtration rate [GFR] +25)

Advantages
- Highly effective
- Tolerated well, e.g. patients resume work earlier than after radiotherapy, because of less fatigue
- Convenient to administer
- Salvage treatment highly effective

Disadvantages
- Unnecessary and possibly harmful treatment to approximately 80% of unselected patients (those without retroperitoneal micro-metastases).
- Insufficient long-term observation

The most appropriate treatment may be chosen according the two risk factors most predictive for micrometastases (Warde et al. 2002):
• Rete testis invasion
• Size of the primary tumour (>4cm)

Consensus on treatment

Following the Spanish Germ Cell Cancer Group's recommendations, we advise surveillance for patients with expected high compliance and without risk factors with treatment reserved for relapse (Aparicio et al. 2003).

Patients with expected low compliance and/or presence of one or both risk factors are advised to undergo adjuvant treatment.
Valid adjuvant treatment strategies:
• Radiotherapy
• Carboplatin

We prefer one course of carboplatin (AUC x 7).

Clinical stage II

Clinical stage II disease, i.e. presence of retroperitoneal lymph node metastases, may be considered as advanced disease and treated by cisplatin-based chemotherapy as described in Chapter 4.6, Testicular cancer: prognosis and management of advanced disease, p.296.

However, non-bulky (<5cm) retroperitoneal lymph node metastases may be effectively treated by:

Radiotherapy
• Stage IIA, i.e. masses <2cm: 30Gy
• Stage IIB, i.e. masses 2–5cm: 36Gy
• *Approach*: 2Gy/day and 5 fractions/week
• *Target*: para-aortic lymph nodes
• Shielding of contralateral testis
• Field size borders:
  • Upper upper edge T11
  • Lower: upper border of ipsilateral acetabulum
  • In CS IIA, same lateral borders as in CS I.

• In CS IIB, lateral borders are modified to cover lymph nodes with a 1.5 cm safety margin

Relapse-free survival at 6 years is 95% for CS IIA and 89% for CS IIB and most patients with relapse are cured by cisplatin-based chemotherapy (Classen et al. 2003).

However, the risk of metastatic disease outside the radiation field increases with stage. We treat our CS II patients preferentially with cisplatin-based chemotherapy (see p.296.)

Further reading

Albers P. Management of stage I testis cancer. *Europ Urol* 2007; **51**:34–44.

Aparicio J, Garcia del Muro X, Maroto P, *et al*. Multicenter study evaluating a dual policy of post-orchiectomy surveillance and selective adjuvant single-agent carboplatin for patients with clinical stage I seminoma. *Ann Oncol* 2003; **14**:867–872.

Classen J, Schmidberger H, Meisner CS, *et al*. Radiotherapy for stages IIA/B testicular seminoma: Final report of a prospective multicenter clinical trial. *J Clin Oncol* 2003; **21**:1101–6.

de Wit R. Fizazi K. Controversies in the management of clinical stage I testis cancer. *J Clin Oncol* 2006; **24**:5482–92.

European Germ Cell Cancer Consensus group. European Consensus Conference on Diagnosis and Treatment of Germ Cell Cancer: A Report of the Second Meeting of the European Germ Cell Cancer Consensus Group (EGCCCG): Part II. *Eur Urol* 2008; **53**:497–513.

Fossa SD, Horwich A, Russell JM, *et al*. Optimal planning target volume for stage I testicular seminoma: A Medical Research Council randomized trial. Medical Research Council Testicular Tumor Working Group. *J Clin Oncol* 1999; **17**:1146

Jones, WG, Fossa SD, Mead GM, *et al*. Randomized trial of 30 versus 20 Gy in the adjuvant treatment of stage I Testicular Seminoma: a report on Medical Research Council Trial TE18, European Organisation for the Research and Treatment of Cancer Trial 30942 (ISRCTN18525328). *J Clin Oncol* 2005; **23**:1200–8.

Oliver RTD, Mason MD, Mead GM, *et al*. Radiotherapy versus single-dose carboplatin in adjuvant treatment of stage I seminoma: a randomised trial. *Lancet* 2005; **366**:293–300.

Warde P, Specht L, Horwich A, *et al*. Prognostic factors for relapse in stage I seminoma managed by surveillance: a pooled analysis. *J Clin Oncol* 2002; **20**:4448–52.

Testicular cancer: management of low stage non-seminoma

Orchiectomy

Orchiectomy is usually the first step of treatment of testicular cancer (TC) and should be performed within one week after diagnosis. However, in patients with advanced life-threatening TC, orchiectomy should not delay cisplatin-based chemotherapy (EGCCCG 2008a).

Organ-sparing surgery may be considered in case of:
- Bilateral testicular cancer
- Small (<2cm) solitary tumour
- Sufficient endocrine function
- Benign tumour
- Treatment at experienced centre

Clinical stage I

Approximately 80% of non-seminoma patients present without detectable metastases, i.e. CS I disease (Horwich et al. 2006). Approximately 20–50% of these harbour micrometastases in the retroperitoneal lymph nodes (Albers 2007). Disease-specific survival rate approaches 100%, independent of which of the following three management strategies are applied (de Wit et al. 2006):
- RPLND (retroperitoneal lymph node dissection)
- surveillance and treatment in case of relapse
- adjuvant cisplatin-based chemotherapy

Retroperitoneal lymph node dissection (RPLND)

RPLND is the only approach providing both staging and cure for the majority of patients. In the hands of an experienced surgeon, i.e. an urologist performing at least 10 RPLNDs per year, this operation has low morbidity. Originally, all the retroperitoneal soft tissue within the diaphragm, ureters, and large iliac vessels was removed. Characterization of the typical landing zones, i.e. the area of primary lymph drainage, allowed for removal of distinct templates for left- and right sided testicular cancers.

After nerve-sparing (NS) RPLND, which aims to identify and preserve sympathetic nerves, only a few patients (<10%) will experience retrograde ejaculation, the most common complication.

Approach
- Laparatomy
- Preparation of the retroperitoneal space
- Identification and preservation of sympathetic nerves and ganglions
- Removal of all tissue of the respective template (which includes numerous lymph nodes)

Advantages
- Curative for the vast majority of patients
- Accurate staging
- Low acute morbidity
- Only way to get rid of subsequent complications from teratoma such as growing teratoma or malignant differentiation
- Only way to 'control of the retroperitoneum', the most frequent site of late relapses
- Abdominal CT scans not needed during follow-up
- Long observation data

Disadvantages
- Unnecessary treatment of approximately 50% of unselected patients (those without retroperitoneal micrometastases)
- Outcome depends largely on the surgeon's experience
- Disease outside the template is left untreated
- Risk of surgery-related complications such as infections, bowel perforation

Laparoscopic RPLND may reduce surgery-related complications such as lymphocoele, bowel complications, infections, chylous ascites and blood loss. However, lymph nodes between or behind the large vessels cannot be removed by this approach. This technique should only be used in a study setting since its efficacy both in terms of diagnostic and curative intent remains doubtful.

Surveillance

Surveillance aims to avoid unnecessary and potentially harmful treatment in about 50% of patients. Compliance to a strict follow-up protocol is prerequisite for this approach. MGCT metastases are thereby detected at an early stage, amenable to chemotherapy, surgery or the combination of both.

Approach
- Frequent follow-up visits for the first 2–3 years with decreasing frequency later on (see Chapter 4.6, Testicular cancer: follow-up and rare testicular tumours, p.304).
- Finding of metastases by radiological or clinical examination or by tumour marker elevation prompts:
- Salvage treatment by cisplatin-based chemotherapy and/or surgery.
- Unfortunately, surveillance has not been investigated in randomized trials and the long-term risk/benefit ratio remains uncertain.

Advantages
- Avoidance of treatment and its toxicities to approximately 50% of unselected patients.
- Salvage treatment highly effective.

Disadvantages
- Long follow-up, including CT abdominal examinations.
- Requires high degree of compliance and experience by patients and physicians, respectively.
- Psychologically demanding.

Adjuvant chemotherapy

Cisplatin-based chemotherapy as adjuvant treatment of CSI non-seminoma consists of two courses of BEP (bleomycin, etoposide, cisplatin—see p.296).

Approach
Two courses of BEP.

Advantages
- Abolishes small non-teratomatous MGCT systemically.
- Lower dose of cytotoxic drugs than required for stage 2 or higher.
- Convenient to administer.
- Usually well tolerated.

Disadvantages
- Unnecessary and harmful treatment to approximately 50% of patients (those without retroperitoneal micro-metastases).
- Insufficient long-term observations, e.g. the risk of late relapses, treatment-induced malignancies, cardiovascular disease, etc. remains unknown.
- Teratoma is left in place.
- Possible selection of chemotherapy-resistant MGCT cells may complicate treatment at relapse.

Recommendations
Optimal management of clinical stage I non-seminoma remains controversial. However, most experts agree that identification of risk factors and tailoring of treatment accordingly should be pursued. Until now only one risk-factor for micrometastases has been broadly accepted:
- Vascular invasion (VI) of the primary tumour
Approximately every second patient with VI harbours micrometastases and adjuvant (prophylactic) treatment remains advised in patients with VI:
- 2 cycles of BEP
- NS-RPLND

If poor compliance is anticipated or if the prospect of watchful waiting appears too distressing for the patient, adjuvant treatment is indicated. Most European experts favour 2 cycles of BEP as opposed to NS-RPLND (EGCCCG 2008b). Most US American experts favour NS-RPLND due to possible chemotherapy-induced long-term complications such as cardiovascular disease and second malignancies.

Absence of VI is associated with a relapse rate of 14–22% and surveillance is the recommended treatment strategy.

Clinical stage II
Small (<2cm) retroperitoneal lymph nodes metastases represent stage IIA and such patients may be cured by primary RPLND alone or by chemotherapy.

Larger retroperitoneal lymph nodes, i.e. stage IIB/C are treated like advanced non-seminoma by cisplatin-based chemotherapy (see p.296).

Further reading
Albers, P. Management of stage I testis cancer. *Eur Urol* 2007; **51**:34–44.

European Germ Cell Cancer Consensus group. European Consensus Conference on Diagnosis and Treatment of Germ Cell Cancer: A Report of the Second Meeting of the European Germ Cell Cancer Consensus group (EGCCCG): Part I. *Eur Urol* 2008a; **53**:478–96.

European Germ Cell Cancer Consensus group. European Consensus Conference on Diagnosis and Treatment of Germ Cell Cancer: A Report of the Second Meeting of the European Germ Cell Cancer Consensus Group (EGCCCG): Part II. *Eur Urol* 2008b; **53**:497–513.

de Wit R, Fizazi, K. Controversies in the management of clinical stage I testis cancer. *J Clin Oncol* 2006; **24**:5482–92.

Horwich, A, Shipley, J, Huddart, R. Testicular germ-cell cancer, *Lancet* 2006; **367**:754–65.

Testicular cancer: follow-up and rare testicular tumours

Follow-up

Follow-up in patients with TC aims primarily at early detection of relapses. Follow-up protocols, i.e. frequency and recommended examinations at each visit, are guided by the pattern of relapse, which is determined by.
- Histology (seminoma vs. non-seminoma)
- Extent of disease (stage and prognostic factors)
- Treatment received

Approximately 2–3% of the patients develop a new primary cancer in the contralateral testis (Fossa et al. 2005). Careful clinical examination of the remaining testis is important at every visit. Additionally, self-examination offers a means for early detection. Therefore each patient should be instructed in testicular self-examination:
- During warm shower or bath (relaxation of scrotal skin)
- Roll the testicle gently between thumb and fingers
- Lumps in or on the side of the testicle?
- (Should be smooth and firm)
- Bumps/lumps require professional examination

As presented in the section on survivorship issue (see p.306) treatment-induced late effects are an important concern. Hypogonadism, sexual dysfunction, cardiovascular disease and its known risk factors, neurological symptoms, and fatigue should be addressed during follow-up.

Follow-up aids the early detection of three complications:
- Relapsing disease
- New primary disease
- Late effects

Despite the importance of an optimal follow-up routine, evidence-based recommendations for follow-up are scarce—except for seminoma stage I. We will focus on the principles behind follow-up.

Stage I seminoma

These patients comprise a large group since about 80% of patients with seminoma present with stage I disease .The following recommendations are based on retrospective analysis of the clinical course of >5500 patients (Martin et al. 2007).

Surveillance
Follow-up schedule:
- 1st and 2nd year 3 x annually
- 3rd and 4th twice annually
- 5th –10th year once annually
- Cease thereafter

Investigations:
- History and physical examination
- HCG, AFP, and LDH serum levels
- CT abdomen + pelvis
- CXR

Radiotherapy
Follow-up schedule:
- 1st –3rd year: twice annually
- 4th –6th years: once annually
- Cease thereafter

Investigations:
- History and physical examination
- HCG, AFP and LDH serum levels
- CXR
- CT pelvis (after para-aortic radiation, not necessary after extended field)

Carboplatin
Follow-up schedule:
- 1st –3rd year: twice annually
- Further recommendations not yet possible

Investigations:
- History and physical examination
- HCG, AFP, and LDH serum levels
- CXR
- CT abdomen + pelvis

Stage I non-seminoma

Stage I non-seminoma may be treated by different strategies resulting in different risk profiles which must be taken into account. As in stage I seminoma, the risk of relapse is higher during surveillance than after adjuvant treatment. With surveillance, 95% of relapses occur during the first 5 years (Daugaard et al. 2003) and two CT examinations (at 3 and 12 months) after orchiectomy are considered sufficient (Rustin et al. 2007).

Surveillance
Follow-up schedule:
- 1st year: 4–12 x annually
- 2nd year: 4–6 x annually
- Decreasing intensity thereafter, e.g. twice annually until 5th year
- Cease thereafter

Investigations:
- History and physical examination
- HCG, AFP, and LDH serum levels
- CT abdomen at 3 and 12 months
- CT pelvis at 3 and 12 months—if prior scrotal violation or inguinal operation
- CXR

Chemotherapy/RPLND
Follow-up schedule:
- 1st year: 4–6 x annually
- 2nd year: 3–4 x annually
- 3rd –5th twice annually
- Once annually thereafter until 10 years

Investigations:
- History and physical examination
- HCG, AFP, and LDH serum levels
- CXR (twice annually sufficient)
- RPLND removes need for CT abdomen
- Only after chemotherapy: CT abdomen at 3 and 12 months
- Only after chemotherapy- if prior scrotal violation or inguinal operation: CT pelvis at 3 and 12 months

Advanced disease, postchemotherapy (Table 4.6.13)

Follow-up protocol is similar to that of non-seminoma after adjuvant chemotherapy. History and physical examinations are performed in conjunction with HCG, AFP, and LDH

Table 4.6.13 Suggested visits according to time after treatment

Years after treatment	1	2	3	4	5	6–10
Suggested visits annually	~6	~4	~3	~3	~2	~1

serum levels. CT or MRI is usually done during the first year in both seminoma and non-seminoma patients. Patients with non-seminoma may harbour teratoma which may grow after several years. Therefore repeated CT scans are usually performed, e.g. at year 3 and 5 and follow-up should be for at least 10 years. An intensified protocol should, however, be followed if there are residual masses, which could not be removed. Residual seminoma masses may be identified by positive PET scans (De Santis et al. 2004).

Furthermore, these patients have usually received at least three courses of cisplatin-based chemotherapy. Complications from long-term treatment-induced toxicities, (see p.306) may be prevented by timely diagnosis and treatment. Evaluation of the following issues annually during follow-up is recommended:
• Hormonal disturbance
• Sexual dysfunction
• Components of the metabolic syndrome
• Cardiovascular disease
• Neurotoxicity

After formal follow-up is completed, every patient should be referred to a GP or cardiologist for regular controls, which should be scheduled at least every 5 years.

Rare testicular tumours

Approximately 5% of all testicular tumours are of the following types:

Sex cord-stromal tumours
Leydig cell tumour
• Composed of testicular interstitial (Leydig) cells
• Associated with androgen and/or oestrogen secretion
• May cause precocious physical and sexual development in prepubertal boys

• Feminization and gynaecomastia is observed in adult males
• Ninety per cent are benign, 10% malignant
• Orchiectomy alone is almost always adequate

Sertoli cell tumour
• Composed of Sertoli cells
• Occurs in males, usually <40 years
• Endocrine effects are uncommon
• Orchiectomy alone is adequate

Germ cell tumour
Spermatocytic seminoma
• Composed of seminoma cells
• Does not develop from TIN
• Occurs in older males (50–70 years),
• Does not metastasize
• Orchiectomy alone is adequate

Lymphoma or *metastases* from carcinomas, e.g. prostate cancer, may be encountered in older males. The remaining testicular tumour types are exceedingly rare and descriptions are given in textbooks of urological pathology.

Further reading

Daugaard G, Petersen PM, Rorth M. Surveillance in stage I testicular cancer. *APMIS* 2003; **111**(1):76–85.

De Santis M, Becherer A, Bokemeyer CS, *et al.* 2-18 fluoro-deoxy-D-glucose positron emission tomography is a reliable predictor for viable tumor in post-chemotherapy seminoma: an update of the prospective multicentric SEMPET Trial. *J Clin Oncol* 2004; **22**(6):1034–9.

Fossa, SD, Chen JB, Schonfeld SJ, *et al.* Risk of contralateral testicular cancer: A population-based study of 29515 US men. *J Nat Cancer Inst* 2005; **97**(4):1056–66.

Martin JM, Panzarella T, Zwahlen DR, *et al.* Evidence-based guidelines for following stage 1 seminoma. *Cancer* 2007; **109**(11):2248–56.

Rustin GJ, Mead GM, Stenning SP, *et al.* Randomized trial of two or five computed tomography scans in the surveillance of patients with stage I nonseminomatous germ cell tumors of the testis: Medical Research Council Trial TE08, ISRCTN56475197—The National Cancer Research Institute Testis Cancer Clinical Studies Group. *J Clin Oncol* 2007; **25**(11):1310–15.

Testicular cancer: fertility issues and survivorship

Fertility issues and sexuality

Conclusions about treatment-related impairment of fertility must take into account reduced fertility before TC diagnosis as implied by the concept of the testicular dysgenesis syndrome (Paduch 2006). In addition, treatment can have considerable impact on the fatherhood rate. Brydoy et al. (2005) demonstrated a decreasing rate of first post-treatment paternity among 554 testicular cancer survivors (TCSs) correlating with treatment intensity (Fig. 4.6.2).

Endocrine hypogonadism increases with treatment intensity as well. Despite these sexual limitations, sexual satisfaction is higher among young long-term survivors after TC than in age-matched males of the general population (Dahl et al. 2007).

> **Key points**
> - Fertility is probably impaired before development and subsequent treatment of TC.
> - Fatherhood-rate decreases by treatment intensity
> - Most long-term testicular cancer survivors are, despite limitations, sexually satisfied

Preservation of fertility

Fertility preservation is an important aspect which must be discussed with the patient before treatment (Magelssen et al. 2006). Retroperitoneal lymph node dissection (RPLND) may damage sympathetic nerves and thereby lead to retrograde ejaculation. Chemotherapy and infradiaphragmatic radiotherapy (if the testis is not shielded) may impair spermatogenesis transiently or permanently.

Therefore, all TC patients should be routinely offered cryopreservation before treatment initiation. At our institution approximately one out of three patients takes advantage of this opportunity. However, most post-treatment children of TC survivors are fathered by natural means.

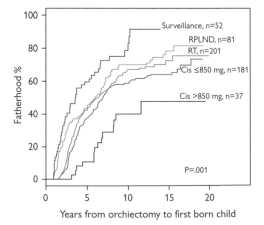

Fig. 4.6.2 Actuarial post-treatment paternity rates in each treatment group for patients who attempted conception without the use of cryopreserved semen from Brydoy et al. (2005) with permission of the publishers. Copyright © (2008), American Medical Association. All Rights reserved. Cis, cisplatin; RT, radiotherapy.

> **Key points**
> - RPLND may lead to retrograde ejaculation
> - Chemo- and radiotherapy may impair spermatogenesis
> - Semen cryopreservation should be offered to all patients

Long-term side effects of treatment

Second cancers

Non-germ-cell cancers might be induced by radiation, chemotherapy, or both. A retrospective analysis of 40,000 TC survivors from 14 national cancer registries showed increased RR for cancer development among TCSs respectively of: 4.0 stomach; 3.6 pancreas; 3.4 mesothelioma; 2.7 bladder; 2.0 colon; 1.7 oesophagus; 1.5 lung. The risk of cancer development 40 years after treatment of 35-year-old patients with seminoma and non-seminoma was 36% and 31% respectively, considerably higher rates than the 23% in the normal population (Travis et al. 2005). The RR for solid tumours attributed to chemotherapy, radiotherapy, and the combination of both was 2.0, 1.8, and 2.9, respectively. An increased risk of second cancers was observed 10 years after treatment and remained after 35 years of treatment. Similar figures were reported by a Dutch research team after 17 years of observation after treatment. The risk of a second malignancy was approximately at least doubled after radio- or chemotherapy as opposed to surgery—a risk increase comparable to that of smoking. Leukaemia may be induced by etoposide, especially after doses >2g and occurs mainly during the first decade after treatment (EGCCCG 2008).

Increased risk of second primary cancers:
- For at least 35 years, probably life-long
- 2-fold with radio- or chemotherapy
- 2-fold with smoking
- 3-fold with the combination of radio- and chemotherapy

Cardiovascular disease (CVD)

CVD related long-term mortality is higher in TCSs than in the general population (Fossa et al. 2007). The relative risk for subsequent myocardial infarction is approximately 1.5–1.9 after chemotherapy compared to surgery only (van den Belt-Dusebout et al. 2006).

Important risk factors for CVD among long-term TCSs:
- Hypertension
- Dyslipidaemia
- Thickening of the blood vessel intima
- BMI increase
- Metabolic syndrome

Compared to healthy controls TCSs who had received chemotherapy had increased levels of fibrinogen, von Willebrand factor, high-sensitivity C-reactive protein, plasminogen activator inhibitor, and tissue-type plasminogen activator (Nuver et al. 2004).

Raynaud-like phenomena

Chemotherapy-related Raynaud-like phenomena had already been reported before the introduction of cisplatin and are usually ascribed to the use of bleomycin. Vinblastine may aggravate bleomycin-induced angiopathy. Bolus infusion of bleomycin as opposed to continuous infusion is associated with a higher incidence of Raynaud's phenomenon. Cisplatin and radiotherapy may also contribute to cold-induced vasospasm. Chemotherapy-related Raynaud's phenomenon may be associated with erectile dysfunction.

Neuro- and ototoxicity

Multiple sites and functions of the nervous system may be compromised by cancer and its treatment.

Paresthesiae are a common symptom of neurotoxic cancer drugs including:
• Vinca-alkaloids
• Cisplatin
• Taxanes
and:
• Radiotherapy

Chemotherapy of TC is usually based on cisplatin and includes bleomycin, etoposide, or vinblastine. Cisplatin-induced neurotoxicity is limited to sensory function and does not impair motor function. Although axonal damage has been related to cisplatin, the principal patho-physiological effect is thought to be due to degeneration of the dorsal nerve ganglion where this drug accumulates.

Cisplatin-induced ototoxicity represents a distinct feature of neurotoxicity and is presumably caused by selective damage to the outer hearing cells.

Symptoms:
• Tinnitus
• Hearing impairment, especially of high frequencies, i.e. > 4000 Hz

Not only the cumulative dose of cisplatin, but also the peak serum concentration is important for ototoxicity, since use of cisplatin 50mg/m^2 over 2 days increased the prevalence of tinnitus and hearing impairment compared to 20mg/m^2 over five days (Fossa et al. 2003a).

Nephrotoxicity

Both radiotherapy and cisplatin-based chemotherapy lead to long-term impairment of renal function in 20–30% of TCSs (Fossa et al. 2002). Reduced renal elimination of cisplatin and bleomycin might increase the risk of other toxicities, e.g. bleomycin-related pneumonitis.

Lifestyle interventions and personality traits

The patient himself should be informed about the importance of adopting a healthy lifestyle, particularly with regard to
• Smoking cessation
• Weight control
• Physical activity

Smoking has a comparable impact on the risk of second malignancies and CVD as radio- or chemotherapy (van den Belt-Dusebout et al. 2007).

Psychosocial well-being

Anxiety, but not depression, is more prevalent among TCSs than the general population (Fossa et al. 2003b).

Fatigue is the subjective experience of tiredness and lack of energy. TCSs report a higher level of fatigue than the general population. Long-term survivors of Hodgkin lymphoma are, however, even more fatigued and the reasons for these differences remain unclear (Fossa et al. 2003b).

Further reading

Brydoy M, Fossa SD, Klepp O, et al. Paternity following treatment for testicular cancer. J Natl Cancer Inst 2005; **97**:1580 8.

Dahl AA, Bremnes R, Dahl O, et al. Is the sexual function compromised in long-term testicular cancer survivors? Eur Urol 2007; **52**:1438–47

European Germ Cell Cancer Consensus Group. European Consensus Conference on Diagnosis and Treatment of Germ Cell Cancer: A Report of the Second Meeting of the European Germ Cell Cancer Consensus Group (EGCCCG): Part II. Eur Urol 2008; **53**:497–513.

Fossa SD, Aass N, Winderen M, et al. 2002, Long-term renal function after treatment for malignant germ-cell tumours. Ann Oncol 2002; **13**:222–8

Fossa SD, de Wit R, Roberts JT, et al. Quality of life in good prognosis patients with metastatic germ cell cancer: A prospective study of the European Organization for Research and Treatment of Cancer Genitourinary Group/Medical Research Council Testicular Cancer Study Group (30941/TE20)207. J Clin Oncol 2003a; **21**:1107–18.

Fossa SD, Dahl AA, Loge JH. Fatigue, anxiety, and depression in long-term survivors of testicular cancer. J Clin Oncol 2003b; **217**:1249–54.

Fossa SD, Gilbert E, Dores GM, et al. Noncancer causes of death in survivors of testicular cancer. J Natl Cancer Inst 2007; **99**:533–544.

Magelssen H, Brydoy M, Fossa SD. The effects of cancer and cancer treatments on male reproductive function. Nat Clin Pract Urol 2006; **3**:312–322.

Nuver J, Smit AJ, Sleijfer DT, et al. Micro albuminuria, decreased fibrinolysis, and inflammation as early signs of atherosclerosis in long-term survivors of disseminated testicular cancer. Eur J Cancer 2004; **40**:701–6.

Paduch DA. Testicular cancer and male infertility. Curr Opin Urol 2006; **16**:419–27.

Travis LB, Fossa SD, Schonfeld SJ, et al. Second cancers among 40,576 testicular cancer patients: focus on long-term survivors. J Natl Cancer Inst 2005; **97**:1354–65.

van den Belt-Dusebout A, Nuver J, de Wit, R, et al.Long-term risk of cardiovascular disease in 5-year survivors of testicular cancer. J Clin Oncol 2006; **24**:467–75.

van den Belt-Dusebout A., de Wit R, Gietema JA, et al. Treatment-specific risks of second malignancies and cardiovascular disease in 5-year survivors of testicular cancer. J Clin Oncol 2007; **25**:4370–8.

Internet resources

American Cancer Society: http://www.cancer.org

Cancer Help UK: http://www.cancerhelp.org.uk/help/default.asp?page=2665

National Cancer Institute: http://www.cancer.gov/cancertopics/types/testicular/

Penile cancer: introduction

Epidemiology

- Penile cancers account for <1% of all cancers in men, with an annual incidence of 1.5/100,000 in Western Europe. Incidence is greater in Africa, Asia, and South America, particularly in areas of low socioeconomic status.
- Peak age of occurrence is 60–80 years. Penile cancer is extremely rare in men <40 years.
- Incidence of penile cancer is generally falling, perhaps due to improved socioeconomic conditions.

Aetiology

- Risk factors for penile cancer include HPV infection (types 16 and 18), smoking, and previous carcinoma in situ (CIS)
- Circumcision is protective, although adequate hygiene with prepuce retraction confers similar benefit.
- Some reports suggest high rates of cervical cancer in female partners of men with penile cancer, lending support to the link with HPV infection.

Pathology

- Premalignant conditions include condylomata acuminate, leukoplakia (chronic irritation), and balanitis xerotica obliterans.
- Epithelial lesions with cytological changes of malignancy confined to the epithelium with no evidence of local invasion or metastases are known as CIS. Three distinct lesions have been described, but these may be variants of the same condition:

Bowen disease (CIS): solitary, grey plaque with shallow ulceration on the skin of shaft/scrotum. Approximately 10% progress to invasion.

Erythroplasia of Queryat: single/multiple shiny red plaques on glans/prepuce, with a velvety appearance. As many as a third progress to invasion.

Bowenoid papulosis: multiple pigmented plaques (very similar in appearance to Bowen disease) but tends to be in a younger age group and associated with HPV 16. Rarely becomes malignant.

- Invasive carcinoma: the majority (>90%) are SCCs. They range from well-differentiated exophytic papillomas to poorly differentiated ulcerative lesions.
- Verrucous carcinoma is an indolent variant which can present with bulky cauliflower-like lesions, accounting for approximately 5% of penile cancers. It is well differentiated and does not spread to lymph nodes.
- Other rare malignancies of the penis include melanoma, sarcomas (particularly Kaposi's sarcoma), BCCs, and metastases from bladder, prostate, or bowel primary tumours.

Clinical features

- Penile cancers present as erythematous patches, exophytic growths, nodules, or ulcers. There may be associated discharge from the prepuce.
- The differential diagnosis includes sexually transmitted diseases, CIS, balanitis or condylomata.
- In patients with phimosis, the presentation may be with distal swelling of the penis. A dorsal slit or circumcision may be required for adequate examination and assessment.

Diagnosis

- Diagnosis is made by clinical appearance, biopsy of the lesion, and histological assessment. Investigations should include a full blood count, urea and electrolytes, and liver function tests.
- The inguinal, pelvic, and abdominal lymph nodes should be imaged with a CT or MRI scan. Clinically enlarged inguinal nodes can be assessed with FNA or biopsy. An MRI scan of the pelvis with an artificial erection may be useful in assessing cavernosal invasion.
- Ultrasonography may be useful in measuring the thickness of the lesion, and also in assessing groin lymph nodes.
- A CXR is usually considered sufficient for distant staging unless there is suspicion of disease elsewhere.
- It is sensible to photograph the lesion before treatment for future reference.

Staging (Table 4.6.14)

Table 4.6.14 Staging of penile cancer

Stage		
I	T1N0	Invasion of sub-epithelial tissue
II	T2N0	Invasion of corpora cavernosa
	T1/2N1	Single superficial inguinal lymph node involvement
III	T3N0/1	Invasion of urethra/prostate
	T1–3N2	Multiple or bilateral superficial inguinal nodes
IV	T4N0–2	Invasion of adjacent structures
	T1–4N3	Deep inguinal or pelvic nodes involved
	M1	Distant metastases

Penile cancer: management

Management of non-invasive disease
- CIS can be treated with topical 5-FU, local excision, laser surgery, electro-dissection, or superficial radiotherapy.
- Topical 5-FU is applied twice a day. Patients should be warned to avoid contact with their hands and to abstain from sexual intercourse during the treatment.

Management of invasive disease
Principles of management
- The management of invasive disease is primarily surgical. The traditional approach of amputation has been superseded by more conservative techniques when possible.
- The aim of treatment is for complete removal of the tumour with adequate margins and control of regional lymph nodes whilst leaving behind a functional penis.
- Radiotherapy is an alternative and potentially organ-sparing technique.

Role of surgery
For very small foreskin lesions, circumcision and laser surgery can be curative.

For other T1/2 lesions of the glans, a glansectomy or partial amputation may suffice. Tumours are usually excised to 1.5–2cm of normal tissue proximal to the invasive margin. Recent reports suggest margins of 1cm are sufficient.

For larger tumours, particularly if the urethra is involved, total amputation is required. A perineal urethrostomy is formed. In cases where there is involvement of the scrotum or perineum, total emasculation is required, sometimes also involving a cystoprostatectomy and urinary diversion.

Radiotherapy
Both EBRT and brachytherapy techniques are employed. There are no randomized trials comparing outcomes of surgery and radiotherapy, but amputation with good margins has the best long-term outcome with 5-year survival approaching 90%. However, radiotherapy has a 30% long-term failure rate. For this reason, primary radiotherapy tends to be reserved for patients unfit for surgery, with locally advanced disease and fixed inguinal lymphadenopathy or those who refuse total amputation. Circumcision should be performed in all patients, even if treated with radiotherapy.

If disease is limited to the glans, electron-beam radiotherapy gives good dose distributions. A lead cut-out is fashioned with a 2cm margin around the tumour and Perspex ® or bolus is placed over the cut-out section to ensure that the skin surface dose is 100%.

For more extensive disease, photon irradiation is appropriate. A common technique is using two lateral opposing fields with the penis held between two halves of a wax block. The block acts as an immobilization device and also as bolus to achieve adequate dose at the penis. The testes and groin are shielded with lead. The CTV for radiotherapy should include tumour with a 2cm margin and the entire circumference of the penile skin. The conventional dose is 60–64Gy in 30–32 daily fractions using 4–6MV photons.

Alternatively a CT planned volume using two lateral oblique beams can be employed.

If there is residual disease following radiotherapy, surgical excision should be considered as a salvage treatment.

Side effects of radiotherapy to the penis
Early
- Mucositis
- Oedema of the prepuce
- Local infections
- Dysuria
- Difficulty with micturition

Late
- Telangiectasia/superficial necrosis
- Stenosis of the urethral meatus
- Deep fibrosis
- Loss of sexual function

Brachytherapy
As with EBRT, the local recurrence rates with brachytherapy are greater than with surgery, although there is the option of salvage surgery at recurrence. Patients are circumcised and catheterized before treatment. Brachytherapy is generally only suitable for T1/2N0 tumours of <4cm in size.

Two techniques are in use:
- The mould technique employs two Perspex ® cylinders, the outer of which is loaded with iridium-192 wires. The device is worn for 8–10 hours per day for 1 week, giving a typical dose of 60Gy. Although reproducibility is poor with this technique, it is useful for superficial lesions and a relatively low dose to the urethra results in a low incidence of urethral stenosis. High-dose rate brachytherapy can also be delivered with this method.
- The interstitial technique involves insertion of radioactive implants under general anaesthetic. The implants are inserted at right angles to the penis, which is supported by foam blocks. One or two planes (at 20–30mm separation) with 2–3 sources each (at 12–15mm separation) are usually required. The target volume for treatment is the tumour with a 1–2cm margin and this is treated with 65Gy to the 85% isodose over 1 week using the Paris system. A 2mm lead shield is applied to the testes. Use of stilboestrol should be considered to prevent erections during the week of treatment. Local control rates of up to 90% have been reported for T1 tumours.

Management of lymph nodes
- 50% of patients with clinically enlarged nodes are found to have only reactive changes with no evidence of tumour involvement.
- Although inguinal lymphadenectomy should be considered for patients with enlarged nodes, the probability of lymph node involvement is very dependent on T stage and grade.
- FNA and cross-sectional imaging may be of help in identifying truly positive nodes and some investigators recommend sentinel lymph node biopsy (SLNB) with the aim of avoiding the complications of lymphadenectomy. However a negative SLNB does not preclude future development of lymph node metastases and patients at

moderate or high-risk may still benefit from prophylactic nodal treatment.

- There is controversy over the need for bilateral dissection, but prophylactic contralateral dissection is appropriate if the one side is heavily involved (some clinicians suggest contralateral dissection if more than two nodes are involved).
- There is also a role for prophylactic lymph node dissection in patients without clinically palpable nodes. In prophylactic lymph node dissection studies, 20–30% of patients with clinically uninvolved nodes are found to have histological involvement.
- Patients with grade 3 or T2 or greater tumours have a particularly high risk of occult lymph node involvement (>80% in some series) so prophylactic lymph node dissection should be considered in the absence of clinically involved nodes. Other predictors of lymph node involvement include lymphovascular invasion, corporal involvement, and DNA ploidy.
- Delayed lymph node dissection is not as effective as early prophylactic treatment.
- Although superficial lymphadenectomy is associated with a low morbidity rate, block dissection of the deep inguinal nodes has high morbidity (up to 80% will experience problems including lymphoedema, wound infection, necrosis, seroma and vessel damage) so should be avoided in well-differentiated stage 1 tumours.
- The value of pelvic node dissection is unproven.
- In patients with large or fixed nodal disease, preoperative inguinal radiotherapy (45–50Gy in 2Gy daily fractions) or chemotherapy can be considered to downsize the nodes prior to dissection.
- Radiotherapy is also an option as prophylaxis in clinically node negative patients in place of surgery. There is a risk of femoral neck fracture after radiotherapy.
- Neither surgery nor radiotherapy is curative when there is gross involvement of the pelvic lymph nodes, and

treatment becomes palliative. In these cases it may be best to avoid the morbidity of dissecting the groin nodes, but palliative radiotherapy to prevent ulceration and leg oedema might be appropriate.

Chemotherapy

SCC of the penis is relatively responsive to chemotherapy, although responses tend to be short-lived. Small studies/case series suggest that adjuvant chemotherapy can improve the long-term survival of patients with radically resected positive nodes. There may also be a role for primary neoadjuvant chemotherapy in patients with fixed inguinal metastases. There are reports that up to 50% of these can be made resectable.

Possible chemotherapy regimens include cisplatin and 5-FU or cisplatin, methotrexate, and bleomycin.

There have been reports of combination chemoradiotherapy in early stage penile cancer, for example with bleomycin. Given the success of chemoradiotherapy in head and neck, anal, and cervical SCCs one might expect benefit in penile cancer, but experience is limited and primary surgery remains the treatment of choice.

Prognosis

Overall 5-year survival rates for cancer of the penis are 70%. Nodal status is the major determinant of prognosis. The 5-year DFS rates of patients with N0 and N+ disease are approximately 80% and 30% respectively.

Palliative treatment

For unfit patients or those with locally advanced disease, palliative treatment with EBRT is an option. A typical dose schedule is 21Gy in 3 fractions administered over one week.

Web resource

Emedicine urology—penile cancer: http://www.emedicine.com/med/topic3046.htm

Cancer of the ureter and renal pelvis

Introduction

Urothelial tumours of ureters and renal pelvis account for 5% of all urothelial tumours. The majority of tumours of the upper urinary tract are transitional cell carcinomas (TCC). However, they are rarer than bladder cancers, with approximately 3000 new diagnoses per year in the USA. Histologically 90% are TCC and 10% are SCCs.

Clinical features and investigations

Gross haematuria is the first symptom in >75% of patients. It can be followed or accompanied by colic and flank pain if the tumour itself or blood clots cause obstruction of the ureter. Sometimes patients describe passing blood clots, a symptom which is rare in lower tract bleeding. Urine cytology is not very sensitive for low-grade tumours. However, sensitivity increases for high-grade tumours up to 70%.

Normally, staging is performed using helical CT scans with iodinated contrast medium. MRI may be performed in patients who are sensitive to contrast. If renal function is poor or compromised, retrograde pyelography is the imaging method of choice. Complete staging in patients with aggressive (> grade I) or advanced (> stage I) disease should include chest CT, and imaging of the abdomen and pelvis for possible hepatic or retroperitoneal lymph node metastases. Isotope renal scanning estimates of kidney function should be proposed to calculate residual function when standard treatment is radical nephrectomy and ureterectomy.

Treatment

Surgery

Standard treatment for patients with TCC of the ureter and renal pelvis of all grades and stages is radical nephro-ureterectomy, involving complete resection of the kidney, perirenal fat, Gerota's fascia, en bloc resection of the ureter to the urinary bladder. When the vena cava or renal veins are involved, thrombus extraction and/or partial vena cava dissection may be mandatory. Traditionally, open surgery has been performed, but a laparoscopic approach is now routinely used. Special attention should be paid because invasive TCC has the capacity to seed, implant, and proliferate if spilled in the abdomen. In patients at high risk of severe renal insufficiency following surgery, physicians should consider other surgical therapies. Percutaneous endoscopic surgery of renal pelvic and calyceal TCC has been developed as a treatment option in selected patients with poor renal function and with medical conditions not permitting open surgery. However, due to the technical complexity and high risk of tumour seeding and the difficulty of resection, vigilant follow up is required. Recurrence is very common.

Adjuvant combined modality therapy

The proper treatment for invasive TCC of the upper urinary tract is nephro-ureterectomy, although 5-year survival is only 0–30%. Metastatic disease seems more frequent than local relapse and extrapolation from experience in advanced bladder cancer suggests that cisplatin-based chemotherapy may be useful. EBRT has been used as adjuvant therapy with unclear results. Local control may be better, but studies are limited in predicting survival due to the small patient numbers in phase II trials. Because of this and the relatively low frequency of disease, data to guide physicians managing local relapse after nephro-ureterectomy are scanty. If local relapse is bulky and metastases present elsewhere, palliative chemotherapy is the treatment of choice. On the other hand, when relapse appears isolated and the patient is fit, other approaches than systemic chemotherapy may occasionally be considered. The recurrence may be reduced in size with a pre-operative radiotherapy dose of 30–45Gy given with sensitizing chemotherapy. An attempt at debulking and possible intraoperative radiation therapy (IORT) directly onto the tumour bed or unresectable mass may be considered.

Chemotherapy

The biology of upper urinary tract TCC is considered identical to bladder TCC. Chemotherapy regimens are, therefore, the same as those recommended for advanced or metastatic bladder cancer. Standard treatment is cisplatin-based combination therapy using gemcitabine and cisplatin or methotrexate, vinblastine, doxorubicin, and cisplatin. Like bladder cancer, upper urinary tract TCC is highly responsive to chemotherapy, most often however, with a short median duration of response.

Summary

- Tumours of the renal pelvis and the ureter are rare. Accurate diagnosis, surgical recognition, and effective local treatment are difficult.
- Haematuria is the most common symptom.
- Urinary cytology may be somewhat less sensitive than in bladder cancer.
- Spiral CT scan is the most useful imaging tool.
- Surgical treatment with new laparoscopic and robotic techniques has changed the approach to this disease.
- Both chemotherapy and radiation therapy seem to be important in extending survival, yet published data are insufficient to fully support these approaches and carefully planned trials are needed.

Further reading

Raman JD, Scherr DS. Management of patients with upper urinary tract transitional cell carcinoma. *Nat Clin Pract Urol* 2007; **4**(8):432–43.

Sanderson KM, Rouprêt M. Upper urinary tract tumour after radical cystectomy for transitional cell carcinoma of the bladder: an update on the risk factors, surveillance regimens and treatments. *BJU Int* 2007; **100**(1):11–16.

Cervical cancer: epidemiology, screening, and pathology

Epidemiology

Cervical cancer is a serious health problem, with nearly 520,000 women developing the disease each year worldwide of whom 443,000 are women in developing countries (Parkin et al. 2005).

There are many risk factors from epidemiological to analytical implicated in the development of cervical cancer.

Human papilloma virus (HPV) has emerged as the principal sexually transmitted causal agent in the development of cancer of the uterine cervix. Almost all women who develop cervical cancer are infected with an oncogenic HPV type, more frequently with type 16 or 18 and to a lesser extent with other oncogenic types. In addition to HPV, cofactors such as parity, use of oral contraceptives, tobacco smoking, immunosuppression, infection with other sexually transmitted diseases, and poor nutrition have been associated with the development of cervical cancer. Age of first sexual intercourse, lifetime number of sexual partners, history of sexually transmitted infections, and other characteristics of sexual activity are linked to the likelihood of becoming infected with HPV and are considered important for the progression of HPV-infected lesions to cervical cancer (Das et al. 2000; National Cancer Registry Programme 2006). An analysis of the pooled data from 11 case–control studies from nine countries (all but two of which were developing countries) involving 1918 women with cervical cancer found that eight HPV types—16, 18, 31, 35, 45, 52, and 58—account for almost 95% of cervical cancers (Muñoz et al. 2003).

Cervical cancer screening

The main goal of screening is to reduce the incidence and mortality. For cancer of the cervix, screening has been shown to be effective in the early identification of a preneoplastic stage, leading to early treatment and thereby reducing the mortality. Cervical cancer is preventable and it should be a high priority in all National Cancer Control Programmes. There are different methods of screening for cervical cancer. Cervical cytology (Pap smear) screening programmes were found to be successful in reducing cervical cancer incidence and it is recommended by the WHO that women in the age group 35–64 years should undergo regular Pap smear screening (see p.22). Various cost-effective methods have been evaluated for implementation in developing countries.

1. Unaided visual inspection: naked eye visualization of the cervix without acetic acid application by health workers, widely known as 'downstaging'.
2. Visual inspection after application of acetic acid (VIA): naked eye visual inspection of the cervix after application of 3–5% acetic acid.
3. VIA with magnification (VIAM): visual inspection with acetic acid using magnification devices.
4. Visual inspection after application of Lugol's iodine (VILI)
5. HPV DNA testing

All these mentioned primary screening methods have been systematically evaluated in cross-sectional, cluster randomized controlled and cost-effectiveness studies. It was found that screening with VIA was the least expensive option, but it also detected fewer cases of CIN 2/3+ than other methods; its long-term cost-effectiveness will depend on the long-term benefits of early detection. Cytology was more effective at detecting cases than VIA but was also more expensive. Although HPV testing is a positive, highly sensitive and reliable approach, a large range in sensitivity was observed in these studies, possibly due to variations in the quality of specimen collected, reference standards and the type of methods employed for HPV detection. Therefore, strong quality controlled procedures must be employed for accurate HPV diagnosis (Sankaranarayanan et al. 2004, 2005, 2007; Legood et al. 2005).

Current studies indicate that VIA reduces the mortality from cervical cancer by 35%. In the absence of a cytology network, and with a high cost for HPV testing, VIA seems to be a feasible alternative in reducing the incidence and mortality of cervical cancer.

In developing/underdeveloped countries, due to a lack of resources and trained manpower, screening is mainly opportunistic. Patients visiting the hospital are often screened with the Pap smear test and thus evaluation is based on such methods. However, information based on such methods may not be true for the general population. For the general population, VIA seems to be a feasible alternative for triaging, followed by appropriate interventions depending on the level of expertise available at referral centres.

Natural history and pathology

Most cervical carcinomas arise at the squamo-columnar junction of the ectocervix and endocervix. The greatest risk of neoplastic transformation coincides with periods of greatest metaplastic activity. Virally-induced atypical squamous metaplasia developing in this region can progress to higher-grade squamous intraepithelial lesions (SILs). These dysplasias undergo spontaneous regression in 25–38%, persist in 50–60%, and progress to invasive cancers in 2–14%. Once tumour breaks through the basement membrane, it may penetrate the cervical stroma directly or through vascular channels. Invasive tumours may develop as exophytic growths protruding from the cervix into the vagina or as endocervical lesions that can cause massive expansion of the cervix. From the cervix, tumour may extend superiorly to the lower uterine segment, inferiorly to the vagina, or into the paracervical spaces by way of the broad or uterosacral ligaments. Tumour may become fixed to the pelvic wall by direct extension or by coalescence of central tumour with regional adenopathy.

Cervical cancer usually follows a relatively orderly pattern of metastatic progression, initially to primary-echelon nodes in the pelvis and then to para-aortic nodes and distant sites. Even patients with locoregionally advanced disease rarely have detectable haematogenous metastases at initial diagnosis of their cervical cancer. The most frequent sites of distant recurrence are lung, extrapelvic nodes, liver, and bone.

Histopathological types:
- Cervical intraepithelial neoplasia, grade III
- Squamous cell carcinoma *in situ*
- Squamous carcinoma: keratinizing, non-keratinizing & verrucous
- Adenocarcinoma In Situ
- Adenocarcinoma In Situ, endocervical type
- Endometrioid adenocarcinoma
- Clear-cell adenocarcinoma

- Adenosquamous carcinoma
- Adenoid cystic carcinoma
- Small cell carcinoma
- Undifferentiated carcinoma

Squamous and adenocarcinomas account for 90–95% of cervical cancers. Although most of these cancers are treated with radiotherapy according to the stage, early operable (stage Ib/IIa) adenocarcinomas are best treated with radical surgery followed by appropriate adjuvant therapy as indicated. Similarly, cisplatin based systemic therapy forms the mainstay in small cell and undifferentiated cancers.

Further reading

Das BC, Gopalkrishna V, Hedau S, et al. Cancer of the uterine cervix and human papilloma virus infection. *Curr Science* 2000; **78**:52–63.

Legood R, Gray A M, Mahe C, et al. Screening for cervical cancer in India: How much will it cost? A trial based analysis of the cost per case detected. *Int. J. Cancer* 2005; **117**:981–98.

Muñoz N, Bosch FX, de Sanjose S, et al. Epidemiologic classification of human papillomavirus types associated with cervical cancer. *N Engl J Med* 2003; **348**(6):518–27.

National Cancer Registry Programme. *Consolidated report of the Population-based Cancer Registries 2001–2004*. New Delhi: Indian Council of Medical Research, 2006.

Parkin DM, Bray F, Ferlay J, et al. Global Cancer Statistics 2002. *Cancer J Clin* 2005, **55**:74–108.

Sankaranarayanan R, Somanathan T, Sharma A, et al. Accuracy of conventional cytology: Results from a multicentre screening study in India. *J Med Screen* 2004; **11**:77–84.

Sankaranarayanan R, Nene BM, Dinshaw KA, et al. on behalf of the Osmanabad District Cervical Screening Study Group. A Cluster Randomised Controlled trial of Visual, Cytology and Human Papilloma Virus screening for Cancer of Cervix in Rural India. *Int J Cancer* 2005; **116**:617–23.

Sankaranarayanan R, Esmy PO, Rajkumar R, et al. Effect of visual screening on cervical cancer incidence and mortality in Tamil Nadu, India: a cluster-randomized trial. *Lancet* 2007; **370**:398–406.

Cervical cancer: clinical features, investigations, staging, and prognosis

Clinical features

Pre-invasive disease is usually detected during routine cervical cytological screening. Early invasive disease may not be associated with any symptoms and may be an incidental finding during examination for uterine bleeding or detected during screening examinations. The earliest symptom of invasive cervical cancer is usually abnormal vaginal bleeding, often post-coital. This may be associated with a clear or foul-smelling vaginal discharge. Pelvic pain may result from coexistent pelvic inflammatory disease or from loco-regionally invasive disease. Flank pain may be a symptom of hydronephrosis, often complicated by pyelonephritis. The triad of sciatic pain, leg oedema, and hydronephrosis is almost always associated with extensive pelvic wall involvement by tumour. Patients with very advanced tumours may have haematuria or incontinence from a vesicovaginal fistula caused by direct extension of tumour to the bladder. Lower limb DVT, severe back ache, and bone pain in the lumbar region may all be presenting symptoms due to lymph nodal masses in the pelvis or para-aortic regions.

Cachexia, cough, jaundice, and left supraclavicular nodal mass may result from distant metastasis.

Pretreatment evaluation and staging

Pretreatment evaluation

- Complete physical and gynaecological examination (examination under anaesthesia, EUA).
- FBC, biochemistry: to rule out anaemia and renal impairment.
- Biopsy—punch, knife, colposcopy-guided or conization: for histopathological diagnosis.
- CXR: to rule out comorbid conditions and general anaesthesia evaluation.
- Ultrasonography abdomen and pelvis: to assess kidneys (rules out hydronephrosis) and can identify gross nodal disease.
- CT scan abdomen and pelvis.
- MRI pelvis (preferred modality to assess primary tumour)/whole body PET scan (optional).

Table 4.7.1 FIGO staging of carcinoma of cervix (2009)

FIGO stage	Categories	TNM
	Primary tumour cannot be assessed	TX
	No evidence of primary tumour	T0
0	Carcinoma *in situ* (pre-invasive carcinoma)	Tis
I	Cervical carcinoma confined to uterus (extension to corpus should be disregarded)	T1
IA	Invasive carcinoma diagnosed only by microscopy.	T1a
	All macroscopically visible lesions—even with superficial invasion—are stage IB/T1b	
IA1	Stromal invasion not >3.0mm in depth and ≤7.0mm in horizontal spread	T1a1
IA2	Stromal invasion >3.0mm and not >5.0mm[a] with a horizontal spread ≤7.0mm	T1a2
IB	Clinically visible lesion confined to the cervix or microscopic lesion greater than IA2/T1a2	T1b
IB1	Clinically visible lesion ≤4.0cm in greatest size	T1b1
IB2	Clinically visible lesion >4cm in greatest size	T1b2
II	Tumour invades beyond the uterus but not to pelvic wall or to lower third of the vagina	T2
IIA	Without parametrial invasion	T2a
IIB	With parametrial invasion	T2b
III	Tumour extends to pelvic wall and/or involves lower third of vagina and/or causes hydronephrosis or non-functioning kidney	T3
IIIA	Tumour involves lower third of vagina with no extension to pelvic wall	T3a
IIIB	Tumour extends to pelvic wall and/or causes hydronephrosis or non-functioning kidney	T3b
IVA	Tumour invades mucosa of bladder or rectum and/or extends beyond true pelvis[b]	T4
IVB	Distant metastasis	M1

[a] Note: The depth of invasion should not be >5mm taken from the base of the epithelium, either surface or glandular, from which it originates. The depth of invasion is defined as the measurement of the tumour from the epithelial-stromal junction of the adjacent most superficial epithelial papilla to the deepest point of invasion. Vascular space involvement, venous or lymphatic, does not affect classification.

[b] Note: The presence of bullous edema is not sufficient to classify a tumour as T4.

- Cystoscopy/sigmoidoscopy/barium enema/IVU: if clinical suspicion of bladder, rectal or ureteric involvement.

Staging
The FIGO (International Federation of Gynecology and Obstetrics) staging of cervical cancer (2009) is given in Table 4.7.1. Staging is done by EUA jointly by gynaecological, surgical, and radiation oncologists.

Stage grouping
In cases treated by surgical procedures, the pathologist's findings in the removed tissues can be the basis for extremely accurate statements on the extent of disease. The findings should not be allowed to change the clinical staging, but should be recorded in the manner described for the pathological staging of disease. The TNM nomenclature is appropriate for this purpose. (Table 4.7.2)

Table 4.7.2 Carcinoma of the cervix uteri—stage grouping

FIGO	UICC		
Stage	T	N	M
0	Tis	N0	M0
IA1	T1a1	N0	M0
IA2	T1a2	N0	M0
IB1	T1b1	N0	M0
IB2	T1b2	N0	M0
IIA	T2a	N0	M0
IIB	T2b	N0	M0
IIIA	T3a	N0	M0
IIIB	T1	N1	M0
	T2	N1	M0
	T3a	N1	M0
	T3b	Any N	M0
IVA	T4	Any N	M0
IVB	Any T	Any N	M1

Salient features of FIGO staging
- Staging of cervical cancer is based on clinical evaluation. The clinical staging must not be changed because of subsequent findings.
- When there is doubt as to which stage a particular cancer should be allocated, choice of the earlier stage is mandatory.
- Suspected bladder or rectal involvement should be confirmed by biopsy and histological evidence.
- Conization or amputation of the cervix is regarded as a clinical examination. Invasive cancers so identified are to be included in the reports.
- FNA of scan-detected suspicious lymph nodes may be helpful in treatment planning.

Prognosis
FIGO stage is the single most important prognostic factor for survival and pelvic disease control rates in cervical cancer. Clinical tumour diameter is also strongly correlated with prognosis for patients treated with radiation or surgery. For patients with more advanced disease, other estimates of tumour bulk—such as the presence of medial versus lateral parametrial involvement in FIGO stage IIB tumours or the presence of unilateral versus bilateral parametrial or pelvic wall involvement—have also been correlated with outcome. Lymph node metastasis is also an important predictor of prognosis. For patients treated with radical hysterectomy for stage IB disease, survival rates are usually reported as 85–95% for patients with negative nodes and 45–55% for those with lymph node metastases. Also, the number of nodes dissected and positivity rates have a bearing on the outcome after surgery. Survival rates for patients with positive para-aortic nodes treated with extended-field radiotherapy vary from 10–50% depending on the extent of pelvic disease and para-aortic lymph node involvement. For patients treated with radical hysterectomy, other histological parameters that have been associated with a poor prognosis are LVSI (lymphovascular space invasion), deep stromal invasion (10mm or more, or >70% invasion) and parametrial extension. The serum concentration of SCC antigen appears to correlate with the stage and size of squamous carcinomas, the presence of lymph node metastases, and the presence of recurrent disease. However, its role as an independent prognostic factor is not yet established.

Cervical cancer: primary management

A thorough evaluation of the locoregional disease extent and correct staging of the disease is essential before deciding on the appropriate treatment. The factors which influence the choice of local treatment include tumour size, stage, histological features, evidence of lymph node involvement, risk factors for complications of surgery or radiotherapy, and patient choice.

Stage 0 cervical cancer (carcinoma *in situ*)

Extent of the disease is the most important factor in the treatment decision. The other factors that also influence the treatment decision include age of the patient, fertility preservation, and other medical conditions.

Ectocervical lesions:
• Loop electrosurgical excision procedure (LEEP)
• Laser therapy
• Conization
• Cryotherapy

Endocervical canal involved:
• Laser or cold-knife conization: to preserve the uterus and avoid radiation.
• Total abdominal or vaginal hysterectomy for the post-reproductive age group and is particularly indicated when the neoplastic process extends to the inner cone margin.
• For medically inoperable patients, a single intracavitary insertion to a dose of 80Gy vaginal surface dose may be used (Grigsby and Perez 1991).

Stage IA: also labelled as superficially invasive cervical cancers (see Fig. 4.7.1)

Stage IA1: micro-invasive (diagnosed only under microscopy), not >3mm depth and no wider than 7mm. The treatment options are:
• Conization
• Total abdominal hysterectomy
• Brachytherapy

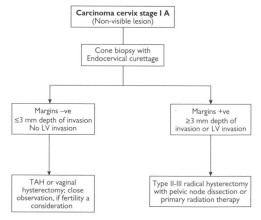

Fig. 4.7.1 Treatment algorithm for Stage IA.
With permission from Tata Memorial Centre, EBM Guidelines, Volume IV 2005.

Conization

In patients with IA1 disease if no vascular or lymphatic channel invasion is noted, and the margins of the cone are negative, conization alone may be appropriate in patients wishing to preserve fertility (Sevin et al. 1992).

Total hysterectomy (abdominal or vaginal)

In patients with IA1 lesion with no vascular or lymphatic involvement, the frequency of lymph node disease is very low and hence lymph node dissection is not required. The ovaries can be preserved in young women (Sevin et al. 1992).

Intracavitary brachytherapy alone

In IA1 lesions if no capillary lymphatic space invasion is noted, the frequency of lymph node involvement is sufficiently low that EBRT is not required. One or two intracavitary insertions may be considered up to a dose of 100–125Gy at the vaginal surface in women who are not fit for surgery (Grigsby and Perez 1991).

Stage IA2: 3.1–5.0mm below the basement membrane (BM) and <7mm in transverse dimension. The treatment options are:
• Radical hysterectomy (type II) with pelvic node dissection
• Radiation therapy

Radical hysterectomy (type II–III) with pelvic node dissection has been recommended (Jones et al. 1993) because of a reported risk of lymph node metastasis of up to 10%. However, a study suggests that the rate of lymph node involvement in this group of patients may be much lower and questions whether conservative therapy might be adequate for patients believed to have no residual disease following conization (Creasman et al. 1998). Radical hysterectomy with node dissection may also be considered for patients where the depth of tumour invasion was uncertain due to invasive tumour at the cone margins.

The options for fertility conservation if it is desired are:
• Large cone biopsy plus extraperitoneal or laparoscopic pelvic lymphadenectomy
• Radical trachelectomy and extraperitoneal or laparoscopic pelvic lymphadenectomy

Radiation therapy: radical intracavitary radiotherapy or intracavitary plus external pelvic irradiation may be considered in women who are not fit for surgery (Grigsby and Perez 1991).

Stage IB and IIA (see Fig. 4.7.2)

Similar cure rates are obtained with either a surgical or radiotherapeutic treatment approach for stage IB squamous carcinoma of the cervix (Landoni et al. 1997). The choice between initial surgical or radiotherapeutic management depends upon the age of the patient, desire to preserve ovarian function, comorbid conditions, and patient choice.

Stage IB1

The treatment options are:
• Radical hysterectomy (type III) with pelvic node dissection
• Radical radiotherapy (see later)

Radical hysterectomy (type III) and bilateral pelvic lymphadenectomy involves removal of the entire uterus, upper third of vagina, bilateral parametria, uterosacral,

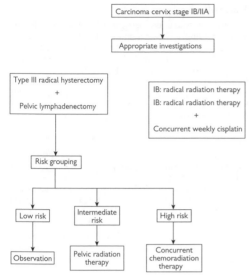

Fig. 4.7.2 Treatment algorithm for FIGO stage IB/IIA cervical cancer. With permission from Tata Memorial Centre, EBM Guidelines, Volume IV 2005.

uterovesical ligaments, and bilateral pelvic lymph nodes. Bilateral salpino-oophrectomy is discretionary.

Radiotherapy: external-beam pelvic irradiation combined with intracavitary applications, which together deliver the dose of equivalent to 80Gy to point A. Point A is a point 2cm from central line and 2cm above ovoids.

Stage IB2 and IIA (see Fig. 4.7.3)
The treatment options include:
• Radical hysterectomy (type III) and bilateral pelvic lymphadenectomy ± adjuvant therapy as indicated
• Radical radiation therapy (external plus intracavitary).
• Concomitant chemoradiation (radiation therapy + weekly cisplatin)

Adjuvant therapy after radical surgery
High risk: lymph node metastases, +ve surgical margins, parametrial extension (any one).

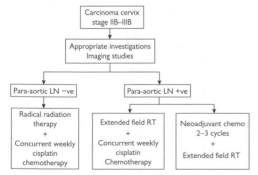

Fig. 4.7.3 Treatment algorithm for FIGO stage IIB–IIIB cervical cancer.
With permission from Tata Memorial Centre, EBM Guidelines, Volume IV 2005.

Adjuvant chemoradiation with external pelvic radiation therapy and concurrent weekly cisplatin chemotherapy is recommended if any one of the listed factors is seen on final histopathology. The risk of recurrence after radical surgery is increased with the presence of positive nodes, positive parametria, or positive surgical margins. Adjuvant concurrent chemoradiation (using 5FU + cisplatin or cisplatin alone) improves survival compared with pelvic irradiation alone in such patients (Peterset al. 2000).

For patients who inadvertently have a hysterectomy for invasive cervical cancer, completion surgery is advocated. However immediate second surgery is not practical so these patients should be considered as high risk and treated with adjuvant chemoradiation, although radical radiotherapy alone may be acceptable if combined chemoradiation is not possible.

Intermediate risk: deep invasion of cervical stroma, lymphovascular space invasion, tumour size >4cm (any two factors)

Adjuvant radiotherapy is recommended if at least two of the listed factors are seen on final histopathology. The risk of recurrence is also increased in patients with uninvolved nodes but with large tumour volume, capillary–like space (CLS) involvement, and outer one-third invasion of the cervical stroma. Adjuvant whole pelvic irradiation reduces the local failure rate and improves PFS compared with patients treated with surgery alone (Sedliset al. 1999).

Low risk: all other patients with none of the previously mentioned risk factors (high and intermediate).

No adjuvant therapy recommended.

Radical radiotherapy
A combination of external-beam pelvic irradiation, covering the uterus, parametria, and pelvic nodes, and intracavitary irradiation, primarily for the central disease, is used. The aim is to deliver a dose equivalent of 80Gy to point A. The planned radical radiation/concomitant chemoradiation should be completed within 8 weeks without significant treatment breaks. Prolonged overall treatment time is associated with poor outcome (Perezet al. 1995).

Cervical cancer is commonest and presents with advanced disease in places where radiotherapy technological solutions are not so readily available and conventional radiotherapy planning methods are still therefore the most useful. However where three-dimensional imaging and treatment planning are available, the outcome may be improved for patients because of a reduction in treatment associated side effects.

Conventional radiotherapy technique
1. External radiation
Using conventional fractionation, a dose of 40–50Gy in 20–25 fractions over a period of 4–5 weeks is recommended. Use of a two- or four-beam arrangement, corner shields, and a special midline block (after 20Gy), helps in reducing the dose to rectum, bladder and small bowel during external radiation.
Radiation portals: two-/four-beam technique
   AP–PA fields:
• Superior border: L5–S1 interspace
• Inferior border: below obturator foramina (or lower for vaginal involvement)
• Lateral border: 1.5cm lateral to pelvic brim

Lateral fields:
• Superior/inferior borders: same as AP–PA portals
• Anterior border: anterior to pubis symphysis
• Posterior border: S2–S3 level

2. Intracavitary brachytherapy

Brachytherapy plays a very important role in obtaining high cure rates with minimum complications. A good intracavitary insertion delivers a very high radiation dose to the cervix, upper vagina, and medial parametria without exceeding the tolerance doses for rectum and bladder. The randomized trials comparing low dose rate (LDR) with high dose rate (HDR) brachytherapy in carcinoma of the cervix have shown that the two modalities are comparable in terms of local control and survival (Patel et al. 1994; el-Baradie et al. 1997; Orton et al. 2001; Hareyama et al. 2002).Thus, either LDR or HDR brachytherapy may be used, taking into account the availability of equipment and other logistics of treatment delivery. HDR brachytherapy can be done as a day procedure in contrast to approximately 20 hours of continuous LDR treatment requiring an overnight inpatient stay. When intracavitary treatment alone is used for radical radiotherapy (for stage I and II), due to radiobiological considerations, 5 applications of HDR (each giving 7Gy to point A) are required in contrast to 2 applications of LDR (each giving 30Gy to point A) to maintain low complication rates. HDR is being increasingly used as the control rates are comparable to LDR and the toxicity is slightly less.

When intracavitary radiotherapy is used after EBRT, a single application of LDR (27–30Gy to point A) after completion of EBRT or 2–3 weekly applications of HDR (7–9Gy to point A) starting from the second week of EBRT are used.

Three-dimensional radiotherapy technique

1. External beam radiotherapy

Three-dimensional and intensity modulated radiotherapy (IMRT) are increasingly being used in cervical cancer. These techniques allow for further sparing of normal tissues and IMRT can also be used to differentially escalate the dose of radiotherapy to high-risk disease (Taylor and Powell 2008). The target volumes are defined on planning CT scan as follows:

• Gross tumour volume (GTV)—is defined by EUA and imaging. MRI is superior to CT scan in defining GTV. Stromal and parametrial invasions are best demonstrated on T2-weighted MRI scan.
• Clinical target volume (CTV)—consists of the uterine body, upper vagina, parametria, and proximal uterosacral ligament in all patients. Further inclusion of vagina and pelvic ligaments in the CTV is based on the findings from the EUA. CTV also includes all the nodal regions at risk of metastasis which are parametrial, external iliac, internal iliac, obturator, and distal common iliac nodes. Inguinal nodes are included in the CTV if disease extends to the lower vagina, and presacral nodes are included if there is posterior tumour extension. Since it is difficult to identify lymph nodes on the planning CT scan, the lymph nodes are defined using major pelvic blood vessels as a surrogate target. In practice, in node-negative patients, the nodal CTV is marked as a 7–10mm margin around contrast enhancing-blood vessels. In cases of radiologically visible nodal disease, a margin of 10–15mm is added to the nodal disease
• Planning target volume (PTV)—is delineated by adding a margin of 15mm around the uterus and cervix and 7–10mm around the nodal CTV. The PTV should be covered by 95% of the prescribed dose.

2. Brachytherapy

Recently it has been recognized that brachytherapy planning using three-dimensional imaging yields better dose optimization. Based on three-dimensional planning, using CT scan and/or MRI compatible applicators, the Gynaecological GEC/ESTRO working group has put forward some recommendations for volume definition and dose–volume parameters (Haie-Meder et al. 2005; Potter et al. 2006). Cumulative dose–volume histograms (DVH) are essential for the evaluation of complex dose distribution.

Definitions of volumes of cervical cancer brachytherapy

The target volumes are delineated after the insertion of applicators and using CT and/MRI the following treatment volumes are defined:

• High-risk CTV (HR-CTV): indicates the residual macroscopic disease with highest risk of local recurrence. The intent is to deliver the highest possible dose of radiotherapy to eradicate all residual macroscopic disease.
• Intermediate-risk CTV (IR-CTV: indicates an area with previous macroscopic disease but with at most residual microscopic disease at the time of brachytherapy. The aim is to deliver at least 60Gy to this volume.
• Low-risk CTV (LR-CTV): denotes area with potential microscopic disease.

The organs at risk contoured should include bladder, rectum, and sigmoid.

Dose prescription

The prescription dose is planned to cover the target as completely as possible. The doses at point A (right, left and mean), D100 for GTV and D90 for HR-CTV and IR CTV should be calculated. Doses to organs at risk should be reported in terms of $D_{0.1cc}$, D_{1cc} and D_{2cc}. For details of 3D brachytherapy for cervical cancer please refer to Gynaecological GEC-ESTRO recommendations (Haie-Meder et al. 2005; Potter et al. 2006).

Concurrent chemoradiation with cisplatin chemotherapy

Five randomized phase III trials of radical RT alone versus concurrent cisplatin-based chemotherapy and RT, and their meta-analysis have shown an absolute benefit in OS and PFS with chemoradiotherapy in patients with stage IB2 to IVA disease as well as in high-risk patients after hysterectomy (Keys et al. 1999; Morris et al. 1999; Thomas 1999; Whitney et al. 1999; Green et al. 2001, 2005; Lukka et al. 2002; Rose et al. 2007). While these trials are somewhat heterogeneous in data, stage of disease, suboptimal doses of radiation, non-uniform usage for chemotherapeutic drugs, and different schedules and doses of cisplatin, a significant survival benefit for this combined approach is still shown. The risk of death from cervical cancer was decreased by 30–50% by concurrent chemoradiation. Based on these results, the NCI has recommended that 'strong consideration should be given to the incorporation of concurrent cisplatin-based chemotherapy with radiation therapy in women who require radiation therapy for treatment of cervical cancer especially in early stage disease'. However, the most recent trial (Pearcey et al. 2002) did not find any additional survival benefit of concurrent weekly cisplatin. The major criticism of this study was that nearly two-thirds of the patients with CT + RT had a low haemoglobin, which was not corrected during radiotherapy.

Concurrent chemoradiation as the new standard of care is reinforced by the results of a population-based study from Ontario which showed that there was a significant improvement in OS at the population level concordant with the widespread adoption of CT-RT (Pearcey et al. 2002). The last meta-analysis of concurrent chemoradiation data is from the Cochrane Database Systematic Review. Collated data from 24 trials and 2491 patients strongly suggested the benefit of adding chemotherapy for both DFS and OS with absolute benefits of 10% and 13% respectively. Due to statistical heterogeneity there was some suggestion that the benefit is greater in stages 1 and 2 (Green et al. 2005).

While chemoradiotherapy is perhaps the new standard of care, it is worth remembering that these results were obtained in a trial setting, in women from affluent countries who had better nutrition, PS, and renal parameters compared with the majority of patients from a lower socioeconomic status and with more advanced disease. Therefore in women with medical or social reasons which may preclude combined modality treatment, radical radiotherapy alone without compromising the doses and duration can still be considered as the gold standard treatment approach.

Stages IIB, IIIA, and IIIB

Radiotherapy remains the mainstay of treatment for advanced stages. Platinum-based concomitant chemoradiation improves survival and the pros and cons of this approach have been discussed earlier. Both the Cochrane and Canadian meta-analysis have to a large extent tried to address the role of concomitant chemoradiation, but in all these trials, Stage III carcinoma of the cervix accounted for only 30–35% of cases and evaluation with optimal radiation schedules and comparison of late toxicities still remains incomplete.

The planned radical radiation/concomitant chemoradiation should be completed within 8 weeks without significant treatment breaks. Prolonged overall treatment time results in poor outcomes (Perez et al. 1995).

Radiation therapy doses

Stage IIB: the radical radiation therapy, including external radiation technique, portals and doses, and intracavitary radiation delivered, is similar to that described earlier for stage IB/IIA.

Stage IIIA: the dose of EBRT is 50Gy to the whole pelvis over 5 weeks with 2Gy fractionation. Whenever possible, a midline block should be used after 40Gy. The radiation portals are similar except that the inferior border is placed 2cm beyond the lower vaginal disease or at the introitus. An LDR intracavitary application with tandem and ovoids to a dose of 30Gy to point A is recommended. Patients, in whom standard ICA is not feasible due to residual disease extending below the upper third of the vagina, an intracavitary application using a tandem and cylinders to a dose of 15–25Gy to point A (depending on rectal dose) is recommended.

Stage IIIB: the dose of EBRT is 50Gy to the whole pelvis over 5 weeks with 2Gy fractionation. Whenever possible, a midline block should be used after 40Gy. Intracavitary application with low dose rate (one application of 30Gy to point A) or high dose rate (three applications of 7Gy to point A each every week, starting from the third or fourth week of external radiation) is recommended.

Stage IVA

The management of patients with stage IVA disease (invasion of bladder and or rectum) has to be individualized, taking into account the extent of bladder/rectal involvement, parametrial infiltration, renal function, and the patient's PS. The treatment options include:
- Neoadjuvant chemotherapy or concurrent chemoradiotherapy
- Palliative radiotherapy/chemotherapy
- Pelvic exenteration
- BSC/palliative care

Neoadjuvant chemotherapy or concurrent chemoradiotherapy: selected patients with good general and renal status and not suitable for surgical exenteration can be treated with this approach with radical intent.

Palliative radiotherapy/chemotherapy: the majority of stage IVA patients who have a poor PS and extensive local disease are best treated with palliative radiotherapy/chemotherapy. The major symptoms which can be palliated are vaginal bleeding, profuse discharge, and low back pain due to local disease. A short palliative regime of 30Gy in 10 fractions over 2 weeks or 30Gy/3#/60 days (10Gy/every month x 3#) is generally used and in a few patients who respond very well, this is followed by an intracavitary application. Palliative chemotherapy is discussed below.

Surgical exenteration: selected patients with stage IV disease who have no or minimal parametrial invasion may be treated with primary exenterative surgery, the extent of which (anterior, posterior or total) depends on the extent of the lesion.

BSC/palliative care: patients with poor general condition, and/or extensive local disease such as fistulae may be offered best supportive care alone.

Stage IVB

No standard chemotherapy regimen is proven in patients with stage IVB cervical cancer. Various single-agent chemotherapy drugs have been used with varying response rates in phase I and II studies (cisplatin + ifosfamide or cisplatin + paclitaxel). Radiotherapy can be used for palliation of central disease or symptomatic distant metastasis. The role of systemic therapy is discussed later under recurrent cervical cancer.

Para-aortic nodes: extended field radiotherapy has been reported to produce long-term disease control in women with microscopic or small volume (<2cm) lower para-aortic nodes (below L3) with acceptable complication rates when the radiation dose did not exceed 50Gy and the lymphadenectomy was performed by an extraperitoneal rather than the transperitoneal route (Vigliotti et al. 1992; Varia et al. 1998). In the RTOG randomized trial (Rotman et al. 1995), the 10-year OS was improved from 44% with pelvic radiation to 55% with pelvic plus prophylactic para-aortic radiation in 367 women with stage IB1 and IIA disease. Grade 4 and 5 radiation toxicities at 10 years, however, increased from 4% to 8% with para-aortic irradiation. Patients with positive common iliac or para aortic nodes may be treated by extended field radiation with or without chemotherapy.

Further reading

Creasman WT, Zaino RJ, Major FJ et al. Early invasive carcinoma of the cervix (3 to 5mm invasion): risk factors and prognosis. A Gynecologic Oncology Group Study. *Am J Obstet Gynecol* 1998; **178**:62–5.

el-Baradie M, Inoue T, Murayama S, et al. HDR and MDR intracavitary treatment for carcinoma of the uterine cervix. A prospective randomized study. Strahlenther *Onkol* 1997; **173**:155–62.

Green JA, Kirwan JM, Tierney JF, et al. Survival and recurrence after concomitant chemotherapy and radiotherapy for cancer of the uterine cervix: a systematic review and meta-analysis. Lancet 2001; 358:781–6.

Green J, Kirwan J, Tierney J, et al. Concomitant chemotherapy and radiation therapy for cancer of the uterine cervix. Cochrane Database Syst Rev 2005; 3:CD002225.

Grigsby PW, Perez CA. Radiotherapy alone for medically inoperable carcinoma of the cervix: stage IA and carcinoma in situ. Int J Radiat Oncol Biol Phys 1991; 21:375–8.

Haie-Meder C, Van Limbergen E, Barillot I, et al. Recommendations from Gynaecological (GYN) GEC-ESTRO Working Group (I): concepts and terms in 3D image based 3D treatment planning in cervix cancer brachytherapy with emphasis on MRI assessment of GTV and CTV. Radiother Oncol 2005; 74:235–45.

Hareyama M, Sakata K, Oouchi A, et al. High-dose-rate versus low-dose-rate intracavitary therapy for carcinoma of the uterine cervix: A Randomized Trial. Cancer 2002; 94:117–24.

Jones WB, Mercer GO, Lewis JL, et al Early invasive carcinoma of the cervix. Gynecol Oncol 1993; 51:26-32.

Keys HM, Bundy BN, Stehman FB, et al. Cisplatin, radiation, and adjuvant hysterectomy compared with radiation and adjuvant hysterectomy for bulky stage IB cervical carcinoma. N Engl J Med 1999; 340:1154–61.

Landoni F, Maneo A, Colombo A, et al. Randomized study of radical surgery versus radiotherapy for stage Ib-IIa cervical cancer. Lancet 1997; 350:535–40.

Lukka H, Hirte H, Fyles A, et al. Concurrent cisplatin-based chemotherapy plus radiotherapy for cervical cancer–a meta-analysis. Clin Oncol 2002; 14(3):203–12.

Morris M, Eifel PJ, Lu J, et al. Pelvic radiation with concurrent chemotherapy compared with pelvic and para-aortic radiation for high-risk cervical cancer. N Engl J Med 1999; 340:1137–43.

Orton.CG. High-dose-rate brachytherapy may be radiobiologically superior to low-dose rate due to slow repair of late-responding normal tissue cells. Int J Radiat Oncol Biol Phys 2001; 49(1):183–9.

Patel FD, Sharma SC, Negi PS, et al. Low dose rate vs. high dose rate brachytherapy in the treatment of carcinoma of the uterine cervix: a clinical trial. Int J Radial Oncol Biol Phys 1994; 28:335–9.

Pearcey R, Brundage M, Drouin P, et al. Phase III trial comparing radical radiotherapy with and without cisplatin chemotherapy in patients with advanced squamous cell cancer of the cervix. J Clin Oncol 2002; 20:966–72.

Pearcey R, Miao Q, Kong W, et al. Impact of adoption of chemora-diotherapy on the outcome of cervical cancer in Ontario: results of a population-based cohort study. J Clin Oncol. 2007; 25(17):2383–8.

Perez Ca, Grigsby PW, Castro-Vita H, et al. Carcinoma of uterine cervix: I. Impact of prolongation of treatment time and timing of brachytherapy on outcome of radiation therapy. Int J Radiat Oncol Biol Phys 1995; 32:1275–88.

Peters WA, Liu PY, Barrett RJ, et al. Concurrent chemotherapy and pelvic radiation therapy compared with pelvic radiation therapy alone as adjuvant therapy after radical surgery in high-risk early-stage cancer of the cervix. Clin Oncol 2000; 18(8):1606–13.

Potter R, Haie-Meder C, Van Limbergen E, et al. Recommendations from Gynaecological (GYN) GEC-ESTRO Working Group (II): concepts and terms in 3D image based 3D treatment planning in cervix cancer brachytherapy – 3D volume parameters and aspects of 3D image-based anatomy, radiation physics, radiobiology. Radiother Oncol 2006; 78:67–77.

Rose PG, Ali S, Watkins E, et al. Long-term follow-up of a rand-omized trial comparing concurrent single agent cisplatin, cispla-tin-based combination chemotherapy, or hydroxyurea during pelvic irradiation for locally advanced cervical cancer: a Gynecologic Oncology Group Study. Gynecologic Oncology Group. J Clin Oncol 2007; 25(19):2804–10.

Rotman M, Pajak TK, Choi K, et al. Prophylactic extended-field irra-diation of para-aortic lymph nodes in stages IIB and bulky IB and IIA cervical carcinomas. Ten-year treatment results of RTOG 79–20. JAMA 1995; 274:387–93.

Sedlis A, Bundy BN, Rotman MZ, et al. A randomized trial of pelvic radiation therapy versus no further therapy in selected patients with stage IB carcinoma of the cervix after radical hysterectomy and pelvic lymphadenectomy: A Gynecologic Oncology Group Study. Gynecol Oncol. 1999; 73(2):177–83.

Sevin BU, Nadji M, Averette HE, et al. Microinvasive carcinoma of the cervix. . Cancer 1992; 70:2121–8.

Taylor A, Powell MEB. Conformal and intensity-modulated radio-therapy for cervical cancer. Clin Oncol 2008; 20:417–25.

Thomas GM. Improved treatment for cervical cancer-concurrent chemotherapy and radiotherapy. N Engl J Med 1999; 340:1198–200.

Varia MA, Bundy BN, Deppe G. Cervical carcinoma metastatic to para-aortic nodes: extended field radiation therapy with con-comitant 5-fluorouracil and cisplatin chemotherapy: a Gynecologic Oncology Group study. Int J Radiat Oncol Biol Phys 1998; 42(5):1015–23.

Vigliotti AP, Wen BC, Hussey DH, et al. Extended field irradiation for carcinoma of the uterine cervix with positive periaortic nodes. Int J Radiat Oncol Biol Phys 1992; 23:501–9.

Whitney CW, Sause W, Bundy BN, et al. Randomized comparison of fluorouracil plus cisplatin versus hydroxyurea as an adjunct to radiation therapy in stage IIB-IVA carcinoma of the cervix with negative para-aortic lymph nodes: a Gynecologic Oncology Group and Southwest Oncology Group study. J Clin Oncol 1999; 17:1339–48.

Cervical cancer: management of recurrence

Management of patients who relapse after primary treatment:

Treatment decisions should be based on the PS of the patient, the site of recurrence and/or metastases, the extent of metastatic disease, and the prior treatment.

Therapeutic options for local relapse after primary surgery (see Fig. 4.7.4)

Relapse in the pelvis following primary surgery may be treated by either radical radiation or pelvic exenteration. Radical irradiation (concurrent chemotherapy) may offer long-term control for a substantial proportion of those with isolated pelvic failure after primary surgery. Radiation dose and volume should be tailored to the extent of disease; 50Gy in 25 fractions should be delivered to microscopic disease and using field reductions 64–66Gy should be delivered to the GTV. Where disease is metastatic or recurrent in the pelvis after failure of primary therapy and not curable, a trial of chemotherapy with palliative intent or symptomatic care is indicated. Cisplatin is the single most active agent for the treatment of cervical cancer. The expected median time to progression or death is 3–7 months (Table 4.7.3).

Local recurrence after primary radiotherapy

Selected patients with resectable recurrences should be considered for pelvic exenteration. The only potentially curative treatment after primary irradiation is pelvic exenteration. Patients should be selected carefully; those with resectable central recurrences that involve the bladder and/or rectum without evidence of intraperitoneal or extra pelvic spread and who have a dissectable tumour-free space along the pelvic sidewall are potentially suitable. The triad of unilateral leg oedema, sciatic pain and ureteral obstruction almost always indicates unresectable disease on the pelvic sidewall, and palliative measures are indicated. This surgery should be undertaken only in centres with suitable facilities and expertise for this surgery and only by teams who have the experience and commitment to look after the long-term rehabilitation of these patients. The prognosis is better for patients with a disease-free interval greater than six months, a recurrence 3cm or less in diameter, and no sidewall fixation. The five-year survival for patients selected for treatment with pelvic exenteration is in the order of 30–60% and the operative mortality should be < 10%. In carefully selected patients, a radical hysterectomy may be performed. Suitable patients are mainly those whose central tumour is not more than 2cm in diameter.

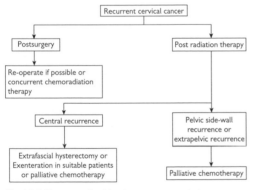

Fig. 4.7.4 Treatment algorithm for recurrent cervical cancer. With permission from Tata Memorial Centre, EBM Guidelines, Volume IV 2005.

Table 4.7.3 Treatment options for locally recurrent cervical cancer after surgery

Locally recurrent cervical cancer following surgery	Evidence
Radiation therapy is indicated in patients with locally recurrent cervical cancer following radical surgery	C
Concurrent chemotherapy with either 5-FU and/or cisplatin with radiation should be considered and may improve outcome	B
Pelvic exenteration may be an alternative (particularly if a fistula is present) to radical radiotherapy and concurrent chemotherapy in selected patients without pelvic sidewall involvement.	C

Cervical cancer: role of chemotherapy

Systemic CT in stage IVB or recurrent disease

Chemotherapy has a palliative role in patients with metastatic or recurrent cervical cancer after failure of surgery or radiotherapy. There are a number of chemotherapeutic agents with activity in metastatic or recurrent cervical cancer. Cisplatin, at present, is considered the most active cytotoxic agent, producing a response rate of 20–30% and a median survival of 7 months. Although the older combination regimens failed to show an improvement in survival compared with cisplatin alone, the use of newer combinations has shown promise. In a phase III GOG study, paclitaxel + cisplatin were superior to cisplatin alone in terms of response, PFS and sustained QoL but not for overall survival. In another GOG study the combination of topotecan + cisplatin was superior to cisplatin alone for response, PFS and OS (Long et al. 2005). Therefore selected patients with recurrent or metastatic disease of good PS could be offered one of the newer combination regimens. For others, single-agent cisplatin and BSC continue to be appropriate choices (Table 4.7.4).

Distant metastases: should be treated with palliative intent with chemotherapy or radiotherapy or symptomatic and supportive care only. Symptoms of recurrent/metastatic cervical cancer may include pain, leg swelling, anorexia, vaginal bleeding, cachexia, and psychological problems among others. The coordinated efforts of a team of professionals are optimal; this may include gynaecological oncologists, radiation and medical oncologists, palliative care physicians, specialized nursing staff, psychologists, and possibly stoma therapists. Relief of pain and other symptoms, with comprehensive support for the patient and her family, are paramount. Local treatment with radiation therapy is indicated to sites of symptomatic involvement in patients with metastatic disease for alleviation of symptoms including pain arising from skeletal metastases, enlarged para-aortic or supraclavicular nodes, and symptoms associated with cerebral metastases. In view of the shortened life expectancy of patients with metastatic cervical cancer, palliative radiotherapy should be given using larger fractions over shorter periods of time than used conventionally for radical treatments.

Further reading

Long HJ 3rd, Bundy BN, Grendys EC, *et al.* Randomized phase III trial of cisplatin with or without topotecan in carcinoma of the uterine cervix: A Gynecologic Oncology Group Study. *J Clin Oncol* 2005; **23**(21):4626–33.

Table 4.7.4 Systemic chemotherapy for metastatic (stage IV B) or recurrent cervical cancer

Systemic chemotherapy in metastatic cervical cancer	Evidence
Cisplatin is the single most active agent	B
The response rate (31%) with 100mg/m^2 cisplatin is higher than that with 50mg/m^2 (21%) but is not associated with any improvement in PFS or OS	B
Response rates to chemotherapy are consistently higher in patients with good PS and extrapelvic disease, and low in previously irradiated sites.	C
Newer combinations of cisplatin with either paclitaxel or topotecan have shown better outcome	B

Cervical cancer: treatment-related morbidity

Complications can be broadly divided into acute, subacute, and late. Acute complications manifest during treatment, subacute occur at 3–6 months and late appear 6 months after treatment. These could be divided according to the principal treatment modality used.

Surgery

The acute intraoperative and immediately postoperative complications include blood loss, ureterovaginal fistula (<2%), vesicovaginal fistula (<1%), paralytic ileus (1–2%), and postoperative fever (20–30%) secondary to DVT, pulmonary infection, pelvic cellulitis, urinary tract infection, or wound infection. The subacute complications include lymphocoele formation and lower extremity oedema. All these mentioned complications are increased if patients receive preoperative or postoperative irradiation. The late sequelae are due to extensive pelvic fibrosis which can result in ureteric obstruction, hydronephrosis, small bowel obstruction, or perforation.

Radiation therapy

During pelvic radiotherapy, most patients experience mild fatigue and mild to moderate diarrhoea which responds to antidiarrhoeal medications, and some experience bladder irritation. These acute symptoms are increased when RT is combined with concurrent chemotherapy or uses extended fields. Patients receiving concurrent chemotherapy may additionally have haematological or renal toxicity (cisplatin).

The late sequelae following radiation therapy which have been seen most frequently affect rectum, bladder, and small bowel. These depend on the duration of follow-up, type of treatment modalities used, and estimated radiation doses to these organs. Reported grade III/IV late sequelae (toxicities requiring hospital admission or intervention) range from 5–15%.

Late rectal sequelae in the form of chronic tenesmus, telangiectasia and profuse bleeding, rectal ulceration, and strictures have been reported (5–8%). These are usually seen during the 18–36 months follow-up period. Treatment options include sucralfate enema, steroid enema, argon plasma coagulation (APC), laser therapy, formalin applied to affected mucosa, or diversion colostomy.

Late bladder complications may occur in the form of continous haematuria, necrosis, or rarely vesicovaginal or urethra-vaginal fistulae. The incidence of symptomatic grade III/IV late toxicities after radical radiation is 4–8%. Hyperbaric oxygen therapy within 6 months of onset of haematuria may produce a good therapeutic response.

Late small bowel sequelae in the form of chronic enteritis, subacute intestinal obstruction, perforation, or strictures can be encountered. The reported incidence of symptomatic grade III/IV late toxicities after radical radiation is 3–12%. These sequelae are greater in patients undergoing radical surgery especially transperitoneal pelvic lymphadenectomy and adjuvant radiation ± chemotherapy.

Most patients treated with radical radiotherapy have telangiectasia and fibrosis of the vagina, resulting in significant vaginal shortening especially in elderly, postmenopausal women and those with extensive tumours treated with a high dose of radiation. These to some extent can be overcome by counselling for regular sexual activity and vaginal dilatation exercises.

Cervical cancer: newer approaches

Laparoscopic and robot-assisted surgeries are being explored only at research centres and should only be carried out by those with expertise.

In the past 10–15 years, there has been rapid progress in radiation delivery techniques in parallel with advances in technology and imaging. Newer external radiation techniques such as intensity modulated radiation therapy (IMRT), image guided radiation therapy (IGRT), and PET-CT guided radiation have also been explored in cervical cancers. However, these need further validation and at present there is no convincing evidence for their use. In cervical cancer brachytherapy, the four three-dimensional imaging modalities that are most commonly used are ultrasound, MRI, CT, and PET depending on the availability at various institutions. The GEC-ESTRO recommendations (Haie-Meder et al. 2005) have recently been adopted in the USA and in Europe as a standard method of communication between centres using three-dimensional imaging at the time of brachytherapy. These recommendations describe a gross tumour volume, which encompasses T2 bright areas in the cervix; the high-risk clinical target volume (HR-CTV), which encompasses the entire cervix and all visible or palpable disease at the time of brachytherapy; and the intermediate-risk (IR-CTV), which is a 1cm margin around this high-risk CTV plus the initial sites of involvement. The intermediate-risk CTV includes vaginal extension at the time of diagnosis that may have significantly decreased over time, and requires subtracting the normal tissues. The group also recommends starting with the standard method of dose prescription, either to point A or to the 60Gy reference volume, and then adjusting the loading pattern and dwell times to ensure comprehensive target coverage. All patients should have the D90, D100, and V100 recorded for the high-risk CTV (Potter et al. 2004). At this time, treatment of the full length of the tandem is recommended with modification if necessary of only the top dwell position based on dose to the sigmoid colon

To summarize, the treatment of patients with cervical cancer demonstrates the radiation oncologists' skill in a MDT of radiologists, medical and surgical oncologists, anaesthetists, physicists, dosimetrists, radiation technologists, and nurses.

Cervical cancer research

HPV DNA as the primary biomarker for early detection of pre-cancer lesions and triaging

Direct detection of HPV DNA in cervical specimens may offer an alternative or complementary methodology to population-based cytological screening. It has been reported that HPV test results are more sensitive than Pap smears in detecting high-grade lesions in older women (Schiffman et al. 2000; Wright et al. 2000). PCR detection of HPV DNA by L1 consensus primers and typing by HPV type-specific primers should be performed to detect the presence of high-risk HPVs. The most widely used MY9 and MY11, L1 consensus primers are capable of detecting about 27 HPV types which include all 15 HR-HPVs (HPV 16, 18, 31, 35, 39, 45, etc.) and 6 LR-HPVs (Gravitt et al. 1998). Since most HPV infections in women are transient and only a minority of women infected with HPV develops persistent infection that may evolve into squamous intraepithelial lesions, triaging of women infected with HR-HPV and management of cofactors such

as inflammation and infection of the reproductive tract is recommended. Studies also support the potential utility of HPV testing for effective triaging of Pap smears of atypical squamous cells of undetermined significance (ASCUS) and atypical glandular cells of undetermined significance (AGUS). It may therefore have a potential role in primary screening of populations in which Pap smears have not been sufficiently effective.

HPV E6 and E7 protein detection in the severe dysplastic and invasive carcinoma

Since two early genes E6 and E7 are the two main viral transforming genes that are invariably retained in almost all cervical cancers, detection of these two viral onco-proteins can serve as important biomarkers of severe dysplastic and invasive cervical cancers and progression of the disease.

Viral load and integration

A link between HPV viral loads and integrated viral genome into the host cell is considered a risk for the progression of pre-cancer to invasive cancer (Lillo et al. 2005). The significantly higher HPV load detected in women with high-grade cervical dysplasia, as well as the dramatic difference in the load after surgical removal of the lesion, suggest that HPV load is a possible prognostic marker of HSILs. Integration of the viral DNA to host cell genome is another biomarker as persistent HPV infection causes integration of viral DNA, leading to tumourigenic transformation.

Secondary biomarkers in the detection of cervical cancer

A number of molecular markers have been found to show early signs of alteration at the onset of the disease which may be useful in predicting the disease course at an early stage. To quote a few:

- p53 has been found to be unregulated, increasing with the grade of lesions, suggesting that p53 abnormality is an early event in cervical carcinogenesis.
- c-fos protein specifically shows exclusive high expression with the increasing severity of lesions and in cancer.
- Fra-1 is expressed in normal cervical tissue and its expression diminishes as the lesion progresses from pre-cancer to cancer.
- The p50 subunit of NF-kB shows enhanced expression in relation to disease progression.
- p16, the cyclin D/cdk inhibitor is overexpressed as the cancerous lesion proceeds to a more aggressive one.
- The NOTCH 1 family of proteins are found to be highly expressed from CIN III onwards.
- Rb protein has been found to be downregulated in poorly differentiated carcinoma, suggesting its important role in differentiation.
- Telomerase activation is a relatively early event in cervical carcinogenesis and is mostly correlated with the grade of the cervical lesion, HR-HPV status (HPV16 and 18 subtypes), and clinical staging.

However, there has been no breakthrough in translational research which has revolutionized the treatment strategies in cervical cancer. Nevertheless, there has been substantial research into targeted therapies which may have a future role in the clinical setting.

Further reading

Gravitt PE, Peyton CL, Apple RJ, *et al.* Genotyping of 27 Human Papilloma Virus Types by using L1 consensus PCR products by single-hybridization, reverse line blot detection method. *J Clin Microbiol* 1998; **36**:3020–7.

Haie-Meder C, Potter R, Van Limbergen E, *et al.* Recommendations from Gynaecological (GYN) GEC-ESTRO Working Group (I): concepts and terms in 3D image based 3D treatment planning in cervix cancer brachytherapy with emphasis on MRI assessment of GTV and CTV. *Radiother Oncol* 2005; **74**(3):235–45.

Lillo FB, Lodini S, Ferrari D, *et al.* Determination of human papilloma virus (HPV) load and type in high-grade cervical lesions surgically resected from HIV-infected women during follow-up of HPV infection. *Clin Infect Dis* 2005; **40**:451–7.

Potter R, Dimopoulos J, Kirisits C, *et al.* Recommendations for image-based intracavitary brachytherapy of cervix cancer: the GYN GEC ESTRO Working Group point of view: in regard to Nag, *et al.* (*Int J Radiat Oncol Biol Phys* 2004; **60**:1160e1172). *Int J Radiat Oncol Biol Phys* 2005; **62**(1):293–5. Author reply 5–6.

Schiffman M, Herrero R, Hildesheim A, *et al.* HPV DNA testing in cervical cancer screening: results from women in a high-risk province of Costa Rica. *JAMA* 2000; **283**:87–93.

Wright TC Jr, Denny L, Kuhn L, *et al.* HPV DNA testing of self-collected vaginal samples compared with cytologic screening to detect cervical cancer. *JAMA* 2000; **283**(1):81–6.

Endometrial cancer

Endometrial cancers are amongst the most common female cancers in developed countries. In the UK, endometrial cancer is the fifth most common female cancer. Primary endometrial cancer arises from the glandular epithelium of the endometrium. Endometrial cancer comprises a number of different histological subtypes. These differ in their molecular characteristics, clinical behaviour and impact on prognosis.

Incidence/epidemiology
- Incidence of endometrial cancer is 2.2–22 per 100,000 worldwide.
- There is significant geographical variation in incidence with higher incidence in developed Western societies.
- Endometrial cancer is the most common gynaecological cancer in the USA with an incidence of 22 per 100,000.
- UK incidence is 15.6 per 100,000.
- The incidence of endometrial cancer is highest in postmenopausal women.
- The median age at presentation is 61 years.
- 20–25% of women with endometrial cancer are premenopausal.
- Approximately 5% of women with endometrial cancer are <40 years of age.
- Epidemiological data from the USA suggests that there may be differences dependent on ethnic background with a significantly higher incidence in Caucasian women compared to Afro-Caribbean women.
- The incidence of endometrial cancer has been gradually increasing although mortality rates have generally declined.

Aetiology/risk factors
The majority of endometrial cancers are endometrioid in type (approximately 75%). These tumours often arise from a precursor lesion, severe atypical hyperplasia, and are associated with excessive endogenous or exogenous unopposed oestrogen stimulation. Up to 50% of women diagnosed with severe atypical hyperplasia are found to have invasive endometrial carcinoma on the hysterectomy specimen.

Risk factors for the development of endometrial cancer are:
- Obesity
- Early menarche
- Late menopause
- Prolonged anovulation
- Polycystic ovarian syndrome (Stein–Leventhal syndrome)
- Nulliparity
- Infertility
- Diabetes mellitus
- Hypertension
- Unopposed oestrogen therapy
- Tamoxifen use
- Oestrogen-secreting ovarian granulosa cell tumour
- Hereditary predisposition—hereditary non-polyposis coli (HNPCC)

Tamoxifen
- Tamoxifen use is associated with an increased risk of endometrial abnormalities e.g. benign polyps, non-atypical hyperplasia, atypical hyperplasia, and malignancy.

- Any histological type of endometrial carcinoma can arise on a background of tamoxifen use.

Hereditary non-polyposis coli
- Less than 5% of endometrial cancers are hereditary. Most hereditary endometrial cancers arise in women with HNPCC (also known as Lynch syndrome). HNPCC is an inherited autosomal dominant disorder arising from germline mutations in one or more mismatch repair genes (hMSH2; hMLH1; hMSH6; PMS1 and PMS2) leading to microsatellite instability (MSI).
- Women with HNPCC have a 40–60% lifetime risk of developing endometrial cancer.
- Approximately 50% of women with HNPCC present with endometrial cancer as their index cancer rather than colorectal cancer
- Clinical criteria (the Amsterdam II criteria) have been developed to aid in the identification of at-risk individuals.
- Women identified as being at high risk are referred for genetic counselling. Modified Bethesda criteria are used to pre-screen women for MSI testing and immunohistochemistry (IHC) on tumour tissue.
- More than 90% of women with HNPCC-related cancers will have MSI on testing compared to 10% of sporadic cancers. Where a gene is mutated, IHC will be negative for expression of that gene.
- Risk-reducing surgery (hysterectomy) is currently the only proven method of preventing endometrial cancer in women with HNPCC. Surveillance colonoscopy is indicated due to the high risk of developing colorectal cancer.
- See 'Risk factors for HNPCC' box, p.329.

Clinical features.

> **Key points: history**
> - Postmenopausal bleeding is the most common presentation. Up to 10% women will be diagnosed with endometrial cancer.
> - Persistent postmenopausal vaginal discharge may indicate pyometra associated with intrauterine pathology.
> - Premenopausal women may describe a significant change in menstrual pattern, e.g. increasingly heavy or irregular bleeding.
> - May present following the identification of abnormal endometrial cells noted incidentally on cervical cytology.
> - Pain is not a significant feature.
> - Presentation with the effects of metastatic disease is uncommon.

> **Key points: examination**
> - Examination with a bivalve speculum may identify a cervical lesion or cervical extension of an endometrial lesion.
> - Bimanual pelvic examination may reveal an enlarged uterus but is often normal.
> - Rectal examination should be performed to assess operability if parametrial extension of tumour is suspected on vaginal examination.

Risk factors for HNPCC

Amsterdam II criteria for identifying individuals at high risk of HNPCC
- Three or more relatives diagnosed with HNPCC-related cancers (colorectal cancer, endometrial cancer, cancers of the small bowel, ureter, or renal pelvis) one of whom is a first-degree relative of the other two.
- Colorectal cancer involving at least two generations.
- One or more of the previously listed cancers diagnosed at <50 years of age.

Modified Bethesda criteria for selecting patients for microsatellite instability testing
- Individuals in families that satisfy the Amsterdam II criteria.
- Individual of any age with two HNPCC-related cancers (including synchronous and metachronous colorectal cancers or extracolonic cancers).
- Diagnosis of colorectal cancer at any age with a first-degree relative with colorectal cancer and/or HNPCC-related extracolonic cancer and/or colorectal adenoma (one of the cancers diagnosed at age <50 and the adenoma diagnosed at <40).
- Diagnosis of colorectal or endometrial cancer when <50 years.
- Right-sided colorectal cancer with a solid/cribriform pattern on histology diagnosed at age <50 years.
- Colorectal cancer with signet-ring morphology diagnosed at age <50 years.
- Colorectal adenomas diagnosed at age <40 years.

Endometrial cancer: diagnosis, screening, and pathology

Diagnosis

Ultrasound scan

- The initial investigation of women with postmenopausal bleeding is transvaginal ultrasound scan.
- Data from meta-analyses of trials indicate that endometrial thickness of >5mm on transvaginal ultrasound scan has a 96% sensitivity and 62% specificity for endometrial cancer.
- 7–8% of postmenopausal women with an endometrial thickness of >5mm have endometrial cancer.
- The negative predictive value of an endometrial thickness of <5mm is 98%.
- The incidence of endometrial cancer where the endometrial thickness is <5mm is <0.5–1.7%.
- Women with endometrial thickness of ≥5mm require endometrial biopsy.
- Women on tamoxifen commonly have benign subendometrial changes that mimic endometrial thickening on ultrasound scan. Ultrasound is therefore not discriminatory in the investigation of abnormal bleeding on tamoxifen. Women with bleeding on tamoxifen treatment should undergo hysteroscopy and endometrial sampling.

Endometrial sampling/hysteroscopy

- Ultrasound scan is not helpful in diagnosing endometrial cancer in premenopausal women as specific cut-off levels for endometrial thickness do not accurately predict or exclude endometrial cancer. Premenopausal women with significant menstrual abnormalities should be investigated by endometrial biopsy ± hysteroscopy.
- 'Blind' endometrial sampling is accurate in diagnosing endometrial cancer where at least 50% of the uterine cavity is involved.
- Small or focal lesions may be missed by blind endometrial biopsy and hysteroscopy is recommended where focal thickening is seen on ultrasound scan.
- Most women (approximately 80%) have outpatient endometrial sampling and/or hysteroscopy. A minority of women require investigation under general anaesthesia (dilatation, hysteroscopy, and curettage).

Screening

- There is no population screening programme for endometrial cancer and no evidence from randomized trials to support the implementation of such a programme.
- Women with HNPCC are offered annual screening with transvaginal ultrasound scan and endometrial sampling although the efficacy of screening in these women is unproven.
- There is currently no evidence to support routine endometrial screening for asymptomatic women taking tamoxifen although abnormal bleeding should prompt urgent investigation.

Pathology

Tumour classification

- Primary endometrial cancers arise from the glandular epithelial elements within the endometrium. Different histological subtypes are recognized and classified according to the WHO classification, based on cell type and pattern (see box).
- Endometrial cancers are rarely metastatic from other tumours. Tumours most commonly reported to metastasize to the endometrium are breast carcinomas. Metastases from lung, gastric, colorectal, ovary, and melanomas are reported in the literature.
- Endometrioid carcinoma is the most common type of primary endometrial cancer (>75%).
- Less common types include serous, clear cell, and carcinosarcoma (previously called malignant mixed Müllerian tumour—see Chapter 4, Uterine sarcomas, p.342).
- Carcinosarcomas contain both an epithelial and a sarcomatous component. Molecular evidence indicates that carcinosarcomas are metaplastic carcinomas rather than sarcomas. These have now been reclassified as epithelial tumours although they have a prognosis similar to that of uterine sarcomas.
- Elements of different histological types may coexist in a single tumour. These cancers are classified as mixed tumours.

WHO classification of epithelial tumours of the uterine corpus

Primary tumours

- Endometrioid adenocarcinoma:
  - Secretory variant
  - Villoglandular variant
  - Ciliated cell variant
  - With squamous differentiation (this is distinct from squamous carcinoma)
- Mucinous adenocarcinoma
- Serous adenocarcinoma
- Clear cell adenocarcinoma
- Squamous cell carcinoma
- Transitional cell carcinoma
- Small cell carcinoma
- Undifferentiated carcinoma
- Mixed cell carcinoma

Tumours metastatic to the endometrium
Note: the WHO classification does not currently include carcinosarcoma although molecular evidence indicates that this is an epithelial tumour rather than a mesenchymal tumour.

Molecular features

Different histological subtypes of endometrial cancer exhibit different molecular characteristics suggesting different developmental pathways. Based on molecular differences, endometrial cancers can be broadly classified into two main groups, type I and type II tumours.

Type I tumours have the following characteristics:
- Grade 1 and 2 endometrioid tumours.
- Frequently arise in association with atypical hyperplasia, a precursor lesion.
- Associated with the risk factors shown listed earlier in this chapter under 'Aetiology/risk factors'.

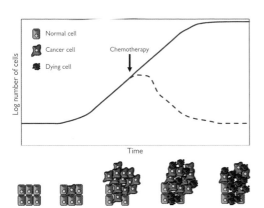

Plate 1 Growth curve depicting the growth of cancer cells and the impact chemotherapy can have.

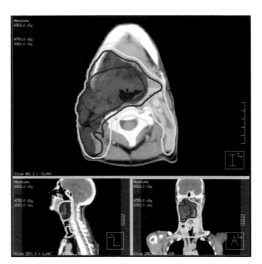

Plate 2 IMRT contours.

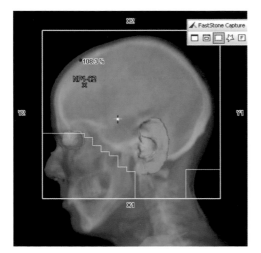

Plate 3 Standard radiotherapy portals fields used for delivery of prophylactic cranial radiotherapy. The lens and oral cavity are shielded to reduce toxicity.

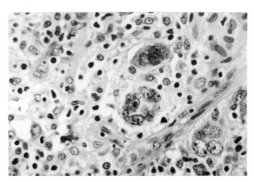

Plate 4 Histological staining of an affected lymph node reveals the typical giant Hodgkin and Reed–Sternberg (H-RS) cells.

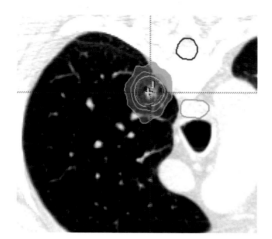

Plate 5 Stereotactic radiotherapy for stage I NSCLC. Dose distributions achieved in high-dose stereotactic radiotherapy for a paravertebral tumour. Using nine non-coplanar beams, a dose of 12Gy was prescribed per fraction to the 80% isodose (light green). Rapid dose-fall off results in <20% of the prescribed dose to the contoured oesophagus and spinal cord. The biological effective dose achieved is 180Gy, which contrasts to the 66–7Gy typically delivered using conventional radiotherapy.

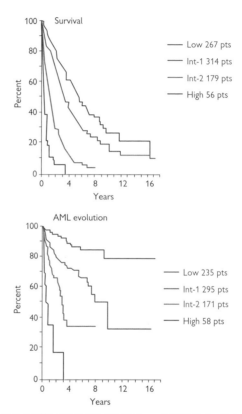

Plate 6 IPSS score predicts clinical outcome in MDS. Kaplan–Meier curves of patient survival (top panel) and freedom from acute myeloid leukemia (AML) evolution (bottom panel) in patients with myelodysplastic syndrome (MDS) according to their classification by the International Prognostic Scoring System (IPSS) for MDS. Reprinted with permission from Greenberg et al. International scoring system for evaluating prognosis in myelodysplastic syndromes. *Blood* 1997: **89**:2079–88.

- Frequently exhibit mutations in the PTEN tumour suppressor gene, K-ras oncogene, and mismatch repair genes.
- Frequently exhibit ER and PgR although these are seen less often in grade 3 disease.
- Are generally associated with a better prognosis overall than type II tumours.

Type II tumours generally have the following characteristics:
- Non-endometrioid tumours, e.g. serous, clear cell, grade 3 endometrioid tumours.
- Not associated with excess or unopposed oestrogens or other typical risk factors for type I tumours.
- Frequently arise in older postmenopausal women.
- Arise on a background of atrophic endometrium.
- Recent evidence suggests the possible existence of a precursor lesion for serous tumours, endometrial intraepithelial carcinoma (EIN).
- Mutations of the p53 tumour suppressor are common in type II tumours.
- Have a tendency to early extrauterine spread despite minimal invasion of the myometrium.
- Spread often occurs intraperitoneally with omental involvement.
- Are generally associated with a worse prognosis than type I tumours.

Tumour grade
- Tumour grade is assessed for all endometrioid endometrial cancers.

- Serous and clear cell tumours and carcinosarcomas are considered high-grade tumours as are undifferentiated tumours.
- There are several grading systems. In the UK the FIGO grading system is used.
- The FIGO system is based upon architectural abnormalities and is determined by the extent to which recognizable glands comprise the tumour compared to solid areas. Significant cytological abnormality upgrades the tumour.
- Tumours are graded 1–3 with grade 1 tumours being low grade.
- Tumour grade is correlated with the risk of lymph node metastasis.

Pattern of spread (see also 'Staging')
- Direct extension into myometrium and cervix.
- Transtubal metastasis to ovaries and peritoneal cavity.
- Lymphatic metastasis to pelvic lymph nodes.
- Para-aortic nodal involvement can arise directly via the lymphatic channels draining the upper uterus.
- Para-aortic involvement is less common in the absence of pelvic node metastasis.
- Lymphatic and haematogenous spread to vagina.
- Haematogenous spread to lungs.
- Serous and clear cell carcinomas have a tendency to early intraperitoneal spread.

Endometrial cancer: investigations, staging, and prognosis

Investigations

Once the diagnosis of endometrial cancer has been made, further investigations are required in order to exclude extra-abdominal metastases and prepare the patient for treatment which is usually surgery. Thorough pretreatment evaluation is essential as women with endometrial cancer are often elderly and/or have other significant comorbidity. Routine measurement of the serum tumour marker CA125 is not indicated as this is neither sensitive nor specific enough to provide staging or prognostic information.

Minimum investigations are:
- Full blood count
- Serum urea and electrolytes
- Serum liver function tests
- CXR

Examination under anaesthesia

EUA is indicated to determine operability where locally advanced tumour is suspected on outpatient examination. Cystoscopy is indicated where bladder invasion is suspected.

Magnetic resonance imaging

MRI is commonly used to evaluate depth of tumour invasion into the myometrium as this is related to the risk of lymph node metastasis. Pelvic lymphadenopathy may be assessed although nodal metastasis cannot be reliably excluded on MRI.

Despite the common use of MRI, there is little evidence of benefit for routine pelvic MRI in women where the disease appears clinically confined to the uterine corpus. MRI may be used to evaluate the cervix where there is clinical suspicion of cervical involvement with tumour. Published series suggest that MRI findings accurately predict cervical extension and depth of myometrial invasion in 92% of cases.

In the UK, MRI is usually performed in order to identify women at high risk of extrauterine disease so that surgery can be performed by a specialist gynaecological oncologist.

MRI is used in the evaluation of suspected central pelvic recurrence.

Computed tomography

CT is inferior to MRI in the evaluation of myometrial invasion but is used in the evaluation of the upper abdomen and/or thorax where there is a higher risk of extrapelvic metastases, e.g. serous carcinoma, carcinosarcoma.

CT is required for radiotherapy treatment planning (see Chapter 4, Role of radiotherapy, p.336), and is used in the evaluation of possible abdominal and extra-abdominal recurrence.

Table 4.7.5 Five-year survival according to FIGO stage

Stage	Approximate 5-year survival (%)
I	85
II	75
III	45
IV	25

> **FIGO staging of endometrial cancer**
>
> *I: tumour confined to the corpus uteri*
> - IA: tumour confined to the endometrium (including endocervical gland involvement)
> - IB: myometrial invasion <50%
> - IC: myometrial invasion ≥50%
>
> *II: tumour invades cervical stroma but not extending beyond the uterus*
>
> *III: extension beyond myometrium*
> - IIIA: carcinoma involves serosa of uterus or adnexae, or positive ascites, or positive peritoneal washings
> - IIIB: vaginal involvement, either direct or metastatic
> - IIIC1: pelvic node involvement
> - IIIC2: para-aortic lymph node involvement with or without positive pelvic lymph nodes
>
> *IV: further spread*
> - IVA: carcinoma involving the mucosa of the bladder or rectum
> - IVB: distant metastases and involvement of other abdominal or inguinal lymph nodes

Positron emission tomography

^{18}FDG-PET does not have an established role in the management of endometrial cancer at present. A small study of women previously treated for endometrial or cervical carcinoma showed that ^{18}FDG-PET was an accurate method of locating the site of disease recurrence. Further studies evaluating ^{18}FDG-PET in recurrent endometrial cancer are needed before it can be incorporated into routine practice.

Staging

Endometrial cancers are staged according to the FIGO staging system (see box) which is based on both surgical findings and histopathology.

Prognosis

Endometrial cancer has a better overall prognosis than other cancers of the female genital tract. The 5-year survival rate across all stages is approximately 80% (Table 4.7.5). This is due to early presentation with most women having stage I disease. Long-term outcomes for women with stage III/IV disease are significantly poorer.

Table 4.7.6 Five-year survival for women with stage I disease according to grade and depth of myometrial invasion

Depth of myometrial invasion (stage)	Survival at 5 years (%)		
	FIGO grade 1	FIGO grade 2	FIGO grade 3
No invasion (Ia)	96	92	85
<50% invasion (Ib)	95	90	69
>50% invasion (Ic)	81	70	42

Prognosis varies considerably depending on:
• Depth of myometrial invasion (Table 4.7.6)
• Stage
• Grade
• Histological subtype
• Age >60 years was an adverse prognostic factor in a large randomized trial of adjuvant radiotherapy versus radiotherapy alone) (Creutzberg et al. 2000).

Further reading

Creutzberg CL, van Putten WLJ, Koper PCM, *et al.* Surgery and postoperative radiotherapy versus surgery alone for patients with stage-1 endometrial carcinoma: multicentre randomised trial. *Lancet* 2000; **355**(9213):1404–11.

Endometrial cancer: role of surgery

Surgery is the cornerstone of treatment for endometrial cancer and may be supplemented by adjuvant treatment. The majority of women have stage I disease at diagnosis (70–75%). Up to 15% of women have stage II cancer, and a further 10–15%, stage III or IV disease.

Surgery provides:

1. Prognostic information, i.e. staging.
2. Therapeutic benefit.
3. Palliation of vaginal bleeding and pelvic pain in cases of incurable metastatic disease.
4. Curative resection of locally recurrent disease.

Surgery for stage I disease

Total abdominal hysterectomy and bilateral salpingo-oophorectomy

A standard surgical approach where disease is confined to the uterine corpus on examination is total hysterectomy and bilateral salpingo-oophorectomy with peritoneal washings (for cytology). This may be performed through a midline laparotomy or a transverse suprapubic incision.

Lymphadenectomy

The role of lymphadenectomy in endometrial cancer surgery is a controversial issue. Full pelvic and para-aortic lymphadenectomy is required for FIGO staging although the therapeutic role of lymphadenectomy has been debated for a considerable time. Many surgeons selectively perform lymphadenectomy in cases where the risk of lymph node metastasis is high e.g. deep myometrial invasion on MRI or grade 3 tumour on endometrial biopsy. Historically, studies that demonstrated benefit from lymphadenectomy were generally retrospective and prone to selection bias.

The UK MRC trial, ASTEC (A Study in the Treatment of Endometrial Cancer) is the only large, adequately powered randomized study to address the role of lymphadenectomy in clinical stage I endometrial cancer (Kitchener et al. 2005). Women with clinical stage 1 disease were randomized to lymphadenectomy versus no lymphadenectomy. Most women had endometrioid histology.

The data from ASTEC show that:

- Lymphadenectomy does not improve survival in women with clinical stage I endometrial cancer (89% survival with lymphadenectomy compared to 88% for women who did not have lymphadenectomy (Kitchener et al. 2005).
- Lymphadenectomy is associated with higher morbidity and mortality.

There have been no large randomized trials evaluating the role of lymphadenectomy in non-endometrioid endometrial cancers. A large series of 148 cases of fully staged serous endometrial cancers indicated that survival in true stage Ia and Ib disease was approximately 80% at 5 years. Similar results were seen for clear cell cancers. This may reflect understaging in other studies. Randomized trials evaluating the role of lymphadenectomy and adjuvant treatment in non-endometrioid cancers are required. Currently lymphadenectomy is indicated in these tumours.

Omentectomy/omental biopsy

Omental biopsy/infracolic omentectomy may be performed in cases of serous endometrial cancer. Although omentectomy is not specifically featured in the FIGO staging system, serous tumours have a tendency to upper abdominal metastasis even when there is minimal myometrial invasion. Omental biopsy/omentectomy is associated with relatively little morbidity and many surgeons consider this to be a standard part of surgery for serous tumours.

Laparoscopic surgery for endometrial cancer

Laparoscopically-assisted vaginal hysterectomy and bilateral salpingo-oophorectomy (LAVH/BSO) or total laparoscopic hysterectomy and bilateral salpingo-oophorectomy (TLH/BSO) may be performed.

Laparoscopic lymphadenectomy and/or omental biopsy/omentectomy may be performed if indicated. There is no difference in the lymph node yield between laparoscopic and open surgery.

Retrospective studies suggest similar DFS compared with open surgery. Lower blood loss and postoperative morbidity is reported in a number of studies, both retrospective and prospective. The Gynecologic Oncology Group (GOG)-LAP2 study randomized >2000 women to laparoscopic staging and surgery for endometrial cancer versus laparotomy. Women with clinical stage I–IIa disease were recruited. Survival data are not yet mature although preliminary results indicate fewer complications, decreased hospital stay, and improved QoL scores in women who had laparoscopy.

Vaginal hysterectomy

In the case of severe comorbidity that prevents safe general anaesthesia for abdominal surgery, vaginal hysterectomy alone may be performed under regional anaesthesia. Vaginal hysterectomy (with or without adjuvant radiotherapy) can achieve 5-year survival rates of 80–90% in very obese and/or medically compromised women (Chan et al. 2001).

Surgery for stage II disease

Women with clinical stage IIb endometrial cancer may be treated with radical hysterectomy, BSO, and lymphadenectomy. The ureters are dissected free of the parametrial and paracervical tissues to provide a sufficient margin of tumour-free tissue around the uterine isthmus and cervix. A cuff of upper vagina of 2cm is taken to ensure a tumour-free vaginal margin of tissue. Due to the extensive dissection around the bladder, ureter, and uterosacral ligaments, bladder dysfunction is common. Bladder drainage with an indwelling catheter is needed for 7–10 days.

Morbidity is significantly higher following radical hysterectomy than standard hysterectomy and a significant proportion of women will not be considered fit enough for radical surgery. In practice many surgeons perform a standard hysterectomy and adjuvant radiotherapy is given postoperatively.

- The USA SEER database shows improved 5-year survival (93%) following radical hysterectomy alone compared to standard hysterectomy (83%) alone for women with stage II endometrial cancer.
- There are no data from randomized trials to suggest that radical hysterectomy alone is superior to standard hysterectomy followed by adjuvant radiotherapy.
- Radical hysterectomy with adequate tumour-free margins and negative nodes can be curative without the addition of adjuvant radiotherapy.

• Stage IIa endometrial cancer is usually diagnosed following hysterectomy and thus there are no specific recommendations for radical surgery.

Surgery for advanced endometrial cancer (stages III/IV)

Women with advanced disease are a heterogeneous group. Prognosis varies considerably within this group according to substage, i.e. women with stage IIIa disease have a better prognosis than those with stage IIIb or IIIc disease.

• Stage III–IV disease is usually managed by surgery with adjuvant radiotherapy and/or chemotherapy and/or hormonal therapy depending on extent of disease and the general health of the patient.

• If locally advanced disease is suspected, EUA should be performed to determine operability. If the patient is considered inoperable initially, primary radiotherapy can be given and surgery considered secondarily following a clinical response.

• Good control of pelvic disease with palliation of vaginal bleeding and pelvic pain can be achieved by hysterectomy and adjuvant treatment even when distant metastases are present. The role of more aggressive debulking surgery in advanced disease is uncertain.

Complications of surgery

Complications may be general complications, that are seen with any surgical procedure, or specific to pelvic surgery.

General
• Haemorrhage
• Pulmonary complications—pneumonia, atelectasis
• Urinary infection
• Urinary retention
• Wound infection

• Thromboembolism—DVT, PE
• Haematoma

Specific to abdominopelvic surgery
• Bladder injury.
• Ureteric injury.
• Bowel injury.
• Damage to major pelvic and abdominal blood vessels with major haemorrhage, e.g. at lymphadenectomy.
• Neurological damage—genitofemoral and obturator nerves at risk during pelvic lymphadenectomy.
• Postoperative ileus.
• Bladder dysfunction: more common with radical hysterectomy due to disruption of autonomic nerves in uterosacral ligaments.
• Pelvic lymphocysts and lymphoedema following pelvic lymphadenectomy.
• Hernia formation, e.g. through abdominal wound or vagina.
• Ureteric fistula—secondary to ischaemia. Usually occurs as a late complication and is more common after radical hysterectomy followed by pelvic irradiation.

Most complications are more common following radical surgery. Prophylactic antibiotics should be administered at the time of surgery and thromboprophylaxis used perioperatively and until the patient is fully mobile.

Further reading

Chan JK, Lin YG, Monk BJ, *et al*. Vaginal hysterectomy as primary treatment of endometrial cancer in medically compromised women. *Obstet Gynecol* 2001; **97**(5 Part 1):707–11.

Kitchener HC RC, Swart AMC, Amos CL. ASTEC (surgery component): a study in the treatment of endometrial cancer. A randomized trial of lymphadenectomy in the treatment of endometrial cancer. ESGO 2005. *Int J Gynecol Cancer* 2005; **15**(Suppl 2):77 [Abstract 00094].

Endometrial cancer: role of radiotherapy

Radiotherapy is useful in the following situations:
- Adjuvant treatment after surgery
- Primary radical treatment
- Radical treatment of pelvic recurrence
- Palliation of advanced/metastatic disease

Adjuvant radiotherapy

Radiotherapy is most commonly used as adjuvant treatment following surgery for women at high risk of disease recurrence. The aim is to treat occult metastases in order to prevent recurrence and improve survival. It can be delivered by:
- EBRT, or
- Vaginal brachytherapy (directly to the vaginal vault)

Women may be treated with EBRT, brachytherapy, or both depending on the clinical situation. EBRT is given to encompass the site of the original tumour and the draining lymph nodes and is given where the risk of lymphatic metastasis is increased. The total treatment dose is usually given as a sequence of short daily treatments (fractions) over several weeks e.g. a total dose of 40Gy may be given in 20 fractions over 4 weeks.

Brachytherapy to the vaginal vault is delivered as sealed radioactive sources inserted into the vagina within specially-designed sheaths. The sources are introduced into the sheaths by remote after-loading systems.

Selective application of adjuvant radiotherapy

The benefit of adjuvant radiotherapy in endometrial cancer has been studied in a number of trials. A randomized trial of adjuvant EBRT versus surgery alone, PORTEC, showed that locoregional recurrence was significantly reduced from 14% to 4% (p<0.001) in women who received radiotherapy and also demonstrated age >60 years to be a poor prognostic factor for recurrence. Survival was not however, improved in women who had radiotherapy (Creutzberg et al. 2000)

A meta-analysis of trials of radiotherapy in endometrial cancer confirmed that radiotherapy does not improve survival in women at low and intermediate risk of recurrence (Johnson et al. 2007). There was a survival advantage of 10% for women with high risk disease, i.e. stage Ic, grade 3 endometrioid cancer treated with radiotherapy compared to surgery alone. Mortality was increased in women who received radiotherapy.

Vault brachytherapy may prevent pelvic recurrence and could be associated with less morbidity than EBRT. This is being evaluated in the PORTEC2 study.

Indications for adjuvant radiotherapy

Indications for postoperative adjuvant radiotherapy are shown in the box.

Radical radiotherapy

May be used as primary treatment in early endometrial cancer where comorbid conditions prevent surgery. Cure rates of >65% can be achieved although the risk of recurrence is high (20%). Primary surgery is therefore advocated wherever possible.

Primary radiotherapy is also indicated in cases of locally advanced cancer where the tumour is inoperable at presentation. EBRT and brachytherapy (intracavitary radiotherapy) are given. Surgery can be considered secondarily if there is a clinical response.

Indications for postoperative radiotherapy in endometrial cancer

- Any age with IC/grade 3 endometrioid carcinoma
- Aged 60 or older with IA-B/grade 3 endometrioid carcinoma
- Aged 60 or older with IC/grade 1–2 endometrioid carcinoma
- Stage II endometrioid cancer treated with standard or 'simple' hysterectomy
- Stage I non-endometrioid cancer with any myometrial invasion
- Stage II non-endometrioid cancer
- Stage III/IV endometrial cancer

Treatment of pelvic recurrence

Radiotherapy is a curative option for non-irradiated women with pelvic recurrence. The cure rate is better for women with isolated central pelvic recurrence than for women with pelvic side-wall disease.

Outcome for recurrent disease depends upon:
- Location of recurrence
- Disease-free interval
- Previous administration of radiotherapy

Palliative radiotherapy

Radiotherapy is an effective palliative treatment and may be used for:
- Problematic vaginal bleeding
- Vaginal metastases
- Symptomatic para-aortic metastases
- Bone pain secondary to bone metastases
- Cerebral metastases

Radiotherapy toxicity

Side effects are common following radiotherapy treatment. These are caused by the effects of ionizing radiation on normal tissues within the treated field. Some organs, e.g. small bowel, have a lower tolerance to radiotherapy than others. Modern radiotherapy techniques, such as three-dimensional conformal radiotherapy, enable more precision so that a maximum dose can be given to the tumour whilst keeping the dose to healthy surrounding tissues to a minimum.

Radiotherapy toxicity may manifest as acute effects or late effects, some months or even years after treatment. Side effects range from mild to severe. Mild to moderate late side effects occur in approximately 25% of women who receive adjuvant treatment. The risk of side effects is increased where both EBRT and brachytherapy are used.

The risk of severe toxicity is dependent on total dose of radiation given as well as the fractionation schedule. The following factors also increase the risk of severe side effects:
- Large treatment volume
- Previous pelvic or abdominal surgery

- Inflammatory conditions affecting the pelvis, e.g. ulcerative colitis.
- Conditions that impair the vascular supply to pelvic/abdominal organs e.g. severe arteriopathy.

Early effects

Early or acute effects are seen during treatment and affect approximately 60% of women. These usually resolve within 4–6 weeks following completion of treatment. These are:
- Abdominal cramps
- Frequent bowel movements
- Diarrhoea
- Urinary frequency
- Urinary urgency
- Skin irritation
- Fatigue

Late effects

Severe late effects are less common and include:
- Radiation proctitis
- Radiation cystitis
- Ischaemic bowel
- Small bowel obstruction
- Bowel/ureteric fistulae
- Vaginal stenosis
- Lower limb lymphoedema

- Insufficiency fractures of the sacrum
- Femoral neck fractures secondary to avascular necrosis
- (Rarely) development of malignancy within the irradiated field (usually sarcomas)

Severe toxicity was reported in 2% of irradiated women in the PORTEC study (Creutzberg et al. 2000). Severe late effects are more common in women who have had radical surgery (including lymphadenectomy) followed by radiotherapy.

Some late effects may respond to conservative measures e.g. steroid enemas for radiation proctitis. Where these are unsuccessful or where the complication is very severe or life-threatening, surgery may be required e.g. bowel resection. There is a higher risk of anastomotic breakdown as irradiated bowel and ureter are poorly vascularized. Colostomy or urinary diversion may therefore be required.

Further reading

Creutzberg CL, van Putten WLJ, Koper PCM, *et al.* Surgery and postoperative radiotherapy versus surgery alone for patients with stage-1 endometrial carcinoma: multicentre randomised trial. *Lancet* 2000; **355**(9213):1404–11.

Johnson N, Cornes P. Survival and recurrent disease after postoperative radiotherapy for early endometrial cancer: systematic review and meta-analysis. *Int J Obstet Gynaecol* 2007; **114**(11):1313–20.

Endometrial cancer: role of chemotherapy and hormonal agents

Chemotherapy

Indications for chemotherapy

- Adjuvant treatment of advanced disease (stage III/IV) following surgery.
- Primary treatment of widely disseminated disease at presentation or where surgery or radical radiotherapy is not possible.
- Adjuvant treatment of high-risk, early stage disease.
- Palliation of extrapelvic recurrence.
- Chemotherapy is most commonly used in the treatment of advanced or recurrent disease. Increasingly, chemotherapy is used in the adjuvant setting for women with early stage non-endometrioid cancers when the risk of systemic disease is considered to be high.

Cytotoxic chemotherapy with single agent activity

- Anthracyclines, e.g. doxorubicin, epirubicin
- Alkylating agents, e.g. cisplatin, carboplatin
- Taxanes, e.g. paclitaxel
- Topoisomerase inhibitors, e.g. topotecan, etoposide
- Vinca alkaloids, e.g. vincristine
- Anti-metabolites e.g. 5-FU

The most active single agents in advanced or recurrent endometrial cancer are anthracyclines, platinum-containing alkylating agents (e.g. carboplatin), and paclitaxel. Most responses are partial and short-lived.

Combination chemotherapy

A systematic review and meta-analysis of chemotherapy in advanced, recurrent and metastatic endometrial cancer concluded that intense combination chemotherapy regimens significantly improve DFS. The gain in survival is modest, of the order of 3 months (Humber et al. 2007). The median OS following chemotherapy for advanced and recurrent disease is 7–10 months. Regimens that combine an anthracycline or taxanes with cisplatin are associated with better response rates although this is at the expense of increased severe toxicity. The use of combination chemotherapy may therefore be limited by poor PS and advanced age in this patient group.
The most common combinations used are:

- Cisplatin + doxorubicin
- Carboplatin + paclitaxel

Cardiotoxicity is a side effect of doxorubicin. This is an important consideration when considering treatment for women who are often elderly and may have coexisting cardiorespiratory problems. A combination of carboplatin and paclitaxel is generally less toxic than doxorubicin-containing combinations.

Chemotherapy in the adjuvant treatment of early stage, high-risk endometrial cancer

A number of women with completely resected early stage disease are at increased risk of distant metastases. These include women with:

- Deep myometrial invasion (Ic)
- Grade 3 endometrioid disease
- Serous or clear cell carcinoma
- Involvement of the uterine isthmus/cervix
- Lymphovascular invasion (LVSI)

Trials evaluating adjuvant chemotherapy in endometrial cancer have included women with different stages of disease. The results from different studies are conflicting although they indicate that the incidence of distant metastases is reduced in women receiving chemotherapy compared with pelvic radiotherapy. There is evidence however that chemotherapy does not prevent pelvic recurrence.

In the EORTC 55591 study of chemotherapy in women with high-risk, early stage disease, four cycles of chemotherapy were given in addition to pelvic irradiation. DFS and OS was significantly improved in those women who received chemotherapy.

The forthcoming PORTEC3 trial will address the role of concurrent chemoradiation and adjuvant chemotherapy compared to pelvic radiotherapy alone in women at high risk of recurrence including those with serous or clear cancers stage Ib and greater.

Currently chemotherapy is considered in women deemed to be at high risk for distant recurrence including those with serous and clear cell carcinomas with any degree of myometrial invasion. Radiotherapy is usually given in addition where the risk of pelvic recurrence is high. The results of further randomized trials will be needed in order to understand fully the role of adjuvant chemotherapy in early stage disease.

Hormonal agents

Systemic hormonal therapy is used to palliate symptoms in advanced and recurrent endometrial cancer. Hormonal treatments are associated with a favourable side-effect profile compared to many cytotoxic drugs and are therefore useful in medically unfit women where the goal of treatment is palliation.

Progestogens

- Progestogen treatment has no benefit in the adjuvant treatment of endometrial cancer (Martin-Hirsch et al. 2000).
- Response rates with oral progestogens are approximately 10–25% in published studies of women with advanced and recurrent disease.
- Recommended regimens are medroxyprogesterone acetate 200–400mg daily or megestrol acetate 40–320mg daily in divided doses.
- Low grade, slow growing tumours are most likely to respond.
- The median progression-free duration is approximately 4 months. Median OS of approximately 10 months is reported. Downregulation of PgRs shortens the duration of response.
- High-grade tumours often lack PgRs and therefore the beneficial effect may be limited. Tamoxifen and other selective ER modulators have been used in some studies with the aim of recruiting receptors and increasing the duration of response to progestogens. Median duration of response is similar to that seen with progestogens alone.

Gonadotrophin-releasing hormone (GnRH) analogues

- GnRH analogues may provide benefit in progestogen-refractory advanced or recurrent disease.

- GnRH analogues downregulate receptors in the pituitary gland and the resulting decrease in gonadotrophin levels leads to a fall in circulating oestrogen levels.
- Complete and partial responses to treatment are seen with monthly injections of goserelin acetate 3.6mg and PFS of several months has been reported.

Aromatase inhibitors
- These drugs decrease oestrogen levels by blocking the aromatase enzyme.
- Response rates in phase II studies are low (approx. 9%) and duration of response limited.

Further reading

Humber CE, Tierney JF, Symonds RP, *et al.* Chemotherapy for advanced, recurrent or metastatic endometrial cancer: a systematic review of Cochrane collaboration. *Ann Oncol* 2007; **18**(3):409–20.

Martin-Hirsch PL, Jarvis G, Kitchener H, *et al.* Progestagens for endometrial cancer. *Cochrane Database Syst Rev* 2000; **2**:CD001040.

Endometrial cancer: recurrence and metastasis

The rate of recurrence of endometrial cancer is related to stage of disease. The overall rate of recurrence is 7–18%.

Recurrence may occur locally, in the pelvis or at distant sites. The pattern of recurrence is influenced by the histological subtype and previous treatment modalities used.

A higher proportion of patients with disease relapse following adjuvant pelvic radiotherapy have recurrence at distant sites. Conversely, pelvic recurrence appears to affect a higher proportion of women who receive adjuvant chemotherapy alone for high-risk disease.

Serous carcinomas have a tendency to intraperitoneal spread and more aggressive histology, e.g. carcinosarcoma, predisposes to distant disease.

Symptoms that may indicate recurrence
- Vaginal bleeding/persistent abnormal vaginal discharge
- Pelvic pressure symptoms
- Unilateral leg swelling or neuropathic pain
- New onset central abdominal pain or back pain
- Symptoms from distant metastases are dependent on the affected organ(s)

Treatment options for recurrent and metastatic endometrial cancer
Treatment depends on the site(s) of recurrence, previous treatments used and PS of the patient.

Surgery
Surgery is a curative option for previously irradiated women with a single recurrence at the vaginal vault. It is vital that other sites of disease are excluded by appropriate imaging, e.g. CT/MRI before embarking on surgery. Pelvic exenteration may be required in order to obtain tumour-free resection margins and if the bladder or bowel are involved with the tumour. Significant morbidity is 60–80% in some series and published perioperative mortality rates are as high as 16%. Careful patient selection is therefore very important.

Radiotherapy
Generally, women with pelvic recurrence who have not previously been exposed to pelvic radiation are treated with radiotherapy. Isolated pelvic recurrence is curable and approximately 65% of women survive for at least 5 years after treatment with combined EBRT and vaginal brachytherapy: the cure rate is lower for women with pelvic side wall disease (see Chapter 4, Endometrial cancer: role of radiotherapy, p.336).

Radiotherapy may be used with palliative intent in cases of extrapelvic disease, e.g. for pain from bony metastasis.

Chemotherapy
See Chapter 4, Endometrial cancer: role of chemotherapy and hormonal agents, p.338.

Chemotherapy is indicated as adjuvant treatment in cases of distant metastasis and extrapelvic recurrence. Administration of chemotherapy may be limited by performance status in some cases.

Hormonal treatment
See Chapter 4, Endometrial cancer: role of chemotherapy and hormonal agents, p.338.

Hormonal treatment can provide good palliation with acceptable side effects in recurrent and widely metastatic disease although the duration of effect is limited. Oral progestogens are used most commonly.

Symptomatic measures
Treatment of symptoms associated with incurable recurrence is important, including the appropriate use of effective analgesia. Vaginal bleeding from advanced inoperable tumour or recurrent disease may respond to oral tranexamic acid, 3–4g daily in divided doses. Uterine artery embolization has also been used with good effect to treat acute haemorrhage from inoperable uterine tumours.

Uterine sarcomas

- Uterine sarcomas represent a rare group of malignancies the most common of which are leiomyosarcoma (LMS) and endometrial stromal sarcoma (ESS).
- Carcinosarcomas (CS), previously known as mixed Müllerian tumours, were historically included within uterine sarcoma trials but these have now been reclassified as aggressive carcinomas. They are included here only as much of the early literature does not separate them from other uterine sarcomas and as the US NCCN treatment guidelines include them within sarcoma.

Incidence/epidemiology
- Incidence of uterine sarcoma 0.5–3.3 per 100,000 worldwide (including CS).
- USA SEER databases give incidences of 0.64/100,000 for LMS and 0.19/100000 for ESS and <0.05/100,000 for other subtypes.
- UK incidence is 1/100,000 for all subtypes combined. LMS and CS are 2–3 times more common in black women than Caucasians.
- Median age at presentation is 50 years.

Aetiology
- Previous pelvic radiotherapy (5–10% of LMS in one study).
- Tamoxifen exposure (0.17 per 1000 women treated but higher in CS) has been identified as a causative agent in a minority of patients.

Clinical features
- Depend on the stage at presentation and the histological subtype and grade of the tumour.
- In localised disease, patients may present with increased vaginal and post menopausal bleeding
- Many uterine sarcomas are found unexpectedly at the time of routine hysterectomy.
- On vaginal examination a polypoidal lesion or mass protruding through the cervical os may be evident.
- Patients with advanced disease may present with an abdominal mass, abdominal pain or symptoms of systemic disease such as lethargy, anorexia and weight loss.
- Nodal disease is rare in uterine sarcomas but inguinal nodes should be excluded on examination.

Diagnosis
- Ultrasound or MRI is often performed because of increased vaginal bleeding and a mass may be visible. MRI is the local imaging of choice (see Fig. 4.7.5).
- Multiple benign leiomyomata may be visible and it may not be possible to distinguish LMS from the benign lesions.
- ESS are seen as infiltrative lesions.
- CS often present as large heterogenous polypoid structures which bulge though the cervical os.
- Pelvic and para-aortic nodes can be seen in CS but are rare in ESS and LMS.
- Biopsy may be performed prior to surgery but only examination of the entire uterus postoperatively gives an accurate diagnosis. In particular, LMS are rarely diagnosed on preoperative biopsy.
- Biopsy of CS often only reveals the epithelial component.

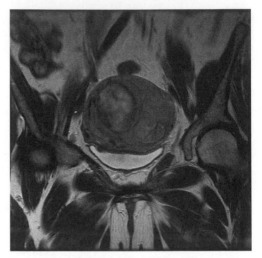

Fig. 4.7.5 Coronal section MRI scan showing extensive uterine sarcoma.

Pathology
- ESS are comprised of cells which resemble those of the stromal component of the myometrium. They grow outwards into the myometrium from the endometrium. Recently ESS have been reclassified. ESS (previously termed low-grade ESS) tend to have a more indolent course and a high incidence of ER positivity. This is distinct from undifferentiated uterine sarcoma, an aggressive malignancy (previously high-grade ESS).
- LMS originate from the myometrium but are often large and protrude into the endometrium. They are predominantly high-grade lesions with a high mitotic rate.
- CS are tumours which have both an epithelial and sarcomatous component. The epithelial component is most commonly endometroid or serous papillary. Sarcomatous components can be homologous (e.g. leiomyosarcoma) or heterologous (e.g. chondrosarcoma). CS have been found to be monoclonal entities in which the epithelial component is frequently seen in metastatic lesions. For this reason they have been reclassified as aggressive carcinomas. Their prognosis, however, more accurately reflects that of sarcomas and a recent study suggested that they should not be included in clinical trials with other epithelial endometrial cancers. They account for up to 43% of patients in early studies in uterine sarcoma.

Hormone receptors
- A significant proportion of uterine sarcomas express oestrogen (ER) or progesterone (PgR) receptors, although the degree of expression varies according to histology. The degree of ER and PgR expression is less than that seen in breast cancer.
- Low-grade ESS usually express PgR. ER expression is most commonly seen in ESS and oestrogen-lowering

therapy has been used as a treatment option. Eighty per cent ESS were positive for ER alpha, none for ER beta and 90% for PgR (Chu 2003)

- Up to 87% of LMS have positive staining for ER and 80% for PgR (Kelley 2004) and this may be functional in intermediate and low-grade LMS.

> **Author tips**
>
> Check ER and PgR status of uterine sarcomas. If strongly positive, oestrogen replacement therapy would be inadvisable.

Uterine sarcomas: management

Molecular features

- Apart from ER and PgR there is sparse data on the molecular biology of these tumours.
- KIT staining has been seen in 44% ESS overall which included undifferentiated tumours. Of low-grade true ESS 22% were KIT positive and 71% of undifferentiated cases expressed KIT. No mutations have been found and there was no correlation with PFS or OS.

Staging

Staging is according to the FIGO staging system and is based on surgical findings, although it does not reflect prognosis as well as endometrial carcinoma.

- Stage I: disease confined to uterine corpus
- Stage II: disease involving the cervix
- Stage III: disease spread to pelvic organs
- Stage IV: disease outside the pelvis

Prognosis

- Prognosis in uterine sarcomas is significantly worse than epithelial endometrial cancer of comparable stage.
- In a SEER study of 1396 LMS patients, 5-year survivals of 75.8% for stage I, 60.1% for stage II, 44.9% stage III, and 28.7% for stage IV were described (Kapp 2008).
- Low-grade ESS have an 80% 5-year survival but an increased risk of long-term relapse even 20 years after diagnosis.
- Undifferentiated uterine sarcoma (previously termed high-grade ESS) have a very aggressive course with a 5-year survival around 30%.
- The 5-year survival for early stage CS is in the order of 50%.

Prognostic factors

- In LMS the factors associated with a poor prognosis were found to be higher grade, increasing age, no definitive surgery, and increasing stage.
- Poor prognostic factors in ESS were high mitotic count, high grade (which would make them undifferentiated) and race (African American) in one study although the majority of these patients also had high grade/undifferentiated disease.

Patterns of relapse

- In ESS pelvic recurrence is more common although distant relapses to the lungs can occur.
- In LMS pelvic and extra pelvic recurrences can occur. Extra pelvic metastases in LMS can occur in the liver, lung, lymph nodes, and bone.
- CS recur locally in the pelvis, throughout the peritoneum (as in epithelial ovarian cancer), in the lymph nodes, and in the lungs.
- Brain metastases are rare in all subgroups. The patterns of relapse can be affected by treatment.
- Extra pelvic relapse has been shown to be more frequent in those who have had adjuvant radiotherapy.

Principles of management

Surgery remains the mainstay of uterine sarcoma treatment but there is a role for radiotherapy in some cases and developments have been made in systemic treatments.

Surgical

- Standard surgical approach is a total abdominal hysterectomy and bilateral salpingo-oophorectomy.
- A single study has shown no improvement in survival for LMS with or without oophorectomy but it is clear from the strong ER positivity of most of the remaining uterine sarcomas that oophorectomy remains an essential part of their surgery.
- Lymph node sampling or removal is advocated in CS but not for leiomyosarcomas or undifferentiated endometrial stromal sarcomas.
- Lymphadenectomy in ESS remains controversial as lymph node metastases have now been reported in several studies.
- Surgery also has a role in the management of isolated relapse or in resection of limited metastases as for other soft tissue sarcomas.
- For resection of metastases there should be no evidence of disease elsewhere and a significant disease-free period with evidence of stable or slowly progressive disease.
- Resection of metastases in rapidly progressive disease is not advocated.

Role of radiotherapy

- External beam palliative radiotherapy is used extensively for symptomatic metastases in all uterine sarcomas.
- Treatment in the adjuvant setting, particularly for early stage disease, is more controversial.
- There are no large randomized controlled trial studies but several retrospective studies have shown a benefit in local control with adjuvant pelvic radiotherapy with doses of 40–50Gy.
- In ESS most studies have combined ESS with undifferentiated uterine sarcoma. There appears to be a benefit in pelvic control but this may be due to selection bias.
- In LMS there is conflicting evidence with studies showing both a benefit and lack of benefit of adjuvant radiotherapy.
- A very small number of retrospective studies have shown a survival benefit of adjuvant radiotherapy but the majority of these were for CS.
- The peritoneal spread of CS led to the use of whole abdominal irradiation (WAI) in some studies. A recent GOG trial compared WAI with cisplatin and ifosfamide chemotherapy as adjuvant treatment and found them both to be equally efficacious, although there was no control treatment-free arm.
- There is an ongoing EORTC trial of adjuvant radiotherapy in stage I and II high-grade uterine sarcomas as these are the most controversial group to treat.

Role of chemotherapy: adjuvant

- The evidence for adjuvant chemotherapy in uterine sarcomas comes from (i) extrapolation from other soft tissue sarcoma studies (ii) retrospective studies of all uterine sarcomas including all subgroups, and CS (iii) smaller studies within specific subgroups.
- In the largest meta-analysis published on adjuvant chemotherapy in soft tissue sarcomas, an overall benefit

of PFS and time to distant metastases was seen with doxorubicin containing chemotherapy. There was also a trend towards improved survival although this did not reach statistical significance. Only one study in the meta-analysis included patients with uterine sarcoma and this did not show a survival benefit.

- An EORTC trial examining the role of adjuvant doxorubicin and ifosfamide in soft tissue sarcomas, presented at ASCO in 2007, did not show a survival benefit.
- Retrospective studies have shown no significant benefit with chemotherapy in early stage resected uterine sarcomas.
- Several studies in CS have shown a benefit to ifosfamide and cisplatin containing chemotherapy although there have been no comparisons without treatment.
- Gemcitabine with docetaxel is effective in advanced LMS, and showed an improvement in PFS compared with historical controls.

Role of chemotherapy: metastatic
In the advanced setting chemotherapy has an established role in the treatment of most uterine sarcomas.
- Originally the agents used were those which had the highest response rates in soft tissue sarcomas (ifosfamide and doxorubicin).
- Recent studies suggest that different agents have specific roles in certain histological subtypes.
- In low-grade ESS, chemotherapy is rarely effective with response rates <10%. Many of these respond to hormonal manipulation.
- In undifferentiated (high-grade ESS) sarcomas ifosfamide has the highest response rate (33% in a phase II GOG study) although the duration of response is limited to a few months.
- Doxorubicin has also shown a response rate (RR) up to 19% in undifferentiated uterine sarcoma.
- In LMS doxorubicin has provided response rates of 16–25% but responses lasted <6 months.
- Ifosfamide has a limited RR in LMS (<10%).
- An ongoing EORTC trial is studying the potential benefit of ifosfamide and doxorubicin compared with doxorubicin alone.
- Gemcitabine has shown activity in LMS, both as a single agent (RR 21% in a GOG study of 44 women) and combined with docetaxel.
- The combination of gemcitabine/docetaxel has shown RRs up to 53% in pretreated LMS with improvement in OS up to 18 months. Trials are underway to assess the combination as first-line treatment.
- In CS trials the most active single agents have been ifosfamide (39%), cisplatin (19%), paclitaxel (18%), and doxorubicin (10%). The most effective agents used in combination have been cisplatin with ifosfamide (RR 45%), although there are uncontrolled series which show a 35% RR to carboplatin and paclitaxel.

Hormonal treatments
Currently there is no prospective trial which has examined the role of hormone therapy in uterine sarcomas.
- The strong ER and PR expression of low-grade ESS has been studied to see if it affects survival.
- Oestrogen replacement therapy and tamoxifen have both been found to be associated with poorer outcome (Chu 2003; Pink 2006)
- Treatment with progestins was found to be beneficial. There are reports of activity with AIs.
- One study showed only a 30% positivity for LMS and no survival benefit (Leitao 2004), but another study of LMS showed a survival benefit for patients with >10% ER expression (Akhan 2005).
- There are anecdotal case reports of response but these require to be validated in the context of a clinical trial.

Further reading
Adjuvant chemotherapy for localised resectable soft tissue sarcoma of adults: meta-analysis of individual data. Sarcoma meta-analysis collaboration. *Lancet* 1997; **350**:1647–54.

Akhan S, Yavuz E, Tecer A, et al. The expression of Ki-67, p53, estrogen and progesterone receptors affecting survival in uterine leiomyosarcomas. *Gynecol Oncol* 2005; **99**(1):36–42.

Chu M, Mor G, Lim C, et al. Low-grade endometrial stromal sarcoma: hormonal aspects. *Gynecol Oncol* 2003; **90**(1):170–6.

Hensley M, Blessing J, Degeest K, et al. Fixed dose gemcitabine plus docetaxel as second line therapy for metastatic uterine leiomyosarcoma: a GOG phase II study. *Gynecol Oncol* 2008; **109**(3):323–8.

Kapp D, Shin J, Chan J. Prognostic factors and survival in 1396 patients with uterine leiomyosarcomas: emphasis on impact of lymphadenectomy and oophorectomy. *Cancer* 2008; **112**(4):820–30.

Kelley T, Borden E, Goldblum J. Estrogen and progesterone receptor expression in uterine and extrauterine leiomyosarcoma: an immunohistochemical study. *Appl Immunohistochem Mol Morphol* 2004; **12**(4):338–41.

Krasner C. Aromatase inhibitors in gynaecologic cancers. *J Steroid Biochem Mol Biol* 2007; **106**(1–5):76–80.

Leitao M, Soslow R, Nonaka D, et al. Tissue microarray immunohistochemical expression of estrogen, progesterone, and androgen receptors in uterine leiomyomata and leiomyosarcoma. *Cancer* 2004; **101**(6):1455–62.

Park J, Kim D, Suh D, et al. Prognostic factors and treatment outcomes of patients with uterine sarcoma: analysis of 127 patients at a single institution. *J Cancer Res Clin Oncol* 2008; **134**(12):1277–87.

Pink D, Lindner T, Mrozek A, et al. Harm or benefit of hormonal treatment in metastatic low-grade endometrial stromal sarcoma: single centre experience with 10 cases and review of the literature. *Gynecol Oncol* 2006; **101**(3):464–9.

Wolfson A, Brady M, Rocerato T, et al. A GOG randomised phase III trial of whole abdominal irradiation (WAI) vs. cisplatin-ifosfamide and mesna (CIM) as post surgical therapy in stage I-IV carcinosarcoma of the uterus. *Gynecol Oncol* 2007; **107**(2):177–85.

Internet resource
Sarcoma UK offers information and access to a growing support network for sarcoma patients and their carers: http://www.sarcoma-uk.org

Epithelial ovarian cancer: introduction, pathology, and clinical features

Introduction

Epidemiological studies from the USA indicate that ovarian cancer occurs in 1 in 57 women and is the fourth leading cause of cancer accounting for 16,000 deaths per year. There are few specific symptoms and signs of this disease and as a result the majority of cases are diagnosed at an advanced stage when the prognosis is generally poor, with 5-year survival rates of around 45% (Jemal et al. 2006).

There are three major types of ovarian cancers: epithelial (90%), germ cell (5%), and sex cord stromal tumours (5%) (Cannistra et al. 2004). Epithelial ovarian tumours are derived from the surface epithelium and the vast majority are sporadic (90–95%).; 15% of epithelial tumours are of borderline malignant potential and the remainder are invasive cancers.

Risk factors

Hormonal and environmental factors

The median age of diagnosis of epithelial ovarian cancer is 63 (SEER, see 'Internet resources'). Epidemiological risk factors include nulliparity, early menarche, and late menopause, possibly due to more frequent ovulations, which predisposes to malignant transformation (Ozals et al. 2004). There have been conflicting reports about exposure to fertility drugs, dietary factors, talcum powder, and asbestos.

Hereditary predisposition

About 10–15% of all epithelial ovarian cancers have a hereditary predisposition (Rubin et al. 1998), most commonly within the breast-ovarian cancer family syndrome due to mutations in BRCA 1 and BRCA 2 (Garber and Offit 2003). Features that may indicate a hereditary syndrome include early onset breast cancer (age <50 years), presence of ovarian cancer, male breast cancer, and an Ashkenazi Jewish ancestry. A small percentage of families have an excess of ovarian cancer without any cases of breast cancer and they represent site-specific ovarian cancer families, a unique phenotype of the hereditary breast-ovarian syndrome (Reedy et al. 2002). These cancers have been linked to the BRCA 1 mutation. A woman with one first-degree relative with ovarian cancer with no hereditary features has a lifetime risk of 5% of developing ovarian cancer.

BRCA 1 and BRCA 2

The products of the BRCA 1 and 2 genes function as DNA repair proteins (Scully et al. 1996). In the general population the prevalence of carriers is 1 in 500 individuals. However in certain ethnic groups, such as the Ashkenazi Jews, this increases to 1 carrier in 40 individuals (King et al. 2003). The lifetime risk of ovarian cancer in women with the BRCA 1 mutation is about 40% and in those with the BRCA 2 mutation from 10–20% (King et al. 2003).

Hereditary non-polyposis colon cancer

Ovarian cancer can also be found in families as part of the HNPCC or Lynch II syndrome (Lindor et al. 2006). This syndrome develops from inherited mutations in DNA mismatch repair genes (Lindor et al. 2006). At-risk individuals have an increased lifetime risk of ovarian cancer (12%), colon cancer (70%), endometrial cancer (40–60%), and gastric cancer (Lindor et al. 2006).

It is important to identify women at high risk of ovarian cancer in order to discuss risk-reducing strategies. This may take the form of increased surveillance with regular examination, CA125 measurements and transvaginal ultrasound scan (Aletti et al. 2007). However there is no evidence that increased surveillance detects ovarian cancer at an early stage and bilateral salpingo-oophorectomy (BSO) is generally recommended in women known to have germline mutations in BRCA 1 or 2 at the age of around 35–40 years, depending on the affected gene and the age of onset of ovarian cancer in the family (Aletti et al. 2007). Prophylactic BSO reduces the risk of ovarian cancer by >90% in these patients, although there remains approximately a 5% risk of primary peritoneal cancer two decades after BSO (Finch et al. 2006).

Screening

Unfortunately the symptoms and signs of ovarian cancer are fairly non-specific and many patients therefore present with advanced incurable disease. Early stage disease has an excellent prognosis after optimal therapy (ICON-1 2003) and better detection of early disease is therefore a key goal in reducing mortality from ovarian cancer. To date there is no evidence that a screening programme for ovarian cancer improves survival (Einhorn et al. 1992). However, there are two large randomized studies currently ongoing in post menopausal women to evaluate the role of transvaginal ultrasound and/or CA125 measurements in screening and mortality reduction (Hassan et al. 2000; UKCTOCS, see 'Internet resources').

Pathology

There are several histological subtypes of epithelial ovarian cancer: serous adenocarcinoma (43%), mucinous adenocarcinoma (15%), endometrioid adenocarcinoma (22%), clear cell adenocarcinoma (5%), Brenner tumours, mixed (≥2 of the 5 major types of epithelial cancer) or undifferentiated tumours (14%) and intraperitoneal cancer (Ozals et al. 2005).

Serous carcinomas, histologically resembling cells lining the fallopian tube, are the most common type of epithelial ovarian cancer and are particularly associated with BRCA mutations. They tend to be high-grade tumours and behave aggressively. Mucinous tumours resemble cervical or intestinal cells and are more common in younger women. These tumours are usually unilateral (75–80%), benign and often may not secrete CA 125. Endometrioid cancers are similar to cells of the uterine lining and may occur as a result of endometriosis. Clear cell carcinomas are relatively uncommon, but occur most frequently in women in the fourth decade and in 50% of cases there is associated endometriosis. Although often of an early stage, clear cell carcinomas are relatively chemoinsensitive and have a worse prognosis.

Clinical features

Key features of the history and examination of ovarian cancer are shown below If symptoms persist for >2–3 weeks further investigations are warranted.

Further reading

Aletti GD, Gallenberg MM, Cliby W, *et al*. Current management strategies for ovarian cancer. *Mayo Clinic Proceedings* 2007; **82**:751–70.

Cannistra SA. Cancer of the ovary. *N Engl J Med* 2004; **351**:2519–29.

Einhorn N, Sjovall K, Knapp RC, *et al*. Prospective evaluation of serum CA 125 levels for early detection of ovarian cancer. *Obstet Gynecol* 1992; **80**:14–18.

Finch A, Beiner M, Lubinski J, *et al*. Hereditary Ovarian Cancer Clinical Study Group. Salpingo-oophorectomy and the risk of ovarian, fallopian tube and peritoneal cancers in women with BRCA 1 or BRCA 2 mutation. *JAMA* 2006; **296**:185–92.

Garber J E, Offit K. Hereditary cancer predisposition syndromes. *J Clin Oncol* 2005; **23**:276–92.

Hassan MA, Fagerstrom RM, Kahane D C, *et al*. Prostate, Lung, Colorectal and Ovarian Cancer Screening Trial Project Team. Design and evolution of the data management systems in the Prostate, Lung, Colorectal and Ovarian (PLCO) Cancer Screening Trial. *Control Clin Trials* 2000; **21**(6 suppl):329S–348S.

International Collaborative Ovarian Neoplasm 1 (ICON 1) and European Organisation for Research and Treatment of Cancer Collaborators-Adjuvant Chemotherapy in Ovarian Neoplasm (EORTC-ACTION). International Collaborative Ovarian Neoplasm Trial 1 and Adjuvant Chemotherapy in Ovarian Neoplasm Trial: two parallel randomised phase III trials of adjuvant chemotherapy in patients with early stage ovarian carcinoma. *J Natl Cancer Inst* 2003; **95**:105–12.

Jemal A, Siegel R, Ward E, *et al*. Cancer Statistics 2006. *CA Cancer J Clin* 2006; **56**:106-130.

King MC, Marks JH, Mandell JB. New York Breast Cancer Study Group: Breast and ovarian cancer risks due to inherited mutations in BRCA 1 and BRCA 2. *Science* 2003; **302**:643–6.

Lindor NM, Petersen GM, Hadley DW, *et al*. Recommendations for the care of individuals with an inherited predisposition to Lynch syndrome: a systematic review. *JAMA* 2006; **296**:1507–17.

Ozals RF, Bookman MA, Connolly DC, *et al*. Focus on epithelial ovarian cancer. *Cancer Cell* 2004; **5**:19–24.

Ozols RF, Rubin SC, Thomas GM, *et al*. Epithelial ovarian cancer. In: Hoskins WJ, Perez CA, Young RC, *et al*. (eds) *Principles and Practice of Gynecologic Oncology*, 4th edition, pp.895–987. Philadelphia, PA: Lippincott Williams and Wilkins, 2005.

Reedy M, Gallion H, Fowler JM, *et al*. Contribution of BRCA 1 and BRCA 2 to familial ovarian cancer: a Gynaecologic Oncology Group study. *Gynecol Oncol* 2002; **85**:255–9

Rubin SC, Blackwood MA, Bandera C, *et al*. BRCA 1, BRCA 2 and hereditary non-polyposis colorectal cancer gene mutations in an unselected ovarian cancer population: relationship to family history and implications for genetic testing. *Am J Obstet Gynecol* 1998; **178**:670–7.

Scully R, Ganesan S, Brown M, *et al*. Location of BRCA 1 in human breast and ovarian cancer cells [letter]. *Science* 1996; **272**:123–6.

Internet resources

National Cancer Institute SEER. Cancer of the ovary. Cancer stat fact sheets. Available at http://seer.cancer.gov

UK Collaborative Trial of Ovarian Cancer Screening: http://www.ukctocs.org.uk

Epithelial ovarian cancer: investigations, staging, and prognosis

Special investigations
- Serum CA125: is raised in 80% of epithelial ovarian malignancies. Beware of false positive results such as endometriosis, benign ovarian cysts, pelvic inflammatory disease, and first trimester pregnancy, cirrhosis, and other malignancies.
- Transvaginal ultrasound: shows a complex ovarian mass with solid and cystic components.
- CT scan: chest, abdomen, and pelvis to assess extent of metastatic spread.
- MRI scan: pelvis.
- Staging/diagnostic laparoscopy

Differential diagnosis
The differential diagnosis of an adnexal mass includes benign ovarian tumours and cysts, endometriosis, and ovarian cancer. The diagnosis can be more difficult in patients with metastatic disease and malignancies of the upper and lower GIT tract can also present with similar symptoms and signs. A serum CA125: CEA ratio >25 is strongly indicative of an ovarian rather than a GI primary. The immunohistochemical cytokeratin profile of biopsy

samples is often very helpful in confirming the diagnosis; a typical profile would include CK 7 positivity and CK 20 negativity.

Staging
The most commonly employed staging system is the FIGO system (see Table 4.7.7), which is based on surgical findings taken at laparotomy (Ozols et al. 2005) Comprehensive staging (total abdominal hysterectomy (TAH), BSO, omentectomy, tumour debulking, peritoneal washings and biopsies, lymph node resection/sampling) is essential as this determines the need for further therapy, which strongly impacts on survival. It is evident that patients presenting with early stage (stage I) disease have an excellent 5-year survival in excess of 80%. Unfortunately the majority of patients present with stage 3 and 4 disease and the 5-year survival is then <20%.

Further reading
Ozols RF, Rubin SC, Thomas GM, *et al.* Epithelial ovarian cancer. In: Hoskins WJ, Perez CA, Young RC, *et al.* (eds) *Principles and Practice of Gynecologic Oncology*, 4th edition, pp.895–7. Philadelphia, PA: Lippincott Williams and Wilkins, 2005.

Table 4.7.7 FIGO staging and prognosis (Ozols et al. 2005)

FIGO stage	Description	Proportion of cases (%)	5-year survival (%)
1	Tumour confined to ovaries	–	–
1a	Tumour confined to one ovary-capsule intact. No tumour on ovarian surface. No malignant cells in ascites/washings	19.3	92.1
1b	Tumour limited to both ovaries, capsule intact. No tumour on ovarian surface. No malignant cells in ascites/washings	2.7	84.9
1c	Tumour on 1 or both ovaries, capsule ruptured or tumour on ovarian surface, or malignant cells in ascites/washings	8.1	82.4
2	Tumour involves 1 or both ovaries with pelvic extension.	-	-
2a	Extension and /or implants in uterus and/or tubes.	2.7	69.0
2b	Extension to other pelvic organ.	4.2	56.4
2c	2a/2b with positive malignant cells in the ascites or positive peritoneal washings.	3.0	51.4
3	Tumour involves 1 or both the ovaries with microscopically confirmed peritoneal metastases outside the pelvis and/or regional lymph node metastasis.	–	–
3a	Microscopic peritoneal metastasis beyond the pelvis.	6.9	39.3
3b	Macroscopic peritoneal metastasis beyond the pelvis ≤2 cm in greatest dimension..	6.6	25.5
3c	Peritoneal metastasis beyond the pelvis ≥2 cm in greatest dimension and/or regional lymph nodes metastasis.	18.0	17.1
4	Distant metastasis beyond peritoneal cavity.	28.3	11.6

(Liver capsule metastasis is stage 3, liver parenchymal metastasis is stage 4. Malignant pleural effusion must be confirmed on cytology)

Epithelial ovarian cancer: early stage disease

Principles of treatment
- Optimal surgical cytoreduction
- Adjuvant chemotherapy in high-risk patients

Surgery
Confirmation that a patient has early stage disease confined to the pelvis at diagnosis is essential as recommendations for postoperative treatment are dependent on accurate surgical staging. There is evidence that a significant proportion of women are understaged from a study by Young and colleagues that restaged 100 consecutive patients with a diagnosis of stage 1A–IIB ovarian cancer (Young et al. 1983). This study found that 31% of women were upstaged and that in fact 77% of these patients had stage III disease.

Chemotherapy
Two large randomized trials (ICON 1 and the Adjuvant Chemotherapy in Ovarian Neoplasm Trial), compared chemotherapy with observation only in high risk patients with early stage disease (ICIN 2003; Trimbos et al. 2003) Combined analysis demonstrated survival rates of 82% vs. 74% with chemotherapy and observation respectively. Furthermore those patients with high-risk stage 1 disease who relapsed had survival rates which were comparable to those of patients with stage III disease (ICIN 2003; Trimbos et al. 2003) The current recommendations are that high-risk patients with early stage disease should receive adjuvant chemotherapy.

The GOG 157 study compared 3 versus 6 cycles of paclitaxel (175mg/m^2) and carboplatin (AUC 7.5) in high-risk patients with stage I and II ovarian cancer (Bell et al. 2006). Five-year survival rates were similar in the 3-cycle (81%) and 6-cycle (83%) arms. This study indicates that after optimal surgery in high-risk patients the majority of benefit is derived in the first 3 cycles of treatment and with the subsequent 3 cycles there is only a modest increase in survival but a significant increase in toxicity. In practice, adjuvant chemotherapy is not recommended in the majority of patients with well-differentiated stage 1A (or 1B) ovarian cancer. However in patients with early stage disease with poor prognostic features (such as high-grade poorly differentiated tumours, stage 1C or stage II disease) carboplatin-paclitaxel chemotherapy is desirable (usually 3–6 cycles).

Further reading
Bell J, Brady MF, Young RC, et al. Randomised phase III trial of three versus six cycles of adjuvant carboplatin and paclitaxel in early stage epithelial ovarian carcinoma: A Gynecologic Oncology Group study. *Gynecol Oncol* 2006; **102**:432–9.

International Collaborative Ovarian Neoplasm (ICON) Collaborators. International Collaborative Ovarian Neoplasm (ICON) Trial 1: a randomised trial of adjuvant chemotherapy in women with early stage ovarian cancer. *J Natl Cancer Inst* 2003; **95**:125–32.

Trimbos JB, Parmar M, Vergote I, et al. International Collaborative Ovarian Neoplasm trial 1 and Adjuvant Chemotherapy in Ovarian Neoplasm Trial: two parallel randomised phase III trials of adjuvant chemotherapy in patients with early stage ovarian carcinoma. *J Natl Cancer Inst* 2003; **95**:105–12.

Young RC, Decker DG, Wharton JT, et al. Staging laparotomy in early ovarian cancer. *JAMA* 1983; **250**:3072–6.

Epithelial ovarian cancer: advanced stage disease

Principles of treatment
- Optimal surgical debulking
- Carboplatin-based chemotherapy

Surgery

Treatment of advanced stage ovarian cancer involves a multidisciplinary approach. Initial surgery permits accurate diagnosis, thorough staging and optimal surgical cytoreduction of metastatic disease. The extent of residual disease after primary surgery has been shown to be the most important predictive factor for survival in patients with advanced ovarian malignancy (Bristow et al. 2002). Optimal debulking for advanced disease is defined as removal of all disease measuring ≥1cm in diameter. Studies have consistently indicated that specialist gynaecologic oncology surgeons are more likely than general surgeons to perform optimal surgery for ovarian cancer (McGowen et al. 1985; Nguyen et al. 1993). A recent study also showed that debulking operations and lymph node dissections were more likely to be performed by specialist surgeons (Earle et al. 2006). Current NICE guidelines recommend that all women with ovarian cancer be referred to a specialist gynaeoncology centre for their initial surgery.

The standard of multidisciplinary care is maximal debulking surgery followed by chemotherapy. However in certain cases, chemotherapy may be given first, followed by so-called interval debulking surgery (after three courses of chemotherapy). Trials of this approach have given conflicting results, and the precise role of neoadjuvant therapy in the initial treatment of patients with advanced disease is currently being evaluated in the CHORUS study, which randomizes patients to receive either upfront surgery or neoadjuvant chemotherapy followed by delayed surgery.

Chemotherapy

Despite advances in therapy the majority of patients with stage 3 and 4 disease will not be cured. The primary goal of treatment in this group of patients is to prolong survival by the addition of chemotherapy following (or prior to) optimal surgical debulking. The two major drug types to consider first are platinum agents and taxanes.

The role of cisplatin in combination therapy was determined by studies in the early eighties. Decker and colleagues demonstrated improved survival rates with a combination of cyclophosphamide and cisplatin versus cyclophosphamide alone (52% versus 19% respectively) (Decker et al. 1982). A GOG study also demonstrated that the addition of cisplatin to cyclophosphamide and doxorubicin led to an increase in median and overall survival (15.7 versus 9.7 months) (Omura et al. 1986). Further studies confirmed that the inclusion of doxorubicin in cisplatin containing combination regimens did not confer additional survival benefit, and until the early 1990s cyclophosphamide/cisplatin represented the standard of care (Bertelsen et al. 1987; Omura et al. 1989).

Paclitaxel was initially shown to be an active agent in patients with platinum-resistant ovarian cancer with response rates of 24% (McGuire et al. 1989). The GOG 111 study in the USA compared cisplatin and paclitaxel to cisplatin, cyclophosphamide in patients with stage 3 and 4 disease and demonstrated superior response rates (73% vs. 60%), PFS (18 vs. 13 months), and median survival

(38 vs. 24 months) for the cisplatin and paclitaxel regimen (McGuire et al. 1989). The OV-10 study (an international trial) also confirmed the superiority of paclitaxel and cisplatin over cyclophosphamide and cisplatin, and so in the mid 1990s paclitaxel-cisplatin became an acceptable standard (Piccart et al. 2000). Various paclitaxel infusion schedules have been tested and it has been shown that the 3-hour treatment has comparable efficacy to the 24-hour infusion and is associated with less myelosuppression, but increased neurotoxicity (Eisenhauer et al. 1994). A number of studies, including GOG 158 have demonstrated that cisplatin and carboplatin have similar efficacy in combination with paclitaxel (Neijt et al. 2000; du Bois et al. 2003; Ozols et al. 2003). In the GOG study median PFS and overall survival were similar in the two arms of the study (6 cycles of paclitaxel 135mg/m^2 for 24 hours plus cisplatin 75mg/m^2 vs. paclitaxel 175mg/m^2 over 3 hours and carboplatin AUC 7.5) (Ozols et al. 2003). Thus paclitaxel combined with carboplatin became the accepted standard of care. Recently the GOG 182-ICON 5 studies have also demonstrated that the addition of an additional agent, such as gemcitabine, liposomal doxorubicin or topotecan to paclitaxel-carboplatin did not improve PFS (Bookman et al. 2006).

Two studies in advanced disease, ICON 3 and GOG-32, provided a counter-intuitive result in that both showed that the results of single-agent carboplatin (or cisplatin) treatment were equivalent to those of paclitaxel combined with carboplatin (or cisplatin). These results are not fully explained, but an overall meta-analysis of the four first-line trials (GOG-111, OVO-10, GOG 32, and ICON 3) does demonstrate an advantage, albeit relatively modest, of the two drug combination. Nevertheless, it is generally agreed that of the 2 drugs, platinum exerts the major effect, and for many cases single agent carboplatin represents an appropriate first line treatment (Sandercock et al. 2002).

Due to ease of administration (outpatient) and equivalent efficacy the combination of 3-hour paclitaxel (rather than the 24-hour schedule) together with carboplatin is widely used as first-line therapy for patients with high-risk early stage disease and in those with advanced disease at presentation (du Bois et al. 2005). There is also evidence that docetaxel may be as efficacious in combination with carboplatin in the initial treatment of patients with all stages of ovarian cancer. Data from a randomized study comparing docetaxel-carboplatin with paclitaxel-carboplatin as first-line therapy demonstrated that the two regimens were similar in terms of PFS (15 vs. 14.8 months respectively, p = 0.707) and objective tumour response rates (58.7% vs. 59.5% respectively). However, the docetaxel-carboplatin arm was associated with less grade 2 and higher neurotoxicity than the paclitaxel-containing arm (11% vs. 30% respectively, p <0.001), but significantly more grade 3 to 4 neutropenia (94% vs. 84% respectively, p <0.001). Global QoL scores were similar in both treatment groups, although a number of symptom scores favoured docetaxel (Vasey et al. 2004).

Chemotherapy in patients with advanced disease is usually administered after initial optimal debulking surgery. In selected cases a neoadjuvant approach may be adopted, in which chemotherapy is given prior to surgery. These cases include those with advanced stage IV disease and those in poor general medical condition.

Intraperitoneal chemotherapy

Advanced ovarian cancer is often confined to the peritoneal cavity. There have been several studies addressing this issue, as well as a recommendation regarding the use of intraperitoneal chemotherapy from the NCI (Alberts et al. 1996; Markman et al. 2001; Armstrong et al. 2006; Bankhead 2006). However no intraperitoneal regimen has been compared to the current standard of care, intravenous carboplatin and paclitaxel. Currently intraperitoneal chemotherapy is not recommended outside of clinical trials.

Further reading

Alberts DS, Liu PY, Hannigan EV, et al. Intraperitoneal cisplatin plus intravenous cyclophosphamide versus intravenous cisplatin plus intravenous cyclophophosphamide for stage III ovarian cancer. *N Engl J Med* 1996; **335**:1950–5.

Armstrong DK, Bundy BN, Alberts DS, et al. Gynecologic Oncology Group. Intraperitoneal cisplatin and paclitaxel in ovarian cancer. *N Engl J Med* 2006; **354**:34–43.

Bankhead C. Intraperitoneal therapy for advanced ovarian cancer: will it become standard care? *J Natl Cancer Inst* 2006; **98**(8):510–12

Bertelsen K, Jakobsen A, Anderson JE, et al. A randomised study of cyclophosphamide and cis-platinum with or without doxorucin in advanced ovarian carcinoma. *Gynecol Oncol* 1987; **28**:161–9.

Bristow RE, Tomacruz RS, Armstrong DK, et al. Survival effect of maximal cytoreductive surgery for advanced ovarian cancer during the platinum era: a meta analysis. *J Clin Oncol* 2002; **20**:1248–59.

Bookman M A. GOG0182-ICON5: 5-arm phase III randomised trial of paclitaxel (P) and carboplatin (C) vs combination with gemcitabine (G), PEGliposomal doxorubicin (D), or topotecan (T) in patients with advanced stage epithelial ovarian (EOC) or primary peritoneal (PPC) carcinoma [abstract]. *J Clin Oncol* 2006; **24**:5002.

Decker DG, Fleming TR, Malkasian GD Jr, et al. Cyclophosphamide plus cis-platinum in combination: treatment program for stage III or IV ovarian carcinoma. *Obstet Gynaecol* 1982; **60**:481–7.

du Bois A, Luck HJ, Meier W, et al. Arbeitsgemeinschaft Gynaekologische Onkologie (AGO) Ovarian Cancer Study Group. A randomised clinical trial of cisplatin/paclitaxel versus carboplatin/paclitaxel as first line treatment of ovarian cancer. *J Natl Cancer Inst* 2003; **95**:1320–9.

du Bois A, Quinn M, Thigpen T, et al. 2004 consensus statements on the management of ovarian cancer: final document of the 3rd International Gynecologic Cancer Intergroup Ovarian Cancer Consensus Conference (GCIC OCCC 2004). *Ann Oncol* 2005; **16**(suppl 8):viii7–viii12.

Earle CC, Schrag D, Neville BA, et al. Effect of surgeon speciality on processes of care and outcomes for ovarian cancer patients. *J Natl Cancer Inst* 2006; **98**(3):172–80.

Eisenhauer EA, ten Bokkel H Swenerton KD, et al. European-Canadian randomised trial of paclitaxel in relapsed ovarian cancer: high dose versus low dose and long versus short infusion. *J Clin Oncol* 1994; **12**:2654–66.

Markman M, Bundy BN, Alberts DS, et al. Phase III trial of standard dose intravenous cisplatin plus paclitaxel versus moderately high dose carboplatin followed by intravenous paclitaxel and intraperitoneal cisplatin in small volume stage III ovarian carcinoma: an intergroup study of the Gynecologic Oncology Group, Southwestern Oncology Group and Eastern Co-operative Oncology Group. *J Clin Oncol* 2001; **19**:1001–7.

McGowen L, Lesher L P, Norris H J, et al. Misstaging of ovarian cancer. *Obstet Gynecol* 1985; **65**:568–72.

McGuire WP, Rowinsky EK, Rosenshein NB, et al. Taxol: an unique antineoplastic agent with significant activity in advanced ovarian epithelial neoplasms. *Ann Intern Med* 1989;**111**:273–9.

Neijt JP, Engelholm SA, Tuxen MK, et al. Exploratory phase III study of paclitaxel and cisplatin versus paclitaxel and carboplatin in advanced ovarian cancer. *J Clin Oncol* 2000; **18**:3084–92.

Nguyen HN, Averette HE, Hoskins W, et al. National survey of ovarian carcinoma, part V: the impact of physicians' speciality on patients' survival. *Cancer* 1993; **72**:3663–70.

Omura G, Blessing JA, Ehrlich CE, et al. A randomised trial of cyclophosphamide and doxorubicin with or without cisplatin in advanced ovarian carcinoma: a Gynecologic Oncology Group Study. *Cancer* 1986; **57**:1725–30.

Omura GA, Bundy BN, Berek JS, et al. Randomised trial of cyclophosphamide plus cisplatin with or without doxorubicin in ovarian carcinoma: a Gynecologic Oncology Group Study. *J Clin Oncol* 1989; **7**:457–65.

Ozols RF, Bundy BN, Greer BE, et al. Phase III trial of carboplatin and paclitaxel compared with cisplatin and paclitaxel in patients with optimally resected stage III ovarian cancer: a Gynecologic Oncology Group study. *J Clin Oncol* 2003; **21**:3194–200.

Piccart MJ, Bertelsen K, James K, et al. Randomised intergroup trial of cisplatin-paclitaxel versus cisplatin-cyclophosphamide in women with advanced epithelial ovarian cancer: three year results. *J Natl Cancer Inst* 2000; **92**:699–708.

Sandercock J, Parmar MK, Torri V, et al. First line treatment for advanced ovarian cancer: paclitaxel platinum and the evidence. *Br J Cancer* 2002; **87**(8):815–24.

Vasey PA, Jayson GC, Gordan A, et al. Phase III randomised trial of docetaxel-carboplatin versus paclitaxel-carboplatin as first line chemotherapy for ovarian carcinoma. *J Natl Cancer Inst* 2004; **96**(22):1682–91.

Epithelial ovarian cancer: recurrent disease

Principles of management

Repeat chemotherapy, based on the treatment-free interval. It is now well established that the time to relapse after platinum-based therapy is a powerful predictor of future response to chemotherapy (platinum/non-platinum regimens) and OS. Patients with a platinum-free interval of <6 months (platinum-resistant disease) generally have lower response rates to subsequent chemotherapy and a poorer prognosis compared to patients with platinum sensitive disease (treatment free interval >6 months) (Gore et al. 1990; Kavanagh et al. 1995).

Repeat surgery in selected cases.

Chemotherapy

Although the majority of patients with advanced stage disease achieve a complete clinical remission with first-line therapy, disease will recur and the 5-year survival rate for this group is around 30% (Ozols 2006). It is important to recognize that while the median PFS has not changed in recent years (16–22 months), the median survival has improved (to 36–60 months), i.e. patients can expect to live longer after their first relapse than before.

The twin aims of therapy in this group of patients are therefore prolongation of survival and symptom control. A number of factors, such as the platinum sensitivity, the number of prior treatments, the potential cumulative toxicities of therapy, the patient's overall fitness (PS), disease volume and symptoms impact on the decision to retreat patients with recurrent disease. At recurrence immediate treatment is not required in women who are asymptomatic as there is no evidence that early administration of chemotherapy impacts positively on survival (Ozols 2005). A recent randomized trial reported a similar OS (41 months since completion of initial treatment) for patients who had second-line chemotherapy based on an increase in CA125 compared with patients who had chemotherapy started only after development of physical symptoms of relapse (which occurred an average of 5 months after CA125 rise) (Rustin and van der Burg 2009). The platinum-free interval is an important predictor of response to chemotherapy and thus prognosis. Patients with a treatment-free interval of >24 months had response rates of around 60% following re-treatment with platinum (Gore 2001).

Two randomized studies have demonstrated the benefit of combination chemotherapy in patients with platinum-sensitive recurrent disease (Parmar et al. 2003; Pfisterer et al. 2006). The ICON 4 study compared single-agent carboplatin with paclitaxel and carboplatin and demonstrated a 2-year survival rate of 50% vs. 57%, favouring combination chemotherapy (Parmer et al. 2003). The Arbeitsgemeinschaft Gynaekologische Onkologie (AGO) group compared carboplatin alone with gemcitabine plus carboplatin and showed response rates of 30.9% vs. 47.2% and median survival of 5.8 vs. 8.6 months (Pfisterer et al. 2006). In both studies combination therapy was associated with a modest overall increase in toxicity. Other combinations being considered in this context include carboplatin with liposomal doxorubicin (see later) and randomized trials in platinum-sensitive disease are ongoing.

As alternatives to platinum, a range of agents, including liposomal doxorubicin, topotecan, taxanes, gemcitabine and oral etoposide have shown activity. Paclitaxel, at a dose of between 135mg/m^2 and 175mg/m^2 (3 weekly) has shown response rates of 24–30% in patients with platinum resistant disease (Thigpen et al. 1994). Interestingly, a phase II study has demonstrated that if given weekly (80mg/m^2) response rates of around 20% can be achieved even in those patients with platinum and paclitaxel (3-weekly schedule) resistant disease (Markman et al. 2006). Further data comparing weekly vs. 3-weekly carboplatin and paclitaxel are awaited.

Topotecan has also been established as an active agent in ovarian cancer, with response rates of 12.4% in patients with platinum insensitive disease and 19.2% in those with platinum sensitive disease (Bookman et al. 1998). However, the standard (1.5mg/m^2) 5-day regimen is associated with significant bone marrow suppression, particularly in heavily pre-treated patients. A number of non-comparative studies in patients with recurrent disease have demonstrated that lower doses (1–1.25mg/m^2) or weekly schedules can be employed to reduce toxicity, whilst maintaining response rates (Gronlund et al. 2002; Bhoola et al. 2004).

In a phase II study liposomal doxorubicin at a dose of 50mg/m^2 (4-weekly) has shown response rates of 26% in patients with platinum and taxane resistant disease (Muggia et al. 1997). However at this dose toxicity, particularly palmer plantar erythrodysaesthesia, is often a limiting factor. Several studies have demonstrated that doses of 40mg/m^2 at 4-weekly intervals achieve response rates of 10–15% with a substantially improved adverse effect profile, which is essential in the palliative setting (Markman et al. 2000; Rose et al. 2001; Thigpen et al. 2005). In a randomized study of liposomal doxorubicin and topotecan overall response rates (19.7% vs. 17%) and survival (60 vs. 56.7 weeks) were statistically similar (Gordan et al. 2001). Many clinicians favour liposomal doxorubicin in patients with platinum-resistant disease because of ease of administration.

Hormones

Hormonal therapies have also been investigated in patients with recurrent ovarian cancer. A trial of high-dose megestrol acetate in a small group of patients with advanced disease has shown response rates of 10% (Veenhof et al. 1994). In a trial of tamoxifen in recurrent disease a complete response rate of 3.2% and partial responses of 6.4% were seen. However, response rates did not correlate with receptor status (Weiner et al. 1987). A more recent study with letrozole suggested that the potential of response could be predicted by quantitative analysis of hormone receptors (Smyth et al. 2007).

Surgery

Studies have demonstrated that for selected patients, surgery to resect recurrence is of benefit. The DESKTOP (Descriptive Evaluation of preoperative Selection KriTeria for Operability in recurrent OVARian cancer) trial set about to determine the criteria for selecting those patients who would derive the most benefit from surgery in relapsed ovarian cancer (Harter et al. 2006). This retrospective analysis of 267 patients determined that a combination of performance status, early FIGO stage initially and no residual disease after first cytoreductive surgery, and absence of ascites could predict complete resection in 79% of patients. Only complete resection was associated with prolonged survival in patients with recurrent disease. The importance of all these criteria for optimal patient selection for surgery in recurrent disease remains to be verified in the prospective AGO-DESKTOP II study.

Novel therapeutic approaches

There is increasing focus on agents that target specific molecular pathways within cancer cells. Angiogenesis in ovarian cancer cells is VEGF driven and agents such as bevacizumab, a recombinant humanized monoclonal antibody have shown activity in women with recurrent ovarian and primary peritoneal carcinoma. In the GOG 170 bevacizumab was given as a single agent to women with relapsed disease; 21% responded and 40% had a survival of 6 months or more (Burger et al. 2005). The main toxicities associated with bevacizumab include hypertension, increased bleeding tendency, and bowel perforation, which may be of particular concern in patients with extensive intra-abdominal cancer. Further studies are required to elucidate the role of bevacizumab in the initial treatment of ovarian cancer and its efficacy is currently being evaluated in patients who have been optimally debulked in the ongoing ICON 7 study.

Further reading

Bhoola SM, Coleman RL, Herzog T, et al. Retrospective analysis of weekly topotecan as salvage therapy in relapsed ovarian cancer. Gynecol Oncol 2004; **95**:564–9.

Bookman MA, Malmstrom H, Bolis G, et al. Topotecan for the treatment of advanced epithelial ovarian cancer: an open labelled phase II study in patients treated after prior chemotherapy that contained cisplatin or carboplatin and paclitaxel. J Clin Oncol 1998; **16**:3345–52.

Burger RA, Sill M, Monk BJ, et al. Phase II trial of bevacizumab in persistent or recurrent epithelial ovarian cancer (EOC) or primary peritoneal cancer (PPC): Gynecologic Oncology Group (GOG) Study [abstract]. J Clin Oncol 2005; **23**:5009.

Gordon AN, Fleagle DN, Guthrie D, et al. Recurrent epithelial ovarian cancer: a randomised phase III study of pegylated liposomal doxorubicin versus topotecan. J Clin Oncol 2001; **19**:3312–22.

Gore M. Treatment of relapsed epithelial ovarian cancer: In Perry MC (ed) American Society of Clinical Oncology: 2001 Educational Book, pp.468–76. Alexandria, VA: American Society of Clinical Oncology, 2001.

Gore ME, Fryatt I, Wiltshaw E, et al. Treatment of relapsed carcinoma of the ovary with cisplatin or carboplatin following initial treatment with these compounds. Gynecol Oncol 1990; **36**:207–11.

Gore M. Treatment of relapsed epithelial ovarian cancer: In Perry MC (ed) American Society of Clinical Oncology: 2001 Educational Book, pp.468–76. Alexandria, VA: American Society of Clinical Oncology, 2001.

Gronlund B, Hansen HH, Hogdall C, et al. Efficacy of low dose topotecan in second line treatment for patients with epithelial ovarian cancer. Cancer 2002; **95**:1656–62.

Harter P, Bois A, Hahmann M, et al. Surgery in recurrent ovarian cancer: the Arbeitsgemeinschaft Gynaekologische Onkologie (AGO) DESKTOP OVAR trial. Ann Surg Oncol 2006; **12**:1702–10.

Kavanagh J, Tresukosol D, Edwards C, et al. Carboplatin reinduction after taxane in patients with platinum refractory epithelial ovarian cancer. J Clin Oncol 1995; **13**:1584–8.

Markman M, Kennedy A, Webster K, et al. Phase II trial of liposomal doxorubicin (40 mg/m^2) in platinum/paclitaxel refractory ovarian and fallopian tube cancers and primary carcinoma of the peritoneum. Gynecol Oncol 2000; **78**:369–72.

Markman M, Blessing J, Rubin SC, et al. Phase II trial of weekly paclitaxel (80mg/m^2) in platinum and paclitaxel resistant ovarian and primary peritoneal cancers: a Gynecologic Oncology Group study. Gynecol Oncol 2006; **101**:436–40.

Muggia FM, Hainsworth JD, Jeffers S, et al. Phase II study of liposomal doxorubicin in refractory ovarian cancer: antitumour activity and toxicity modification by liposomal encapsulation. J Clin Oncol 1997; **15**:987–93.

Ozols RF. Treatment goals in ovarian cancer. Int J Gynaecol Cancer 2005; **1**(suppl 1):3–11.

Ozols RF. Systemic therapy for ovarian cancer: current status and new treatments. Semin Oncol 2006; **33**(2 suppl 6):S3–S11.

Parmar MK, Ledermann JA, Colombo N, et al. Paclitaxel plus platinum based chemotherapy versus conventional platinum based chemotherapy in women with relapsed ovarian cancer. The ICON 4/AGO-OVAR-2.2 trial. Lancet 2003; **261**:2099–106.

Pfisterer J, Plante M, Vergote I, et al. Gemcitabine plus carboplatin compared with carboplatin in patients with platinum-sensitive recurrent ovarian cancer: an intergroup trial of the AGO-OVAR, the NCIC CTG, and the EORTC GCG. J Clin Oncol 2006; **24**:4699–707.

Rose PG, Maxson JH, Fusco N, et al. Liposomal doxorubicin in ovarian, peritoneal, and tubal carcinoma: a retrospective, comparative study of single agent dosages. Gynecol Oncol 2001; **82**:323–8.

Rustin GJ, van der Burg ME. A randomized trial in ovarian cancer (OC) of early treatment of relapse based on CA125 level alone versus delayed treatment based on conventional clinical indicators (MRCOV05/EORTC 55955 trials). J Clin Oncol 2009; **27**:18s(suppl; abstr 1)

Smyth JF, Gourley C, Walker G, et al. Antiestrogen therapy is active in selected ovarian cancer cases: the use of letrozole in estrogen receptor-positive patients. Clin Cancer Res 2007; **13**(12):3617–22.

Thigpen JT, Blessing JA, Ball H, et al. Phase II trial of paclitaxel in patients with progressive ovarian cancer after platinum-based therapy: a Gynecologic Oncology Group study. J Clin Oncol 1994; **12**:1748–53.

Thigpen JT, Aghajanian CA, Alberts DS, et al. Role of pegylated liposomal doxorubicin in ovarian cancer. Gynecol Oncol 2005; **96**:10–18.

Veenhof CH, van der Burg ME, Nooy M, et al. Phase II study of high dose megestrol acetate in patients with advanced ovarian carcinoma. Eur J Cancer 1994; **30A**:697–98.

Weiner SA, Alberts DS, Surwit EA, et al. Tamoxifen therapy in recurrent epithelial ovarian carcinoma. Gynecol Oncol 1987; **27**:208–13.

Epithelial ovarian cancer: palliative care issues

The 5-year survival rates of women with ovarian cancer are around 45%; however, many will experience multiple disease relapses during this period and contend with significant morbidity (Booth et al. 1989). Response rates to chemotherapy decline with subsequent treatments and there comes a point where toxicity will outweigh therapeutic benefit and supportive or palliative care only will be most appropriate for patients.

Due to the extensive spread of ovarian cancer within the abdominoperitoneal cavity, bowel obstruction is a major end of life complication. One study demonstrated that in 62 patients, within the last 3 months of life, bowel obstruction occurred in 13 patients. Once a provisional diagnosis of bowel obstruction has been made, a CT scan may be useful to determine the site of obstruction. Initial conservative measures to rest the bowel such as withholding oral intake and nasogastric tube suction should be instituted. A multidisciplinary approach is often required and a surgical opinion should also be sought early on. However in many patients there are multiple levels of obstruction and surgery may not be feasible. Other factors that also need to be taken into consideration are the patient's overall condition, the aggressiveness of disease, disease extent, and the availability of further chemotherapy. There are some data to suggest that there are no survival differences in chemotherapy-refractory patients treated surgically or conservatively (von Gruenigan et al. 2003). If surgery is not possible or is considered to be inappropriate, other palliative measures such as stent placement to expand the bowel may be considered in selected patients (Baron et al. 2005).

However, in the majority of patients medical management with a combination of octreotide, corticosteroids, analgesia, and antiemetics is often more appropriate. Octreotide, a somatostatin analogue that blocks certain gut hormones that increase intestinal secretions such as vasointestinal peptide (VIP), at a dose of between 600–800mcg has been shown to provide symptom palliation by bowel decompression (Mercadante et al. 1993). Dexamethasone (8mg/day IV or SC) improved pain, nausea, and vomiting in 9 of 13 patients with bowel obstruction, an effect most likely to be due to its well-described antiemetic and anti-inflammatory effects (Phillip et al. 1999). Adequate analgesia (often a subcutaneous morphine infusion) and antiemetics are also required in the medical management of these patients, although metoclopramide should be avoided because of its effects on bowel motility (von Gruenigan et al. 2003).

Often the most distressing feature of inoperable bowel obstruction for patients and their families will be the inability to maintain oral intake. Multiple randomized studies have demonstrated that in advanced disease parental nutrition does not improve QoL or improve survival and therefore its use is not advocated in patients with advanced ovarian cancer who have inoperable bowel obstruction (American College of Physicians 1989; Barber et al. 1998; Whitworth et al. 2004).

Conclusion

It is evident that ovarian cancer may present non-specifically and that early diagnosis is associated with better overall survival. A multidisciplinary approach is required at all stages in the diagnosis and management of patients with early and advanced stages of disease. The mainstay of treatment is often a combination of surgery and chemotherapy, and improvements in the treatment of relapsed disease have led to overall increases in life expectancy. However, recurrent disease is ultimately fatal, and expert palliative care is essential. Novel therapeutic approaches including antiangiogenic agents and molecular targeted therapy show considerable promise for improvements in the near future.

Further reading

American College of Physicians. Parental nutrition in patients receiving cancer therapy. *Ann Intern Med* 1989; **110**:734–6.

Barber MD, Fearon KC, Delmore G, et al. Should cancer patients with incurable disease receive parenteral or enteral nutritional support? *Eur J Cancer* 1998; **34**:279–85.

Baron TH. Colonic stenting: technique, technology and outcomes for malignant and benign disease. *Gastrolintest Endosc Clin N Am* 2005; **15**:757–71.

Booth M, Beral V, Smith P. Risk factors for ovarian cancer: a case control study. *Br J Cancer* 1989; **60**:592–8.

Mercadante S, Spoldi E, Carcni A, et al. Octreotide in relieving gastrointestinal symptoms due to bowel obstruction. *Palliat Med* 1993; **7**:295–9.

Phillip J, Lickiss N, Grant PT, et al. Corticosteroids in the treatment of bowel obstruction on a gynaecological oncology unit. *Gynecol Oncol* 1999; **74**:68–73.

von Gruenigan VE, Frasure HE, Reidy AM, et al. Clinical disease course during the last year in ovarian cancer. *Gynecol Oncol* 2003; **90**:619–24.

Whitworth MK, Whitfield A, Holm S, et al. Doctor, does this mean that I am going to starve to death? *J Clin Oncol* 2004; **22**:199–201.

Malignant ovarian germ cell tumours: introduction

Overview

Ovarian germ cell tumours (OGCT) are derived from embryonic germ cells and may undergo germinomatous or embryonic differentiation. They account for 20–25% of all ovarian tumours, the vast majority of which are benign teratoma. Malignant ovarian germ cell tumours (MOGCT) account for <5% of all ovarian cancers. OGCTs occur at one-tenth the frequency of testicular germ cell tumours.

Although rare, MOGCT occur in children and young women. Dysgerminoma, immature teratoma, yolk sac tumours, and mixed germ cell tumours make up >90% of all malignant germ cell tumours. Embryonal carcinoma, choriocarcinoma, and polyembryoma make up the remaining 5–10% and have the worst outcome.

Epidemiology

The incidence of MOGCT is 0.41 per 100,000 in the USA and 0.2 per 100,000 in the UK. MOGCT occur more frequently in Asian and black women than Caucasians (3:1). Peak incidence is in young women or adolescent girls and the median age at presentation is 18.

Aetiology

The exact aetiology is unknown. Five per cent of dysgerminomas are associated with phenotypic females who have constitutional cytogenetic abnormality of all or part of the Y chromosome. These include pure gonadal dysgenesis (46XY), mixed gonadal dysgenesis (45X, 46XY), or complete androgen insensitivity (testicular feminization, 46XY). In these patients dysgerminomas may develop within a gonadoblastoma (a benign ovarian tumour composed of germ cell and sex cord stroma)

Pathology

Germ cell tumour histologies mimic the developing embryo and are classified according to degree and character of cellular differentiation. The most recent version of the WHO classification classifies germ cells into three categories: primitive germ cell tumours, biphasic or triphasic teratoma, and monodermal teratoma and somatic-type tumours associated with dermoid cysts.

Primitive germ cell tumours

Dysgerminomas (33%) are pale and lobulated tumours composed of monotonous undifferentiated cells. Patients often present with abdominal enlargement and pain due to torsion or rupture.

Yolk sac tumours or endodermal sinus tumours (15%) are smooth tumours with a haemorrhagic and necrotic surface. Histology shows a range of histological patterns: polyvesicular vitelline tumours, glandular and hepatoid variants. Patients often present with abdominal pain and a pelvic mass. Tumour growth can be rapid, and pain may be acute, mimicking appendicitis. Spread is to the peritoneum and omentum, para-aortic lymph nodes, and liver.

Embryonal tumours (4%) are made up of pluripotent epithelial-like cells resembling those of the embryonic disc, with syncytiotrophoblastic cells and sometimes mesenchymal tissue. Tumours appear haemorrhagic and necrotic and display papillary or gland-like structures. They most commonly present with an abdominal or pelvic mass. Over 50% have hormonal abnormalities such as precocious puberty, irregular vaginal bleeding, amenorrhoea, or hirsutism.

Primary choriocarcinoma of the ovary is very rare. Tumours show extra-embryonic differentiation. It is distinguished from gestational choriocarcinoma by lack of paternal DNA.

Polyembryona is also very rare. Morphologically these tumours resemble normal embryo.

Mixed germ cell tumours (5%) are most commonly composed of dysgerminoma and yolk sac tumours. Teratocarcinomas are a combination of teratoma and embryonal carcinoma. Tumours with a component of dysgerminoma are bilateral in 10% of cases.

Biphasic or triphasic teratoma

Immature teratoma (36%) consists of variable amounts of tissue resembling early neural tissue, cartilage, bone, muscle, etc. It is graded according to the proportion of tissue containing immature neural elements: I, II, and III if they have 0–1, 2–3, and ≥4 low-power fields (x40) containing immature neuroepithelium respectively.

Monodermal highly specialized teratoma

These are composed mainly (i.e. 50%) of one mature tissue element. The two most common types are Struma ovarii, comprised of thyroid tissue, and carcinoid. Less than 5% of cases are malignant.

Somatic type tumours associated with biphasic or triphasic teratoma

Approximately 1% of mature cystic teratomas will undergo malignant degeneration. Squamous cell carcinoma is the most common secondary tumour. However, melanoma, sarcoma, adenocarcinoma and others have been reported. Treatment is as for that of the secondary tumour histiotype.

Immunohistochemical and molecular features

Placental alkaline phosphatase (PLAP) is expressed in >95% of cases of dysgerminoma. OCT 3/4 is a marker for pluripotency and is expressed in all dysgerminomas and embryonal carcinomas. C-kit (CD117) is expressed in 87% of dysgerminomas.

Eighty one per cent of dysgerminoma and other primitive germ cell tumours show gains in chromosome 12p.

Clinical features

- Abdominal pain (>85%). Particularly associated with rapidly growing tumours, i.e. dysgerminoma and endodermal sinus tumours (50% have symptoms of <1 week's duration).
- Abdominal distension (35%).
- Acute abdominal pain due to rupture, torsion, or haemorrhage (10%).
- Precocious puberty in premenarchal patients associated with increased β-hCG and/or oestrogen secretion, particularly choriocarcinoma.
- Abnormal vaginal bleeding (10%) in postmenarchal patients with increased β-hCG and/or oestrogen production.
- Hirsutism if there is androgen secretion (some embryonal tumours).
- Primary amenorrhea, undeveloped or absent secondary sexual characteristics, ambiguous genitalia secondary to gonadal dysgenesis.

Examination

- Abdominal and/or adnexal mass (85% of patients).
- Ascites (20%).

- Lymphadenopathy—common route of dissemination of dysgerminoma.
- Signs of distant spread—hepatomegaly, decreased air entry on chest examination, bony tenderness, particularly choriocarcinoma, yolk sac tumour.

Investigations

The initial investigation of women with pain and/or abdominal mass is an abdominal ultrasound and transvaginal ultrasound depending on position. In suspected cases of germ cell tumours, serum tumour markers (AFP, β-hCG, LDH) should be estimated in addition to CA125 for an undiagnosed pelvic mass. Other investigations include:

- FBC, urea and electrolytes, liver function tests, calcium.
- CXR.
- CT abdomen/pelvis if U/S does not show characteristics of dermoid cyst.
- MRI if CT contraindicated or for further imaging if indicated.
- Karyotyping for premenarchal patient with an ovarian mass.
- Lung function tests for those likely to require adjuvant chemotherapy including bleomycin.

Diagnosis

Tumour markers

AFP and β-hCG can be used for diagnosis, to monitor response to treatment, and in post-treatment surveillance. Up to 5% of patients with dysgerminoma have elevated β-hCG due to the presence of multinucleated syncytiotrophoblastic giant cells. However, a β-hCG level of >100 IU/L or an elevated AFP suggests the presence of non-dysgerminomatous elements in the tumour. Most endodermal sinus tumours secrete AFP. Polyembryoma may secrete both AFP and β-hCG. Immature teratomas may secrete AFP (30%) and choriocarcinomas always produce β-hCG.

LDH is raised in 88% of cases and is associated with high tumour burden.

Imaging

Most MOGCT are unilateral with the exception of dysgerminomas, which are bilateral in 10–15% of cases. Dysgerminoma appears as a multiloculated solid mass divided by fibrovascular septa on CT and MRI. There may be areas of high or low signal intensity due to fresh blood. Calcification is rare in dysgerminoma. Non-dysgerminoma appears as a large irregular heterogeneous mass lesion with solid and cystic components which may contain calcifications (40%), foci of fat, and areas of haemorrhage. All types of MOGCT can be associated with abdominal lymphadenopathy, peritoneal or omental disease and liver metastasis.

There are no studies of use of PET in OGCT; however, clinical uses of PET scan in testicular germ cell tumours may be applicable to MOGCT.

Staging

MOGCT are staged according the FIGO staging for ovarian cancer (see Chapter 4, Epithelial ovarian cancer: investigations, staging, and prognosis, Table 4.7.7, p.348). Unlike epithelial ovarian cancer, most malignant germ cell tumours present at an early stage: 60–70% stage I, 25–30% stage II and stage III, and rarely stage IV.

Further reading

Gershenson DM. Management of ovarian germ cell tumors. *Clin Oncol* 2007; **25**:2938–43.

Pectasides D, Pectasides E and Kassanos D. Germ cell tumours of the ovary. *Cancer Treat Rev* 2008; **34**:427–41.

Malignant ovarian germ cell tumours: management

General principles of surgery

Staging laparotomy follows the same principles as for epithelial ovarian cancer. Fertility preservation can be achieved even in extensive and metastatic disease without compromising the chances of cure. Patients with dysgerminoma have an increased risk of bilateral disease and should have a biopsy of the contralateral ovary. Patients with dysgenetic gonads and Y chromosome should have both ovaries removed, but the uterus may be left *in situ* for future assisted reproduction. The contralateral ovary should be carefully examined and biopsied if necessary. The role of routine lymphadenectomy is not defined.

Primary surgery

Surgery as the initial management is aimed at establishing the diagnosis, staging, and complete removal or optimal debulking of the tumour. Fertility-sparing surgery with unilateral salpingo-oophorectomy is the standard in young women with tumours confined to the ovary. For patients with advanced disease wishing to preserve fertility, optimal debulking is attempted with preservation of the contralateral ovary, fallopian tube, and uterus. Total hysterectomy and unilateral oophorectomy is appropriate for most women who have completed their family.

Role of optimal cytoreduction

Although optimal cytoreduction is recommended whenever feasible, the role of such surgery is less well defined than for epithelial ovarian cancer. Morbidity considerations may take greater precedence in attempting optimal debulking of germ cell tumours compared with epithelial ovarian tumours. Though there are no randomized studies, retrospective series show a survival benefit for women with less bulky or completely resected disease. The largest series have shown DFS of 65–68% for patients who have had completely resected disease compared with 28–34% who have not. However, patients with dysgerminomas do uniformly well regardless of residual disease with long-term survival and in them optimal debulking may be less important.

Second-look laparotomy

In those with complete primary debulking and normal radiology and serum markers following chemotherapy, second-look laparotomy is not recommended due to the low incidence of viable residual tumour. Laparotomy is negative in >95% of patients with non-dysgerminomas and approaches 100% for dysgerminoma.

A second-look procedure would be recommended for a subset of patients with a teratoma (pure or mixed) and persistent radiological abnormalities and normal serum tumour markers to avoid growing teratoma syndrome. This syndrome results from continued growth of mature teratoma, which may cause local compressive symptoms or rarely undergo malignant transformation. Immature teratoma may undergo a transformation to benign mature teratoma following chemotherapy—a process known as chemotherapeutic retroconversion which is almost exclusive to this histiotype.

For patients with non-teratoma germ cell tumours at diagnosis and residual disease postchemotherapy, second-look laparotomy is not currently standard since viable tumour is uncommon and surgery has not been proved to alter outcome.

For residual or progressive malignant disease following primary chemotherapy, the role of salvage surgery has not been established and chemotherapy remains the standard of care with the exception of immature teratoma (see secondary cytoreduction) for which surgery and chemotherapy may be the treatment of choice.

Neo-adjuvant chemotherapy

MOGCT usually present at an early stage, and as for epithelial ovarian tumours, primary debulking is the standard of care. Published data about neoadjuvant chemotherapy is sparse.

Postoperative management strategies

Stage IA dysgerminoma and stage IA, grade 1 immature teratoma are treated adequately with surgery alone followed by surveillance. The recurrence rate is relatively low at 15–25%, and recurrences can be effectively salvaged with chemotherapy. The overall cure rate for stage IA dysgerminoma with surveillance is 97%.

All other patients are treated with postoperative chemotherapy.

Radiotherapy, has a limited, if any, role now but may still be an option for women with contraindications to chemotherapy, or in those who decline chemotherapy.

Extending surveillance strategies

It has been proposed that surveillance is extended to patients with stage IA disease other than dysgerminoma, including grade II immature teratoma. Results of small studies have supported this approach; however, acceptance of surveillance into standard practice awaits validation in larger studies.

Adjuvant chemotherapy

Chemotherapy overview

Before the introduction of cisplatin based chemotherapy in the 1970s, long-term survival was <50% for MOGCT. With current platinum-based regimens 95–100% of patients with early disease, and 75–80% of patients with advanced disease are long-term survivors. For patients with dysgerminoma, the prognosis is even better with cure rates of >95% even in advanced disease.

The platinum-based regimen bleomycin, etoposide, and cisplatin (BEP) is the gold standard postoperative treatment.

In the largest study of adjuvant BEP, a GOG study by Williams et al., 93 patients with stages I–III completely resected non-dysgerminomatous MOGCT received 3 cycles of adjuvant 5-day BEP (bleomycin 30IU IV weekly, etoposide 100mg/m^2 for days 1–5, cisplatin 20mg/m^2 days 1–5 q21). Of these, 89 (96%) remained continuously disease-free at a median follow-up of 38.6 months. Two patients developed secondary haematological malignancies. This compares with the results of a previous series showing DFS of 78% (n = 54) in patients treated with VAC.

Attempts to omit bleomycin from chemotherapy for metastatic testicular germ cell regimens, or replace cisplatin with carboplatin resulted in inferior outcomes. These results have been extrapolated to chemotherapy regimens for MOGCT.

Patients are considered to have received an optimal regimen if they have received one containing cisplatin and bleomycin.

3-day BEP

A 3-day modified bleomycin, etoposide and cisplatin (mBEP) regimen appears feasible and effective based on a study in 48 patients with stages I–IV MOGCT (bleomycin 15mg IV days 1–3, etoposide 120mg/m^2 IV days 1–3, and cisplatin 40mg/m^2 IV days 1–3 + G-CSF q21). Patients received either 3 courses of mBEP (completely resected stages I–III) or 4 courses (incompletely resected or stage IV). DFS at 5 years was 96%. Two of the 10 patients with suboptimally debulked non-dysgerminomatous tumour experienced progressive disease. All 22 patients with stage I or II disease, and all 13 patients with dysgerminoma remained free of disease.

The described study utilized a lower dose of bleomycin to avoid lung toxicity compared with 3-day BEP regimen used for testicular germ cell tumours (bleomycin 30IU, days 2, 8, 15, etoposide 165mg/m^2 days 1–3 and cisplatin 50mg/m^2 days 1–2 q21). Although 5-day BEP remains the gold standard many have moved to the 3-day testicular BEP regimen for completely resected germ cell tumours. Some centres choose to substitute a lower dose of etoposide (120mg/m^2 days 1–3) and/or of bleomycin (10–15IU). However, there is no randomized trial to guide such a practice.

Alternative adjuvant regimens

Attempts are underway to evaluate less toxic regimens in patients with curable disease and more effective treatments for advanced disease.

• Carboplatin and etoposide:

Carboplatin and etoposide have been evaluated as a less toxic regimen for those with completely resected stage IB–III dysgerminoma. The GOG study evaluated adjuvant chemotherapy with 3 courses of carboplatin (400mg/m^2 on day 1) and etoposide (120mg/m^2 on days 1–3 every 4 weeks) in 42 patients. None of the 39 evaluable patients developed recurrence at a median follow-up of 7.8 years. The regimen was well tolerated and has the advantage of minimal neurotoxicity compared with BEP.

Although promising, carboplatin and etoposide awaits validation and has not replaced adjuvant BEP as standard treatment for dysgerminoma. However, it may be considered as an alternative to BEP for stage IB–III dysgerminoma patients for whom minimizing toxicity is critical or where reducing the number of treatment days is important.

• Carboplatin:

A single cycle of carboplatin (or surveillance) is accepted treatment for stage I testicular dysgerminoma. It is not known if a subset of patients with MOGCT may be cured with one course of single agent carboplatin.

• POMB-ACE/POMB-ACE-PAV:

Similar results as obtained with adjuvant BEP have been reported for patients with OGCT receiving cisplatin, vincristine, methotrexate, bleomycin–actinomycin D, cyclophosphamide and etoposide (POMB-ACE), though there are no direct comparisons. This regimen allows early exposure to the cytotoxic drugs in order to minimize the development of drug resistance. A study of 113 patients showed 10-year DFS of 82%. These survival figures are lower than published using BEP and other regimens (87–97%); however a higher proportion of patients in this study had stages II–IV (80% vs. 31–69%).

POMB-ACE is used instead of BEP as adjuvant treatment for poor prognosis tumours in some UK centres.

The POMB-ACE-PAV regimen includes additionally cisplatin, dactinomycin, and vinblastine. In a retrospective study of 20 patients (14 of whom had stages II–IV disease) who received this adjuvant regimen, 95% were disease-free at a median of 66 months. There were no treatment related deaths in either study.

Other treatments developed for intermediate and poor prognosis testicular germ cell tumours using dose intensified and broadened regimens have also been used to treat MOGCT, though patient numbers remain small.

Practical considerations for chemotherapy

• Treatment should start within 7–10 days of surgery.
• Dose reductions or delays are not indicated unless serious complications have arisen as a consequence.
• Full doses of chemotherapy should be administered at the scheduled time, regardless of white blood cell count.
• Febrile neutropenia rate with 5- and 3-day BEP is approximately 10%.
• Haematopoietic support is given in the first instance, as reductions in dose intensity may compromise cure.

Number of courses

Unlike in testicular tumours where validated risk stratification determines the type and number of cycles of chemotherapy, the optimal number of courses of chemotherapy for malignant OGCT is unclear.

Patients with completely resected stage IB–III non-dysgerminomatous tumours should receive 3–4 cycles of adjuvant BEP. Results from a GOG study suggest that 3 cycles are probably sufficient; however in the absence of randomized controlled trials, many would treat only completely resected stage I non-dysgerminomas with 3 cycles, and completely resected stage II–IV with 4 cycles. Dysgerminomas are treated similarly, though the outlook is better still. Given the chemosensitivity of dysgerminoma, 3 cycles would appear sufficient treatment for stage I completely resected dysgerminoma, with 4 cycles reserved for stage II–IV. For patients receiving 4 cycles, bleomycin is commonly omitted after cycle 3 (total cumulative dose 270 IU) to avoid lung toxicity. Total doses of >300 IU are associated with increased risk of lung toxicity in patients receiving BEP for testicular germ cell tumours.

Patients with incompletely resected disease or stage IV non-dysgerminomatous tumours are treated with 4 cycles of 5-day BEP. Adopting the principles of treatment from other chemosensitive tumours, common practice is to continue chemotherapy for 2 cycles after tumour markers return to normal. Up to 6 cycles may be needed depending on serum tumour marker status, bulkiness of residual disease, and histology. In those with initially raised tumour markers, failure to achieve a negative tumour marker status at 4 cycles is generally considered a failure of response. This should be treated as chemorefractory disease with salvage chemotherapy (see later).

Malignant ovarian germ cell tumours: prognosis, surveillance, and management of recurrence

Prognostic factors

The most important prognostic factors are:

• Histiotype: dysgerminoma has the best prognosis among all histological types in all studies with cure rates of >95% even in advanced disease. There is a poor prognosis for yolk sac tumour and choriocarcinomas with <30% cure for advanced stages.
• Stage: see Table 4.7.8.

Other reported prognostic factors include:

• Amount of residual tumour (≤2cm) following primary surgery
• Raised tumour markers at diagnosis: 1 year survival of 90% for patients with raised β-hCG and AFP compared with 50% for those with normal markers.
• Grade of immature teratoma in addition to stage has been reported to be important. Five-year survival is 91% for grades I and II compared with 25% for those with grade III.
• For endodermal sinus tumours, stage and size of residual tumour are important prognostic factors.

Post treatment surveillance

Ninety per cent of relapses occur within 2 years. Dysgerminomas may recur late, up to 10 years after primary treatment. Patients are followed by serial measurement of tumour markers, radiological and clinical assessment. AFP and β-hCG are routinely measured for all patients even if not initially raised since occasionally recurrences may start to produce tumour markers. Clinical assessment, measurement of serological markers and radiological assessment with CT chest/abdomen/pelvis every 3 months for the first 2 years, 6-monthly for 3 years, then annually to 5 years is recommended for non-dysgerminomatous tumours, and to 10 years for dysgerminomas (NCCN).

Management of relapsed and refractory tumours

Approximately 20% of advanced germ cell tumours will be resistant to treatment or will relapse at a later stage.

For patients failing primary treatment, either with persistent, progressive, or relapsed disease, described in the literature as chemorefractory, the outlook is poor. Previous descriptions of 50% long-term survival are probably an overestimate due to suboptimal primary treatment and small sample sizes. More recent studies suggest much lower long-term survival rates.

Table 4.7.8 Five-year survival for all MOGCT

FIGO Stage	5-year survival overall
I	100%
II	85
III	79
IV	71

Murugaesu et al. (2006) showed a 10% long-term survival amongst the 20 patients who relapsed following primary surgery and optimal chemotherapy. All patients were treated with salvage chemotherapy, including high dose chemotherapy (HDCT) in 4 cases. This compares unfavourably with long-term survival rates for relapsed testicular germ cell tumours of approximately 25%.

For patients relapsing >4 weeks after completion of chemotherapy (platinum sensitive), salvage chemotherapy regimens have been based on those used for testicular germ cell tumours, and incorporate ifosfamide and platinum. Active regimes include paclitaxel, ifosfamide and cisplatin (TIP); etoposide, ifosfamide, and cisplatin (VIP); and vinblastine, ifosfamide, and cisplatin (VeIP), or BEP for those who have not previously received this regimen.

Disease which shows an incomplete response to first-line chemotherapy or relapses within 4 weeks of completing cisplatin chemotherapy has been described as either platinum-resistant or platinum-refractory. This group of patients rarely show long-term survival with conventional dose chemotherapy. These patients should be referred to a tertiary centre for consideration of alternative regimens. Although there are no positive randomized controlled trials, case series of testicular germ cell tumours favour HDCT with peripheral stem cell support. A recently published retrospective series showed DFS of 55% in patients with incomplete response to primary treatment (n = 100) (Einhorn 2007). All patients also had surgery for residual disease after chemotherapy. Response rates compared favourably with VIP in the platinum sensitive group.

Patients failing second-line conventional dose chemotherapy should also be considered for HDCT.

For patients with recurrent or resistant disease after multiple lines of chemotherapy or HDCT, responses rates of between 10–20% are seen with single agents such as oral etoposide, paclitaxel, gemcitabine, and oxaliplatin.

Salvage surgery

The value of salvage surgery in OGCT remains unclear. Although there are no randomized controlled trials to address this question, survival rates compare favourably with those seen in patients treated for relapse with chemotherapy alone and evidence suggests that salvage surgery is an important component of management of relapse.

In a retrospective study carried out by Li et al. (2007) of 34 patients who underwent salvage cytoreductive surgery, 5-year survival was 61% in the optimally cytoreduced group (≤1cm), compared with 14% in the sub-optimally cytoreduced tumours. Most patients (two-thirds) had recurrent disease, the remainder having progressive or persistent disease. All cases were treated with chemotherapy following surgery

Another study of 20 patients (14 with progressive disease, 3 persistent and 3 recurrent), 60% had long-term DFS following salvage surgery (and chemotherapy for most). For those patients in whom optimal debulking was achieved (≤2cm) there was a trend towards better survival (64% vs. 25%).

For testicular teratoma patients, relapses at >2 years are generally considered relatively chemoresistant and are treated with surgery first, followed by chemotherapy. It is not known if the same is true for OGCTs.

Issues of survivorship

Secondary malignancies

A dose-related risk of leukaemia is associated with administration of etoposide. Those treated with 3 or 4 cycles of BEP will receive <20,000mg/m^2, with an risk of <0.5% of leukaemia. Patients requiring extended treatment or salvage chemotherapy will often receive>2000mg/m^2, with an increase in the associated risk of malignancy of up to 5%.

Fertility and teratogenesis

Most studies do not suggest an adverse effect on fertility or increased risk of teratogenesis following fertility preserving surgery and chemotherapy for MOGCT.

One study of 71 patients reported that 87% of patients receiving chemotherapy were menstruating at follow-up compared with a control group of 83.2% (Gershenson 2007).

Studies report success rates of 68–100% in those trying to conceive. From the available evidence, fertility may be unaffected or marginally affected by treatment for MOGCT. The risk of premature menopause is estimated at 3%.

Most studies do not report any birth defects among babies born to women following treatment for germ cell tumours: three studies report no birth defects among a total of 49 babies born to women treated for MOGCT. In the study carried out by Zanetti et al. (2001) the rates of malformation were slightly higher than the general population (3%). However there was no difference among women who were and were not treated with chemotherapy (7.1% and 7.3% respectively). Miscarriages were in the expected range for the general population.

Prospective reporting of reproductive and sexual function suggests that there is some increase in gynaecologic symptoms and diminution in sexual pleasure following treatment for MOGCT. However survivors tended to have stronger more positive relationships with their partners (Gershenson 2007).

In summary, with fertility preservation, the majority of patients regain normal menstrual function after treatment for malignant OGCT and a significant proportion will be able to conceive. There is no evidence to suggest treatment predisposes to early pregnancy loss or congenital malformation of the fetus.

Conclusion

MOGCTs are rare tumours, the majority of which occur at a critical point in the development of young women. Most patients can be treated with fertility-preserving surgery.

Even in patients with metastasis at presentation, the aim of surgery is fertility preservation with maximal cytoreduction. All patients except those with adequately staged FIGO stage IA dysgerminoma and stage IA grade I immature teratoma should receive postoperative chemotherapy with the BEP regimen which gives a 95% cure rate for stage I and 75% cure rate for advanced disease. For patients whose disease relapses, salvage with conventional TIP, VIP, or VeIP produces long-term survival in 10–50%. Those with primarily platinum-resistant disease should be referred to a tertiary referral centre for consideration of HDCT. Most of these young patients will recover menstruation within 2–6 months of completing their chemotherapy and provided they have not had radical surgery, most of these patients should be able to complete their families normally. The incidence of other late effects such as secondary leukaemia is also rare in those treated with BEP but increased in the few who require a greater number of cycles of BEP or salvage chemotherapy.

Further reading

Dimopoulos, MA, Papdimitriou D, Hamilos G, et al. Treatment of ovarian germ cell tumours with a 3-day bleomycin, etoposide, and cisplatin regimen: a prospective multicenter study. *Gynecol Oncol* 2004; **95**:695–700.

Einhorn LH, Williams SD, Chamness A, et al. High-dose chemotherapy and stem-cell rescue for metastatic germ-cell tumors, *N Engl J Med* 2007; **357**:340–8.

Gershenson DM. Management of ovarian germ cell tumors. *Clin Oncol* 2007; **25**:2938

Gershenson DM, Miller AM, Champion VL, et al. Reproductive and sexual function after platinum-based chemotherapy in long-term ovarian germ cell tumor survivors: a Gynecologic Oncology Group Study, *J Clin Oncol* 2007; **25**:2792–7.

Li J, Yang W, Wu X. Prognostic factors and role of salvage surgery in chemorefractory ovarian germ cell malignancies: a study in Chinese patients, *Gynecol Oncol* 2007; **105**:769–75.

Murugaesu N, Schmid P, Dancey G, et al. Malignant ovarian germ cell tumors: identification of novel prognostic markers and long-term outcome after multimodality treatment, *J Clin Oncol* 2006; **24**:4862–6.

Williams SD, Blessing JA, Liau S-Y, et al. Adjuvant therapy of ovarian germ cell tumours with cisplatin, etoposide and bleomycin: a trial of the Gynecologic Oncology Group. *J Clin Oncol* 1994; **12**:701–6

Zanetta G, Bonazzi C, Cantu M, et al. Survival and reproductive function after treatment of malignant germ cell ovarian tumors, *J Clin Oncol* 2001; **19**:1015–20.

Sex cord-stromal tumours

Introduction and classification

Sex cord-stromal tumours (SCST) account for approximately 7% of all primary malignant ovarian neoplasms, and generally present early, have an indolent course, and favourable prognosis. Table 4.7.9 gives the classification of SCSTs.

Granulosa cell tumours

Granulosa cell tumours (GCTs) are the most common malignant SCST accounting for 70% of cases. They are considered to be low-grade malignancies.

Adult granulosa cell tumours

Adult GCT account for 95% of all GCTs. The incidence of GCT in developed countries varies from 0.4–1.7 cases per 100,000. They commonly present at 40–60 years of age (median 50 years).

There are no clearly identifiable risk factors. Macroscopically adult GCT are large (median size 12cm), unilateral tumours (92–98%), often multicystic. Microscopically cells are round and pale, with classic 'coffee-bean' grooved nuclei, or Call–Exner bodies. Inhibin staining is the most sensitive and specific immunohistochemical marker for GCT. Approximately 95% of tumours stain positive for inhibin compared with 10–20% of metastatic epithelial carcinomas. These tumours are characterized by slow growth, early stage at presentation, and a late relapse. The overall prognosis is excellent, with long-term survival of 75–90%, attributable mainly to early stage at presentation.

Clinical presentation

Common presenting symptoms are:
- Abnormal vaginal bleeding due to hormonal secretion. Up to 70% of GCTs secrete oestriol and up to 40% of patients will have oestrogenic symptoms. Androgens are only rarely secreted.
- Abdominal pain and distension due to tumour size.

Table 4.7.9 Classification of sex cord-stromal tumours

Granulosa-stromal cell tumours:
Granulosa:
Adult type
Juvenile type
Thecoma-fibroma group:
Thecoma
Fibroma-fibrosarcoma
Sclerosing stromal tumour
Sertoli stromal cell tumours, androblastomas:
Sertoli cell tumours
Sertoli–Leydig cell tumour
Gynandroblastoma
Sex cord tumour with annular tubules
Steroid (lipid) cell tumours: stromal luteoma, Leydig cell tumour, unclassified
Unclassified

Less common presenting symptoms are acute abdominal pain due to haemorrhagic rupture of the tumour into the abdominal cavity (15%), or torsion, isosexual precocious pseudopuberty in premenarchal girls as a result of hormonal secretion; and infertility as a result of inhibin secretion. Rarely patients present with virilization or hirsutism if androgen secretion is present.

Investigations and diagnosis

Surgery is required for a definitive diagnosis. Ultrasound and tumour markers may support the diagnosis if it is suspected preoperatively. Discovery of a synchronous endometrial cancer on preoperative endometrial biopsy may inform discussion on fertility-sparing surgery.

Ultrasound: most GCTs are large multilocular-solid masses with a large number of locules, or solid masses of heterogenous echogenicity. Haemorrhagic components are common. All women with abnormal bleeding should have a transvaginal ultrasound.

Tumour markers:
- Inhibin is the most useful clinical tumour marker and is raised in 95–100% of patients with GCT. However, it is not specific for GCT and can be raised in epithelial ovarian cancer.
- Oestriol is raised in 70% of patients.
- Müllerian-inhibiting substance (MIS) is highly specific and sensitive, but is not routinely available.

Endometrial biopsy: if GCT is suspected preoperatively, endometrial biopsy should be carried out since endometrial hyperplasia is present in 25–50% of patients, and endometrial adenocarcinoma in 5–10% of patients with GCT as a result of hyperoestrogenism. GCT associated endometrial cancers are generally early stage, low-grade tumours.

Treatment

Surgery is the cornerstone of SCST management, both for primary treatment and relapsed disease, because of their characteristic localized presentation and slow growth.

Surgical treatment for early stage tumours is total abdominal hysterectomy and bilateral salpingo-oophorectomy (TAH-BSO). Pelvic and para-aortic lymphadenectomy is not required as part of routine staging, since the risk of involvement is low. Complete surgical staging is recommended, and the FIGO staging system is used, as for epithelial ovarian tumours. An endometrial curettage must be carried out to rule out concomitant endometrial carcinoma if an endometrial biopsy was not performed preoperatively. For advanced disease, complete cytoreduction is the goal, as for epithelial ovarian cancer.

Fertility-sparing surgery is an option for women of childbearing age with stage IA–C disease wishing to preserve fertility or avoid oestrogen therapy.

Adjuvant therapy

For most patients with stage I disease and no high-risk features (tumour rupture, stage IC, size >10–15cm, and ≥4 to 10 mitoses per 10 HPF), the long-term survival is >90%, and surgery alone may be sufficient. The National Comprehensive Cancer Network (NCCN) guidelines recommend consideration of adjuvant platinum-based chemotherapy (or radiotherapy for limited disease) for women with high-risk stage I disease. Ruptured stage IC is the most clearly validated of the proposed high-risk factors, and most (but not all) would advocate adjuvant chemotherapy for stage IC tumours. Some authors suggest treatment with the less toxic carboplatin and paclitaxel, or carboplatin rather than BEP (bleomycin, etoposide, and cisplatin) for stage I (see later).

Based on some retrospective evidence, many studies recommend adjuvant chemotherapy for patients with completely resected stage II–IV disease. NCCN guidelines recommend platinum-based chemotherapy; 3–4 cycles of BEP or 6 cycles of carboplatin/paclitaxel are the preferred regimens.

Radiotherapy may be an option for limited disease, if chemotherapy is undesirable or contraindicated, though the exact benefit is not quantified.

Recurrent disease or metastatic disease

Patients with recurrent disease should be considered for secondary tumour-reductive surgery if the disease-free interval has been prolonged, and particularly if disease is localized to the intraperitoneal space of the pelvis. Multifocal disease may also be considered for surgery. Though survival benefit is unproven, postoperative platinum-based chemotherapy is usually given following surgery for relapse. BEP has been the most commonly used regimen for those who have not previously received this regimen. Carboplatin and paclitaxel is used in those who have received BEP previously or as an alternative to BEP. In patients with completely resected disease treated with chemotherapy, PFS is measured in years, and although most will eventually relapse, long-term DFS may be seen in around 15–20%.

Diffuse/unresectable disease is generally treated with chemotherapy. BEP (if not previously used) and carboplatin and paclitaxel may be the most appropriate regimens with similar response rates of 60–70%. For patients with measurable relapsed disease treated with BEP, complete pathological response at second-look laparotomy is seen in 37–46% of patients. Other platinum-based chemotherapy options include etoposide/cisplatin (EP), cyclophosphamide/adriamcyin, cisplatin (CAP), and single-agent platinum.

Radiotherapy is occasionally used to treat localized or symptomatic disease, since clinical responses and even long-term DFS have been seen in women with recurrent disease, particularly after surgery.

Overexpression of FSH receptors in some tumours, and secretion of oestrogen suggests a rationale for treatment of these tumours with hormonal agents. The GnRH analogue leuprolide has perhaps been the most widely used, given at 7.5mg IM every 4 weeks or 22.5mg IM every 3 months. A response rate of 40% has been reported in one small series; however, others have failed to find a benefit. Other hormonal treatments with reported activity include oral megestrol acetate 160mg daily, tamoxifen, alternating biweekly cycles of megestrol 40mg twice daily for 2 weeks with tamoxifen 10mg twice daily for 2 weeks, and aromatase inhibitors.

Follow-up

Because of their tendency for late recurrence, long-term surveillance is required. The median time to relapse is 4–6 years. Common sites of recurrence are the upper abdomen (55–70%) and pelvis (30–45%). Approximately 15% of relapses occur at >10 years with the longest interval to relapse recorded being 40 years after diagnosis.

There is no consensus about a surveillance policy. Follow-up must include history, physical examination with pelvic examination, and the tumour marker including inhibin and oestriol (if raised initially).

In patients who have had fertility-sparing surgery, additional imaging is often carried out, including pelvic ultrasound every 6 months with annual CT scan of the abdomen and pelvis.

Prognosis

The prognosis of GCT depends upon the stage of disease at diagnosis and the presence of residual disease after surgery. Survival according to stage is shown in Table 4.7.10.

Juvenile granulosa cell tumours

Juvenile GCTs are a variant of GCTs that tend to occur in younger women, and have a different histopathology and natural history from adult GCT.

Approximately 90% of juvenile GCTs occur in prepubertal girls. They are unilateral (95%) and macroscopically similar to adult GCT. Juvenile GCTs almost always secrete hormones and the majority of patients present with symptoms of isosexual puberty due to hyperoestrogenism. Occasionally, patients present with virilization as a result of androgen-secreting tumours.

The same guidelines for surgical staging and preservation of fertility apply to juvenile GCT as their adult counterpart. Surgical staging is particularly important since, although the overall cure rate is 95%, this is because almost all tumours present as stage I. Advanced-stage juvenile GCT are aggressive and less responsive to chemotherapy and radiotherapy, with short times to relapse. Combined small series show 25% survival for stage II–IV with relapse and death occurring within 3 years.

There is no consensus for adjuvant chemotherapy treatment of stage I disease. Some recommend platinum-based chemotherapy for all tumours of stage IB or greater, others for any 'natural' stage IC (i.e. preoperative rupture or ascites), or alternatively for stage IC and a high mitotic index (≥20 per 10 HPF).

In advanced disease, adjuvant chemotherapy appears to contribute to long-term DFS, and should be given for stages II–IV. BEP is the most frequently used regimen, though carboplatin with paclitaxel has also been used, mainly for stage I disease.

For patients who relapse, surgery, radiotherapy, and chemotherapy have all been used; however, few durable responses are seen. Responses have been seen with a number of different platinum and non-platinum containing regimes, notably BEP, paclitaxel, and carboplatin. Hormone treatment with leuprolide has demonstrated stable disease in a number of cases.

Thecoma-fibroma tumours

This group of SCST includes thecomas, fibromas, fibrosarcomas, and sclerosing stromal tumours. Classification into distinct thecoma or fibroma categories may not always be possible as they represent a spectrum of tumours. All of these tumours are benign except the rare fibrosarcomas.

Table 4.7.10 Survival according to stage

FIGO stage	5-year survival	10-year survival
I	90–100%	84–95%
II	55–75%	50–65%
III and IV	22–50%	17–33%

Thecoma

Most thecomas secrete hormones, usually oestrogen (sometimes androgens), and up to 20% of women will present with synchronous endometrial cancer; therefore all women should have preoperative or intraoperative endometrial sampling if they undergo fertility-sparing surgery. For others and postmenopausal women, TAH and BSO is the treatment of choice and is curative.

Fibroma/fibrosarcoma

Fibromas are the most common SCST. They are non-secreting tumours. The association of ovarian fibroma with ascites and/or pleural effusion is known as Meigs' syndrome. Meigs' syndrome may be associated with a raised CA125. Ovarian fibromas may occur in associated with basal cell carcinoma as part of Gorlin's syndrome. Treatment is with unilateral oophorectomy, or cystectomy to preserve the ovary.

Cellular fibromas are a rare subtype of fibroma which show evidence of hypercellularity, mitoses (≥4 per 10 HPF) and nuclear atypia, and are considered tumours of low malignant potential. Oophorectomy is sufficient for diagnosis and cure.

Fibrosarcomas are rare aggressive tumours with marked cellularity, moderate to marked nuclear atypia, and ≥4 mitotic figures per 10 HPF. They treated as for other sarcomas with surgery ± chemotherapy ± radiotherapy.

Sclerosing stromal tumour

These are rare benign tumours treated by excision and unilateral salpingo-oophorectomy (USO).

Sertoli stromal-cell tumours (androblastoma)

Sertoli stromal-cell tumours are a rare group accounting for <0.2% of malignant ovarian tumours. They are characteristically differentiated towards testicular structures, and may be pure Sertoli cell tumours or mixed Sertoli–Leydig tumours.

Pure Sertoli cell tumours

Sertoli cell tumours are diagnosed in young women and are invariably stage I, unilateral, and secrete oestrogen. Only one death has been recorded.

Sertoli–Leydig cell tumours

These occur in women in their teens and 20s, with a mean age at diagnosis of 25 years. They can behave in a benign or malignant fashion depending on the degree of differentiation.

Sertoli–Leydig cell tumours are subclassified into five subtypes: well differentiated, intermediate, poorly differentiated, retiform, and mixed. Most tumours are low grade. Some Sertoli–Leydig cell tumours contain heterologous elements, which are associated with a poorer prognosis. Overall, 20% behave in a malignant fashion (metastasize or recur).

The majority present at stage I (97–98%) and are large (mean 16cm) and unilateral (95%). They commonly secrete androgens, and patients present with symptoms of androgen excess, abdominal swelling, or pain. A small number of Sertoli–Leydig cell tumours produce inhibin or AFP.

Since most patients present with unilateral stage I disease, fertility-sparing surgery may be carried out in those of childbearing age with a normal appearing contralateral ovary and uterus. Full surgical staging should be carried out as for epithelial ovarian cancer. Stage is the most important predictor of outcome. In patients with poorly differentiated tumours of any stage, stage IC or greater, or with heterologous elements, adjuvant platinum-chemotherapy seems

reasonable in view of the higher risk of recurrence, though there are no randomized controlled trials to demonstrate a benefit. BEP or carboplatin and paclitaxel are the most commonly used regimens.

Case series have shown rates of recurrence of 0%, 10%, and 60% for well differentiated, intermediate, and poorly differentiated tumours respectively. Tumours with heterologous elements have a 20% risk of recurrence. Two-thirds of recurrences will occur within the first year, and only 5% will occur after 5 years. Follow-up is with physical examination, including pelvic examination and with serum testosterone, AFP, and inhibin. For patients who relapse, platinum-based chemotherapy is the mainstay of treatment.

Sex cord tumour with annular tubules (SCTAT)

SCTAT represent 6% of SCST. They are intermediate between GCT and the Sertoli cell tumour, but are a distinct entity. Histologically, they are characterized by simple or complex ring-shaped tubules and may be benign or malignant. Risk of malignancy is determined by whether they are associated with Peutz–Jeghers syndrome (see following section). Almost all secrete oestrogens, and the most common presentation is with abnormal uterine bleeding.

SCTAT without Peutz–Jeghers syndrome

Non-PJS associated SCTAT are unilateral, large and uncalcified and have a significant risk of malignancy. They are seen most frequently in women in their 20s, and present most commonly with abnormal uterine bleeding, and less frequently with abdominal pain, or isosexual puberty in the younger age group.

Approximately 20% of patients will have metastatic disease at the time of diagnosis. Surgical staging and treatment follow the same principles as for other malignant SCTAT. GCT or Sertoli–Leydig cell tumour markers may be used for follow-up. In relapsed patients, responses to platinum-based chemotherapy have been seen, though optimal treatment has not been determined.

SCTAT associated with Peutz–Jeghers syndrome

These account for one-third of cases, and usually present in women in their 30s. Tumours are typically small (<3cm), multifocal, bilateral, calcified, and are always benign. Tumours are often asymptomatic. Up to 15% of patients will have associated malignant adenoma of the cervix, and hence should have cervical screening. The cervical imaging may reveal a multicystic mass, in the absence of positive cytology or colposcopy. Any cervical masses should be evaluated by excisional biopsy.

Treatment of SCTAT associated with Peutz–Jeghers syndrome is by unilateral oophorectomy, with total hysterectomy for those with malignant adenoma of the cervix. Consideration should be given to a prophylactic hysterectomy for those in whom cervical screening has been negative, with ongoing screening for those who do not have a hysterectomy.

Gynandroblastoma

Gynandroblastoma is a very rare tumour accounting for <1% of SCST, consisting of a combination of granulosa and Sertoli or Sertoli–Leydig cell elements (with at least 10% of the minor component). They are usually large and benign (one malignant case reported), and occur in women between the ages of 16–65. Most (60%) secrete androgens and produce virilization. Testosterone may be converted peripherally to oestrogen causing abnormal vaginal bleeding. Patients should have surgical staging because of the potential for tumours to behave like either their granulosa or Sertoli-stromal component. Unilateral salpingo-oophorectomy is the appropriate treatment for women of childbearing age.

Steroid or lipid cell tumours

There are three types of steroid or lipid cell tumours; stromal luteomas, Leydig cell tumours, and steroid cell tumours not otherwise specified (NOS). Together they account for <0.1% of all ovarian tumours.

Stromal luteomas **and** *Leydig cell tumours* **are** small, benign tumours occurring most commonly in postmenopausal women. They do not require surgical staging or postoperative treatment. In younger patients of childbearing age, fertility-preserving surgery should be carried out.

Steroid cell tumours NOS are the most common type of steroid cell tumours (accounting for 50–60%). They present at an earlier age (mean 43 years), are large (average size 8.5cm), and may be bilateral. They can be malignant and aggressive and for this reason intraoperatively discovered steroid cell tumours should be staged and aggressively cytoreduced. In the largest series, 43% with metastasis at presentation have recurred. Fertility-preserving surgery may be carried out in fully staged, stage IA patients. The strongest prognostic factor other than stage is the mitotic count. Over 90% of tumours with >2 mitoses per 10 HPF are malignant. Based on other possible prognostic factors, some experts recommend platinum-based chemotherapy for pleomorphic tumours, those with an increased mitotic count, and for large or advanced tumours.

Borderline ovarian tumours

Introduction

Borderline ovarian tumours are also known as carcinomas of low malignant potential, or atypical proliferative tumours. They account for 15% of ovarian tumours, with overall survival of 80–90%. They generally occur at a younger age than epithelial ovarian cancer, with an average at diagnosis of 40–60 years, 15 years earlier than epithelial ovarian cancer.

Aetiology

Borderline tumours have similar epidemiological and reproductive risk factors to their malignant counterpart. There appears to be a protective effect from increasing parity (40–70% risk reduction) and lactation (50% reduction in risk). Reports on the effect of the contraceptive pill have been conflicting.

Clinicopathological features

Pathological criteria for a borderline tumour include a lack of obvious stromal invasion, and the presence of mitotic activity and nuclear abnormalities intermediate between benign and malignant tumours of a similar cell. Histological subtypes of borderline tumours are:
• Serous (50%)
• Mucinous (46%)
• Endometrioid, clear cell and transitional cell (4%).

The most common presentations of borderline tumours are abdominal pain or pressure and abdominal distension. Approximately 25% will present asymptomatically as an incidental finding on clinical or radiological examination. Uncommon presentations include abnormal pre-menstrual bleeding, torsion, haemorrhage, or weight loss.

Serous borderline tumours: approximately 70% will present at stage I, 10% stage II, 20% stage III, and <1% stage IV. The mean size is 10cm. Tumours are bilateral in 40% of cases. Survival for stage I tumours is virtually 100%. Survival for advanced stage tumours with non-invasive implants is 95%, whereas survival for tumours with invasive implants is 66%.

Non-invasive implants are more common (90%) and behave in a benign fashion, whereas invasive implants are less common (10%) and behave like low-grade serous carcinomas. Micropapillary features are present in 6–18% of serous borderline tumours and strongly predict for invasive implants, increasing the risk from 6% to 49%, and thus serve as a marker for invasive carcinoma. Peritoneal implants may originate as metastasis from the primary ovarian tumour, or from multicentric endosalpingiosis. There is molecular evidence to support both origins.

Mucinous borderline tumours: almost all present as stage I (95–100%), and are unilateral (>90%). Implants are generally not seen, and their presence should suggest the possibility of a misclassified mucinous carcinoma. Extra-ovarian implants may be encountered in the endocervical subtype of mucinous tumour, which is also bilateral in 13–40% of cases.

Endometrioid, clear cell and Brenner borderline tumours are almost always unilateral. Extraovarian implants have not been well characterized due to their rarity.

Diagnosis

Accurate preoperative diagnosis is difficult. CA125 is raised in 40% of stage I and 90% of advanced stage borderline ovarian tumours, but lacks specificity. Appearances on ultrasound range from unilocular cysts to masses with solid and cystic components.

Staging

Staging is according to the FIGO system as for ovarian carcinomas.

Treatment

Surgery

Surgery is the cornerstone for borderline tumour management, diagnosis, and treatment.

When intraoperative frozen sections on an undiagnosed pelvic mass reveal a borderline tumour, full surgical staging, as for epithelial carcinomas, is generally recommended, and results in an upstaging of approximately 25%. There is no indication for a wedge biopsy of a clinically uninvolved contralateral ovary as micrometastases have not been recorded.

The necessity for pelvic and para-aortic sampling is debated, since even advanced tumours have a good prognosis. One meta-analysis has shown 98% survival at 6.5 years in those with lymph node involvement. A metaplastic rather than metastatic process was suggested as one explanation. The best approach has yet to be determined.

Proper surgical staging helps with better prognostication, discovery of occult invasive implants, and the avoidance of underdiagnosis (or rarely overdiagnosis) on frozen section. Upgrading of frozen sections to invasive cancer following final histopathology has been reported to be as high as 30%, while downgrading rates reported are around 5–10%. Reasons for high underdiagnosis rates include sampling errors due to the large size of the tumour, and the difficulty in assessing invasion in mucinous tumours on frozen section. Mucinous tumours should therefore always have a full staging and the patient should have an appendicectomy.

For women with borderline tumours who wish to preserve their fertility, USO with staging is the first choice of conservative treatment as the recurrence rates are lower than for cystectomy. USO is considered appropriate and safe for clinical stage IA disease, and may be carried out even in advanced disease in the presence of a normal contralateral ovary, though this is more controversial.

One retrospective study carried out in early stage disease showed recurrence rates of 7% for USO and 23% for cystectomy. Comparative recurrence rates for radical surgery with TAH/BSO are 0–5%. Involvement of the resection margin following cystectomy is almost always associated with persistence or recurrence of tumours. Unlike most other tumours, almost all recurrences of borderline tumours can be salvaged surgically, often with further conservative surgery. Fatality rates following recurrence are 0–5%.

Despite retrospective data indicating equivalent survival for patients having USO and ovarian cystectomy, because of the high salvage rates, many would reserve cystectomy for patients with bilateral disease wishing to preserve fertility. Patients having any form of conservative surgery should be prepared for increased surveillance, with physical examination, ultrasound scan, and CA125.

Patients with advanced disease should have a complete cytoreduction, and studies have demonstrated that patients with gross residual disease are at increased risk of recurrence and death.

Adjuvant treatment

The use of adjuvant chemotherapy is controversial and there are no randomized controlled trials to demonstrate a benefit from adjuvant chemotherapy. Most experts would recommend adjuvant treatment for patients with invasive implants, since these represent small foci of invasive carcinoma, and their prognosis is poorer. Regimens used are as for epithelial ovarian cancer, with 6 courses of carboplatin ± paclitaxel.

Unexpected postoperative diagnosis of borderline tumours

Sometimes an unexpected diagnosis of borderline tumour is made postoperatively, in which case a decision is required as to whether to carry out re-exploration for surgical staging. There is no consensus. Most would try to avoid a second operation, except perhaps in cases of micropapillary borderline tumours, where the risk of invasive implants is higher. Careful follow-up is suggested for patients who have not been fully staged with clinical examination, CA125, and CT.

For patients who have had simple cystectomy for a supposed benign cyst, and without staging, again there is no consensus. Some would suggest re-exploration and surgical staging only when complete macroscopic exploration has been not been carried out, or there has been a spillage, the borderline lesion is on the outside of the cyst, or the margins are involved. Again, close follow-up should be carried out for those who are not restaged.

Residual or recurrent disease

Surgery should be considered whenever possible for recurrent disease, since in most cases disease is slow growing, and is thought to be comparatively resistant to other modalities.

Studies have shown that patients with optimally reduced disease at secondary cytoreduction have significantly better survival. Borderline tumours are thought to be relatively resistant to chemotherapy, hormonal treatment, and

radiotherapy because of the low percentage of actively dividing cells.

Response rates appear highest for platinum-based chemotherapy and are in the order of 25–40%. There are no randomized trials to demonstrate a benefit of chemotherapy in recurrent disease; nevertheless chemotherapy is usually considered for unresectable disease, or for tumours with a rapid growth rate which are symptomatic. Median survival from the time of first relapse is 7–8 years.

Fertility

Case series suggest that women who have had fertility-sparing surgery have a high probability of successful reproduction, though in some cases this may require ovulation induction or IVF. There is no evidence that pregnancy or fertility treatments increase the risk of recurrence in patients who have had fertility-sparing surgery

Follow-up

There is no consensus on follow-up schedules. Patients with surgically staged stage IA borderline tumours do not require any further follow-up. The suggested follow-up for other patients includes monitoring every 3–6 months for 5 years, followed by annual review. Patients should have a physical examination including pelvic examination and CA125 estimation.

Patients who have undergone fertility-sparing surgery are at increased risk of relapse and should be monitored by transvaginal ultrasound in addition.

Prognosis

Stage and subclassification of extraovarian disease into invasive and non-invasive implants are the most important prognostic factors for serous borderline tumours (Table 4.7.11).

Other uncommon ovarian tumours

Carcinosarcoma or malignant mixed Müllerian tumours

These account for <1% of ovarian neoplasms. They occur commonly in women in their 60s. Most present at an advanced stage (75%). They are aggressive tumours, with a poor prognosis. Treatment is with cytoreductive surgery, as for epithelial ovarian tumours, followed by postoperative chemotherapy. Chemotherapy regimens are as for those used in the more common MMMT of the uterus (see Chapter 4, Uterine sarcomas, p.342) with ifosfamide and cisplatin-based regimens or carboplatin and paclitaxel. The median survival is 1 year.

Small cell carcinoma of the ovary

This is an aggressive tumour, occurring predominantly in young women. Approximately 50% will have localized disease at presentation. Two-thirds of cases have hypercalcaemia. Patients should have TAH/BSO staging and tumour reduction. The role of adjuvant chemotherapy and radiotherapy is unclear; however, in view of their aggressive

Table 4.7.11 Survival for borderline ovarian tumours according to stage

Stage	5-year	10-year
I	99	97
II	98	90
III	96	88
IV	77	69

nature, chemotherapy is recommended and radiotherapy may be considered to improve local control. Cisplatin and etoposide (EP), or vincristine, adriamycin and cyclophosphamide (VAC) are the most commonly used regimens. Case series show DFS of 33% for stage IA, 10% survival for stage IC and 6.5% survival for stages II–IV.

Further reading

Brown J, Gershensen D.M. Treatment of rare ovarian malignancies. In: Eifel PJ, Gershenson DM, Kanavagh JJ, et al. (eds) *MD Anderson Cancer Care Series, Gynecological Cancer*, Vol. 5, pp.207–25. New York: Springer, 2006.

Colombo N, Parma G, Zanagnolo V, Insinga A. Management of ovarian stromal cell tumors. *J Clin Oncol* 2007; **25**:2944–51.

Miller K, McCluggage W.G. Prognostic factors in ovarian adult granulosa cell tumour. *J Clin Pathol* 2008; **61**:881–4.

Pectasides D, Pectasides E, Psyrri A. 2008. Granulosa cell tumour of the ovary. *Canc Treat Rev* 2008; **34**:1–12.

Schumer, ST, Cannistra, SA. Granulosa cell tumour of the ovary. *J Clin Oncol* 2003; **21**:1180–9.

Seidman JD, Kurman RJ. Ovarian serous borderline tumors: a critical review of the literature with emphasis on prognostic indicators. *Prog in Path* 2000; **31**:531.

Internet resources

National Comprehensive Cancer network: http://www.nccn.org

Society of Obstetricians and Gynaecologists of Canada—clinical practice guidelines: http://www.sogc.org/guidelines/

Gestational trophoblastic disease

Introduction

Gestational trophoblastic disease (GTD) is a rare complication of pregnancy. It includes a spectrum of interrelated tumours arising from tissues of placental origin. These include: hydatidiform mole (complete and partial), invasive mole, choriocarcinoma, and placental site trophoblastic tumour (PSTT).

Gestational trophoblastic neoplasia (GTN) is a term used to describe persistent GTD and gestational trophoblastic tumours (GTT). GTN encompasses invasive mole, choriocarcinoma, and PSTT.

GTN is the most curable gynaecologic neoplasm largely due to its sensitivity to chemotherapy; however, occasional patients still die. During the last 50 years, there have been major improvements in the diagnosis and treatment including:
1 Introduction of chemotherapy.
2 Improved precision and sensitivity of human chorionic gonadotrophin (hCG) assay.
3 Development of prognostic risk score assessments which help to individualize treatment.

Despite its rarity, GTD remains an important disease for clinicians to diagnose because, if it is recognized and treated appropriately, it is almost always curable with preservation of fertility.

In the UK, patients diagnosed with GTD are registered at one of three reference centres, Ninewells Hospital in Dundee, Weston Park Hospital in Sheffield, and the Charing Cross Hospital in London, for serial estimation of hCG concentration. Most molar pregnancies resolve spontaneously after evacuation of the uterus; however, 15% of complete moles and 0.5% of partial moles need chemotherapy (Newlands 2003).

Epidemiology and aetiology

Epidemiology

Hydatidiform mole is the commonest variant of GTD and its incidence varies between different regions of the world and even between different areas within the same country. In the UK it is around 1.5 per 1000 live births. Fifteen per cent of complete moles develop into *invasive mole*.

The incidence of *choriocarcinoma* is highly variable. For example, its incidence following term delivery is 1 per 50,000, while 3% of complete moles may develop into choriocarcinomas. Unlike complete moles there are no clear geographical trends in the incidence of choriocarcinoma; however, the effect of age remains important.

PSTT is an uncommon but important variant of GTD. It is thought to constitute about 1% of all trophoblastic tumours.

Aetiology

Maternal age Complete moles are more common in women who become pregnant at <16 years or >40 years. Partial moles are not age related.
Previous pregnancies History of previous molar gestation increases the risk of a subsequent occurrence by a factor of 10.
Ethnicity Incidence of molar pregnancy varies between different ethnic groups. Women of Asian origin have at least a 2-fold increase in risk.
Diet Evidence is conflicting; however, deficiencies in protein and vitamin A derivatives are most commonly implicated.

Pathology

Hydatidiform mole

Hydatidiform moles can be categorised either complete or partial on the basis of gross morphology, histopathology and karyotyping (see Tables 4.7.12 and 4.7.13).
Complete moles (see Fig. 4.7.6) are characterized by:
- Lack of identifiable embryonic or fetal tissues.
- Swollen villi surrounded by diffuse trophoblastic hyperplasia.
- 46XX karyotype (occasionally 46XY) and molar chromosomes are entirely of paternal origin.
- Macroscopically the cystic villi have the appearance of clusters of grapes.

Invasive moles have the same histological appearance of complete mole but with invasion of the underlying tissues.

Table 4.7.12 Features of complete mole and partial mole

	Complete	Partial
Fetal or embryonic tissues	Absent	Present
Hydatidiform swelling of chorionic villi	Diffuse	Focal
Trophoblastic hyperplasia	Diffuse	Focal
Scalloping of chorionic villi	Absent	Present
Karyotype	46XX; 46XY	69XXY; 69XYY

Table 4.7.13 Summary of pathological features

Abnormality	Embryo	Hydrops	Trophoblast
Partial mole	Yes	Focal	Some excess
Complete mole	No	Extensive	Marked excess
Invasive mole	No	Extensive	Marked excess
Choriocarcinoma	No	No villi	Neoplastic
PSTT	No	No villi	Neoplastic

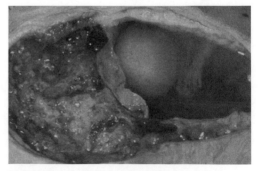

Fig. 4.7.6 Twin pregnancy showing coexisting normal fetus and complete mole.

Partial moles are characterized by:
• Chorionic villi of varying size with focal hydatidiform swelling.
• Identifiable embryonic or fetal tissues.
• Focal trophoblastic hyperplasia
• Triploid karyotype (69 chromosomes) with two sets of paternal haploid genes and one set of maternal haploid genes.

Choriocarcinoma
Choriocarcinomas are characterized by:
• Absence of chorionic villi.
• Sheets of anaplastic cytotrophoblast and syncytiotrophoblast.
• Macroscopically they are soft, purple, and largely haemorrhagic.

Placental site trophoblastic tumour (PSTT)
PSTT consists mainly of intermediate trophoblasts and few syncytial elements hence secreting less hCG hormone. Macroscopically, it is largely necrotic.

Clinical features
Complete hydatidiform mole (CHM)
The clinical presentation of molar pregnancies has changed over the last 50 years. In the 1960s and 1970s, excessive uterine size, anaemia, hyperemesis, thyrotoxicosis, early pregnancy pre-eclampsia, cystic ovarian enlargement (theca lutein cyst), and metastatic disease were common. These presentations still occur, particularly in less developed countries. In developed countries they are less common.

Abnormal bleeding in early pregnancy is the most common presenting symptom occurring in up to 97% of cases. Uterine enlargement greater than expected for gestational age is still seen in over a quarter of the patients. Most cases are diagnosed in the first trimester of pregnancy by ultrasound scanning (see Fig. 4.7.7) (Hancock and Tidy 2002).

Partial hydatidiform mole (PHM)
• Usually does not have the clinical features associated with complete mole.
• In general, patients present with symptoms and signs of incomplete or missed miscarriage.
• Diagnosis often made after histological review of curettings.

Gestational trophoblastic neoplasia (GTN)
Up to 20% of trophoblastic diseases persist and patients usually present with irregular vaginal bleeding and/or elevated serum β-hCG. Excessive uterine enlargement, theca lutein ovarian cysts, and markedly elevated hCG are the main predictors of persistent trophoblastic disease. Maternal age, DNA ploidy status and use of oral contraceptives are other factors.

Table 4.7.14 Incidence of common metastatic sites (%)

Lungs	78–93%
Vagina	5–16%
Pelvis	4–7%
CNS	8–15%
Liver	10%
Bowel, kidney, spleen	<5%
Other	<5%

Metastatic disease occurs in 4% of patients after evacuation of complete molar pregnancy and rarely after other pregnancies. Metastases of choriocarcinoma have been reported in every body site and bleeding often occurs (sites of metastatic spread are shown in Table 4.7.14). Pulmonary metastases may be asymptomatic or present with signs of PE. CNS lesions may produce subtle neurological symptoms or acute symptoms of intracranial haemorrhage. Choriocarcinoma should be considered in any premenopausal woman presenting with metastatic disease with unknown primary.

Further reading
Hancock, BW, Tidy JA. Current management of molar pregnancy. *J Reprod Med* 2002; **47**(5):347–54.

Newlands, E. Presentation and treatment of gestational trophoblastic disease (GTD) and gestational trophoblastic tumour (GTT) in the UK. In: Hancock BW, Newlands ES, Berkowitz RS, *et al.* (eds) *Gestational Trophoblastic Disease* pp.229–47. London: Chapman and Hall, 2003.

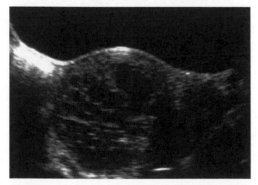
Fig. 4.7.7 Ultrasound scan of pregnant uterus showing complete mole.

Gestational trophoblastic disease: diagnosis, staging and prognosis

Initial management

Women with suspected molar pregnancy should undergo pelvic ultrasound scan, serum hCG measurement, and CXR.

In complete moles, ultrasound scan may show a classical snowstorm appearance. The ultrasound scan picture of partial moles is more complex.

The primary treatment of patients with suspected molar pregnancy is evacuation of the uterus by an experienced gynaecologist.

Suction curettage is the method of choice for evacuation of complete mole. Medical termination of complete mole, including cervical preparation, should be avoided where possible and oxytocic agents should only be commenced after uterine cavity is evacuated due to the risk of embolization of trophoblastic tissue.

In partial moles, suction curettage may be limited by the presence of fetal parts and therefore medical termination may be necessary.

Sometimes it is difficult to diagnose molar pregnancy prior to uterine evacuation; therefore, it is recommended that all products of conception obtained after medical or surgical evacuation of the uterus and from therapeutic terminations with no fetal tissue should undergo histological examination.

It should be remembered that persistent GTD can occur after any pregnancy. Therefore, women with persistent vaginal bleeding after non-molar pregnancy should undergo pregnancy test to exclude persistent GTD. Persistent GTD should be considered in women developing acute respiratory or neurological symptoms after any pregnancy.

Registration and assessment

Since 1973 there has been a national registration system in the UK for all cases of molar pregnancy. According to their geographical location, patients are registered and followed-up by one of three UK centres at Weston Park Hospital, Sheffield; Charing Cross Hospital, London; and Ninewells Hospital, Dundee.

Once registered, patients and their gynaecologists receive an information package and, if uneventful, the patient will be followed-up for 6 months. Follow-up involves periodic assays of urine and/or serum hCG initially weekly reduced to monthly depending on the rate of hCG fall (RCOG 2004).

The return to normal of hCG after uterine evacuation can reliably predict the likelihood of subsequently developing persistent GTD. If the level of hCG has fallen to normal within 8 weeks of uterine evacuation then marker follow-up can safely be reduced to 6 months in total since it has been shown that these women are highly unlikely to subsequently require chemotherapy. However, if hCG remains elevated beyond 8 weeks, follow up is continued until the hCG level is normal and for 6 months thereafter.

Patients with persistent trophoblastic disease (PTD) in the UK are treated either in Sheffield or London.

Persistent gestational trophoblastic disease

The need for treatment is identified by evidence of persistent disease activity, which is unlikely to resolve spontaneously. In the UK only 5–8% of patients require chemotherapy whilst in Europe this figure is 12–15% and in

North America 20–30%. These differences are explained by the different criteria for treatment among different centres.

Second uterine evacuation may be performed provided that:
• HCG elevation is low
• There is a significant amount of intrauterine abnormal tissue on repeat ultrasound scan.

Further evacuations are contraindicated as they are associated with increased rate of uterine perforation, haemorrhage, and infection without reducing the need for subsequent chemotherapy.

About 15–20% of complete moles and 0.5% of partial moles ultimately require chemotherapy. The indications for chemotherapy in the UK are shown in Table 4.7.15.

Patients who fulfil the treatment criteria are admitted promptly to the nearest treatment centre. They require careful assessment of the extent of the disease prior to initiation of treatment and have:
• Complete history and physical examination.
• Blood tests:
  Endocrine: β-hCG, thyroid function.
  Haematology: full blood count.
  Biochemistry: liver and renal function.
• Imaging:
  CXR
  CT scan of thorax.

Other assessments should be performed as clinically indicated (see CNS assessment section).
• Central review of the histopathological specimen.

Prior to commencing treatment, prognostic risk score is calculated for each new patient using the FIGO-adapted WHO prognostic scoring system (Table 4.7.16). This has evolved over a number of years since Bagshawe's 1976 scoring system. It is hoped that adherence to this internationally agreed system will facilitate future comparisons between management strategies employed in different centres. The risk score is obtained by adding the individual scores for each prognostic factor. Patients then are categorized either low (score ≤6) or high (score ≥7) risk for treatment purposes (Hancock 2003).

Patients also should be staged according to FIGO criteria because this will encourage objective comparisons of data among centres here in the UK and internationally (Table 4.7.17).

Table 4.7.15 Indications for chemotherapy

Serum hCG >20,000 IU/L after one or two uterine evacuations
Static or rising hCG levels after one or two uterine evacuations
Persistent hCG elevation 6 months postuterine evacuation
Persistent vaginal bleeding with raised hCG levels
Pulmonary metastasis with static or rising hCG levels
Metastasis in liver, brain, or GI tract
Histological diagnosis of choriocarcinoma

Table 4.7.16 FIGO-adapted WHO prognostic scoring system

Score	0	1	2	4
Age(years)	<40	>40	NA	NA
Antecedent pregnancy	Mole	Abortion	Term	NA
Interval months from index pregnancy	<4	4–<7	7–<13	≥13
Pretreatment serum hCG concentration (IU/L)	<10^3	10^3–<10^4	10^4–<10^5	≥10^5
Largest tumour size (including uterus) cm	<3	3–<5	≥5	NA
Site of metastasis	Lung	Spleen, kidney	Gastrointestinal	Liver, brain
Number of metastases	NA	1–4	5–8	>8
Previous failed chemotherapy	NA	NA	Single drug	≥ 2 drugs

NA, not applicable

Table 4.7.17 FIGO staging system

Stage I	Disease confined to uterus
Stage II	GTD extends beyond uterus but is limited to genital structures
Stage III	GTD extends to lungs, with or without known genital tract involvement
Sage IV	All other metastatic sites.

Main changes from previous WHO scoring system are:
- ABO blood group risk factors are eliminated.
- Risk factor for liver metastases is upgraded from 2 to highest score of 4.
- PSTT is excluded.

Central nervous system assessment

It is recognized that persistent GTD can readily metastasize to the brain. The risk of brain metastasis is greater in patients with:
- High risk score (≥7)
- Multiple pulmonary metastases
- β-hCG levels >50,000 IU/L

It is therefore recommended that patients with any of these criteria should undergo CT or MRI scan of the head, and a lumbar puncture. Provided there is no clinical evidence of increased intracranial pressure, lumbar puncture allows estimation of hCG levels in cerebrospinal fluid (CSF). An abnormal value is interpreted when ratio with serum hCG level is >1 in 60.

Counselling and communication

It is important that all patients who are admitted to a trophoblastic disease centre are treated by staff who are experienced in the management of this disease.

The majority of the patients are both anxious and depressed due to one or more of the reasons listed which should be addressed prior to any treatment:
- They have had a recent pregnancy which resulted in both 'miscarriage' and their disease.
- They are diagnosed with a disease that is malignant or potentially malignant.
- Fears about the side effects of chemotherapy, particularly nausea, vomiting, and alopecia.
- The majority of these patients are in their reproductive age and have concerns about their fertility, sexual life, and future pregnancies.

Key points
- Hydatidiform moles should be evacuated by an experienced gynaecologist using suction curettage. Cervical priming and oxytocics should be avoided.
- Registration with the supraregional centre is mandatory.
- hCG is an excellent marker for monitoring treatment of GTD, with the exception of PSTT.
- Patients with GTD should only be treated by experienced staff

- They have worries about how their families can cope with their treatment, especially if they have young children.

These patients need continuous emotional support during the treatment and even once the treatment is concluded.

We found that having a dedicated specialist nurse who counsels and follows-up the patients from their admission through treatment and finally their discharge helps considerably in providing this support.

Further reading

RCOG. *The Management of Gestational Trophoblastic Neoplasia* (38). London: RCOG, 2004.

Hancock BW. Staging and classification of gestational trophoblastic disease. *Best Pract Res Clin Obstet Gynaecol* 2003; **17**(6):869–83.

Gestational trophoblastic disease: low risk

Principles of management

Low-risk GTD patients are those who have a risk score of ≤6 according to WHO/FIGO classification (this includes the old WHO low risk 0–4 and intermediate 5–6).

The majority of low-risk patients have disease that is limited to the pelvis; however, occasional patients have metastases (invariably to the lungs).

Patients with low-risk GTD (Fig. 4.7.8) have been successfully treated with single-agent chemotherapy.

There are large numbers of regimens used worldwide to manage low-risk GTD. The choice depends on the geographic location, training, and experience and to a lesser extent, cost, and patient choice.

The most widely used single agents worldwide for low-risk GTD are methotrexate and dactinomycin. Many protocols have been reported for the administration of these agents.

In the UK, patients with low-risk GTN are treated with intramuscular low-dose methotrexate with oral folinic acid rescue as described by Bagshawe et al. (1989) (see 'Sheffield low-dose methotrexate regimen' box).

Sheffield low-dose methotrexate regimen

- Intramuscular methotrexate on alternate days for four doses.
- Oral folinic acid on alternate days.
- Seven days' rest between treatment cycles.

In general, this schedule is well tolerated provided the patient has normal renal function and maintains adequate hydration during treatment, since methotrexate is excreted through the urine. In our experience although about 60–70% of the patients experienced side effects to methotrexate treatment these were mainly mild and <10% developed significant side effects. Occasional patients develop methotrexate-induced liver damage requiring change of treatment (Table 4.7.18).

Methotrexate has two major advantages over other cytotoxic agents in that it does not cause alopecia and its long-term safety profile is excellent. There have been no recorded second malignancies in our experience.

The other major drug used in the treatment of low-risk disease is dactinomycin. Historically it was a 5-day treatment repeated every 14 days. This resulted in grade 3/4 alopecia and GI dysfunction. In an attempt to manage the side-effect profile of this regimen better, it has largely been

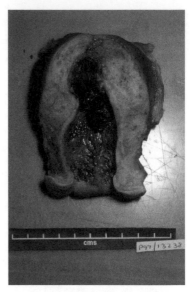

Fig. 4.7.8 Uterus showing penetrative invasive mole.

replaced by the 'pulse' dactinomycin regimen that employs bolus dose ($1.25mg/m^2$) repeated every 2 weeks.

Dactinomycin may provide slightly higher cure rates than methotrexate. Therefore, most centres use it as a second-line treatment when methotrexate is inappropriate either due to resistance or toxicity.

The Chinese have used flurouracil for several decades mainly because of its low cost. In the last decade etopside has been reported to be highly effective in this disease, administered either orally or paranterally.

Other agents like 6-mercaptopurine and cisplatin are rarely used in the treatment of low-risk GTN due to concerns about their acute and chronic toxicity.

Low-risk metastatic GTN

Patients with low-risk metastatic GTN have been treated successfully with single-agent chemotherapy, using methotrexate or dactinomycin. In the UK all patients with low-risk GTN receive single-agent methotrexate, whether they have metastases or not. However, in the USA, the approach is often more aggressive and some patients with

Table 4.7.18 Side effects from methotrexate treatment (Khan et al. 2003)

Side effect	Mild (%)	Severe (%)	Comments
Mucositis /stomatitis	25%	<1%	Analgesic mouth wash (Difran®) and low-dose corticosteroids
Conjunctivitis	25%		Hypromellose eye drops
Pleuritic chest pain	9–24%	1.2%	Simple analgesia. Avoid NSAIDs*
Skin rash	3%	1%	
Vaginal bleeding	15–20%	2%	
Haematological	<1%	<1%	

* Non-steroidal anti-inflammatory drugs

low-risk metastatic GTN might be treated with combination chemotherapy.

Specific management

Relapsed or resistant low-risk disease

Approximately 10–20% of patients with non-metastatic low-risk disease will develop methotrexate resistance and need salvage chemotherapy with or without surgery to achieve remission. The incidence is higher in patients with metastatic low-risk GTD and can be up to 30–50%. Treatment strategies vary on how to deal with this scenario. In the UK, patients who develop resistance to methotrexate but with a low β-hCG level are changed to single-agent dactinomycin, routinely given in bolus dose regimen (see 'Sheffield low-risk salvage regimen' box). Those with high β-hCG are changed to combination chemotherapy; in Sheffield they receive methotrexate, etoposide, and dactinomycin (MEA) while in London they receive etoposide, methotrexate, dactinomycin/cyclophosphamide and vincristine (EMA/CO).

Sheffield low-risk salvage regimen

- Dactinomycin intravenous infusion.
- Etoposide intravenous infusion.
- These drugs are given daily and for 3 days.
- Seven days' rest between treatment cycles.

Role of hysterectomy

Though the majority of patients are cured with chemotherapy alone, hysterectomy continues to play an important role in the management of persistent GTD, especially in those countries where there are problems with patient surveillance and provision of chemotherapy.

In the developed world, the two commonest indications for hysterectomy are:
- To control excessive vaginal bleeding before or following the start of chemotherapy.
- The management of GTN which is resistant to chemotherapy.

Where the disease is limited to the uterus and the patient desires sterilization, hysterectomy can be integrated into the management plan as this was found to reduce the amount of chemotherapy needed to achieve remission and salvage those who developed resistance to chemotherapy.

Hysterectomy for GTD may be a difficult procedure. Arteriovenous malformations following chemotherapy, presence of extrauterine disease, and the involvement of adjacent organs and vessels can complicate the procedure. Surgery should therefore be performed by experienced surgeon and anaesthetist.

Follow-up

During treatment

Prior to each cycle of treatment, β-hCG, full blood count, renal and liver function tests are checked.

Following completion of treatment

Once the treatment is concluded serum β-hCG is measured:
- Weekly for the first 6 weeks.
- Monthly for the subsequent 6 months
- If remains normal; follow-up, with periodic urine hCG, for life.

Contraception

All patients are advised to avoid the use of oestrogen-containing oral contraceptive pills (OCP) whilst hCG levels are elevated as there is a theoretical risk of inducing metastatic or drug resistance disease. Combined OCP may be used again once the hCG levels have returned to normal.

All patients also advised to avoid using intrauterine contraceptive devices (IUCD and coil) until normal menstrual cycle is established.

Pregnancy

Patients are advised not to conceive for at least 12 months from the conclusion of their treatment. There is risk of teratogenicity resulting from cytotoxic chemotherapy and secondly the risk of recurrent GTD is greatest during this time.

Communication with referring gynaecologist and GP

As minimum, formal summaries are sent after conclusion of the first and final treatment cycles with periodic updates as appropriate.

Further reading

Bagshawe KD, Dent J, Newlands ES, et al. The role of low-dose methotrexate and folinic acid in gestational trophoblastic tumours (GTT). Br J Obstet Gynaecol 1989; **96**(7):795–802.

Khan F, Everard J, Ahmed S, et al. Low-risk persistent gestational trophoblastic disease treated with low-dose methotrexate: efficacy, acute and long-term effects. Br J Cancer 2003; **89**(12):2197–201.

Internet resource

International Society for the Study of Trophoblastic Diseases: http://www.isstd.org

Gestational trophoblastic disease: high risk

Principles of management

Patients categorized as having high-risk GTD (with prognostic score ≥7) are more likely to have tumour resistant to single-agent chemotherapy. Therefore, they should be treated with combination chemotherapy from the start with or without adjuvant surgery.

Since the early 1970s, various combination chemotherapy regimens for treating high-risk GTN have been used, such as MAC (methotrexate, dactinomycin, and cyclophosphamide or chlorambucil), EMA/CO (etoposide, methotrexate and dactinomycin/cyclophosphamide and vincristine), EMA (etoposide, methotrexate and dactinomycin), CHAMOCA (cyclophosphamide, hydroxyurea, dactinomycin, methotrexate, vincristine, and doxorubicin). Although these regimens are effective, they all result in unavoidable side effects.

At the Sheffield centre in the UK, high-risk patients receive a regimen consisting of moderate-dose intravenous methotrexate with folinic acid, alternating after weekly rest with dactinomycin and etoposide (MEA) (see 'Sheffield high-risk GTD regimen' box); 75% of patients receiving this regimen had full remission. The regimen is well tolerated; however, the higher dose of methotrexate means that particular care is required with renal and liver function.

At the Charing Cross centre in the UK, an alternative regimen is used consisting of intravenous etoposide, methotrexate, and dactinomycin for 2 days followed by cyclophosphamide and vincristine (EMA/CO) 1 week later; 78% of patients receiving this regimen had full remission.

In the USA patients with high-risk GTN are treated either with EMA/CO or MAC chemotherapy together with radiotherapy or surgery.

In treating high-risk GTN particular caution should be employed in those with widespread pulmonary metastases who are at a higher risk of developing respiratory failure following starting chemotherapy. This could occur as a result of tumour necrosis and oedema and may be ameliorated by administration of dexamethasone. Reduction of the initial dose of chemotherapy does not seem to protect against this potentially lethal complication. Respiratory failure may also be due to other causes including the possibility of a venous embolism and should be treated accordingly. Mechanical ventilation should be avoided as the high airway pressure can trigger fatal pulmonary haemorrhage.

Treatment toxicity

The majority of the patients are cured irrespective of the chemotherapy regimen used; however, associated toxicity varies between different chemotherapies.

EMA/CO is associated with higher levels of grade III/IV anaemia, neutropenia, and thrombocytopenia compared with MEA. Both regimens can result in grade II/III nausea (EMA/CO 23%, MEA 15%). The incidences of stomatitis and skin rash are similar in both regimens. MAC chemotherapy is associated with significant myelotoxicity which can be life threatening in about 6% of patients.

Specific management

Relapsed or resistant high-risk disease

Failure of first-line chemotherapy in high-risk patients is a more difficult situation since there is no chemotherapy regimen with guaranteed good outcome. About 20–30%

> **Sheffield high-risk GTD regimen**
>
> *Arm A*
> - *Methotrexate* intravenous infusion in normal saline.
> - *Folinic acid* commencing 24 hours after the start of methotrexate. Eight doses administered in total and the first four given by intravenous injection.
>
> *Arm B*
> - *Dactinomycin* intravenous infusion in normal saline over 1 hour.
> - *Etoposide* intravenous infusion in normal saline over 1 hour.
>
> Arms A and B are repeated sequentially with 7 days of rest interval between them.

of high-risk patients will develop resistance to first-line chemotherapy or relapse after treatment and need salvage treatment.

In general, salvage treatment with alternative agents (especially cisplatin) is needed for failed initial combination chemotherapy (see 'Sheffield salvage protocol for high-risk patients' box). Patients who develop resistance to EMA/CO are commonly treated with EP/EMA (P is cisplatin). The EP/EMA regimen is difficult to administer owing to both myelosuppression and the fact that even minor impairment of renal function caused by cisplatin can escalate the toxicities associated with methotrexate (El-Helw and Hancock 2007).

> **Sheffield salvage protocol for high-risk patients**
>
> - *Cisplatin* intravenous infusion, three times daily.
> - *Etoposide* intravenous infusion, once daily.
> - *Cyclophosphamide* intravenous infusion, only on the first day.
> - Repeat cycles should be administered at a 7–10 day interval

Salvage surgery to remove the resistant disease, for example, hysterectomy, thoracotomy, or craniotomy, may occasionally be required.

Role of surgery

Surgery during the treatment of high-risk GTN is employed in selected patients with drug-resistant disease. Thoracotomy with pulmonary wedge resection is the commonly performed procedure. Hysterectomy after careful exclusion of other sites of metastatic disease may benefit selected patients. Women with high-risk GTN may undergo surgery for removal of primary tumour or metastases, or for the management of metastatic complications, such as haemorrhage or infection. A careful evaluation for the extent of the disease should be carried out prior to proceeding with surgery. Prompt regression of β-hCG within 1 or 2 weeks of the surgical procedure predicts favourable outcome.

Long-term complications of treatment

Patients treated with combination chemotherapy are at a higher risk of developing secondary tumours, such as myeloid leukaemia, colon and breast cancer. Multiple-agent chemotherapy may result in premature menopause.

Follow-up

See follow-up for low-risk GTN.

Further reading

El-Helw LM, Hancock BW. Treatment of metastatic gestational trophoblastic neoplasia. *Lancet Oncol* 2007; **8**(8):715–24.

Internet resource

International Society for the Study of Trophoblastic Diseases: http://www.isstd.org

Gestational trophoblastic disease: special situations

Pulmonary metastases (Fig. 4.7.9)

Respiratory failure from pulmonary metastases is a rare but potentially lethal problem. If the patient is breathless at rest before treatment their respiratory function is likely to deteriorate further when they start chemotherapy. Other risk factors for developing respiratory failure include cyanosis, pulmonary hypertension, anaemia, and >50% lung opacification. Mortality rates of 100% have been reported in such patients and reducing the initial dose of chemotherapy does not seem to protect against the development of respiratory failure.

Due to increased risk of haemorrhage, extracorporeal perfusion techniques and avoidance of mechanical ventilation are recommended.

Brain/central nervous system disease (Fig. 4.7.10)

It is recognized that persistent GTD can readily metastasize to the brain, with an incidence as high as 8–15%. When CNS metastases are present the prognosis is at its worst. The risk of CNS metastases is increased with increased risk score, multiple pulmonary metastases, and when β-hCG level is >50,000 IU/L.

Patients with CNS metastases require coordinated multimodality treatment to achieve the optimal outcome.

Treatment of CNS metastases differs between centres. In the UK, chemotherapy with or without surgery or stereotactic radiotherapy are standard management while in USA radiotherapy is often used simultaneously with systemic chemotherapy. Brain irradiation has a dual advantage of both being tumourocidal and haemostatic.

In the UK, as an alternative to brain irradiation, systemic chemotherapy regimens (EMA/CO in Charing Cross and MEA in Sheffield) were modified by increasing the dose of systemic methotrexate and including intrathecal methotrexate to ensure maximum penetration of the drug to the CNS (see 'Sheffield treatment for established CNS disease' box).

Craniotomy is reserved for patients with resectable cerebral metastases prior to chemotherapy or to evacuate intracranial haematoma or in cases where a patient develops resistance to chemotherapy, provided that there is no active disease elsewhere. Irrespective of treatment approach in both sides of the Atlantic, cure rates are similar and range from 60–80%.

Some centres advise administering intrathecal methotrexate for patients considered to be at high risk of

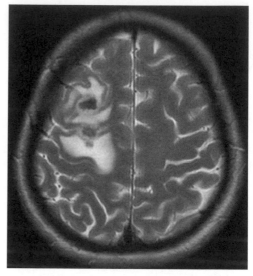

Fig. 4.7.10 CT scan showing brain haemorrhagic metastases of choriocarcinoma

CNS metastases. However, in a study from Sheffield this was found not to be necessary (Gillespie et al. 1999).

Other sites of metastasis

Liver metastases are an ominous feature and reported survival rates are poor. There is also substantial risk of hepatic bleeding especially during the first course of chemotherapy. Irradiation of the whole liver, in conjunction with chemotherapy has been advocated to reduce the risk of serious haemorrhage, but there is no conclusive evidence. Selective hepatic artery occlusion has been shown to be effective in controlling liver haemorrhage from choriocarcinoma. Hepatic resection might be necessary to control bleeding or to excise resistant foci.

Metastatic trophoblastic tumours to the vagina are highly vascular and friable and can cause acute spontaneous haemorrhage. If the patient develops acute bleeding, surgical intervention might be necessary to control haemorrhage.

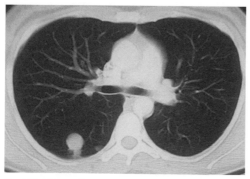

Fig. 4.7.9 CT scan of lung showing metastatic choriocarcinoma.

Sheffield treatment for established CNS disease

Arm A
- *Methotrexate* infusion over 24 hours.
- *Folinic acid* commencing at the end of methotrexate infusion given by intravenous injection or orally.

Arm B
- *Dactinomycin* intravenous infusion.
- *Etoposide* intravenous infusion.
- *Intrathecal methotrexate*.

Arms A and B are repeated sequentially with seven day rest interval between them.

Placental site trophoblastic tumour (PSTT)

PSTT is a rare and unique form of GTN. It arises from intermediate cytotrophoblast at the implantation site following any type of pregnancy. It has various clinical presentations, most commonly vaginal bleeding and its clinical course is unpredictable.

Unlike other forms of GTN, PSTT have little syncytiotrophoblast and therefore secrete less β-hCG. β-hCG levels correlate neither with the volume nor with the malignant behaviour of the tumour. Some tumours secrete human placental lactogen (hPL) and if elevated, serial measurement of serum levels may serve as a tumour marker.

Most PSTTs are confined to the uterus; however, 30% of patients have metastases at time of diagnosis. Unlike other forms of GTD the WHO risk score is of little help.

After careful metastatic work-up, hysterectomy is the best mode of treatment for patients with disease limited to the uterus. However, patients with metastatic PSTT cannot be cured with surgery alone and treatment with multi-agent chemotherapy is required. Data from the Charing Cross suggest EMA/EP as the best regimen while in Sheffield patients are treated primarily with MAE. Other centres use EMA/CO.

PSTT have better prognosis when:
- Tumour is limited to uterus.
- Antecedent pregnancy is <4 years.
- Absence of distant metastases at time of diagnosis.

Twin molar pregnancy

The coexistence of normal intrauterine pregnancy and GTD (usually CHM) is rare and it occurs in <1 in 200 molar pregnancies. This situation poses both diagnostic and therapeutic dilemmas. It is often diagnosed late, associated with reduced live birth and increased risk of complications like pre-eclampsia and bleeding. In addition, the need for chemotherapy is greater than other molar pregnancies regardless of whether the pregnancy was terminated or allowed to proceed to term.

The guidance in the UK is that 'if twin pregnancy is associated with a partial mole then it would be allowed to proceed; in the case of association with complete mole then the pregnancy may proceed after appropriate counselling'.

Ectopic molar pregnancy

As with normal pregnancy, hydatidiform mole could occur with ectopic pregnancy, most commonly in the fallopian tubes. Their presentation and management is similar to non-ectopic molar pregnancy. Once suspected, histopathology should be reviewed at special centres to avoid overdiagnosis and in confirmed cases registration to a special centre and strict follow-up is essential.

Fertility issues

After successful treatment of molar pregnancy (with preserving reproductive organs) patients should expect normal reproduction. Only 1–2% of these patients will subsequently develop another molar pregnancy (60-fold increased risk). Therefore, all patients with history of molar pregnancy should have:
- First trimester ultrasound scan to confirm normal gestation.
- β-hCG measurement 6 weeks after completion of pregnancy to exclude persistent trophoblastic tissues.

It appears that the obstetric outcomes for patients with history of molar pregnancy are no different from those who have no such history. Neither low- nor high-risk treatments affect fertility or congenital abnormality rates in subsequent pregnancies.

Contraception

Following chemotherapy, women are advised not to conceive for at least 12 months after the conclusion of their treatment.

In the UK, all patients with GTD are advised to avoid the use of oestrogen containing oral contraceptives while β-hCG levels are still elevated since there is a theoretical risk of inducing metastases or drug-resistance. Combined oral contraceptives can be used once β-hCG levels have returned to normal. However, in North America clinicians consider the risks of early further pregnancy are higher than the risks of oral contraceptives and therefore are willing to recommend these during the first year of remission. There is agreement that intrauterine contraceptive devices should be avoided until hCG levels become normal due to the risk of uterine perforation and bleeding.

Key points

- Respiratory failure should be considered imminent in patients with multiple pulmonary metastases, high hCG, and cyanosis.
- CNS metastasis is a poor prognostic sign and needs multimodality treatment.
- Surgery is the primary treatment for patients with PSTT; however, chemotherapy is essential in those with metastases.
- FIGO staging or WHO prognostic score cannot be applied to PSTT.
- Women should avoid pregnancy for 1 year after chemotherapy. The majority will conceive with no increased rate of congenital malformation.

Further reading

Bagshawe KD, Dent J, et al. The role of low-dose methotrexate and folinic acid in gestational trophoblastic tumours (GTT). *Br J Obstet Gynaecol* 1989; **96**(7):795–802.

El-Helw LM and Hancock BW. Treatment of metastatic gestational trophoblastic neoplasia. *Lancet Oncol* 2007; **8**(8):715–24.

Gillespie, AM, Siddiqui N, et al. Gestational trophoblastic disease: does central nervous system chemoprophylaxis have a role? *Br J Cancer* 1999; **79**(7–8):1270–2.

Hancock, BW. .Staging and classification of gestational trophoblastic disease. *Best Pract Res Clin Obstet Gynaecol* 2003; **17**(6):869–83.

Hancock, BW and Tidy JA. Current management of molar pregnancy. *J Reprod Med* 2002; **47**(5):347–54.

Khan F, Everard J, et al. Low-risk persistent gestational trophoblastic disease treated with low-dose methotrexate: efficacy, acute and long-term effects. *Br J Cancer* 2003; **89**(12):2197–201.

Newlands E. Presentation and treatment of gestational trophoblastic disease (GTD) and gestational trophoblastic tumour (GTT) in the UK. In: Hancock BW, Newlands ES, Berkowitz RS, et al. (eds) *Gestational Trophoblastic Disease 2nd ed*, London: Chapman and Hall, 2003. pp.229–47.

RCOG. *The Management of Gestational Trophoblastic Neoplasia* (38). London: RCOG, 2004.

Internet resource

International Society for the Study of Trophoblastic Diseases: http://www.isstd.org

Cancers of vulva and vagina

Vulval cancer

Epidemiology

The incidence of vulval cancer appears to be increasing. Despite this, cancer of the vulva is rare, with approximately 1022 new cases being diagnosed in the UK each year.

Aetiology

Age

It tends to be seen in older women, with 80% of cases occurring in the >60 years age group. The increased incidence of vulval cancer may reflect the increased life expectancy. However, there also appears to be an upward trend of younger women (<50 years of age) being diagnosed with the disease.

Human papilloma virus

HPV has been found to be responsible for approximately 30–50% of vulval cancers and up to 80% of vulval intraepithelial neoplasias (VINs). It is now widely accepted that the development of vulval cancer is linked with the persistence of high risk subtypes of HPV, mainly, 16, 18, and 31. HPV has also been found to be associated with multicentric disease of the lower genital tract, and concurrent lesions can be found in the vulva, cervix, vagina, and anus in patients infected with HPV.

Immunosuppression

Women with coexisting medical conditions that result in suppression of the immune system also appear to be at increased risk of developing vulval cancer. These include women infected with HIV, and those on immunosuppressive medication, for example, women with renal transplants.

Smoking

Studies have shown an association between smoking and the development of vulval tumours. The pathogenesis is thought to be due to the increased likelihood of persistent HPV infection, the direct damage of cells by the toxins found in tobacco, or alterations in local or cell-mediated immunity.

Chronic skin conditions and inflammation

Several chronic skin conditions predispose women to developing vulval cancer, and include lichen sclerosus, lichen planus, and Paget's disease. Of these, lichen sclerosus is the most common, with a 4–7% risk of malignancy. Studies suggest that the majority of vulval cancers will have lichen sclerosus, squamous cell hyperplasia, or differentiated VIN in the adjacent epidermis. Lichen planus is thought to coexist and possibly cross-over with lichen sclerosus, and may have a similar risk of malignancy.

Vulvar intraepithelial neoplasia (VIN)

The pathology and natural history of VIN is different from that of cervical intraepithelial neoplasia (CIN) and certainly more complicated. The evidence to show that VIN is linked with vulval cancer is based on clinical cancer developing with adjacent VIN, occult cancers found within areas of VIN, and reports of VIN progressing to cancer. The risk of developing vulval cancer in women is approximately 5–8%, and is more likely in women with high-grade VIN or VIN with high-grade multicentric disease.

Lifestyle and social background

It has been suggested that obesity may increase the risk of vulval cancer, while women who eat foods rich in vitamin A are reportedly less likely to develop it. However, more research is required to substantiate these claims. Squamous cell carcinomas are also said to be associated with poverty, nulliparity, early menopause, condylomata, and granulomatous inflammation.

Pathology

The majority of vulval cancers are squamous cell in origin; however, melanomas, basal cell carcinomas, adenocarcinomas, undifferentiated carcinomas, sarcomas, and metastatic tumours from a variety of primary sites have also been reported in the literature.

Squamous cell carcinoma

This is by far the most common type of vulval cancer and is responsible for approximately 90% of all cases. It tends to be less aggressive, in the sense that it tends to develop slowly over years. Furthermore, adequate treatment and follow-up of VIN can reduce the risk of cancer development. Verrucous carcinomas are a slow growing type of squamous cell carcinoma, and as its name suggests have the appearance of a large wart.

Vulval melanoma

After squamous cell carcinoma this is the second commonest type of vulval cancer. Vulval melanomas cause 4% of all vulval cancers.

Adenocarcinoma

Paget's disease of the vulva can predispose to vulval adenocarcinoma, and is found in 1–2% of women with vulval cancer.

Sarcomas

Sarcomas are responsible for <2% of all cancers of the vulva. They tend to be aggressive and therefore grow quickly. There are several different types of sarcomas that can affect the vulva. These include leiomyosarcomas, rhabdomyosarcomas, angiosarcomas, neurofibrosarcomas, and epithelioid sarcomas.

Screening

Education

At present, a screening programme for vulval cancer does not exist. However, vigilance for any early warning signs and symptoms of vulval cancer is important. Women should be educated about self-examination, and healthcare professionals are advised to examine the vulva during routine cervical smear taking.

Vulval cytology

Vulval cytology obtained either using liquid-based cytology or the traditional Papanicolaou method may provide a clinically useful non-invasive method of screening for vulval cancer, although at present, this remains a research tool. Biopsy and histology continue to remain the gold standard for diagnosis.

Clinical features

The most common symptoms that women with vulval cancer present with include itch or irritation, pain and soreness, a thickened, raised area of discoloration, an open sore or ulcer, vaginal discharge or bleeding, a lump or swelling. It is important to remember, however, that these symptoms can be common, and the majority of these women will not have vulval cancer.

Diagnosis and staging

The size and location of the lesion should be documented, and any involvement of adjacent structures such as vagina, urethra, base of bladder, or anus, should be duly noted. Diagnosis of vulval cancer is made on clinical suspicion and confirmed by biopsy and histology. Vulval cancer is staged surgicopathologically using the FIGO classification, and not clinically.

Vulval cancer spreads by direct extension to involve adjacent structures such as the vagina, urethra, and anus; by lymphatic channels to the inguinal and femoral nodes, and haematogenously to distant sites including the lungs, liver, and bone. Lymphatic metastases tend to occur earlier than haemotogenous spread, with the overall incidence of lymph node metastases reported to be approximately 30%. Haematogenous spread tends to occur late, and is rare in the absence of nodal metastases.

Vaginal cancer

Epidemiology

Primary vaginal cancer constitutes 2% of female genital tract cancers, and Cancer Research UK estimates that approximately 240 new cases are diagnosed annually. It causes approximately 100 deaths in the UK each year and is responsible for 1 out of every 1000 cancers diagnosed in women. Advances in diagnosis and treatment have made cure rates comparable to those of cervical cancer.

Aetiology

Age

Vaginal cancer tends to be most commonly seen in older women between the ages of 60–70 years, with >70% of cases occurring in this group. Vaginal cancer (clear cell carcinoma) in younger women is more common in those whose mothers were administered diethylstilboestrol during pregnancy.

Human papilloma virus

It is well established that the development of both pre-invasive and invasive vaginal cancer is associated with persistent infection with high risk oncogenic subtypes of HPV, especially 16.

Cervical intraepithelial neoplasia or cervical cancer

Up to 30% of women with primary vaginal cancer have a history of in situ or invasive cervical cancer treated in the preceding 5 years.

Vaginal intraepithelial neoplasia (VAIN)

VAIN is less common than CIN, and the relationship between VAIN and the development of invasive vaginal cancer remains unclear, but appears to be multifactorial.

Chronic conditions

A previous history of chronic vaginal irritation, the use of ring pessaries, and previous treatment with radiotherapy have been shown to be associated with the development of vaginal cancer.

Social background

When compared to both healthy women and those with in situ disease, women with invasive disease have been found to be less well educated, have lower income, are more likely to have five or more lifetime sexual partners, have an early age at first intercourse, and be current smokers at diagnosis.

Pathology

Squamous cell carcinoma

Due to the close proximity of the cervix to adjacent structures, 80% of vaginal cancers are due to direct extension of adjacent tumours (e.g. cervical) or mestastases (e.g. endometrial). Of the 20% that originate in the vagina (primary vaginal cancer), the most common histological type is squamous cell in origin, and accounts for >90% of cases. The association between the development of squamous cell vaginal carcinoma following either cervical or vulvar carcinoma reinforces the correlation between HPV and the development of multicentric disease.

Adenocarcinoma

Most women with vaginal adenocarcinomas tend to be >50 years, with the exception of clear cell carcinoma. Clear cell adenocarcinoma is very uncommon, and is almost always associated with an exposure to diethylstilboestrol in utero. It is unusual before the age of 13, and most commonly presents between the ages of 17–22. Early stage disease is often curable but more advanced disease can result in both haematogenous and lymphatic metastases.

Papillary adenocarcinoma tends to arise from the connective tissue surrounding the vagina, and is less likely to spread via the lymphatics.

Adenosquamous carcinomas are also known as mixed epithelial tumours, and tend to be more aggressive. They are extremely rare and are found in up to 2% of women diagnosed with vaginal carcinoma.

Malignant melanoma

Malignant melanomas of the vagina are found in about 2% of women with vaginal cancer. They are more likely to develop in women in the fifth decade of life, and in the lower third of the vagina. Vaginal melanomas are harder to treat compared to malignant melanomas of the vulva, and the most important factor for survival appears to be tumour size. The prognosis of patients with primary malignant melanoma is poor regardless of the primary method of treatment (surgery, radiotherapy, or both).

Small cell carcinoma

These tumours are also known as oat cell carcinomas. They are extremely rare, with only 20 cases reported worldwide.

Sarcoma botyroides

This vaginal tumour is extremely uncommon and is almost exclusively found in children under the age of 5 years. It arises from the lamina propria of the vagina and is of mesenchymal origin.

Screening

Vaginal cancer does not fulfil the WHO screening criteria, and therefore a national screening programme for vaginal cancer does not exist. Detecting and treating women with a history of CIN, VIN, and those undergoing cervical screening can prevent vaginal cancer developing.

Clinical features

Patients generally remain asymptomatic in both the pre-invasive and early stages of vaginal cancer, and tumours are most commonly detected during routine cervical screening. Cancer Research UK estimates that up to 20% of women with vaginal cancer remain asymptomatic at presentation.

In general, 80–90% of women will present with one of more of the following symptoms: intermenstrual, postcoital or postmenopausal bleeding, offensive or blood-stained discharge, dyspareunia, vaginal irritation, or a vaginal mass. In more advanced disease, women may also complain of pelvic pain, constipation, difficulty in micturition, and lower limb oedema.

Women with a history of HPV infection, CIN, or VAIN are at an increased risk of developing vaginal cancer and adequate follow-up of these women should be arranged.

Diagnosis and staging

The diagnosis of primary vaginal cancer is made by histology and clinical examination. FIGO classifies vaginal tumours depending on their site of involvement. Tumours extending to the external cervical os should be deemed cervical cancers, while tumours involving the vulva should be classified as vulval cancers. This emphasizes the necessity for, and vigilance during, the staging process, which incorporates an examination under anaesthesia, cystoscopy, proctoscopy, and sigmoidoscopy, depending on the site of the lesion.

Although the staging of vaginal cancer is made clinically, the concurrent use of radiological imaging allows an assessment of the tumour size and extent to be made. A combination of these influence the type of treatment the woman is offered, i.e. surgery versus radiotherapy. MRI provides a greater degree of resolution enabling the boundaries of the tumour to be assessed with greater accuracy.

The use of integrated PET/CT in gynaecological malignancies has increased in recent years, evolving into a potential method of assessing treatment response and disease progression.

PET/CT has been shown to be of value in the primary staging of untreated advanced cervical cancer, in helping to identify the cause of post-treatment elevation of tumour markers, and in the assessment of recurrent cervical cancer. Significantly fewer studies have been carried out using PET/CT in the staging, assessment of tumour progression, and response to treatment in vaginal cancer due to the relative rarity of the disease.

Further reading

Daling JR, Madeleine MM, Schwartz SM, et al. A population-based study of squamous cell vaginal cancer: HPV and cofactors. Gynecol Oncol 2002; **84**:263–70.

Lai CH, Yen TC, Chang TC. Positron emission tomography imaging in gynaecologic malignancy. Curr Opin Obstet Gynecol 2007; **19**:37–41.

Podratz PC, Symmonds RE, Taylor WF, et al. Carcinoma of the vulva: analysis of treatment and survival. Obstet Gynecol 1983; **61**:63–74.

Robboy SJ, Duggan MA, Kurman RJ. The female reproductive system. In: Rubin E, Farber JL. Pathology, 3rd edition pp. 962–1027. Philadelphia, PA: Lippencott-Raven, 1999.

Internet resource

Cancer Research UK: Vulval Cancer—available from http://www.cancerreseachuk.org/.

Management of vulval cancer

Principles of management

The management of women with vulval cancer should be undertaken by the MDT within a gynaecological cancer centre. It allows development of expertise and experience, and has been shown to improve the clinical outcome for this group of women. Management should be individualized, as there is no 'standard' form of management for every woman.

Surgery

The aim of surgery in the management of vulval cancer is to remove sufficient tissue to prevent local recurrence. This is achieved with an adequate resection margin of at least 1cm. The choice of surgery as the primary form of treatment depends on whether it is felt that an adequate margin can be achieved (i.e. the stage and site of disease) and the woman's clinical condition. Groin lymphadenectomy allows the disease to be staged, identifies both microscopic and macroscopic metastases, and removes all nodal disease, thereby reducing the risk of groin recurrence. The radicality of surgery depends on the size and location of the primary lesion, with radical vulvectomy being reserved for large tumours, and wide local excision for smaller ones.

The radical vulvectomy employs a triple incision technique, in which the groin node dissections are performed through separate incisions to the excision of the primary lesion. On the other hand, a butterfly (en bloc) incision is indicated in circumstances where, due to tumour site and size, a triple incision procedure would not allow complete removal of disease. However, skin bridge recurrences between the tumour and the groins in early stage disease appear to be uncommon.

Radical vulvectomies involving triple incisions are associated with a shorter operating time, less blood loss, a shorter hospital stay and less wound morbidity compared to en bloc dissection, although, stage for stage and site for site, there is no significant difference in the recurrence rate, overall or DFS between the two procedures. To date, there have been no randomized trials comparing the triple incision technique to the butterfly incision.

Early-stage disease

Lesions <2cm in diameter that are confined to the vulva or perineum with stromal invasion of ≤1mm (FIGO stage 1A), can be managed by wide local excision without groin node dissection. This is because the risk of lymph node metastases is negligible (<1%). If the lesion is central, and the resection margin comes to within 1cm of the midline, bilateral groin node dissection should be carried out. In order to reduce the risk of recurrence, groin node dissection should involve removal of both the superficial inguinal as well as the deep femoral nodes. To date, there is no evidence to favour the use of prophylactic groin irradiation over primary surgery in early stage disease.

Advanced disease

Although the main form of treatment in women with advanced disease tends to be radiotherapy (see later), a small group of carefully selected patients can still benefit from surgical intervention. In those women with extensive disease where it is felt that adequate resection margins can be achieved, surgery in the form of radical vulvectomy, bilateral groin node dissection and pelvic exenteration, or ano-vulvectomy with formation of end colostomy can be carried out with good results. The overall 5-year survival rate in women with locally advanced disease treated by radical ano-vulvectomy has been reported to be 62%, and is comparable to that reported in other series of similar patients treated with other modalities.

Lateral lesions

Tumours are considered lateral if the lesion with a 1-cm margin does not impinge upon any midline structure such as the clitoris, urethra, vagina, perineal body and anus. In these tumours, only ipsilateral groin node dissection may be performed. However, if the ipsilateral nodes are positive, contralateral lymphadenectomy should then be recommended.

Other lesions

Excision of other skin lesions such as VIN or lichen sclerosus should be considered as they may contain foci of invasion. The depth of tissue that needs to be removed is much more superficial than if malignancy is suspected.

Radiotherapy

Radiotherapy may be given as a primary form of treatment in those women with larger, more advanced lesions involving bladder or rectum, or who are considered unsuitable for surgery. It may also be used as an adjunct to surgery in patients who have inadequate surgical resection margins, or lymph node involvement. There appears to be improved survival in women with positive margins who receive adjuvant radiotherapy compared to those who do not.

Several published studies suggest that adjuvant radiotherapy should be recommended in women with two or more nodal micrometastases in either groin, one macrometastasis (>5mm), or extra-capsular spread in any node. In these situations, external beam radiotherapy should be administered to the pelvis and groins. It is uncertain, however, whether unilateral or bilateral adjuvant radiotherapy should be given to the groins in women with unilateral positive groin nodes.

In the radical setting small fraction sizes are required to avoid unacceptable toxicity. 1.7Gy may be considered the optimum but some centres will use 1.8Gy with a reduced total dose. Radical treatment usually requires an initial dose of 45–50Gy to the primary and nodal sites followed by either a second phase limited to the primary lesion, or brachytherapy to this area. Adjuvant therapy to the inguinal and lower pelvic nodes can be given using larger fraction sizes of up to 2Gy daily to avoid prolonged treatment times.

Chemotherapy

The role of chemotherapy in the management of vulval cancer remains unclear. It has been used in combination with radiotherapy as a form of adjuvant treatment in women with node-positive disease, those with inoperable or unresectable tumours, or in women presenting with recurrence.

Although platinum and 5-FU have also been used in the management of recurrent vulval disease, there appears to be little consensus as to how best to integrate chemotherapy into the management of vulvar cancer. The choice of chemotherapy depends on the patient's age and performance status. As yet, the use of postoperative adjuvant chemotherapy is unproven.

Chemoradiotherapy

Chemoradiation is a more recent advance in both the neoadjuvant and adjuvant treatment of vulvar cancer. This has involved the use of single-agent cisplatin or cisplatin and 5-FU, in combination with radiotherapy. There continues to be some discrepancy regarding the efficacy of chemoradiotherapy in treating vulval cancer, as some studies have shown a reduction in the local relapse rate, improved PFS and OS, while others have not.

Prognosis

Prognosis appears to depend on both nodal status and the size of the primary lesion. In the absence of lymph node involvement, the 5-year survival for vulval cancer exceeds 80% (all stages). This decreases to approximately 50% with inguinal node involvement, and to 10–15% with pelvic node metastases. The rate of nodal positivity appears to rise with increasing tumour depth. Furthermore, the incidence of vulval recurrence has also been shown to be related to the measured disease-free surgical margin on the histological specimen.

Post-treatment issues

The major complications related to surgery include wound breakdown, wound infection, lymphocyst formation, and lymphoedema. The morbidity related to groin wound infection, necrosis, and breakdown has been reported in up to 85% of patients who have had a butterfly incision. This is reduced to 44% if a triple incision is carried out, with major wound breakdown occurring in 14% of women.

Forty per cent of patients develop lymphocysts following groin lymphadenectomy, which, if large and problematic, can be managed by incision and drainage. The incidence of lymphocyst formation appears to increase with early and greater mobilization. Lymphoedema is a later complication, with an incidence of 62–69% following groin node dissection. The onset of lymphoedema occurs within 3 months in 50% of women, and in up to 85% of women by 12 months.

The development of complications following treatment with radiotherapy depends on several factors such as dose, dose per fraction, the size of the radiation field, the radiation dose rate, the woman's general health, and associated treatments such as surgery and chemotherapy. These complications include vulval soreness, skin blistering, diarrhoea, urinary frequency, and the formation of fistulae (rectovaginal, vesico-vaginal, and entero-vaginal). The incidence of lower limb lymphoedema is also greater in those women who have been treated by surgery including lymphadenectomy, and adjuvant radiotherapy (groin and pelvis). In this group of patients, the prevalence of lymphoedema has been shown to be approximately 47%.

Many women who have been diagnosed with cancer, even when successfully treated, have a fear of recurrence. Follow-up clinics (at least up to 5 years initially), nurse specialists, and self-help groups can be very supportive and reassuring. However, as contact with the medical and nursing team becomes less common as the woman continues to recover, this can also be a source of anxiety for some. Sexual dysfunction is a consequence for many women diagnosed with and treated for a gynaecological cancer, and vulvar cancer is certainly no exception.

Recurrence and management

Recurrent vulval cancer appears to correlate most closely with the number of positive groin nodes. The recurrence rate for invasive squamous cell carcinoma of the vulva appears to range from 15–33%. The most common sites of recurrence include the vulva (69.5%), groin nodes (24.3%), the pelvis in 15.6%, and distant metastases in 18.5%.

Local vulval recurrences carry a better prognosis compared with groin or distant metastases, as these lesions tend to be more amenable to surgical excision. Groin recurrences are difficult to manage, and although radiotherapy would be the preferred first option, surgical excision should be considered in patients who have already received groin irradiation.

Recent advances

Sentinel lymph node biopsy

The concept of sentinel node biopsy is based on the assumption that the first node to receive lymphatic drainage from the malignant tumour should be the first site of metastatic spread. In vulval cancer, if the sentinel node is free of the disease, so should the entire lymphatic basin of the groin be. The benefit of sentinel node biopsy is the reduction in the need for a complete groin node dissection in women who do not have metastatic disease, with a resulting fall in the associated morbidity. Recent studies show that the sentinel node is best identified through a combination of methylene blue dye, technetium, and the use of a hand-held gamma probe.

Sentinel node dissection has been reported to have an approximately 98% detection rate with a false negative rate of 0% in patients with early stage disease. The ability to identify bilateral sentinel inguinal lymph nodes appears to be related to the proximity of the tumour to the midline.

Further reading

Ansink A, van der Velden J, Collingwood M. Surgical interventions for early squamous cell carcinoma of the vulva. *Cochrane Database Syst Rev* 2000; **2**:CD002036.

Dhar KK and Woolas RP. Lymphatic mapping and sentinel node biopsy in early vulvar cancer. *BJOG* 2005; **112**:696–702.

Nyberg RH, Iivonen M, Parkkinen J, et al. Sentinel node and vulvar cancer: a series of 47 patients. *Acta Obstet Gynecol Scand* 2007; **86**:615–19.

Stehman FB, Bundy BN, Dvoretsky PM, et al. Early stage I carcinoma of the vulva treated by ipsilateral superficial inguinal lymphadenectomy and modified radical hemivulvectomy: a prospective study of the Gynecologic Oncology Group. *Obstet Gynecol* 1992; **79**:490–7.

van der Velden J and Ansink A. Primary groin irradiation vs primary groin surgery for early vulvar cancer. *Cochrane Database Syst Rev* 2000; **3**:CD002224 [update in Cochrane Database Syst Rev 2001; **4**:CD002224].

Management of vaginal cancer

Principles of management

Women with vaginal cancer should be managed in a cancer centre within a MDT setting. Vaginal cancer can be effectively treated, and when found in early stages can be curable. Factors to be considered when planning treatment for vaginal cancer are the stage, size, and location of the lesion; the presence or absence of the uterus; whether there has been previous pelvic irradiation; and the fitness of the woman. The management of each woman must therefore be individualized accordingly.

In women who have had a previous hysterectomy, 62% of women developed cancer in the upper third of the vagina, compared to 34% of women who had not had a hysterectomy.

Surgery

Surgical treatment of vaginal carcinoma can be curative in carefully selected women with early stage (I, small stage II) disease, and in women with stage IV disease in whom exenterative surgery is planned. Surgery is the treatment of choice if clear excision margins are achievable. However, the proximity of the bladder and the rectum can make vaginectomy potentially problematic.

In stage I disease, lesions at the apex, particularly on the posterior vaginal wall, may be treated with a partial vaginectomy or extension of a radical hysterectomy. More superficial lesions may be treated by wide local excision. Lesions that lie in the upper part of the vagina can be treated by radical hysterovaginectomy with removal of the parametria and paracolpos. In women who have had a previous hysterectomy, an upper vaginectomy and parametrectomy can be performed, although care must be taken to ensure adequate resection margins. Both procedures should also include bilateral pelvic node dissection.

In stage II disease, surgery should be reserved for those women with minimal extension outside the vaginal wall, and those with lesions in sites that would allow a procedure less aggressive than a radical vaginectomy.

Pelvic exenteration is rarely performed as a primary procedure, except in stage IVa disease. In these instances, the type of exenterative procedure performed will depend on the affected organs (bladder, rectum, or both). In these women, extension of the lesion to the pelvic side walls, or distant sites of metastases must be excluded prior to surgery if long-term cure is to be achieved.

Radiotherapy

Radiotherapy continues to remain the treatment modality of choice unless clear resection margins can be obtained. The proximity of the vagina to the bladder and rectum can potentially limit treatment options and increase the risk of complications to these organs. More recent advances include improvements in reducing the complications following radiotherapy by conforming the treatment volume to reduce the dose to the bowel and bladder.

In early stage disease, intracavitary radiation may be used, while both intracavitary and external irradiation are required for larger and more advanced lesions. The use of both external irradiation and brachytherapy in treating vaginal cancer has been shown to achieve excellent results. Furthermore, it also allows vaginal preservation, albeit a reduced functional capacity.

Women with advanced disease tend to be treated with chemoradiation rather than by radiotherapy alone (see following section). Prognosis in these women tends to be poorer compared to those with early stage disease, and although surgical salvage may be required, primary radiotherapy does not appear to have any advantage over surgery.

Chemoradiotherapy

Much of the current evidence in the use of chemoradiotherapy in managing women with vaginal cancer stems from studies in cervical cancer. As much of the aetiology of the two diseases is similar, it is not unreasonable to extrapolate such data. Several large randomized trials have demonstrated the use of chemoradiation in treating women with advanced cervical cancer with good results. The use of platinum-containing regimens, namely, cisplatin and 5-FU-cisplatin, have been shown to improve overall and PFS in women with advanced disease (stage IIb, III, and IVa cervical carcinoma), bulky stage 1B disease, and high-risk early stage cervical carcinoma. Other studies have also shown an initial response rate as high as 60–85% with the concurrent use 5-FU, mitomycin, and cisplatin alongside radiotherapy. The longer-term benefits, however, have been more variable.

Chemotherapy alone appears to offer little benefit in the management of advanced (stage III and IV) disease.

Prognosis

The reported overall 5-year survival rate for vaginal cancer is 44%, which is poorer than that for both cervical and vulval cancer. Prognosis depends not only on the stage and location of the disease, but age, symptomatology, and differentiation. Women who present over 60 years of age, who are symptomatic at the time of diagnosis, have lesions in the middle and lower third of the vagina, and have poorly differentiated tumours, appear to have a poorer prognosis. The extent of involvement of the vaginal wall is also significantly correlated to survival, and the stage of disease in women with vaginal squamous cell carcinoma.

Post-treatment issues

Several complications can occur following the treatment of vaginal cancer. Following surgical resection of the tumour, vaginal scarring and stenosis can be particularly problematic in sexually active women. It is estimated that approximately 20% of vaginal carcinomas are diagnosed in women <50 years of age. Feelings of depression, grief, stress, and sexual dysfunction are frequently experienced by women following treatment for a gynaecological malignancy. This highlights the role of nurse specialists and psychosexual counsellors in the continuing care of these women.

Problems with urinary retention can occur in those who have undergone radical total vaginectomy. In patients who have received neoadjuvant radiotherapy, surgery can also result in the development of bladder and bowel fistulae.

Women who require adjuvant radiotherapy often undergo a 'radiation menopause' if premenopausal, which can also result in 'thinning' of the vaginal mucosa. Hormone replacement therapy may have a role in some women.

Recurrence and management

The factors that affect the risk of recurrence are increased tumour bulk (specified by size in centimetres or FIGO stage), tumour site (upper lesions faring better), and tumour circumferential location (lesions involving the posterior wall faring worse). The major pattern of relapse appears to be pelvic. Increased tumour bulk increases the likelihood of metastatic relapse, as does failure to achieve local control of the tumour.

Recurrent vaginal cancer carries a grave prognosis, with most cases presenting within 2 years of primary treatment. The 5-year survival rate following recurrence is approximately 12%. In centrally recurrent vaginal cancers, there may be a role for pelvic exenteration or further radiotherapy. Studies have not shown any benefit to using either cisplatin or mitoxantrone in recurrent or advanced disease, and chemotherapy does not appear to play a role in the management of these women.

Recent advances

HPV vaccine
Women who have had a previous anogenital cancer, especially cervical cancer, have a higher risk of developing vaginal cancer. Many of the risk factors for the development of cervical cancer also increase the risk of vaginal cancer. HPV, especially type 16, has been found to play a role in the aetiology of vaginal cancer. Evidence supporting HPV vaccination in vaginal cancer is limited and extends from studies in cervical cancer. The anticipated reduction in the incidence of cervical cancer in women who have been vaccinated against the oncogenic subtypes of HPV is likely to result in a similar fall in the number of women who develop vaginal cancer.

Sentinel node detection
Sentinel node detection using technetium-labelled nanocolloid has been demonstrated in patients with primary and recurrent vaginal carcinoma. There appears to be a strong correlation between sentinel node status and histological findings at lymphadenectomy. Determining sentinel node status in women with vaginal cancer may have a role in planning treatment, when decisions between the benefits of radical surgery versus chemoradiotherapy/radiotherapy must be made.

Further reading

Carter J, Rowland K, Chi D et al. Gynecologic cancer treatment and the impact of cancer-related infertility. *Gynecol Oncol* 2005; **97**:90–5.

Chu AM, Beechinor R. Survival and recurrence patterns in the radiation treatment of carcinoma of the vagina. *Gynecol Oncol* 1984; **19**:298–307.

Malmstrom H, Simonson E, Trope C. Primary invasive squamous cell carcinoma of the vagina. *Acta Obstet Gynecol Scand* 1989; **68**:411–15.

Tewari KS, Cappuccini F, Puthawala AA, et al. Primary invasive carcinoma of the vagina: treatment with interstitial brachytherapy. *Cancer* 2001; **91**:758–70.

van Dam P, Sonnemans H, van Dam P-J, et al. Sentinel node detection in patients with vaginal carcinoma. *Gynecol Oncol* 2004; **92**:89–92

Basal cell carcinoma

Introduction

Basal cell carcinoma (BCC) is a slow growing, locally invasive (hence called rodent ulcer) malignant epidermal skin tumour. The exact incidence is difficult to obtain although there is a worldwide trend in increasing incidence. Approximately 1 million new cases are diagnosed per year in the USA.

Aetiology

The most important aetiological factors appear to be UV exposure and genetic predisposition.

- BCC is common in the sun-exposed area of the head and neck. Some studies suggest intermittent brief holidays may cause a higher risk than occupational exposure to sunlight.
- BCC is a feature of a number of genetic conditions such as Gorlin's syndrome (basal cell naevus syndrome), Basex syndrome, and Rombo syndrome. In Gorlin's syndrome which is due to mutations in the tumour suppressor PTCH gene, hundreds of BCCs can develop.
- Other risk factors include increasing age, male gender, fair skin, immunosuppression, vaccination scars and arsenic exposure. Sunscreen use and low fat diet are thought to be protective.

Pathology

The common histological subtypes are superficial, nodular, and morpheoic (sclerosing). Other variants include micronodular, infiltrative, and basosquamous BCC which are aggressive with high risk of local recurrence. Perivascular and perineural invasion are also associated with aggressive tumours. BCC infiltrate tissues in a three-dimensional fashion. Lymph node metastasis is extremely rare except in those with multiple recurrences or uncontrolled primary tumour.

Clinical features

Clinical suspicion arises when there is any friable non-healing lesion on the skin. Some lesions manifest with brief bleeding and complete healing followed by recurrence of the lesion.

The common growth patterns are nodular, superficial, multifocal, and morphoeic. The sites affected are head and neck (52%), trunk (27%), upper limb (13%), and lower limb (8%)

- Nodular BCC, the commonest clinical subtype, occurs on the skin of the head and neck region of elderly patients. It presents as a shiny, pearly, telangiectatic papule or nodule. The pearly appearance becomes more prominent during skin stretching. Radially arranged dilated capillaries are often seen across the surface of lesion. With ongoing growth, tumour ulceration can occur which leads to central umbilication of the lesion with a raised rolled border. Islands of pigments can also be seen.
- Superficial BCC occurs on the trunk or limbs of young people. It presents as a well-defined, erythematous, scaling or slightly shiny macular lesion. Stretching the lesion causes an increase in the degree of erythema, highlights the shiny surface and reveals a peripheral thread-like pearly rim or islands of pearliness distributed throughout the lesion. These lesions will progressively enlarge

and may reach 5–10cm in diameter. Biopsy is needed prior to definitive treatment.

- Morphoeic SCC typically presents as a pale scar and palpation reveals firm induration which extends more widely and deeply than is evident on inspection. It slowly enlarges to reach a large size. Biopsy is necessary.
- Pigmented BCC are nodular BCCs with increased melanization leading to an appearance of a hyperpigmented translucent papule.

Examination

Clinical examination should be done in a well-lit area with the aid of a magnifier. Whole skin and regional nodal examination are necessary.

Diagnosis

Diagnosis is often clinical. Biopsy is indicated when there is clinical suspicion of an alternative diagnosis or if histological subtype may influence treatment decision. Punch or shave biopsy may be appropriate. Imaging of the local area, e.g. by CT, may be indicated when there is suspicion of bone involvement and deep infiltration (particularly for a lesion close to the embryonic fusion lines such as the nasal vestibular region, or pre- and postauricular regions).

Treatment

Treatment is aimed at eradication of tumour with acceptable cosmetic and functional outcome. A number of treatment options are available for BCCs (see 'Treatment modalities in BCC' box) and the choice of treatment in small BCCs depends on various factors (see 'Treatment of choice in BCC' box). Radiotherapy is indicated when cosmetic and/or functional outcome is better with radiotherapy compared with surgery and when there is a need to avoid complex plastic surgery.

Surgery

Wide excision (WE)

WE of simple lesions needs a 2–3mm margin whereas complex lesions, clinically poorly defined lesions, and recurrent disease need a margin of 3–5mm. An adequate microscopic margin is 0.5mm. Excision of the primary BCC should extend to fat to ensure adequate tumour control.

The most appropriate management after incomplete excision is debatable. The treatment options include re-excision, Mohs micrographic surgery (MMS), or radiotherapy. Adjuvant radiotherapy improves 5-year recurrence-free survival from 61–91%. Observation is an option for frail elderly patients where further surgery and radiotherapy may not be appropriate.

Mohs' micrographic surgery

During this procedure, the tumour is excised and the entire peripheral and deep margins are examined by frozen section for residual tumour. Mapping and staining of excised tissue and a specialized tissue sectioning procedure enable precise localization of residual tumour and the process of excision continues until the margin is tumour free. It offers better histological analysis of tumour margin with maximal conservation of tissue compared with surgical excision. MMS is the treatment of choice for tumours with poorly defined borders (morphoeic), recurrent tumours, extensive disease, aggressive histological subtype, incompletely excised tumours and BCCs at high-risk anatomical sites (mask area of face, scalp, embryonic fusion planes, periorbital area and eyelid). In these situations, MMS offers better chances of cure than excision.

Curettage and desiccation
It is suitable for small lesions (<2cm) where >95% cure can be achieved. However it is highly operator dependent. It is not recommended for morphoeic BCC, tumours >2cm, and recurrent BCC.

Cryosurgery
During cryotherapy BCC is destroyed with a clinically normal margin. However, it lacks the benefit of histological confirmation of a complete tumour removal. The best reported results are around 99% at 5 years. An important adverse outcome of cryotherapy is the obscuring of tumour recurrence by fibrous scar tissue.

Topical imiquimod (5% cream)
Imiquimod is believed to act by boosting T helper 1 type immunity by inducing various cytokines. In superficial BCC, it is reported to result in 73–75% histological clearance.

Photodynamic therapy (PDT)
PDT involves activation of a photosensitizing drug by visible light to produce activated oxygen species that destroy the cancer cells. Though there is good initial clearance (88%) with one or multiple treatments, the recurrence rates are higher (up to 31%). Hence it is recommended only for situations in which established treatments are not feasible.

Radiotherapy
Radiotherapy results in 93–95% 10-year control rate for BCC of ≤2cm. Radiotherapy details are given in the 'Radiotherapy for skin cancer' box.

Recurrence
Recurrence is common with mid-face and pre-auricular lesions, tumours >2cm, and aggressive subtypes. Two-thirds of recurrences occur within 2 years of primary treatment and 20% occur in 2–5 years. Recurrences after non-surgical treatment are generally treated with surgical resection followed by plastic surgical repair. Recurrence after surgical treatment can be treated with surgery or radiotherapy.

The rate of recurrence depends on the mode of primary treatment. MMS has the lowest recurrence rate (1%). The reported recurrence rates with other treatments are: standard excision 10%, curettage and dessication 7.7%, radiotherapy 8.7%, and cryotherapy 7.5%.

Prognosis
Overall 10-year control rate is >90%. A number of factors influence prognosis. The important prognostic factors are size, depth of invasion, histological subtype (morphoeic, infiltrative, and basosquamous have higher recurrence rates), completion of excision (incomplete excisions have a 30% recurrence rate), site of disease (disease around nose, eyes and ears have higher recurrence rates), and presence of perineural spread.

Further reading
Ceilley RI, Del Rosso JQ. Current modalities and new advances in the treatment of basal cell carcinoma. *Int J Dermatol* 2006; **45**:489–98.

Neville JA, Welch E, Leffell DJ. Management of nonmelanoma skin cancer in 2007. *Nat Clin Prac Oncol* 2007, **4**:462–9.

Telfer NR, Colver GB, Morton CA. Guidelines for the management of basal cell carcinoma. 2008. *Br J Dermatol* **159**:35–48.

Veness MJ. The important role of radiotherapy in patients with non-melanoma skin cancer and other cutaneous entities. *J Med Imaging Rad Oncol* 2008; **52**:278–86.

Internet resources
British Association of Dermatologists: http://www.bad.org.uk
National Comprehensive Cancer Network: http://www.nccn.org
Skin Cancer Foundation: http://www.skincancer.org

Treatment modalities in BCC
Surgical excision
- WE
- MMS

Surgical destruction
- Curettage and desiccation
- Cryosurgery
- Carbon dioxide laser

Non-surgical destruction
- Topical immunotherapy with imiquimod
- Photodynamic therapy
- Radiotherapy

Treatment of choice in BCC
Surgery and radiotherapy (RT) are effective treatments for small and less invasive tumours. Large and deeply invasive lesions are treated with surgery with or without postoperative radiotherapy.
RT favoured in:
- Mid-face, nasal, inner canthus, lower eye lid, lip commissures (better function)
- Multiple superficial lesions difficult to excise (better cosmesis)
- Patients >70 years (long-term toxicity is less of an issue)
- Patients who wish to avoid surgery
- Patients prone to keloid formation

Surgery is the choice in:
- Readily excisable lesions in those <70 years
- Lesions in hair-bearing areas or overlying lacrimal gland
- Recurrence after RT
- Multifocal disease especially with dysplastic skin
- Upper eye lid tumours (better function)
- Dorsum of the hand (better function)
- Below knee and other sites of poor vascularity (problem with healing and function)
- Invasion to bones and joints*

*Cartilage invasion is not an absolute contraindication to radiotherapy. Radiotherapy is, however, avoided in large pinna lesions with extensive, inflamed, or painful cartilage invasion.

Radiotherapy for skin cancer

Consent
- Acute reactions involve dermatitis and mucositis which resolve by 6 weeks following treatment.
- Late effects involve thinning of skin, alopecia, loss of sweating, change in colour, telangiectasia, and fibrosis.

Position and immobilization: depends on the site

Type of radiation: depends on depth of penetration needed and type of underlying tissue:

Depth of penetration
- ≤5mm deep lesion—superficial X-ray
- >5mm–2cm deep lesion—orthovoltage X-ray or low energy electrons (4–6MeV)
- >2cm tumour—high energy electrons or photons

Underlying tissue
- Bone—electrons are preferable to avoid increased absorbed dose from orthovoltage X-rays.
- Air cavities (e.g. near sinuses)—X-rays or photons preferred as dosimetry is difficult with electrons

Treatment volume
- Well-defined BCC: 5mm margin around macroscopic tumour
- Ill-defined BCC and SCC: 10mm margin

Beam shaping
Custom-made lead cut out for X-rays and end frame cut-out for electrons. Crenellation of the margin of a round cut out gives a better cosmesis by blurring the edge of the radiation reaction.

Radiotherapy dose
BCC is thought to be more radiosensitive than SCC. Equivalent doses for BCC and SCC and a rough guide for selection of fractionation regimens are as follows:

BCC	SCC	Patient/tumour characteristic
60Gy/30 fractions	60–66Gy/30–32 fractions	<70 years, >3cm tumour
50Gy/20 fractions	55Gy/20 fractions	<70 years, >3cm tumour
40Gy/15 fractions	40Gy/10 fractions	>70 years + <3cm tumour
40.5Gy/9 fractions	45Gy/9 fractions	>70 years + <3cm tumour
32.5Gy/5 fractions	32.5Gy/5 fractions	>70 years + <3cm tumour
12–15Gy/1 fraction	12–15Gy/1 fraction	selected elderly patients

Special considerations

Electron planning
- Electron beam field is defined by 50% isodose and the 90% is 3–5mm inside the field. The PTV needs to be enclosed within 90% isodose which needs a 5mm larger electron applicator than defined by PTV.
- At higher energies, isodoses close to the surface bow inwards which necessitates 1cm larger applicator diameter than the defined PTV to ensure homogenous dose to the tumour
- Surface dose increases with electron energy, such that there is a need for bolus for lower energies
- Bolus is also used to bring up high dose to surface to avoid radiation to underlying critical structures.
- Stand-off effect: fill the area with bolus/calculate correction

Normal tissue shielding
- Lower eyelid and canthi tumours need corneal shielding.
- Lip tumours need buccal shields.
- Shields used with electrons should be coated with wax to absorb scattered radiation.
- When treated with electrons tumours in the pinna and nasal regions need wax coated lead plugs in the external auditory canal and nose respectively to minimize normal tissue damage.

Squamous cell carcinoma

Introduction

Squamous cell carcinoma (SCC) is the second most common skin cancer constituting 20% of skin malignancies. The incidence appears to be increasing and males are more commonly affected.

Risk factors include exposure to ionizing or ultraviolet radiation, immunosuppression, scars, chronic wounds, smoking, and arsenic exposure. Congenital conditions such as oculocutaneous albinism and xeroderma pigmentosum are also associated with increased risk of SCC. It is common in sun exposed areas and hence sun screen is protective.

Pathology

In situ SCC (Bowen's disease) is limited to the epidermis and presents as a flat scaling pink lesion with irregular borders. There is no risk of metastasis, although progression to invasive SCC occurs in 3–11% of cases.

In situ SCC of the glans penis (erythroplasia of Queyrat) has 20% risk of metastasis and 30% can progress to invasive disease.

Invasive SCC is composed of a collection of atypical keratocytes which invade the dermis and deeper structures. Other histological variants are:

- Adenoid SCC: can metastasize in 3–19% and is associated with rapid local growth
- Adenosquamous SCC: shows squamous appearance superficially and glandular appearance deeply. These are aggressive tumours.
- Spindle cell SCC: appears as ulcerated nodules or exophytic tumours and may be difficult to distinguish from sarcoma histologically. These tumours are aggressive with a tendency to perineural invasion and metastasis (25%).
- Verrucous SCC: appears like a large wart. These are slow growing, locally invasive, and do not metastasize.
- Keratoacanthoma: appears as a rapidly growing nodule with a central keratin plug. True lesions can undergo spontaneous regression but most are now viewed as SCC.

Clinical presentation

Typical presentation is a raised pink papule or plaque with erosion or ulceration. In advanced cases SCC presents as large ulcerated masses with bleeding. Metastasis is primarily to the regional nodes (2–6%). The head and neck region is the commonest site in men whereas the upper limb followed by head and neck are the commonest sites in females. Only 8% of SCC arise on the trunk.

Examination should include the whole skin and regional lymph nodes.

Diagnosis

Tissue biopsy is essential for diagnosis. CT scan helps to detect regional lymph nodes. FNA of the enlarged lymph node under radiological guidance is advised. Open surgical biopsy should be avoided. The role of sentinel node biopsy is evolving.

Staging

- T1: ≤2cm in greatest dimension
- T2: >2–5cm in greatest dimension
- T3: >5cm in greatest dimension
- T4: tumour invades deep extradermal structures
- N1: regional nodal metastasis
- M1: distant metastasis

Treatment

Three factors that influence treatment of SCC are: the need for removal of tumour locally, the possibility of 'in-transit' metastasis, and regional nodal metastasis. Treatment options include:

- Surgical excision
- Radiotherapy—used a primary treatment and adjuvantly after surgery
- MMS

Ablative techniques such as cryotherapy and curettage and electrodessication are generally not recommended for invasive SCC as these do not allow histological confirmation of adequate excision margin.

Surgery

Surgery is aimed at complete removal of the tumour and of any metastasis. Low risk tumours of <2cm are excised with a minimal margin of 4mm whereas tumours of >2cm size, high risk tumours (grade 2–4, in high-risk locations such as ear, lip, scalp, eyelids, and nose) and those extending into subcutaneous tissue need a minimum margin of 6mm or more. Depth of excision should be through normal underlying fat. The accepted minimal microscopic margin is >1mm.

Mohs micrographic surgery

MMS is indicated in high-risk tumours and recurrences. MMS allows a high cure rate with minimal tissue destruction. High-risk SCC include lesions of >2cm, depth of >4mm, and Clark level IV or V, tumour involvement of muscle, nerve or bone, scar carcinomas, high-grade (3–4) tumours, and tumours on ear and lip.

Tumours involving periocular and periauricular regions, recurrent tumours, tumours with poorly defined margins and recurrences after radiotherapy are best treated with MMS.

Management of lymph nodes

The treatment of metastatic lymph nodes is primary surgery. Elective lymph node dissection is not routinely advised. There is some evidence that it may have a role in tumours of >8 mm in depth. Patients with recurrent thick (>4mm) lesions in the vicinity of the parotid (temple, forehead and preauricular area) are also considered for elective nodal treatment.

Radiotherapy

Principles of primary radiotherapy and treatment guidelines are same as those for BCC (see Chapter 4.8, Basal cell carcinoma, p.386). Five-year control rate with radiotherapy is comparable with surgery with >93% for T1 lesions, 65–85% with T2, and 50–60% with T3–4 lesions. Radiotherapy is indicated after incomplete excision when further surgery is not contemplated, as incomplete excision leads to 50% local recurrence.

Postoperative radiotherapy to the primary tumour site is considered for patients with high-risk disease after complete excision. High-risk disease includes: tumour invasion beyond subcutaneous tissue (T4), recurrent disease, margin <5mm, perineural invasion (major or minor nerve), lymphovascular invasion, in-transit metastases, and nodal metastasis. Indications for postoperative radiotherapy after primary surgical management of metastatic lymph nodes are:

- ≥3cm node
- ≥2 positive nodes in neck and ≥3 nodes in axilla and groin
- Extranodal tumour extension
- Close or positive margin
- Skin involvement
- Major nerve involvement
- Parotid node metastases
- After salvage surgery for recurrent nodal metastases

The role of postoperative chemoradiotherapy for high-risk SCC is being evaluated. Palliative radiotherapy is used in metastatic disease to obtain symptom relief.

Chemotherapy
In patients with distant metastasis from SCC, cisplatin-based chemotherapy is the most effective. A commonly used combination is cisplatin with adriamycin, which has an overall response rate of >80% with complete response rate of 30%. However, survival is generally <2 years.

Recurrence

Most recurrences occur within 2–3 years. Treatment is individualized based on the extent of recurrence and previous treatment.

The reported recurrence rate with various treatments are as follows: MMS 3.1%, surgical excision 8.1%, and radiotherapy 10%.

Prognostic factors

- Grade of differentiation: grade 3–4 lesions are twice as likely to recur and three times as likely to metastasize than grade 1–2 lesions.
- Histological type: spindle cell carcinoma and adenosquamous carcinoma have a high risk of recurrence and metastasis.
- Location of tumour: scalp, lips, pinna, nose, and genital lesions have a high risk of metastasis.
- Tumour size: risk of recurrence and metastasis increases with size of the tumour. Risk of recurrence is twice (15% vs. 7%) and risk of metastasis is 3-fold (30% vs. 9%) in tumours >2cm compared with tumours of <2cm.

- Depth of invasion: tumours with of depth <2mm seldom metastasize whereas those with >4mm have a high risk of recurrence and metastasis.
- Perineural invasion: occurs in 2.5% of tumours and its presence indicates a high risk of local recurrence (up to 50%) and distant metastasis (up to 35%).
- After lymphadenectomy, prognosis depends on number of positive nodes and presence of extranodal spread.
- Recurrence: local recurrence increases rate for further recurrence (25%) and lymph node metastasis (30%)
- Tumours in immunosuppressed patients and those arising from scars have a poor prognosis.

Outcome

Local control rate for SCC is 10–15% lower than for a similarly sized BCC.

Bowen's disease (*in situ* SCC)

Bowen's disease presents as a slow-growing erythematous plaque. Surgery, topical treatment, and radiotherapy are the options for treatment. Radiotherapy dose is 40–50Gy in 10–20 fractions using 100–150KV superficial X-rays and results in 95–100% local control.

Keratoacanthoma

Keratoacanthoma presents as a rapidly enlarging lesion with a central keratin plug. Histologically, it is difficult to distinguish from SCC. In up to 20% of patients spontaneous regression can occur over 6–12 weeks. Treatment options include early excision and radiotherapy (similar to SCC).

Further reading

Motley R, Kersey P, Lawrence C. Multiprofessional guidelines for the management of the patient with primary cutaneous squamous cell carcinoma. *Br J Plast Surg* 2003; **56**:85–91.

Neville JA, Welch E, Leffell DJ. Management of nonmelanoma skin cancer in 2007. *Nature Clin Prac Oncol* 2007; **4**:462–9.

Veness MJ. The important role of radiotherapy in patients with non-melanoma skin cancer and other cutaneous entities. *J Med Imaging Radiat Oncol* 2008; **52**:278–86.

Internet resources

British Association of Dermatologists: http://www.bad.org.uk
National Comprehensive Cancer Network: http://www.nccn.org
Skin Cancer Foundation: http://www.skincancer.org

Merkel cell carcinoma

Introduction

Merkel cell carcinoma (MCC) is a rare aggressive neuroendocrine tumour of the skin. The estimated incidence is 0.44 per 100,000 people. The incidence is lower in the black population. The average age at presentation is 69 years. Males are more commonly affected (2:1 ratio). MCC commonly affects sun exposed areas of the body with 50% occurring in the head and neck region (especially the periorbital region), 40% occurring in the extremities, and the rest in the trunk.

Aetiology

The exact aetiology is not known. The reported risk factors include UV exposure, previous skin cancers and haematological malignancies, immunosuppression, and HIV infection. Both UVB and UVA are implicated in the causation. With renal transplantation the estimated risk is 0.13 per 1000 person-years and the transplant associated MCC tends to be aggressive. The relative risk of developing MCC in individuals with acquired immunodeficiency is approximately 13.

Pathology

Histologically these tumours consist of small blue cells which are usually ovoid with scanty cytoplasm and fine granular nuclei. There will be numerous mitoses and apoptotic figures. The triad of vesicular nuclei with small nucleoli, abundant mitoses, and apoptosis is highly suggestive of MCC. There are three histological patterns: intermediate type which is the most common followed by small cell, and the classic trabecular type.

MCC express neuroendocrine markers (NSE, synaptophysin, and chromogranin) and cytokeratin markers (cytokeratin 20 and CAM 5.2.). CK 20 staining showing a 'perinuclear dot' pattern of cytokeratin is pathognomonic for MCC. S100 and LCA are negative; 95% of MCC express CD117. TTF-1 is negative in MCC and positive in small cell lung cancer.

The minimal immunohistochemical panel for the primary tumour should preferably include CK-20 and TTF-1 where as that for node biopsy should include CK-20 and pancytokeratins (AE 1/AE3).

Differential diagnosis includes poorly differentiated small cell neoplasms such as small cell carcinoma, lymphoma, and melanoma.

Clinical features

MCC present as red or violaceous nodules with a shiny surface, often with overlying telangiectasia. Spread through dermal lymphatics can result in the development of satellite lesions. One-third of patients have regional nodal metastases at presentation and 50% develop distant metastases. Liver, lung, bone, and brain are the common sites of distant metastasis.

Diagnosis and staging

Initial evaluation includes clinical examination of the whole skin surface and regional nodes. Imaging includes CT scan of the relevant nodal region as well as chest and liver, especially in node positive patients. Blood tests include full blood count and biochemistry.

Studies of octreotide scanning show a sensitivity of 78% and specificity of 96%, but they are not used clinically. FDG PET is also being used but not routinely.

Staging

The new AJCC staging system is as follows:

Stage I
Tumours ≤2cm in maximum diameter:
- IA: pathologically negative nodes
- IB: clinically negative nodes

Stage II
Tumour >2cm in maximum diameter:
- IA: pathologically negative nodes
- IB: clinically negative nodes
- IC: tumour invades muscle, fascia, bone or cartilage and no nodal involvement

Stage III
Involvement of regional lymph nodes/ in transit metastasis:
- IIIA: micrometastasis in node
- IIIB: macrometastasis or in transit metastasis

Stage IV
Distant metastasis.
Note: 70–80% patients present with stage I–II, 10–30% with stage III, and 1–4% with stage IV disease.

Treatment

Stage I and II disease

Patients with clinically node-negative disease are treated with WE of the primary tumour (2–3cm margin –due to the risk of dermal lymphatic spread) and sentinel node biopsy (SNB). An excision margin of <2cm leads to 29% risk of local recurrence. SNB should be carried out at the same time as that of WE to avoid disturbance of the lymphatic drainage. If radiotherapy is to be used as an adjuvant treatment, the adequacy of surgical margin becomes less important. Approximately 30% patients have nodal disease on SNB. Mohs surgery is also an option for the treatment of the primary tumour.

Since there is a high risk of recurrence (46–76%), regional lymph nodes are generally treated electively with surgery or radiotherapy. Recently SNB has been used to identify micrometastasis. In the absence of nodal metastasis (negative on immunohistochemistry) no further treatment may be necessary (see later). Patients with positive SNB are treated with completion lymphadenectomy and/or radiotherapy. There is no proven survival advantage with prophylactic nodal dissection; however some experts advise nodal dissection in high-risk tumours such as those >2cm, with mitotic rate >10/HPF, histological evidence of lymphatic permeation and small cell histological pattern.

Though some experts advise aggressive surgery alone, most authors recommend routine postoperative radiotherapy to the primary site with a generous margin of 3–5cm (to ensure dermal lymphatics are treated). Based on retrospective reviews, adjuvant radiotherapy reduces local failure from 39% to 26% and the regional failure from 46% to 22%.

Radiotherapy to the nodal bed may be avoided in immunohistochemically proven-negative SNB. However, it may be considered if there is any risk of false negative SNB such as previous surgery and failure to perform immunohistochemistry on SNB. After lymph node dissection, postoperative radiotherapy may be avoided for axillary and groin disease to prevent significant risk of lymphoedema, unless there is multiple node involvement and/or presence of more than focal extracapsular extension.

In view of the risk of rapid repopulation after surgery, radiation should be started as soon as the wound is healed.

Radiotherapy dose to the primary tumour area ranges from 45–60Gy using 1.8–2Gy per fraction depending on the extent of the resection margin and residual disease. Nodal bed radiotherapy is given to a dose of 45–60Gy depending on the extent of the nodal involvement.

Radiotherapy alone can be used in the primary treatment as the tumour is radiosensitive.

There is no proven role for adjuvant chemotherapy in stage I–II disease.

Stage III disease

Stage III disease is treated with surgery of the primary lesion and nodal dissection. All patients receive postoperative radiotherapy (50–60Gy). Adjuvant chemotherapy may be considered. In a small study, concomitant chemoradiotherapy and adjuvant chemotherapy has resulted in a 3-year overall survival of 76%. The chemotherapy regimen is similar to that used for small cell lung cancer.

Stage IV disease

Stage IV disease is associated with a median survival of 9 months. The common sites of metastases are liver, bone, lung, brain, and skin. Platinum-based chemotherapy yields a short-lived complete response of 44% and partial response of 11%. The combination of cyclophosphamide, doxorubicin (or epirubicin) and vincristine has an overall response of 76% with 35% complete response, whereas the combination of platinum and etoposide results in 60% response rate with 36% complete response.

Follow-up

Most recurrences (90%) in MCC occur within 2 years of diagnosis and the median time of recurrence is about 8 months. This necessitates frequent follow-up to detect recurrences early. NCCN recommends follow-up every 1–3 months for the first year, 3–6 months for the second year, and annually thereafter. The follow-up programme should include history and physical examination with a complete skin and regional lymph node examination.

Prognosis

Stage is the most important prognostic factor. The 5-year DFS of stage I disease is 81%, stage II 67%, stage III 52%, and stage IV 11%. The median survival with node-negative disease is 40 months whereas that of node-positive disease is 11 months. The median survival of patients with distant metastases is 9 months.

Other poor prognostic factors include tumour >2cm, age >60 years, and lack of adjuvant radiotherapy.

Further reading

Bichakjian CK, Lao CD, Sandler HM. Merkel cell carcinoma: critical review with guidelines for multidisciplinary management. *Cancer* 2007; **110**:1–12.

Eng TY, Boersma MG, Fuller CD, *et al*. A comprehensive review of the treatment of Merkel cell carcinoma. *J Clin Oncol* 2007; **30**:624–36.

Henness S, Vereecken P. Management of Merkel tumours: an evidence based review. *Curr Opin Oncol* 2008; **20**:280–6.

Poulsen M. Merkel cell carcinoma of the skin. *Lancet Oncol* 2004; **5**:593–9.

Rockville Merkel Cell Carcinoma Group. Merkel cell carcinoma: recent progress and current priorities on etiology, pathogenesis, and clinical management *J Clin Oncol* 2009; **27**:4021–6.

Internet resources

Merkel cell carcinoma information: http://www.merkelcell.org/
National Comprehensive Cancer Network: http://www.nccn.org

Malignant skin adnexal tumours

Introduction

Malignant skin adnexal tumours represent 0.2% of skin cancers. These tumours generally exhibit a high risk of local recurrence and can be aggressive.

There is no consensus on the ideal classification of these tumours and a summary of histopathological classification is given in the box.

Many of the malignant skin appendage tumours arise from their benign counterpart. These tumours present as longstanding single or multiple lesions which start to grow rapidly. Multiple tumours can often be due to inherited (autosomal dominant) conditions and are usually associated with various cutaneous and non-cutaneous pathologies. The anatomical distribution of various subtypes depends on the normal distribution of the adnexal structures from which the tumours arise.

Surgery is the definitive treatment for localized tumours. Wide local excision is the standard surgery and in some tumours MMS is being evaluated. Patients with clinically enlarged nodes need regional lymphadenectomy whilst the role of elective lymphadenectomy is controversial. A few case series have reported the role of sentinel node biopsy.

Adjuvant radiotherapy is individualized based on the surgical margins, type of tumour, and risk of locoregional recurrence. Radiotherapy is also useful in a palliative setting.

A small number of patients present with metastatic disease and treatment is based on the fitness of patient, the site of disease, and symptoms. Various chemotherapy regimens have been used with varying success.

Sweat gland carcinomas

General features and management

Sweat gland carcinomas are traditionally divided into eccrine and apocrine carcinoma (see box). Sweat gland carcinomas are common on the head and neck, trunk and extremities (eccrine carcinoma), and axilla (apocrine carcinoma). These tumours exhibit an initially indolent growth followed by rapid progression including distant metastasis. The common sites of distant metastases include lungs, liver, and bone.

Surgery is the treatment of choice which involves WE and MMS is currently being evaluated.

Patients with clinically positive nodes need regional lymphadenectomy. The role of elective lymph node dissection is still controversial; some authors recommend it for patients with undifferentiated tumours and recurrent lesions. Results from small case series suggest that SNB is useful in detecting regional nodal metastasis in sweat gland carcinoma. However, it is not used routinely.

The role of adjuvant treatment with radiotherapy is unknown. However some authors recommend postoperative radiotherapy in cases of tumour of >5cm, deep infiltration, close (<1mm) or positive margin, high-grade tumours, perineural infiltration, dermal lymphatic invasion, ≥4 positive nodes, and extranodal invasion. Radiotherapy management is the same as for SCC of the skin (see Chapter 4.8, Squamous cell carcinoma, p.390).

There is no accepted chemotherapy regimen for advanced sweat gland carcinoma. Cisplatin/5-FU-based chemotherapy regimens are commonly used. Other reported treatments include: methotrexate; bleomycin; a combination of doxorubicin, cyclophosphamide, vincristine, and bleomycin; paclitaxel and cetuximab.

Prognostic factors include size, histological type, and presence of metastasis. Reported 10-year DFS is 56% in node-negative patients and 9% in node-positive patients.

Classification of malignant skin appendage tumours

Tumours with apocrine differentiation
- Adenoid cystic carcinoma
- Ductal carcinoma
- Apocrine adenocarcinoma
- Hidradenocarcinoma papilliferum
- Malignant mixed tumour
- Mucinous carcinoma
- Syringocystadenocarcinoma papilliferum
- Signet ring cell carcinoma
- Extramammary Paget disease

Tumours with eccrine differentiation
- Aggressive digital papillary adenoma and adenocarcinoma
- Cylindrocarcinoma
- Eccrine carcinoma
- Hidranocarcinoma
- Microcycstic adnexal carcinoma
- Polymorphous sweat gland carcinoma
- Porocarcinoma
- Spiradenocarcinoma

Tumours with sebaceous differentiation
- Sebaceous carcinoma
- Neoplasms in Muir–Torre syndrome

Tumours with follicular differentiation
- BCC with follicular differentiation
- Pilomatrical carcinoma
- Trichilemmal carcinoma

Subtypes of sweat gland tumours

Tumours with apocrine differentiation

These tumours present as non-tender single or multiple, firm rubbery or cystic masses with red to purple overlying skin.

- *Apocrine carcinoma*: an aggressive tumour presenting as solitary or multiple lesions in the axilla or anogenital area. Nodal metastasis and visceral metastasis can occur.
- *Ductal carcinoma*: commonly occurs in elderly men as a solitary nodule in the axilla. Local recurrences and regional and distant metastases are common.
- *Hidradenocarcinoma papilliferum:* these tumours often arise from a pre-existing benign lesion in the anogenital region in middle-aged women. It presents as a solitary ulcerated nodule. Regional and distant metastases can occur.
- *Malignant mixed tumour:* often arises in the trunk or extremities of middle aged women. It often presents as a solitary non-ulcerated or subcutaneous lesion. Lymph node metastasis is common. Surgical excision with prophylactic nodal dissection with or without adjuvant radiotherapy is the treatment.

- *Mucinous carcinoma*: is a rare low-grade tumour presenting as a solitary slow growing lesion in elderly men in the head and neck region. Metastases are rare.
- *Syringocystadenocarcinoma*: usually arises from a long-standing benign lesion. It commonly involves the scalp of adult women. The usual presentation is a sudden enlargement of a long-standing nodule or papule. Regional lymph node metastases are common.

Tumours with eccrine differentiation
These tumours have a wider bodily distribution than apocrine tumours and no specific distinctive clinical features.
- *Aggressive digital papillary adenoma and adenocarcinoma*: both occur usually in middle aged adults in acral locations and have a high risk of local recurrence (50%). Adenocarcinoma also has a tendency for distant metastasis (up to 40%) which occurs mainly in the lungs (>70%). These tumours present as a firm tan-grey to white-pink rubbery nodule usually over the volar surface of the space between the nail bed and the distal interphalangeal joint.
Lymphovascular spread is the only prognostic factor for predicting metastasis.
Radical excision or preferably digital amputation is the treatment of choice. SNB has been shown to be useful in a small case series. Lymphadenectomy is needed for nodal disease. Close follow with clinical examination and CXR is recommended for at least 10 years.
- *Cylindrocarcinoma*: occurs in the middle aged and elderly and is common in women. These tumours present as a rapidly growing ulcerated or bleeding nodule on the scalp. Tumour spread is by local destructive invasion and nodal and distant metastases.
- *Hidranocarcinoma*: occurs as a solitary ulcerated nodule on the head and neck, trunk, or extremities of middle-aged or elderly people. Local recurrence is common even after optimal local treatment.
- *Microcystic adnexal carcinoma*: is a locally destructive carcinoma often present as a sclerotic or indurated plaque with an intact dermis. The usual sites of involvement are mid face and lip. Wide local excision and Mohs surgery are the treatments of choice. Surgery is associated with a local recurrence rate of 50–60%. These are thought to be radioresistant tumours.
- *Porocarcinoma*: is the malignant counterpart of poroadenoma occurring in the elderly. It usually presents as a partially ulcerated, verrucous plaque or polypoid tumour on the lower extremities, head and neck, and trunk. Up to 20% develop local recurrence and regional recurrence can also occur. Surgery is the treatment of choice. Metastatic porocarcinoma is thought to be resistant to radiotherapy and chemotherapy.
- *Spiradenocarcinoma*: presents in the middle-aged and elderly as a single large nodule on the extremities, trunk, and abdomen. Since it arises usually from a benign counterpart, patients often give a history of a long-standing nodule with recent increase in size and other associated symptoms. Locoregional recurrences are common and 20% develop distant metastasis. Surgery is the treatment of choice.

Sebaceous carcinoma
General features and management
Sebaceous carcinomas commonly occur in women and are divided into ocular or extraocular type. The ocular type presents as a small solitary papule or nodule on the eyelids in the elderly. One-third of these patients have regional nodal metastasis (preauricular or cervical) and 5-year survival is 20%.

Surgical excision or MMS is the primary treatment of choice. Radiotherapy may be indicated for high-risk patients such as those with a positive tumour margin after excision and extensive nodal involvement. However, the risk of potential damage to ocular structures needs to be considered. Elderly patients may be treated with primary radiotherapy delivering >55Gy. Thirty-six per cent of patients develop local recurrence and 20–25% patients die of this cancer.

Extraocular tumours present as a yellowish, often ulcerated nodule on the head and neck region, foot, or genital region of elderly people. These tumours rarely metastasize to lymph nodes or viscera. Surgery is the treatment of choice; either WE or MMS.

Muir–Torre syndrome
This is an autosomal dominant disorder manifesting with various sebaceous tumours and visceral malignancy, usually colonic carcinoma but also cancers of ovary, uterus, and other GI sites. A single sebaceous tumour is adequate for the diagnosis if associated with internal tumours, but lesions are often multiple.

Skin appendage tumours with follicular differentiation
Histopathological features of these tumours resemble different portions of a normal hair follicle, hair shaft and/or perifollicular fibrous sheath.
- *Basal cell carcinoma with follicular differentiation*: this differs from BCC by occurring only on the face as a small circumscribed lesion and histologically it shows BCC with follicular differentiation features.
- *Pilomatrical carcinoma*: usually arise on the skin in the head and neck region (60%) in the elderly. These tumours are locally aggressive (>60% recurrence with surgery alone) but can also metastasize to lungs, bones, and lymph nodes. Lower limb tumours have more aggressive behaviour. WE is the treatment of choice. The role of radiotherapy and chemotherapy is not known.
- *Trichilemmal carcinoma*: usually present in older individuals as a solitary, exophytic or polypoidal nodule over sun-exposed areas. It usually presents as a long-standing nodule with a rapid growth phase. It has a non aggressive course with local damage only and is therefore treated with WE alone.

Further reading
Perna AG, Smith MJ, Krishnan B, *et al*. Primary cutaneous adnexal neoplasms and their metastatic look-alikes. *Pathol Case Rev* 2007; **12**:61–9.

Cutaneous melanoma: introduction, clinical features, and staging

Epidemiology

Melanoma is the most aggressive form of skin cancer. Its incidence is increasing worldwide. In Europe, its incidence has risen by 3–8% per year since the 1960s. The lifetime risk of melanoma in the UK is 1 in 147 for men and 1 in 117 for women. In Australia, the risks are significantly higher with lifetime risks of 1 in 25 for men and 1 in 35 for women. OS rates have improved due to early detection but survival of higher stage disease has improved very little in the past 10 years.

The peak incidence of melanoma occurs in middle age (40s) with <10% occurring in childhood, although the rates in those <20 years have increased by over 3% in the past 10 years. More than 25% of cases occur in people <45 years of age.

Aetiology

A number of factors are associated with increased risk of malignant melanoma:

- Ultraviolet sun radiation (especially UVB) is the main risk factor for the development of cutaneous melanoma. People with a history of blistering sunburn have a 2.5 times higher risk of melanoma. Other surrogate markers of sun sensitivity such as freckling (RR 2.5), burn without tanning (RR 1.7), red hair (RR 2.4), and blue eyes (RR 1.6) also confer an increased risk.
- People with a strong family history and multiple atypical moles are at the greatest risk of melanoma. Familial melanoma accounts for 10–15% of all patients. With one first-degree relative with melanoma the risk doubles and with ≥3 affected first-degree relatives there is a 35–70-fold increase.
- Mutation in chromosome 9p21 tumour suppressor gene, cycline dependent kinase inhibitor 2A (CDKN2A) accounts for 40% of hereditary melanomas, and CDK4 gene mutations confer a 60–90% lifetime risk of melanoma. CDKN2A mutation also increases the risk of pancreatic cancer (15% lifetime risk).
- B-RAF is a serine/threonine kinase which is a major player in the Ras-Raf-Mek-Erk mitogen activated protein kinase signalling transduction pathway that regulates cell growth, proliferation, and differentiation in response to various growth factors, cytokines, and hormones. BRAF mutation occurs in 66% of melanomas and >80% of melanoma associated with intermittent sun exposure have BRAF or NRAS mutations. Acral melanoma is not associated with either mutation.
- Mutation of melanocortin 1 receptor (MC1R) gene may contribute to the red hair/fair skin melanoma. MC1R mutation increases the risk of melanoma by 2–4-fold and there is also an increased risk of non-melanoma skin cancer.
- Xeroderma pigmentosa shows 600–1000-fold increase in skin cancers including melanoma.
- BRCA2 mutation increases risk of melanoma by 2.5–8-fold.
- Naevi: multiple benign naevi (>100) as well as multiple aypical naevi increase the risk of melanoma (RR 11).
- Immunosuppression: transplant recipients (RR 3) and patients with AIDS (RR 1.5) have increased risk of melanoma.

- Previous melanoma: those with a previous melanoma have a 2–10% risk of a further melanoma which increases further with two previous melanomas.

Pathology

There are four histological variants of cutaneous melanoma:

- Superficial spreading is the most common type (70%) occurring in the fourth to fifth decade of life. This often arises within a pre-existing naevus and is surrounded by a zone of atypical melanocytes that may extend beyond the visible border of the lesion. It is common on the intermittent sun exposed areas—lower extremities of women and back in men.
- Nodular melanoma (10–15%) presents as a symmetrical, uniform dark blue-black lesion. The median age at presentation is 53 years. Most common site is the trunk and these tumours show rapid evolution. Amelanotic nodular melanomas are often misdiagnosed.
- Lentigo maligna melanoma (10–15%) usually occurs on the sun-exposed areas of the head and neck and hands. Clinically these are large (often >3cm) flat lesions with areas of dark brown or black discoloration. These lesions arise from the premalignant lesion called Hutchinson's freckle.
- Acral-lentigenous melanomas, as the name suggests (acral-distal), occur on the palms, soles, and subungual regions. These lesions occur with the same frequency in whites and non-whites (2–8% of melanoma in whites and 40–60% melanoma of non-whites). These lesions can be easily misdiagnosed as subungual haematoma.
- Desmoplatic melanoma is a locally aggressive variant occurring in the sixth to seventh decade of life and men are commonly affected. It is common on the sun-exposed head and neck region.

The histology of melanomas is very variable depending on the specific subtype and primary site. Typically, the pathologist should report the type of melanoma, greatest thickness, radial or vertical growth phase, excision margins, and immunohistochemical staining pattern. Immunohistochemical stains used in melanoma include S100 (the most frequently used but it also stains benign melanocytes), HMB-45, Mitf, MART-1, and tyrosinase.

Clinical presentation

Patients usually present with new skin lesions or change in an existing skin lesion.

Initial evaluation includes a detailed history of duration of the lesion, duration in the change of appearance of lesion, previous history of sun exposure, sun burn, skin cancers, and immunosuppressive treatment and family history of melanoma.

Clinical assessment includes detailed examination and a clinical photograph of the lesion, full skin examination, and examination for lymphadenopathy and hepatomegaly. Clinical signs of melanoma include itching, bleeding, ulceration, or changes in a pre-existing mole. ABCDE features help to distinguish early melanoma from a benign mole:

- A: asymmetry
- B: border irregularity

- C: colour variation
- D: diameter of >6mm
- E: evolution (change in lesion)

However, >50% of melanomas arise *de novo* and may not have the ABCDE features.

Diagnosis

Investigations

In the absence of clinical evidence of regional lymph node involvement (i.e. stage I and IIa–b) or symptoms of distant metastases, there is no indication for any staging investigations. In patients with thick primary tumours (>4mm), CT scan may be useful to rule out metastatic disease. Studies show that a routine CXR revealed metastasis in only 0.1% whereas 15% showed false positivity. Similarly CT scan showed metastasis in 1.3% while false positivity was 16%.

Patients with an ulcerated lesion of >4mm (stage IIC) have an unfavourable outcome with median survival of 40%, which is lower than stage IIIA and hence a staging work-up similar to that for stage III disease is advised.

All patients with evidence of nodal metastasis (including micrometastasis) need staging investigations with full blood count, liver function tests, serum LDH, CXR, and CT scan of chest, abdomen, and pelvis.

PET/CT is more sensitive than anatomical imaging. Sensitivity is highest for metastases that are >1cm (≥90%), but can be useful in smaller deposits up to 0.6mm.

Tissue diagnosis

Excision biopsy to include 2–5mm of clinical margin of normal skin with a cuff of subdermal fat is the standard procedure. This helps to confirm diagnosis and provide guidance for subsequent management based on Breslow thickness (mm). Full-thickness incisional biopsy from the thickest part of the lesion is acceptable as a mode of diagnosis in certain anatomical areas (e.g. face, ear, palm/sole) and for large lesions. Shave and punch biopsies are not recommended.

The pathology report should include Breslow thickness, Clark level (for lesions ≤1mm), presence of ulceration, mitotic index (0 or $\geq 1/mm^2$), lateral and deep margin (mm) size, presence of satellite lesions, vascular invasion, nodal disease, and extranodal spread. Evidence of regression, tumour-infiltrating lymphocytes, vertical growth phase, and angiolymphatic invasion are useful prognostic factors.

Staging

Breslow thickness and ulceration are the two most important prognostic factors of localized disease. Clark level was considered as an independent prognostic factor for melanoma of <1mm thickness. Mitotic index is being introduced into the new TNM AJCC staging system which is related to prognosis (Table 4.8.1). M1a includes distant skin, subcutaneous, or nodal metastases with a normal LDH. M1b is lung metastases with a normal LDH and M1c is any other metastases with or without a raised LDH level.

Table 4.8.1 Staging of malignant melanoma (data from AJCC Staging 2009)

Stage IA	**T1a** N0M0	Breslow thickness ≤1.00mm with no ulceration and mitosis <1/mm²
Stage IB	**T1b**N0M0	Breslow thickness ≤1.00mm with ulceration or mitosis ≥1/mm²
	T2a NoM0	Breslow thickness 1.01–2.00mm without ulceration
Stage IIA	**T2b**N0M0	Breslow thickness 1.01–2.00mm with ulceration
	T3aN0M0	Breslow thickness 2.01–4.00mm without ulceration
Stage IIB	**T3b**N0M0	Breslow thickness 2.01–4.00mm with ulceration
	T4aN0M0	Breslow thickness >4.00mm without ulceration
Stage IIIA	T1–4a**N1a**M0	Micrometastasis in 1 node after SNLB
	T1–4a**N2a**M0	Micrometastasis in 2–3 nodes after SLNB
Stage IIIB	**T1–4b**N1aM0	Breslow thickness >4.00mm with ulceration
	T1–4bN2aM0	
	T1–4a**N1b**M	Clinically detectable metastasis in 1 node
	T1–4a**N2b**M	Clinically detectable metastasis in 2–3 node
	T1–4a**N2c**M	In transit metastases/satellites without metastatic nodes
Stage IIIC	T1–4bN1bM0	
	T1–4bN2b/cM0	
	Any T **N3**M0	≥4 metastatic nodes or matted nodes or intransit metastases/satellites with metastatic nodes
Stage IV	Any T any N **M1**	Distant skin, subcutaneous or nodal metastases with normal LDH (M1a) Lung metastases with normal LDH (M1b) All other visceral metastases with normal LDH or elevated LDH (M1c)

Further reading

Balch CM, Gershenwald, JE, Soong, SJ, *et al*. Final version of 2009 AJCC melanoma staging and classification. *J Clin Oncol* **27**:6199–206.

MacKie RM, Hauschild A, Eggermont AMM. Epidemiology of invasive cutaneous melanoma. *Ann Oncol* 2009; **20**(suppl 6):vi1–vi7.

Meyle KD, Guldberg P. Genetic factors for melanoma. *Hum Genet* 2009; **126**:499–510.

Internet resource

http://www.melanomaprognosis.org

Cutaneous melanoma: management of non-metastatic disease

Primary surgery

Surgical excision with an adequate margin is the primary treatment of choice for patients with no distant metastasis. The margin is the clinically measured margin during surgery rather than the histopathological margin. The extent of the margin depends on the depth of the melanoma and may need to be adjusted for cosmetic or functional reasons. Based on randomized studies, the recommended margins are: 1cm for lesions <1mm in depth, 1–2cm for lesions 1–2mm in depth, and 2cm for lesions >2mm in depth. Depth of excision is at least up to the muscle fascia, a more superficial excision is inadequate and a more deep excision does not improve outcome.

Though there are no conclusive clinical trials, a margin of 5mm is recommended for melanoma *in situ* and wider margin is recommend for desmoplastic melanoma because of its increased risk of local recurrence due to contiguous subclinical spread.

The long axis of excision should be in the direction of the lymphatic drainage and parallel to the long axis of the limb to reduce the risk of lymphoedema.

MMS is not advisable for the treatment of melanoma. It may have a role in ill-defined *in situ* melanoma of the lentigo maligna type and possibly desmoplastic melanoma.

Management of regional lymph nodes

The role of elective lymph node excision for node-negative disease has been debated for several years. Although initial retrospective studies showed a survival benefit with this approach, four randomized studies failed to show any survival advantage. Debate on the role of elective node dissection has been subsumed by emergence of the sentinel node (SN) concept.

Sentinel node biopsy (SNB)

The SN is the node to which the lymph initially drains from a tumour before passing to the other regional nodes. In theory the SN is most likely to contain tumour cells and if none are present in this node, it is unlikely that other lymph nodes are involved.

The risk of SN metastasis in melanoma depends on the thickness of the lesion. A tumour of <0.75mm thick has 1% SN positivity; 0.75–1mm has 5%; and 1mm thickness has 8% risk which steadily increases with increasing depth reaching 30% risk with 4mm thickness. A lesion >4mm thick has a 40% risk.

Although SN positivity is proven to have strong correlation with survival (90% 5-year survival for SN negative vs. 56% for SN positive), the role of lymph node dissection for SN-positive disease is still evolving. Many agree that there is no proven OS benefit from the routine application of SN biopsy in patients with cutaneous melanoma. However, there is some suggestion that it may increase the DFS. The recently reported MSLT-1 study was designed to assess the outcome of patients with occult metastases detected by SNB compared with those who received wide local excision alone. This study reported no OS benefit but better DFS, a secondary endpoint of the study. However, there is some controversy about the interpretation of this trial data.

There is no data on the role of SLN in predicting overall survival in these patients.

In practice, patients with lesions >4mm thick have a predicted incidence of SN positivity of 30–40%. Hence it is reasonable to offer SNB in this group of patients to provide prognostic information and selection into clinical trials. SNB may also be offered to selected patients with melanoma >1mm or Clark IV to provide staging and prognostic information.

SNB should be performed before wide local excision.

In patients with positive SNB the current practice is completion lymphadenectomy. However it is not known whether this will improve survival. The ongoing MSLT-II trial aims to examine the benefit of complete dissection on survival by randomizing patients with SN positive melanoma to undergo either complete nodal dissection or observation.

Management of positive nodes

Patients with metastatic lymph node disease are treated with regional node dissection if feasible and up to 13–59% of these patients do not develop metastatic disease. There is a significant risk of lymphoedema (especially with groin dissections) and patients should wear compression stockings for many months.

Lymph node dissection in melanoma patients should be undertaken only by surgeons with specialist training for such operations. This is because even after a complete dissection, there is a significant risk of recurrence in the nodal basin, necessitating a thorough formal dissection.

A dissection can only be deemed thorough if it includes levels I–III in the axilla and a complete clearance of the femoral triangle nodes in the groin. Ilioinguinal dissection may be indicated if there is evidence of pelvic nodes on imaging, gross involvement of inguinal nodes, or microscopic involvement of ≥3 inguinal nodes.

A therapeutic neck node dissection may include a superficial parotidectomy if clinically indicated. Even after such a dissection, there is up to 28% recurrence in the neck. Hence postoperative radiotherapy may be considered in high-risk lymph node disease (see later).

Adjuvant treatment

Adjuvant radiotherapy

There is no proven role for radiotherapy after complete excision of primary cutaneous melanoma. Adjuvant radiotherapy should be considered for close or positive margin when a re-excision is not feasible.

More than 20% of patients with melanomas of >2mm thickness have positive SNB and in patients with positive nodes, there is ≥20% risk of local recurrence after a complete node dissection. Several factors such as the number of lymph nodes involved (>3), size of lymph nodes (>3 cm), location (cervical), and presence of extracapsular extension (ECE) are shown to increase the risk of regional recurrence. ECE is the single most important risk factor.

A number of retrospective studies suggested some potential benefit with adjuvant radiotherapy for high-risk nodal disease. A phase II study of 234 patients treated with 45–50Gy in 2Gy fractions reported a 7% regional recurrence rate if there are any high-risk factors of extranodal extension, >3 nodes, recurrent disease in dissected nodal basin, or peroperative tumour spill (Burmeister et al. 2006). The interim analysis of a phase III randomized study of surgery alone vs. surgery followed by 48Gy in 20 fractions in 248 patients with macroscopic nodal disease has shown that radiotherapy improves lymph node field control with no impact on overall survival. Radiotherapy reduced the incidence of in-field recurrence from 20% to 5%.

Risk of recurrence varies with the location of tumour. In patients with high-risk cervical node metastasis (≥2 nodes, extranodal extension, node of ≥3cm in size, and recurrence in previously dissected neck), use of adjuvant radiotherapy is associated with regional control of 90%. Similar benefit is also seen with high-risk axillary nodal disease. However, the benefit of radiotherapy in high-risk inguinofemoral metastasis is inconsistent (Guadagnolo 2009).

Though there is a general consensus that radiotherapy improves regional control in high-risk nodal disease, the definitions of high-risk disease vary. The commonly used radiation fractionations are 48Gy in 20 fractions over 4 weeks and 30Gy in 5 fractions in 2.5 weeks. However, the shorter course of radiotherapy can result in a higher risk of lymphoedema.

Adjuvant systemic treatment

No trial has shown a survival benefit for adjuvant chemotherapy in localized malignant melanoma. Due to the activity of immune treatment in advanced melanoma, several trials have examined the role of interferon and vaccines in the adjuvant treatment of melanoma. A pooled analysis of three ECOG studies showed that adjuvant high-dose interferon improves relapse-free-survival (about 10% at 5 years) but not OS in patients with a high-risk resected melanoma. This group included patients with lesions ≥4mm thick with no nodal involvement and melanoma involving regional nodes or in transit metastasis. High dose interferon (20 MIU/m^2 IV 5 days per week for 4 weeks, 10 MIU/m^2 SC 3 days a week for 48 weeks) is an approved treatment for stage IIB/III melanoma in the USA and Europe. However, high-dose interferon is associated with a number of side effects such as acute constitutional symptoms, chronic fatigue, headache, weight loss, nausea, myelosuppression, and depression and most patients will require dose modifications during treatment. A recent study suggested that 15 MIU IV 5 days per week for 4 weeks is equivalent to and better tolerated than 10 MIU SC 3 days a week for 48 weeks (Gogas et al. 2007)

An EORTC trial (18961) examining the role of a ganglioside vaccine (GM2) in the adjuvant treatment of high-risk melanoma showed no benefit and there were concerns that patients may have done worse than with no treatment which lead to an early termination of this trial (Eggermont et al. 2008).

Primary radiotherapy

Radiotherapy has no role as a primary modality treatment except in elderly patients with extensive or unresectable lentigo maligna.

Ongoing studies

An ECOG study is evaluating the role of adjuvant high-dose IFN in patients with stage II and III disease compared with observation alone.

The EORTC 18991 trial will evaluate the role of 5 years of pegylated IFN-α2b compared with observation alone.

The EORTC 18081 study will assess the role of pegylated IFN in high-risk stage II patients with ulcerated melanoma.

A number of antiangiogenic agents and immunomodulators are undergoing further investigations. The AVASTIN-M study in the UK is evaluating the role of adjuvant bevacizumab in high-risk melanoma whereas the anti-CTLA-4 antibody, ipilimumab will be investigated as an adjuvant treatment in the EORTC 18071 study.

Further reading

Burmeister BH, Smithers BM, Burmeister E, et al. A prospective phase II study of adjuvant postoperative radiation therapy following nodal surgery in malignant melanoma-Trans Tasman Radiation Oncology Group (TROG) Study 96.06. Radiother Oncol 2006; 81:136–42

Eggermont AM, Suciu S, Ruka W, et al. EORTC 18961: Post-operative adjuvant ganglioside GM2-KLH21 vaccination treatment vs. observation in stage II (T3-T4N0M0) melanoma: 2nd interim analysis led to an early disclosure of the results. J Clin Oncol 2008; 26:A9004.

Eggermont AM, Testori A, Marsden J, et al. Utility of adjuvant systemic therapy in melanoma. Ann Oncol 2009; 20(6s):vi30–4.

Gogas H, Dafni U, Bafaloukos D, et al. A randomized phase III trial of 1 month versus 1 year adjuvant high-dose interferon alfa-2b in patients with resected high risk melanoma. J Clin Oncol 2007; 25:A8505.

Guadagnolo BA and Zagars GK. Adjuvant radiotherapy for high-risk nodal metastases from cutaneous melanoma. Lancet Oncol 2009; 10:409–16.

Henderson MA, Burmeister B, Thompson JF, et al. Adjuvant radiotherapy and regional lymph node field control in melanoma patients after lymphadenectomy: Results of an intergroup randomized trial (ANZMTG 01.02/TROG 02.01). J Clin Oncol 2009; 27(18s):Abstr LBA9084.

Phan GQ, Weber JS, Sondak VK, et al. Sentinel lymph node biopsy for melanoma: indications and rationale. Cancer Control 2009; 16:234–9.

Internet resources

Australian cancer network Melanoma guideline, Available from: http://www.cancer.org.au

National Comprehensive Cancer Network: http://www.nccn.org

Cutaneous melanoma: management of metastatic disease

Metastatic melanoma has a poor prognosis. Most patients with non-visceral metastases survive up to 18 months whereas the median survival of those with visceral involvement or an elevated serum LDH is 4–6 months. Lymph node and skin metastases in the absence of other metastases have the best prognosis (up to 18 months). Those with lung metastases in the absence of other visceral disease have an intermediate prognosis (up to 12 months median survival). Those with other visceral disease have a median survival of <6 months which is limited further in the presence of a high and rapidly increasing LDH. Patients with liver metastases from a primary uveal melanoma have a particularly poor prognosis usually limited to <3 months.

Treatment of melanoma metastases depends on the site of disease, whether or not it is localized and the overall fitness of the patient. Treatment can be with surgery, radiotherapy, systemic therapies, or BSC.

Role of surgery
In the presence of an isolated metastasis, especially if the patient has a long disease-free interval, e.g. 1 year, surgery may be the best option. The most common sites for surgical resection are skin, brain, and lung. Resection of liver metastases is not usually performed as liver metastases are associated with such a poor prognosis. Appropriate staging is important in these patients who undergo surgical resection. PET scans have been used to exclude further distant disease, especially if complex surgery is planned, e.g. resection of cerebral metastases.

Patients with up to three visceral metastases are candidates for surgical resection and the 5-year survival can be >20% after complete resection of lung metastases and 28–41% after complete resection of GI metastases. Similarly patients with solitary brain metastases can also be candidates for resection. Adjuvant radiotherapy is often used in some of these patients, especially after resection of cerebral metastasis.

Role of radiotherapy
Brain metastasis
Radiotherapy may be considered after surgical resection of a solitary metastasis. Treatment options include whole brain radiotherapy (WBRT; 20Gy in 5 fractions or 30Gy in 10 fractions), stereotactic radiosurgery, or a combination of both. The optimal radiotherapy in this situation is yet to be defined. The best reported median survival is in the region of 10–12 months.

For patients with poor prognosis brain metastasis (multiple metastases, extracranial disease and poor PS), options include WBRT (median survival 3.4 months), steroids, and BSC (median survival 2.1 months).

A number of phase II studies have addressed the role of chemotherapy in brain disease. Temozolomide yielded a median survival of 3.5 months. With concurrent radiotherapy, temozolomide showed a median survival of 8 months.

Metastasis at other sites
Palliative radiotherapy is useful in bone metastasis and spinal cord compression not amenable to surgical decompression (see p.584). Skin metastases which are rapidly enlarging and about to ulcerate can also be treated with palliative radiotherapy.

Systemic treatments
Systemic treatments evaluated include chemotherapy, immunotherapy or a combination of both. Many targeted molecules are under evaluation (see p.401).

Chemotherapy
Dacarbazine is the standard intravenous chemotherapy drug for metastatic melanoma with a response rate of 10–20% and a complete response rate of <3%. The median duration of response is 3–6 months. It is given 3–4-weekly at doses of 850–1000mg/m^2 with nausea as the main side effect.

Temozolamide is an oral analogue of dacarbazine and crosses the blood–brain barrier but is more expensive and has shown no improvement in response rate compared with dacarbazine. PFS (1.9 vs. 1.5 months p = 0.012) and median survival (7.7 months vs. 6.4) with temozolomide are comparable to DTIC.

Other agents and response rates are given in Table 4.8.2.

There is no evidence that combination chemotherapy regimens are superior to single-agent drugs in terms of response rates or survival. However, there were higher rates of grade 3–4 toxicities with combination chemotherapy.

Table 4.8.2 Response rates (%) for single agents in metastatic melanoma

Agent	% response rate (CR + PR)
Dacarbazine	20
Temozolamide	21
Carmustine (BCNU)	18
Lomustine (CCNU)	13
Cisplatin	23
Carboplatin	16
Vinblastine	13
Paclitaxel	18
Docetaxel	15

Immunotherapy
Immunotherapies used in metastatic melanoma include IFNA and interleukin-2 (IL-2). IFN is a pleiotropic cytokine with a potential anti-tumour effect. IL-2 is a cytokine produced by CD4 + T lymphocytes. Its exact antitumour action is not known, but is thought to be due to stimulation and recruitment of natural killer cells and induction of other cytokines.

Immunotherapy with high dose IL-2 or IFNA has shown response rates of 10–21% with a rare chance of complete response. Toxicities include hypotension, capillary leak syndrome, sepsis, and renal failure.

Combination of chemotherapy and immunotherapy
Combining chemotherapy with an immune modulator has been assessed in several clinical trials. A meta-analysis of nine randomized studies showed that a combination of chemotherapy with IL-2 or IFN improved response rate

(RR 1.52; 95% CI 1.24–1.87; p <0.0001), but did not translate into a survival benefit (Hamm et al 2008).

In summary, no drug or combination of drugs has shown a significant response rate and survival benefit over single-agent dacarbazine. Hence, it remains the standard drug in metastatic melanoma; but patients should be entered into clinical trials where possible.

Isolated limb perfusion and isolated limb infusion

In some cases widespread metastases do not occur but there may be disseminated skin metastases in a limb which cover an area too large for radiotherapy. In these patients, if systemic treatment is not feasible, isolated limb perfusion (ILP) with TNF-A and melphalan or melphalan alone under hypothermic conditions can establish good local control. This is only performed in a limited number of centres but can provide good clinical benefit.

Isolated limb infusion (ILI) is a simpler method of regional drug delivery which has similar response rate and duration of response as that of ILP. The reported response rate is 90% with a complete response of 60–70%. In approximately 50% of responders, the response may be sustained for a year, which may obviate or delay the need for palliative amputation.

Radiofrequency ablation

For some patients with limited systemic disease but in whom surgery is not possible, RFA has been used for liver and lung metastases. In general they should be <5cm in size and accessible to the RFA catheter used. Complications include bleeding and pneumothorax.

Newer agents

Given the risk of recurrence and poor outcomes with systemic treatment in metastatic disease, new agents are being developed to target specific pathways involved in melanoma. The most promising approaches are antiangiogenic agents (e.g. bevacizumab, thalidomide, lenalidomide), Bcl-2 antisense therapy, B-RAF inhibitors, and cytotoxic T lymphocyte associated antigen 4 (CTLA-4) monoclonal antibody therapy.

Studies are ongoing to assess the potential benefit of bevacizumab in resected stage III and stage IV disease.

Bcl-2 is an anti-apoptotic protein, which is increased in up to 80% of melanoma. Chemotherapy resistance in melanoma is thought to be related to overexpression of Bcl-2. A phase III study of dacarbazine alone vs. a combination of dacarbazine with oblimersen (an inhibitor of Bcl-2 mRNS translation) showed increased response rate (13% vs. 7% p = 0.006) and prolonged DFS (78 vs. 49 days p = 0.0003) but with no improvement in OS.

Sorafenib, a TKI which has activity against BRAF, has been shown to improve response rates when combined with chemotherapy, although no survival benefit was observed. Agents with more specific BRAF activity are being developed.

Since many tumour cells present self-antigens, the immune system of the body cannot effectively eliminate tumours. T regulatory cells are thought to play an important role in inducing such tolerance and downregulating immune responses to tumour antigens by expressing a receptor called CTLA-4. CTLA-4 inhibits T cell responses in an ongoing immune response by suppressing a co-stimulatory signal which is important for T cell activation. Experimental studies showed that anti-CTLA4 monoclonal antibody resulted in the regression of tumour growth in mice and enhancement of chemotherapy cytotoxicity. Following favourable results in phase II trials, the ongoing EORTC trial 18071 is comparing DTIC with or without ipilimumab, an anti-CTLA4 monoclonal antibody. Another phase III study is comparing ipilimumab with or without a peptide vaccine as second-line therapy.

Prognostic factors and survival

Clinical stage is the most important prognostic factor. In patients with localized melanoma (stage I and II), Breslow thickness, ulceration, and mitotic index are the important prognostic factors. Other reported prognostic factors include lymphocytic infiltration, regression, vascular invasion, and cell type.

In stage III disease, the most important determinant of prognosis is the number of lymph nodes involved. In stage IV disease, increasing number of metastatic sites, visceral metastasis, high LDH level, and poor PS are associated with reduced survival.

Five-year survivals by stage are IA >95%, IB 90%, IIA 78%, IIB 65%, IIC 45%, IIIA 63%, IIIB 45–60%, IIIC 25–30%, and IV 5–18%.

Follow-up

After surgery all patients should be followed-up because of the risk of further melanomas as well as nodal or systemic recurrence; 80% of recurrences develop in the first 3 years. Full skin and nodal examination should be carried out and abdominal examination to exclude hepatomegaly. For high-risk patients (>IA) blood tests to examine LDH, liver function tests, and FBC may be carried out.

For stage I disease 6-monthly follow-up for 5 years and yearly thereafter is necessary. Patients with stage II and III disease are followed up 3–4-monthly for 5 years and yearly thereafter.

For ocular melanoma an ultrasound scan of the liver and CXR should be carried out at least annually. At the point of nodal recurrence, reassessment with CT is suggested prior to surgery and 6–12 months later. For those who have had metastatic disease resected, a CT several months later is recommended along with close follow-up. All patients, especially those who have had nodal disease or metastases, should be warned about the symptoms of spinal cord compression.

Recurrent disease

Melanoma can recur as locoregional disease, metastatic disease, or a combination of both.

Locoregional recurrence

Locoregional recurrence occurs in the anatomical region from the primary site to the regional lymph nodes. It can occur as local recurrence at the primary site, as in-transit metastasis or satellitosis due to lymphatic and or haematogenous metastasis or regional lymph node metastasis. Local recurrence at primary site can be either regrowth of incompletely excised primary melanoma involving the excision site scar or graft (called persistent melanoma) or local metastasis at the primary site.

Persistent melanoma is distinguished from local metastasis by histological features of presence of an epidermal component with or without a dermal component, full range of dermal growth patterns, lymphocytic inflammation, full range of cell types, variable mitotic rate, fibrosis in the zones of regression, and in desmoplasia.

Persistent melanoma is treated with complete excision with the same recommended margin as that for primary melanoma. Adjuvant radiotherapy should be considered if there is a close or positive margin and further surgery is not feasible.

Local metastasis, in transit metastasis and satellitosis are recurrences with poor prognosis and a high risk of distant metastases. The aim of treatment is local control. Treatment options include excision, cryotherapy, laser therapy, intralesional drugs, radiotherapy, and chemotherapy

Patients with multiple, rapidly progressive lesions involving limbs can be treated with regional drug therapy using ILP or ILI.

Patients with distant metastatic recurrence are managed similarly to those with metastasis at presentation.

Genetic testing

Predictive gene testing for an inherited mutation in CDKNA2A (located at 9p21) should be considered for:

• Patients with ≥3 melanomas in aggregate in first-degree or second-degree relatives on the same side of the family or

• Families with ≥3 cases of melanoma or pancreatic cancer on the same side of family or
• Individuals (in low incidence countries) with ≥3 primary melanomas.

Further reading

Leachman S, Carucci J, Kohlmann W, et al. Selection criteria for genetic assessment of patients with familial melanoma. J Am Acad Dermatol 2009; 61;677.

Hamm C, Verma S, Patrella T, et al. Biochemotherapy for the treatment of metastatic malignant melanomas: A systemic review. Cancer Treat Rev 2008; 34:145–56.

Lui P, Cashin R, Machado M, et al. Treatment for metastatic melanoma: synthesis of evidence from randomized trials. Cancer Treat Rev 2007; 33:665–680

Hersey P, Bastholt L, Chiarion-Sileni V, et al. Small molecules and targeted therapies in distant metastatic disease. Ann Oncol 2009; 20(suppl 6):vi35–40.

Non-cutaneous melanoma

Ocular melanoma

Ocular melanoma is a rare subtype of melanoma which can be either uveal (choroid, iris, and ciliary body) or conjunctival. Most commonly it occurs in the choroid but <5% occur in the iris. The aetiology is uncertain but there are some studies which suggest a link with UV radiation. The risks are higher in those who have had cutaneous melanoma, pale iris colour, or who have a family history of ocular melanoma. The staging system differs from that of cutaneous melanoma (see Shields et al. 2009).

Poor prognostic factors include age >60, size, and involvement of the ciliary body. Although often localized at presentation they have a high risk (10–80% depending on number of prognostic factors) to spread to the liver, often several years after successful treatment of the primary. Long-term survival is <35% even with successful treatment of the primary.

Surgery used to be the standard treatment but radiotherapy has replaced this in most cases. Radiotherapy can be administered by external beam, as a radioactive plaque (e.g. iridium-192) or with protons or other charged particles. Local control rates are similar with each technique. The vision is often lost in the irradiated eye with other complications including cataracts, glaucoma, retinopathy, and vitreous haemorrhage.

Treatment of metastases in ocular melanoma has shown that they tend to have a lower response rate to chemotherapy and immunotherapy than cutaneous melanoma and are more rapidly progressive.

Due to their propensity for metastases (especially liver and lung) which can be delayed, follow-up includes imaging of the liver and lungs in addition to LDH and liver function tests. Combined follow-up with ophthalmologists is required.

Mucosal melanoma

Mucosal melanomas constitute <3% of all melanomas. The most common sites of presentation are the head and neck (up to 50%), female genital tract (mostly vulva, 25%), and anorectal region (20%). The remainder occur in very rare sites such as other areas of the GI tract, Eustachian tube, and salivary glands.

They occur later in life (50–70s) than cutaneous melanoma, are more common in non-Caucasians, and slightly more common in men than women. They tend to present late as they are essentially hidden from sight and have a very poor prognosis. Over the years, the incidence of mucosal melanoma has remained relatively stable, unlike cutaneous melanoma.

Diagnosis is by full-thickness biopsy of the suspicious lesion.

The treatment of choice is surgical resection with clear margins but this is often difficult due to location of the tumour.

Radiotherapy has been used to try to improve local control but has not shown an improvement in survival and is not a standard practice. A study using carbon ions to minimize local morbidity showed good local control but 5-year survival was still <30%. Chemotherapy with standard drugs for cutaneous melanoma has been tried with similar success. Nodal disease occurs to a greater extent than in ocular melanoma so regional nodal groups should always be examined at follow-up.

Head and neck mucosal melanoma

Mucosal melanoma of the head and neck region accounts for <1% of all head and neck melanoma. The median age of presentation is 60 years and males are commonly affected. The commonly affected sites are nasal and oral cavities. The most common presentations are bleeding, anaemia, or local symptoms such as pain. There is no specific staging system.

Complete surgical excision is the treatment of choice. Head and neck melanoma has a tendency to recur locoregionally before developing distant metastasis and hence many clinicians consider radiotherapy as an adjuvant after surgery, though there is no evidence for improvement in either local control or survival. Only one small study found a small improvement in local control.

In patients where surgery is not feasible, primary radiotherapy may be used which leads to tumour regression in up to 80% but with poor local control and survival compared with surgery. Five-year survival is <30% which reduces to <20% if lymph nodes are involved.

Female genital tract melanoma

Vulval melanoma

Vulval melanoma accounts for <1% of gynaecological malignancies. Age at presentation is late 60s. The common histological types are lentiginous melanoma and nodular melanoma. Most patients present with a mass and/or bleeding, pruritus, and pain. One-third of patients have regional metastasis and one-fourth have distant metastasis at presentation.

Prognostic factors include tumour thickness, ulceration, and nodal status.

Surgery is the treatment of choice. Superficial lesions can be treated with wide excision. Central and thick lesions require aggressive surgery with bilateral vulvectomy with inguinal lymphadenectomy.

Overall 2-year survival is 50% with >70% for patients with a lesion <1mm thick but <20% with nodal involvement.

The role of SNB is being evaluated.

Vaginal melanoma

Vaginal melanoma most commonly occurs in the lower third and patients usually present with advanced disease. Complete surgical removal is the treatment of choice. A high risk of local recurrence in spite of an aggressive approach to treatment is the norm.

Anorectal melanoma

Anorectal melanoma comprises <1% of anorectal tumours. The median age of presentation is 60 years with a slight female preponderance. The usual presenting symptoms are bleeding, discomfort or mass. Twenty per cent of patients have regional nodal metastasis and another 20–40% present with distant metastasis. Tumours are usually >4mm thick and thickness, nodal metastases, and histological type are not reliable prognostic factors.

Evaluation includes endoscopic ultrasound and staging CT scan of chest, abdomen, and pelvis.

If an adequate margin can be achieved, wide local excision with sphincter preservation is the best treatment option. One-third of patients need abdominoperineal resection to accomplish a complete resection.

Patients with nodal metastases need lymphadenectomy at the time of the definite surgery of the primary tumour.

Currently SNB is not recommended as there is no evidence supporting its role and there is no established relationship between outcome and lymph node status.

The majority of patients relapse with metastatic disease within 2 years, the commonest sites being lung (>50%) followed by liver, brain, and GI tract. The management of metastatic disease is similar to that for metastatic cutaneous melanoma.

Patients without nodal metastasis have a median survival of 30 months and 5-year survival of 35%. With metastatic nodal disease the median survival is 20 months, whereas with distant metastatic disease it is 12 months.

Further reading

Krengli M, Jereczek-Fossa BA, Kaanders JH, et al. What is the role of radiotherapy in the treatment of mucosal melanoma of the head and neck? Crit Rev Oncol Haematol 2008; **65**:121–8

Meleti M, Mooi WJ, Leemans CR, et al. Oral malignant melanoma: A review of literature. Oral Oncol 2007; **43**:116–21.

Patrick RJ, Fenske NA, Messina JL. Primary mucosal melanoma. J Am Acad Dermatol 2007; **56**:828–34.

Piura B. Management of primary melanoma of the female urogenital tract. Lancet Oncol 2008; **9**:973–81.

Shields CL, Shields JA. Ocular melanoma: relatively rare but requiring respect. Clinic Dermatol 2009; **27**:122–33

Bone tumours: introduction

Primary malignant tumours of bone are rare and comprise a large number of histological subtypes.
- The most common are osteosarcoma, Ewing's family of tumours, and chondrosarcoma. Each of these has further subgroups which will be discussed in detail under their subheadings.
- The remaining subgroups are exceptionally rare and include the presentation of spindle cell sarcoma of bone e.g. malignant fibrous histiocytoma (MFH), within the bone as a primary lesion. MFH of bone is treated as other primary bone tumours (Bramwell et al. 1999).

Epidemiology
- Osteosarcoma peaks in adolescence with a second peak in the >65-year age group.
- Ewing's sarcoma peaks at age 10–15 years but can occur at all ages.
- Chondrosarcoma increases in incidence with age >40 years.

Incidence
- There are 650 cases of bone sarcomas per year in USA.
- 12 per million cases of childhood osteosarcoma per year (UK).
- 5 per million childhood Ewing's sarcoma per year (UK).
- <2 per million chondrosarcoma rising to 7 per million in those >70 years (UK).

Aetiology and risk factors
Most primary bone tumours arise spontaneously without a predisposing risk factor. However for each subgroup there are recognized risk factors.

Osteosarcoma (Figs. 4.9.1 and 4.9.2)
- Prior radiotherapy (3% cases) with a time interval of 14 years (range 4–40 years).
- Chemotherapy with alkylating agents, especially if with anthracyclines and radiotherapy.
- Paget's disease (1%).
- Chronic osteomyelitis (<1%).
- Genetic e.g. Li–Fraumeni, hereditary retinoblastoma, Rothmund–Thomson syndrome.

Ewing's sarcoma (see Fig. 4.9.3; also see Figs. 4.9.7–9, p.414–415)
- Rarely after treatment for primary cancer in childhood.

Chondrosarcoma (Fig. 4.9.4)
Increased risk in those with hereditary multiple exostosis or enchondromatosis syndromes (e.g. Maffucci syndrome). Presentation is at an earlier age in these groups.

Further reading
Bramwell V, Steward W, Van der Eijken JW. Neoadjuvant chemotherapy with doxorubicin and cisplatin in MFH of bone. *J Clin Oncol* 1999; **17**(10):3260–9.

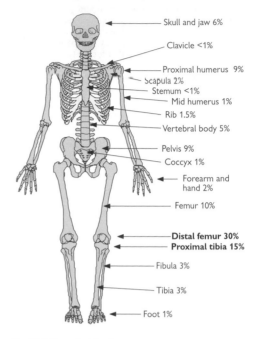

Fig. 4.9.1 Sites of origin of osteosarcomas.

Skull and jaw 6%
Clavicle <1%
Proximal humerus 9%
Scapula 2%
Sternum <1%
Mid humerus 1%
Rib 1.5%
Vertebral body 5%
Pelvis 9%
Coccyx 1%
Forearm and hand 2%
Femur 10%
Distal femur 30%
Proximal tibia 15%
Fibula 3%
Tibia 3%
Foot 1%

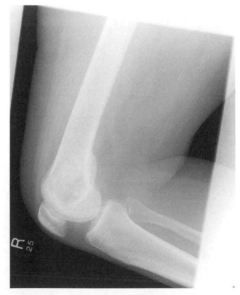

Fig. 4.9.2 X-ray of osteosarcoma of distal femur.

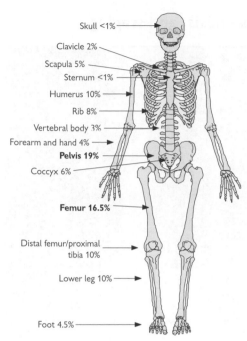

Skull <1%
Clavicle 2%
Scapula 5%
Sternum <1%
Humerus 10%
Rib 8%
Vertebral body 3%
Forearm and hand 4%
Pelvis 19%
Coccyx 6%

Femur 16.5%

Distal femur/proximal
tibia 10%

Lower leg 10%

Foot 4.5%

Fig. 4.9.3 Sites of origin of Ewing's sarcomas.

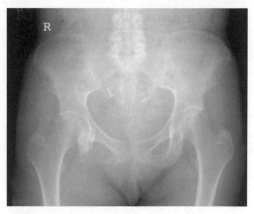

Fig. 4.9.4 X-ray of chrondrosarcoma eroding into pubis.

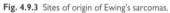

Bone tumours: clinical features, diagnosis, and staging

Clinical features

There are some features which are common to many types of bone tumour:

- Localized bone pain usually present for several months.
- Pain at night or at rest.
- Often a previous injury to the region has been noted and can result in delay in diagnosis.
- In advanced disease, systemic symptoms may be present. These include fever, weight loss, and lethargy. They occur more often in Ewing's sarcoma than any other bone sarcoma.

Diagnosis

- An X-ray of the affected area may be suggestive of a diagnosis but the majority of patients will require a diagnostic biopsy.
- Biopsy should only be performed by a specialist sarcoma surgeon who will take into account possible future surgery and will minimize the risks of tumour spread to the skin or adjacent structures.
- Open incisional biopsy is usually performed but a core biopsy may be appropriate.
- Fine needle biopsies are not suitable for primary diagnosis but can be used to confirm metastatic disease.
- Biopsy is often performed under radiological guidance (fluoroscopy or ultrasound).
- Adequate drainage of the biopsy site is necessary as haematomas can also act to spread disease.
- The biopsy tract is often marked by clips to ensure it is removed at the time of definitive surgery.

Staging

Adequate staging includes:

- Optimal imaging of the primary site (MRI) and the entire bone to exclude intra-medullary skip metastases.
- CT scan of the chest to exclude pulmonary metastases. For PNETs arising in the lower half of the body, a CT of the pelvis and abdomen can be considered as there may be lymph node involvement.
- Bone scintigram to exclude bone metastases. If a CT-PET scan is performed to exclude soft tissue metastases, a bone scintigram will not be required.
- Whole body MRI on STIR sequence has been shown to be effective in detection of bone metastases which may not be visible with other forms of imaging.
- Bone marrow aspirate for the Ewing's family of tumours.
- Blood tests including LDH and ALP which have prognostic value in Ewing's tumours and osteosarcomas respectively.

AJCC staging for bone tumours

Primary tumour (T)

- TX: primary tumour cannot be assessed
- T0: no evidence of primary tumour
- T1: tumour ≤8cm in greatest dimension
- T2: tumour >8cm in greatest dimension
- T3: discontinuous tumours (skip lesions) in the primary bone site

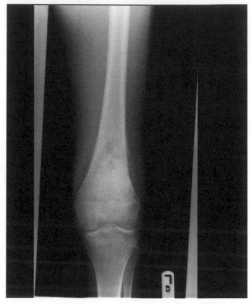

Fig. 4.9.5 X-ray of the femur showing an osteosarcoma in the distal femur. Note the bone expansion with lifting of the periosteum and overlying soft tissue reaction

Regional lymph nodes (N)

- NX: regional lymph nodes cannot be assessed
- N0: no regional lymph node metastasis
- N1: regional lymph node metastasis

Distant metastasis (M)

- MX: distant metastasis cannot be assessed
- M0: no distant metastasis
- M1: distant metastasis
- M1a: lung
- M1b: other distant sites

Histological grade (G)

- GX: grade cannot be assessed
- G1: well differentiated—low grade
- G2: moderately differentiated—low grade
- G3: poorly differentiated—high grade
- G4: undifferentiated—high grade
- Note: Ewing's sarcoma is classified as G4

Stage grouping

- Stage IA: T1N0M0G1,2 low grade
- Stage IB: T2N0M0G1,2 low grade
- Stage IIA: T1N0M0G3,4 high grade
- Stage IIB: T2N0M0G3,4 high grade
- Stage III: T3N0M0, any G
- Stage IVA: any TN0M1a, any G
- Stage IVB:
  Any T, N1, any M, any G
  Any T, any N, M1b, any G

Internet resources

Support groups and information

Sarcoma UK offers information and access to a growing support network for sarcoma patients and their carers

http://www.sarcoma-uk.org

Email: info@sarcoma-uk.org

Bone Cancer Research Trust provides information, support and counselling services for those with primary bone cancer and their families

http://www.bonecancerresearch.org.uk

Email: info@bonecancerresearch.org.uk

Bone tumours: non-metastatic osteosarcoma

Osteosarcoma is the most common type of bone cancer accounting for up to 35% of all primary bone tumours.

Incidence and age
There is a wide variation in incidence according to age.
- It has a peak incidence in those aged 15–19 at a rate of 1 per 100,000.
- Overall incidence is 0.2 per 100,000.
- Smaller second peak incidence occurs over the age of 65 associated with Paget's disease.

Presentation
Pain is the most common presenting symptom (especially at night or at rest). Pain is often associated with a recent injury. Systemic symptoms are rare, unlike Ewing's sarcoma.

Risk factors
- Previous radiotherapy. Most common secondary malignancy following treatment for childhood cancer.
- Chemotherapy, especially alkylating agents and anthracyclines. Increased risk is dose dependent. Chemotherapy plus radiotherapy.
- Paget's disease, although occurs in ≤1% patients with Paget's disease.
- Hereditary conditions (see later).

Genetics and biology
Several genetic syndromes predispose patients to the development of osteosarcoma. The most well known are:
- Hereditary retinoblastoma due to a germline mutation in the retinoblastoma (Rb) gene on the long arm of chromosome 13. The relative risk of osteosarcoma is 500 times for limb osteosarcomas and 2000 for skull osteosarcomas following irradiation for retinoblastoma.
- Li–Fraumeni syndrome in which there is a germline mutation in the p53 tumour suppressor gene. These patients have a RR of 15 for osteosarcoma at all sites.
- Several rarer syndromes which involve deficiencies of DNA repair mechanisms are also associated with a moderately increased risk of osteosarcoma including Werner, Bloom, and Rothmund–Thomson syndromes.
- Unlike Ewing's sarcomas and many soft tissue sarcomas there are no characteristic chromosomal translocations, although loss of heterozygosity in the region of both Rb and p53 have been described.
- A significant number of osteosarcomas express IGF1-R which is being explored as a therapeutic target.

Subtypes of osteosarcoma
Osteosarcomas are characterized as primary bone tumours in which there is a significant component of osteoid bone in addition to a malignant stromal environment. Several subtypes exist defined by the presence, absence, or relative amount of other components. Most (90%) are high-grade intramedullary tumours which fall into the following categories
- Osteoblastic osteosarcoma (50%)
- Fibroblastic osteosarcoma (25%)
- Chondroblastic osteosarcoma (25%)

Further variants exist with distinct histologies
- Telangiectatic osteosarcomas which are high grade and very vascular. They appear lytic on X-ray. Previously thought to be more aggressive than intramedullary tumours but a recent study shows the same survival if given the same treatment.
- Small cell osteosarcoma which may resemble EFT (Ewing's family of tumours) but will not have the same genetic abnormalities or immunohistochemistry profile.
- Malignant fibrous histiocytoma of bone which lacks the osteoid component but responds to the same treatment as intramedullary osteosarcoma (Bramwell 1999).
- Juxtacortical osteosarcomas which subdivide into low grade (paraosteal and periosteal) and high grade. Treatment differs from that for intramedullary tumours as surgery alone may be used in low-grade juxtacortical tumours.
- Extraosseous osteosarcomas which are extremely rare (<0.5% osteosarcomas in McCarter study). They are high-grade lesions which occur deep in the extremities of older patients with an OS of 50% at 5 years. They may occur as a secondary malignancy.

Principles of management
Surgery
- Complete surgical resection by specialist sarcoma orthopaedic surgeons is required for the best outcome.
- Limb-sparing surgery has evolved significantly in the past 30 years such that amputation is used less often.
- Extending endoprostheses have been developed to minimize the number of surgeries a growing child or young adult may require.

Chemotherapy
- Before the 1980s all patients with apparently localized disease had surgery but only 20–30% survived over 5 years. Most died of disseminated disease suggesting the presence of micrometastases in apparently early disease.
- A pivotal study showed that giving adjuvant chemotherapy improved survival from 17% to 66% (Link 1986).
- Neoadjuvant chemotherapy was subsequently developed to allow time to plan surgery. A study showed neoadjuvant therapy to be as efficacious as adjuvant chemotherapy (Goorin 2003).
- Methotrexate at doses up to $12g/m^2$ is used in addition to cisplatin and doxorubicin in younger patients and has been found to increase tumour necrosis.
- The bacterial cell wall mimic muramyl tripeptide (MTP) improved 6-year survival to 78% in primary osteosarcomas when added to chemotherapy (Meyers 2008).

Radiotherapy
Radiotherapy is markedly inferior to surgical resection of the primary tumour in terms of OS but has been used in patients who decline or who are unable to have surgery.

Prognosis/prognostic factors
Several factors have been associated with a poor prognosis which include:
- Age <14 years or >40 years.

- Poor response (<90% necrosis) to neoadjuvant chemotherapy.
- Pathological fracture.
- Large tumour volume, which is also associated with lung metastases.
- Metastases at presentation with bone metastases having a worse prognosis than lung metastases.
- Primary tumours which are axial or extraosseous.
- Secondary osteosarcoma
- Raised ALP or LDH.
- Increased Cadherin 11 expression.

Other factors are not associated with prognosis such as proliferative index. The expression of c-erbB-2 has been shown to have no relation to prognosis in some studies but poor prognosis in others.

Further reading

Bacci G, Ferrari S Bertoni F, et al. Predictive factors of histologic response to primary chemotherapy in osteosarcoma of the extremity. *J Clin Oncol* 1998; **16**(2):658–63.

Bramwell V, Steward WP, Van der Eijken JW, et al. Neoadjuvant chemotherapy with doxorubicin and cisplatin in MFH of bone. *J Clin Oncol* 1999; **17**(10):3260–69.

Burrow S, Andrulis I Pollak M, et al. Expression of IGF-1 and IGF-2 in primary and metastatic osteosarcoma. *J Surg Oncol* 1998; **69**(1):21–7.

Clark J, Dass C and Choong P. A review of clinical and molecular prognostic factors in osteosarcoma. *J Cancer Res Clin Oncol* 2008; **134**:281–297.

Goorin AM, Schwartzentruber DJ, Devidas M, et al. Presurgical chemotherapy compared with immediate surgery and adjuvant chemotherapy for non metastatic osteosarcoma. *J Clin Oncol* 2003; **21**:1574.

Link MP, Goorin AM, Miser AW, et al. The effect of adjuvant chemotherapy on relapse-free survival in patients with osteosarcoma of the extremity. *New Eng J Med.* 1986; **314**:1600–6.

McCarter M, Lewis J, Antonescu CR, et al. Extraskeletal osteosarcoma: analysis of outcome of a rare neoplasm. *Sarcoma* 2000; **4**:119–23.

Meyers PA, Schwartz CL, Krailo M, et al. Osteosarcoma: the addition of MTP to chemotherapy improves survival. *J Clin Oncol* 2008; **26**(4):633–8.

Rosen G, Caparros B, Huvos AG, et al. Preoperative chemotherapy for osteogenic sarcoma. *Cancer* 1982; **49**(6):1221–30.

Bone tumours: metastatic and recurrent osteosarcoma

Metastatic osteosarcoma
- 11.4% osteosarcoma patients have metastases at the time of presentation (Kager 2003).
- OS at 5 years ranges from 10–50%.
- Metastases can occur in the lungs (see Fig 4.9.6), bone, and bone marrow. Lymph node and brain metastases are exceptionally rare.
- Isolated pulmonary metastases have the best prognosis and bone metastases the worst prognosis.
- Up to 30% of patients with lung metastases survive >10 years with a combination of surgery, multi-agent chemotherapy, and occasionally radiotherapy.

Principles of management
Although the chance of cure is small, patients particularly with limited and potentially resectable lung metastases should be treated aggressively with chemotherapy and surgery.

For those with large numbers of lung metastases or bone metastases, chemotherapy and radiotherapy can provide good palliation.

Chemotherapy
- The most effective agents are cisplatin, doxorubicin, methotrexate, and ifosfamide.
- Response rates are 20–40% although some tumours and metastases may not reduce in size. Calcification can occur in responding lung metastases.
- If metastases are present at diagnosis, combination chemotherapy should be used, as it is for localized disease. In younger patients, cisplatin, doxorubicin, and methotrexate can be used. In older patients methotrexate is often omitted because of increased toxicity.
- If the patient has relapsed with metastases within 1–2 years of the original treatment, the same chemotherapy

is unlikely to be useful. In these cases ifosfamide with or without etoposide can be effective but is less so than chemotherapy given for metastases at presentation.
- High-dose methotrexate with folinic acid rescue can be effective if previously treatment was with cisplatin and doxorubicin alone.
- High-dose ifosfamide ($12–15g/m^2$) can be effective.
- High-dose treatment with stem cell rescue has shown no improvement in survival.
- Gemcitabine and docetaxel, a combination which has proved effective in some soft tissue sarcomas, is being investigated for activity in advanced osteosarcoma.
- Trials are underway to evaluate biological agents such as IGF1-R.
- Immunotherapy may have a role and the use of liposomal muramyl tripeptide-phosphatidyl-ethanolamine has been shown to produce a survival benefit in the adjuvant setting (Meyers et al. 2008).

Surgery
Surgery in the metastatic setting should either be
- Aimed at palliation of symptoms, e.g. resection of a large primary extremity tumour with low volume lung metastases, *or*
- Performed with the intention of cure, e.g. resection of lung metastases

Lung metastases should be evaluated for resectability in conjunction with thoracic surgeons. Resection may follow chemotherapy.

Radiotherapy
Although osteosarcomas are relatively radioresistant tumours, radiotherapy has been successfully used:
- To control bone pain.
- In addition to chemotherapy and surgery, e.g. following resection of lung metastases some groups advocate whole lung radiotherapy as well as chemotherapy.
- To provide local control for some patients with advanced metastatic disease for whom resection of the primary tumour is inappropriate.

In one review of 39 patients with high-risk, metastatic or recurrent disease, 76% had clinical benefit from radiotherapy. The 4-year survival of the group was 39% (Mahajan 2008). The median radiation dose was 30Gy in 10 fractions with a range of 10–70Gy in 4–35 fractions.

Recurrent osteosarcoma
Approximately 40% of patients treated for a primary osteosarcoma will have recurrence either locally or with metastatic disease. Those who recur locally only have a better prognosis than those with distant disease, but prognosis is worse than at initial presentation.

Management
Management of local recurrence can involve chemotherapy, surgery or radiotherapy.
- If chemotherapy is given, unless a significant time has passed (at least 1 year), the same chemotherapy is unlikely to be beneficial due to the development of tumour resistance.
- Drugs are the same as those used for metastatic disease. Ifosfamide and etoposide can be effective, especially if not given previously.

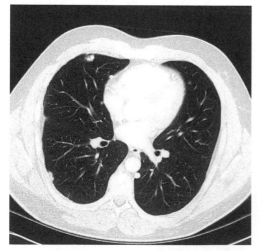

Fig. 4.9.6 Axial CT scan showing lung metastases from osteosarcoma. Typically these can be peripheral or pleural (causing bloody pleural effusions) or can be calcified. A calcified metastasis is seen at the top of the figure in the right lower lobe.

- Surgery may be possible but limb-sparing surgery is less likely for local recurrence of extremity tumours.
- Radiotherapy may be useful for local control but is less effective than surgery.

Metastatic and recurrent osteosarcoma

Over 11% of recurrent osteosarcomas present with metastases and 40% with initially isolated disease relapse. Although the overall prognosis of these patients is poor, approximately 10–30% have a prolonged survival, predominantly those with resectable disease. Treatment should be aimed at cure for those with limited disease and effective palliation for those with more extensive disease. Chemotherapy has a primary role for these patients but surgery and radiotherapy also provide significant benefit.

Further reading

Kager L, Zoubek A, Pötschger U, *et al.* Cooperative German-Austrian-Swiss Osteosarcoma Study Group. Primary metastatic osteosarcoma: presentation and outcome of patients treated on neoadjuvant Cooperative Osteosarcoma Study Group protocols. *J Clin Oncol.* 2003; **21**(10):2011–18.

Mahajan A, Mahajan A, Woo SY, et al. Multimodality treatment of osteosarcoma: radiation in a high-risk cohort. *Pediatr Blood Cancer* 2008; **50**(5):976–82.

Meyers PA, Schwartz CL, Krailo M, *et al.* Osteosarcoma: the addition of muramyl tripeptide to chemotherapy improves overall survival. *J Clin Oncol* 2008; **26**(4):633–8.

Bone tumours: Ewing's sarcoma

Introduction
- Described by James Ewing in 1921.
- Part of a spectrum of tumours called Ewing's sarcoma family of tumours (EFT). EFT includes primitive neuroectodermal tumour (PNET) and Askin's tumour of the chest.

Incidence
- EFT comprise 3% paediatric and adolescent malignancies in USA and UK and are the second most common bone malignancy.
- Median age at diagnosis is 14 years although they can occur at any age.
- Highest in Caucasians with very low incidence in other racial groups.
- There is a male predominance with a 1.5:1 male: female ratio.

Presentation
- Most common site is long bone (53%) or axial skeleton (47%). Within presentations in the long bones, 52% occur distally and 48% proximally.
- Presenting symptoms in local disease are of pain, gradually increasing and worse at night (wakes from sleep).
- Median delay from symptoms to diagnosis is 6–9 months (Simpson 2005).
- An associated soft tissue mass may be seen and is sometimes confused for a sign of infection; 25% have a soft tissue primary.
- Pelvic lesions are the most likely to present with metastatic disease (they are often large before being detected).
- Systemic symptoms may be present and are associated with advanced disease. Symptoms include fever, weight loss, lethargy.
- 25% of patients have metastases at presentation.
- Subclinical metastases are present in 80–90% with apparently localized disease

Prognostic factors
Poor prognosis is associated with metastases at presentation, especially non-pulmonary metastases, pelvic or axial primary site, size >8cm, raised LDH, and age over 14 years (Cotterill et al 2000; Rodriguez-Galdino et al 2007).

Genetics
- EFT consistently have reciprocal translocations, usually between the *EWS* gene on chromosome 22 and FLI-1 on chromosome 11.
- t(11;22)(q24;q12) occurs in >85%.
- Other variants place EWS with other genes such as t(21;22)(q22;q12) EWS-ERG translocation which occurs in up to 10%.
- Due to consistency of the translocations these are used in diagnosis, either with cytogenetics, FISH, or PCR.

Diagnosis and staging
Initial X-ray may show:
- A characteristic destructive lesion within the bone with periosteal reaction (onion skin appearance).
- A soft tissue reaction (see Fig. 4.9.7).
- A pathological fracture (15%).

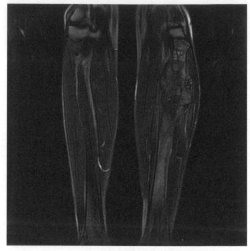

Fig. 4.9.7 Coronal section MRI (STIR sequence) of leg showing Ewing's sarcoma of left fibula with extensive soft tissue component.

Biopsy should be performed to confirm the diagnosis and exclude infection which in some cases may look similar radiologically. Biopsy should be:
- Performed by a sarcoma specialist to allow for the tract to be removed during definitive surgery.
- Of significant size such as a core or rarely operative biopsy. FNA cytology is not suitable for diagnosis but may be used to confirm relapse or metastases in a patient with confirmed EFT.
- Sent for histology, microbiology and cytogenetics or molecular pathology.

Staging should be performed to help direct treatment
- MRI of primary lesion and remainder of that bone to exclude intramedullary skip lesions (Fig. 4.9.8)
- CT chest, bone scan (Fig. 4.9.9), bone marrow biopsy.
- Blood tests including LDH.
- Whole body MRI (STIR) may be considered to exclude occult bone metastases in otherwise localized disease.

Management of localized disease
- Without systemic treatment >80% with apparently localized disease will die of distant relapse.
- Multimodality treatment including chemotherapy, surgery, and/or radiotherapy is required.

Surgical management
- Should be undertaken by a sarcoma specialist.
- Aim for limb-sparing surgery if possible but need clear margins. Margins may be defined by compartment or joint. If joint involved joint replacement may be required. Pelvic tumours are the most difficult to resect especially if involve the sacrum (sacral nerve involvement).
- Usually after induction chemotherapy to assess response and reduce risk of relapse.

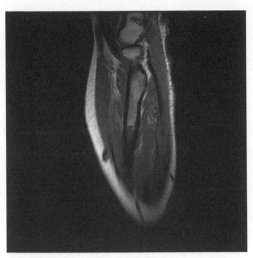

Fig. 4.9.8 MRI of left forearm showing Ewing's sarcoma of proximal radius with extensive intramedullary component but no soft tissue involvement.

Chemotherapy
- Combination chemotherapy pre- and postoperatively is usually given.
- Alkylating agents have highest response rate and have been combined with doxorubicin, vincristine, actinomycin D, and etoposide.
- International cooperation has allowed trials in this rare tumour with groups such as Intergroup Ewing's Sarcoma Study (IESS) which produced a series of trials.
- IESS-III showed that alternating ifosfamide and etoposide with vincristine, doxorubicin and cyclophosphamide improved survival from 54 to 69% in localized disease (Grier et al. 2003).
- High-dose treatment in localized low-risk disease has not been shown to improve survival.
- Response to chemotherapy at the time of surgery reflects prognosis.
- Stratifying treatment according to risk is under investigation in the EURO-EWING 99 trial. Low-risk patients are randomized between standard treatment and less intense treatment. High-risk/metastatic patients are randomized between standard treatment and high-dose with stem cell rescue.

Radiotherapy for localized disease
Unlike osteosarcomas, EFT are radiosensitive and prior to chemotherapy, radiotherapy was a principal method of achieving disease control.
- Used as a primary method of local control in unresectable tumours, e.g. large pelvic tumours.
- Only used in addition to surgery with positive margins or significant soft tissue involvement.
- Studies have shown radiotherapy to have a worse outcome than surgery for local control but there may be some selection bias in that large pelvic tumours are more likely to be unresectable and be treated with radiotherapy alone compared with smaller limb tumours.

- Doses of 45–55Gy have been used. The lower dose has been found inadequate for local control and higher doses have been associated with second malignancy.
- Modern techniques of IMRT, tomotherapy, and protons may reduce early and late side effects.

Prognosis in localized disease
Prognosis in localized disease has improved significantly since the introduction of chemotherapy.
- With combination chemotherapy and surgery or radiotherapy 5-year survival is 70%.

Management of advanced disease
Chemotherapy
Some patients with limited pulmonary metastases may still be cured of their disease and many studies have examined the role of dose intensification to improve survival.
- The same combination chemotherapy agents are used in advanced disease as in localized disease.
- As mentioned earlier, the benefit of high-dose treatment is being examined within the EURO-EWING 99 trial.

Surgery in advanced disease
- Surgery of the primary lesion may still be appropriate with limited pulmonary metastases if these respond to initial chemotherapy.
- Surgery may also be necessary for local control, especially if highly symptomatic.

Radiotherapy in advanced disease
Radiotherapy can be used to treat either the primary tumour or metastatic lesions in advanced disease.
- The dose (radical or palliative) used for the primary will depend on the extent of other disease.
- Bilateral low-dose lung radiotherapy can be used as an adjunct to chemotherapy in responding patients with lung metastases.
- Unilateral lung irradiation is used for symptomatic bulky chest wall lesions.
- Palliative radiotherapy is used for painful bony metastases, including those causing spinal cord compression.

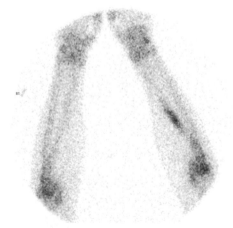

Fig. 4.9.9 Localized bone scan of Ewing's sarcoma of radius (same case as Fig. 4.9.8).

Prognosis of advanced disease

- With limited lung metastases and treatment with chemotherapy plus surgery or radiotherapy 5-year survival of 20–40% can be expected.
- With more extensive disease 5-year survival falls to <25%.
- All patients who are fit enough should be treated with combination chemotherapy initially as some will have prolonged responses.

Recurrence and management

- Recurrence usually occurs within the first 2–5 years and few of these patients survive.
- Relapse after 5–10 years is associated with a survival similar to that of advanced disease at presentation.
- After 10 years few patients relapse but it does occur. Late relapses have been reported in association with persistent infection and pregnancy.
- Treatment depends on the nature of relapse (local/systemic), nature of initial chemotherapy, and time from the end of primary treatment.
- Local recurrence in a limb previously treated with radiotherapy may be treated with surgery and chemotherapy.
- Isolated lung metastases after a long treatment interval may be suitable for surgical resection and further chemotherapy.
- To date, high-dose regimens remain experimental in this group.
- Type of chemotherapy depends on the initial regimen but ifosfamide and etoposide have shown some activity (Miser et al. 2004). A broad phase II trial in paediatric

patients showed that 6/17 patients responded to a combination of cyclophosphamide and topotecan (Saylors et al. 2001).
- Trials of new agents such as insulin growth factor 1 receptor antagonists are underway.

Further reading

Cotterill SJ, Ahrens S, Paulussen M, et al. Prognostic factors in Ewing's tumour of bone: analysis of 975 patients from the European Intergroup Cooperative Ewing's sarcoma study group. J Clin Oncol 2000; **18**:3108–14.

Daldrup-Link HE, Franzius C, Link TM, et al. Whole body MR for detection of bone metastases in children and young adults. Am J Roentgenol 2001; **177**(1):229–36.

Furth C, Amthauer H, Denecke T, et al. Impact of whole-body MRI and FDG-PET on staging and assessment of therapy response in a patient with Ewing sarcoma. Pediatr Blood Cancer 2006; **47**(5):607–11.

Grier HE, Krailo MD, Tarbell NJ, et al. Addition of ifosfamide and etoposide to standard chemotherapy for Ewings sarcoma and PNET. N Engl J Med 2003; **348**(8):694–701.

Miser JS, Krailo MD, Tarbell NJ, et al. Treatment of metastatic Ewing's sarcoma or PNET: evaluation of combination ifosfamide and etoposide. J Clin Oncol 2004; **22**:2873–6.

Rodriguez-Galindo C, Liu T, et al. Analysis of prognostic factors in wing Sarcoma family of tumours. Cancer. 2007; **110**:375–84.

Saylors RL, Stine KC, Sullivan J, et al. Cyclophosphamide plus topotecan in children with recurrent or refractory solid tumours: a pediatric oncology group phase II study. J Clin Oncol 2001; **19**(15):3463–9.

Simpson P, Reid R, Porter D. Ewing's sarcoma of the upper extremity: presenting symptoms, diagnostic delay and outcome. Sarcoma 2005; **9**(1/2):15–20.

Bone tumours: rare tumours

Chondrosarcoma

• See Fig. 4.9.10.
• Comprise <12% bone tumours.
• Third most common malignant bone tumour.
• More common over the age of 40.
• There are several subtypes including peripheral, central, dedifferentiated, mesenchymal, juxtacortical, and clear cell variants.
• The most common sites are pelvis (Fig. 4.9.10), axial skeleton, and proximal limbs.
• As with other bone tumours, axial tumours have a worse prognosis than extremity tumours.
• Aetiology unknown. Some patients have a history of osteochondroma or enchondroma (Ollier's disease). Rare genetic condition resulting in multiple exostoses (Mafucci syndrome) also confers increased risk.
• Presents with mass which may be painful or painless or with symptoms due to local disease.
• Systemic symptoms are rare except with widely disseminated disease.
• Diagnosis may be suggested from plain X-rays but MRI should be undertaken for suspected sarcomas. Chondrosarcomas frequently exhibit calcification. MRI can also be used to assess soft tissue extension. The lesion often has a cauliflower-like appearance.
• As with other bone tumours an adequate biopsy should be performed at a specialist centre with sarcoma expertise.
• Local staging is determined by MRI with a CT scan of the chest to exclude lung metastases. PET is of no known benefit in staging these tumours.
• Staging system is as for other bone tumours.
• There are 3 grades of tumour from well to poorly differentiated. Five-year survival is >90% for a localized grade 1 tumour but reduces to 25% for a grade 3 tumour.
• The primary modality of treatment is surgery. Chemotherapy and radiotherapy have limited activity in chondrosarcoma but have been used for palliation in

Table 4.9.1 Staging for giant cell tumours of bone

Stage I	Benign latent giant cell tumours
	No aggressive activity
Stage II	Benign active giant cell tumours; imaging studies demonstrate alteration of cortical bone structure
Stage III	Locally aggressive tumours
	Imaging studies demonstrate a lytic lesion surrounding medullary and cortical bone
	There may be indication of tumour penetration through the cortex into the soft tissues

some cases. Proton therapy has shown some recent success. Dedifferentiated chondrosarcomas may respond to chemotherapy.

Giant cell tumour

• Reported as distinct entity by Jaffe and Lichtenstein in 1940.
• Less than 5% primary bone tumours.
• Most are benign but up to 10% can be malignant and 5% develop lung metastases.
• Malignant tumours are often secondary to radiotherapy.
• Peak age at presentation is 20–50 years.
• Most frequent sites are distal femur, proximal tibia, and distal radius.
• Can also occur in fibula, distal tibia, pelvis, and spine.
• Presentation is usually due to pain as most occur near joint site. Pain increases with activity. Five to 10% are associated with a pathological fracture; 20% associated with a joint effusion.
• Radiologically can be distinguishable from other bone tumours on X-ray as they have an expansile lytic area ('soap bubble appearance') which is located close to the epiphysis. MRI is used to assess soft tissue and intramedullary extension.
• Staging should include chest CT scan as there is a possibility of lung metastases.
• A bone scintigram will show increased tracer uptake in the region of the tumour.
• Staging of giant cell tumours differs from other bone tumours (see Table 4.9.1).
• Surgery is the most effective treatment but often the whole tumour cannot be removed without leaving a residual deficit in the bone. This space is filled with bone graft material. Adding bone cement to the graft may reduce the risk of recurrence from 45% to <30%. Additional local treatments include cryotherapy and chemical adjuvants.
• Embolization is often used prior to surgery, especially for sacral tumours, to prevent excessive blood loss at the time of surgery.
• Radiotherapy can be used for these tumours but there is a risk up to 15% of secondary malignancy.
• Other trial treatments include denosumab, a monoclonal antibody to RANK ligand, and use of the drug interferon.

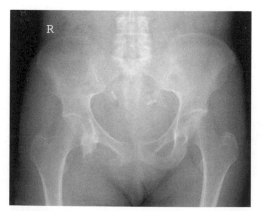

Fig. 4.9.10 X-ray of the pelvis showing a chondrosarcoma arising from the right pubis with local bone destruction. Note the presence of the tips of ureteric stents in the bladder.

• Lung metastases may resolve after treatment of primary or can be resected.

Primary bone lymphoma

• Otherwise known as primary non-Hodgkin lymphoma (NHL) of bone.
• Mean age at presentation is 40–45 years.
• Males are affected almost twice as much as females.
• Presentation is with bone pain not relieved by rest and systemic ('B') symptoms (weight loss, fever, night sweats) are well described.
• Can present as a localized, solitary destructive lesion (stage IE), with associated local lymph node (stage IIE) or widespread bony disease (stage IV).
• X-rays show diffuse medullary mottling with lytic areas. MRI does not show a consistent picture as the appearance depends on the degree of fibrosis in the lesion.
• Bone biopsy should be performed with the same care and expertise as for other bone tumours. Immunohistochemistry should include lymphoid markers as this will affect treatment options.
• Staging should involve a CT of chest, abdomen, and pelvis to exclude distant nodal disease. PET is useful in excluding distant metastases but its role in assessment of primary lymphoma of bone in the absence of metastases has not been evaluated.
• Unlike most bone tumours, primary treatment is not surgery. Chemotherapy with CHOP- like regimens has proved most effective, with or without rituximab.
• For localized disease in adults, EBRT has been used with doses up to 40Gy with or without a boost of 10Gy to the tumour bed.
• In children excellent tumour control and survival rates are achieved in 90% with chemotherapy alone.
• There is a significant risk of secondary malignancy if anthracyline chemotherapy and radiotherapy are used as treatment.
• Pathological fracture and osteonecrosis may also occur if radiotherapy is combined with chemotherapy or doses >50Gy are used.

• Surgery is usually restricted to stabilization following impending or actual fracture.
• Prognosis is better in those aged <40, with localized disease and treated with combination therapy.
• Poor prognostic factors include pathological fracture and multifocal disease.

Langerhans cell histiocytosis of bone (eosinophilic granuloma)

• Incidence 0.5 per million per year.
• Predominantly in children 5–10 years with a 2:1 male: female ratio.
• One manifestation of a rare syndrome that includes pituitary involvement, skin abnormalities, interstitial lung disease, and lytic bone tumours.
• Most common site is the skull followed by vertebra, femur, humerus, and ribs.
• Presents with painful swelling, spinal cord compression, or reduced joint movement.
• Can be isolated (>50%) or multiple lesions (<30%).
• Biopsy is necessary for diagnosis with immunohistochemical staining for CD1a and S100.
• Treatment may include corticosteroid injection, surgery, radiotherapy, and radiofrequency ablation.

Further reading

Beal K, Allen L, Yahalom J. Primary bone lymphoma: treatment results and prognostic factors with long term follow up of 82 patients. *Cancer* 2006; **106**(12):2652–6.

Corby RR, Stacy GS, Peabody TD, *et al*. Radiofrequency ablation of solitary eosinophilic granuloma of bone. *Am J Roentgenol*. 2008; **190**(6):1492–4.

Lipton A, and Jun S. RANKL inhibition in the treatment of bone metastases. *Curr Opin Support Palliat Care* 2008; **2**(3):197–203.

Ramadan K, Shenkier T, Sehn LH, *et al*. A clinicopathological retrospective study of 131 patients treated with primary bone lymphoma. *Ann Oncol* 2007; **18**(1):129–35.

Windebank K. Advances in the management of histiocytic disorders. *Paediatr Child Health* 2008; **18**(3):129–135.

Soft tissue sarcomas: introduction, clinical features, diagnosis, and staging

Soft tissue sarcomas represent a rare collection of hetero-geneous tumours characterized by malignant growth of mesenchymal tissue.

Different subgroups can be divided by genetics, pathology, anatomical location, and clinical behaviour.

Incidence/epidemiology
• Less than 1% of malignant tumours with an incidence of 30 per million per annum.
• Median age at presentation depends on histological subtype. For example, rhabdomyosarcomas are most common in children and adolescents, whereas leiomy-osarcomas predominate over the age of 40.

Aetiology
• Most cases arise de novo with no obvious predisposing factor.
• Known predisposing factors include familial cancer syndromes, prior radiotherapy and/or chemotherapy, chronic lymphoedema, or infection. Polyvinyl chloride is associated with angiosarcoma of the liver.
• Familial cancer syndromes include Li–Fraumeni, heredi-tary retinoblastoma, familial GIST tumours. Malignant peripheral nerve sheath tumours (MPNST) are more common in neurofibromatosis with inherited muta-tions in NF1 associated with a 10% lifetime risk of MPNST. Desmoid tumours and aggressive fibromatosis occur in those with APC gene mutations associated with FAP.

Pathology
• There are >80 subtypes of soft tissue sarcoma. The most common are leiomyosarcoma, liposarcoma, synovial sarcoma, rhabdomyosarcoma, fibrosarcoma (several subtypes), MPNST, and alveolar soft part sarcoma.
• These are named after their supposed tissue of origin (e.g. leiomyosarcoma) or tissue which they most obvi-ously resemble (e.g. liposarcoma).
• Many soft tissue sarcomas are characterised and classi-fied according to specific gene rearrangements.
• WHO guidelines classify them according to malignant potential in addition to morphology.

Clinical features
Presentation depends on the stage of disease and histo-logical subtype of sarcoma.
• 9/10 soft tissue masses will be benign.
• Risk factors for malignancy are:
  >5cm
  Deep to deep fascia
  Rapid growth
  Painful
• However, malignant tumours can be more superficial, painless, and < 5cm.
• Systemic symptoms (fever, weight loss, anorexia, breath-lessness) may be present in advanced disease, particu-larly if associated with extensive chest disease.

Diagnosis
Because of their rarity and the need for complex manage-ment, sarcomas should be managed by specialist centres from diagnosis to treatment. Differential diagnoses may include infection, metastatic disease, and lymphoma.
• Correct diagnosis requires an adequate biopsy which, as for bone tumours, should not compromise later surgery.
• In some cases when the mass is small and relatively superficial an excision biopsy can be undertaken.
• Biopsies are usually performed under image guidance (ultrasound or CT if deep).
• Samples should be sent to microbiology if infection is suspected.
• Pathology should be reviewed by an experienced sarco-ma pathologist. Due to the difficulty of diagnosis even with immunohistochemistry, specialist techniques such as cytogenetics and PCR may also be used to identify translocation specific sarcomas.

Staging
Staging should include:
• MRI of primary to evaluate extension of tumour.
• CT scan of chest to exclude lung metastases.
• In certain rare subgroups (rhabdomyosarcoma, synovial sarcoma, clear cell and epithelioid sarcomas), nodal disease may occur and therefore regional CT scanning may be appropriate (see Fig. 4.9.11).
• The role of bone scintigraphy is less established in soft tissue sarcomas than for bone sarcomas. PET has not been evaluated (except for GIST) in sufficient soft tissue sarcomas.
• Several staging systems exist, the most frequently used of which are the AJCC and Memorial–Sloan Kettering (MSK).

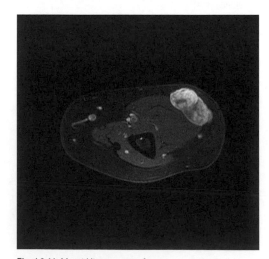

Fig. 4.9.11 Myxoid liposarcoma of arm.

- AJCC staging can be used online (see 'Internet resources').
- AJCC does not include histology or site which limits its use. It should not be used for non-extremity sarcomas.

Soft tissue sarcoma AJCC staging

The AJCC has designated staging by the four criteria of tumour size, nodal status, grade, and metastasis (TNGM).

Grade and TNM definitions

Tumour grade (G)
- GX: grade cannot be assessed
- G1: well differentiated
- G2: moderately differentiated
- G3: poorly differentiated
- G4: poorly differentiated or undifferentiated

Primary tumour (T)
- TX: primary tumour cannot be assessed
- T0: no evidence of primary tumour
- T1: tumour ≤5cm in greatest dimension:
  T1a: superficial tumour
  T1b: deep tumour
- T2: tumour ≥5cm in greatest dimension:
  T2a: superficial tumour
  T2b: deep tumour

(Note: superficial tumour is located exclusively above the superficial fascia without invasion of the fascia; deep tumour is located either exclusively beneath the superficial fascia, or superficial to the fascia with invasion of or through the fascia, or both superficial yet beneath the fascia. Retroperitoneal, mediastinal, and pelvic sarcomas are classified as deep tumours.)

Regional lymph nodes (N)
- NX: regional lymph nodes cannot be assessed
- N0: no regional lymph node metastasis
- N1: regional lymph node metastasis (note: presence of positive nodes (N1) is considered stage IV)

Distant metastasis (M)
- MX: distant metastasis cannot be assessed
- M0: no distant metastasis
- M1: distant metastasis

AJCC stage groupings

Stage I
Stage I tumour is defined as low-grade, superficial, and deep.
- G1T1aN0M0
- G1T1bN0M0
- G1T2aN0M0
- G1T2bN0M0
- G2T1aN0M0
- G2T1bN0M0
- G2T2aN0M0
- G2T2bN0M0

Stage II
Stage II tumour is defined as high-grade, superficial, and deep.
- G3T1aN0M0
- G3T1bN0M0
- G3T2aN0M0
- G4T1aN0M0

- G4T1bN0M0
- G4T2aN0M0

Stage III
Stage III tumour is defined as high-grade, large, and deep.
- G3T2bN0M0
- G4T2bN0M0

Stage IV
Stage IV is defined as any metastasis to lymph nodes or distant sites.
- Any G, any TN1M0
- Any G, any TN0M1

Common subgroups of soft tissue sarcoma

Leiomyosarcoma
- Any site of body.
- Commonest subtype of uterine sarcoma.
- Most common sites of metastases are lung, except in uterine (liver). Soft tissue and bone metastases also occur.
- Chaotic karyotype.
- Variable grade and sensitivity to chemotherapy.

Liposarcoma
- Different subtypes with considerable differences in behaviour and management.
- Myxoid or round cell
- Arise in limbs and spread to soft tissues (retroperitoneum, mediastinum).
- Propensity for bone metastases (especially spine) in up to 17% (Schwab et al 2007) which may only be visualized on MRI. They are chemosensitive, e.g. to doxorubicin and trabectedin.
- Characteristic balanced translocation t(12;16) TLS-CHOP (Antonescu et al 2000).
- Well differentiated, often abdominal. Tend to recur locally not systemically. Chemo-resistant.
- Dedifferentiated tend to occur in the retroperitoneum or abdomen. High-grade, chemo-resistant tumours. They have characteristic genetics with abnormalities in CDK4/MDM2 (Italiano et al 2008).

Synovial sarcoma
- Predominantly in children and younger adults.
- Better prognosis in those aged 1–10 years.
- Most common sites are limbs and trunk.
- Chemosensitive, especially to ifosfamide.
- Metastases predominantly in lungs.
- Balanced translocation t(X;18) between SYT and SSX1 or SSX2.

Prognosis

Different prognostic factors predict for local and systemic recurrence.
- Size and grade best predict distant recurrence and OS.
- Other factors which predict survival include age, anatomical site, and histological subtype.
- Retroperitoneal and visceral tumours carry a worse prognosis than extremity tumours as, like EFT, they can grow to a very large size before they are detected.
- Specific tumour subtypes such as MPNST and leiomyosarcoma have a poorer OS.

- Increased proliferative activity as assessed by immunocytochemical stains has shown a correlation with poorer survival in at least three studies.
- In synovial sarcomas, a translocation-specific sarcoma, several studies have shown a poorer prognosis in SYT-SSX1 gene fusion tumours than SYT-SSX2. However other studies have not confirmed this finding.
- Involved resection margins and age >50 are worst for local recurrence.
- Specific histological tumour types with a higher rate of local recurrence include MPNST and fibrosarcomas.

- Nomograms have been developed, and validated, which help to predict survival based on these features. The best known is the MSK nomogram which can be found online (see 'Internet resources')

Further reading

Antonescu C, Elahi A Humphrey M, et al. Specificity of TLS-CHOP rearrangement for classic myxoid liposarcoma: absence in predominantly myxoid well differentiated sarcomas. J Mol Diagn 2000; 2(3):132–8.

Italiano A, Bianchini L, Keslair F, et al. HMGA2 is the partner of MDM-2 in well-differentiated and dedifferentiated liposarcomas whereas CDK4 belongs to a distinct inconsistent amplicon. Int J Cancer 2008; 122(10):2233–41.

Schwab J, Boland P, Guo T, et al. Skeletal metastases in myxoid liposarcoma: an unusual pattern of distant spread. Ann Surg Oncol 2007; 14(4):1507–14.

Schwab J, Boland P, Antonescu C, et al. Spinal metastases from myxoid liposarcoma warrant screening with magnetic resonance imaging. Cancer 2007; 110(8):1815–22.

Internet resources

AJCC staging online: https://www.protocols.fccc.edu/fccc/pims/staging/sarcoma.html

MSK nomogram: http://www.mskcc.org/mskcc/html/443.cfm

Soft tissue sarcomas: management of localized disease

Surgical resection with wide margins remains the treatment of choice for soft tissue sarcomas. Radiotherapy has a role in high-grade tumours and those with involved resection margins. Chemotherapy remains controversial in the adjuvant setting but may have a role in specific subgroups.

Surgery

Surgery from biopsy to definitive resection should be performed at a specialist sarcoma centre.

Resection must extend beyond the tumour to a wide margin.

An involved resection margin is the most important factor which predicts risk of recurrence. In two studies of patients who had surgery and radiotherapy, local recurrence was increased from 3–12% to 19–36% with uninvolved versus involved margins.

Margins must be defined in terms of compartments and fascial or skin borders as well as distance. For example, reporting a negative skin margin when the involved skin overlying the sarcoma has been removed represents a clear margin.

Although amputation and compartmentectomy reduce local recurrence rates compared with local resection, morbidity is significant. Surgery should be discussed within a sarcoma MDT to ensure morbidity is minimized with the use of radiotherapy if required.

Radical resection or combining radiotherapy with resection can reduce local recurrence to <10%. In specialist sarcoma centres amputation rates are <5% whilst maintaining good local control.

Amputation may be necessary in some cases because of -involvement of vital structures, usually blood vessels, preventing radical resection.

Radiotherapy

Although surgery is the primary curative modality for soft tissue sarcomas, radiotherapy has a significant role in the prevention and treatment of local recurrence. Many soft tissue sarcomas are radiosensitive. The doses required (>60Gy) are higher than those used for many epithelial cancers due to the aggressive nature of many sarcomas. There is no evidence that radiotherapy improves OS.

The use of radiotherapy should be discussed in the context of a MDT but the following are appropriate reasons for post-operative radiotherapy
• High-grade tumour
• Deep tumour
• Size >5cm
• Positive margins when re-resection is not possible
• Local recurrence which has been re-resected

For some patients who are unfit for surgery or in whom resection is technically not feasible, radiotherapy may be considered as a primary treatment modality. However, unless the tumour is very small and superficial, local control will not be as good as with surgery.

Limb sarcoma radiotherapy presents several challenges:
• Positioning and immobilizing the limb to ensure consistent placement and accurate dose to the tumour bed. Immobilization aids are used and the contralateral limb must be placed away from the treatment field.
• A wide 2cm margin is usually added to account for limb movement.

• Adequate dose must be delivered to the tumour bed but must not cross the fascial compartment to avoid lymphoedema. The risk of morbidity due to fibrosis, which significantly affects mobility, increases with treatment volume and dose.

Chest wall sarcoma presents other challenges:
• The tumour may be close to the heart or spinal cord making planning complex and potentially limiting doses delivered.
• Many sarcomas follow the pleural contour of the chest wall making it difficult to avoid significant lung volumes within the treatment field.

Other specific regions such as head and neck or retroperitoneal sarcomas pose their own problems which are discussed elsewhere (head and neck, STS special types, retroperitoneal).

Preoperative and postoperative radiotherapy

Postoperative radiotherapy is usually planned in two phases to take into account possible tumour spillage at the edge of the surgical procedure and then to focus on the central tumour bed. Planning must take into account pre-operative scans to estimate tumour location, but should also encompass the surgical edges. Preoperative radiotherapy allows a single phase approach. An ongoing trial, VORTEX, is examining the possibility of reducing the volume of the postoperative treatment comparing a single phase treatment with a standard two-phase approach.

Radiotherapy has traditionally been given postoperatively but there are potential benefits to giving preoperative radiotherapy
• Smaller treatment volume (and possibly dose)
• Tumour visible on planning scan
• Reduction of tumour before surgery allowing a less morbid and complete operation
• Reduction in significant late toxicity such as limb oedema, joint restriction, and fibrosis.

The concerns about preoperative radiotherapy are:
• It may affect interpretation of histology
• It is associated with greater wound complications postoperatively (O'Sullivan 2002). This study was stopped early due to a significant increase in acute wound complications (17% to 35%). Local control and overall survival was equivalent in the two groups, and further follow-up showed a reduction in late morbidity with preoperative radiotherapy.

Sarcomas represent one of the ideal tumour types for which IMRT and tomotherapy can provide accurate planning, conformal dose delivery, and reduced long-term morbidity.

Adjuvant chemotherapy

The use of adjuvant chemotherapy in soft tissue sarcomas remains controversial and is compounded by:
• Different histological subtypes of sarcoma with varied chemosensitivities being grouped together in the majority of studies
• The development of new chemotherapy agents which may have greater efficacy in specific subgroups but have not yet been studied in the adjuvant setting, e.g. gemcitabine/docetaxel in leiomyosarcomas.

- The rarity of the disease and need for international collaboration in trials which has only relatively recently been achieved.

There are some sarcomas, which tend to predominate in the paediatric setting, in which adjuvant treatment has been shown to be useful, e.g. rhabdomyosarcomas and the extra-skeletal Ewing's tumours such as PNETs. However, for the majority there is no consensus concerning the use of adjuvant chemotherapy.

A large meta-analysis provides some guidance (Sarcoma meta-analysis collaboration 1997). A meta-analysis of 1568 patients from 14 trials which used doxorubicin-containing chemotherapy showed a statistically significant improvement in local and distant recurrence if adjuvant chemotherapy was given. There was a trend towards an improved OS of 4% at 10 years, but this was not statistically significant.

The best evidence for adjuvant chemotherapy appeared to be for large (> 8cm), high- grade extremity sarcomas, but there was no absolute benefit for any specific subgroup.

Criticisms of the meta-analysis note the fact that many patients were included with tumours now known to be truly chemo-insensitive (e.g. GISTs) or which have been reclassified (e.g. carcinosarcomas). Recurrent tumours were also included. Some studies used only doxorubicin whereas others included additional drugs. The dose of doxorubicin was also variable from 50–90mg/m^2 although it is known that doses <60mg/m^2 are rarely effective in metastatic sarcoma.

With the development of ifosfamide, which has shown good activity in the treatment of metastatic sarcomas, three subsequent trials examined the role of combined adjuvant anthracycline and ifosfamide.

A study of 104 patients with large or recurrent sarcomas, many of whom were thought to have tumours of chemosensitive histologies (e.g. synovial sarcoma) were randomized to surgery alone versus intensive ifosfamide and epirubicin (Ferrari 2004). Although initial results showed an improvement in OS this difference was not statistically significant on longer follow-up.

Another trial randomized 88 patients with high-risk extremity sarcomas to standard treatment (43) or chemotherapy (45). The chemotherapy could be either epirubicin (26) or epirubicin combined with ifosfamide (19). In this study the 5-year survival was increased from 47% to 72%. (Petroli 2002)

An international multicentre EORTC study randomized 351 patients to standard treatment versus ifosfamide with doxorubicin. Over half had high-grade extremity tumours, 40% of which were >10cm. A preliminary analysis has shown no statistically significant difference between the two groups in either local recurrence rates or OS (Woll 2007). This trial did include some low-grade tumours and many non-extremity tumours but they were balanced between the two arms of the trial.

There have also been a number of retrospective reviews, some of which have shown a benefit, particularly for ifosfamide-containing chemotherapy, although others have not. A few studies have concentrated on tumours which are more chemosensitive in the metastatic setting such as synovial sarcoma.

The 5-year metastasis-free survival was found to improve from 48% to 60% for the 61 patients of 215 with synovial sarcoma who received adjuvant chemotherapy in one study. However other studies have shown an initial benefit for chemotherapy in the first 12–24 months which is not sustained.

In many of these retrospective studies the outcome may have been affected by the fact that the majority of the patients who received chemotherapy had tumours of higher risk because of factors such as recurrence, size >10cm, and grade.

The use of adjuvant chemotherapy is not, therefore, routinely recommended outside a clinical trial, but the studies mentioned here should be discussed with patients in their particular situations.

Hyperthermia

Hyperthermia in conjunction with neoadjuvant chemotherapy with etoposide, ifosfamide, and doxorubicin has shown an improvement in local control from 16.2 months to 31.7 months after a median follow-up of 24.9 months in a phase III trial (Issels 2007).

Treatment recommendations

Surgery remains the mainstay of treatment for soft tissue sarcoma. This should be performed by specialist sarcoma surgeons and clear margins should be the aim. Radiotherapy is recommended for the majority of cases except low-grade tumours which have been excised with a wide margin. The role of adjuvant chemotherapy for most subgroups remains controversial but could be considered within the context of a clinical trial.

Outcome

The prognosis for soft tissue sarcomas depends on the histological subtype, size at presentation, grade of tumour, and age of the patient. This is highlighted in more detail for the most common subtypes of sarcoma.

Further reading

Davis AM, O'Sullivan B, Bell RS, et al. Preoperative versus postoperative radiotherapy in soft tissue sarcoma of the limbs. Lancet 2002; 359:2235–41.

Ferrari A, Gronchi A Casanova M, et al. Synovial sarcoma: a retrospective analysis of 271 patients of all ages treated at a single institution. Cancer 2004; 101:627–34.

Issels R, Abdel-Rahman S, Wendtner C-M, et al. Neoadjuvant chemotherapy combined with regional hyperthermia for locally advanced primary or recurrent high risk soft tissue sarcomas: long term results of a phase II study. Eur J Cancer 2001; 37:1599–608.

Issels R, Lindner LH, Wust P, et al. Regional hyperthermia improves response and survival when combined with systemic chemotherapy in the management of locally advanced, high grade soft tissue sarcomas. J Clin Oncol 2007; 25(18S):A10009.

O'Sullivan B, Davis AM, Turcotte R, et al. Preoperative versus postoperative radiotherapy in soft-tissue sarcoma of the limbs: a randomised trial. Lancet 2002; 359(9325):2235-41.

Petrioli R, Coratti A, Correale P, et al. Adjuvant epirubicin with or without ifosfamide for adult soft tissue sarcoma. Am J Clin Oncol 2002; 25:468–473.

Sarcoma meta-analysis collaboration. Adjuvant chemotherapy for localised resectable soft tissue sarcoma of adults: meta-analysis of individual data. Lancet 1997; 350:1647–54.

Woll P, van Glabbeke M, Hohenberger P, et al. Adjuvant chemotherapy with doxorubicin and ifosfamide in resected soft tissue sarcomas. Interim analysis of a randomised phase III trial. J Clin Oncol 2007; 25(18S):10008.

Soft tissue sarcomas: management of locally advanced and metastatic disease

The presentation of sarcoma can be with locally advanced or metastatic disease (see Fig. 4.9.12). In the majority of cases this presentation carries a very poor prognosis. In other cases patients present with limited metastatic disease some time after their initial treatment for localized sarcoma and the prognosis is slightly better in this situation. In both cases treatment options depend on PS, comorbidities, and histological subtype of sarcoma.

Median survival with metastatic disease is 12–14 months.

Chemotherapy
Systemic treatment with chemotherapy can be useful but its role is more complex than in other malignancies:
- There is little evidence that chemotherapy prolongs survival but it can provide significant benefits in symptom control.
- Tumours with a high response rate to chemotherapy (often high grade) do not necessarily have a better prognosis than those with a lower response rate.
- Response rates as determined by RECIST criteria often do not reflect symptomatic benefit or disease control, especially in response to certain agents such as trabectadin.
- Different tumour types show different responses to chemotherapy in general and to specific drugs. The most chemosensitive tumours are synovial sarcoma, myxoid liposarcoma, and childhood rhabdomyosarcoma. Extraskeletal Ewing's tumours are also chemosensitive. The most chemo-resistant tumours are dedifferentiated liposarcoma, alveolar soft part sarcoma, GIST, low-grade liposarcoma, and clear-cell sarcoma.
- Trials of chemotherapy in advanced sarcoma, as in the adjuvant setting, have been hampered by inclusion of many resistant histological subtypes including GIST.
- Doxorubicin is a standard first-line agent with response rates of 20–25%. Doses <60mg/m^2 have been shown to

be ineffective and >75mg/m^2 to have increased toxicity without clinical benefit.
- Ifosfamide is often used as a second-line agent and has a response rate of 25% overall.
- A review of an unselected group of patients with metastatic soft tissue sarcoma treated with doxorubicin-based chemotherapy showed a clinical benefit of 45% with a 6-month PFS (Karavasilis 2008).
- An EORTC trial is assessing whether a combination of doxorubicin and ifosfamide is more effective than doxorubicin alone.
- In general, combination chemotherapy has been shown to improve response rates up to 46% but with no improvement in PFS or OS and with increased toxicity.
- Combination chemotherapy does have a role in tumours of childhood and adolescence such as rhabdomyosarcoma and extraskeletal Ewing's.
- High dose treatment with stem cell rescue has shown no survival benefit.

Combined doxorubicin/ifosfamide chemotherapy
There are a few special circumstances in which combined chemotherapy may be used first-line:
- Life-threatening progressive disease.
- Preoperatively to downstage tumour and aim for resection.
- Unassessable advanced disease, e.g. retroperitoneal liposarcoma.

Specific chemotherapy and histology
Recent studies have shown that some chemotherapy agents are more effective in particular tumours:
- Taxanes and liposomal doxorubicin have been shown to be effective in angiosarcoma.
- Gemcitabine and docetaxel initially showed activity in uterine leiomyosarcoma (Hensley 2004) but also give a response rate up to 30% in other leiomyosarcomas (Maki 2007).
- Trabectedin has been shown to be effective in the treatment of liposarcomas, especially myxoid liposarcomas. It also has a >30% response rate in previously treated leiomyosarcomas and some activity in other sarcomas. Although complete and partial responses are rare, disease stabilization with a median duration of response of 16.5 months was reported in one study (Le Cesne 2005). The median survival was 13.9 months in a study comparing 3-weekly with weekly therapy when used as third-line therapy (Demetri et al 2009).

Surgery
Despite the poor median OS with metastatic disease a small group of patients have a prolonged survival. The majority of these have disease which is amenable to surgery. Most of these patients will have isolated lung metastases or isolated intra-abdominal recurrence.

Pulmonary metastatectomy
Criteria for consideration of pulmonary metastatectomy are:
- No other sites of disease (including primary site).
- Complete resection appears possible.

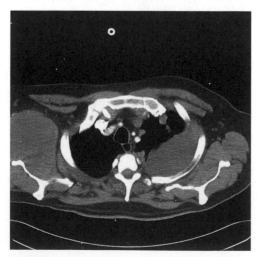

Fig. 4.9.12 Synovial sarcoma of scapula with pleural effusion and lung metastases.

- Long disease-free interval (preferably at least 18 months).
- Slowly progressive disease.
- Low number of metastases, preferably in one lung.

No randomized trial has evaluated the benefit of surgical resection of lung metastases but the 5-year survival of patients selected using strict criteria is up to 40%.

The actual number of metastases which can be removed varies according to each institution but the prognosis decreases as the number of metastases increases.

- In a single institutional study of 274 patients, having more than one lung metastasis, poor prognostic factors were shown to be metastases >2cm and a short disease-free interval of <18 months. Patients with all three factors had 0% chance of survival at 5 years compared with 60% survival if none of the factors were present.

Other surgery for locally advanced or metastatic sarcoma
Other situations in which surgery is considered in advanced sarcoma include isolated abdominal recurrence, as occurs with retroperitoneal sarcomas (see p.428) and soft tissue metastases elsewhere. As for lung metastases there are criteria which apply to the appropriateness of further surgery:
- Isolated disease
- Resectable
- Long disease-free interval
- Slow growing
- Patient fit for surgery

In addition, consideration must be made for previous surgery and radiotherapy as this will affect the potential success and morbidity of the surgery. For this reason, multiple retroperitoneal surgeries are usually avoided.

Resection of liver metastases, other than for GIST, is performed rarely and there is little evidence that it is of benefit either in terms of survival or symptom control.

Chemotherapy after surgical resection
Since the development of metastases by definition confirms systemic disease, chemotherapy pre- or postoperatively may be considered. However, there are no trials to show that this is of benefit and the guidance is as that for adjuvant chemotherapy for sarcomas. It may be appropriate in paediatric type tumours such as rhabdomyosarcoma or synovial sarcoma, where young patients with advanced disease appear to have a better prognosis than adults with equivalent stage disease. It has also been suggested that giving chemotherapy before surgery allows evaluation of disease biology but this can also be assessed by a short interval CXR or CT scan.

Radiotherapy
The majority of soft tissue sarcomas are radiosensitive and radiotherapy can be an effective tool in disease and symptom control. Doses used, as with radical radiotherapy in sarcoma, range from 45–66Gy.

It may be used:
- To treat inoperable recurrence, particularly isolated recurrence and for chemoresistant tumours.
- Where there is skin infiltration.
- Over a chest drain site used to drain a malignant effusion.
- Following chemotherapy which may have reduced the tumour bulk (smaller field) but the symptoms are still present or likely to recur rapidly.

- If there is spinal cord compression or impending spinal cord compression.
- To relieve painful bone metastases.

Isolated limb perfusion
Some patients present with a massive limb sarcoma which may involve several compartments, neurovascular structures, or be inoperable due to other patient factors. This can occur as the initial presentation or as recurrence. These locally advanced tumours are often accompanied by significant symptoms and may be too large to be encompassed within a radiotherapy field. For some patients systemic chemotherapy may not be appropriate due to comorbidities or histological subtype. For some there may be an option of isolated limb perfusion therapy (ILP)
- ILP involves isolating the circulation of the limb affected before perfusing it with recombinant TNFα and melphalan.
- Although this is a localized treatment it is associated with systemic symptoms such as fever and tachycardia.
- In some patients surgery is then possible. In a small meta-analysis, limb salvage was obtained in 57–86% of patients. ILP was associated with the highest limb salvage rate and lowest complication rate (Noorda 2004).
- It is only available in a small number of specialist centres.

Treatment recommendations
- Metastatic soft tissue sarcomas should be managed by a MDT of sarcoma specialists who can discuss all available options.
- Where possible, and clinically indicated, surgery should be performed for isolated recurrence or metastasis as this appears to be associated with the best survival.
- Chemotherapy can give effective symptom control in many sarcomas but an understanding of the specific differences in histological subtypes is required. There is no evidence that combination chemotherapy improves survival but it is useful in special situations and in adolescent sarcomas.
- Radiotherapy should be used for specific indications.
- Isolated limb perfusion may be of benefit for a subgroup of patients.

Further reading
Demetri GD, Schuetze S, Blay J, et al. Long-term results of a randomized phase II study of trabectedin by two different dose and schedule regimens in patients with advanced liposarcoma or leiomyosarcoma after failure of prior anthracyclines and ifosfamide. *J Clin Oncol* 2009; **27**:15S:A10060.

Hensley ML, Anderson S, Soslow R, et al. Activity of gemcitabine plus docetaxel in leiomyosarcoma (LMS) and other histologies: Report of an expanded phase II trial. *J Clin Oncol* 2004; **22**(14s):9010.

Karavasilis V, Seddon BM Ashley S, et al. Significant clinical benefit of first-line palliative chemotherapy in advanced soft-tissue sarcoma. *Cancer* 2008; **112**:1585–91.

Le Cesne A, Blay JY Judson I, et al. 2005; Phase II study of ET-743 in advanced soft tissue sarcomas. *J Clin Oncol.* **23**(3):576–84.

Maki RG, Wathen JK Patel SR, et al. Randomized phase II study of gemcitabine and docetaxel compared with gemcitabine alone in patients with metastatic soft tissue sarcomas. *J Clin Oncol* 2007; **25**(19):2755–63.

Soft tissue sarcomas: special situations issues and future directions

Retroperitoneal sarcoma (Fig. 4.9.13)

Retroperitoneal sarcomas are a subgroup of soft tissue sarcomas but are discussed separately here due to specialized management.

- Incidence is 3 per million per annum.
- Represent 13% of soft tissue sarcomas.
- Most common histologies at this site are liposarcoma and leiomyosarcoma.
- Rarely present with symptoms until quite large. Many found incidentally when scanned for other reasons.
- Symptoms usually due to large mass such as abdominal swelling, leg swelling distal to the mass, pain if paraspinal or femoral nerve roots are involved.
- Median presenting size is 15cm.

Diagnosis

Diagnosis is often suggested by CT scan appearances, which may also indicate an alternative diagnosis such as lymphoma or germ cell tumour.

- If operable a biopsy may not be performed and the tumour is resected en masse to prevent tumour seeding the biopsy tract. Alternatively if the diagnosis is uncertain, a biopsy may be requested in collaboration with the surgeons who will perform the operation.
- If not operable a biopsy must be obtained to ensure correct management of an unsuspected alternative diagnosis.
- Sufficient material must be obtained to perform immunohistochemistry to exclude lymphoma, carcinoma, and germ cell tumours.
- Ideally samples should be sent for molecular analysis to characterize histology further, which may affect their future management.

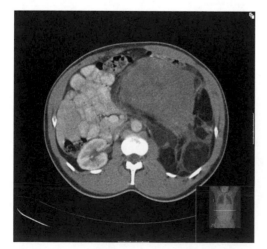

Fig. 4.9.13 Large retroperitoneal mixed liposarcoma showing elements of myxoid differentiation (posteriorly). In these tumours the kidney is often displaced across the midline.

Staging

Staging should include a CT scan of chest (to exclude pulmonary metastases), and abdomen and pelvis (to examine resectability). In retroperitoneal tumours, MRI often adds little information. Bone scintigrams and PET scans have not been demonstrated to be of value in these tumours.

The staging system used is often the AJCC system for limb sarcomas but this is of limited value given the usual size at presentation.

Surgery

Surgery is the treatment of choice and should be performed in a centre with sufficient experience in retroperitoneal surgery. Surgery is complex and may require resection of other structures such as kidney (20% cases), spleen, or bowel. Vascular involvement and metastatic disease are the two most common reasons for inoperability.

Clear resection margins should be the aim. If disease is found at the margins at histological review, re-resection should be attempted if technically feasible.

Chemotherapy

Adjuvant chemotherapy is not standard treatment in these tumours and in one retrospective study was associated with worse outcome (Singer 1995).

In advanced disease chemotherapy has been used to aim for operability but there is no evidence it improves OS.

In metastatic disease or inoperable recurrence, chemotherapy may have a role but is dependent upon histology. Response according to histology is similar to that for other soft tissue sarcomas. Leiomyosarcomas may respond to doxorubicin, ifosfamide, or gemcitabine with docetaxel. Myxoid liposarcomas may also respond to doxorubicin, ifosfamide, and trabectedin. Dedifferentiated and low-grade liposarcomas are essentially chemoresistant, although a recent trial shows some response to trabectedin (Morgan 2007).

Radiotherapy

Postoperative

Postoperative radiotherapy has not been shown to be of benefit in a randomized clinical trial. Several small retrospective or non-randomized studies have shown an improvement in local recurrence rates by up to 30% in completely resected tumours (Stoeckle 2001). However, there was no improvement in OS.

In those cases where postoperative resection margins are involved, radiotherapy may be considered although the proximity of vital structures (kidney, small bowel) may limit the ability to deliver a sufficient dose. There are no randomized controlled trials examining the role of radiotherapy in this setting but a retrospective review including 17 patients with retroperitoneal tumours showed that local control appeared to be improved with radiotherapy. Doses of 64Gy are needed. This is technically challenging in this location but may be achievable with IMRT.

Preoperative

The presence of a large tumour provides some protection to the critical surrounding tissues (kidney, small bowel) if radiotherapy is given preoperatively. This allows higher doses to be administered to the tumour and it is technically easier to plan radiotherapy with the tumour *in situ*.

Two prospective pilot studies were combined (Pawlik 2006) and showed that in 54 patients given radiotherapy preoperatively for primary disease with a median dose of 45Gy (range of 18–50.4Gy), the 5-year recurrence-free survival was 60% and OS was 61%. Survival was improved with doses >45Gy. Some patients were also treated concurrently with preoperative doxorubicin. One study used postoperative brachytherapy but this was associated with significant bowel toxicity and was not continued.

A few pilot studies have also examined the possibility of intraoperative radiotherapy with postoperative radiotherapy. This has shown good local control rates but may be associated with additional toxicities such as damage to the ureters.

Prognosis

Prognostic factors associated with improved survival (in this order) are:
• Complete resection with uninvolved margins
• Grade of tumour
• No metastatic disease

In general, retroperitoneal tumours have a worse prognosis than other soft tissue sarcomas of the same histology. This is taken into account in the MSK nomogram (see 'Internet resource').

Further reading

Demetri GD, Schuetze S, Blay J, *et al*. Long-term results of a randomized phase II study of trabectedin by two different dose and schedule regimens in patients with advanced liposarcoma or leiomyosarcoma after failure of prior anthracyclines and ifosfamide. *J Clin Oncol* 2009; **27**(15s):A10509

Pawlik TM, Pisters P, Mikula L, *et al*. Long-term results of two prospective trials of preoperative external beam radiotherapy for localized intermediate or high grade retroperitoneal soft tissue sarcoma. *Annals Surg Oncol* 2006; **13**(4):508–17.

Singer S, Corson J, Demetri GD, *et al*. Prognostic factors predictive of survival for truncal and retroperitoneal soft tissue sarcoma. *Ann Surg* 1995; **221**(2):185–95.

Stoeckle E, Coindre JM, Bonvalot S, *et al*. Prognostic factors in retroperitoneal sarcoma: a multivariate analysis of a series of 165 patients. *Cancer* 2001; **92**:359–68.

Internet resource

MSK nomogram: http://www.mskcc.org/mskcc/html/443.cfm

Gastrointestinal stromal tumour

GISTs are a rare subgroup of soft tissue sarcomas which can occur anywhere in the GI tract (Fig. 4.9.14).
- Incidence is 15 per million per year for all GISTs and 3–4 million per year for high-grade GISTs.
- A small number are associated with a familial GIST syndrome in which there are germ line mutations in the KIT gene.
- Rare paediatric cases are usually wild type with no KIT mutation and tend to have a more indolent course.
- The most common sites are stomach (50%) and small bowel (25%).
- Rarely, they can occur in the colon (10%), omentum, peritoneum and mesentery (7%), or oesophagus (5%).
- Presentation is most commonly with anaemia, abdominal mass, or as an incidental finding at endoscopy but abdominal pain can occur with larger tumours. Bowel obstruction is rare even with small bowel tumours.
- Patterns of spread include liver metastases (most common) and peritoneal metastases. Bone metastases occur rarely and late, often after years of treatment. Lung metastases (unlike other soft tissue sarcomas) are exceptionally rare. Nodal metastases are also uncommon.

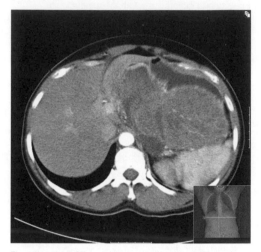

Fig. 4.9.14 Axial CT scan showing a large gastric GIST arising from the greater curvature of the stomach and compressing the stomach lumen.

Diagnosis and staging
- Diagnosis of GIST is often suspected at endoscopy or on CT scan due to the shape and location of the lesion. Biopsy preoperatively may not be necessary in these circumstances and the disease should be staged to determine operability. CT scan of the primary area and the liver is required. A PET scan is also useful as this may show small peritoneal or liver metastases undetectable by CT scan. Endoscopic ultrasound for upper GI GISTs may also be useful.

Pathology and genetics
- The cell of origin is thought to be a precursor to the pacemaker cells of the GI tract, the interstitial cells of Cajal.
- The morphology can be spindle cell (70%), epithelioid (20%), or mixed type (10%).
- 95% of GISTs express c-KIT or the CD117 antigen.
- Mutations in the KIT gene occur in >90% of cases. The exons most commonly affected are:
  Exon 11 (66%)
  Exon 9 (13%)
  Exon 13 (1.2%)
  Exon 17 (0.6%)
- In those cases with *KIT* mutations constitutive activation of the KIT receptor occurs. Activation of KIT is thought to be pathogenetic in familial and sporadic cases.
- In an additional 7% of GISTs, mutations within the PDGFRA gene are found. These are more frequently associated with an epithelioid morphology and with primary site in the stomach. These tend to have a more indolent behaviour.

Factors predicting malignant potential in GIST
The malignant potential of GISTs has been shown to be related to size of the tumour, mitotic rate, and location of the primary. Table 4.9.2 shows the NIH consensus criteria for establishing risk based on size and mitotic count (Fletcher 2002). All GISTs should be regarded as potentially malignant.

Other features now shown to affect risk of aggressive behaviour are:
- Primary site: duodenal and small bowel GISTs are more aggressive than those with arising in the stomach. This has been incorporated into a modified risk stratification (Miettinen and Lasota 2006).
- Tumour rupture spontaneously or at surgery.
- Location of the KIT mutation has been evaluated in several studies. Some have shown mutations in exon 9 to have a more aggressive course than exon 11. Mutations within codons 562–579 in one study and 557–558 in another were associated with a higher risk of metastases.
- See following section for responsiveness to drugs according to mutation.
- Male gender (Rutkovsky 2010).

Management
- Definitive curative treatment is only possible with resection of the primary tumour in the absence of metastases.

Table 4.9.2 Risk of aggressive behaviour in GISTs according to NIH consensus criteria

Risk	Size of tumour	Mitotic count
Very low risk	< 2cm	< 5 per 50 HPF
Low risk	2–5 cm	< 5 per 50 HPF
	< 5cm	6–10 per 50 HPF
Intermediate risk	5–10 cm	< 5 per 50 HPF
	>5 cm	>5 per 50 HPF
High risk	>10 cm	Any mitotic rate
	Any size	>10 per 50 HPF

HPF, high power fields

- High-risk (and intermediate-risk) tumours are, by definition, at risk of relapse after a clear resection. Several trials (e.g. EORTC 62024, ACOZOG-Z9001) are examining the use of imatinib (see later) in the adjuvant setting. Early results suggest an improvement in relapse-free survival in the high-risk group but it is not yet known if this translates into an improvement in OS.
- Patients with inoperable primary tumours who do not have metastases may be rendered operable by the use of imatinib.
- Patients with metastatic disease should be treated initially with imatinib 400mg per day. Imatinib is a tyrosine kinase inhibitor (TKI) which blocks signalling via KIT by binding to the ATP-binding pocket which is essential for phosphorylation and activation of the KIT receptor.
- The median time to progression for metastatic disease on imatinib is 2 years.
- Imatinib should be continued without a break (except for toxicity) until progression. It has been shown that interrupting treatment is associated with progression, although many patients respond again after reintroduction of imatinib. The impact of interruption of imatinib on survival is uncertain.
- At progression, dose escalation to 800mg per day may enable temporary control of disease in 30–35% cases with a median time to progression of 4 months.
- For patients with an isolated liver metastasis who have responded to imatinib, local hepatic resection or radiofrequency ablation may be considered.
- Sunitinib malate is a multitargeted TKI which has shown activity in GISTs which have progressed on imatinib. The median PFS in this clinical situation is 6 months (Demetri et al. 2006); 68% patients achieved a partial response or stable disease on sunitinib.
- Other TKIs which have shown activity in GIST but are not in routine use are nilotinib, valatinib, and AMG-706.

Assessment of response

- Assessment of response in GIST is performed by CT scanning but it has been shown that size criteria of response as defined by RECIST are suboptimal for measuring the activity of imatinib in these tumours.
- FDG-PET can detect reduction in tumour activity within days of commencing imatinib or can visualize small liver metastases which may not be visible on CT scan. Similarly it can detect increased activity should the tumour develop resistance (new mutations) once on imatinib.
- Early response to treatment may not be associated with a significant size change. Choi (2007) described alternative criteria to evaluate GIST response. A 15% reduction

in tumour density or 10% unidimensional reduction in tumour size was a better predictor of response than RECIST. Choi's criteria have been shown to correlate better with survival than RECIST.

Location of mutations and response to TKIs

There is a correlation between location of KIT or PDGFRA mutation and response to imatinib or sunitinib:
- Patients with an exon 11 KIT mutation have a greater chance of response to imatinib (67–84%) than those with an exon 9 (40–48%) or no (0–39%) mutation at a dose of 400mg per day.
- Exon 11 responses were also of a longer duration (576 days) than exon 9 (308 days) or those without a mutation (251 days).
- Higher-dose imatinib (800mg per day) has been shown to be of greater benefit in PFS in patients with exon 9 mutations.
- Of the 7% patients with PDGFRA mutations, tumour with the commonest mutation (D842V) is resistant to imatinib but others may respond.
- Sunitinib has been shown to be more effective against exon 9 mutant GIST than standard dose imatinib and also appears to be effective against wild-type disease. Secondary mutations that confer resistance to imatinib occur more commonly after prolonged exposure (hence in exon 11 mutant tumours) and may respond to sunitinib.

Further reading

Choi H, Charnangavej C Faria SC, et al. Correlation of CT and PET in patients with metastatic GIST treated at a single institution with imatinib: proposal of new CT response criteria *J Clin Oncol* 2007; **25**:1753–9.

Demetri G, van Oosterom A, Garrett CR, et al. Efficacy and safety of sunitinib in patients with advanced GIST after failure of imatinib. *Lancet* 2006; **368**:1329–38.

Demetri G, von Mehren M, Blanke CD, et al. Efficacy and safety of imatinib mesylate in advanced GISTs. *N Engl J Med* 2002; **347**(7):472–80.

Fletcher C, Berman J Corless C, et al. Diagnosis of GIST: a consensus approach. *Int J Surg Pathol* 2002; **10**:81–9.

Hirota S, Isozaki K, Moriyama YY, et al. Gain of function mutations of c-KIT in human GISTs. *Science* 1998; **279**(5350):577–80.

Judson I. Imatinib in advanced GIST: when is 800mg the correct dose? *Curr Opin Oncol* 2008; **20**:433–7.

Miettinen M, Lasota J. GISTs: pathology and prognosis at different sites. *Sem Diag Pathol* 2006;**23**:70–83.

Rutkovsky P, Bylina E, Wozniak Z, et al. Validation of Joensuu risk criteria for primary resectable gastrointestinal stromal tumors: ASCO abstract 10018 2010.

Future directions in soft tissue sarcoma

The development of molecularly targeted therapy for GIST in the form of imatinib and sunitinib has raised the hope that other sarcomas will prove similarly treatable. However, whereas the target in GIST is an activating mutation in KIT or PDGFRA resulting in an altered receptor tyrosine kinase, which can be inhibited by a small molecule, the majority of sarcomas with a defined molecular abnormality have a balanced translocation resulting in multiple alterations in gene expression. Most of these are not easily amenable to pharmaceutical intervention. Nevertheless, work is ongoing to exploit this information for new drug development.

Meanwhile, other, more generic approaches such as inhibition of angiogenesis, are showing promise in the management of sarcomas, and monoclonal antibodies have facilitated the inhibition of previously inaccessible targets such as the insulin-like growth factor 1 receptor, which is difficult to target owing to its close homology with the insulin receptor. This approach is showing promise in the management of both bone and soft tissue sarcomas and may also prove useful in the treatment of imatinib-refractory GIST.

As new targets emerge there is genuine hope that other diseases will indeed prove to be amenable to molecularly targeted therapy.

Hodgkin disease: introduction

Origin and history

Hodgkin's lymphoma (HL), now called Hodgkin disease, is one of the neoplastic diseases of the lymphatic tissue. In 1832, Thomas Hodgkin first described the disease in his historic paper entitled 'On Some Morbid Appearances of the Absorbant Glands and Spleen'. In 1898 and 1902 Carl Sternberg and Dorothy Reed contributed the first microscopic descriptions of the pathognomonic Hodgkin and Reed–Sternberg (H-RS) cells (Fig. 4.10.1). At that time Dorothy Reed wrote: *the treatment for this disease is dismal. All patients die within 3–4 years. Even if you resect the tumour totally, it will recur and grow even faster than before…*

Hodgkin had already assumed that it was an autonomous lymphatic process rather than an inflammatory condition, autoimmune process, or infectious disease like tuberculosis. Despite fragments of evidence for the malignant nature of HL for a very long period of time, the malignant clonal origin of H-RS cells from germinal centre-derived B lymphocytes was shown only recently (Kuppers and Rajewsky 1998). However, the mechanisms that drive the proliferative activity and the causes that hinder the cells from undergoing apoptosis, programmed cell death in the germinal centre, are still not fully understood.

Early in the disease process, HL is typically restricted to the lymph nodes. Lymphatic structures are often breached with progression of disease, which then results in organ involvement, mainly of the bone marrow, liver, or lungs. Without effective treatment, the classic form of HL is fatal. However, since the first descriptions of HL, therapeutic strategies have developed from surgery, herbs, and arsenic acid to sophisticated stage- and risk-adapted treatment regimens including modern polychemotherapy and radiotherapy. Currently about 80% of patients achieve long-term DFS, rendering this entity one of the most curable human cancers.

For patients with newly diagnosed HL, current treatment strategies aim at maintaining the high standard of cure reached for all stages and further improving outcome. At the same time, efforts are made to minimize or prevent therapy-induced complications, such as infertility, cardiopulmonary toxicity, and secondary malignancies. Ongoing trials for patients with early stage disease try to define the minimal treatment needed for cure with the least acute and long-term toxicity. Over the last few years, there has been a trend towards combining chemo- and radiotherapy. Recent studies have predominantly investigated lower doses and smaller fields of radiation and a possible reduction of chemotherapy in terms of number of drugs or cycles given. For patients with advanced stage disease, new schedules of established drug combinations with higher dose density and intensity have been developed, which are currently being evaluated in clinical trials. Furthermore, ongoing studies are trying to use new diagnostic tools, such as PET with 6FD-glucose to enable a response adapted therapy. Detection of early response during chemotherapy or of a satisfactory response after chemotherapy might allow reduction of treatment cycles or render consolidation radiation unnecessary.

Depending on previous treatment given, approaches for relapsed HL consist of radiotherapy, chemotherapy, and high-dose chemotherapy followed by autologous stem cell transplantation. In recent years, the introduction of effective salvage high-dose therapy and a better understanding of prognostic factors have remarkably improved the management of relapsed HL. For multiply pretreated patients, radioimmunoconjugates, monoclonal antibodies and more recently small molecules targeting signal transcription pathways have demonstrated some clinical efficacy; most of these approaches, however, are still experimental.

Histology

The WHO classification defines two types of HL: 1) classical type of HL (cHL) with the subtypes of nodular sclerosis (NS), mixed cellularity (MC), lymphocyte depleted (LD), and lymphocyte-rich classical HL (LRCHL); 2) nodular lymphocyte predominant HL (nLPHL). There is a great variation in the frequency of occurrence between the different subtypes (Harris et al. 1999) (Table 4.10.1).

Epidemiology

In the Western world, the annual incidence of HL is about 2–3 per 100,000 persons at risk, and has remained remarkably constant over the last decades (EUCAN online database). As a result of clinical progress in recent years, the mortality rate has dropped, particularly in the 1990s, from earlier rates >2 to a current mortality rate of about 0.5 per 100,000. In Asia, HL occurs only at a very low rate of about 0.6/100,000, but Asians who migrate to Western countries will develop HL as frequently as locally born natives.

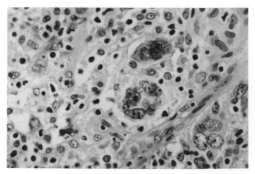

Fig. 4.10.1 Histological staining of an affected lymph node reveals the typical giant Hodgkin and Reed–Sternberg (H-RS) cells (see also colour plate section).

Table 4.10.1 WHO classification of Hodgkin lymphoma. Extracted and modified from Harris et al. (1999)

	Frequency
Classical Hodgkin lymphoma:	
Nodular sclerosis Hodgkin lymphoma (grades 1 and 2)	60–70%
Mixed cellularity Hodgkin lymphoma	20–30%
Lymphocyte-rich classical Hodgkin lymphoma	3–5%
Lymphocyte-depleted Hodgkin lymphoma	0.8–1%
Nodular lymphocyte-predominant Hodgkin lymphoma	3–5%

More men than women develop HL with a ratio of 1.4:1. Four out of five males and three out of four females develop HL before the age of 60, which is very early compared to most other malignancies. In industrialized countries, the age at onset has historically shown two peaks, one in the third decade and a second for patients >50 years. However, in more recent analyses, the second peak seems to have disappeared, because Non-Hodgkin lymphomas (NHLs) were misclassified mainly as lymphocyte-depleted HL in the past.

There is a noteworthy difference in the timing of onset of HL between developing and industrialized countries: in developing countries, the disorder usually appears during childhood and the incidence decreases with age, whereas in industrialized countries the first peak is seen in young adulthood. Furthermore, in economically developed countries the early occurrence of HL is often related to better maternal education, early birth order, low number of siblings and playmates, and single-family dwellings. The incidence of HL by age also depends upon histological subtype. Among young adults, the most common subtype is nodular-sclerosing (NS) HL occurring at a higher frequency than the mixed-cellularity (MC) subtype. The frequency of MC increases with age, while NS subtypes reach a plateau in the group >30 years of age.

Pathophysiology

For a long time HL was considered an infectious disease, as indicated by its former designation 'lymphogranulomatosis'. The giant mono- and multinucleated H-RS cells typically account for <1% of the affected tissue in classical HL, which made systematic analyses difficult in the past. The detection of their malignant clonal origin in microdissected cells by polymerase chain reaction was demonstrated only recently. H-RS cells are derived from germinal-centre B cells in >90% of cases. However, in a small group of patients the H-RS cells exhibit T-cell characteristics.

HL can basically be distinguished from other types of malignant lymphoma by the presence of characteristic types of tumour cells, H-RS cells, in a background of non-neoplastic cells such as lymphocytes, histiocytes, neutrophils, eosinophils, and monocytes. The histological subclassification of HL considers both the morphology and immunophenotype of the H-RS cells and the composition of the cellular background. The WHO classification differentiates between the classical form of HL with CD30-positive H-RS cells and the nodular lymphocyte predominant form of HL (LPHL) with CD20-positive lymphocytic and histiocytic (L&H) cells. In classical HL, immunophenotyping demonstrated that H-RS cells stain positive for CD15 in about 80% and for CD30 in about 90% of cases. The activation of B-cell antigens has only been reported in few cases. In contrast, in NLPHL, the L&H cells are scattered in the nodular structures and are usually CD45-positive. They express B-cell associated antigens such as CD20 in 98% of cases, but also express CD19,

CD22, CD79a, and EMA; however they lack CD15 and CD30 expression.

Despite enormous efforts and progress in basic research, many key questions concerning transforming events and pathways, oncogenic viruses, and the exact mechanism(s) by which H-RS cells proliferate and resist apoptosis in the germinal centre still remain unanswered. Some reports suggest that NFκB is a central effector of malignant transformation in classical HL by downregulation of an anti-apoptotic signalling network. LMP1 as an EBV encoded gene may also induce tumorigenesis by triggering NFκB-activation.

Viral infections (e.g. EBV) have been implicated in the pathogenesis of HL by several studies (Jarrett and MacKenzie 1999). Patients with a medical history of EBV-related mononucleosis have a 2–3-fold increased risk of developing HL. In about 50% of cases of classical HL in Western countries, EBV DNA is present in the H-RS cells, predominantly in the MC subtype. In contrast, patients of low socioeconomic status and those from developing countries show EBV-positive H-RS cells in about 90% of cases.

However, since EBV is not present in the tumour cells of a substantial proportion of patients in the Western world, other viruses might be involved in the transformation process of HL in these cases. To date, the role of other viruses in the pathogenesis of HL is uncertain and other transforming mechanisms must also be taken into account.

Genetic components seem to contribute to the appearance of this malignancy. Family members of patients affected by HL are at a 3–9-fold increased risk of developing the same disease. Furthermore, the analysis of monozygotic twin pairs and the remarkable proportion in which both twins are affected strongly supports the idea of HL as a genetically imbalanced disorder. However, no specific mechanism of inheritance or evidence for a genetic translocation unique to cases of familial HL have been identified so far and familial HL only appears to play a role in a small subset of HL patients.

Further reading

Harris NL, Jaffe ES, Diebold J, et al. The World Health Organization classification of neoplastic diseases of the hematopoietic and lymphoid tissues. Report of the Clinical Advisory Committee meeting, Airlie House, Virginia, November, 1997. *Ann Oncol* 1999; **10**:1419–32.

Jarrett RF, MacKenzie J. Epstein-Barr virus and other candidate viruses in the pathogenesis of Hodgkin's disease. *Semin Hematol* 1999; **36**:260–9.

Kuppers R, Rajewsky K. The origin of Hodgkin and Reed/Sternberg cells in Hodgkin's disease. *Annu Rev Immunol* 1998; **16**:471–93.

Internet resource

EUCAN online database: Incidence and mortality data on Hodgkin's disease: 1998 estimates, version 5.0—available at: www.dep.iarc.fr/eucan/eucan.htm

Hodgkin disease: clinical features, diagnosis, and staging

Clinical features

In most cases, swollen indolent lymph nodes localized in the cervical or supraclavicular region (60–70%) are noticed first, but axillary or inguinal lymph nodes can also be affected. Almost two-thirds of patients with newly diagnosed classical HL have radiographic evidence of intra-thoracic involvement Symptoms caused by a large mediastinal mass include a feeling of pressure, cough, venous congestion, or even dyspnoea owing to tracheal compression or pericardial or pleural effusions. Hepato- or splenomegaly may indicate hepatic or splenic involvement, but affected organs can also be of normal size. In advanced stages, adjacent regions such as lung, pericardium, chest wall or bone are affected and patients sometimes suffer from bone pain, neurological, or endocrinological symptoms. Compared with NHL, bulky infradiaphragmatic lesions with obstructive symptoms are rare in HL. Bone marrow involvement occurs in <10% of newly diagnosed patients. The frequency of involvement of different anatomical sites in untreated patients is shown in Table 4.10.2.

About 40% of patients, especially those with initial abdominal involvement or advanced stage disease, report systemic symptoms ('B-symptoms') which are defined as fever >38°C, drenching night sweats, or weight loss >10% within the previous 6 months (with no other cause). Other symptoms include pain at the site of nodal involvement shortly after drinking alcohol, pruritus, or fatigue. Compared with classical HL, nodular LPHL usually begins as a localized, slowly-growing and rather benign entity with involvement of only one peripheral nodal region, usually a cervical, axillary or inguinal lymph node.

Diagnosis and staging

The physical examination should include a thorough inspection and palpation of possibly involved nodal regions, as well as thoracic auscultation and examination of the abdomen, liver, and spleen, and the spine. An excisional biopsy of a suspicious lymph node should be performed to confirm the initial diagnosis of HL. Adequate material should be obtained but 'debulking' to reduce tumour mass does not improve the prognosis. The assessment of bone marrow is important for disease staging and to evaluate normal bone marrow function prior to therapy.

Accurate staging procedures and assessment of risk factors are essential to allocate patients to appropriate treatment groups. Clinical staging (CS) methods have become less invasive in recent years. They usually include CXR, abdominal sonography, CT scans of the neck, thorax, abdomen and pelvis, bone marrow biopsy and bone marrow or skeletal radionuclide imaging. In some cases, additional procedures including MRI, PET, or a liver biopsy may be indicated. Pathological staging procedures such as laparotomy or splenectomy to assess occult infradiaphragmatic disease are no longer used routinely. They are associated with possible acute or long-term side effects, such as an overwhelming postsplenectomy infection (OPSI) syndrome. Furthermore, better imaging techniques and the introduction of systemic chemotherapy for most patients with early stage disease have restricted invasive measures to a very few patients for whom the initial diagnostic findings give conflicting or unclear results.

The differential diagnosis of HL includes all types of benign or malignant lymph node swelling due to infectious or reactive disease or to other types of lymphoma or solid tumours. Infectious lymphadenopathy can be of bacterial

Table 4.10.2 Anatomical sites of disease involved in untreated patients with Hodgkin lymphoma. Modified from Gupta et al. (1999)

Anatomical site	Involvement (%)
Waldeyer's ring	1–2
Cervical nodes	60–70
Axillary nodes	30–35
Mediastinum	50–60
Hilar nodes	15–35
Para-aortic nodes	30–40
Iliac nodes	15–20
Mesenteric nodes	1–4
Inguinal nodes	8–15
Spleen	30–35
Liver	2–6
Bone marrow	1–4
Total extranodal	10–15

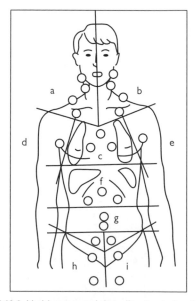

Fig. 4.10.2 Nodal regions and their allocation to lymph node areas; Regions above the diaphragm: Waldeyer's ring, upper cervical/nuchal/submental/cervical region, supraclavicular region, infraclavicular region (area a/b); upper/lower mediastinal region, lung hilum (area c); axillary region (area d/e). Regions below the diaphragm: spleen and spleen hilum, liver hilum, coeliac region (area f); mesenteric and para-aortic region (area g); iliac region (area h/i); inguinal region (area k/l).

Table 4.10.3 The Cotswolds staging classification for Hodgkin lymphoma

Cotswolds staging classification	
Stage I	Involvement of a single lymph node region or lymphoid structure (e.g. spleen, thymus, Waldeyer's ring) or involvement of a single extralymphatic site (IE)
Stage II	Involvement of 2 or more lymph node regions on the same side of the diaphragm; localized contiguous involvement of only 1 extranodal organ or site and lymph node region(s) on the same side of the diaphragm (IIE)
	The number of anatomical regions involved should be indicated by a subscript (e.g. II3)
Stage III	Involvement of lymph node regions on both sides of the diaphragm (III),which may also be accompanied by involvement of the spleen (IIIS) or by localized contiguous involvement of only one extranodal organ site (IIIE) or both (IIISE)
	III1: with or without involvement of splenic, hilar, coeliac, or portal nodes
	III2: with involvement of para-aortic, iliac, and mesenteric nodes
Stage IV	Diffuse or disseminated involvement of 1 or more extranodal organs or tissues, with or without associated lymph node involvement

Designations applicable to any disease stage	
A	No symptoms
B	Fever (temperature, > 38°C), drenching night sweats, unexplained loss of 10% of body weight within the preceding 6 months
X	Bulky disease (a widening of the mediastinum by more than one-third or the presence of a nodal mass with a maximal dimension >10cm)
E	Involvement of a single extranodal site that is contiguous or proximal to the known nodal site
CS	Clinical stage
PS	Pathological stage (as determined by laparotomy)

Modified from Lister et al. (1989).

(e.g. purulent or tuberculous), viral (e.g. EBV, HIV, CMV), fungal (e.g. coccidomycosis) or parasitic (e.g. toxoplasmosis) origin. Reactive lymphadenopathy can be associated with sarcoidosis as well as other diseases of the soft tissues or the skin or can be drug-induced (e.g. by diphenylhydantoin). Malignant causes include metastases from other solid tumours, leukaemias or NHL. The differential diagnosis between certain types of HL and NHL can be very challenging and should be performed by an experienced haematopathologist. Occasionally, a composite lymphoma, comprising both HL and NHL, is diagnosed.

HL patients are usually treated according to stage and risk factors. The histological subtype—except the lymphocyte predominant type—does not influence the treatment decision. The stage of HL at diagnosis is determined according to the Ann Arbor classification depending on the number of nodal regions involved and their distribution on one (stage I+II) or both (stage III) sides of the diaphragm (Fig. 4.10.2) or on organ involvement (stage IV). The presence (B) or absence (A) of systemic symptoms further characterizes severity of disease. Clinical, biological, and serological risk factors further influence the choice of treatment. The Cotswolds modification (proposed in 1989 during a meeting held in the Cotswolds, England) of the Ann Arbor classification uses information from staging and treatment collected over 20 years (Lister et al. 1989). Information about prognostic factors such as mediastinal mass, other bulky nodal disease, extranodal extension of disease, and the extent of subdiaphragmatic disease is included in this classification (Table 4.10.3).

Generally, patients with clinical stage I and II without risk factors are allocated to the early-stage favourable group, and those with risk factors to the early-stage unfavourable group. Patients with stage III and IV disease are assigned to the advanced-stage risk group. Besides stage and B-symptoms, most groups have included larger tumour burden as a relevant prognostic factor (bulky disease >10cm or a large mediastinal mass ≥1/3 of thoracic diameter).

However, there are still small differences in the definition of risk factors used and the classification of certain subgroups of HL patients among the different study groups in Europe and the USA. In the USA, patients are usually

Table 4.10.4 Definition of treatment groups according to different study groups in Europe and the USA

Treatment group	EORTC/GELA	GHSG	NCIC/ECOG
Early-stage favourable	CS I–II without risk factors (supradiaphragmatic)	CS I–II without risk factors	Standard risk group: favourable CS I–II (without risk factors)
Early-stage unfavourable (intermediate)	CS I–II with ≥1 risk factors (supradiaphragmatic)	CS I, CSIIA ≥1 risk factors; CS IIB with C/D but without A/B	Standard risk group: unfavourable CS I–II (at least 1 risk factor)
Advanced stage	CS III–IV	CS IIB with A/B; CS III–IV	High risk group: CS I or II with bulky disease; intra-abdominal disease; CS III, IV
Risk factors (RF)	A: large mediastinal mass B: age ≥50 years C: elevated ESR* D: ≥4 involved regions	A: large mediastinal mass B: extranodal disease C: elevated ESR* D: ≥3 involved areas	A: ≥40 years B: not NLPHL or NS histology C: ESR ≥50mm/hour D: ≥4 involved nodal regions

ECOG, Eastern Cooperative Oncology Group; EORTC, European Organization for Research and treatment of Cancer; GELA, Groupe d'Etude des Lymphomes de l'Adulte; GHSG, German Hodgkin Lymphoma Study Group; NCIC, National Cancer Institute of Canada

*Erythrocyte sedimentation rate (≥ 50mm/hour without or ≥30mm/hour with B-symptoms).

either allocated to early or advanced stages. More patients, even with low tumour burden, are included in the advanced stage group. These patients then receive more therapy than in other groups, which must be considered when comparing the data (Table 4.10.4).

Prognostic factors define the likely outcome of the disease for an individual patient at diagnosis. Such analysis may be used to inform a patient, or in the context of clinical trials to describe the study population or guide data analysis. For the clinician, the most important use of prognostic factors is to select appropriate treatment strategies. There are two major determinants for dividing HL patients according to a risk- or prognosis-adapted therapeutic approach: stage, and systemic symptoms. A third clinically relevant factor used in USA is massive local tumour burden (bulk >10cm or large mediastinal mass ≥1/3 of thoracic diameter).

In an attempt to define more precisely the risk for patients with advanced HL, a variety of clinical and laboratory parameters have been analyzed to construct a prognostic index. The International Prognostic Score (IPS) consists of seven factors that have been shown to be significantly related to an unfavourable prognosis when present at initial diagnosis : serum albumin <4g/dL, haemoglobin <10.5g/dL, male sex, age <45 years, stage IV disease, leukocytosis >15.000/mm^3, lymphocytopaenia <600/mm^3, and/or <8% white-cells (Hasenclever and Diehl 1998).

Prognostic factors may be used to identify patients either for treatment intensification or treatment reduction. Reduction may be achieved by creating a modified protocol or by including these patients in the early stage group.

Intensification by early high-dose chemotherapy with haematological stem-cell support has not shown a clinically relevant long-term survival benefit compared with conventional treatment. Since clinical and biological factors so far have not been able to select patients with advanced stage disease who will progress during therapy or experience an early relapse, new molecular, genetic or biological parameters that reliably predict response and outcome are awaited.

Further reading

Gupta RK, Gospodarowicz MK, Lister TA. Clinical evaluation and staging of Hodgkin's disease. In: Mauch PM, Armitage JO, Diehl V, et al. (eds) *Hodgkin's Disease*, Chapter 15. Philadelphia, PA: Lippincott Williams and Wilkins, 1999.

Hasenclever D, Diehl V. A prognostic score for advanced Hodgkin's disease. International Prognostic Factors Project on Advanced Hodgkin's Disease. *N Engl J Med* 1998; **339**:1506–14.

Lister TA, Crowther D, Sutcliffe SB, et al. Report of a committee convened to discuss the evaluation and staging of patients with Hodgkin's disease: Cotswolds meeting. *J Clin Oncol* 1989; **7**:1630–6.

Hodgkin disease: treatment of early stage disease

Definition and prognostic groups

According to current knowledge, risk adapted therapy can be stratified into three groups: early favourable, early unfavourable, and advanced stage cases. Patients in the early-stage favourable group are those with clinical stage I and II disease at diagnosis without risk factors (Table 4.10.3, p.437). Those with certain risk factors are allocated to the early-stage unfavourable group (see Table 4.10.4, p.437).

Early-stage favourable HL

Radiotherapy

In the treatment of early stages, extended-field radiotherapy (EFRT) was considered standard treatment for a long time. The EF strategy delivers radiation to all initially involved and adjacent lymph node regions, leading to large irradiation fields compared with involved-field radiotherapy (IFRT), which is restricted to the initially involved lymph node regions only. With the successful introduction of MOPP and ABVD chemotherapy for advanced stages in the 1980s, the shift from radiation alone to additional chemotherapy in early stages was accelerated by the recognition of long-term toxicity and mortality related to large radiotherapy fields and doses. Longer follow-up of patients who underwent EFRT showed the development of severe late effects as competing causes of death, including heart failure, pulmonary dysfunction, and secondary malignancies. Furthermore, though complete remission was generally achieved, there was a high risk of relapsing from first-line treatment when EFRT alone was given. Two different strategies were explored to prevent these relapses: either using even more intensive radiotherapy or adding chemotherapy for early favourable stages to control occult lesions. The latter strategy produced better outcomes and at the same time enabled reduction of radiotherapy to the involved-field for this risk group.

Thus radiotherapy alone is almost obsolete, with one exception: patients with a first diagnosis of nodular lymphocyte predominant subtype of HL (LPHL) clinical stage IA without risk factors are usually not included in ongoing trials for classical HL. On the basis of the very favourable prognosis of this subtype, European groups currently recommend treatment with 30Gy IFRT only. This less toxic strategy seems to produce similar responses for LPHL IA patients to those obtained with combined modality treatment. Experimental approaches for these patients focus on the humanized monoclonal anti-CD20 antibody rituximab which has given impressive results in relapsed LPHL and is currently being evaluated in a GHSG phase-II study in selected IA LPHL patients. Compared with LPHL IA patients, advanced LPHL stages at initial diagnosis have less favourable outcomes and are therefore treated according to protocols used for classical HL.

Chemoradiotherapy and chemotherapy

Most centres and groups in Europe and the USA have now accepted combined modality treatment, consisting of 2–4 cycles of ABVD, followed by 20–30Gy IFRT as the standard of care for early favourable stage disease. Several randomized studies have confirmed the superiority of combined modality treatment over radiotherapy alone. Other trials were conducted to investigate and reduce radiation fields and dose and, likewise, to decrease chemotherapy drug combinations and duration of treatment.

The Southwest Oncology Group (SWOG) demonstrated that patients treated with combined modality therapy consisting of 3 cycles of doxorubicin and vinblastine followed by subtotal lymphoid irradiation (STLI) had a markedly superior outcome in terms of freedom from treatment failure than those receiving STLI alone (FFTF: 91% vs. 81% at 3 years). Another study from Milan showed that STLI can be effectively replaced by IFRT after short duration ABVD chemotherapy, while maintaining the same PFS (97%) and OS (93%) at 5 years. The European Organization for Research and Treatment of Cancer (EORTC) and the Groupe d'Etude des Lymphomes de l'Adulte (GELA) demonstrated that combined modality with either 6 courses of EBVP (H7F trial) or 3 of MOPP/ABV (H8F trial) followed by IFRT yielded a significantly better event-free survival than that achieved by subtotal nodal irradiation alone. The aim of their H9F trial was to evaluate a possible dose reduction of radiotherapy (36Gy or 20Gy or no radiotherapy) after administering 6 cycles of EBVP. However, the arm without radiotherapy was closed prematurely due to a higher relapse rate than expected. Although EBVP was used instead of ABVD in this setting, the use of chemotherapy alone in early favourable stages should currently still be regarded as experimental. Another recent randomized trial by Straus et al. for non-bulky, asymptomatic stage I–III HL failed to demonstrate any superiority of ABVD+RT over ABVD alone; however, the total number of patients was small and all patients received 6 cycles of ABVD, even those in clinical stage I and II without risk factors.

A combined modality approach was also used in the HD7 trial by the German Hodgkin Study Group (GHSG). In this trial, 2 cycles of ABVD plus EFRT were shown to be superior to EFRT alone in terms of FFTF (88% vs. 67% at 7 years). Overall survival was equal in both arms due to effective salvage treatment. Further improvement in treatment, because of the already excellent long-term survival rates, seems difficult. Thus, strategies to reduce drug dose and toxicity while maintaining efficacy are being pursued. In the subsequent HD10 trial of the GHSG, a possible reduction in chemotherapy from 4 to 2 cycles of ABVD and/or IFRT from 30Gy to 20Gy was evaluated. In the interim analyses, no significant differences in FFTF and OS have been detected so far between those receiving 4 or 2 cycles of ABVD between patients receiving different doses of radiotherapy (30Gy vs. 20Gy), but final results are awaited. The aim of the ongoing GHSG HD13 trial was to omit the presumably less effective drugs, bleomycin or dacarbazine, from the ABVD regimen and patients were randomized between 2 cycles of ABVD, ABV, AVD or AV followed by 30Gy IFRT. However the arms without dacarbazine (ABV and AV) were closed prematurely for safety reasons because more progressive disease was seen in these arms. Future trials will try to incorporate PET as a tool to help to evaluate early response and reduce chemotherapy or avoid radiation for some patients with very good prognosis.

Early-stage unfavourable HL

Patients with early-stage unfavourable (intermediate) HL are generally treated with combined modality treatment. However, the ideal chemotherapy and radiation regimens have not yet been clearly defined. Optimization of therapy in this risk group is being attempted by reducing radiation doses and field sizes in a similar manner to that for early favourable stages.

Several trials seem to indicate that the reduction of field size does not compromise the efficacy of treatment. A trial from Italy comparing STLI with IFRT after 4 cycles of ABVD in patients with early favourable and unfavourable stages reported a similar treatment outcome in both arms. In the H8U trial, the EORTC randomized patients between 6 cycles of MOPP/ABV + 36Gy IFRT, 4 cycles of MOPP/ABV + 36Gy IFRT, and 4 cycles MOPP/ABV + STLI. There was no difference between the groups in terms of response rates, failure-free survival, or overall survival. The largest trial investigating radiotherapy reduction was conducted by the GHSG: in the HD8 trial, patients were randomized to 2 alternating cycles of COPP/ABVD plus radiotherapy to either extended (arm A) or involved field (arm B). Final results at 5 years did not show any significant differences between the two arms in terms of FFTF (86% and 84%) and overall survival (91% and 92%), but more toxicity was reported in patients treated with EFRT. A NCIC/ECOG trial by Meyer et al. argues in favour of combined modality treatment rather than ABVD alone in unfavourable non-bulky stage IA/IIA HL. Furthermore, a recent retrospective analysis by Vassilakopoulos et al. supports the use of approximately 30Gy IFRT after a good response to ABVD, a strategy that has been adopted in the ongoing GHSG and EORTC trials.

In early-unfavourable stages, efforts were made to improve the efficacy of chemotherapy by altering drugs and schedules as well as the number of cycles. In the past, alternation or hybridization of a MOPP-like regimen with ABVD did not produce better outcomes when compared with ABVD alone. Furthermore, studies in advanced stage HL indicated that ABVD alone is equally effective and less myelotoxic than alternating MOPP/ABVD, and both are superior to MOPP alone. Thus, a combined modality treatment consisting of 4 courses of ABVD followed by 30Gy IFRT is considered standard treatment for patients with early-stage unfavourable HL. Despite the excellent initial remission rates obtained with ABVD and radiotherapy, approximately 15% of patients with early unfavourable stages relapse within 5 years and about another 5% suffer from primary progressive disease. These outcomes are similar to those in patients with advanced stage disease, treated with more intense regimens. Thus, study groups are currently evaluating regimens for the early unfavourable group that have been previously tested for the treatment of advanced stages.

In their ongoing intergroup trial #2496, the ECOG and SWOG are assessing whether the Stanford V regimen (12 weeks) is superior to 6 cycles of ABVD. In another approach, 4 cycles of ABVD and 4 cycles of BEACOPP-baseline were compared by the EORTC-GELA (H9U trial) and by the GHSG (HD11 trial). In addition, two large trials analyzed whether 4 cycles of combined modality treatment were equally effective as 6 cycles (EORTC: H8U and H9U trial). In the H9U trial, recently reported by the EORTC and GELA, patients were randomly assigned to 6 cycles of ABVD, 4 cycles of ABVD, or 4 cycles of BEACOPP-baseline, followed by 30Gy IFRT in all arms. After a median follow up of 4 years, no significant difference was observed between the three different treatment arms with respect to EFS or OS. Interim results of the GHSG trial HD11 demonstrate equal FFTF and OS for all patients. At 3 years, there was no difference with respect to outcome, either between the ABVD and BEACOPP-baseline arms or between the 30Gy and 20Gy IFRT. Although it must be remembered that these are relatively early data, there is, nevertheless, no evidence for changing treatment from 4 to 6 cycles of ABVD or for recommending 4 cycles of BEACOPP-baseline in this group of patients. However, the low FFTF in this risk group led the GHSG to a further intensification of treatment. In the ongoing HD14 trial for early-unfavourable stages, the BEACOPP escalated regimen was introduced, which has shown high efficacy in the treatment of advanced HL. Patients are currently being randomized to 2x BEACOPP escalated + 2x ABVD or 4x ABVD followed by 30Gy IFRT. In future trials, the GHSG is trying to optimize the BEACOPP regimen to be more effective. Involved node radiotherapy with even smaller fields will be compared in a randomized setting with IFRT. The EORTC is using PET to try to apply a risk-adapted schedule.

Outcome

Currently, combined modality treatment strategies including 2–4 cycles of ABVD chemotherapy followed by 30Gy radiotherapy to the involved field is the standard treatment for patients with early stages of HL at diagnosis. Patients in the early-favourable group achieve an FFTF of more than 90% and an OS of about 95% at 5 years. Patients in the early unfavourable group have an FFTF of about 84% and an OS of 91%.

Further reading

Bar Ad V, Paltiel O, Glatstein E. Radiotherapy for early stage Hodgkin's lymphoma: a 21st century perspective and review of multiple randomized clinical trials. *Int J Radiat Oncol Biol Phys* 2008; **72**(5):1472–9.

Fermé C, Eghbali H, Meerwaldt JH, et al. Chemotherapy plus involved-field radiation in early-stage Hodgkin's disease. *N Engl J Med* 2007, **357**:1968–71.

Hodgkin disease: treatment of advanced disease

Definition

Patients in the advanced stage risk group are those with clinical stage III and IV disease at diagnosis or special risk factors according to Table 4.10.4 (see p.437), which slightly differ between the various European and US study groups.

Prognosis

Before the introduction of combination chemotherapy, >95% of patients with advanced HL succumbed to their disease within 5 years. The remission rates achieved with MOPP were a major breakthrough and MOPP was subsequently used successfully for many years for advanced-stage disease, with long-term remission rates of nearly 50%. The regimen was then replaced by ABVD, after a series of large multicentre trials had proved the superiority of ABVD and alternating MOPP/ABVD over MOPP alone. Hybrid regimens such as MOPP/ABV were only as effective as alternating MOPP/ABVD and even rapidly alternating multidrug regimens such as COPP/ABV/IMEP did not result in better outcome. However, more acute toxicity and a higher incidence of leukaemia were reported after the MOPP/ABV combination as compared with ABVD. At present, ABVD is regarded as the standard regimen against which all new combinations must be tested in the future. However, a long-term follow-up report of 123 patients previously treated with ABVD for advanced HL revealed a failure free survival of only 47% and an overall survival of 59% after 14.1 years.

Treatment options

Chemotherapy

Different study groups have tried to improve these rates by developing new regimens with additional drugs and by increasing dose intensity and dose density with the support of colony-stimulating factors and modern antibiotics. These new approaches include multidrug regimens such as Stanford V, MOPPEBVCAD, VAPEC-B, ChlVPP/EVA, and various BEACOPP variants. The schemes and their drug combinations are listed in Table 4.10.5.

Stanford V was developed as a short-duration, reduced-toxicity programme and is given weekly over 12 weeks. Consolidating radiotherapy to sites of initial disease was used. With an estimated 5-year FFP of 89% and OS of 96%, it seemed to be a promising strategy when used at a single centre. However, a prospective randomized multicentre comparison with MOPPEBVCAD and ABVD showed that Stanford V was clearly inferior in terms of response rate (76 versus 89 and 94%) and PFS (73 versus 85 and 94%) and ABVD was still the best choice when it was combined with optional, limited irradiation. These conflicting results may be partly explained by the use of less radiotherapy in the randomized setting and better treatment quality in single-centre studies. The Manchester group developed VAPEC-B, an abbreviated 11-week chemotherapy programme and conducted a randomized comparison with the hybrid ChlVPP/EVA. After 5 years, EFS and OS were significantly better with ChlVPP/EVA than with VAPEC-B (EFS: 78% versus 58%; OS: 89 versus 79%).

The GHSG HD9 trial compared COPP/ABVD, BEACOPP-baseline and BEACOPP-escalated. Results from 1195 randomized patients showed a clear superiority of escalated BEACOPP over BEACOPP-baseline and COPP/ABVD at 5 years. The follow-up data at 7 years confirmed

these results: with a median follow-up of 82 months, the FFTF and OS rates were 67% and 79% in the COPP/ABVD group, 75% and 84% in the BEACOPP baseline group, and 85% and 90% in the BEACOPP-escalated group. The subsequent GHSG HD12 trial aimed at de-escalating chemotherapy and radiotherapy by comparing 4 courses of BEACOPP-escalated with 4 courses of escalated and 4 courses of baseline BEACOPP, with or without consolidation radiation to initial bulky and residual disease. In an interim analysis at a median follow-up of 30 months, the FFTF was 88% and OS 94% for the whole cohort. There is no significant difference between the arms so far, but final results are awaited. In the ongoing HD15 trial, patients are randomized between 8 courses of BEACOPP-escalated, 6 courses of BEACOPP-escalated, or 8 courses of BEACOPP-14, which is a time-intensified variant of BEACOPP-baseline. Additional radiotherapy is only given for residual lesions ≥2.5cm positive by PET. The question whether escalated BEACOPP is superior to ABVD alone in a randomized setting is currently being evaluated in an intergroup trial initiated by the EORTC (#20012). Here, 8 cycles of ABVD are being compared with 4 cycles of BEACOPP-escalated plus 4 cycles of BEACOPP-baseline.

Further intensification of first-line therapy in high-risk patients by directly administering high-dose chemotherapy and autologous stem cell transplantation after 4 instead of 8 cycles of ABVD did not improve outcome compared with conventional treatment. BEACOPP chemotherapy is generally associated with more haematological toxicity, sterility, and secondary leukaemia when compared with ABVD.

Table 4.10.5 Chemotherapy regimens used in HL

Regimen	Drug combination
MOPP	Mechlorethamine, Oncovin (vincristine), Procarbazine, Prednisone
COPP	Cyclophosphamide, Oncovin (vincristine), Procarbazine, Prednisone
ABVD	Adriamycin (doxorubicin), Bleomycin, Vinblastine, Dacarbazine
EBVP	Epirubicin, Bleomycin, Vinblastine, Prednisone
VAPEC-B	Vincristine, Adriamycin (doxorubicin), Prednisolone, Etoposide, Cyclophosphamide, Bleomycin
ChlVPP/EVA	Chlorambucil, Vinblastine, Procarbazine, Prednisolone, Etoposide, Vincristine, Adriamycin (doxorubicin)
MOPPEBVCAD	Mechlorethamine, Oncovin (vincristine), Procarbazine, Prednisone, Epidoxorubicin, Bleomycin, Vinblastine, CCNU (Lomustine), Alkeran, Vindesine,
Stanford V	Mechlorethamine, adriamycin (doxorubicin), vinblastine, vincristine, bleomycin, etoposide, prednisone
BEACOPP(baseline, escalated or 14)	Bleomycin, Etoposide, Adriamycin (doxorubicin), Cyclophosphamide, Oncovin (vincristine), Procarbazine, Prednisone

Nevertheless, cardiotoxicity and pulmonary side effects are similar with both regimens, especially when combined with radiotherapy. A combination of gemcitabine and bleomycin in a BEACOPP variant (BAGCOPP) resulted in severe pulmonary toxicity and should be avoided.

Combined modality therapy

The role of consolidation radiotherapy after effective chemotherapy in the treatment of patients with advanced HL is still being investigated. A meta-analysis by Loeffler et al. comparing combined modality approaches and chemotherapy alone reported equal tumour control and even better OS in patients treated with chemotherapy alone. Therefore, randomized trials are currently evaluating the impact of radiotherapy after effective chemotherapy for advanced HL. A study conducted by the EORTC indicated that consolidation IFRT did not result in better outcome in patients who had already achieved a complete remission after 6–8 cycles of MOPP/ABV, although radiotherapy may be beneficial to patients with partial remissions. Longer follow-up of the GHSG HD12 trial and the ongoing HD15 trial may help to define the role of radiotherapy for residual disease. In ongoing studies, such as the HD15 trial, PET scanning is not only used to demonstrate tumour activity in residual masses after chemotherapy but also to assess response to chemotherapy. There are data from small trials by Hutchings et al. suggesting that early PET scan during chemotherapy may discriminate between responders and non-responders and thus have a potential role in response-adapted strategies. This approach will be investigated in larger randomized GHSG and EORTC studies.

Elderly patients with HL

Although the general health and performance status of elderly patients with HL may vary considerably, the age at diagnosis remains an unfavourable risk factor, particularly for patients with advanced stage disease. For most study groups, patients are considered 'elderly' if they are >60 years. Factors such as more aggressive disease, more frequent diagnosis of advanced stage, comorbidity, poor tolerance of treatment, failure to maintain dose intensity, shorter survival after relapse, and death due to other causes contribute to the poorer outcome of elderly patients. A retrospective analysis of GHSG trials showed that elderly patients have a poorer risk profile, more treatment-associated toxicity, a lower dose-intensity, and higher mortality as major factors for poorer outcome. Generally, elderly patients without major comorbidities who are sufficiently fit to tolerate standard therapy have a treatment outcome comparable to that of younger patients. In the HD9$_{elderly}$ trial of the GHSG, patients aged 66–75 years with advanced stage HL were treated with either COPP/ABVD or BEACOPP baseline. Tumour control appeared to be better with the BEACOPP regimen, but toxicity was higher, resulting in no differences in FFTF or OS.

Whenever possible, elderly patients should be treated with a doxorubicin-containing regimen. Large radiotherapy fields should be avoided. Whether or not the results of new approaches such as ChlVPP-ABV, ODBEP, PVAG, BACOPP, or VEPEMB would be superior compared with ABVD or equally good with less toxicity is currently a matter of speculation due to the lack of randomized studies.

Outcome

In many centres, 6–8 cycles of ABVD plus consolidation radiotherapy to residual disease is considered the gold standard for patients with advanced stage HL. In spite of higher toxicities, the GHSG recommends BEACOPP escalated for patients <60 years due to significantly better outcomes. With ABVD, Stanford V and MOPPEBVCAD the 5-year failure-free survival rates were 78%, 54%, 81%. Corresponding 5-year OS rates were 90%, 82%, and 89%. With BEACOPP escalated, freedom from treatment failure and OS rates of 87% and 91% have been observed at 5 years.

Further reading

Diehl V, Engert A, Re D. New strategies for the treatment of advanced stage Hodgkin's lymphoma. *Hematol Oncol Clin North Am* 2007; **21**(5):897–914.

Klimm B, Diehl V, Engert A. 2007. Hodgkin's lymphoma in the elderly: a different disease in patients over 60. *Oncology* **21**(8):982–90.

Zekri JM, Mouncey P, Hancock BW. Trials in advanced Hodgkin's disease: more than 30 years experience of the British National Lymphoma Investigation. *Clin Lymphoma* 2004; **5**(3):174–183.

Hodgkin disease: management of recurrence

Treatment options

The majority of patients achieve complete remission with current first-line treatment. Patients who relapse still have a chance of being cured with adequate salvage treatment. Depending on first-line therapy, there are various treatment options. Conventional chemotherapy is usually the treatment of choice for patients who relapse after initial radiotherapy only. In contrast, options for those who relapse after prior chemotherapy include salvage radiotherapy for strictly localized relapse in previously non-irradiated areas, salvage chemotherapy, or high-dose chemotherapy (HDCT) followed by autologous stem cell transplantation (SCT). Other experimental options, such as allogeneic SCT and monoclonal antibodies are being evaluated for multiply pretreated patients. Depending on the duration of remission after first-line treatment, most study groups categorize failures into three subgroups: early and late relapses of HL and primary progressive HL.

Recurrence after radiotherapy

Salvage radiotherapy alone offers an effective treatment option for a selected subset of patients with relapsed HL. This applies to patients with localized relapses in previously non-irradiated areas. In a retrospective analysis from the GHSG database including 624 relapsed or refractory HL patients, 100 patients were eligible to receive salvage radiotherapy alone: the 5-year freedom from second failure (FF2F) and OS rates were 28% and 51%, respectively. Prognostic factors for OS were B-symptoms, stage at relapse, performance status, and duration of first remission in limited stage relapses. Conventional chemotherapy is the treatment of choice for patients who relapse after initial radiotherapy for early-stage disease. The survival of these patients is equal to that of patients with advanced stage HL initially treated with chemotherapy.

Recurrence after chemotherapy

The best treatment for recurrent HL after primary chemotherapy is high-dose chemotherapy. A number of conventional salvage protocols have been developed during the last decade. However, long term follow-up data are scarce since most of the patients achieving complete (CR) and partial remission (PR) immediately proceeded to HDCT with autologous SCT. Overall response rates with conventional salvage therapy ranged from 60–80%, but <30% of patients achieve a lasting remission. Patients relapsing after >2 cycles of polychemotherapy should be treated with HDCT at relapse. The best treatment for patients relapsing after 2 cycles of treatment plus IFRT remains to be defined. A recent analysis of patients relapsing after 2 cycles of ABVD and IFRT showed best and equal results from treatment with either 8 cycles of BEACOPP escalated or HDCT with autologous SCT at relapse.

Younger patients relapsing after initial chemotherapy are usually treated with HDCT and peripheral blood SCT. This strategy has been shown to produce 30–65% long-term DFS. So far, two randomized trials have demonstrated the superiority of HDCT followed by autologous SCT over conventional chemotherapy. The British National Lymphoma Investigation (BNLI) reported that patients with relapsed or refractory HL receiving high-dose BEAM with autologous SCT fared significantly better than those treated with conventional dose mini-BEAM. The 3-year

EFS was 53% versus 10% for those treated with conventional chemotherapy. In the HD-R1-trial of the GHSG, chemosensitive patients relapsing after initial chemotherapy were randomized between 4 cycles of Dexa-BEAM and 2 cycles of Dexa-BEAM followed by BEAM and autologous SCT. The final results at 5 years demonstrated a higher FF2F in the transplanted group than in the group receiving conventional salvage-chemotherapy (55% vs. 34%).

The HDR2 pilot study conducted by the GHSG evaluated the feasibility and efficacy of sequential HDCT in 102 patients with relapsed or refractory HL. Treatment consisted of 2 cycles of DHAP followed by sequential high-dose chemotherapy with cyclophosphamide, methotrexate plus vincristine, and etoposide. The final myeloablative course was BEAM followed by peripheral blood SCT. With a median follow-up of 30 months, FF2F and OS rates were 59% and 78%, respectively. In multivariate analysis, response after DHAP and duration of first remission were prognostic factors for FF2F and OS. Based on the promising results of this study, the GHSG started a prospective European intergroup trial (HD-R2) to compare the effectiveness of 2 courses of DHAP followed by BEAM with the intensified sequential strategy in a randomized setting. Patients with histologically confirmed early relapsed HL and patients in second relapse with no prior HDCT were included.

The reduction of tumour volume before HDCT followed by autologous SCT is an important variable affecting outcome in relapsed and refractory HL. A brief tumour-reducing programme with 2 cycles of DHAP given at short intervals supported by G-CSF was shown to be both effective and well-tolerated in patients with relapsed and refractory disease. Therefore, this regimen was chosen for the HD-R2 study instead of previously used regimens such as Dexa-BEAM which were associated with severe treatment-related toxicity and mortality before the dose reduction of etoposide. Furthermore, the DHAP regimen can be used to collect stem cells successfully in most HL patients.

For patients with primary progressive disease during induction treatment or within 3 months after the end of first-line therapy, conventional salvage chemotherapy has given disappointing results in the vast majority of patients. Reasons for not proceeding to HDCT include insufficient stem cell harvest, poor PS, and older age. The effectiveness of HDCT and autologous SCT for patients with biopsy-proven primary refractory HL was also shown by the Memorial Sloan–Kettering Cancer Center, New York in a study of 75 consecutive patients who were treated with HDCT and autologous SCT. At a median follow-up of 10 years for surviving patients, the EFS, PFS, and OS rates were 45%, 49%, and 48% respectively. Chemosensitivity to standard-dose second-line chemotherapy was predictive of better survival.

The success of HDCT followed by autologous SCT does not only depend on obvious factors such as tumour burden or chemosensitivity. A prognostic score based on treatment outcome of patients with relapsed HL also identified the time to relapse, the clinical stage at relapse and the presence of anaemia as independent risk factors.

Recurrence after HDCT and autologous SCT

Depending on the patient's physical condition there are several options. In some patients, allogeneic SCT is a choice; however, it cannot yet be considered an alternative standard treatment in patients with relapsed HL. So far, the advantages of a potential graft-versus-lymphoma effect were offset by a very high transplant-related mortality (TRM) of >50%. As shown by a matched-pair analysis by Sureda et al. TRM might be significantly reduced by employing reduced-intensity conditioning (RIC). A recent study by Peggs et al. using RIC in 49 HL patients showed the potential for durable responses in patients who have previously had substantial treatment for HL. The low non-relapse-related mortality suggests that allo-transplants should be considered earlier in the course of disease. Allogeneic SCT following RIC might thus become an appropriate strategy in selected subgroups of young poor-risk patients; however, the number of patients treated is still small, requiring further clinical studies to define clear indications.

Depending on age, number and character of relapses, previous therapies and presence of concomitant diseases, it should be carefully evaluated whether a curative or a palliative approach is appropriate. A palliative regimen can achieve satisfactory pain control, improve general condition, and lead to partial, sometimes long-lasting, remissions. Drugs such as gemcitabine, vinorelbine, vinblastine, idarubicin, or etoposide are mostly given as monotherapy which can be combined with corticosteroids. The most promising alternative is gemcitabine which proved to be a effective and well tolerated drug, even for patients with multiple relapses of HL in a phase-II study.

Experimental strategies in the treatment of HL include passive immunotherapy based on monoclonal antibodies to specifically target malignant cells and active immunotherapy with modulation of cellular response by cytokines, tumour vaccines or gene transfer. HL seems to be an ideal target for antibody-based therapeutic approaches since H-RS cells express specific surface antigens such as CD25 and CD30 in large amounts. Approaches involving antibody-based agents have given promising results in experimental HL models and have demonstrated some clinical efficacy in patients with advanced refractory HL. Clinical phase I/II trials with unmodified humanized or human monoclonal antibodies are ongoing. These antibodies either induce target cell death by direct interaction or antibody-dependent cellular or complement-dependent cytotoxicity. Different approaches evaluated clinically include use of bispecific immunotoxin constructs, and radioimmunoconjugates. More recently, small molecules and fully human antibodies, e.g. against CD30, have given promising results.

However, it seems unlikely that patients with resistant disease and with larger tumour masses can be cured by any of these approaches. Future strategies aim at combining conventional chemo- and/or radiotherapy for debulking, and experimental therapies with biological agents to kill residual H-RS cells and thus prevent relapses.

Outcome

For patients with relapsed HL, outcome rates have been significantly improved with the use of high-dose therapy and autologous SCT. For patients with chemosensitive relapse, the FF2F is about 55% and the OS 71% at 5 years.

Despite all clinical progress, prognosis still poor for patients with primary refractory disease or for some patients who cannot be treated with a curative approach at diagnosis or relapse owing to age, concomitant disease or organ impairment.

Further reading

Brice P. Managing relapsed and refractory Hodgkin's lymphoma. *Brit J Haematol* 2008; **141**(1):3–13.

Canellos GP. Relapsed and refractory Hodgkin's lymphoma: new avenues? *Hematol Oncol Clin North Am* 2007; **21**(5):929–41.

David KA, Mauro L and Evens AM. Relapsed and refractory Hodgkin lymphoma: transplantation strategies and novel therapeutic options. *Curr Treat Options Oncol* 2007; **8**(5):352–74.

Josting A, Nogova L, Franklin J, et al. Salvage radiotherapy in patients with relapsed and refractory Hodgkin's lymphoma: a retrospective analysis from the German Hodgkin Lymphoma Study Group. *J Clin Oncol* 2005; **23**:1522–9.

Sieniawski M, Franklin J, Nogova L, et al. Outcome of patients experiencing progression or relapse after primary treatment with two cycles of chemotherapy and radiotherapy for early-stage favorable Hodgkin's lymphoma. *J Clin Oncol* 2007; **25**:2000–5.

Hodgkin disease: long-term toxicities and fertility issues

Surveillance and long-term toxicities

During the follow-up period of HL patients, attention should be paid to two crucial areas. First, more than two-thirds of relapses occur within 2.5 years and >90% within 5 years after initial treatment. The patient should therefore be given a schedule for follow-up visits and examinations (Table 4.10.6). Second, a number of long-term toxic effects related to treatment of HL can occur. They include minor disorders such as endocrine dysfunction, long-term immunosuppression, and viral infections. Serious impairments include lung fibrosis from bleomycin and irradiation, myocardial damage from anthracyclines and irradiation, sterility, growth abnormalities in children, opportunistic infections, psychological and psychosocial problems, and fatigue. Potentially fatal effects include the OPSI syndrome after splenectomy or spleen irradiation, and secondary neoplasms. Acute myeloid leukaemia and myelodysplastic syndrome are mostly observed within the first 3-5 years and secondary NHL mainly at 5–15 years after initial treatment. Solid tumours, such as lung or breast cancer can also occur decades after initial treatment and sometimes multiple tumours develop.

Fertility issues

Because of the substantially improved long-term survival in young patients with HL undergoing chemotherapy, preservation of fertility becomes an increasingly important issue. Regimens such as COPP, MOPP, or BEACOPP containing alkylating agents such as procarbazine or cyclophosphamide often lead to therapy-induced infertility, whereas ABVD is less gonadotoxic. For men cryopreservation of semen prior to therapy is possible; however, strategies for women are less clear. A birth after ovarian cryopreservation and reimplantation has been reported. Nevertheless, reproductive technologies, including ovarian cryopreservation with auto- or xenotransplantation as well as in vitro maturation of thawed primordial follicles, followed by fertilization and embryo transfer have not yet been successfully established.

Data on co-treatment to preserve ovarian function is still scarce. A retrospective analysis of the GHSG demonstrated that the rate of therapy-induced amenorrhoea is higher in women receiving 8 cycles of escalated BEACOPP than in women treated with ABVD alone, COPP/ABVD or standard BEACOPP. Moreover, amenorrhoea after therapy was most pronounced in women with advanced-stage HL, in those >30 years at treatment, and in women who did not take oral contraceptives during chemotherapy. Administration of oral contraceptives or gonadotropin-releasing hormone agonists (goserelin) during chemotherapy may possibly result in lower rates of ovarian failure, but larger studies are awaited.

Further reading

Blumenfeld Z, Dann E, Avivi I, et al. Fertility after treatment for Hodgkin's disease. Ann Oncol 2002; 13(Suppl 1):138–47.

Demeestere I, Simon P, Emiliani S, et al. Fertility preservation: successful transplantation of cryopreserved ovarian tissue in a young patient previously treated for Hodgkin's disease. Oncologist 2007; 12(12):1437–42.

Friedman DL, Constine LS. Late effects of treatment for Hodgkin Lymphoma. J Natl Compr Canc Netw 2006; 4(3):249–57.

Hodgson DC. Hodgkin lymphoma: the follow-up of long term survivors. Hematol Oncol Clin North Am 2008; 22(2):233–4.

Table 4.10.6 Information for HL patients concerning follow-up examinations (extracted and modified from the current GHSG trial protocol HD15 for treatment of advanced-stage HL)

Examination time point	1st year			2nd–4th year	5th year onwards
	Month 3	Month 6	Month 12	Every 6 months	Annually
Physical examination	X	X	X	X	X
Case history	X	X	X	X	X
Laboratory tests:					
Blood count and differential distribution	X	X	X	X	X
ESR, CRP	X	X	X	X	X
TSH	X	X	X	X	X
CTª (if PR)	Xª		X		
CXR (if no CT)	X		X	Xᵇ	X
Lung function		X			
Abdominal ultrasound	X		X	Xᵇ	X

ª Further CT scans are recommended according to findings in final restaging and follow-up

ᵇ Imaging examinations annually.

CRP: C-reactive protein; ESR: erythrocyte sedimentation rate; TSH: thyroid stimulating hormone

Non-Hodgkin lymphoma: introduction and pathology

Introduction

Non-Hodgkin lymphomas (NHLs) are a group of lymphoid malignancies of varying subtypes with a range of clinical behaviours and treatment strategies. It has a high incidence in Europe, USA, and Australia and lowest incidence in Asia. Around 8450 new cases are diagnosed per year in the UK and 65,980 cases in the USA. The median age is 65 although aggressive B-cell lymphomas are the predominant NHL in younger adults. The male: female ratio is 1.5:1.

Aetiology

The aetiology of NHL is largely unknown. Autoimmune disease and immunodeficiency are known to predispose to NHL. Sjögren's disease (associated with marginal zone lymphomas of salivary gland) and rheumatoid arthritis are linked with NHL. Immunodeficiency (both acquired and inherited) and solid organ transplantations increase the risk of NHL. In patients with AIDS, NHL is the second most common malignancy, and its incidence is declining due to antiretroviral therapy. A number of infective agents are associated with various types of NHL. These include:

- Epstein–Barr virus (EBV): associated with post-transplant immunoproliferative disorders, immunodeficiency associated lymphomas (e.g. HIV associated primary CNS lymphoma), Burkitt lymphoma, etc.
- Human herpesvirus 8 (HHV-8): associated with primary effusion lymphoma, and plasmablastic lymphoma in Castleman disease.
- Human T-lymphotropic virus 1 (HTLV-1): associated with adult T-cell lymphoma/leukaemia.
- Hepatitis C virus (HCV): associated with extranodal and splenic marginal zone B-cell lymphoma.
- *Helicobacter pylori*: associated with gastric marginal zone B-cell lymphoma of MALT type. Eradication of *H. pylori* can lead to regression of this type of lymphoma.

There is some evidence of a link with agricultural work, farming, and forestry. This occupational risk of lymphoma is possibly attributable to organo-chlorine based pesticides. Prior radiotherapy and chemotherapy also increase the risk of NHL.

Pathology

The cell of origin is different for each subtype of lymphoma. Classification is by the updated WHO modification of the REAL (revised European and American lymphoma) classification system which is broadly divided into B cell, T cell/natural killer (NK) cell, and Hodgkin disease. Immunophenotyping has a significant role in the classification of NHL. Table 4.10.7 gives a summarized classification showing common varieties of NHL, and their cytogenetic and molecular characteristics. B-cell lymphomas constitute >90% of NHL, and T-cell lymphomas approximately 10%. Immunohistochemistry based on the expression of cell surface antigens and immunoglobulin proteins, which in turn depends on the type of lymphocyte and its stage of differentiation, is important diagnostically and to determine causality. B-cell lineage is indicated by pan B cell markers (CD22, CD19, and CD20) and T-cell lineage by T-cell markers (CD3, CD2, CD7, CD4, and CD8). Immunophenotyping using flow cytometry is used in the subclassification of NHL. The markers of mature B-cell NHL include surface Ig heavy and light chains, CD79a,

CD19, CD20, and CD22. Antibodies such as CD5, CD10, CD23, and cyclin D1 are used to subtype NHL (see Table 4.10.7). In the majority of lymphomas there is good reproducibility (>85%) in the diagnoses except in Burkitt-like lymphoma, lymphoplasmacytic lymphoma, and marginal zone B-cell lymphoma of nodal type (<60%).

Chromosomal translocations and molecular rearrangement are commonly used to confirm diagnosis. The most common chromosomal abnormality in NHL is t(14;18)(q31;q21), which is found in >80% of follicular lymphomas and > 25% of diffuse large B-cell lymphoma. Follicular lymphoma and diffuse large B-cell lymphoma constitute >50% of adult NHL. Other common chromosomal translocations and molecular arrangements are shown in Table 4.10.8.

The REAL classification is important for management and prognostication. Based on biological behaviour there are three categories of NHL: indolent (low grade), aggressive, and highly aggressive.

- Indolent lymphomas usually occur in older adults and are characterized by a waxing and waning course. Follicular, small lymphocytic, mantle cell, and lymphoplasmacytic lymphomas are included in this group. More than 80% of patients with indolent lymphomas present with advanced stage disease with a high risk of involvement of bone marrow. Some of the tumours can transform to high-grade, large-cell lymphoma. Indolent lymphomas are not curable.
- Aggressive lymphomas can occur in any age group. These tumours are fast growing and untreated are fatal within a year or two. Diffuse large B-cell lymphomas and some of the T/NK cell lymphomas fall into this category. Patients can present with all stages of disease and bone marrow involvement indicates a poor prognosis. Approximately 70–80% of patients achieve complete remission (CR) with combination chemotherapy of whom two-thirds are cured.
- Burkitts' and lymphoblastic lymphomas constitute the highly aggressive category of NHL. These subtypes are common in children and young adults and are very fast growing. These tumours present with advanced stage and a high incidence of bone marrow and CNS involvement. With combination chemotherapy some patients with these tumours can be cured, especially those who present with an early stage.

Assessing response to treatment in NHL

Standardized response assessment criteria are important in facilitating and comparing clinical studies. Recent guidelines for response assessment in NHL incorporate PET scan, immunohistochemistry, and flow cytometry. PET is recommended routinely for diffuse large B-cell lymphoma as a staging investigation as well as 6–8 weeks after completion of treatment to assess response to treatment.

Complete response (CR) in NHL is defined as the complete disappearance of all evidence of disease including negative PET scan if it was positive before treatment, and clear bone marrow. Partial response (PR) is defined as the regression of measurable disease and no new disease. Persistence of one or more PET-positive areas is also included in partial response. Progressive/relapsed disease (PD) is defined as appearance of a new nodal lesion of >1.5cm in any axis, an increase of a previously involved

Table 4.10.7 WHO–REAL classification of NHL

Type of NHL	Biological behaviour	Immunohistochemistry
B-cell neoplasms (>90%)		
Precursor B- cell neoplasms		
Precursor B lymphoblastic leukaemia/ lymphoblastic lymphoma	Highly aggressive	B cell marker (CD19, PAX-5) positive TdT+, CD99+, CD10+ Rearrangement of Ig heavy chain gene
Mature B cell neoplasms (83%)		
CLL/small lymphocytic lymphoma (17%)	Low grade	CD20+, CD3−, CD10−, CD5+, CD23+
Lymphoplasmacytic lymphoma (0.9%)	Low grade	
Splenic marginal zone lymphoma (0.4%)	Low grade	
Extranodal marginal zone lymphoma of MALT type (3.8%)	Low grade	
Nodal marginal zone B cell lymphoma (1.5%)	Low grade	CD20+, CD3−, CD10−, CD5−, CD23−
Follicular lymphoma (12%)	Low grade	CD20+, CD3−, CD10−, CD5−, CD23−
Mantle zone lymphoma (2.2%)	Low grade	CD20+, CD3−, CD10+, CD5−
Diffuse large B cell lymphoma (23%)	High grade	CD20+, CD3−, CD10−, CD5+, CD24−, PRAD1+
Mediastinal large B-cell lymphoma (0.1%)	Favourable group, of DLBCL	CD20+, CD3−
Burkitt lymphoma (1.4%)	Highly aggressive	CD20+, CD3−, CD10−, CD5−, Tdt−
T-cell and NK-cell neoplasms (7%)		
Precursor T-cell and NK-cell neoplasms (0.9%)	Highly aggressive	CD20−, CD3+, CD30+, CD15−, EMA+, ALK+
Precursor T-lymphoblastic leukaemia/ lymphoblastic lymphoma		
Peripheral T-cell and NK-cell neoplasms (3.8%)		
T-cell prolymphocytic leukaemia (0.1%)	Low grade	
Aggressive NK-cell leukaemia (0.2%)	High grade	
Adult T-cell lymphoma/leukaemia (0.1%)	Highly aggressive	
Mycosis fungoides/Sézary syndrome (1.5%)	Low grade(MF)	
Primary cutaneous anaplastic large cell lymphoma (0.3%)	Low grade	
Peripheral T-cell lymphoma (1.4%)	High grade	
Anaplastic large cell lymphoma (1%)	Different behaviour (e.g. nodal disease aggressive and skin disease indolent)	CD30+

Table 4.10.8 Cytogenetic characteristics of common varieties of NHL

Type of NHL	Cytogenetic abnormality	Genes involved
Mature B-cell neoplasms:		
CLL/small lymphocytic lymphoma	17p13 del	TP53
Lymphoplasmacytic lymphoma	t(9;14)(p13;q32)—50%	pax-5
Splenic marginal zone lymphoma	7q21–32 deletion	CDK6
Extranodal marginal zone lymphoma of MALT type	t(11;18)(q21;q21)—50%	api2/mlt
Nodal marginal zone B cell lymphoma	t(1;14)(p22;q32)	bcl-10
Follicular lymphoma	t (14;18)(q32;q21)—90% t (2;18)(p11;q21) t(18;22)(q21;q11)	bcl-2
Mantle zone lymphoma	t(11;14)(q13;q32)—70%	bcl-1/cyclin D1
Diffuse large B cell lymphoma	der (3)(q27) – 35%, t(14;18) (q32;q21)	bcl-6 bcl-2
Mediastinal large B-cell lymphoma (0.1%)	9p gain	REL
Burkitt lymphoma (1.4%)	t(8;14)(q24;q32)—80% t(2;8)(p11;q24)—15% t(8;22)(q24;q11)	c-myc
T-cell and NK-cell neoplasms:		
Anaplastic large cell lymphoma	t(2;5)(p23;q35)—70–80%% t (1;2)(q25;p23)—10–20%	npm/alk tpm3/alk

area by ≥50%, or the appearance of a PET-positive lesion. Patients whose disease does not satisfy the definition of CR, PR, or PD are considered to have stable disease (SD).

Further reading

Chan JKC. Tumours of the lymphoreticular system. In: Fletcher CDM (ed) *Diagnostic Histopathology of Tumours*, Volume 2, 3rd edition, pp.1139–361, Philadelphia, PA: Elsevier, 2007.

Juweid ME, Stroobants S, Hoekstra OS, *et al.* Use of positron emission tomography for response assessment of lymphoma: consensus of the imaging subcommittee of the International Harmonization Project in Lymphoma. *J Clin Oncol* 2007; **25**:571–8.

Cheson BD, Pfistner B, Juweid ME, *et al.* Revised response criteria for malignant lymphoma. *J Clin Oncol* 2007; **25**:579–86.

Non-Hodgkin lymphoma: clinical features, diagnosis, staging, and prognosis

Clinical features

The clinical presentation of patients with NHL is extremely variable.

Patients most commonly present with a painless lymph node enlargement. In indolent lymphoma, lymphadenopathy may wax and wane. Other symptoms are due to specific organ involvement, e.g. abdominal pain due to obstruction by bulky disease, spinal cord compression, etc.

Constitutional symptoms, known as B symptoms (fever >38°C, night sweats, unintended weight loss of >10% of body weight during the last 6 months) occur in up to 50% of patients.

Diagnosis

The most important step in treating patients with NHL is an accurate histopathological diagnosis.

Diagnosis of NHL and its subtypes is based on the histopathological evaluation of an adequate sample of tissue preferably obtained with an excisional lymph node biopsy or a generous incisional biopsy of an involved organ. Adequate histological diagnosis mainly depends upon a sufficient amount of tissue. If the material is non-diagnostic, rebiopsy must not be deferred.

FNA is not appropriate for the initial diagnosis of lymphoma. However, it may be sufficient to establish relapse or confirm involvement of organs when in doubt.

An image-guided core biopsy is discouraged but can be performed if there is no easily accessible lymph node, e.g. where there is retroperitoneal involvement.

Diagnostic standards for the classification of malignant lymphomas are laid down in the 2008 edition of the WHO classification of haematopoietic tumours. Conventional histological examination of paraffin-embedded sections, immunohistochemistry, and genetic tests (FISH analyses, cytogenetics, molecular genetics, e.g. PCR) are mandatory to provide an accurate diagnosis. At present, gene-expression profiling is not part of routine clinical practice.

Staging

Once the diagnosis of NHL is established, detailed staging must be undertaken to determine sites of involvement by the lymphoma. This is the basis for the choice of the most appropriate therapy.

Initial evaluation of a patient with NHL should include a careful history and clinical examination. The presence or absence of constitutional symptoms should be noted. The performance status of the patient should be assessed using Karnofsky or ECOG score.

A complete physical examination should be done with particular attention to location and size of enlarged lymph nodes including Waldeyer's ring and size of the liver and spleen.

Laboratory studies should include a complete blood count with careful examination of a peripheral blood smear to evaluate for the presence of circulating lymphoma cells. Serum biochemical tests should include an assessment of renal and hepatic function and the uric acid level. LDH can identify patients with a high tumour mass and is a prognostic factor in indolent and aggressive lymphomas.

Serological testing for HIV and hepatitis should be performed before starting therapy.

A bone marrow biopsy with aspiration is essential in all cases. Although bilateral biopsy has been reported to increase the sensitivity of detection of bone marrow infiltration, a unilateral biopsy of at least 1.5cm in length is generally sufficient. The clinical relevance of bone marrow involvement detected only by flow cytometry has not been demonstrated.

Standard imaging studies include CT scans of the neck, chest, abdomen, and pelvis, as well as other apparently involved sites. The major criterion for recognition of nodal involvement is that of size. Detection of lymphoma in normal sized lymph nodes is not possible.

PET scans are not routinely used for initial staging in NHL but play a role in the response assessment in HL and aggressive lymphomas. Use of this technology is still in flux and further studies are needed to determine the role of PET in the initial staging.

A diagnostic lumbar puncture is recommended in patients with neurological symptoms or in patients presenting with sinus or testicular involvement.

Colonoscopy should be performed in mantle cell lymphoma, which often involves the bowel. Gastroduodenal endoscopy and endoscopic ultrasound are mandatory in gastric MALT lymphomas.

If anthracyclines are included in the treatment regimen, an echocardiogram should be performed.

Other diagnostic procedures may be useful in specific patients.

Based on the results of the diagnostic procedures, patients are assigned to an Ann Arbor stage I–IV. The suffix A or B reflects the absence or presence of constitutional symptoms.

Prognosis

Clinical prognostic markers

The International Prognostic Index (IPI) has been developed based on data from patients with aggressive lymphoma who were treated with an anthracyclin-containing regimen. Based on the IPI, patients with diffuse large B-cell lymphoma can be stratified into four different prognostic groups: low risk (IPI 0–1), low–intermediate risk (IPI 2), high-intermediate risk (IPI 3), and high risk (IPI 4–5). Prognostic factors associated with a poor prognosis include age >60 years, advanced anatomical stage, poor PS, involvement of more than one extranodal site, and elevated serum LDH. The most important factor is age, because it also influences the ability to tolerate dose-intensified therapy. Based on these factors, response rate and survival can be predicted. In low risk patients, tumour bulk was recently identified as an additional unfavourable prognostic factor.

Introduction of treatment with rituximab improved prognosis in all four risk groups, but the IPI retained its clinical relevance.

To date, the IPI remains the most important prognostic marker and should be applied to all patients with diffuse large B cell lymphoma.

The IPI can also be applied to indolent lymphomas, but the FLIPI score (Follicular Lymphoma International Prognostic Index) has been shown to be more discriminatory.

The FLIPI score comprises five adverse factors: age >60 years, advanced stage, haemoglobin level <12.0g/L, elevated serum LDH, and involvement of more than four extranodal sites. The FLIPI defines three risk groups: low risk (0–1 adverse factor), intermediate risk (2 adverse factors), and poor risk (≥3 adverse factors).

Minimal residual disease has proven to be predictive of prolonged PFS after autologous stem cell transplantation in follicular lymphoma. With a median molecular follow-up of 75 months, an 88% incidence of relapse was observed among patients never attaining molecular remission. In contrast, relapse incidence was only 8% among patients attaining a durable molecular remission.

Molecular prognostic markers

Most clinical risk factors are based on surrogate markers. Molecular genetic analysis adds important information for lymphoma biology and prognosis.

Gene expression profiling in diffuse large B-cell lymphoma allows differentiation between a germinal centre B-cell (GCB) and an activated B-cell (ABC) type. These two subgroups can be considered distinct diseases. In the GCB type the cell of origin is a germinal centre B cell and in the ABC type it is a postgerminal centre B cell. Oncogenic mechanisms seem to be different in both groups and explain the robustness of the detection in several studies.

The clinical outcome is much better in the GCB type with a 5-year-survival of 60% versus 35% in the ABC type. The prognostic difference between GCB and ABC was recently confirmed for rituximab-containing treatment regimens.

An immunohistochemistry-based classifier which focuses on CD10, bcl-6, and MUM1 as a surrogate for gene-expression based classification could not be confirmed in several recent studies.

In follicular lymphoma, molecular features of the non-malignant immune cells present in the tumour seem to be predictive of survival. Two gene expression signatures were used to construct a survival predictor. These signatures allowed patients to be divided into four quartiles with widely disparate median lengths of survival independently of clinical prognostic variables. A T-cell activation signature was associated with a favourable prognosis whereas a macrophage/dendritic cell signature correlated with poor survival.

Further reading

Matasar MJ, Zelenetz AD. Overview of lymphoma diagnosis and management. *Radio Clin North Am 2008*; **46**(2):175–98. See related articles in the same issue.

Sehn LH. Optimal use of prognostic factors in non-Hodgkins lymphoma. Hematology *Am Soc Haematol Educ Program* 2006; **1**:295–302.

Teruya-Feldstein J. Getting the diagnosis right in NHL: role of immunohistochemistry and molecular diagnostic testing. *J Natl Compr Canc Netw* 2008; **6**(4):422–7.

Non-Hodgkin lymphoma: treatment of low-grade disease

By far the most prevalent subtype of low-grade lymphoma is follicular lymphoma, the second most common B-cell lymphoma in the Western world. Follicular lymphoma accounts for approximately 20% of all lymphomas with an annual incidence of 2 per 100,000. The clinical course of follicular lymphoma is highly variable and characterized by a continuous pattern of relapse. Most patients present with advanced disease and median survival is 10–15 years from diagnosis. Spontaneous regression occasionally occurs.

Transformation to an aggressive histological type occurs in up to 40% and is associated with a poor prognosis.

The histological subtype FL grade IIIA/B (as distinguished from the subtype I/II with low numbers of blastic cells) behaves like an aggressive lymphoma and should thus be treated like a diffuse large B-cell lymphoma.

Over the last three decades, chemotherapy alone has not resulted in a significant improvement of OS in advanced stages. However, the introduction of monoclonal antibodies in the treatment of follicular lymphoma does improve the long-term outcome of these patients and may ultimately lead to improved OS.

Early stage

Only about one-third of patients with follicular lymphoma present initially with limited stages I and II or stage III limited (with up to five involved lymph nodes). Patients with stage II and bulky disease should be treated like patients with advanced disease. Radiotherapy with conventionally fractionated doses of 36–44Gy has shown curative potential and is the treatment modality of choice in this group of patients. In a German retrospective study, OS was 70% and DFS 63% at 10 years, respectively. Out-of-field recurrence rate was 34%. In several studies there was no relevant difference in OS between extended field and involved field radiotherapy. Superiority of total lymphoid radiation has not been demonstrated so far.

In patients with early stage disease and large tumour burden, systemic immunochemotherapy before radiation therapy might be effective but there are no data from randomized trials.

Advanced stage

In patients with advanced disease stage III and IV, no curative treatment is yet established.

To date, there are three clinical trials which could not demonstrate a survival benefit for early initiation of chemotherapy compared with deferred treatment.

In a prospective study of the National Cancer Institute from 1983, 104 patients with newly diagnosed follicular lymphoma were randomly assigned to a 'watch and wait' strategy or to immediate multiagent chemotherapy with ProMACE-MOPP followed by total nodal irradiation. In a study update from 1997, no difference in survival between the two arms was reported.

In a more recent study conducted by the French GELF study group, delay of treatment until clinically relevant progression was compared with immediate treatment with prednimustine, an oral alkylating agent, or alfa-interferon. The OS rate at 5 years was not inferior when treatment was deferred. These data were confirmed in a British National Lymphoma Investigation randomized trial comparing immediate chemotherapy with chlorambucil with delayed treatment. Median OS in the observation arm was 6.7 years compared with 5.9 years in the treatment arm at a median follow-up of 16 years. Importantly, in the observation group, the chance of not needing chemotherapy at 10 years was 19% and even 40% in patients >70 years.

In summary, all three trials show conclusive evidence that the policy of watch and wait in patients with asymptomatic advanced follicular lymphoma is effective and appropriate.

Therefore, the goal of treatment in these patients must be to improve their quality of life and delay the impact of treatment-related toxicity. Based on this data, treatment in advanced follicular lymphoma should be initiated only when lymphoma-associated symptoms occur.

In practice, treatment is indicated most frequently due to potential or actual local compressive disease or impairment of organ function, bulky disease, constitutional symptoms or rapid disease progression. Other indications are bone marrow infiltration with consequent haematopoietic impairment, massive hepatosplenomegaly, or transformation to an aggressive lymphoma.

The most widely used single-agent cytotoxic drugs in the treatment of follicular lymphoma are chlorambucil, an alkylating drug, and purine analogues, namely fludarabine. For chlorambucil, there are many different treatment schedules. The overall response rate is approximately 50–75%, but CRs are rare. With fludarabine alone, CR can be achieved in 30%. However, the stem cell toxicity of fludarabine must be considered when a stem cell harvest is planned.

Several different combination chemotherapy regimens have been developed yielding higher complete response rates compared with single agents. CVP (cyclophosphamide, vincristine, and prednisolone) and CHOP both are popular regimens and result in higher response rates and better freedom from progression, but there is no evidence so far for improved OS.

Bendamustine is another drug that has shown substantial activity alone or in combination. In a randomized phase II trial, bendamustine, vincristine and prednisone (BOP) was compared with COP in 164 patients with indolent lymphoma. The rate of CR was 22% with BOP and 20% with COP. The projected 5-year survival rate was 61% with BOP and 46% with COP.

In a recent trial, fludarabine alone achieved higher overall response and CRs (38.6% vs. 15%) compared with CVP. Time to treatment failure and OS were not different. Fludarabine-containing regimens have demonstrated very high rates (>80%) of CR in several trials. In a phase II trial from the NHL co-operative study group, 60 newly diagnosed patients were treated with 6 cycles of fludarabine, cyclophosphamide, and mitoxantrone (FCM). Complete response was achieved in 77% and partial response in 10%. Notably, 25 out of 36 patients achieved a molecular response. The 4-year estimated probabilities of OS and failure-free survival were 78.2% and 45%, respectively.

Combined chemoimmunotherapy with the monoclonal anti-CD20 antibody rituximab is a promising treatment option in advanced follicular lymphoma. There are four randomized trials demonstrating superiority of the addition of rituximab to different chemotherapy regimens in terms of EFS and (presumably also, but not proven so far) OS in first-line treatment. However, there is no indication that this is a curative approach.

In relapsed patients, there are two trials evaluating the efficacy of rituximab added to chemotherapy in rituximab-naive patients. In both trials, EFS and OS were improved with rituximab. These results were confirmed in a recent meta-analysis including 1943 patients from seven randomized trials with follicular lymphoma, mantle cell lymphoma, or other indolent lymphomas. Long-term outcome was significant better for rituximab-containing treatment in primary and relapsed disease.

Because of the high relapse rate in follicular lymphoma, maintenance therapy with different agents was investigated for improving outcome. Interferon-alpha has been shown to prolong OS when given as maintenance therapy but its toxicity profile precluded widespread use.

Over the past few years it has been shown in two large randomized trials that rituximab maintenance has a clear clinical benefit in relapsed or refractory follicular lymphoma after induction with chemotherapy alone and rituximab plus chemotherapy. In the EORTC trial 20981, 465 patients were initially randomized to 6 cycles of CHOP or R-CHOP. Responders were randomized to maintenance with rituximab once every 3 months for a maximum of 2 years or observation. Rituximab maintenance yielded an impressive improvement of median PFS from second randomization of 51.5 months versus 14.9 months with observation. OS was improved with 85% at 3 years versus 77% and the hazard ratio was 0.52. In a second prospective randomized trial of the GLSG, patients with recurring or refractory FL and MCL were randomized to 4 courses of FCM alone or combined with rituximab. Responders were randomized to rituximab-maintenance comprising 2 further courses of 4-times-weekly doses of rituximab after 3 and 9 months. Response duration was significantly prolonged by maintenance therapy after R-FCM and PFS was doubled. OS was improved with 82% versus 55% at 3 years.

In conclusion, both trials demonstrated that rituximab maintenance therapy significantly prolongs OS in relapsed follicular lymphoma with a low rate of clinically relevant side effects.

The role of consolidating autologous stem cell transplantation in first remission was evaluated in three randomized trials from the pre-rituximab era. In conclusion, none of these studies could show a relevant improvement in long-term outcome. In addition, the risk of secondary neoplasms after stem cell transplantation has to be considered.

Multiple studies have also shown the efficacy of radioimmunotherapy (RIT) both as a single agent and in combination with chemotherapy. By conjugating a radioisotope to an anti-CD20 antibody, radiation is directly delivered to the tumour cell. Ibritumomab tiuxetan, a yttrium-90 labelled radio-immunoconjugate, is registered in Europe to treat relapsed follicular lymphoma. One recently presented trial has demonstrated a significant benefit for ibritumomab consolidation after initial chemotherapy without rituximab. Other studies are underway looking at personalized vaccines and oral targeted therapies that work by inhibiting the enzyme SKY kinase (e.g. biovax ID and fostamatinib).

Treatment recommendations

In patients presenting with stage I and II disease without bulky disease, radiotherapy is the treatment of choice with curative potential.

To date there is no standard treatment in advanced follicular lymphoma. To achieve long PFS, rituximab in combination with chemotherapy such as CHOP, CVP, or FCM should be administered. Rituximab monotherapy or single-agent chemotherapy is an alternative in elderly patients with comorbidities. Rituximab maintenance significantly prolongs PFS in relapsed patients, whereas it remains investigational in primary disease. Ibritumomab tiuxetan with or without prior re-induction is an effective and safe treatment in first and subsequent relapses. The role of autologous transplantation in relapse is being evaluated in clinical trials.

Further reading

Czuczman MS, Weaver R, Alkuzweny B, et al. Prolonged clinical and molecular remission in patients with low grade or follicular non-Hodgkin's lymphoma treated with rituximab plus CHOP chemotherapy: 9 year follow-up. J Clin Oncol 2004; **22**(23):4711–6.

Mac Manus MP, Hoppe RT. Is radiotherapy curative for stage I and II low grade follicular lymphoma? Results of a long term follow-up study of patients treated at Stanford University. J Clin Oncol 1996; **14**(4):1282–90.

Vidal L, Gafter-Gvilli A, Leibovici L, et al. Rituximab maintenance for the treatment of patients with follicular lymphoma: systematic review and meta-analysis of randomized trials. J Natl Cancer Inst 2009; **101**(4):248–55.

Non-Hodgkin lymphoma: mantle cell lymphoma

In patients with mantle cell lymphoma, conventional chemotherapy remains a non-curative approach.

Median OS in the pre-rituximab era has been reported to be 3–4 years without a chance of cure. However, in a retrospective single-centre study including an unselected patient population from 1997–2007, the median OS was 7.1 years (95% CI 78–92%). An analysis of the GLSG also showed an improvement of OS in mantle cell lymphoma from 2.7 to 4.8 years during the last 3 decades.

Thus, the prognosis of patients with mantle cell lymphoma appears to be improving with the introduction of rituximab and more aggressive treatment strategies.

First-line therapy

As a result of the aggressive clinical course of mantle cell lymphoma, a watch and wait strategy is not generally recommended, although in selected asymptomatic patients it may have a role.

There is no standard first-line treatment for mantle cell lymphoma.

The most widely used baseline regimen in mantle cell lymphoma is CHOP, although a major benefit of anthracycline-containing over non-anthracycline-containing combinations (i.e. COP or MCP) could not be demonstrated in two randomized trials.

The GLSG performed a randomized trial comparing combined cyclophosphamide, vincristine, doxorubicin, and prednisone (CHOP) chemotherapy with combined mitoxantrone, chlorambucil, and prednisone (MCP) chemotherapy as first-line therapy. Overall response rate was slightly but not significantly higher after CHOP. However, no significant differences were observed in the time to treatment failure or in OS.

In a randomized phase III trial, combined immunochemotherapy with R-CHOP as initial therapy resulted in a significantly higher overall response rate (ORR 94% vs. 75%) and CR rate (34% vs. 7%). However, no differences were observed for PFS and OS. In fact, R-CHOP gives a higher remission rate than CHOP alone but the remission seems not to be durable.

Fludarabine-containing regimens are effective in the first-line setting as well as in relapsed disease but are hampered by their stem cell toxicity.

Cladribine has also shown single-agent activity in a large cohort of patients with untreated and relapsed mantle cell lymphomas, achieving a response rate of 58%.

In a French phase II study with 27 patients, CHOP was followed by DHAP if CHOP failed to induce CR. After four cycles of CHOP, only 2 patients (7%) obtained a complete response. The other 25 patients received DHAP and in this group a response rate of 92% was observed. In this study, CHOP plus DHAP appeared to be more effective than CHOP alone.

Several different approaches are being tested to try to improve the results of conventional therapy:

One such approach uses dose-intensified induction regimens. In a recent update of a M.D. Anderson Cancer Center phase II trial, rituximab plus hyper-CVAD alternating with high-dose methotrexate/cytarabine in newly diagnosed mantle cell lymphoma showed a 5-year failure-free survival and OS rate of 48% and 65%, respectively. Median follow-up was 4.8 years. The complete remission rate (CR/CRu) was 87%. Among patients <65 years, the 5-year failure-free survival was 60%. Patients with disease of blastoid morphology had a 7-year survival rate of 47%. Although the remissions were more durable compared to those obtained with R-CHOP there was no plateau in failure-free survival curves.

However, in a multicentre trial of the Southwest Oncology Group (SWOG) these data could not be replicated completely. The rate of CR was lower with 58% compared to 87% and nearly half of the patients (48%) could not complete therapy because of toxicity. PFS at 2 years of 63% was also lower than reported in the M.D. Anderson trial.

Second-line therapy

So far, no optimal second-line therapy has been defined.

FCM, a fludarabine-containing regimen in combination with rituximab, has been shown to be highly active in relapsed mantle cell lymphoma. OR and CR rates were improved and OS was significantly prolonged compared to FCM alone. Hence, the addition of rituximab to FCM significantly improved the outcome of relapsed mantle cell lymphoma.

In a German phase II study, patients with relapsed or refractory mantle cell lymphoma were treated with bendamustine, a nitrogen mustard compound, and rituximab. The CR rate was 50% and the median PFS was 18 months at a median follow-up of 20 months.

In a phase II study with 155 patients with relapsed mantle cell lymphoma, bortezomib was administered for up to 17 cycles. Response rate in 141 assessable patients was 33% including 8% CR/CRu. Median duration of response was 9.2 months. The most common adverse event of grade 3 or higher was peripheral neuropathy (13%). Bortezomib has recently been approved for treatment of relapsed mantle cell lymphoma in the USA.

RIT has been investigated in two ongoing phase II trials in relapsed mantle cell lymphoma. Overall response rate was 30–40% but the duration of response was short.

Postremission therapy

Another strategy to improve long-term outcome in mantle cell lymphoma focuses on postremission therapy, either consolidation or maintenance therapy.

In a prospective randomized trial of the European MCL Network, early consolidation by myeloablative radiochemotherapy followed by autologous stem cell transplantation in first remission was compared to alpha-interferon maintenance. PFS was significantly prolonged with a median of 39 months compared with 17 months. Three-year OS was 83% after ASCT versus 77% in the IFN group. This study shows that consolidating transplantation is likely to improve PFS but longer follow-up is needed to determine the effect on OS.

The value of high-dose cytarabine in first-line therapy is currently being investigated in a clinical trial of the European MCL Network for younger patients. In this randomized, prospective multicentre trial, the efficacy of 6 courses R-CHOP followed by myeloablative radiochemotherapy and autologous stem cell transplantation is being compared to alternating treatment with 3 courses R-CHOP and 3 courses R-DHAP followed by high-dose cytarabine-containing myeloablative radiochemotherapy and autologous stem cell transplantation.

Maintenance rituximab therapy is another possibility for post remission therapy.

In a multicentre phase II pilot study from the Wisconsin Oncology Network, rituximab and a modified hyperCVAD regimen without methotrexate and cytarabine was administered for 4–6 cycles as induction therapy followed by rituximab maintenance therapy consisting of four weekly doses every 6 months for 2 years. The overall response rate was 77% and the complete response rate was 64%. With a median follow-up time of 37 months in surviving patients, the median PFS was 37 months and the median OS was not reached. The major toxicity was myelosuppression.

New drugs

Temsirolimus, an inhibitor of the mammalian target of rapamycin kinase (mTOR), has shown activity in a phase II trial conducted by the North Central Cancer Treatment Group. Twenty-nine patients with relapsed or refractory MCL received temsirolimus 25mg intravenously every week as a single agent for at least 6 cycles. The overall response rate was 41% with 1 complete response and 10 partial responses. The median time to progression was 6 months. Haematological toxicities were the most common toxicities observed (50% grade 3).

Everolimus is another oral mTOR inhibitor which also showed activity with relapsed mantle cell lymphoma. The response rate was 29% in a small cohort of 14 patients.

The immunomodulatory agent thalidomide in combination with rituximab produced responses in 13 of 16 patients. Lenalidomide has also shown antitumour activity in a preliminary report producing a 53% response rate in 15 relapsed patients.

Treatment recommendations

Optimal initial treatment in mantle cell lymphoma is an unsettled issue. The only curative treatment option is offered by allogeneic transplantation.

In the absence of more comprehensive data from phase III trials, R-HyperCVAD seems to be a promising option in younger patients (< 60 years) without significant comorbidity.

In elderly patients (>60 years) R-CHOP is a very reasonable alternative due to its lower toxicity.

Consolidating autologous stem cell transplantation in first remission improves PFS in eligible younger patients.

Rituximab maintenance therapy seems to be a therapeutic alternative particularly in elderly patients.

In relapsed patients, fludarabine-containing regimens, bendamustine and bortezomib seem to be effective.

Further reading

Kahl BS, Longo WL, Eickhoff JC, et al. Maintenance rituximab following induction chemo-immunotherapy may prolong progression-free survival in Mantle cell lymphoma: a pilot study from the Wisconsin Oncology Network. Ann Oncol 2006; **17**(9):1418–23.

Martin P, Chadburn A, Christos P, et al. Outcome of deferred initial therapy in Mantle-cell lymphoma. J Clin Oncol 2009; **27**(8):1209–13.

Schmidt C, Dreyling M. Therapy of mantle cell lymphoma: current standards and future strategies. Hematol Oncol Clin North Am 2008; **22**(5):953–63.

Non-Hodgkin lymphoma: the role of stem cell transplantation in aggressive disease

Autologous stem cell transplantation

Haematopoietic stem cell transplantation has become the standard treatment for younger patients with a first chemosensitive relapse of aggressive lymphoma.

In the PARMA trial from 1995, a total of 215 patients with relapses of NHL were treated with salvage therapy of two courses of conventional chemotherapy. Responders were randomly assigned to receive four more courses of chemotherapy plus radiotherapy or high-dose chemoradiotherapy and autologous bone marrow transplantation. The response rate was 84% after bone marrow transplantation and 44% after chemotherapy without transplantation at a median follow-up of 63 months. At 5 years, OS was 53% and 32% respectively. In this trial, high-dose chemotherapy and autologous bone marrow transplantation was shown for the first time to be superior to conventional salvage chemotherapy in NHL relapse.

In another analysis of the PARMA trial, it could be clearly shown that patients with a high IPI at relapse benefit most from high-dose chemotherapy. Patients with a low IPI did not benefit from autologous transplantation compared with conventional chemotherapy. The role of autologous stem cell transplantation in relapse after rituximab-containing front-line treatment has not been determined. Recent data from the CORAL trial indicate a significantly worse outcome for patients with previous rituximab treatment.

However, the value of high-dose chemotherapy followed by autologous stem cell transplantation in first-line treatment of patients with high-risk features is still an unsettled issue. A number of trials addressing the role of stem cell transplantation in this setting have given conflicting results.

In a recent Cochrane database meta-analysis, fifteen randomized trials with a total of 3079 patients were included. Despite a higher rate of CRs in the group with high-dose chemotherapy, there was no significant difference in EFS and OS compared with conventional chemotherapy. Therefore, this treatment should not be given even to patients with high-risk disease outside controlled clinical trials.

Allogeneic stem cell transplantation

The role of allogeneic transplantation in the management of patients with aggressive lymphoma is a matter of intense debate.

In contrast to indolent lymphomas, there is still no general agreement about the existence of a clinically meaningful graft-versus-lymphoma effect. However, there are some observations which support the existence of such an effect.

In a prospective trial comparing autologous with allogeneic transplantation, there was a significantly lower relapse rate after allogeneic transplantation. Furthermore, T-cell depleted stem cell grafts have a negative impact on the relapse rate. Responses to donor lymphocyte infusion (DLI) have also been reported in aggressive lymphomas. Assessment of study results is difficult because most of the clinical trials are hampered by small patient numbers, different conditioning regimens, and short follow-up.

Due to the limited amount of clinical data, there are no routine indications for allogeneic stem cell transplantation in aggressive lymphoma outside clinical trials

In general, there are two major advantages of allogeneic stem cell transplantation over autologous stem cell transplantation: first tumour contamination from re-infused autologous stem cells is avoided and second there is a postulated allogeneic graft-versus-lymphoma effect. The major disadvantages of allogeneic transplantation are the high treatment-related mortality as well as graft-versus-host disease.

Allogeneic transplantation appears to be superior to autologous transplantation in terms of producing a lower relapse rate but this effect is impaired by a high treatment-related mortality. The toxicity of myeloablative regimens is substantial and is up to 40%.

Prognosis of patients resistant to first-line therapy, with an early relapse within 12 months after primary therapy or relapse after autologous transplantation remains very poor. These patients seem to be candidates for allogeneic transplantation.

In an EBMT registry matched study, myeloablative allogeneic transplantation was compared with autologous transplantation in 255 patients (median age 27 years) with aggressive lymphoma. OS in the allogeneic transplantation group was 41% at 4 years. Median OS was 1 year. Despite a lower relapse rate compared to autologous transplantation (47 vs. 51% at 5 years) outcome was relatively poor because of the high treatment-related mortality (33%). For low levels of acute graft-versus-host disease, a trend towards improved OS was seen. Status at transplant showed a significant effect on OS in multivariate analysis.

To exploit the graft-versus-lymphoma effect, to decrease treatment-related mortality, and to increase the upper age limit of eligible patients, reduced-intensity conditioning (RIC) regimens have been developed in the last decade.

Because the effect of RIC is mainly based upon graft-versus-lymphoma effect, rigorous tumour debulking before transplantation is essential.

While results with RIC in patients with chemosensitive disease are acceptable, results in refractory disease are not satisfactory.

There have been several reports of RIC for aggressive lymphoma in the last few years.

In an analysis of the Lymphoma Working Party of the EBMT from 2002, the outcome of RIC for 188 patients with lymphoma was reported, including 62 patients with aggressive histology disease. 48% of patients had undergone prior autologous transplantation. Conditioning consisted of fludarabine-containing regimens in most cases (84%). The OS rate at 2 years for patients with aggressive lymphoma was 46.7% compared to 65% in indolent lymphomas. The treatment-related mortality at 1 year was substantially higher at 36% than that reported in other studies. Patients >50 years and those with more than three lines of prior therapy had a significant higher TRM than younger patients.

The progression rate was very high (78.8% at 2 years) and PFS was only 13% at 2 years compared with 21% and 54% respectively in indolent lymphoma.

By multivariate analysis only chemosensitivity was associated with PFS. Patients with chemoresistant disease achieved only a poor response and frequently had progressive disease.

These data suggest that the graft-versus-lymphoma effect is not sufficient to control chemoresistant disease in aggressive lymphoma. In these patients, more intensive regimens are required to achieve adequate disease control prior to transplantation.

A more recent retrospective study assessed the role of conditioning intensity on outcome among patients with lymphoma and chronic lymphocytic leukaemia given either myeloablative or non-myeloablative conditioning regimens. Forty patients in the non-myeloablative group and 51 patients in the myeloablative group had high-grade histology.

Patients with aggressive lymphoma had similar outcomes to those with indolent lymphoma—higher non-relapse mortality and mortality after myeloablative conditioning. Conversely, relapse risk was lower although, these differences were not statistically significant.

Patients without significant comorbidities had comparable PFS and OS in both groups. These patients tolerated both conditioning regimens equally well, whereas patients with comorbidity experienced a lower non-relapse mortality and a better survival after non-myeloablative conditioning.

Further reading

Greb A, Bohlius J, Schiefer D, *et al*. High-dose chemotherapy with autologous stem cell transplantation in the first line treatment of aggressive non-Hodgkin lymphoma (NHL) in adults. *Cochrane Database Syst Rev* 2008; **1**:CD004024.

Khouri IF. Reduced–intensity regimens in allogenic stem cell transplantation for non-Hodgkin lymphoma and chronic lymphocytic leukaemia. Hematology *Am Soc Hematol Educ Program* 2006; **1**:390–7.

Wrench D, Gribben JG. Stem cell transplantation for Non-Hodgkin's lymphoma. *Hematol Oncol Clin North Am* 2008; **22**(5):1051–79.

Cutaneous Non-Hodgkin lymphomas

Epidemiology

Primary cutaneous lymphomas present in the skin without evidence of extracutaneous disease at the time of diagnosis. This group of lymphomas has to be differentiated from secondary involvement of the skin by primary systemic lymphomas.

The annual incidence is 0.5–1 per 100,000 with a much higher overall prevalence because most primary cutaneous lymphomas are indolent malignancies with a long survival.

Primary cutaneous lymphomas differ considerably in their clinical course and outcome from systemic lymphomas. They are classified according to the WHO–EORTC classification (2005).

According to this classification, primary cutaneous lymphomas are generally divided into lymphomas with an indolent or an aggressive clinical course.

Approximately 75% of primary cutaneous lymphomas are T-cell lymphomas of which nearly two-thirds are mycosis fungoides (MF) and Sézary syndrome (SS).

Primary cutaneous CD30+ lymphoproliferative disorders are the second most common group of cutaneous T-cell lymphomas. This group includes primary cutaneous anaplastic large cell lymphoma and lymphomatoid papulosis. Both entities can only be differentiated by their clinical course.

The remaining group of primary cutaneous T-cell lymphomas constitutes <10% of all cases and is very heterogeneous in terms of clinicopathological features. Prognosis of this group is poor.

Primary cutaneous B-cell lymphomas are less common than primary cutaneous T-cell lymphomas and represent approximately 25% of all primary cutaneous lymphomas.

In the WHO–EORTC classification three main subtypes can be distinguished: primary cutaneous marginal zone B-cell lymphoma, primary cutaneous follicle centre B-cell lymphoma, and primary cutaneous diffuse large B-cell lymphoma, leg-type.

Clinical features

MF typically presents with erythematous patches, plaques, and tumours usually in areas not often exposed to sunlight. Most patients have multiple lesions and ulceration can occur. The lesions can be atrophic and dyspigmented. The course of the disease is indolent.

The lesions of MF can be classified into four groups: T1 and T2 with patches and plaques affecting less or more than 10% of body surface, T3 with tumours >1cm and T4 with erythroderma affecting >80% of body surface.

In T1 disease outcome is excellent and patients with T2 disease also have a median OS of more than 10 years.

Patients with erythrodermic MF have a median survival of 5 years and those with visceral involvement have an even worse survival of only 1 or 2 years.

SS is defined as an erythrodermic cutaneous T-cell lymphoma with haematological evidence of leukaemic involvement and can be preceded by MF. Sézary cells are atypical cerebriform mononuclear cells circulating in the peripheral blood. However, morphological features alone are prone to interobserver variability. Therefore, diagnosis of SS should be made primarily on the basis of objective molecular or flow cytometric evidence of a clonal abnormal T-cell population in the peripheral blood.

The clinical behaviour of the disease is aggressive.

MF and SS are classified according to the TNMB staging system.

Primary cutaneous marginal zone B-cell lymphoma and primary cutaneous follicle centre B-cell lymphoma usually show an indolent clinical behaviour.

The former presents characteristically with violaceous solitary or multiple papules or nodules located mainly on the extremities. Spontaneous resolution may occur. In some cases, association with *Borrelia burgdorferi* has been reported.

Primary cutaneous follicle centre B-cell lymphoma preferentially involves the head and trunk with solitary or grouped plaques and tumours. The presence of multiple lesions is not of prognostic importance.

In both entities, transformation into a diffuse large B-cell lymphoma is extremely rare.

Cutaneous relapses are common in both types. However, extracutaneous dissemination rarely occurs.

The 5-year survival is excellent, >95% in both entities.

In contrast, primary cutaneous diffuse large B-cell lymphoma, leg-type, behaves aggressively and affects predominantly elderly patients. This entity typically presents as red solitary or multiple nodules on the leg but can also rarely be found at other sites. Both cutaneous relapses and extracutaneous dissemination are frequent.

With a 5-year survival of only 50%, prognosis is significantly worse than in the other two entities.

Management of cutaneous T-cell lymphoma

In patients with early stages of MF, topical therapy with mechlorethamine or bexarotene, superficial radiotherapy and phototherapy (PUVA) are appropriate treatment options.

Patients with more advanced disease will require some form of systemic treatment. Total skin electron beam therapy (TSEBT) is appropriate in patients with generalized thickened plaques or tumorous disease due to its depth of penetration. The rate of complete response is >80% but the long-term outcome is not affected. TSEBT should be followed by an adjuvant therapy such as mechlorethamine or PUVA.

Patients with erythroderma are difficult to manage.

Patients without evidence of circulating peripheral cells are suitable candidates for low-dose PUVA. Initial doses must be very low to avoid phototoxic reactions.

In patients with leukaemic or nodal involvement systemic treatment usually in combination with topical therapy is required.

Extracorporal photophoresis (ECPP) can be used for patients with erythroderma and a low number of circulating cells. ECCP is usually administered every 4 weeks, but the frequency can be increased to twice monthly.

Systemic therapy with the orally administered retinoid bexarotene can achieve response rates of 50%. Bexarotene is teratogenic. Liver function and serum lipids must be carefully monitored.

MF and SS are relatively chemoresistant diseases. Methotrexate, chlorambucil, and gemcitabine are active agents. Pegylated doxorubicin achieved an overall response rate of 80% in patients with relapsed and refractory MF in one trial. Superiority of one agent has not been shown so far.

Most frequently used combination chemotherapy regimens include cyclophosphamide, vincristine, and prednisone with or without doxorubicin. There are no trials comparing single-agent chemotherapy with combination chemotherapy.

Vorinostat, a novel oral histone deacetylase inhibitor was evaluated in patients with progressive or relapsed MF/SS. An objective response was achieved in 30%. Time to progression was 148 days for all patients and was not reached for responders. Remarkably, vorinostat seems not to be cross-resistant to other agents.

High-dose chemotherapy followed by autologous stem cell transplantation in patients with advanced disease has been shown to induce high response rates in most patients but the responses were predominantly of short duration. In contrast, allogeneic transplantation seems to induce long-term durable remissions of >3 years.

Management of cutaneous B-cell lymphoma

Treatment options include local and systemic treatment modalities.

Due to their indolent course and the excellent outcome in primary cutaneous marginal zone and follicle centre B-cell lymphoma, a watch-and-wait strategy is adequate management in most cases with asymptomatic lesions.

In patients with limited symptomatic skin lesions, local excision or radiotherapy (20–36Gy) are the first choices of treatment. Both modalities result in nearly 100% CR. However, local recurrence or relapse at distant sites occurs in approximately one-half of the patients.

Cutaneous relapses can be treated in the same way as the initial lesion and do not worsen prognosis.

In patients with extensive skin lesions rituximab is the treatment of choice. Treatment schedules vary in different studies, but most patients have been treated with rituximab once weekly for 4–8 weeks.

Oral chlorambucil is a treatment option often used in Europe.

Multiagent chemotherapy is rarely indicated in these types of cutaneous lymphomas with the exception of patients developing extracutaneous disease.

Primary cutaneous diffuse large B-cell lymphoma, leg-type, should be treated like systemic diffuse large B-cell lymphomas.

Non-Hodgkin lymphoma: extranodal involvement

Epidemiology

Primary extranodal NHLs are defined as those that clinically present with a predominant extranodal tumour mass amenable to directed treatment, e.g. by radiotherapy. Regional or distant nodal involvement is common and does not exclude this diagnosis. However, in some cases, primary extranodal disease will be hard to distinguish from secondary spread of a disseminated primary nodal lymphoma.

Extranodal lymphomas occur frequently. The proportion of primary extranodal NHL is approximately 25–30%. Extranodal lymphomas can arise from almost any anatomical site of the body, even from those which normally do not contain lymphoid tissue.

The most common involved sites are the skin, stomach, brain, small intestine, and Waldeyer's ring.

Histologically, nearly 50% of all extranodal lymphomas are diffuse large B-cell lymphomas. It is the most common histological subtype in the testis, brain, bone, thyroid, and sinus.

The majority of the remaining group arise from MALT. This subtype is termed extranodal marginal-zone lymphoma of MALT-type and represents 5–10% of all NHLs. The most commonly involved sites are the stomach, small intestine, orbits, salivary glands, and the lung. Chronic antigenic stimulation from either infectious agents or autoimmune diseases plays a major role in the pathogenesis of MALT lymphoma. For gastric MALT lymphoma, chronic infection with *Helicobacter pylori* has been demonstrated as an aetiological factor. Furthermore, *Borrelia burgdorferi* and *Chlamydia psittaci* may be involved in the pathogenesis of at least a subset of cutaneous and ocular adnexal marginal-zone lymphoma. More recently, immunoproliferative small intestine disease (IPSID) was found to be associated with *Campylobacter jejuni*. Chronic inflammatory diseases such as Sjögren's syndrome in the salivary glands, myoepithelial sialadenitis (MESA), and Hashimoto's thyroiditis have also been associated with MALT lymphoma.

CNS lymphoma

Primary CNS lymphoma may involve the brain, cerebrospinal fluid, and the eyes without systemic involvement. There has been a marked increase in incidence over the last decades in both immunocompromised and immunocompetent hosts. The reason for this increase remains unclear.

Risk factors for development of this tumour are congenital and acquired immunodeficiencies such as iatrogenic immunosuppression in organ allograft recipients and infection with HIV, implicating an important role of the immune system in the pathogenesis of this lymphoma. In immunocompromised patients, EBV genomic DNA can be detected in nearly all cases. In the era of highly active antiretroviral therapy the incidence of HIV-related primary CNS lymphoma has decreased again. However, most patients with CNS lymphoma are immunocompetent. EBV seems not to play a pathogenic role in these patients.

The median age at diagnosis is 60 years in immunocompetent patients and 30 years in HIV patients. Initial symptoms are related to size and site of the tumour lesion. Primary CNS lymphoma often has a rapidly progressive course.

Systemic dissemination is rare. Early diagnosis and rapid initiation of therapy are crucial. The finding of characteristic features on CAT scan and MRI should prompt a stereotactic biopsy. Corticosteroids should be avoided before biopsy whenever possible.

Histologically, tumours are predominantly classified as diffuse large B-cell lymphomas. The growth fraction is usually high with >80% positivity for Ki-67.

Resection of the tumour provides no relevant therapeutic benefit and does not prolong survival.

With a median OS of only 12 months, whole-brain radiation alone does not result in durable tumour control and is associated with a high risk of neurotoxicity in older patients.

High-dose methotrexate with or without whole brain radiation therapy prolongs survival in primary CNS lymphoma patients (>24 months) compared with whole-brain radiation therapy alone. However, the combination of chemotherapy and radiation has been associated with delayed neurotoxicity. Methotrexate-based multiagent chemotherapy alone seems to result in similar survival rates compared with regimens that include whole-brain radiation therapy, although there are no controlled trials. The risk of neurotoxicity is lower in patients treated with chemotherapy alone.

Consequently, patients are often treated with chemotherapy alone, and radiation therapy is deferred until relapse to minimize the risk of treatment-related neurotoxicity. Salvage whole brain radiation therapy is an effective regimen for recurrent and refractory primary CNS lymphoma.

The prognosis of HIV-associated primary CNS lymphoma is generally worse and depends on the CD4+ cell count. Whereas patients with a CD4+ cell count >200/μL can achieve a long-term remission, those with a CD4+ cell count <200/μL do not respond to chemotherapy. These patients may respond to highly active antiretroviral therapy.

Bone lymphoma

In most cases, involvement of the bone is secondary in patients with advanced-stage lymphoma whereas primary bone lymphoma is rare. The presenting symptom is mainly localized bone pain. Depending on the involved site a pathological fracture or spinal cord compression can occur. To establish diagnosis an open biopsy is required. Diffuse large B-cell lymphoma is the most common histological diagnosis.

In a retrospective population-based study of 131 patients with primary bone lymphoma, 79% had diffuse large B-cell lymphoma. The median age was 63 years. OS at 5 and 10 years was 62% and 41%, respectively. Three different prognostic groups (patients <60 years, patients >60 years and IPI 0–3, and IPI 4–5) with significantly different OS at 5 years of 90%, 61%, and 25%, respectively, could be identified. Patients receiving rituximab plus CHOP had a significantly better 3-year PFS than those who received CHOP only (88% vs. 52%).

In conclusion, combined immunochemotherapy with rituximab and CHOP with or without irradiation is the mainstay of therapy in primary bone lymphoma. Radical surgery does not improve outcome.

Testicular lymphoma

Primary testicular lymphoma is a rare disease representing 1–2% of all NHLs.

The estimated annual incidence is 0.2 per 100,000. However, it is the most common malignancy of the testis in men >60 years. In most cases patients present with unilateral painless scrotal swelling.

The vast majority of these lymphomas are diffuse large B-cell lymphomas. Other histological subtypes including Burkitt's and lymphoblastic lymphoma are rare. Histological diagnosis is usually established by initial orchiectomy. In spite of providing local tumour control, orchiectomy alone is not curative.

The diagnostic work-up is the same as for other lymphomas. In approximately 80% of cases at initial presentation, stage I or II is diagnosed. Distant relapses are frequent and occur predominantly in other extranodal tissues like the CNS, the contralateral testicle, the skin, soft tissues, and lung and pleura.

In a retrospective survey by the International Extranodal Lymphoma Study Group (IELSG), prognostic factors and clinical outcome in 373 patients with primary lymphoma of the testis were analysed. The median age of patients was 66 years. Prophylactic intrathecal chemotherapy was given to 18% of patients. Although 80% of all patients had stage I or II disease, clinical outcome was significantly worse than in diffuse large B-cell lymphomas at other sites. The 5-year OS was only 48% and the survival curves did not reach a plateau. Fifty-two per cent of patients relapsed at a median follow-up of 7.6 years. The majority of relapses (72%) occurred at extranodal sites. 15% relapsed in the CNS, mainly in the brain parenchyma up to 10 years after presentation. Advanced disease at diagnosis was a risk factor for CNS relapse. Patients receiving prophylactic intrathecal chemotherapy had better PFS than without. A low IPI, no B-symptoms, the use of anthracyclines, and prophylactic contralateral scrotal radiotherapy were significantly associated with longer survival in multivariate analysis. Recurrence in the contralateral testis was common in patients without prophylactic scrotal radiotherapy. Systemic chemotherapy alone does not seem to be effective in preventing relapses in the contralateral testis because the testis is an immunological sanctuary site.

Benefit from prophylactic cranial radiation has not been clearly shown so far.

The efficacy of CNS and contralateral testicular prophylaxis in addition to combination therapy with rituximab and CHOP was analysed in a prospective single-arm trial conducted by the IELSG. In a preliminary analysis 3-year OS was 86% and 3-year PFS 77%. Recurrence in the contralateral testicle was not seen and the number of CNS relapses was slightly decreased.

Based on these data, patients with primary testicular lymphoma should be treated with 6–8 courses of R-CHOP followed by prophylactic irradiation of the contralateral testis. Although data are not convincing, prophylactic intrathecal therapy should always be considered. The efficacy of prophylactic cranial radiation has not been proven so far.

Further reading

Ekenel M. DeAngelis LM. Treatment of central nervous system lymphoma. *Curr Neurol Neurosci Rep* 2007; **7**(3):191–9.

Ferreri AJ, Reni M. Primary central nervous system lymphoma. *Crit Rev Oncol Hemato* 2007; **63**(3):257–68.

Mohile NA, Abrey LE. Primary central nervous system lymphoma. *Sem Radiat Oncol* 2007; **17**(3):223–9.

Ramadan KM, Shenkier T, Sehn LH, et al. A clinicopathological retrospective study of 131 patients with primary bone lymphoma: a population based study of successively treated cohorts from the British Columbia Cancer Agency. *Ann Oncol* 2007; **18**(1):129–35.

Vitolo U, Ferreri AJ, Zucca E. Primary testicular lymphoma. *Crit Rev Oncol Hematol* 2008; **65**(2):183–9.

Zucca E. Extranodal lymphoma: a reappraisal. *Ann Oncol* 2008; **19**(suppl. 4):iv77–80.

Non-Hodgkin lymphoma: targeted therapy

Newer monoclonal antibodies

Ofatumumab

Ofatumumab is a fully human monoclonal IgG1 antibody targeted at a distinct small loop epitope on the CD20 molecule. The complement-dependent cytotoxicity is stronger than that seen with rituximab.

There are preliminary results from phase I/II trials evaluating ofatumumab in patients with chronic lymphocytic leukaemia and refractory follicular lymphoma and a phase II trial in patients with diffuse large B-cell lymphoma is ongoing.

The safety and efficacy of ofatumumab in relapsed or refractory follicular lymphoma was investigated in a phase 1/2 trial with 40 patients. Fifteen patients had received rituximab as part of prior therapy. Ofatumumab was administered as a 4-weekly infusion in four different dose groups. Of 274 adverse events reported, 190 were related to ofatumumab. Two grade 3 infections were reported. No safety concerns or maximum tolerated dose were identified. The overall response rate ranged from 20–63%. For responders, median time to progression was 32.6 months with a median follow-up of 9.2 months. Currently there is an ongoing trial evaluating ofatumumab in rituximab-refractory patients with follicular lymphoma as well as a phase II trial of up-front chemotherapy with CHOP and ofatumumab in follicular lymphoma.

Epratuzumab

Epratuzumab is a recombinant, humanized monoclonal IgG1 antibody directed against CD22, a 135kD surface protein expressed on mature B cells. CD22 acts as an adhesion molecule and negative regulator of the B-cell receptor signalling complex. After binding of the antibody, CD 22 is endocytosed. The antitumour activity of epratuzumab seems to be mediated predominantly through antibody-dependent cellular cytotoxicity.

In a first single-centre dose-escalation study, safety and efficacy of epratuzumab were evaluated in patients with aggressive NHL. Epratuzumab was administered once weekly for 4 weeks in 56 heavily pretreated patients with diffuse large B-cell lymphoma. Epratuzumab was well tolerated and objective responses were observed in five patients including three complete responses. Median duration of OR was 26.3 weeks, and median time to progression for responders was 35 weeks.

In another multicentre, single-arm study epratuzumab was combined with rituximab in 65 pretreated patients with recurrent or refractory NHL. Epratuzumab was given weekly at 360mg/m^2 intravenously followed by infusion of 375mg/m^2 rituximab for 4 consecutive weeks. The objective response rate was 46%. CR was achieved in 24% of patients with follicular lymphoma and in 33% with diffuse large B cell lymphoma. Median duration of response was 16 months for follicular lymphoma and 6 months for diffuse large B cell lymphoma.

Results from a recent multicentre phase II trial evaluating the combination of epratuzumab and rituximab with CHOP (ER-CHOP) in untreated patients with diffuse large B-cell lymphoma were presented at ASCO in 2008. 107 patients received epratuzumab 360mg/m^2 plus rituximab 375mg/m^2, and CHOP every 3 weeks for 6 cycles. 68% of 104 evaluable patients developed grade 4 neutropenia and grade 3/4 febrile neutropenia was observed in 17%.

The overall response rate was 94% in 34 evaluable patients including 16 complete and 13 partial remissions. EFS at 12 months was 85%.

Further randomized phase III trials are warranted to assess the additional efficacy of epratuzumab in combination with rituximab.

Radioimmunotherapy

RIT is an innovative treatment modality that combines the tumour cell targeting ability of monoclonal antibodies with the cytotoxic effect of radiation by linking a radioisotope to the antibody. Thus, the antibody has its own cytotoxic effect mediated by ADCC and CDCC and similarly functions as a vehicle that carries the radioisotope to the tumour cell. This results in the delivery of radiation directly to the tumour cell. Adjacent tumour cells that did not bind directly to the anti-body can also be destroyed due to the cross-fire effect. B-cell lymphoma cells are especially suitable for RIT because of the abundant and fairly homogeneous expression of CD20 antigen on its surface and its marked radiosensitivity.

Two anti-CD20 RIT agents have been approved by the Food and Drug Administration: ^{90}Y-ibritumomab tiuxetan and ^{131}I tositumomab. The latter is not approved in Europe.

^{90}Y-ibritumomab tiuxetan was the first anti-B-cell radiolabelled antibody approved by the FDA in 2002. ^{90}Yttrium is a pure β emitter and dosing is based solely on body weight. β particles have a range of up to 5mm which is important for the so called cross-fire effect. An initial 'cold' (unlabelled) antibody dose clears the body of normal B-cells so that subsequent doses will be more focused on lymphoma cells. The main toxicity is haematological.

Radiation exposure for medical staff is negligible and treatment can be given on an outpatient basis.

There is a large number of trials evaluating RIT in follicular lymphoma in untreated and relapsed disease.

In a phase III study, RIT with ^{90}Y-ibritumomab tiuxetan was compared with four doses of rituximab weekly in 143 patients with relapsed or refractory follicular or transformed lymphoma. The overall response rate was 80% for RIT compared with 56% for rituximab. A complete response was achieved in 30% and 16%, respectively. Median duration of response was 14.2 months in the ^{90}Y-ibritumomab tiuxetan group versus 12.1 months and time to progression was 11.2 versus 10.1 months. Sixty-four per cent of patients treated with RIT had durable responses of >6 months compared with 47% in the rituximab group.

Kaminski et al. conducted a trial evaluating the efficacy of a single dose of ^{131}I tositumomab in 76 patients with previously untreated good risk follicular lymphoma. The overall response rate was 95%, and 75% achieved a complete response. Median PFS was 6.1 years after a median follow-up of 5.1 years. Haematological toxicity was moderate.

In a phase II trial, 6 cycles of CHOP followed by ^{131}I tositumomab were evaluated in 90 patients with previously untreated, advanced stage follicular lymphoma. The overall response rate was 90%. CR rate after induction treatment with CHOP was only 39% but improved after RIT to 69%. The estimated 2-year PFS was 81% and the 2-year OS 97% at a median follow-up of 2.3 years.

These encouraging results were confirmed in a more recent trial using ^{90}Y-ibritumomab tiuxetan following 6 cycles of fludarabine and mitoxantrone. The estimated 3-year PFS was 76% and the 3-year OS was 100% at a median follow-up of 30 months. Sixty-three per cent of patients had grade 3/4 haematological toxicity.

In diffuse large B-cell lymphoma, Zinzani et al. (2008) conducted a small phase II trial with 20 patients evaluating CHOP plus RIT in untreated elderly patients. ^{90}Y-ibritumomab tiuxetan was given 6–10 weeks after induction treatment. Ninety-five per cent of patients achieved a CR and the estimated 2-year PFS was 75% at a median follow-up of 15 months.

In conclusion, RIT is a highly effective treatment option in untreated and relapsed follicular lymphoma. The treatment is generally well tolerated and produces a high rate of durable remissions.

However, so far there are no data from trials evaluating the efficacy of RIT following rituximab-containing regimens. Furthermore, there are no randomized trials comparing RIT with rituximab-containing chemotherapy salvage regimens in relapsed patients. Therefore, results from ongoing phase III trials are of outstanding interest to demonstrate a substantial benefit in PFS and OS with radio-immunotherapy compared with conventional therapy and 'cold' rituximab.

The role of RIT in aggressive B-cell lymphoma is not yet established.

Bortezomib

Bortezomib is a proteasome inhibitor. The proteasome pathway plays a critical role in the degradation of cellular proteins. By binding to the proteasome's active binding site, bortezomib inhibits the degradation of proteins involved in apoptosis and cell survival. This results in inhibition of cell cycle progression and induction of apoptosis. In mantle cell lymphoma, bortezomib has shown response rates of 30–40% in heavily pretreated patients. Peripheral neuropathy and thrombocytopenia are the main toxicities.

Lenalidomide

Lenalidomide is a derivative of thalidomide. Both are immunomodulatory drugs and inhibit angiogenesis, reduce TNF-alpha production and T-cell activity thereby promoting apoptosis of tumour cells. Lenalidomide has shown modest activity in follicular, T-cell and diffuse large B-cell lymphoma in small phase II trials. In pretreated patients, objective response rates were observed in 25–30%.

Further reading

Kaminsky MS, Tuck M, Estes J, et al. ^{131}I-tositumomab therapy as initial treatment for follicular lymphoma. N Engl J Med 2005; **352**:441–9.

Leonard JP, Martin P, Barrientos J, et al. Targeted treatment and new agents in diffuse large B-cell lymphoma. Semin Hematol 2008; **45**(3 Suppl 2):S11–16.

Sharkey RM, Press OW, Goldenberg DM. Re-examination of radio-immunotherapy in the treatment of non-Hodgkin's lymphoma: prospects for dual targeted antibody/radioantibody therapy. Blood 2009; **113**(17):3891–5.

Sikder MA, Friedberg JW. Beyond rituximab: the future of monoclonal antibodies in B-cell non-Hodgkin lymphoma. Curr Oncol Rep 2008; **10**(5):420–6.

Zinzani PL, Tani M, Fanti S, et al. A phase II trial of CHOP chemotherapy followed by yttrium 90 ibritumomab tiuxetan (Zevalin) for previously untreated elderly diffuse large B-cell lymphoma patients. Ann Oncol 2008; **19**(4):769–73.

Internet resources

European Society for Medical Oncology: http://www.esmo.org

National Comprehensive Cancer Network: http://www.nccn.org

Adult acute lymphoblastic leukaemia

Acute lymphoblastic leukaemia (ALL) is a malignant neoplasm of the lymphocyte precursor, characterized by aberrations in proliferation and differentiation of leukaemic lymphoblasts leading to failure of the normal immune response and decreased production of normal haematopoiesis.

Epidemiology and aetiology
ALL represents <1% of adult cancers, but 25% of all childhood cancers. In adults, the incidence increases with age, being 5 per million in those aged 25–50 and 12 per million in those aged >60 years. ALL occurs slightly more frequently in males than in females.

Although a small percentage of cases are associated with inherited genetic syndromes, and many environmental factors (ionizing radiation, chemicals, electromagnetic fields, viruses) have been investigated as potential risk factors, the cause remains largely unknown.

Clinical features
Initial signs and symptoms reflect bone marrow infiltration and extramedullary disease. Signs of bone marrow failure include anaemia, neutropenia, and thrombocytopenia, clinically responsible for fatigue and pallor, fever, and petechiae, easy bruising, and bleeding. Other signs include weight loss, bone pain, and symptoms due to CNS or other extramedullary infiltration. A mediastinal mass is present in about half of T-cell ALL cases.

Laboratory studies
Peripheral blood
The white blood cell (WBC) count may be abnormally low, within the normal range, or abnormally high. Haemoglobin level and platelet count are generally low and patients may require transfusions.

Bone marrow
A complete morphological and immunological examination of the bone marrow is required to establish the diagnosis of ALL. The French–American–British (FAB) classification, which recognized three subtypes of ALL—L1 (30%), L2 (60%), L3 (10%)—was strictly based on morphology and cytochemistry, whereas the current WHO classification also incorporates immunophenotyping and cytogenetics.

Immunophenotyping
The majority of ALL cases (75%) have phenotypes that correspond to those of B-cell progenitors (CD19, CD22, CD79). Additional subclassification within B-lineage into pro-B ALL, common ALL, pre-B, or mature B is made according to the expression of CD10, cytoplasmic immunoglobulin (Ig) μ heavy-chain proteins, surface or cytoplasmic Igκ or Igλ.

T-cell ALL (25%) is identified by the expression of T-associated surface antigens (CD3, CD7, CD5, or CD2). T-ALL subtypes comprise early T-ALL, thymic (cortical T-ALL CD1a$^+$) and mature T-ALL. ALL blasts coexpress myeloid markers in 15–50% of adults.

Flow cytometry allows the identification of an immunophenotype specific to the leukaemic blasts. This can be used in tandem with molecular techniques for monitoring the level of minimal residual disease (MRD) which correlates with outcome.

Cytogenetic and molecular biology
Genetic alterations are identified in >65% of cases. In addition to standard cytogenetic analysis, molecular techniques (RT-PCR, Southern blot) and FISH can identify translocations that are not detected by routine analysis of the karyotype.

Important genetic alterations in B-lineage ALL include t(9;22) and/or BCR-ABL (30–35%), t(1;19) and/or E2A-PBX1 (3–4%), t(12;21) and/or TEL-AML1 (1–3%), a variety of MLL gene rearrangements: t(4;11) and/or MLL-AF4 (3–4%), or 11q23 aberrations (<5%), and hyperdiploidy defined as >50 and <67 chromosomes or a DNA index of 1.16 or higher.

In T-ALL, elevated expression of HOX11, HOX11L2, SIL-TAL1, and CALM-AF10 is associated with different subtypes. HOX11L2 and SIL-TAL1 + T-ALL have poorer outcomes than thymic T-ALL overexpressing HOX11. Notch1 activating mutations are identified in up to 50% of T-ALL and may be targeted by γ-secretase inhibitors. NUP214–ABL1 aberration is detected in 4% of T-ALL cases and may be targeted by imatinib therapy.

Risk classification
Clinical features (age >50 years, WBC >30G/L in B-lineage), immunophenotyping (pro-B, early-T, mature-T), cytogenetics and molecular biology (t(9;22)/BCR-ABL, t(4;11)/MLL-AF4), and response to treatment (late achievement of response, MRD positivity) have prognostic importance and are used by most study groups in the definition of ALL risk groups: standard risk for those without any risk factors and high risk for those with one or more risk factors. Philadelphia chromosome positive (Ph +) ALL (t(9;22)/BCR-ABL) are allocated to a separate high-risk group since they are eligible for treatment including tyrosine kinase inhibitors.

Treatment
Most of the therapeutic advances in adult ALL have arisen from successful adaptation of ALL treatment strategies in children. However, the current treatments lead to only 30–40% long-term survivors in adult ALL.

Induction chemotherapy
Induction chemotherapy should contain at least vincristine, daunorubicin, prednisone/dexamethasone, and asparaginase. Some groups also administer to all patients or specific subgroups cyclophosphamide, cytarabine, methotrexate, and/or mercaptopurine. Induction therapy can be preceded by a prephase with corticosteroids in order to detect poor responders and to avoid acute tumour lysis syndrome. Intensive combination therapy has resulted in CR proportions of 80–90%. Whereas a limit for intensification of myelotoxic drugs seems to have been reached, intensification with non-myelotoxic drugs (such as vincristine, steroids, or asparaginase) is still possible. Dexamethasone has replaced prednisone for better antileukaemic activity and achievement of higher levels in the cerebrospinal fluid (CSF). In B-precursor ALL, higher doses of anthracyclines may be associated with improved results. Results of T-ALL have improved with the combination of cytarabine and cyclophosphamide added to the conventional drugs. Supportive care is of increasing importance during induction, including the concomitant application of

haematopoietic growth factors throughout chemotherapy. CR is currently morphologically defined as a reduction of blast cells to <5% together with return of marrow cellularity and function to normal levels and the disappearance of all extramedullary manifestations. In the future, an increase of molecular CR rates may be the most important measure for efficacy of induction. Molecular remission may be defined as a level of MRD below the detection limit of clone-specific PCR, which is generally 10^{-4}.

Consolidation chemotherapy
Consolidation therapy is administered after achievement of CR. Consolidation chemotherapy cycles in large studies are very variable. The type, duration, and intensity of consolidation may be adapted to the initial features, the response to prephase, the remission status, and/or level of MRD at the end of induction therapy. Several studies have demonstrated that late modified reinduction improves outcome. In general, it seems that intensive application of high-dose methotrexate is beneficial. There is also an important role for dose intensification of asparaginase. The role of high-dose anthracyclines, podophyllotoxins, and high-dose cytarabine is more questionable. Stricter adherence to protocols with fewer delays, dose reductions, or omission of drugs may be important factors for therapeutic improvement.

Central nervous system treatment
The diagnosis of CNS ALL requires the presence of more than five leukocytes per microlitre in the CSF and the identification of lymphoblasts in the CSF differential cell count. False-negative CSF results may occur in patients with predominantly cranial nerve involvement. Effective CNS prophylaxis not only reduces the risk of isolated CNS relapse but also improves general outcome. CNS prophylaxis includes intrathecal (IT) chemotherapy (methotrexate, cytarabine, steroids), high-dose systemic chemotherapy (methotrexate, cytarabine, asparaginase), and craniospinal irradiation. The use of IT liposomal cytarabine may reduce the number of IT injections and improve efficacy.

Maintenance chemotherapy
After consolidation, maintenance therapy given over 1.5–2 years is still standard in ALL. Omission of maintenance therapy has been associated with shorter DFS rates. Daily doses of mercaptopurine and weekly doses of methotrexate are the backbone of maintenance, and are eventually combined with monthly pulses of vincristine and corticosteroids. No clear advantage has been demonstrated with intensified versus conventional maintenance doses. Patients with mature B-ALL do not require maintenance. In T-ALL, the benefit of maintenance chemotherapy has been questioned.

Allogeneic stem cell transplantation
A myeloablative conditioning regimen followed by rescue with infusion of HLA-matched haematopoietic stem cells is generally used in Ph+ ALL and non-Ph+ high risk ALL. A recent meta-analysis concluded that allogeneic stem cell transplantation (SCT) in first CR is recommended in high-risk but not in standard-risk ALL. The survival rate with matched related allogeneic SCT in first CR is about 50% (range, 20–80%). In large prospective trials, results are similar between allogeneic related SCT and allogeneic matched unrelated (MUD) SCT, with however, higher relapse rates for sibling and higher mortality for MUD SCT. In second CR, the outcome of SCT is superior to that of

chemotherapy. Intensity of therapy before SCT, conditioning regimens, and immunosuppressive therapy after SCT may influence outcomes.

Autologous stem cell transplantation
Autologous SCT is inferior to allogeneic SCT. No significant difference has been detected in several randomized studies between autologous SCT and chemotherapy. Autologous SCT may be of interest in patients with low MRD after induction and/or consolidation, MRD negative stem cell graft and the option to give MRD-based maintenance after autologous SCT.

New therapeutic agents
Advances in the understanding of molecular mechanisms of disease, and the successful model of imatinib in Ph$^+$ disease, have led to the development of several new therapeutic approaches in ALL.

Therapy with monoclonal antibodies is an attractive treatment approach in ALL. Its use may be most promising in the setting of MRD. The anti-CD20 antibody (rituximab) has been successfully integrated into therapy of mature B-ALL. It is also currently being explored in B-precursor ALL and Ph$^+$ ALL. Studies integrating anti-CD52 (alemtuzumab) are also ongoing.

A number of other novel agents are being investigated in relapsed or refractory disease states and include new nucleoside analogues (clofarabine, nelarabine), liposomal agents (liposomal vincristine), or hypomethylating agents (decitabine).

Subset specific approaches

Philadelphia chromosome-positive ALL
New molecular therapeutic strategies with imatinib and other new kinase inhibitors (dasatinib, nilotinib) have led to considerable improvement in the treatment of this unfavourable subgroup. The efficacy of imatinib has been explored with 400–800mg/day as front-line therapy combined with chemotherapy, given either simultaneously or as an alternating regimen. Efficacy analyses based on BCR-ABL transcript levels showed a clear advantage of the simultaneous over the alternating schedule. Adding imatinib to consolidation chemotherapy may increase the proportion of PCR negativity and decrease the relapse rate prior to SCT. A higher proportion of patients can proceed to SCT in first remission. The DFS after transplant at 3 years was 75–80%. These results suggest that imatinib interim therapy might thereby improve the curative potential of SCT in Ph + ALL. Postallogeneic SCT maintenance strategies are also being explored. Imatinib has been used as a treatment for MRD after transplantation in order to abort relapse. New strategies using new tyrosine kinase inhibitors are being developed to overcome resistance to imatinib.

Burkitt's ALL
Outcome with conventional ALL therapy for mature B-ALL was poor, with long-term DFS of <10%. Mature B-ALL is now generally treated in separate studies with short intensive cycles. Hyperfractionation of cyclophosphamide, and use of different non-cross-resistant agents together, formed the basis of many dose-intensive programmes. Intensive early prophylactic IT therapy, in addition to intensive systemic methotrexate and cytarabine, significantly reduced the rate of CNS recurrence. CR is now achieved in about 90% of patients and 2-year DFS rates have increased to 60–80%. Disease recurrence is rare

after the first year in remission. Recent integration of anti-CD20 before each chemotherapy cycle appears very promising with 70–80% OS in preliminary analyses.

ALL in adolescents

Comparisons demonstrate that adolescents with ALL significantly benefit from paediatric rather than adult chemotherapy regimens. Differences in drugs and dose intensity of many chemotherapeutic agents (such as asparaginase, vincristine, corticosteroids, and methotrexate) may explain the superior results with paediatric regimens. Although no major differences were demonstrated in terms of achievement of CR, CR is more rapidly obtained with paediatric regimens. These results have led to new paediatric-inspired therapeutic approaches that might also improve the efficacy of CNS leukaemia prophylaxis.

ALL in the elderly

Increasing age is the most adverse factor for CR rate and is also associated with shorter remissions. The remission rate ranges from 30–70%. The OS at 3 years was estimated to be only 7–19% in patients aged 60 years and older. Older patients with ALL have often been excluded from clinical trials by eligibility criteria. Very few clinical trials have focused on therapies designed specifically for older patients, and fewer still have sufficient numbers to deal with the clinical and biological heterogeneity within this age group.

Salvage therapy

The outcome of salvage therapy remains unsatisfactory. CR rates range from 10–50% and long-term DFS is poor. Regimens are divided into combinations of vincristine, steroids, and anthracyclines, combinations of asparaginase and methotrexate, programmes that integrate high-dose cytarabine, incorporation of new therapeutic agents, and SCT.

Although SCT is superior to chemotherapy with long-term DFS rates of 20–40% in salvage therapy, only 30–40% of patients who achieved a second CR were eligible for SCT and <50% had enough time before disease recurrence to undergo SCT.

Further reading

Faderl S, Jeha S, Kantarjian HM. The biology and treatment of adult acute lymphoblastic leukemia. Cancer 2003; 98:1337–54.

Fenaux P, Bourhis JH, Ribrag V. Burkitt's acute lymphocytic leukemia (L3ALL) in adults. Hematol Oncol Clin North Am 2001; 15:37–50.

Garcia-Manero G, Thomas DA. Salvage therapy for refractory or relapsed acute lymphocytic leukemia. Hematol Oncol Clin North Am 2001; 15:163–205.

Gokbuget N, Hoelzer D. Treatment of adult acute lymphoblastic leukemia. Hematology 2006; 1:133–41.

Gokbuget N, Hoelzer D. Rituximab in the treatment of adult ALL. Ann Hematol 2006; 85:117–19.

Harris NL, Jaffe ES, Diebold J, et al. World Health Organization classification of neoplastic diseases of the hematopoietic and lymphoid tissues: report of the Clinical Advisory Committee Meeting – Airlie House, Virginia, November 1997. J Clin Oncol 1999; 17:3835–49.

Larson RA. Acute lymphoblastic leukemia: older patients and newer drugs. Hematology 2005; 1:131–6.

Sallan SE. Acute lymphoblastic leukemia in adults and children. Myths and lessons from the adult/pediatric interface in acute lymphoblastic leukemia. Hematology 2006; 1:128–32.

Thomas X, Dombret H. Treatment of Philadelphia chromosome-positive adult acute lymphoblastic leukemia. Leuk Lymphoma 2008; 23:1–9.

Yanada M, Matsuo K, Suzuki T, et al. Allogeneic hematopoietic stem cell transplantation as part of postremission therapy improves survival for adult patients with high-risk acute lymphoblastic leukemia. A meta-analysis. Cancer 2006; 106:2657–63.

Adult acute myeloid leukaemia

Acute myeloid leukaemia (AML) is a malignancy that is characterized by infiltration of bone marrow by abnormal haematopoietic progenitors that disrupt normal production of erythroid, myeloid, and/or megakaryocytic cell lines.

Epidemiology and aetiology

AML is diagnosed in people of all ages. The risk increases about 10-fold from age 30 (10 cases per million population) to age 70 (100 cases per million population). Sex distribution (male:female) is approximately 1:1 in patients <60 years, but 2:1 in those ≥60 years. Although the cause of AML in most patients is unknown, several factors are associated with its development: exposure to toxic chemicals (benzene, toluene), prior treatment with antineoplastic cytotoxic agents (alkylating agents, podophyllotoxin derivatives or other inhibitors of DNA topoisomerase II activity), exposure to radiation, and inherited disorders (Fanconi's anaemia) or genetic abnormalities, such as Down's syndrome. This suggests that these factors trigger a malignant transformation through the action of different oncogenes.

Clinical features

Clinical features comprise those caused by a deficiency of normal functioning cells and those due to the proliferation of the leukaemic cell population. Haematological symptoms include anaemia (fatigue), thrombocytopenia (haemorrhage), neutropaenia (infection, fever). Infiltrative disease may include adenopathies, hepatomegaly, splenomegaly, skin or CNS involvement. High WBC count (>100G/L) may be associated with hyperviscosity, intracerebral and/or pulmonary leukostasis, or haemorrhage. This is a poor prognostic factor for early death. Although there are no studies proving an advantage of leukapheresis, this procedure should be carefully considered in those patients.

Older patients may present with myelodysplasia (MDS), an indolent disorder characterized by progressive cytopaenias, which may last for several months or even years before converting into AML.

Laboratory studies

Peripheral blood

The WBC count may be abnormally low, within the normal range, or abnormally high. Haemoglobin level and platelet count are generally low and patients may require transfusions.

Bone marrow

A complete morphological and immunological examination of the bone marrow is required to establish the diagnosis of AML. The FAB classification recognized eight subtypes of AML—M0 minimal myeloid differentiation (3%), M1 poorly differentiated myeloblasts (15–20%); M2 myeloblastic with differentiation (25–30%); M3 promyelocytic (5–10%); M4 myelo-monoblastic (20%); M5 monoblastic (2–9%); M6 erythroblastic (3–5%); M7 megakaryoblastic (3–12%)—strictly based on morphology and cytochemistry (most AML cells have positive reactions to myeloperoxidase and Sudan black stains; esterase stains can differentiate myeloid from monocytic leukaemia; periodic acid–Schiff positivity indicates acute biphenotypic leukaemia or undifferentiated leukaemia with lymphoblastic features). The current WHO classification, that also incorporates cytogenetics, has classified AML into the following groups:
- AML with recurrent cytogenetic abnormalities
- AML with multilineage dysplasia
- AML and MDS, therapy related
- AML not otherwise categorized

Trephine biopsy of bone marrow for histology analysis is not routinely performed, but may be useful in the presence of failure of marrow aspiration.

Immunophenotyping

Myeloid markers include CD13, CD14, CD15, and CD33, with >90% of leukaemia cells demonstrating positivity to some of these antigens. CD34 is also frequently found in AML blasts and is a marker of poor prognosis.

Cytogenetics and molecular biology

Cytogenetic abnormalities are found in >85% of patients by classical cytogenetic and/or molecular analyses (Table 4.10.9).

Table 4.10.9 Cytogenetic abnormalities and associated molecular changes

FAB	Cytogenetics	Molecular biology
M0	t(3;21)(q26;q22) and t(3;3)	EVI1
M2	t(8;21)(q22;q22) t(6;9)(p23;q34)	AML1-ETO DEK-CAN
M3	t(15;17)(q22;q11)	PML-RARα
M4	t(11;V)(q23;V), inv(3q26) and t(3;3)	MLL, DEK-CAN, EVI1
M4Eo	inv(16)(p13;q22) and t(16;16) (p13;q22)	CBFβ-MYH11
M5	t(11;V)(q23;v) t(8;16)	MLL/various
M6	inv(3)(q21;q26) t(3;3)(q21;q26)	MDS1 (EVI1; EAP)
M7	t(1;22)	Unknown

Prognostic factors

Cytogenetic abnormalities at presentation are the most important prognostic factor. Conventional cytogenetic analysis is not always informative. In cases of normal or failed cytogenetic examination, FISH is recommended to detect abnormality such as an MLL fusion transcript. Three cytogenetic groups can be distinguished:
- A favourable group with core binding factor (CBF) leukaemias [inv(16), t(16;16), or t(8;21)], and t(15;17). This group represents at most 10% of patients and involves mainly patients <60 years of age.
- An unfavourable group with monosomies or partial deletions of chromosome 5 and/or 7, or with abnormalities involving ≥3 chromosomes (complex abnormalities. This group constitutes about 30–40% of all patients, on average older (>50–60 years) often with an antecedent haematological disorder or AML related to therapy.

• The remaining 50–60% of patients fall into a group whose prognosis is intermediate.

Research in defining prognostic factors has moved to an examination of molecular markers, beginning with the P-glycoprotein transmembrane transporter proteins, which are the product of the multidrug resistance gene (MDR-1). Most of the studies attempting to overcome MDR-1 have been negative. Unfavourable prognosis is associated with overexpression of specific genes including: the Wilms tumour gene, WT1; the genes for the apoptosis regulators B-cell lymphoma protein, BCL2, and BCL2-associated X protein, BAX; the brain and acute leukaemia cytoplasmic gene, BAALC; the ectropic viral integration site 1 gene, EVI1; the FMS-like tyrosine kinase type 3 gene, FLT3 (especially in the form of internal tandem duplication (ITD); and KIT, ERG, and the mixed-limeage leukaemia gene, MLL. Some mutations confer a more favourable prognosis; most notably, mutations in the gene for CCAAT enhancer binding protein-α (C/EBP-α), CEBPA, and nucleophosmin, NPM1. These prognostic determinants have been particularly important for patients with AML and a normal karyotype, identifying within this group two genotypes, NPM1$^+$ FLT3-ITD$^-$ and CEBPA$^+$ FLT3-ITD$^-$, which are associated with a favourable risk profile, comparable with that of CBF AML. Within the group of patients with CBF leukaemia, a c-Kit mutation identifies a subgroup at high risk of relapse.

Treatment

Rates of therapy-induced mortality increase with increasing age, abnormal organ function, and poor PS. An ambulatory (performance status <3) adult aged <50 years would be expected to have an induction mortality rate of <5–10%. This rate might be 10–20% at age 60 years, 20% at age 70–79 years, and 30–40% at age 80 years and above.

Induction chemotherapy

All induction chemotherapeutic regimens use some combination of an anthracycline (daunorubicin, idarubicin) or mitoxantrone, in conjunction with cytarabine. Typically the anthracycline (daunorubicin at 45–60mg/m²/day) is given for 3 days, whereas cytarabine is given at 100–200mg/m² daily for 7 days by constant infusion. With this regimen, the CR rate for younger adults (≤55–60 years) is 60–80% and the OS rate is approximately 30%. Among older adults (>55–60 years), the CR rate is 40–55%, but there are only 10–15% long-term survivors. Numerous randomized trials have attempted to identify which anthracycline should be combined with cytarabine. The general consensus favours idarubicin, which is generally administered at a dose of 12mg/m² daily for 3 days. Additional drugs may include etoposide, and mercaptopurine. The value of high-dose cytarabine is currently being tested in induction for younger adults. Other strategies to improve the CR rate include combination of fludarabine with cytarabine, sequential therapy followed by high doses of cytarabine, timed sequential chemotherapy, or the addition of growth factors for either haematological support or priming to recruit leukaemia cells into the cell cycle to render them more susceptible to cytotoxic chemotherapy.

Supportive care during remission induction treatment should routinely include red blood cell and platelet transfusions when appropriate, prophylactic oral antibiotics, and empirical broad-spectrum antimicrobial therapy for febrile neutropenic patients.

CR is characterized by a percentage of bone marrow blast cells <5%, calculated on at least 200 nucleated cells in an aspirate sample with marrow spicules, absence of cells with Auer rods, and resolution of peripheral blood cytopenia.

It has been shown that failure to achieve an early response (clearance of blasts to a percentage lower than 10–15% in bone marrow at day 14–16) has an important prognostic value. A second course of induction therapy can be recommended in those patients with persistent leukaemia at early assessment.

Consolidation chemotherapy

Consolidation therapy is administered after achievement of CR. Consolidation chemotherapy may comprise the same drugs used for induction therapy or non-cross resistant drugs. Increasing the intensity of postremission therapy is beneficial in younger adults, but not in older adults. Usually consolidation chemotherapy combines cytarabine at different dosages with other drugs. However, there is no clear advantage with use of one regimen compared to others. The effect of cytarabine dose intensity has been investigated. The advantage associated with more intensive doses of cytarabine (3g/m² x 6 doses) was found to be significant for patients with CBF leukaemia, high-dose cytarabine. For patients with CBF leukaemia, high-dose cytarabine for 3 or 4 courses may provide the highest likelihood of cure. Patients eligible for transplant should receive a shorter consolidation.

The role of post-consolidation maintenance therapy is not clearly defined. Despite several favourable effects on DFS with several schedules of maintenance therapy, there is not enough evidence to support a recommendation.

Allogeneic stem cell transplantation

Considerable progress has occurred in the area of allogeneic SCT, making this option available to a greater number of patients with AML.

Indications for standard allogeneic SCT (Table 4.10.10)

There is a marked diversity in the risk of relapse according to the (cyto)genetic profile. The low rate of relapse following allogeneic SCT has been confirmed in all donor/no donor comparisons but has not translated into a consistent survival advantage. Therefore allogeneic SCT from an HLA-matched family donor represents the best option for prevention of relapse in patients with unfavourable or intermediate AML (except NPM1$^+$ or CEBPA$^+$ and FLT3-ITD$^-$). Age limits have also commonly been part of eligibility criteria for standard allogeneic SCT.

Outcome of allografts beyond first remission is inferior to that in first remission, owing to an increase in both treatment-related mortality (25–35%) and relapse (40–45%).

Table 4.10.10 Indications for standard allogeneic SCT in AML

Prognostic subgroup	First CR	Further CR
Favourable-risk AML		
APL	No	Yes*
CBF	No	Yes*
Intermediate-risk AML	Yes	Yes*
Poor-risk AML	Yes*	Yes*

* Matched family donor or matched unrelated donor

Reduced-intensity conditioning

Despite its wide use, to date there have been no prospective comparative studies. The most important reason for reduced-intensity conditioning is age or significant comorbidity. Reduced-intensity conditioning is a feasible option, but how feasible and how important this is in the management of AML still needs to be established. The best data have come from a multicentre study in the US and Europe, referred as the Consortium Study. The immunosuppression regimen involved minimally toxic total body irradiation of 2Gy, most often with fludarabine before, and a combination of cyclosporine and mycophenolate mofetil after, allogeneic SCT. The regimen was used for both related- and unrelated-donor transplantations. The postgrafting immunosuppression both enhanced engraftment and mitigated serious graft-versus-host disease (GVHD). Serial analyses for chimerism were performed on days 28, 56, 84, 180, and 360 after SCT. The OS rate at 2 years was 48%, and patients receiving SCT during first CR had 2-year OS rates of 44% (related SCT) and 63% (unrelated SCT). Cumulative incidences of acute GVHD (grades 2–4) were 35% at 180 days after related SCT and 42% after unrelated SCT. The probability of chronic GVHD was 36% at 2 years. Engraftment is generally prompt as indicated by the percentages of donor chimerism during the first 180 days after transplantation.

Alternative-donor transplantation

Few matched unrelated donor (MUD) transplantations take place during first CR in AML patients with unfavourable cytogenetics. Patients who did not have a sibling are assigned to MUD, if a donor is available. The risk of GVHD, graft failure, and mortality increases progressively with the number of HLA disparities, emphasizing the importance of high-resolution HLA typing and the selection of donors with preferably no more than one mismatched allele out of 10.

T-cell depleted allogeneic SCT from a haplotype mismatched relative emerges as a viable alternative option for AML patients without matched donors and/or those who urgently need transplantation, especially when the donor shows alloreactivity of natural killer cells towards the recipient.

Cord blood has now become established as a suitable source for haematopoietic transplantation. Even two HLA disparities between donor and recipient can be tolerated for a cord blood transplant. Promising results in terms of reduction of transplant-related mortality have been reported in adults given two different cord blood units. Compared to MUD transplants, several advantages exist: the immaturity of the immune system allowing a less restrictive HLA-compatibility requirement, a shorter time for transplant, the absence of any risk for donors.

Autologous stem cell transplantation

Data about superiority of autologous SCT in first CR over standard dose consolidation are controversial. Autologous SCT has been shown to improve EFS without any effect on OS, compared with consolidation chemotherapy. Five-year OS rates of 45% in high-risk and 64% in favourable-risk patients have been observed. A significant reduction in relapse incidence has been reported in favourable- and intermediate-risk AML. Stem cell harvest is usually performed after the last consolidation chemotherapy cycle. The collection of stem cells is potentially contaminated by clonogenic leukaemia cells surviving previous cytotoxic therapies, so that the efficacy of the treatment is strongly dependent on good *in vivo* purging with chemotherapy. Autologous SCT should be done within a period not exceeding 6 months from first CR. Different non-randomized trials have provided evidence in favour of a reduced relapse rate when *ex vivo* purging with mafosfamide is employed. No evidence supports maintenance chemotherapy after autologous SCT performed in patients with a first CR. Vaccination with high density dendritic cells generated from autologous leukaemic blasts in combination with interleukin-2 administration might elicit anti-leukaemia T cell responses and represents a promising approach in consolidation therapy of patients treated with autologous SCT.

New and targeted therapies

Several novel agents have emerged recently for therapy for AML. Among these are drugs that specifically bind to the surface of the AML blasts such as Mylotarg ® (gemtuzumab ozogamicin). Agents have been designed to inhibit the multidrug-resistant (MDR) protein (PSC-833, Zosuquidar), the enzyme farnesyl transferase (Tipifarnib®), *FLT3* (PKC-412, CEP-701, MLN518, SU11248) and other tyrosine kinases, the processes of angiogenesis (anti-vascular endothelial growth factors: SU5416), apoptosis (BCL-2 antisense oligonucleotide) and methylation (histone deacetylases: decitabine, 5-azacytidine). Cloretazine is a novel sulfonylhydrazine alkylating agent which has recently been reported to be associated with significant efficacy in AML. Lastly, new nucleoside analogues (clofarabine, troxacitabine) have shown activity in AML. The development of these agents, coupled with new insights into the molecular pathogenesis of the disease offers hope for significant progress in the treatment of AML.

Subset specific approaches

Acute promyelocytic leukaemia

Several developments over the past 30 years have made acute promyelocytic leukaemia (APL) the most curable of all types of AML. APL is more frequent in the Mediterranean countries. Chromosome aberrations other than t(15;17), CD56 expression, or short PML/RARα isoform are adverse prognostic factors. A stratification system has been developed that distinguishes low-risk patients with a WBC count <10G/L and platelets >40G/L, high-risk patients with WBC count >10G/L, whereas others are at intermediate risk.

A sizable fraction of patients develop fatal haemorrhages during the diagnostic evaluation. The disease should therefore be managed as a medical emergency, starting supportive measures (frozen plasma, fibrinogen, platelet support) and all-trans retinoic acid (ATRA) therapy to reverse the ongoing coagulopathy. Addition of ATRA to chemotherapy is of clear benefit and represents the current standard approach for newly diagnosed APL. ATRA should be used together with anthracyclines during induction and, probably, during post-remission therapy. Anthracyclines are so effective in APL that there is probably no reason to administer cytarabine. Idarubicin has shown a slight survival advantage when compared with daunorubicin. The ATRA syndrome (25% of patients) is the major toxicity of ATRA and is characterized by fever and leakage of fluid into the extravascular space producing fluid retention, dyspnoea, effusions, and hypotension. It is treated effectively with high doses of methylprednisolone or dexamethasone. Development of a PCR test to detect the characteristic t(15;17) provides a sensitive and highly specific means to detect relapse. The achievement of molecular remission rates of 90–99% in patients receiving at least 2 further cycles of anthracycline-based chemotherapy after induction has led to the adoption of this strategy as the standard for consolidation. Randomized studies have shown a benefit from administering ATRA maintenance intermittently or continuously.

Arsenic trioxide is currently regarded as the best option in the context of relapsing APL. Arsenic trioxide produces CR rates of 80% in relapsed APL and may be more effective than ATRA. Its role in postinduction therapy in newly diagnosed APL is also currently being explored. In second-line therapy, the choice of transplant modality is mainly based on PCR status achieved after reinduction.

AML in the elderly
The intensive induction approach remains the best treatment option for carefully selected patients. This selection process should consider host-related (age, chronic organ dysfunctions, PS, infection at baseline) as well as AML-related (cytogenetics) selection criteria. There is no confirmed postremission strategy in elderly patients once CR has been achieved using standard intensive induction. High-dose consolidation courses, with or without high-dose cytarabine, are usually too toxic to benefit most patients. Beneficial effects associated with prolonged therapy with lower doses of chemotherapy have been reported. Allogeneic SCT after reduced-intensity conditioning is being used with increased frequency from either matched related or unrelated donors. Prolonged maintenance with new agents is being studied.

Further reading
Brunning RD, Matute E, Harris NL, et al. Acute myeloid leukemias. In: Jaffe EJHN, Stein H, Vardiman JW (eds) *World Health Organization Classification of tumors: Pathology and genetics of tumours of haematopoietic and lymphoid tissues*, pp.75–105. Lyon: IARC Press, 2001.

Burnett AK, Knapper S. Targeting treatment in AML. *Hematology* 2007; **1**:429–34.

Cornelissen JJ, Lowenberg B. Role of allogeneic stem cell transplantation in current treatment of acute myeloid leukemia. *Hematology* 2005; **1**:151–5.

Deschler B, Lubbert M. Acute myeloid leukaemia: epidemiology and etiology. *Cancer* 2006; **107**:2099–107.

Dohner H. Implication of the molecular characterization of acute myeloid leukemia. *Hematology* 2007; **1**:412–19.

Estey EH. How I treat older patients with AML. *Blood* 2000; **96**:1670–73.

Gorin NC, Aegerter P, Auvert B, et al. Autologous bone marrow transplantation for acute myelocytic leukemia in first remission: a European survey of the role of marrow purging. *Blood* 1990; **75**:1606–14.

Grimwade D, Walker H, Harrison G, et al. The predictive value of hierarchical cytogenetic classification in older adults with acute myeloid leukemia (AML): analysis of 1065 patients entered into the United Kingdom Medical Research Council AML 11 trial. *Blood* 2001; **98**:1312–20.

Hegenbart U, Niederwieser D, Sandmaier BM, et al. Treatment for acute myelogenous leukemia by low-dose, total-body irradiation-based conditioning and hematopoietic cell transplantation from related and unrelated donors. *J Clin Oncol* 2006; **24**:444–53.

Mayer RJ, Davis RB, Schiffer CA, et al. Intensive postremission chemotherapy in adults with acute myeloid leukemia. *N Engl J Med* 1994; **331**:896–903.

Sanz MA. Treatment of acute promyelocytic leukemia. *Hematology* 2006; **1**:147–55.

Tallman MS. New strategies for the treatment of acute myeloid leukemia including antibodies and other novel agents. *Hematology* 2005; **1**:143–50.

Chronic myeloid leukaemia: introduction

Chronic myeloid leukaemia (CML) is a myeloproliferative disorder characterized by an acquired mutation affecting haematopoietic stem cells. The mutation results in a reciprocal translocation between the long arms of chromosomes 9 and 22, t (9;22)(q34;q11), producing a shortened chromosome 22, first identified in 1960, and termed the Philadelphia (Ph) chromosome (Nowell and Hungerford 1960).

Epidemiology
- CML is rare with an annual incidence of 1.6 per 100,000.
- Median age at diagnosis is 55 years. It is very rare in children and the incidence increases with age.
- There is a slight male preponderance with a male:female ratio of 1.4:1. Females have a survival advantage.

Aetiology
In most patients there is no known aetiological factor. There are no ethnic, geographic, socioeconomic, or hereditary associations. Radiation exposure is the only known aetiological factor predisposing to CML.

Pathology and cytogenetics
The Philadelphia translocation relocates the 3′ segment of ABL, the human homologue of the Abelson murine leukaemia proto-oncogene, encoding a non-receptor tyrosine kinase (TK), from the long arm of chromosome 9 to the 5′ segment of the breakpoint cluster region (BCR) gene in the long arm of chromosome 22. BCR encodes a protein with serine-threonine kinase activity. The resulting fusion gene is translated to a chimeric protein, BCR-ABL, with constitutive leukaemogenic TK activity. Cytokine-independent cell growth and haematopoietic cell transformation are mediated by BCR-ABL through increased transcriptional activity via signal transducer and activator of transcription (STAT)-5 recruitment, enhanced proliferation from RAS activation, and reduced apoptosis secondary to phosphatidylinositol 3-kinase (PI3K)/protein kinase B (Akt) activation.
- Ph chromosome is detected in 95% of patients with CML, 5% of children, and 15–30% of adults with ALL, and 2% of patients with AML.
- Variant Ph chromosome translocations, involving one or more additional chromosomes arise in 5–10% of patients with Ph chromosome-positive CML (Huret 1990). Variant Ph translocations are associated with a similar response to treatment when compared with patients with classic Ph chromosome.
- 5–10% of patients with clinical features typical of CML are Ph chromosome-negative, of whom 30–50% demonstrate the BCR-ABL molecular rearrangement by RT-PCR. These patients have the same outcome as those expressing the Ph chromosome.
- Patients lacking the Ph chromosome and BCR-ABL molecular abnormality are classed as atypical CML, require different treatment, have a different prognosis and should be considered as a separate disease entity (Kurzrock et al. 1990).

Breakpoints within ABL span a region of >300 kb at its 5′ end, and within BCR localize to three main breakpoint cluster regions, resulting in three fusion transcripts, each encoding a BCR-ABL hybrid protein.

- p210$^{BCR-ABL}$, a 210 kd fusion protein occurs in most patients with CML and a third of patients with Ph chromosome-positive ALL. Breakpoint occurs within the major breakpoint cluster region (M-bcr), a 5.8 kb area between BCR exons e12–e16.
- p190$^{BCR-ABL}$ arises very rarely in CML and in two-thirds of patients with Ph chromosome-positive ALL. Breakpoints identified in the minor breakpoint cluster region (m-bcr), spanning an area of 54.4 kb between exons e2′ and e2. It is associated in CML with monocytosis at presentation and worse prognosis than patients with p210.
- p230$^{BCR-ABL}$ is associated with chronic neutrophilic leukaemia, and arises from a breakpoint cluster region (μ-bcr) downstream of BCR exon 19. Reduced TK activity relative to p190$^{BCR-ABL}$ is reflected in a less aggressive clinical course.

Evidence from studies utilizing highly sensitive (10^{-8}) RT-PCR demonstrates the presence of BCR-ABL in up to 30% of healthy individuals, suggesting that BCR-ABL is not the only genetic abnormality involved in the pathogenesis of CML (Bose et al. 1998).

Clinical features
Natural history
Three disease phases are recognized. Patients are classified at diagnosis according to disease stage into chronic phase (CP), accelerated phase (AP) or blastic transformation.
- 90% of patients present in CP. Median duration 3–5 years if not treated with a thymidine kinase inhibitor (TKI). 3–4% annual risk of transformation to BP.
- AP is characterized by increasing maturation arrest, blast count, organomegaly, and clonal evolution. Most frequent secondary chromosomal abnormalities are trisomy 8, monosomy 17, duplicate Ph chromosome; trisomy 19, 21, 17, and deletion 7 are found in <10% of cases. Median survival 1–2 years. Most patients progress to blast phase after 4–6 months.
- Blast phase (BP) resembles acute leukaemia with >20% blasts in peripheral blood or marrow. Lymphoid BP occurs in 20–30%, myeloid in 50%, and undifferentiated in 25%. Median survival is 3–6 months with lymphoid BP.

AP and BP may be combined as advanced phase disease. Different criteria have been proposed to define the three phases of disease (see Table 4.10.11 for WHO criteria). CP and BP are clearly defined, while AP CML remains a somewhat subjective entity in terms of the degree of increasing splenomegaly, marrow fibrosis, and megakaryocytic proliferation. The classification systems provide prognostic information for patients and clinicians, and standardization for clinical trials.

Symptoms and signs
- Insidious onset. Diagnosis often made following incidental finding of leucocytosis on routine full blood count in an asymptomatic patient.
- Non-specific constitutional symptoms of weight loss, night sweats, and low-grade fever characterize the hypermetabolic state.
- Splenomegaly is the most common physical finding. Patients report abdominal discomfort, 'fullness' and early satiety related to splenomegaly and/or hepatomegaly.

Splenic infarction is associated with left upper quadrant pain. Spleen extends ≥5cm below left costal margin in over 50% of patients at diagnosis.

- Hyperviscosity and leukostasis may occur in patients presenting with marked leukocytosis and white blood cells (WBC) >300 × 10^9/L. Fundoscopy may demonstrate papilloedema, fundal haemorrhages and venous obstruction. Priapism, confusion, visual disturbance, cerebrovascular accidents and tinnitus are also reported secondary to leukostasis. Leukapheresis may transiently reduce WBC.
- Suspect transformation to BP if bleeding, petechiae, fever, secondary to infection, and bone pain are prominent symptoms.

Diagnosis

- *Full blood count, peripheral blood film and preferably 1000 cell differential performed by microscopy (Goldman 2007).* High WBC. Left shifted leucocytosis, with all stages of granulopoiesis visible; predominant neutrophils and myelocytes. Mild basophilia and eosinophilia also seen. Platelet count may be elevated, normal, or low. Mild anaemia is common; usually normochromic normocytic.
- *Bone marrow aspirate and trephine biopsy.* Bone marrow markedly hypercellular with expansion of the myeloid cell line and progenitors; all stages of maturation present with myelocyte peak. <10% myeloblasts and promyelocytes in CP. Trephine biopsy allows assessment of fibrosis by reticulin stain.
- *Bone marrow or peripheral blood cytogenetics.* Confirms diagnosis by demonstrating presence of Ph chromosome. May reveal possible additional chromosomal abnormalities. Allows detection of clonal evolution in AP and BP.

Table 4.10.11 WHO criteria for CML AP and BP (Vardiman et al. 2002)

CML AP diagnosed by presence of one or more:

10–19% peripheral blood or bone marrow blasts
≥20% peripheral blood basophils
Platelets <100 x 10^9/L unrelated to therapy,
or >1000 x 10^9/L unresponsive to therapy
Increasing spleen size and WBC unresponsive to therapy
Cytogenetics showing clonal evolution
Megakaryocytic proliferation
Marked bone marrow fibrosis

CML BP diagnosed by presence of one or more:

≥20% peripheral blood or bone marrow blasts
Extramedullary blast proliferation
Large foci or clusters of blasts in bone marrow

- *FISH on bone marrow or peripheral blood cells.* Detects Ph chromosome and can be designed to also allow detection of prognostically important deletions of the derivative chromosome 9, der(9).
- *Real-time quantitative PCR (RQ-PCR) for BCR-ABL transcripts.* Results expressed as ratio of BCR-ABL transcripts to number of copies of control gene (Hughes et al. 2006).
- *Upper abdominal ultrasound/CT scan.* Confirms presence of splenomegaly and/or hepatomegaly.
- *Serum urate level.* Hyperuricaemia associated with marked leucocytosis and high cell turnover.
- *Human leucocyte antigen (HLA) typing at diagnosis on patient and siblings if fit and aged <65 years.*

Differential diagnosis

Leukaemoid reactions secondary to inflammation, infection or malignancy. Absent Ph chromosome, evidence of secondary disorder.
Myeloproliferative disease. Essential thrombocythaemia characterized by absent Ph chromosome and possible presence of Jak2 mutation. Myelofibrosis excluded by Ph chromosome.
Myelodysplasia. Absent Ph chromosome, dysplasia and maturation arrest on bone marrow aspirate and peripheral blood film.
Chronic neutrophilic leukaemia.

Further reading

Bose S, Deininger M, Gora-Tybor J, et al. The presence of typical and atypical BCR-ABL fusion genes in leukocytes of normal individuals: the biologic significance and implications for the assessment of minimal residual disease. *Blood* 1998; **92**:3362–7.

Goldman J. Recommendations for the management of BCR-ABL-positive chronic myeloid leukaemia. BCSH approved document, 2007—available at http://www.bcshguidelines.com

Hughes TP, Deininger M, Hochhaus A, et al. Monitoring CML patients responding to treatment with tyrosine kinase inhibitors: review and recommendations for harmonizing current methodology for detecting BCR-ABL transcripts and kinase domain mutations and for expressing results. *Blood* 2006; **108**:28–37.

Huret JL. Complex translocations, simple variant translocations and Ph-negative cases in chronic myelogenous leukaemia. *Hum Genet* 1990; **85**: 565–8.

Kurzrock R, Kantarjian HM, Shtalrid JU, et al. Philadelphia chromosome negative chronic myeloid leukaemia without breakpoint cluster region rearrangement: a chronic myeloid leukaemia with a distinct clinical course. *Blood* 1990; **75**:445–52.

Nowell PC, Hungerford DA. A minute chromosome in human chronic granulocytic leukaemia. Science 1960; **132**:1497–501

Vardiman JW, Harris NL, Brunning RD, et al. The World Health Organization (WHO) classification of the myeloid neoplasms. *Blood* 2002; **100**:2292–302.

Chronic myeloid leukaemia: staging, prognosis, and treatment

Staging and prognosis

- Accurate identification of disease phase at diagnosis is essential (see 'Natural history' section in Chapter 4, Chronic myeloid leukaemia: introduction, p.474).
- Patients in CP further differentiated according to low, intermediate, and high risk determined by a prognostic score based on clinical and laboratory factors. Most extensively used system is the Sokal score (based on age, spleen size, percentage blasts, and platelet count); later modified, to include basophil and eosinophil counts, as the Hasford score (Sokal et al. 1984; Hasford, 1998). Although the scoring systems were derived from survival figures for patients treated predominantly with busulfan or interferon-alpha, (Sokal and Hasford systems respectively), the data remain relevant to patients treated in the imatinib era.
- Timing and degree of haematological, cytogenetic and molecular response also predicts outcome (Table 4.10.12).
- Additional high-risk factors include deletion der (9), secondary chromosomal abnormalities in Ph-positive cells at diagnosis, clonal evolution, and less than MCyR after 12 months imatinib therapy (see 'Chronic phase' section).

Table 4.10.12 Definitions of response to treatment (Baccarani et al. 2006)

Haematological response (HR)—complete (CHR)	
Platelets	$<450 \times 10^9$/L
WBC	$<10 \times 10^9$/L
Differential	No immature granulocytes
	Basophils <5%

Cytogenetic response (CyR)	
	% Ph-pos metaphases
Complete (CCyR)	0
Major (MCyR)	≤35
Partial (PCYR)	1–35
Minor	36–65
Minimal	66–95
None	>95

Molecular response (MR)	
	BCR-ABL to control gene ratio
Complete (CMR)	Transcripts not detectable
Major (MMR)	≤0.1% Equivalent to 3 log reduction from standardized base-line

Treatment

The treatment of CML has been revolutionized in the last decade with the advent of molecularly targeted TKIs. Imatinib mesylate is a TKI with activity against BCR-ABL, ABL, c-kit, stem cell factor receptor, and platelet-derived growth factor receptor (PDGFR). Imatinib binds to the inactive non-adenosine triphosphate (ATP)-binding conformation of BCR-ABL, stabilizing the kinase in its inactive form. ATP binding is competitively inhibited, preventing substrate phosphorylation, resulting in inhibition of CML cell proliferation and induction of apoptosis.

Chronic phase

- Interferon-alpha was standard therapy for CP CML prior to the discovery of imatinib; other treatment options included myelosuppression with hydroxycarbamide or busulfan.
- Up to 25% of patients achieved CCyR with interferon-alpha (Kantarjian et al. 1995); increasing to 35% with the addition of cytarabine (Guilhot et al. 1997). OS 70% at 5 years.
- 10-year survival of 78% reported in patients achieving CCyR with interferon-alpha (Kantarjian et al. 2003). Thirty per cent of patients in CCyR also achieved CMR; no reported relapses after a median follow-up of 10 years.
- Superiority of imatinib demonstrated by the International Randomized Study of Interferon and STI571 (IRIS) trial in 1106 newly diagnosed patients with CP CML. Estimated CCyR rate at 18 months was 76% in the imatinib group and 14% in the interferon-cytarabine arm (O'Brien et al. 2003).
- Five-year estimated cumulative rate of CCyR was 87%, EFS 83%, and OS 89% in the imatinib group (Druker et al. 2006).
- Cytogenetic and molecular response to TKI therapy shown to predict outcome. In imatinib treated patients, 5-year PFS was 97% in those who had CCyR after 12 months of therapy, 93% for those with PCyR, and 81% for those without MCyR after 12 months; at 60 months, PFS was 100% in patients with CCyR and at least a 3 log reduction in BCR-ABL transcript level after 18 months of treatment (Druker et al. 2006).
- Severe, grade 3/4, adverse effects are rare with imatinib. Myelosuppression occurs most frequently, followed by hepatotoxicity. Less severe side effects are more common. Peripheral and periorbital oedema occurs in 60%, diarrhoea or nausea in around 50%, musculoskeletal pain in 47%, rashes in 40%, and fatigue in 39% (Druker et al. 2006). Teratogenic requiring use of contraception in men and women.
- Imatinib resistance occurs in CP at a rate of <2% per year. Most commonly results from the development of BCR-ABL mutations in the TK domain, particularly the P-loop region responsible for ATP docking. Site of mutation affects degree of imatinib insensitivity; first mutation described, T315I, a threonine to isoleucine substitution at position 315, affects a residue critical in the formation of a hydrogen bond with TKIs and confers complete *in vivo* resistance. Upregulation of BCR-ABL or expansion of the leukaemia clone due to secondary genetic anomalies also confers imatinib insensitivity.

Treatment recommendation

The IRIS trial established imatinib 400mg daily as the medical standard of care for newly diagnosed adult patients in CP (Baccarani et al. 2006; Goldman, 2007).

- Lower doses may predispose to resistance and should be avoided.
- Higher doses, 600–800mg daily, induce more rapid cytogenetic and molecular responses, but are less well tolerated; no evidence of OS advantage. To be tested in latest STI571 Prospective International Randomized Trial (SPIRIT) (see 'Internet resource').
- Indefinite therapy recommended due to reports of relapse on cessation.
- Possible exceptions to first-line imatinib therapy include high-risk disease and low allogeneic haematopoietic stem cell transplantation (allo-HSCT) risk, e.g. a child with an HLA-identical sibling or adult with a syngeneic twin (Goldman et al. 2007). No evidence of deleterious effect on transplant outcome from prior imatinib therapy.

RQ-PCR for BCR-ABL transcripts is the cornerstone for monitoring patients responding to imatinib therapy (Hughes et al. 2006).
- Bone marrow aspirate and cytogenetic assessment for the Ph chromosome should be undertaken routinely, every 3 months until CCyR (Goldman 2007).
- Thereafter, recommend monitoring peripheral blood BCR-ABL transcript levels every 3 months indefinitely (Goldman et al. 2007).
- Annual bone marrow cytogenetic studies may have a role in detecting clonal evolution in Ph-negative cells, although prognostic significance unclear (Baccarani 2006).
- A rise in BCR-ABL transcripts by 0.5–1.0 log necessitates examination of the bone marrow for Ph-positive cells and screening for kinase domain mutations.
- Mutational analysis indicated in patients in CP with inadequate response, or loss of response to treatment, and in patients presenting in advanced-phase disease (Hughes et al. 2006).
- Imatinib failure defined as no HR after 3 months, incomplete HR or no CyR after 6 months, less than PCyR at 12 months, less than CCyR at 18 months, loss of CHR or CCyR, or detection of resistant BCR-ABL mutations (Baccarani et al. 2006). Lack of CHR at 3 months, PCyR at 6 months, CCyR at 12 months or MMR at 18 months, loss of MMR, or clonal evolution in Ph-positive cells represents a suboptimal response.

Imatinib failure or suboptimal response warrants increased dose of imatinib, alternative TKIs or allo-HSCT (Baccarani et al. 2006). Likewise consider alternative therapy in imatinib intolerance.
- *Increased dose imatinib.* Check compliance with 400mg dose. 600–800mg imatinib daily may be effective in mildly resistant mutations.
- *Second generation TKIs.*

Dasatinib is a competitive Src- and ABL-kinase inhibitor, binding active and inactive forms, with 300-fold greater potency than imatinib, licensed for the treatment of imatinib-resistant CML. At 8 months, CHR achieved in 90% and MCyR in 52% of imatinib-resistant or intolerant patients in CP treated with 70mg dasatinib twice daily (Hochhaus et al. 2007). Superior to high-dose imatinib in patients failing imatinib 400mg daily, with MCyR in 52% on dasatinib and 33% for imatinib 800mg (Kantarjian et al. 2007a). Higher discontinuation rate is due to toxicities, including pleural and pericardial effusions.

Nilotinib, a derivative of imatinib, exhibits 30-fold greater *in vitro* potency. In imatinib-intolerant or resistant patients, the 6-month rate of MCyR was 48% (Kantarjian et al. 2007b). Awaiting European licence.

Bosutinib, a dual Src- and ABL-kinase inhibitor active against CML cell lines, undergoing clinical trial.

Early dasatinib and nilotinib data is sufficiently promising that first-line standard of care may change. Currently dasatinib is considered second-line therapy after imatinib failure, although neither dasatinib nor nilotinib are effective in the context of T315I mutations. Alternative second-line therapy is allo-HSCT.

Allo-HSCT
Transplant rates have decreased significantly since the introduction of imatinib. A randomized controlled trial comparing first line best available medical therapy, mainly interferon-alpha, with allo-HSCT showed better survival in the drug-treatment arm (Hehlmann et al. 2007); TKIs will improve outcome further. However, allo-HSCT remains the only current therapy with curative potential in CML. Long-term survival at 20 years reported in 41% of eligible patients undergoing HLA-matched sibling transplants in first CP (Gratwohl et al. 2006). Prognostic risk stratification according to age, duration of disease, phase, donor type, and sex; 5-year OS ranges from 22–72% depending on risk (Gratwohl et al. 1998).

High treatment-related mortality (TRM), lack of suitable sibling donor, and poorer outcome from unrelated donor transplants limit eligibility for allo-HSCT. Reduced intensity conditioning (RIC), shown to have lower TRM, may allow transplants in older patients and those with comorbidities that would otherwise preclude allo-HSCT (Crawley et al. 2005). Registry data for RIC matched-sibling allo-HSCT in older patients (median age 50) shows 3-year overall survival of 30–70% depending on prognostic score (Crawley et al. 2005); long-term outcome remains unknown.

Monitor response following allo-HSCT as for imatinib therapy. Relapse post-transplant may be treated with donor lymphocyte infusions (DLI) with or without imatinib.

Third-line options for resistant patients in CP, ineligible for allo-HSCT, include interferon-alpha, hydroxycarbamide, or experimental agents including aurora kinase inhibitors (MK-0457) preferably in the context of a clinical trial.

Accelerated and blastic phases
Newly diagnosed patients presenting in advanced phase should receive imatinib at 600mg or 800mg daily (Goldman et al. 2007). Median survival with imatinib in BP is only 7.5 months. Responders who have an appropriate donor and are fit for transplant should proceed to allo-HSCT.

Progression to advanced phase CML on imatinib therapy similarly requires use of an alternative TKI and allo-HSCT.

Overall prognosis in CML BC is poor; imatinib achieves CHR in <15% of patients, allo-HSCT results in durable remission in around 10%. Dasatinib has demonstrated CCyR in 20–30% of patients in BC, but responses are short-lived (Cortes et al. 2007).

Further reading
Baccarani M, Saglio G, Goldman JM, *et al.* Evolving concepts in the management of chronic myeloid leukaemia. Recommendations from an expert panel on behalf of the European LeukemiaNet. *Blood* 2006; **108**:1809–20.
Cortes J, Rousselot P, Kim DW, *et al.* Dasatinib induces complete hematologic and cytogenetic responses in patients with

imatinib-resistant or –intolerant chronic myeloid leukaemia in blast crisis. *Blood* 2007; **109**:3207–13.

Crawley C, Szydlo R, Lalancette M, *et al*. Outcomes of reduced-intensity transplantation for chronic myeloid leukemia: an analysis of prognostic factors from the Chronic Leukemia Working Party of the EBMT. *Blood* 2005; **106**:2969–76.

Druker BJ, Guilhot F, O'Brian SG, *et al*. Five-year follow-up of patients receiving imatinib for chronic myeloid leukaemia. *N Engl J Med* 2006; **355**:2404–17.

Goldman J. Recommendations for the management of BCR-ABL-positive chronic myeloid leukaemia. BCSH approved document, 2007—available at http://www.bcshguidelines.com

Gratwohl A, Hermans J, Goldman JM, *et al*. Risk assessment for patients with chronic myeloid leukaemia before allogeneic blood or marrow transplantation: Chronic Leukemia Working Party of the European Group for Blood and Marrow Transplantation. *Lancet* 1998; **352**:1087–92.

Gratwohl A, Brand R, *et al*. Allogeneic hematopoietic stem cell transplantation for chronic myeloid leukemia in Europe 2006: transplant activity, long term data and current results: an analysis by the Chronic Leukemia Working Party of the European Group for Blood and Marrow Transplantation (EBMT). *Haematologica* 2006; **91**:513–21.

Guilhot F, Chastang C, Michallet M, *et al*. French Chronic Myeloid Leukemia Study Group. Interferon alfa-2b combined with cytarabine versus interferon alone in chronic myelogenous leukaemia. *N Engl J Med* 1997; **337**:223–9.

Hasford J, Pfirrmann M, Hehlmann R, *et al*. A new prognostic score for survival of patients with chronic myeloid leukaemia treated with interferon alpha. Writing Committee for the Collaborative CML Prognostic Factors Project Group. *J Natl Cancer Inst* 1998; **90**:850–8.

Hehlmann R, Berger U, Pfirrmann M, *et al*. Drug treatment is superior to allografting as first line therapy in chronic myeloid leukaemia. *Blood* 2007; **109**:4686–92.

Hochhaus A, Kantarjian HM,Baccarani L, *et al*. Dasatinib induces notable hematologic and cytogenetic responses in chronic phase chronic myeloid leukaemia after failure of imatinib therapy. *Blood* 2007; **109**:2303–9.

Hughes TP, Deininger M, Hochhaus A, *et al*. Monitoring CML patients responding to treatment with tyrosine kinase inhibitors: review and recommendations for harmonizing current methodology for detecting BCR-ABL transcripts and kinase domain mutations and for expressing results. *Blood* 2006; **108**:28–37.

Kantarjian HM, Smith I L, O'Brian S, *et al*. The Leukaemia Service. Prolonged survival in chronic myelogenous leukaemia after cytogenetic response to interferon-alpha therapy. *Ann Internal Med* 1995; **122**:254–61.

Kantarjian HM, O'Brien S, Cortes JE, *et al*. Complete cytogenetic and molecular responses to interferon-alpha-based therapy for chronic myelogenous leukaemia are associated with excellent long-term prognosis. *Cancer* 2003; **97**:1033–41.

Kantarjian HM, Pasquini R, Hamerschlak N, *et al*. Dasatinib or high-dose imatinib for chronic-phase chronic myeloid leukaemia after failure of imatinib therapy. *Blood* 2007a; **109**:5143–50.

Kantarjian HM, Giles F, Gattermann N, *et al*. Nilotinib (formerly AMN107), a highly selective BCR-ABL tyrosine kinase inhibitor, is effective in patients with Philadelphia chromosome-positive chronic myelogenous leukaemia in chronic phase following imatinib resistance and intolerance. *Blood* 2007b; **110**;3540–6.

O'Brien SG, Guilhot F, Larson R, *et al*. Imatinib compared with interferon and low-dose cytarabine for newly diagnosed chronic-phase chronic myeloid leukaemia. *N Engl J Med* 2003; **348**:994–1004.

Sokal JE, Cox EB, Baccarani M, *et al*. 1984; Prognostic discrimination in 'good risk' chronic granulocytic leukaemia. *Blood* **63**:789–99.

Internet resource

STI571 Prospective International Randomized Trial (SPIRIT): http://www.spirit-cml.org

Chronic lymphocytic leukaemia: introduction

Chronic lymphocytic leukaemia (CLL) is a malignant clonal expansion of lymphocytes, usually B cells but rarely T cells or natural killer cells. It is considered one of a group of B-cell lymphoproliferative disorders, classified by WHO on the basis of their histopathological appearance. The malignant lymphocytes are commonly identified in the blood, bone marrow, and lymphoid organs. When primarily confined to lymph nodes it is termed small lymphocytic lymphoma (SLL).

Epidemiology

CLL is the most common leukaemia in the Western world. It is seen more frequently with increasing age; however approximately 15% of patients are <50 years when diagnosed. It is twice as common in males than females. In older patients, there is less male excess, and in general the disease is less advanced at diagnosis. CLL is rare in Asian populations, irrespective of lifestyle or geography. Black and white populations have similar incidence (20–30 times more than Asian populations). The overall UK incidence is 3 per 100,000.

Aetiology

There are no environmental factors proven to cause CLL. Proposed risk factors include several viruses and agricultural chemicals.

There is evidence of inherited susceptibility in first- and second-degree relatives with up to 10% of CLL cases considered familial (Houlston et al. 2002). Familial cases tend to occur at an earlier age and with more severe disease in subsequent generations (Yuille et al. 1998).

Pathology and cytogenetics

CLL usually originates in lymph nodes and/or bone marrow and then accumulates in other lymphoid organs. In the marrow, involvement begins as interstitial or nodular infiltrates progressing to diffuse replacement of normal marrow.

Proliferation centres are unique to CLL and SLL. These centres have a high proliferation index with high expression of CD23. They are commonly found in lymph nodes of patients with CLL and in the bone marrow in very active disease. Their presence differentiates CLL from the leukaemic phase of NHL.

Standard cytogenetic analysis is able to identify abnormalities in <50% of CLL cases. This is often because samples lack sufficient cells in metaphase. FISH detects abnormalities in approximately 80% of cases. The commonest abnormalities are listed here. They are neither unique nor specific to CLL and can be seen in other lymphoproliferative disorders.
- 13q deletion: approximately 50% of patients
- 11q deletion: 10–20% of patients
- 12q trisomy: 15–20% of patients
- 17p deletion: 5–10% of patients

17p deletions often result in loss of p53 (17p13) and therefore loss of cell cycle regulation. These patients respond poorly to standard treatment, have a greater tendency to transform, and exhibit shorter survival (Dohner et al. 1995). 11q deletions may involve the ATM gene (11q22–q23), which normally activates p53 in response to DNA damage. 11q23 deletions are more commonly seen in younger patients and are associated with poor outcome (Dohner et al. 1997). Trisomy 12q commonly leads to a higher proliferation rate and disease progression. When 13q deletion is the sole cytogenetic abnormality it confers a better prognosis (Juliusson et al. 1990).

Diagnosis

The differential diagnosis of lymphocytosis includes malignant and several non-malignant conditions including infection. Once lymphocyte clonality is established, CLL must be differentiated from other lymphoproliferative conditions such as mantle cell lymphoma, prolymphocytic leukaemia, marginal zone lymphoma, follicular lymphoma, hairy cell leukaemia, and lymphoplasmacytoid lymphoma.

The diagnostic criteria for CLL are:
- Lymphocytosis $>5 \times 10^9$/L
- Typical morphology
- Typical immunophenotype

In typical CLL, >90% of the cells will be small to medium-sized lymphocytes with clumped chromatin, absent nucleoli and scanty cytoplasm. Atypical CLL (which accounts for up to 15% of cases) can be diagnosed morphologically when >10% of cells are prolymphocytes or >15% are lymphoplasmacytoid and/or have cleaved nuclei. During preparation of the blood film, smear cells are often produced secondary to crushing of lymphocytes. They are characteristic of CLL but may also be seen in viral infections.

Moreau et al. (1997) identified five markers which differentiate between B-cell lymphoproliferative disorders. The markers are:
- Weak SmIg
- Positive CD5
- Positive CD23
- Weak or absent FMC7
- Weak or absent CD79b

Typical CLL will score 4 or 5, atypical CLL 3–5, and other disorders ≤2.
Other commonly used investigations include:
- Direct antiglobulin test—to look for haemolysis
- Serum immunoglobulins
- CXR
- Bone marrow aspirate and trephine
- Lymph node biopsy
- FISH—to exclude t(11;14) which is diagnostic of mantle cell lymphoma and look for p53 mutations
- CT scan—to provide baseline assessment of lymphadenopathy and splenomegaly

Chronic lymphocytic leukaemia: clinical features and staging

Clinical features

CLL is most often diagnosed incidentally. Patients may present with:
- Lymphadenopathy (usually symmetrical and painless)
- Systemic symptoms (weight loss, night sweats, tiredness)
- Symptoms secondary to bone marrow failure

Patients with CLL have immune dysregulation, resulting in higher rates of autoimmune complications especially haemolytic anaemia and immune thrombocytopenia. If the haemoglobin or platelet count is disproportionately low, causes include autoimmune destruction, bone marrow infiltration, and hypersplenism. CLL may be complicated by hypogammaglobulinaemia and frequent infections can occur despite adequate neutrophil counts.

Staging

The two most commonly used clinical staging systems were devised by Binet (Europe) (Binet et al. 1981) and Rai (USA)(Rai et al. 1975). They classify patients into low, intermediate-, and high-risk groups (see Table 4.10.13).

Patients with Binet stage A or Rai stage 0 disease have no bone marrow failure and minimal solid disease. Their median survival is >10 years. This is compared to a median survival of 3–5 years in patient with bone marrow failure, i.e. Binet stage C disease or Rai stage III and IV.

Smoldering CLL is a sub group of Binet stage A disease with haemoglobin >13g/dL, lymphocyte count <30 × 10⁹/L, lymphocyte doubling time >12 months, minimal or no lymph node involvement, and non-diffuse bone marrow infiltration. This confers a significantly better prognosis with 80% of patients alive at 10 years and only 15% showing any signs of progression (Monteserrat et al. 1988).

Up to 5% of patients undergo immunoblastic transformation to a more aggressive malignancy (Richter's syndrome). This resembles diffuse large B cell lymphoma. Transformation is usually seen as rapid enlargement of one lymph node associated with more severe systemic symptoms. The clinical outcome is poor with median survival of approximately 6 months.

Prognostic factors

Lymphocyte doubling time is often used as a threshold for treatment. A doubling time <12 months confers a worse prognosis. Whilst quick and easy to perform, the lymphocyte count can be significantly altered by stresses such as infection.

Other prognostic factors are not yet used routinely. In a patient with advanced disease (Binet C or Rai III/IV) the only marker likely to be of use is FISH for p53. This will alter the choice of first-line treatment. Other cytogenetic abnormalities, as discussed earlier, also affect prognosis. For patients with low- to intermediate-risk disease, prognostic markers may eventually be used to identify patients who should receive early treatment or treatment at higher intensity or longer duration.

Table 4.10.13 Clinical staging systems in chronic lymphocytic leukaemia

Risk	Binet		Rai	
Low	A	<3 lymphoid areas	0	Lymphocytosis only
Intermediate	B	>3 lymphoid areas	I	Lymphadenopathy
			II	Hepato or splenomegaly ± lymphadenopathy
High	C	Hb <10g/dL or platelets <100 × 10⁹/L	III	Haemoglobin < 11g/dL
			IV	Platelets <100 × 10⁹/L

Lymphoid areas are; cervical, axillary, inguinal, hepatomegaly, splenomegaly.

Other causes of anaemia or thrombocytopenia, e.g. hypersplenism, nutritional deficiencies, red cell aplasia, and autoimmune disease must be ruled out.

Normal B cells undergo somatic hypermutation of the IgVH gene, in lymph node germinal centres, after they have been exposed to antigen. There is then selection of B cells with improved antigen binding, a process known as affinity maturation. The median survival of patients with mutated IgVH (i.e. post germinal centre) is 25 years compared to 8 years for patients with unmutated (i.e. pregerminal centre) genes (Hamblin et al. 1999).

Increased levels of ZAP-70 (Crespo et al. 2003) and CD38 (Ghia et al. 2003) are seen in cells with unmutated IgVH. Both ZAP-70 and CD38 are detectable by flow cytometric analysis. This provides a cost and time saving over gene sequencing of IgVH, and therefore CD38 and ZAP-70 may be used as surrogate markers. Their use is currently limited because they require standard assay methods and cut-off values for validation.

β_2 microglobulin, lactate dehydrogenase, serum thymidine kinase, and soluble CD23 (Knauf et al. 1997; Hallek et al. 1999) have all been shown to predict survival in Binet stage A patients.

Chronic lymphocytic leukaemia: treatment

An overview of treatment is given in Fig 4.10.3
Treatment: early stage

Many patients will require no treatment and in many cases do not even require specialist referral. Monitoring of the full blood count every 3–6 months is recommended. Indications for referral include:
- Patient preference
- Systemic symptoms
- Lymphadenopathy/organomegaly
- Lymphocyte doubling time <6 months
- High lymphocyte count
- Cytopenia

In early stage disease, active monitoring should be pursued until the patient fulfils criteria for treatment.

Results from the MRC CLL2 trial (Catovsky et al. 1991) showed that early treatment for patient with Binet stage A disease reduced OS when compared to delayed treatment. A subsequent meta-analysis of trial data shows no difference between early and delayed treatment. Most clinicians chose to delay treatment until one or more of the following are present:
- Progressive marrow failure
- Massive (>10cm)/progressive lymphadenopathy
- Massive (> 6cm)/progressive splenomegaly
- Progressive lymphocytosis (doubling time <6 months)
- Systemic symptoms:
- Weight loss >10% in 6 months
  Fever >38°C for >2 weeks
  Extreme fatigue or night sweats
- Autoimmune cytopenias (this may only require treatment of the autoimmune component not necessarily the leukaemia)

Response criteria

Response criteria published by the National Cancer Institute are included in Table 4.10.14) (Cheson et al. 1996). Responses are complete (CR) or partial (PR). Patients who fulfil all criteria for CR except having lymphoid nodules on bone marrow trephine are termed nodular partial response (nPR).

First-line therapy

For some patients, active treatment is not appropriate due to either comorbidities or personal preference. In these patients, supportive care with blood and platelet support, antibiotics and palliative nursing may be considered.

Chlorambucil

Current first-line therapy in the UK is either chlorambucil alone or fludarabine and cyclophosphamide in combination (FC). The MRC CLL1 trial (Catovsky et al. 1991) showed that chlorambucil was equivalent to anthracyclines (COP regimen). This has been confirmed by meta-analysis. Fludarabine alone produces more responses and longer remissions than chlorambucil but does not provide a survival benefit due to an increase in grade III/IV infections and increased severity of autoimmune haemolytic anaemia. Response to chlorambucil appears to be dose dependent (Jaksic and Brugiatelli 1988). Comparing patients given chlorambucil alone in CLL3 ($60mg/m^2$) versus CLL4 ($70mg/m^2$), 5-year survival increased from 46% to 62% and proportion of patients achieving complete or nodular partial remission rose from 15% to 26.5%. Chlorambucil is an oral agent and is usually given for the first 7 days of a 28-day cycle. Patients will usually receive 6 cycles. There is no evidence to support use in combination with steroid (Han et al. 1973) except in patients with autoimmune complications.

Fludarabine and cyclophosphamide (FC)

Following the results of the LRF CLL4 trial (Catovsky et al. 2007), many now consider FC to be the gold standard first-line treatment. This showed a significant improvement in 5-year PFS from 9% in patients treated with chlorambucil to 33% in patients treated with FC. Toxicity was greater with almost double the number of episodes of severe neutropenia and hospital admissions. Nausea and vomiting, alopecia, and other toxicities were also increased; however, autoimmune haemolytic anaemia was seen less frequently in the FC group. There is no OS benefit despite the improved PFS (5-year OS 61% chlorambucil vs. 54% FC) and therefore a better strategy for many patients may be the less toxic (and significantly cheaper) chlorambucil regimen as first-line therapy, reserving FC for non-responders or as second-line treatment.

Rituximab

Rituximab is a monoclonal antibody against CD20 found on the surface of B cells. It has been successfully used in other B cell malignancies and in the treatment of autoimmune disorders. It has relatively fewer side effects than

Table 4.10.14 National Cancer Institute response criteria in CLL

Criteria	Complete response	Partial response	Progressive disease
Symptoms	None		
Lymph nodes	None	>50% decrease	>50% increase or new nodes
Liver/spleen	Not palpable	>50% decrease	>50% increase
Haemoglobin (untransfused)	>11.0g/dL	>11.0 g/dL or >50% improvement from baseline	
Neutrophils	>1.5 × 10⁹/L	>1.5 × 10⁹/L or >50% improvement from baseline	
Lymphocytes	<4.0 × 10⁹/L	>50% decrease	>50% increase
Platelets	>100 × 10⁹/L	>100 × 10⁹/L or >50% improvement from baseline	
Marrow aspirate	<30% lymphocytes	May be residual lymphoid nodules	
Marrow trephine	No interstitial or nodular infiltrate		

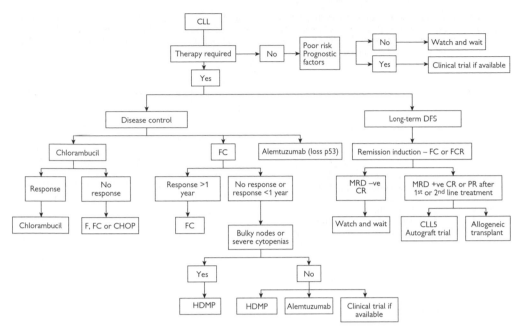

Fig 4.10.3 Overview of CLL treatment. Adapted from British Committee for Standards in Haematology Guidelines on the Diagnosis and Management of Chronic Lymphocytic Leukaemia.

conventional therapy. When given as monotherapy the response is poor. However, data from patients receiving fludarabine and rituximab showed 2-year PFS 67% and OS 93%. This compares favourably to the historical data (Byrd et al. 2005) when fludarabine alone resulted in PFS 45% and OS 81%. More recently rituximab has been combined with fludarabine and cyclophoshomide (FCR) (Hallek et al. 2008) with overall response rates of 95% for FCR and 88% for FC. Patients receiving FCR were almost twice as likely to achieve complete remissions but also experienced more side effects. The 2-year OS was not significantly different, 91% versus 88%. NICE has approved the use of rituximab with FC as first line treatment and for relapsed or refractory disease.

Steroids
Glucocorticoids are used in CLL for nodal disease alongside alemtuzumab, for patients with autoimmune complications and to improve bone marrow function prior to chemotherapy in patients with high tumour burden.

Radiotherapy
Radiotherapy is of limited use in CLL. It is sometimes used for bulky nodes causing compressive symptoms. Splenic irradiation has been used as part of therapy and in CLL1 showed equivalence with chlorambucil

Length of therapy
Chlorambucil is generally given for 6–12 months, FC for up to 6 cycles and alemtuzumab for 3–4 months. These are shortened if patients have significant side effects.

Subsequent therapy
Most patients will enter a period of active monitoring following therapy. Recent data suggests improved survival with better remission independent of the treatment used. Therefore the role of consolidation therapy may become more important. Consolidation may be regular monoclonal antibody, high-dose therapy with autologous stem cell return,

or allogenic stem cell transplantation. Use of maintenance therapy with monoclonal antibodies remains experimental and is currently limited to clinical trials, e.g. MRC CLL207.

The use of high-dose chemotherapy either alone or combined with total body irradiation is designed to provide a deeper remission by increasing tumour cell destruction. This should be considered for all patients in CR and some in PR. Return of autologous stem cells (autografting) allows chemotherapy dose intensification without rendering patients aplastic. While there are no direct comparisons of autografting versus chemotherapy, most patients do well initially but relapse appears inevitable. The improved outcomes following autografting may in part be due to patient selection. There is a treatment related mortality of 5–10% with OS approximately 80% and DFS approximately 55% at 5 years (Dreger et al. 2000).

Allogeneic stem cell transplantation can be used as consolidation and should be considered in patients with poor risk disease, i.e. those with loss of p53 or poor response to first-line therapy. The stem cells may be sourced from matched sibling or unrelated donors. Allogeneic transplantation may be curative and does offer most patients a better long-term survival. The benefits are offset by treatment toxicity and complications such as graft-versus-host disease and CMV reactivation. There is evidence for a graft-versus-leukaemia effect, which allows reduced intensity conditioning and therefore older patients can be considered for this treatment. The graft-versus-leukaemia effect is also able to overcome the effect of ZAP-70 positivity and unmutated IgVH genes on outcome. This is not seen following autologous stem cell return. Transplant related mortality is around 20–40%; however, this is improving with use of reduced intensity conditioning and better supportive care. The 6-year OS is approximately 55–60%. Alemtuzumab is commonly used prior to transplantation and this has been shown to eradicate MRD before the transplant is performed. It has been shown that patients who have received less treatment prior to allogeneic stem cell transplant have better outcomes than those who have received more treatment and therefore use of this treatment option may be best suited to consolidation therapy in first remission.

Second-line therapy

The choice of second-line therapy will depend on what first-line therapy was given and the clinical situation at relapse. In general, patients who had good and long (>12 month) remissions will usually respond again to the same treatment; however, the length of remission will often reduce with subsequent cycles of treatment. Patients refractory to chlorambucil have an overall response of 60–70% with fludarabine as monotherapy. If fludarabine is contraindicated, CHOP chemotherapy may be used. In patients who relapse <12 months after fludarabine monotherapy, FC should be used. In patients refractory or resistant to fludarabine current treatment options are alemtuzumab and/or high-dose methylprednisolone. In these patients there is an overall response of 40% with CR in 10% when treated with Campath alone. Young patients who have an early relapse after treatment should be considered for allogeneic stem cell transplant.

Treatment of complications

In patients with hypersplenism, autoimmune complications, or symptomatic splenic enlargement, splenectomy may prove useful. For autoimmune complications steroids, intravenous immunoglobulin or rituximab may be useful. Patients developing a Richter's transformation have a 40% overall response to CHOP chemotherapy but OS remains poor at <6 months.

Infectious complications remain a significant problem during the treatment of CLL. Patients with hypogammaglobulinaemia and recurrent infections benefit from prophylactic intravenous immunoglobulin infusion. All patients should have annual influenza vaccination unless contraindicated. Patients may develop bronchiectasis and in this case should receive prophylactic antibiotics. Patients receiving alemtuzumab and fludarabine should be given prophylactic co-trimoxazole, acyclovir, and antifungal medication.

Future therapies

There are many ongoing trials looking at when different therapies should be used in CLL and different combinations of agents. In addition several new monoclonal antibodies and chemotherapy drugs are under investigation.

The German CLLSG CLL7 trial is investigating whether patients with early stage (Binet A) but with high risk of progression (defined as one or more unfavourable cytogenetics; unmutated IgVH; elevated serum thymidine kinase; and short lymphocyte doubling time) benefit from immediate or delayed treatment with FCR

The optimum timing for autologous transplantation is yet to be determined. The MRC CLL5 trial is investigating the use of autologous stem cell transplant compared to no further treatment in patients with high-risk CLL reaching CR, very good PR, or nodular PR in either first- or second-line therapy.

For relapsed disease GCLLSG CLL2L is combining alemtuzumab with FC. CLL2O is a phase II trial in patients refractory to fludarabine or with 17p deletion using subcutaneous alemtuzumab and oral dexamethasone prior to allogeneic transplant or alemtuzumab maintenance.

The MRC CLL201 trial, which has closed but not yet reported, has compared the combination of fludarabine, cyclophosphamide, and mitoxantrone with or without rituximab in previously treated patients.

Novel agents

Oblimersen sodium is an antisense molecule to Bcl-2. Bcl-2 is an anti-apoptotic protein that is expressed at high levels in CLL cells. Oblimersen has been used in combination with FC and has been shown to significantly improve the rate of CR/nPR. Lenalidomide is a thalidomide derivative and is both immunomodulatory and anti-angiogenic. It has been used primarily in multiple myeloma. Phase II trials in relapsed/refractory CLL showed an OR of 47% with 9% of patients achieving CR. Flavopiridol inhibits cyclin dependent kinases and therefore can induce cell cycle arrest. It has been shown to have some activity in CLL patients

Further reading

Binet JL, Auquier A, Dighiero G, et al. A new prognostic classification of chronic lymphocytic leukaemia derived from a multivariate survival analysis. *Cancer* 1981; **48**:198–206.

Byrd JC, Rai, K, Peterson BL, et al. Addition of rituximab to fludarabine may prolong progression-free survival and overall survival in patients with previously untreated chronic lymphocytic leukemia: an updated retrospective comparative analysis of CALGB 9712 and CALGB 9011 *Blood* 2005;**105**(1):49–53.

Catovsky D, Richards S, Fooks J, et al. CLL trials in the United Kingdom. The Medical Research Council CLL Trials 1,2,3. *Leuk Lymphoma* 1991; **5**(Suppl.):105–12.

Catovsky D, Richards S, Matutes E, et al. Assessment of fludarabine plus cyclophosphamide for patients with chronic lymphocytic leukaemia (the LRF CLL4 Trial):a randomized controlled trial *Lancet* 2007; **370**:230–9.

Cheson BD, Bennett JM, Grever M, et al. National Cancer Institute-sponsored Working Group guidelines for chronic lymphocytic leukemia: revised guidelines for diagnosis and treatment. *Blood* 1996; **87**:4990–7.

Crespo M, Bosch F, Villamor N, et al. ZAP-70 expression as a surrogate for immunoglobulin-variable-region mutations in chronic lymphocytic leukemia. *N Engl J Med* 2003; **348**:1764–75.

Dohner H, Fischer K, Bentz M, et al. p53 gene deletion predicts for poor survival and non-response to therapy with purine analogs in chronic B-cell leukemias. *Blood* 1995; **85**:1580–8.

Dohner H, Stilgenbauer S, James MR, et al. 11q deletions identify a new subset of B-cell chronic lymphocytic leukaemia characterised by extensive nodal involvement and inferior prognosis. *Blood* 1997; **89**:2516–22.

Dreger P, von Neuhoff N, Sonnen R, et al. Feasibility and efficacy of autologous stem cell transplantation for poor risk CLL. *Blood* 2000b; **96**(Suppl. 1):483a.

Ghia P, Guida G, Stella S, et al. The pattern of CD38 expression defines a distinct subset of chronic lymphocytic leukemia (CLL) patients at risk of disease progression. *Blood* 2003; **101**:1262–9.

Hallek M, Langenmayer I, Nerl C, et al. Elevated serum thymidine kinase levels identify a subgroup at high risk of disease progression in early, nonsmoldering chronic lymphocytic leukemia. *Blood* 1999; **93**:1732–7.

Hallek M, Fingerle-Rowson G, Fink, A-M, et al. Immunochemotherapy with Fludarabine (F), Cyclophosphamide (C), and Rituximab (R) (FCR) Versus Fludarabine and Cyclophosphamide (FC) Improves Response Rates and Progression-Free Survival (PFS) of Previously Untreated Patients (pts) with Advanced Chronic Lymphocytic Leukemia (CLL) ASH 2008; Abstract 325.

Hamblin TJ, Davis Z, Gardiner A et al. Unmutated IgV(H) genes are associated with a more aggressive form of chronic lymphocytic leukemia. *Blood* 1999; **94**:1848–54.

Han T, Ezdinli EZ, Shimaoka K, et al. Chlorambucil vs. combined chlorambucil-corticosteroid therapy in chronic lymphocytic leukemia. *Cancer* 1973; **31**:502–8.

Houlston R, Catovsky D, Yuille M. Genetic susceptibility to chronic lymphocytic leukemia. *Leukemia* 2002; **16**:1008–14.

Jaksic B, Brugiatelli M. High dose continuous chlorambucil vs intermittent chlorambucil plus prednisone for treatment of B-CLL–IGCI CLL-01 trial. *Nouvelle Revue Française d'Hematologie* 1988; **30**:437–42.

Juliusson G, Oscier DG, Fitchett M, et al. Prognostic subgroups in B-cell chronic lymphocytic leukaemia defined by specific chromosomal abnormalities. *N Engl J Med* 1990; **323**:720–4.

Kennedy B, Rawstron A, Haynes A, et al. Eradication of detectable minimal residual disease with Campath-1H therapy results in prolonged survival in patients with refractory B-CLL. *Blood* 2001; **98**(Suppl. 1):365a.

Knauf WU, Ehlers B, Mohr B, et al. Prognostic impact of the serum levels of soluble CD23 in B-cell chronic lymphocytic leukemia. *Blood* 1997; **89**:4241–2.

Monteserrat N, Vinolas N, Reverter JC, et al. Natural history of chronic lymphocytic leukaemia: on the progression and prognosis of early stages. *Nouvelle Revue Française d'Hematologie* 1988; **30**:359–61.

Moreau EJ, Matutes E, A'Hern RP, et al. Improvement of the chronic lymphocytic leukemia scoring system with the monoclonal antibody SN8 (CD79b). *Am J Clin Pathol* 1997; **108**:378–82

Rai KI, Sawitsky A, Cronkite EP, et al. Clinical staging of chronic lymphocytic leukaemia. *Blood* 1975; **46**:219–34.

Rai K, Coutre S, Rizzeri D, et al. Efficacy and safety of alemtuzumab (Campath-1H) in refractory B-CLL patients treated on a compassionate basis. *Blood* 2001; **98**(Suppl.1):365a.

Yuille MR, Houlston RS, Catovsky D. Anticipation in familial chronic lymphocytic leukaemia. *Leukemia* 1998; **12**:1696–8.

Internet resources

BCSH Guidelines: http://www.bcshguidelines.com

Cancerbackup: http://www.cancerbackup.org.uk

Cancer Research UK: http://www.cancerresearchuk.org

Leukaemia Research Foundation: http://www.lrf.org.uk

UKCLL Forum: http://www.ukcllforum.org

NICE: guidance.nice.org.uk/cancer/haematological cancer/ leukaemia

Hairy cell leukaemia

Epidemiology and aetiology

Hairy cell leukaemia is an uncommon B-cell lymphoprolif-erative disorder. The incidence has been estimated as 2% of all forms of lymphoid leukaemias. Patients are predominantly middle aged to elderly adults with a median age of 55 years. The male to female ratio is 4.5:1. There is no known aetiology.

Clinical features

Presenting complaints can be varied and about a quarter of patients are asymptomatic and diagnosed following the incidental finding of splenomegaly or cytopenia. About a quarter may present with fullness or discomfort in the abdomen due to splenomegaly. Another quarter may present with systemic symptoms such as fatigue, weakness, weight loss, and occasionally fever and night sweats. The remaining quarter present with bleeding, bruising, and recurrent infections due to cytopenias.

Diagnosis

Peripheral blood

The main laboratory findings are of cytopenias usually affecting two to three lineages; monocytopenia is a consistent feature. The leucocyte count tends to be low except in the hairy cell variant. Blood film examination shows the characteristic hairy cells which are twice as large as normal lymphocytes with cytoplasmic projections, and an oval or kidney-shaped nucleus with loose chromatin pattern.

Bone marrow

A good length (2–3cm) bone marrow trephine biopsy is important in making the definitive diagnosis of HCL as the infiltration by hairy cells may be patchy and can be missed on small biopsies. The trephine biopsy may show an interstitial or focal pattern of infiltration, with clear zones between the cells. Reticulin is always increased and explains the frequent dry taps. Immunohistochemistry on paraffin sections using CD20 and/or DBA44 and an antibody to tartarate resistant acid phosphatase (TRAP) can be done to confirm hairy cell infiltration.

Immunophenotype

The tumour cells are SIg + and express B-cell associated antigens (CD19, CD20, CD22, CD79a but not CD79b). They are typically CD5-, CD10-, and CD23- and express CD11c (strong), CD25 (strong), FMC7, and CD103. Although no single marker is specific for distinguishing hairy cell from other B-cell lymphomas, strong expression of these markers with CD103, together with the characteristic morphological features are most useful in making the diagnosis.

Genetics

Ig heavy and light chain genes are rearranged in HCL. Although studies are limited, Ig variable region genes are mutated, consistent with a postgerminal centre cell origin. In two-thirds of patients clonal karyotypic abnormalities are present of which 40% abnormalities involve chromosome 5 (Haglund et al. 1994).

Staging and prognostic features

There is no widely agreed system for staging HCL. Historically, heavy disease burden in the form of diffuse marrow infiltration and splenomegaly, with resulting cytopenias, has had prognostic significance. However, with more effective treatment modalities, response to treatment has assumed a much greater prognostic value. The response to splenectomy assessed by an improvement in blood counts has been shown to be a reliable prognostic marker (Jansen 1981). Patients presenting with bulky abdominal lymphadenopathy respond less well to first-line therapy, as this manifestation may represent a degree of transformation of their disease (Catovsky and Foa 1990).

Treatment

Asymptomatic patients can be observed and there is no clear advantage to early treatment. Therapy is indicated only when patients develop significant cytopenias or have systemic symptoms.

The mainstay of treatment of HCL comprises the nucleoside analogues pentostatin (2′ deoxycoformycin, 2-DCF) (Catovsky et al. 1994; Grever et al. 1995) and cladribine (2-chlorodeoxyadenosine, 2-CDA) (Hoffman et al. 1997; Saven et al. 1998). Both agents induce a high rate of complete remission (>80%) and give a 10-year OS rate of 95–100% (Else et al. 2005). Patients achieving a CR with either agent show a significantly longer DFS than those attaining only a PR (>14 years versus 5.5 years). The standard regimens for the administration of these drugs are as follows.

Cladribine

0.1mg/kg/day as a continuous infusion over 7 days, to be repeated at 6 months if CR not achieved.

Alternative schedules using shorter duration of infusions have been used and shown to be equally efficacious and safe but have not been compared with the 7-day infusion in terms of long-term survival.

Pentostatin

4mg/m^2 every 2 weeks until maximal response followed by one or two more doses. Pentostatin should not be used if creatinine clearance <50mL/min and the dose should be halved if 50–60mL/min.

As both these drugs cause lymphopenia, the use of irradiated blood products and cotrimoxazole prophylaxis for *Pneumocystis jirovecii* (*carinii*) pneumonia are recommended for the duration of lymphopenia.

For severely cytopenic patients at presentation, interferon alfa can be given three times a week for a couple of months before starting treatment with purine analogues. Alternatively, G-CSF could be used in neutropenic patients at presentation or during therapy with the nucleoside analogues.

Role of splenectomy

Patients with large spleen and moderate or little bone marrow involvement may have splenectomy first and purine analogues if and when there is evidence of disease progression. It is important to wait for at least 6 months for the full benefits of splenectomy to become apparent, before starting chemotherapy. It is not clear if splenectomy as a debulking procedure improves long-term outcome.

Treatment of relapsed HCL

Eradication of minimal residual disease is possible in HCL, using cladribine followed by rituximab, but whether this leads to a reduced risk of relapse is currently not known (Ravandi et al. 2006).

The majority (70%) of relapsed patients achieve remission after retreatment with cladribine or pentostatin. While the overall response is good, the disease-free interval gets progressively shorter with each course of therapy. In one study, DFS after first-, second-, and third-line treatment with purine analogues was, 'not reached at 14 years', 7.5 years, and 4 years respectively (Else et al. 2005).

Monoclonal antibodies directed against CD20 (rituximab), CD22 (Pseudomonas exotoxin linked anti-CD22 antibody) (Kreitman et al. 2001) and CD25 have been found to be active and well tolerated in patients resistant to treatment with purine analogues. In particular, rituximab may be useful in patients who have failed to respond to two courses of cladribine.

HCL variant

HCL variant is a rare disease in which the bone marrow and spleen histology resemble the typical HCL, but the circulating cells have a round or oval nucleus with a prominent nucleolus and a moderately basophilic villous cytoplasm. Patients typically present with high WCC and monocytopaenia is absent. The cells have a B-cell phenotype and often IgG on the cell membrane, but lack the typical hairy cell antigens such as CD25 and sometimes also CD103, and are often TRAP negative. Differential diagnostic considerations include SLVL and B-PLL. The response to agents effective in typical HCL is usually poor and, as a result the median survival is significantly shorter in the HCL variant.

Further reading

Catovsky D, Foa R. *The Lymphoid Leukaemias*. London: Butterworth, 1990.

Catovsky D, Matutes E, Talavera G. Long-term results with 2' deoxycoformycin in hairy cell leukaemia. *Leuk Lymphoma* 1994; **14**(suppl 1):109–13.

Else M, Ruchlemer R, Osuji N, et al. Long remissions in hairy cell leukaemias with purine analogs: a report of 219 patients with a median follow up of 12.5 years. *Cancer* 2005; **104**: 2442–8.

Haglund U, Juliusson G, Stellan B, et al. Hairy cell leukaemia is characterised by clonal chromosomal abnormalities clustered to specific regions. *Blood* 1994; **83**:2637–45.

Grever M, Kopecky K, Foucar MK, et al. Randomised comparison of pentostatin with interferon alpfa 2a in previously untreated patients with hairy cell leukaemia. An Intergroup Study. *J Clin Oncol* 1995; **13**:974–82.

Hoffman MA, Janson D, Rose E, et al. Treatment of hairy cell leukaemia with cladribine: response, toxicity and longterm follow up. *J Clin Oncol* 1997; **15**:1138–42.

Jansen J. Splenectomy in hairy cell leukaemia. A multicenter retrospective analysis. *Cancer* 1981; **47**:2066–7.

Kreitman RJ, Wilson WH, Robbins D, et al. Efficacy of anti CD22 recombinant immunotoxin BL22 in chemotherapy resistant hairy cell leukaemia. *N Engl J Med* 2001; **345**:241–7.

Ravandi F, Jorgensen JL, O'Brien SM, et al; Eradication of minimal residual disease in hairy cell leukaemia. *Blood* 2006; **2**:4658–62.

Saven A, Burian C, Koziol JA, Piro LD. Long term follow up of hairy cell leukaemia patients after cladribine treatment. *Blood* 1998; **92**:1918–26.

Myelodysplastic syndrome: introduction

The myelodysplastic syndromes (MDSs) are a heterogeneous group of clonal haematopoietic stem cell diseases characterized by dysplasia and ineffective haematopoiesis in one or more of the major cell lineages. The dysplasia may be accompanied by an increase in the myeloblasts in the bone marrow but the number is <20%, which is the requisite threshold recommended for the diagnosis of acute myeloid leukaemia.

Epidemiology and aetiology

MDS occurs predominantly in older adults (median age 70 years), with a non-age incidence of 3 per 100,000 but rising to 20 per 100,000 over age 70 years.

The MDSs occur as primary or *de novo* disorders and an increasing number of therapy-related disease or 'secondary MDS/AML' have been recognized as a result of chemotherapy/radiation therapy for other malignant disorders. In '*de novo*' MDS, possible aetiologies include viruses and exposure to benzene/petrochemicals. Cigarette smoking increases the risk by 2-fold. Some inherited haematological disorders, such as Fanconi's anaemia are also associated with an increased incidence of MDS.

Secondary MDS/AML may represent as many as 10–15% of all MDS and AML diagnosed each year. Two major types are recognized based on the causative agents:

- Alkylating agents/radiation related: usually occur 5–6 years (range of 10–192 months) following exposure to the mutagenic agents. The risk for occurrence is related to the total cumulative dose of the alkylating agent and the age of the patient (Michaels et al. 1985).
- Topoisomerase II inhibitor related: usually has a shorter latency period and develops at a median interval of 33–34 months (range 12–130 months) from the time of institution of the implicated agents. Major agents are etoposide and teniposide but anthracyclines like doxorubicin are also implicated.

Classification

In 2001, WHO published a new classification scheme for MDS (see Table 4.10.15), incorporating the FAB classification with modifications to improve its prognostic value.

Diagnosis

The minimal initial evaluation for patients clinically suspected to have MDS includes a comprehensive history and physical examination, complete blood count with leukocyte differential which usually shows one or more cytopenias, bone marrow aspiration and biopsy with iron stain, and cytogenetic studies, erythropoietin levels, and iron studies (Greenberg et al. 2005).

Other investigations to exclude transient or reactive causes for macrocytic anaemia or isolated cytopenias such as vitamin B12 and folate levels, hepatic and renal functions, screen for viral infections/alcohol/toxins, and thyroid function should be done.

Morphological considerations

Assessment of the degree of dysplasia and hence the diagnosis of MDS requires high-quality smear preparation and staining.

The blood and marrow aspirate smears should be examined for dysplasia, the percentage of blasts and monocytes, and for ringed sideroblasts.

Cells counted as 'blasts' include myeloblasts, monoblasts and megakaryoblasts. Small dysplastic megakaryocytes are not blasts and erythroid precursors are also not counted as blasts except in rare cases of 'erythroleukaemia' in which primitive erythroblasts account for the majority of the cells. In myelomonocytic proliferations, promonocytes are included as 'blast equivalents'. Substitution of the percent of CD34+ cells determined by flow cytometry for a visual blast count on morphology is misleading and is discouraged.

Dyserythropoiesis is manifested principally by alterations in the nucleus including budding, internuclear bridging, karyorrhexis, multinuclearity, and megaloblastoid changes; cytoplasmic features include ring sideroblasts, vacuolization and periodic acid–Schiff positivity, either diffuse or granular.

Dysgranulopoiesis is characterized primarily by small size, nuclear hypolobulation (pseudo Pelger–Huët), and hypersegmentation, hypogranularity, and pseudo-Chediak–Higashi granules.

Megakaryocyte dysplasia may be characterized by hypolobulated micromegakaryocytes, non-lobulated nuclei in megakaryocytes of all sizes, and multiple widely separated nuclei.

The marrow is usually hypercellular or normocellular and the cytopenias result from ineffective haematopoiesis.

A bone marrow biopsy, although not always necessary, can provide valuable diagnostic and prognostic information such as disruption of normal marrow architecture in the form of abnormal localization of immature precursors (ALIPs).

Immunophenotypic considerations

Enumeration of CD 34+ cells by flow cytometry provides diagnostic and prognostic information.

No single abnormality is specific for MDS, but an abnormal light scatter of dysplastic cells, abnormal antigen density, loss of antigens and dys-synchronous expression of antigens that are normally coexpressed during myeloid maturation have all been reported in MDS and may even correlate with the grade of the disease (Stetler-Stevenson et al. 2001)

Cytogenetics and molecular aspects

The importance of cytogenetic abnormalities in the prediction of survival and in assessing the risk of transformation to acute leukaemia is well known and cytogenetic studies have been included in most of the classification and predictive scoring systems developed for MDS (Greenberg et al. 1997). Clonality in MDS is demonstrated by deletional defects, i.e. monosomy 7 occurring in at least two of 30 cells and additional defects, i.e. trisomy 8 occurring in one or more of 30 cells examined. Clonal chromosomal abnormalities are detected in 40–70% of cases of *de novo* MDS cases. Deletions of part or all of chromosome 5 and/or 7 and complex chromosomal abnormalities account for 90% of karyotypic changes in therapy related MDSs (t-MDS).

The *de novo* '5q- syndrome' is recognized as a specific type of MDS which occurs primarily in women, is characterized by normal or increased platelet counts, megakaryocytes with hypolobulated nuclei, refractory macrocytic anaemia, an isolated del(5q) chromosome abnormality, and a favourable clinical course.

Other cytogenetic abnormalities with prognostic significance are included in the IPSS scoring system.

Molecular abnormalities involved in the pathogenesis of MDS are multiple and incompletely understood. However, some of the mechanisms resulting in an imbalance between apoptosis and proliferation pathways are:
- Uncontrolled proliferation: RAS (NRAS), JAK2, PDGRFβ mutations
- Loss of apoptotic mechanisms: p53 mutation
- Differentiation block: c-fms pathway, G-CSF receptor mutations
- Constitutive activation of tyrosine kinases: flt 3 pathway
- Epigenetic mechanisms: methylation of genes like p15, e-cadherin
- Aberrant immune surveillance: increased T regulatory cells
- Aberrant gene 5q-: block of ribosomal protein RPS14 expression.

Specific diagnostic issues

Reactive or transient cytopenias
- Morphologic dysplasia is not specific to MDS
- Reactive dysplasia is seen in conditions like megaloblastic anaemia, exposure to toxins like arsenic and alcohol, and after cytotoxic and growth factor therapy.
- Dyserythropoiesis is common in situations of 'stressed haemopoiesis' like haemolysis, recovery from cytotoxic therapy or transplantation
- Cytogenetic abnormalities or raised percentage of blasts are uncommon.

Unexplained cytopenias
- Unexplained persistent cytopenias with little or no morphologic dysplasia can be a challenging problem and can be seen commonly in older adults.
- If not associated with a clonal cytogenetic abnormality, they should be monitored at regular intervals.
- A small proportion will evolve into MDS- morphologically and cytogenetically

Hypocellular MDS
- A minority of MDS patients have a hypocellular bone marrow (<30% cellularity in patients <60 years old; <20% cellularity in patients ≥60 years old).
- Differentiating between hypocellular MDS and aplastic anaemia (AA) can be very difficult. Features favouring MDS are neutrophils with pseudo Pelger–Huët nuclei and/or hypogranular cytoplasm in blood smears and dysplastic granulopoiesis and megakaryocytopoiesis and normal or raised blasts in the bone marrow.
- Abnormal antigen expression of CD34$^+$ cells measured by multiparameter flow cytometry, the number of HbF containing erythroblasts, and the percentage of Ki-67$^+$ cells, have also been reported to be helpful in separation of AA from MDS.
- Although the identification of a clonal chromosomal abnormality at the time of presentation is generally considered as indicative of MDS, patients with clonal chromosomal abnormalities have been included in some series of AA.
- It is necessary to exclude other diseases with hypocellular bone marrow specimens that may masquerade clinically as AA or MDS, particularly hypocellular AML, hairy cell leukaemia and large granular lymphocytosis.

Myelodysplastic syndrome/myeloproliferative disorders (MDS/MPD)
The MDS/MPD category includes clonal myeloid disorders that have both dysplastic and proliferative features at presentation.
Disorders included in this category of WHO classification are:
- Chronic myelomonocytic leukaemia (CMML)
- Atypical chronic myeloid leukaemia
- Juvenile myelomonocytic leukaemia (JMML)
- Myelodysplastic/myeloproliferative disease, unclassifiable

Table 4.10.15 WHO classification of MDS

Disease	Peripheral blood criteria	Bone marrow criteria
Refractory anaemia	Anaemia, no or rare blasts	Erythroid dysplasia alone, <5% blasts, <15% ringed sideroblasts
Refractory anaemia with ringed sideroblasts	Anaemia, no blasts	Erythroid dysplasia alone, <5% blasts, >15% ringed sideroblasts
Refractory cytopenia with multilineage dysplasia	Cytopenias (bicytopenia or pancytopenia), no or rare blasts, no Auer rods, <1 x 10^9/L monocytes	Dysplasia in >10% of cells in >2 myeloid cell lines, <5% blasts, no Auer rods, <15% ringed sideroblasts
Refractory cytopenia with multilineage dysplasia and ringed sideroblasts	Cytopenias (bicytopenia or pancytopenia), no or rare blasts, no Auer rods, <1 x 10^9/L monocytes	Dysplasia in >10% of cells in >2 myeloid cell lines, <5% blasts, no Auer rods, >15% ringed sideroblasts
Refractory anaemia with excess blasts type 1 (RAEB I)	Cytopenias, <5% blasts, no Auer rods, <1 x 10^9/L monocytes	Unilineage or multilineage dysplasia, 5–9% blasts, no Auer rods
Refractory anaemia with excess blasts type 2 (RAEB II)	Cytopenias, 5–19% blasts, no Auer rods, <1 x 10^9/L monocytes	Unilineage or multilineage dysplasia, 10–19% blasts, occasional Auer rods
Myelodysplastic syndrome unclassified	Cytopenias, no or rare blasts, no Auer rods	Unilineage dysplasia in granulocytes or megakaryocytes, <5% blasts, no Auer rods
Myelodysplastic syndrome associated with isolated del(5q)	Anaemia, <5% blasts, platelet count normal to increased	Normal-to-increased megakaryocytes with hypolobulated nuclei, <5% blasts, no Auer rods, isolated del (5q)

Further reading

Greenberg P, Cox C, LeBeau MM, *et al*. International Scoring System for evaluating prognosis in myelodysplastic syndromes. *Blood* 1997; **89**:2079–88.

Greenberg PL, NCCN panel. National Comprehensive Cancer Network (NCCN) Clinical Practice Guidelines in Oncology-v.1.2005: Myelodysplastic syndromes (Sept 2004) Vol 2005. Chicago, IL: NCCN, 2005.

Michaels SD, McKenna RW, Arthur DC, *et al*; Therapy-related acute myeloid leukaemia and myelodysplastic syndrome: a clinical and morphologic study of 65 cases. *Blood* 1985; **65**:1364–72.

Stetler-Stevenson M, Arthur DC, Jabbour N, *et al*. Diagnostic utility of flow cytometric immunophenotyping in myelodysplastic syndromes. *Blood* 2001; **98**:979–87.

Myelodysplastic syndrome: clinical features, staging, and prognosis

Clinical features

- Signs and symptoms of the disease are those associated with cytopenias, i.e. symptoms of anaemia, bleeding/petechiae with thrombocytopenia, or infections because of neutropenia.
- Many patients can be asymptomatic and MDS is diagnosed on routine screening blood tests.
- Infection remains the principal cause of death in patients with MDS. Although fungal, viral, and mycobacterial infections can occur, they are rare in the absence of concurrent administration of immunosuppressive agents.
- Autoimmune manifestations can be seen in about 14% of MDS patients—the most common are cutaneous vasculitis and monoarticular arthritis.
- Acute febrile neutrophilic dermatosis (Sweet's syndrome) is the most common vasculitic condition in MDS.
- Although connective tissue disorders such as relapsing polychondritis, polymyalgia rheumatica, Raynaud's phenomenon, and Sjögren's syndrome, inflammatory bowel disease, pyoderma gangrenosum, and glomerulonephritis have been reported in association with MDS, a causal relationship has not been established.

Staging and prognosis

- The International Prognostic Scoring System (IPSS) was published in 1997 (Greenberg et al. 1997) In this system, percentage of marrow blasts, specific cytogenetic abnormalities, and number of cytopenias were used in combination to define four risk groups for overall survival and AML evolution: low, intermediate-1, intermediate-2, and high (see Table 4.10.16).
- The overall median survival was 5.7, 3.5, 1.2, and 0.4 years for the four groups respectively (see Fig. 4.10.4).
- The time for disease in 25% of patients in each of the four risk groups to evolve into acute leukaemia was 9.4, 3.3, 1.1, and 0.2 years respectively.
- Although survival of high-risk patients was independent of age, survival of low-risk patients was strongly dependant on age, with median survivals of 11.8, 4.8, and 3.9 years in patients <60, >60, and >70 years of age respectively.
- Most patients with MDS, even intermediate-2 risk group, die because of the consequences of bone marrow failure rather than transformation to AML, while many patients with IPSS high-risk disease would be considered by some already to have AML.
- Other factors have been shown to add significant prognostic information to that provided by the IPSS. One of these is the mutation and/or loss of the heterozygosity of the tumour suppressor gene p53. This defect is commonly noted in MDS, especially in older patients and following exposure to alkylating agents and is associated with complex karyotypic changes, an increased tendency to evolve into AML, reduced responses to chemotherapy, and shorter OS (Christiansen et al. 2001). Other prognostic factors which have been studied are:

  Transfusion dependence (Malcovati et al. 2007)

  CD34 positivity of bone marrow nucleated cells

  Increased expression of the Wilms' tumour gene

Table 4.10.16 The IPSS scoring system for MDS

Prognostic variable	Score value				
	0	0.5	1.0	1.5	2.0
Bone marrow blasts %	<5	5–10	–	11–20	21–30
Karyotype*	Good	Intermediate	Poor		
Cytopenias**	0 or 1	2 or 3			

Scores for risk groups are as follows: Low: 0, INT-1: 0.5–1.0, INT-2: 1.5–2.0; High >2.5

* Karyotype:
- Good: normal, -Y, del(5q), del(20q)
- Poor: complex (>3 abnormalities), or chromosome 7 anomalies
- Intermediate: other abnormalities

**Cytopenias: defined as Hb <10g/dL, absolute neutrophil count <1.5 x 10⁹/L and platelet count <100 x 10⁹/L.

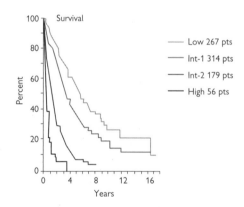

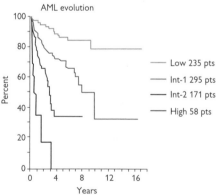

Fig 4.10.4 IPSS score predicts clinical outcome in MDS. Kaplan–Meier curves of patient survival (top panel) and freedom from acute myeloid leukemia (AML) evolution (bottom panel) in patients with myelodysplastic syndrome (MDS) according to their classification by the International Prognostic Scoring System (IPSS) for MDS. Reprinted with permission from Greenberg et al. International scoring system for evaluating prognosis in myelodysplastic syndromes. *Blood* 1997: **89**:2079–88 (see also colour plate section).

Increased serum beta-2 microglobulin concentration

Decreased platelet mass

Abnormal localization of immature precursors (ALIPs).

Further reading

Christiansen DH, Andersen MK, Pederson-Bjergaard J. Mutations with loss of heterozygosity of p53 are common in therapy related myelodysplasia and acute myeloid leukaemia after exposure to alkylating agents and significantly associated with deletion or loss of 5q, a complex karyotype, and a poor prognosis. *J Clin Oncol* 2001; **19**:1405–13.

Greenberg P, Cox C, LeBeau MM, *et al.* International Scoring System for evaluating prognosis in myelodysplastic syndromes. *Blood* 1997; **89**:2079–88.

Malcovati L, Germing U, Kuendgen A, *et al.* Time dependent prognostic scoring system for predicting survival and leukaemic evolution in myelodysplastic syndromes. *J Clin Oncol* 2007; **25**:3503–10.

Myelodysplastic syndrome: treatment

The IPSS score at diagnosis, blood transfusion dependence, bone marrow cellularity and comorbidities of the patient guide management of MDS. Supportive care has previously been the standard of care for patients with MDS and may still be the only care appropriate for some. However, the following key advances in MDS emphasize better outcomes with state-of-the-art treatment leading to supportive care being an important scaffold in the definitive treatment of MDS.

Key advances
- The FDA approval of three drugs, azacitidine, decitabine and lenalidomide, for the treatment of MDS.
- Recognition of transfusion dependence and iron overload as independent adverse prognostic factors that affect overall and leukaemia-free survival (Malcovati et al. 2005).
- The demonstration that treatment of anaemia with erythropoietin stimulating agents (ESAs) or immunosuppression lowers the risk of progression to AML.
- Evidence that the treatment of iron overload also significantly increases overall survival.

Supportive care
This consists of monitoring blood counts, blood product replacement, treatment of infections, and iron chelation.

Indications for supportive care
- Patients not suitable for definitive treatment.
- During and pending a response to definitive treatment.
- Failure to respond or loss of response to active drugs.

Monitoring blood counts
- In low-risk MDS, monitoring blood counts for disease progression may be the only requirement.

Platelet transfusions
- Bleeding may be due to thrombocytopenia or platelet dysfunction (even with normal counts).
- Treatment with platelet transfusions to maintain a threshold of 10×10^9/L if the patient is not septic or bleeding, 20×10^9/L if septic, and higher if surgery is contemplated.
- Immune thrombocytopenia responsive to steroids or danazole may occur with MDS.

Blood transfusions
- Eighty per cent of patients are anaemic at presentation.
- Correctable causes such as iron, vitamin B12, or folate deficiency, thyroid and liver dysfunction, autoimmune haemolytic anaemia, PNH (paroxysmal nocturnal haemoglobinuria) should be excluded.
- Blood transfusions are usually introduced for symptomatic anaemia (Hb ≤8g/dL; higher if there is a history of cardiac impairment).

Iron chelation therapy
- In low-risk MDS, where long-term transfusion therapy is anticipated, iron chelation is recommended when ferritin >1000mcg/L or 25 units of blood have been transfused (Bowen et al. 2003).
- Ophthalmological and audiometric review are prerequisites to commencing desferrioxamine or deferasirox as both can cause sensorineural hearing loss and lenticular opacities.

- Creatinine clearance of at least 60mL/min is necessary before commencing deferasirox
- Desferrioxamine 20–40mg/kg subcutaneously over 12 hours, 5–7 days a week is commenced to achieve a target ferritin of <1000mcg/L. The dose of desferrioxamine is reduced to <25mg/kg once ferritin levels are <2000mcg/L (Bowen et al. 2003).
- Vitamin C 100–200mg daily orally started a month after desferrioxamine enables the iron chelation process.
- Deferasirox (Exjade®, Novartis) an oral iron chelator is commenced at 20–30mg/kg/day (Cappellini et al. 2006; Porter et al. 2008). Renal and liver function monitoring is recommended with the use of deferasirox.

Management of infections
- There is no evidence for a role for prophylactic antibiotics or antifungal drugs.
- G-CSF therapy in severe neutropenia may be used to maintain a neutrophil count $>1 \times 10^9$/L.
- Episodes of neutropenic sepsis are treated as emergencies according to local protocols.

Differentiation therapy
Erythropoietin stimulating agents
- Recombinant human erythropoietin (EPO) or darbepoietin alpha (Aranesp®, its hypersialyated derivative with a longer half-life) can be used to stimulate erythropoiesis in MDS.
- Factors predicting EPO responsiveness include <10% bone marrow blasts; Low or Int-1 IPSS, serum EPO levels <200U/L, transfusion independence, and a short time between diagnosis and treatment (Park et al. 2008).
- The presence of del 5q- with or without additional cytogenetic abnormalities reduces response duration from a mean of 24 months to 12 months but does not affect response rates (Kelaidi et al. 2008; Park et al. 2008).
- Treatment of anaemia with ESAs reduces the risk of progression to AML, and responders to EPO/G-CSF combination have a longer overall survival of 53 months compared with 23 months in non-responders (Balleari et al. 2006).
- Patients are selected on the basis of the ESA predictive score: see Table 4.10.17 (Hellstrom-Lindberg et al. 2003).
- EPO/darbepoietin may be commenced for symptomatic anaemia at Hb between 9–11g/dL
- If the Hb is lower than this, initial transfusion support in addition to an ESA may be necessary.

Table 4.10.17 Predictive score for treatment of MDS with GCSF and EPO

Parameter	Value	Score
Serum erythropoietin	<500U/L	0
	>500U/L	1
Blood transfusions	<2U/month	0
	>2U/month	1

Predicted response rate pre-treatment: score 0=74% score 1=23%, and score 2=7%.

- A front-loading schedule utilizes 30,000–60,000 units of erythropoietin SC per week initially for 6–8 weeks aiming for a target haemoglobin of 12g/dL. If the increment in Hb is <1g/dL in this time frame, GCSF 300mcg SC twice a week is added.
- Lower doses of GCSF 150mcg SC once or twice a week may be sufficient.
- If no response is obtained in a further 8 weeks a de-escalation of EPO should ensue.
- On obtaining a response EPO should be continued at the same dose until the target Hb is reached before lowering the dose.
- Darbepoietin is administered less frequently (weekly to once every 3 weeks) with doses between 150–300mcg/week.
- It is effective in MDS even in patients who have failed EPO therapy. Dosing starts at 300mcg SC once every 1–3 weeks accompanied by G-CSF weekly. The median time to response is usually 6–8 weeks.
- Ferritin levels in ESA treated patients need to be maintained above 100ng/L by parenteral rather than oral supplementation.
- Loss of response to ESAs may accompany disease progression. Variability in EPO manufacturing is a historic cause of loss of response with reticulocytopenia.

Cytokines
- The recombinant human GSF has been used in MDS in combination with erythropoietin or to support neutropenic patients with a neutrophil count <0.5 × 10⁹/L.
- It may be used in neutropenic sepsis.
- Though supportive data is lacking, it may be used to prevent infections in patients who have had previous severe or life threatening infections.

Immunosuppressive treatment (IST)
Autoimmune suppression of haemopoiesis due to cytotoxic T lymphocytes occurs in approximately 50% of patients with MDS (Kochenderfer et al. 2002). This immune component is a potential therapeutic target particularly in hypoplastic MDS.

Antithymocyte globulin with cyclosporine
- Antithymocyte globulin (ATG) with or without cyclosporine evokes haematological improvement in a third of patients (Molldrem et al. 2002; Killick et al. 2003).
- Clinical features predicting response to immune suppressive therapy (IST) include (Saunthararajah et al. 2003):
  Age <60 years
  <6 months of RBC transfusion dependence
  Hypocellular marrow.
  The presence of a PNH clone.
  HLA DR15 phenotype.
- ATG is administered via a central line after a test dose (1mg of ATG in 100mL of normal saline over 1 hour).
- Severe anaphylaxis is a contraindication to treatment with ATG.
- Horse ATG (lymphoglobulin) 15mg/kg/day for 5 days or rabbit ATG (thymoglobulin) 3.75mg/kg/day for 5 days are equivalent treatment doses infused daily over 12–18 hours.

- Reverse barrier nursing, premedication with hydrocortisone and piriton, and daily platelet transfusion to maintain platelets at >30 × 10⁹/L is necessary.
- Prednisolone 1mg/kg is given from day 5 of ATG until day 14 and is rapidly tapered over 5 days to prevent serum sickness.
- Serum sickness manifesting as urticarial rash and joint pains may occur 7–10 days later and responds to 100mg IV hydrocortisone 6-hourly.
- Ciclosporin 5mg/kg is commenced on day 14 after starting ATG to achieve target trough levels of 150–250µg/ml. The median time to a response is 3 months.

Immunomodulatory drugs (IMIDS)
- Thalidomide 100–400mg orally daily yields erythroid responses in 13% of patients, but not neutrophil or platelet responses. Neurotoxicity, fatigue, constipation, and sedation are dose limiting.
- Lenalidomide (derivative of thalidomide CC5013, Celgene Revlimid®) is particularly effective in treating patients with an interstitial deletion of 5q. It is FDA approved for low or Int-1 transfusion dependent MDS with a del 5q.
- Dosing: 10mg daily or 10mg daily for 21 out of 28 days orally as a cycle of treatment. Recurrent cycles of treatment are necessary. Lower dose scheduling of 5mg daily is being studied.
- Teratogenicity is a potential problem and pregnancy tests/contraception are advised in patients with reproductive potential.
- Responses: three trials have established the efficacy of lenalidomide in transfusion dependent MDS who had failed or had a poor predictive score for EPO MDS (List et al. 2005, 2006; Raza et al. 2008).
- The best responses are in patients with a deletion 5q (some with additional cytogenetic abnormalities) who experienced 76% erythroid response and 67% transfusion independence. Accompanying cytogenetic responses occurred in 73%.
- The incidence of response is lower (43% erythroid response) in transfusion dependent Low/Int-1 MDS without del 5q.
- The median duration of response is 2 years.
- Myelosuppression is the predominant toxicity with grade 3 or more neutropenia and thrombocytopenia seen in >50% of patients. GCSF administration may ameliorate this.
- Predictors of response to lenalidomide:
  Interstitial deletion of 5q
  Myelosuppression in the first 8 weeks of treatment
  RBC transfusions <4 units in 8 weeks
  Low-risk IPSS
  Age <70 years
  Low ECOG score
  Cytogenetic response predicts prolonged survival and reduced risk of leukaemic transformation

Epigenetic therapies
Epigenetic changes such as methylation of promoters of genes or deacetylation of histones modulate gene expression reversibly. As these changes are frequent in all cancers

including MDS, they offer a therapeutic target. Epigenetic therapies include the both the DNA methyl transferase inhibitors (DNMTI) and histone deacetylase (HDAC) inhibitors.

DNA methyltransferase inhibitors

- 5-azacytidine-Vidaza ® (Pharmion) and its analogue 5-aza-2'deoxycytidine Decitabine ® (Dacogen) are emerging as first-line therapies for Int-2 and higher MDS.
- FDA approval for 5-azacytidine includes the treatment of all subtypes of MDS whereas 5-aza-2' deoxycytidine has been approved for IPSS Int-1 or higher MDS.
- 5-azacytidine is a pyrimidine analogue that is chemically synthesized and incorporates into both DNA and RNA.
- It can be administered intravenously or subcutaneously.
- The recommended dose is $75mg/m^2$ daily for 7 days every 28 days (constitutes 1 cycle) for at least 4–6 cycles of treatment.
- Local skin reactions (treated with topical steroid cream), and nausea and vomiting (premedicate with granisetron/odansetron) are the commonest side effects.
- Almost all patients develop grade 3–4 neutropenia.
- The transfusion requirements particularly for platelets may increase in the first few cycles and then decrease once a response is obtained.
- Medians of 4–6 cycles of treatment are needed for a response. An increase in platelet counts may be the first sign of a response. Once a response is seen therapy is continued indefinitely.
- In the CALGB 9221 phase III randomized controlled trial 5-azacytidine was compared with best supportive care. Cross over of patients into the 5-azacytidine arm was permitted. An overall response of 60% with 7% CR 16% PR, and 37% haematological improvement (HI) was observed (Silverman et al. 2002).
- The median duration of response was 18 months and a significant disease modifying activity was observed. The time to progression to AML was prolonged by 6 months.
- A phase III randomized controlled trial comparing 5-azacytidine to physicians' choice treatment (best supportive care, or low dose cytarabine $20mg/m^2$ SC for 14 days every 28 days or AML induction chemotherapy) for high-risk MDS (IPSS Int-2 or higher) showed overall survival was significantly prolonged to 24.4 months for patients treated with 5-azacytidine whereas for the comparator arm this was 15 months. The time to progression to AML was prolonged to 26.1 months with 5-azacytidine and transfusion independence was observed in 45% of patients.
- 5-azacytidine should be considered as first-line treatment for patients with high risk MDS.
- Decitabine is an analogue of azacytidine that only incorporates into DNA.
- A low-dose schedule of 20 mg/m^2 IV for 5 days every 4 weeks yielded promising results with 32% CR, 1% PR, and 13% HI in phase I/II studies (Hagop et al. 2007; Kantarjian et al. 2007).
- For both drugs altered doses, schedules of administration and synergistic combinations are being studied.

Histone deacetylase inhibitors

- Chromatin with acetylated (negatively charged) histones is in the open configuration and transcriptionally active.

Deacetylation of histones leads to chromatin being tightly configured and inaccessible to the transcriptional machinery. HDACs prevent deacetylation of histones enabling transcription of genes. The exact mechanism by which this group of drugs is effective in MDS is unclear.

- Sodium valproate, sodium phenyl butyrate and arsenic trioxide and suberoylanilide hydroxamic acid (SAHA) are examples of HDAC inhibitors.
- They have been used as single agents and in combination therapy with DNMTI and Al transretinoic acids (Garcia-Manero et al. 2006; Vey et al. 2006).
- Whilst responses have been achieved, their exact place in the treatment of MDS is to be determined.

Combination therapy

- HDAC inhibitors and DNMTIs are synergistic in their activity *in vitro*.
- *In vivo* combinations of 5-azacytidine and sodium phenyl butyrate, 5-azacytidine with sodium valproate and ATRA and decitabine with sodium valproate and ATRA show promise in phase I/II trials (Gore et al. 2006; Soriano et al. 2007).
- Further randomized trials comparing each agent alone versus an HDAC DNMTI combination are in progress.

Novel therapies

Drugs targeting crucial molecular abnormalities such as N-RAS mutations, PDGFR mutations, and apoptotic pathways are in early trials.

Farnesyl transferase inhibitor

- Farnesylation of RAS enables translocation to the plasma membrane, which is specifically inhibited by a farnesyl transferase inhibitor such as Tipifarnib ® (Johnson and Johnson). In phase I studies, 3/28 patients responded at doses of 600mg orally twice a day for 4 out of 6 weeks. Further evaluation of 82 patients showed that 32% responded (Fenaux et al. 2007).
- Responses were independent of the RAS mutation status.

Imatinib

- Imatinib mesylate (Glivec ® Novartis), a tyrosine kinase inhibitor, is useful in the treatment of chronic myelomonocytic leukaemia associated with eosinophilia, characterized by the presence of a t(5;12) (q33; p13) with an ETV6-PDGFR mutation.
- Treatment with imatinib 400mg orally daily led to clinical responses in 4 weeks followed by molecular responses (Apperley et al. 2002).

Others

- MAPK inhibitors, and TLK 199, a glutathione derivative that can induce haemopoietic differentiation are amongst several drugs in trials.

Chemotherapy

- Conventional AML induction type chemotherapy is used for remission induction in good performance, high-risk MDS particularly when consolidation with an allogeneic stem cell transplant is possible.
- Daunorubicin combined with cytarabine with or without etoposide (DA or ADE) or fludarabine, high dose cytarabine; GCSF and idarubicin (FLAG/FLAG Ida) (Parker et al. 1997) have been used.
- Prolonged time to neutrophil recovery has been a problem with FLAG/Ida and often associated with morbidity such as invasive fungal aspergillosis.

- The role of these chemotherapies and various novel agents is being studied in the NCRN AML 16 trial (see 'Internet resources') open to patients at least 60 years old with RAEB II MDS or AML

Stem cell transplantation

- Despite more treatment options becoming available to patients with MDS, haemopoietic stem cell transplantation remains the only modality with a curative potential.
- Non-myeloablative stem cell transplants that are immunosuppressive rather than myeloablative have enabled transplants in this elderly group of patients.
- For low risk or Int-1 MDS, delaying transplantation until progression and for Int-2 or higher MDS early transplant, are associated with the best life expectancy (Cutler et al. 2004).
- The non-relapse mortality using fludarabine 125mg, busulphan 8mg, and campath 100mg is approximately 10% in the first 100 days and 1-year OS 70% (Ho et al. 2004).
- OS at 3 years varies from 30% for high-risk to 60% for low-risk MDS. Increased risk of relapse, graft-versus-host disease, and infections contribute to morbidity and mortality.
- The AML 16 trial is studying the role of non-myeloablative transplants in elderly patients.

Treatment algorithm

- Risk stratify patient based on their IPSS, transfusion requirement, PS, and comorbidities. Institute supportive care as necessary.
- Low-risk patient if bone marrow hypocellular and <60 years, HLA DR15 or good PS, consider ATG/ciclosporin.
- Normocellular, becoming transfusion dependent, assess EPO/GCSF predictive score to determine a trial of EPO.
- Del 5q- with or without additional cytogenetic abnormalities, lenalidomide is the treatment of choice. Consider lenalidomide for low or Int-1 MDS who have failed EPO therapy.
- Int-2 or higher MDS, treatment with 5-azacytidine should be considered (may be followed by consolidation with an allograft).
- In young and fit patients, AML induction chemotherapy consolidated by an allogeneic stem cell transplant should be considered.
- Eligible patients should be considered for trials of novel agents.

Further reading

Apperley JF, Gardembas M, Melo JV, et al. Response to imatinib mesylate in patients with chronic myeloproliferative diseases with rearrangements of the platelet-derived growth factor receptor beta. N Engl J Med 2002; 347(7):481–7.

Balleari E, Rossi E, Clavio M, et al. Erythropoietin plus granulocyte colony-stimulating factor is better than erythropoietin alone to treat anemia in low-risk myelodysplastic syndromes: results from a randomized single-centre study. Ann Hematol 2006; 85(3):174–80.

Bowen D, Culligan D, Jowitt S, et al. Guidelines for the diagnosis and therapy of adult myelodysplastic syndromes. Br J Haematol 2003; 120(2):187–200.

Cappellini MD, Cohen A, Piga A, et al. A phase 3 study of deferasirox (ICL670), a once-daily oral iron chelator, in patients with beta-thalassemia. Blood 2006; 2107(9):3455–62.

Cutler CS, Lee SJ, Greenberg P, et al. A decision analysis of allogeneic bone marrow transplantation for the myelodysplastic syndromes: delayed transplantation for low-risk myelodysplasia is associated with improved outcome. Blood 2004; 104(2):579–85.

Fenaux P, Raza A, Mufti GJ, et al. A multicenter phase 2 study of the farnesyltransferase inhibitor tipifarnib in intermediate- to high-risk myelodysplastic syndrome. Blood 2007; 109(10):4158–63.

Garcia-Manero G, Kantarjian HM, Sanchez-Gonzalez B, et al. Phase 1/2 study of the combination of 5-aza-2'-deoxycytidine with valproic acid in patients with leukemia. Blood 2006; 108(10):3271–9.

Gore SD, Baylin S, Sugar E, et al. Combined DNA methyltransferase and histone deacetylase inhibition in the treatment of myeloid neoplasms. Cancer Res 2006; 66(12):6361–9.

Hagop M. Kantarjian SOB, Jianqin Shan, et al. Update of the decitabine experience in higher risk myelodysplastic syndrome and analysis of prognostic factors associated with outcome. Cancer 2007; 109(2):265–73.

Hellstrom-Lindberg E, Gulbrandsen N, Lindberg G, et al. A validated decision model for treating the anaemia of myelodysplastic syndromes with erythropoietin + granulocyte colony-stimulating factor: significant effects on quality of life. Br J Haematol 2003; 120(6):1037–46.

Ho AY, Pagliuca A, Kenyon M, et al. Reduced-intensity allogeneic hematopoietic stem cell transplantation for myelodysplastic syndrome and acute myeloid leukemia with multilineage dysplasia using fludarabine, busulphan, and alemtuzumab (FBC) conditioning. Blood 2004; 104(6):1616–23.

Kantarjian H, Issa JP, Rosenfeld CS, DiPersio J, et al. Decitabine improves patient outcomes in myelodysplastic syndromes: results of a phase III randomized study. Cancer 2006; 106(8):1794–803.

Kantarjian H, Oki Y, Garcia-Manero G, et al. Blood results of a randomized study of 3 schedules of low-dose decitabine in higher-risk myelodysplastic syndrome and chronic myelomonocytic leukaemia. 2007; Blood 109(1):52–7.

Kelaidi C, Park S, Brechignac S, et al. Treatment of myelodysplastic syndromes with 5q deletion before the lenalidomide era; the GFM experience with EPO and thalidomide. Leuk Res 2008; 32:1049–53.

Killick SB, Mufti G, Cavenagh JD, et al. A pilot study of antithymocyte globulin (ATG) in the treatment of patients with 'low-risk' myelodysplasia. Br J Haematol 2003; 120(4):679–84.

Kochenderfer JN, Kobayashi S, Wieder ED, et al. Loss of T-lymphocyte clonal dominance in patients with myelodysplastic syndrome responsive to immunosuppression. Blood 2002; 100(10):3639–45.

List A, Kurtin S, Roe DJ, et al. Efficacy of lenalidomide in myelodysplastic Syndromes. N Engl J Med 2005; 352(6):549–57.

List A, Dewald G, Bennett J, et al. Lenalidomide in the myelodysplastic syndrome with chromosome 5q deletion. N Engl J Med 2006; 355(14):1456–65.

Malcovati L, Porta MGD, Pascutto C, I, et al. Prognostic factors and life expectancy in myelodysplastic syndromes classified according to WHO criteria: A basis for clinical decision making. J Clin Oncol 2005; 23(30):7594–603.

Molldrem JJ, Leifer E, Bahceci E, et al. Antithymocyte globulin for treatment of the bone marrow failure associated with myelodysplastic syndromes. Ann Intern Med 2002; 137(3):156–63.

Park S, Grabar S, Kelaidi C, et al. Predictive factors of response and survival in myelodysplastic syndrome treated with erythropoietin and G-CSF: the GFM experience. Blood 2008; 111(2):574–82.

Parker JE, Pagliuca A, Mijovic A, et al. Fludarabine, cytarabine, G-CSF and idarubicin (FLAG-IDA) for the treatment of poor-risk myelodysplastic syndromes and acute myeloid leukaemia. Br J Haematol 1997; 99(4):939–44.

Porter J, Galanello R, Saglio G, et al. Relative response of patients with myelodysplastic syndromes and other transfusion-dependent anaemias to deferasirox (ICL670): a 1-yr prospective study. Eur J Haematol 2008; 80(2):168–76.

Raza A, Reeves JA, Feldman EJ, et al. Phase 2 study of lenalidomide in transfusion-dependent, low-risk, and intermediate-1 risk myelodysplastic syndromes with karyotypes other than deletion 5q. *Blood* 2008; **111**(1):86–93.

Saunthararajah Y, Nakamura R, Wesley R, A simple method to predict response to immunosuppressive therapy in patients with myelodysplastic syndrome *Blood* 2003; **102**(8):3025–7.

Silverman LR, Demakos EP, Peterson BL, *et al*. Randomized controlled trial of azacitidine in patients with the myelodysplastic syndrome: a study of the Cancer and Leukemia Group. *Br J Clin Oncol* 2002; **20**(10):2429–40.

Soriano AO, Yang H, Faderl S, *et al*. Safety and clinical activity of the combination of 5-azacytidine, valproic acid, and all-trans retinoic acid in acute myeloid leukemia and myelodysplastic syndrome. *Blood* 2007; **110**(7):2302–8.

Vey N, Bosly A, Guerci A, *et al*. Arsenic trioxide in patients with myelodysplastic syndromes: A phase ii multicenter study. *J Clin Oncol* 2006; **24**(16):2465–71.

Wijermans PW, Krulder JW, Huijgens PC, *et al*. Continuous infusion of low-dose 5-Aza-2'-deoxycytidine in elderly patients with high-risk myelodysplastic syndrome. *Leukemia* 1997; **11**(1):1–5.

Internet resources

MDS forum: http://ukmdsforum.org/LENALIDOMIDE%20IN%20MDS%20SAFETY_vers4_table.doc

NCCN guidelines for treatment of MDS: http://www.nccn.org/professionals/physician_gls/PDF/mds.pdf

http://www.cancer.gov/cancertopics/pdq/treatment/myelodysplastic/healthprofessional/allpages#Reference4.52

NCRN AML 16 trial: http://www.aml16.bham.ac.uk/

Multiple myeloma

Introduction

Multiple myeloma accounts for approximately 10% of haematological malignancies (Kyle et al. 2004; Rajkumar et al. 2005). In almost all patients disease evolves from an asymptomatic premalignant stage termed monoclonal gammopathy of undetermined significance (MGUS). In some patients, an intermediate asymptomatic premalignant stage referred to as smoldering multiple myeloma (SMM) can be recognized clinically. The diagnosis of active myeloma requires 10% or more clonal plasma cells on bone marrow examination (or biopsy proven plasmacytoma), monoclonal (M) protein in the serum, and/or urine (except in patients with true non-secretory myeloma) and evidence of end-organ damage (hypercalcaemia, renal insufficiency, anaemia, or bone lesions) secondary to the underlying plasma cell disorder.

Epidemiology

The annual incidence is approximately 4 per 100,000. The disease is twice as common in African–Americans compared to Caucasians, and slightly more common in males than females. The median age at diagnosis is 66 years.

Aetiology

The aetiology of myeloma is not known; however, important advances have occurred that shed light on the pathogenesis of the disease. The first pathogenetic event is the establishment of the premalignant phase, MGUS. MGUS is thought to occur as a result of specific cytogenetic events triggered by infection or immunosuppression. The cytogenetic changes associated with MGUS are immunoglobulin heavy chain (IgH) gene translocations (50% of MGUS) or hyperdiploidy (the remaining 50%) (Fonseca et al. 2004).

There are five recurrent IgH translocations seen in MGUS, and they involve fusion of the IgH locus on chromosome 14q32 with one of five partner chromosome loci. The partner chromosome loci and the corresponding genes dysregulated are: 11q13 (CCND1 [cyclin D1 gene]); 4p16.3 (FGFR-3 and MMSET); 6p21 (CCND3 [cyclin D3 gene]); 16q23 (c-maf); and 20q11 (mafB) (Bergsagel et al. 2001). Approximately 50% of MGUS are not associated with IgH translocations, but have evidence of hyperdiploidy, usually of the odd numbered chromosomes with the exception of 13; and the origin of the remaining 5% or fewer of MGUS is not clear (Fonseca et al. 2004).

Once MGUS is established it progresses to myeloma or related malignancy at a constant rate of 1% per year (Kyle et al. 2002). The specific second-hit that initiates this progression is unknown, but several additional cytogenetic events are felt to be important including Ras mutations, p16 methylation, abnormalities involving the myc family of oncogenes, secondary translocations, and p53 mutations. In addition, the bone marrow microenvironment undergoes marked changes with progression, including induction of angiogenesis (Rajkumar et al. 2002), suppression of cell-mediated immunity (Galea et al. 2002), and paracrine loops involving cytokines such as interleukin-6 and VEGF (vascular endothelial growth factor). Lytic bone lesions in myeloma are caused by an imbalance between the activity of osteoclasts and osteoblasts. There is an increase in RANKL (receptor activator of nuclear factor κB ligand) expression by osteoblasts (and possibly plasma cells) accompanied by a reduction in the level of its decoy receptor, osteoprotegerin (OPG) (Roodman et al. 2004). This leads to an increase in RANKL/OPG ratio, which causes osteoclast activation and bone resorption. In addition, there is inhibition of osteoblast differentiation resulting in the type of osteolytic bone destruction without evidence of new bone formation that is characteristic of myeloma.

Clinical features

The most common presenting symptoms of myeloma are fatigue and bone pain (Kyle et al. 2003). Osteolytic bone lesions and/or compression fractures, that can be detected on routine radiographs, MRI, or CT scans, are the hallmark of the disease, and cause significant morbidity (Figs. 4.10.5–7). Bone pain may present as an area of persistent pain or migratory bone pain, often in the lower back and pelvis. Pain may be sudden in onset when associated with a pathological fracture, and is often precipitated by movement. Extramedullary expansion of bone lesions may cause nerve root or spinal cord compression. Anaemia occurs in 70% of patients at diagnosis and is the primary cause of fatigue. Hypercalcaemia is found in one-fourth of patients while the serum creatinine is elevated in almost one–half. Other symptoms may result from infections, hypercalcaemia, painful radiculopathy, or spinal cord compression.

On physical examination, pallor is the most frequent finding. The liver is palpable in about 5% of patients and the spleen in 1%. Tenderness may be noted at sites of bone involvement. Occasionally, extramedullary or bone plasmacytomas may be visible and/or palpable.

Diagnosis

A complete blood count, serum creatinine, and calcium are the essential tests in the diagnostic evaluation of suspected myeloma. A normocytic, normochromic anaemia is present initially in approximately 75% of patients but eventually occurs in almost all patients with multiple myeloma. The serum creatinine value is increased initially in almost half of patients. The major causes of renal insufficiency are light-chain cast nephropathy ('myeloma kidney') and hypercalcaemia. Myeloma kidney is characterized by the

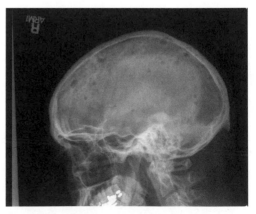

Fig. 4.10.5 Skull radiograph showing multiple lytic lesions in myeloma.

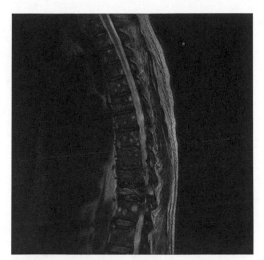

Fig. 4.10.6 MRI sagittal section showing myeloma involving T11 vertebral body with compression fracture.

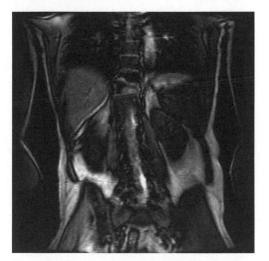

Fig. 4.10.7 MRI coronal section showing myeloma involving T11 vertebral body with compression fracture.

presence of large, waxy, laminated casts in the distal and collecting tubules. The casts are composed mainly of precipitated monoclonal light chains. Hypercalcaemia is present in 15–20% of patients initially.

Myeloma is characterized by the presence of monoclonal immunoglobulins in the serum and/or urine in almost 98% of patients but the presence of M proteins is not diagnostic of myeloma. Conditions such as MGUS, Waldenström macroglobulinemia, amyloidosis are also associated with M proteins and need to be differentiated from myeloma. M proteins can be detected by serum protein electrophoresis (SPEP) in 82% of patients with myeloma, and by serum immunofixation electrophoresis (IFE) in 93% (Kyle et al. 2003). Up to 20% of patients with myeloma lack heavy-chain expression in the M protein, and are considered to have light-chain myeloma. The M protein in

these patients is detected mainly in the urine, and thus addition of urine protein electrophoresis (UPEP) increases the sensitivity of detecting M proteins in patients with myeloma to 98%. The serum free light chain (FLC) assay can be used instead of urine studies when screening for myeloma since it is as sensitive as urine studies in detecting light chain myeloma. Currently only 1–2% of patients with myeloma will have no detectable M on any of these tests; these patients have true non-secretory myeloma.

Plain radiographic examination of all bones including long bones (skeletal survey) is the preferred method of detecting lytic bone lesions in myeloma. Conventional roentgenograms show skeletal abnormalities in almost 80% of patients with myeloma; often these lesions have a characteristic punched-out appearance. Osteoporosis and/ or fractures are also detected by conventional radiography. CT and/or MRI studies are indicated when symptomatic areas show no abnormality on routine radiographs.

A unilateral bone marrow aspiration and biopsy is indicated in all patients with myeloma. By definition, all patients with myeloma should have 10% or more clonal bone marrow plasma cells. If a lower extent of involvement is detected, one is either dealing with an erroneous diagnosis or there is a sampling error due to patchy marrow involvement in which case a repeat marrow biopsy is indicated. Clonal is defined as a kappa/lambda ratio on immunohistochemistry or flow cytometry that is >4:1 or <1:2. Occasionally an entity called 'multiple' solitary plasmacytomas has been described in which there are clearly multiple plasmacytomas on clinical and radiographic examination, but marrow involvement is either minimal or absent.

Based on these tests, myeloma is diagnosed by the following three criteria:
• Clonal bone marrow plasma cells ≥10%, *and*
• Presence of serum and/or urinary monoclonal protein (except in patients with true non-secretory multiple myeloma), *and*
• Evidence of end organ damage that can be attributed to the underlying plasma cell proliferative disorder, specifically:
  Bone lesions: lytic lesions, severe osteopenia or pathological fractures
  Anaemia: normochromic, normocytic with a haemoglobin value of >2g/dL below the lower limit of normal or a haemoglobin value <10g/dL
  Hypercalcaemia: serum calcium >0.25mmol/L above the upper limit of normal or >2.75mmol/L), or
  Renal failure: serum creatinine >1.73 mmol/L)

The main differential diagnosis is between myeloma, MGUS, smoldering myeloma, macroglobulinemia, and primary amyloidosis. These disorders are distinguished from each other using the criteria listed in Table 4.10.18.

MGUS and smoldering multiple myeloma are precursor conditions to myeloma that are asymptomatic and need no therapy. They lack the end-organ damage that is required for the diagnosis of multiple myeloma. MGUS and smoldering myeloma are distinguished from each other because they have different rates of progression to myeloma or related malignancy, 1% per year in the case of MGUS, and approximately 10% per year in the case of smoldering myeloma. Not all patients with an M protein and evidence of possible end organ damage have myeloma. It must be reasonably established that the end-organ damage is likely to be related to the underlying plasma cell disorder rather than an unrelated process. For example, bone lesions in a patient with MGUS due to an unrelated metastatic carcinoma may be mistaken for multiple myeloma. In this case, the presence of a small M protein and <10% plasma cells in the bone marrow makes metastatic carcinoma with an

Table 4.10.18 Diagnostic criteria for myeloma and differentiation from related disorders

Disorder	Diagnostic criteria
Monoclonal gammopathy of undetermined significance (MGUS)	1. Serum monoclonal protein < 3g/dL, and 2. Clonal bone marrow plasma cells <10%, and 3. Absence of end-organ damage such as lytic bone lesions, anaemia, hypercalcaemia, or renal failure that can be attributed to a plasma cell proliferative disorder
Smoldering multiple myeloma (also referred to as asymptomatic multiple myeloma)	1. Serum monoclonal protein (IgG or IgA) ≥3gm/dL and/or clonal bone marrow plasma cells ≥10%, and 2. Absence of end-organ damage such as lytic bone lesions, anaemia, hypercalcaemia, or renal failure that can be attributed to a plasma cell proliferative disorder

Multiple myeloma	1. ≥10% clonal bone marrow plasma cells, and
	2. Presence of serum and/or urinary monoclonal protein (except in patients with true non-secretory multiple myeloma), and
	3. Evidence of end organ damage that can be attributed to the underlying plasma cell proliferative disorder, specifically one or more of the following
	  a. Bone lesions (specifically, lytic lesions, severe osteopaenia or pathologic fractures) or extramedullary plasmacytomas
	  b. Anaemia
	  c. Hypercalcaemia
	  d. Renal failure

unrelated MGUS more likely. If there is any doubt, a biopsy of one of the lytic lesions is needed.

Myeloma is differentiated by kappa/lambda staining from polyclonal reactive plasmacytosis that occurs in conditions such as autoimmune diseases, metastatic carcinoma, chronic liver disease, acquired immunodeficiency syndrome (AIDS), or chronic infection.

Further reading

Bergsagel PL, Kuehl WM. Chromosome translocations in multiple myeloma. *Oncogene* 2001; **20**:5611–22.

Fonseca R, Barlogie B, Bataille R, et al. Genetics and cytogenetics of multiple myeloma: a workshop report. *Cancer Res* 2004; **64**:1546–58.

Galea HR, Cogne M. GM-CSF and IL-12 production by malignant plasma cells promotes cell-mediated immune responses against monoclonal Ig determinants in a light chain myeloma model. *Clinical & Experimental Immunology* 2002; **129**:247–53.

Kyle RA, Therneau TM, Rajkumar SV, et al. A long-term study of prognosis of monoclonal gammopathy of undetermined significance. *N Engl J Med* 2002; **346**:564–69.

Kyle RA, Gertz MA, Witzig TE, et al. Review of 1,027 patients with newly diagnosed multiple myeloma. *Mayo Clinic Proc* 2003; **78**:21–33.

Kyle RA, Rajkumar SV. Multiple myeloma. *N Engl J Med* 2004; **351**:1860–73.

Rajkumar SV, Mesa RA, Fonseca R, et al. Bone marrow angiogenesis in 400 patients with monoclonal gammopathy of undetermined significance, multiple myeloma, and primary amyloidosis. *Clin Cancer Res* 2002; **8**:2210–6.

Rajkumar SV, Kyle RA. Multiple myeloma: diagnosis and treatment. *Mayo Clin Proc* 2005; **80**:1371–82.

Roodman GD. Mechanisms of bone metastasis. *N Engl J Med* 2004; **350**:1655–64.

Internet resources

International Myeloma Foundation: http://www.myeloma.org

Multiple Myeloma Research Foundation: http://www.multiplemyeloma.org

Multiple myeloma: staging, prognosis, and treatment response criteria

Staging

Durie–Salmon Staging

The median survival of myeloma is approximately 4–5 years. However, some patients can live >10 years. Since 1975, the Durie–Salmon staging system has been used as the standard staging system for patients with multiple myeloma (Durie and Salmon 1975). This system provides a simple and practical estimate of tumour burden. Patients were categorized as stage I, stage II, or stage III, depending on the degree of anaemia, hypercalcaemia, levels of M protein in the serum and urine, or bone lesions. In addition, patients without, or with serum creatinine of 2mg/dL or more, were designated A or B. However, this staging system has limitations especially in the categorization of bone lesions.

International Staging System

A new International Staging System (ISS) which is based solely on two readily available laboratory tests, the beta-2-microglobulin and albumin, has replaced the Durie–Salmon staging system (Greipp et al. 2005). It overcomes the limitations of the Durie–Salmon staging, and divides patients into three distinct stages with significantly different outcomes (Table 4.10.19). Patients with stage I, II, and III have median survivals of 62, 44, and 29 months respectively.

The ISS allows outcome in clinical trials to be compared with each other more readily. It is easy to assess and reproducible. The ISS has two important limitations. The first is that it is not useful unless the diagnosis of myeloma has already been made. The ISS has no role in MGUS or smouldering (asymptomatic) multiple myeloma (SMM), and cannot distinguish these two premalignant disorders from myeloma. Secondly, the ISS does not identify an adverse prognostic group that is sufficiently high-risk to warrant a different therapeutic approach.

Prognosis

Age, ISS stage, haemoglobin concentration, creatinine, calcium, albumin, immunoglobulin class subtype, and extent of bone marrow involvement are all significant predictors of survival in myeloma. Plasmablastic morphology, circulating plasma cells, LDH, and CRP are additional independent risk factors for survival. The most important independent predictors of survival are discussed in the following sections.

Performance status

PS is probably the single most powerful predictor of outcome in myeloma, but its value has not been highlighted in the literature. PS is also a key determinant of transplant eligibility. Patients with poor PS are not candidates for stem cell transplantation. PS is assessed usually by the Eastern Cooperative Oncology Group (ECOG) scale, which

Table 4.10.19 International Staging System for myeloma

1 Stage I (serum β-2 microglobulin <3.5mg/L and albumin ≥3.5g/dL): median survival: 62 months)

2 Stage II (not fitting stage I or II): median survival 44 months

3 Stage III (serum β-2 microglobulin ≥5.5 mg/L): median survival 29 months

grades patients from 0–4 based on activity level. Patients who are fully functional are classified as 0, while patients who are bed-ridden are classified as 4. Patients with slight limitations in activity are classified as 1, those with significant limitations but are up and about >50% of waking hours are classified as 2, and those who have some activity but are up and about <50% of time are classified as 3.

In one study, an ECOG PS of 3–4 had a greater adverse impact on outcome (hazard ratio 1.9, 95% CI 1.6–2.4) than any other single variable (Kyle et al. 2003).

Conventional metaphase cytogenetics

Deletion of chromosome 13 detected by conventional metaphase karyotyping has a particularly adverse prognostic effect in myeloma. In a study of 1000 patients with myeloma who received autologous stem cell transplantation (ASCT), the 5-year survival rate was 16% in those with karyotypic deletion 13 (163 patients), compared to 44% in those without the abnormality (830 patients)(p <0.001). Five-year EFS was 0% versus 28% (p <0.001), respectively (Desikan et al. 2000). In contrast, the prognostic value of deletion 13 detected by interphase FISH appears to be almost fully related to coexisting IgH translocations such as t4;14, such that there is minimal effect on outcome in patients who have FISH deletion 13 in the absence of the t4;14 translocation.

The presence of karyotypically detected deletion 13 may have therapeutic implications, since such patients appear to receive minimal benefit from single or tandem ASCT (Desikan et al. 2000). Such patients may have better results with novel therapy.

Although metaphase deletion 13 is one of the best recognized cytogenetic abnormalities associated with poor prognosis, it is now becoming increasingly apparent that hypodiploidy on karyotypic analysis is also a major adverse prognostic factor.

Molecular cytogenetics

Cytogenetic abnormalities are present in most if not all patients with myeloma if sensitive interphase FISH techniques are used. The most common cytogenetic changes include deletion chromosome 13 (30–55% of patients), deletion 17p13.1 (10%), t(11;14)(q13;q32) (15–20%), t(4;14) (p16.3;q32) (15%), and t(14;16)(q32;q23) (5%) (Fonseca et al. 2004).

The presence of t(4; 14) (p16.3;q32), t(14;16)(q32q23), and 17p13 which are detected by interphase FISH (or metaphase spectral karyotype imaging) are associated with a markedly adverse prognosis (Fonseca et al. 2003). The t(4; 14) (p16.3; q32) abnormality results in dysregulation of the fibroblast growth factor receptor 3 (FGFR3) and MMSET; inhibitors of FGFR3 are being developed for targeted therapy in these cases. The t14; 16 translocation dysregulates the c-maf oncogene while deletions involving 17p13 result in p53 inactivation.

Risk-stratification of myeloma

The specific prognostic factors used to stratify patients into high-risk and standard-risk myeloma to guide therapeutic strategy are deletion 13 or hypodiploidy on metaphase cytogenetic studies, deletion 17p- or IgH translocations t(4;14) or t(14;16) on FISH studies. Presence of any one or more of these high-risk factors classifies a

Table 4.10.20 International Myeloma Working Group criteria for response and progression in myeloma

Response category	Response criteria
Complete response (CR)	• Negative immunofixation on the serum and urine, and • Disappearance of any soft tissue plasmacytomas, and • <5% plasma cells in bone marrow
Partial response (PR)	• ≥50% reduction of serum M-protein and • Reduction in 24-hour urinary M-protein by ≥90% or to <200mg per 24 hour
Progressive disease (PD)	Increase of 25% from lowest response value in: • Serum M-component (absolute increase must be ≥ 0.5 g/dL) and/or • Urine M-component (absolute increase must be ≥ 200 mg/24 hour) and/or • Definite development of new bone lesions or soft tissue plasmacytomas or definite increase in the size of existing bone lesions or soft tissue plasmacytomas and/or • Development of hypercalcemia that can be attributed solely to the plasma cell proliferative disorder

patient as having high-risk myeloma. Patients with none of the features are considered to have standard-risk disease. The median survival of high-risk myeloma is only 2–3 years even with tandem stem cell transplantation, compared to >6–7 years in patients with standard-risk myeloma (Rajkumar et al. 2005). In an ECOG clinical trial of 351 patients, the presence of t4;14, t(14;16) or 17p- were associated with the poor prognosis (median survival 25 months) (Fonseca et al. 2003).

Treatment response criteria

Uniform response criteria are required to monitor effectiveness of therapy in patients and to evaluate new drugs and interventions in clinical trials. Several response criteria have been developed for myeloma over the years that define various categories of response and progression. The most commonly used response criteria in the past were those developed by the European Group for Blood and Bone Marrow Transplant/International Bone Marrow Transplant Registry/American Bone Marrow Transplant Registry (EBMT/IBMTR/ABMTR) (Blade et al. 1998). In 2006, the International Myeloma Working Group (IMWG) recognized the need for uniformity and published uniform response criteria that are to be used in future clinical trials and in clinical practice (Durie et al. 2006).

The IMWG uniform response criteria are similar to the EBMT criteria with the following main exceptions: addition of free light chain response and progression criteria, difference in definition of progression for patients in complete response, addition of very good partial response and stringent response categories, elimination of the minor response category. In addition, The IMWG uniform response criteria have clarified that patients in CR need to meet the same criteria for disease progression as other patients not in CR for purposes of calculating PFS and time to progression (TTP). The relapse from CR definition should not be used to define progression in these patients as had been done previously in the EBMT criteria. The immunofixation results used to define CR can vary significantly due to laboratory variation. Thus using relapse from CR criteria would erroneously result in shorter TTP and PFS for CR patients compared to those not in CR with regiments that produce high CR rates.

The major definitions of response and progression are listed in Table 4.10.20.

Further reading

Bladé J, Samson D, Reece D, et al. Criteria for evaluating disease response and progression in patients with multiple myeloma treated by high-dose therapy and haemopoietic stem cell transplantation. Myeloma Subcommittee of the EBMT. European Group for Blood and Marrow Transplant. *Br J Haematol* 1998; **102**:1115–23.

Desikan R, Barlogie B, Sawyer J, et al. Results of high-dose therapy for 1000 patients with multiple myeloma: durable complete remissions and superior survival in the absence of chromosome 13 abnormalities. *Blood* 2000; **95**:4008–10.

Durie BG, Salmon SE. A clinical staging system for multiple myeloma. Correlation of measured myeloma cell mass with presenting clinical features, response to treatment, and survival. *Cancer* 1975; **36**:842–54.

Durie BGM, Harousseau J-L, Miguel JS, et al. International uniform response criteria for multiple myeloma. *Leukemia* 2006; **20**: 1467–73.

Fonseca R, Blood E, Rue M, et al. Clinical and biologic implications of recurrent genomic aberrations in myeloma. *Blood* 2003; **101**:4569–75.

Fonseca R, Barlogie B, Bataille R, et al. Genetics and cytogenetics of multiple myeloma: a workshop report. *Cancer Res* 2004; **64**: 1546–58.

Greipp PR, San Miguel JF, Durie BG, et al. International Staging System for multiple myeloma. *J Clin Oncol* 2005; **23**:3412–20.

Kyle RA, Gertz MA, Witzig TE, et al. Review of 1,027 patients with newly diagnosed multiple myeloma. *Mayo Clinic Proc* 2003; **78**: 21–33.

Rajkumar SV, Kyle RA Multiple myeloma: diagnosis and treatment. *Mayo Clin Proc* 2005; **80**:1371–82.

Internet resources

International Myeloma Foundation: http://www.myeloma.org
Multiple Myeloma Research Foundation: http://www.multiplemyeloma.org

Multiple myeloma: treatment

Untreated patients

The treatment of newly diagnosed multiple myeloma is rapidly evolving (Kyle et al. 2004). The median survival of symptomatic myeloma until recently was approximately 3 years after chemotherapy (Myeloma Trialists' Collaborative Group 1998), and approximately 5 years with high dose therapy with ASCT (Attal et al. 1996). The introduction of thalidomide, bortezomib, and lenalidomide, has prolonged the survival of multiple myeloma significantly (Singhal et al. 1999; Richardson et al. 2003, 2005; Rajkumar et al. 2005a).

The first step in the treatment of myeloma is to exclude MGUS and SMM which do not require therapy. The next step is to determine whether the patient is a potential candidate for stem cell transplantation because initial therapy differs accordingly. Transplant eligibility is determined by a variety of factors including age, PS, and comorbidities. In most countries, age 65 is considered as the upper limit for ASCT.

The third step is risk-stratification into high- and standard-risk myeloma based on specific prognostic markers (Rajkumar et al. 2005b). Presence of deletion 13 or hypodiploidy on metaphase cytogenetic studies, or the presence of deletion 17p- or IgH translocations t(4;14) or t(14;16) on FISH classifies a patient as having high-risk myeloma.

The approach to treatment of symptomatic newly diagnosed multiple myeloma is outlined in Fig. 4.10.8. Table 4.10.21 lists the most common regimens used in the treatment of newly diagnosed myeloma.

Initial treatment of patients eligible for transplantation

It is important to avoid protracted melphalan-based therapy in patients with newly diagnosed myeloma who are considered eligible for ASCT, since it can interfere with adequate stem cell mobilization, regardless of whether an early or delayed transplant is contemplated. Patients who are determined to be candidates for ASCT are typically treated with 2–4 cycles of non-melphalan containing induction therapy followed by stem cell harvest.

Thalidomide plus dexamethasone (Thal/Dex) is one of the most commonly used induction regimens for the treatment of newly diagnosed myeloma. In randomized trials it is superior to dexamethasone alone, and has a response rate of approximately 65–75% (Rajkumar et al. 2006, 2008). DVT, infections, skin rash, and peripheral neuropathy are important adverse effects of Thal/Dex.

Lenalidomide/dexamethasone (Len/Dex) is an alternative to Thal/Dex. Lenalidomide is an immunomodulatory drug that is a safer, more potent analogue of thalidomide. In newly diagnosed myeloma, Len/Dex may be more efficacious (response rate 70–90%) and safer compared with Thal/Dex (Rajkumar et al. 2005a). The most important adverse events are DVT, infections, skin rash, and cytopenias.

Bortezomib plus dexamethasone (Vel/Dex), is a third option for this group of patients, with a response rate of about 70–80%. The most common adverse events are neuropathy, infections, cytopenias, and GI side effects.

Finally, bortezomib–thalidomide–dexamethasone (VTD) has shown high activity (>80% response rate) and can be a useful regimen in patients with acute renal failure due to cast nephropathy in whom a rapid tumour reduction is needed.

A recent randomized trial showed that in newly diagnosed myeloma, low-dose dexamethasone (40mg once a week) is safer and more effective than standard high-dose dexamethasone (Rajkumar et al. 2007). Thus the dose of dexamethasone with Len/Dex, Thal/Dex, VTD, and other regimens in newly diagnosed disease should be approximately 40mg once a week.

Several other induction regimens besides the four listed here have been evaluated, but most are still investigational. Of the four regimens listed, Thal/Dex and Len/Dex have the advantage of oral administration but carry an increased risk of DVT necessitating routine thromboprophylaxis. Len/Dex or Thal/Dex is the preferred choice for most patients. Vel/Dex or VTD are preferred in patients presenting with high-risk myeloma or renal failure.

Initial treatment of patients not eligible for transplantation

Patients who are not transplant candidates are treated with melphalan-based therapy. Melphalan plus prednisone (MP) has for decades been the standard regimen for this group of patients (Myeloma Trialists' Collaborative Group 1998). MP is associated with a response rate of 50% and a median survival of about 3 years. Recently two new combinations have emerged with significantly superior survival compared to MP: melphalan, prednisone, thalidomide (MPT); and bortezomib, melphalan, prednisone, bortezomib (MPV).

Four randomized trials have compared MP with MPT (Facon et al. 2005; Palumbo et al. 2006; Hulin et al. 2007a).

Table 4.10.21 Common regimens used in the treatment of newly diagnosed myeloma

Regimen	Usual dosing schedule*	Approximate response rate in newly diagnosed disease
Thalidomide–dexamethasone (Thal/Dex)	Thalidomide 100–200mg oral, days 1–28 Dexamethasone 40mg oral, days 1, 8, 15, 22, every 28 days Repeated every 4 weeks	65%
Lenalidomide–dexamethasone (Rev*/low–dose Dex)	Lenalidomide 25mg oral, days 1–21 every 28 days Dexamethasone 40mg oral, days 1, 8, 15, 22, every 28 days Repeated every 4 weeks	70%
Bortezomib–Dex (Vel/Dex)	Bortezomib 1.3mg/m^2 intravenous days 1, 4, 8, 11 Dexamethasone 40mg oral, days 1–4, 9–12 Reduce dexamethasone to days 1–4 only after first 2 cycles Repeated every 3 weeks	80%

* Lenalidomide-trade name Revlimid

Table 4.10.21 (Cont'd.)

Regimen	Usual dosing schedule*	Approximate response rate in newly diagnosed disease
Bortezomib–thalidomide–dexamethasone (VTD)	Bortezomib 1.3mg/m^2 intravenous days 1, 4, 8, 11 Thalidomide 200mg oral, days 1–21 Dexamethasone 20 mg day of and day after bortezomib Repeated every 3 weeks	90%
Melphalan–prednisone–thalidomide (MPT)	Melphalan 0.25mg/kg oral, days 1–4 Prednisone 2mg/kg oral, days 1–4 Thalidomide 100–200mg oral, days 1–28 Repeated every 6 weeks	75%
Borteozmib–melphalan–prednisone (VMP)	Melphalan 9mg/m^2 oral, days 1–4 Prednisone 60mg/m^2 oral, days 1–4 Bortezomib 1.3mg/m^2 intravenous, days 1, 4, 8, 11, 22, 25, 29, 32 Repeated every 42 days x 4 cycles followed by maintenance therapy as given below: • Melphalan 9mg/m^2 oral, days 1–4 • Prednisone 60mg/m^2 oral, days 1–4 • Bortezomib 1.3mg/m^2 intravenous, days 1, 8, 15, 22 • Repeated every 35 days x 5 cycles	70%

*Starting and subsequent doses need to be adjusted for PS, renal function, blood counts, and other toxicities

All four trials showed a higher response rate with MPT compared with MP. In two of the four trials, MPT was associated with significantly superior OS (Facon et al. 2007; Hulin et al. 2007b). DVT, cytopenias, infections, and neuropathy are important adverse effects of MPT. Studies are investigating whether efficacy can be further improved by using MPR in place of MPT.

A recent randomized trial showed VMP to be superior to MP in terms of response and overall survival (San Miguel et al. 2007). Cytopenias, infections, and neuropathy are important adverse effects of VMP.

At present, MPT is the preferred regimen for standard-risk patients who are not candidates for transplantation. VMP would be the preferred regimen for high-risk patients who are not candidates for transplantation.

Treatment of high-risk myeloma
Patients with high-risk myeloma tend to do poorly with median overall survival of approximately 2 years even with tandem ASCT. There are two options for these high-risk patients. The first option is to treat patients according to transplant-eligibility as described earlier, but follow such therapy with long-term maintenance therapy. The second option is to consider ASCT followed by non-myeloablative allogeneic transplantation in selected patients.

DVT prophylaxis
DVT is a major complication of thalidomide and lenalidomide based therapy. For most patients, aspirin alone can be used as DVT prophylaxis as long as patients are receiving low-dose corticosteroids (e.g. dexamethasone

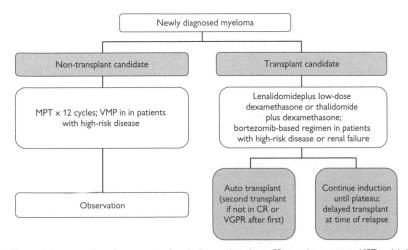

Fig. 4.10.8 Algorithm outlining approach to the treatment of newly diagnosed myeloma. CR, complete response; MPT, melphalan, prednisone, thalidomide; VGPR, very good partial response; VMP bortezomib, melphalan, prednisone.

40mg once a week or prednisone), and provided no concomitant erythropoietic agents are used. On the other hand, patients receiving thalidomide or lenalidomide in combination with high-dose steroids or doxorubicin need higher intensity thromboprophylaxis with coumadin (target INR 2–3) or low-molecular-weight heparin (equivalent of enoxaparin 40mg once daily).

Autologous stem cell transplantation

Although not curative, ASCT improves complete response rates and prolongs median overall survival in myeloma by approximately 12 months (Attal et al. 1996; Child et al. 2003). The mortality rate is 1–2%. Melphalan, 200mg/m^2 is the most widely used preparative (conditioning) regimen for ASCT.

There is little doubt that ASCT prolongs survival in myeloma, but its timing (early versus delayed) is controversial. Survival is similar whether ASCT is done early (immediately following 4 cycles of induction therapy) or delayed (at the time of relapse as salvage therapy) (Barlogie et al. 2003). Overall, given the inconvenience and side effects of prolonged chemotherapy, insurance, and other issues we still favour early ASCT, especially for patients <65 years of age with adequate renal function. However, given effective new agents to treat myeloma, some patients and physicians may choose to delay the procedure. The need for early ASCT is an important question for future clinical trials.

With tandem (double) ASCT, patients receive a second planned ASCT after recovery from the first procedure. Two randomized trials found better EFS and OS in recipients of double versus single ASCT (Attal et al. 2002; Cavo et al. 2004). In both trials, the benefit of a second ASCT was restricted to patients failing to achieve a complete response or very good partial response with the first procedure. A tandem ASCT can be therefore considered in patients who fail to achieve a complete response or very good partial response (>90% reduction in M protein level) with the first ASCT.

Allogeneic transplantation

Conventional allogeneic transplants are unacceptable for most patients due to high treatment-related mortality rates. Non-myeloablative conditioning regimens (mini-allogeneic transplantation) have reduced treatment related mortality rates. Studies are testing ASCT followed by a non-myeloablative allogeneic stem cell transplant in selected patients. A recent randomized trial in patients with deletion 13 and high β2-microglobulin levels did not show significant benefit with this strategy compared to tandem ASCT (Garban et al. 2006). However, in another randomized trial, a significant survival advantage was seen with ASCT followed by a non-myeloablative allogeneic SCT compared with tandem ASCT (Bruno et al. 2007). Thus the role of allogeneic strategies in myeloma remains unresolved, and at this time, these approaches remain investigational.

Maintenance therapy

Recent studies have found a significant improvement in EFS and OS with maintenance thalidomide following transplantation. However, at present no routine maintenance is provided following ASCT for most patients, unless they have high-risk myeloma.

Refractory and relapsing myeloma

Almost all patients with myeloma eventually relapse. If relapse occurs >6 months after stopping therapy, the initial chemotherapy regimen should be reinstituted. Patients who have cryopreserved stem cells early in the disease course can derive significant benefit from ASCT as salvage therapy. In general, patients who have indolent relapse can often be treated with single agents. In contrast, patients with more aggressive relapse often require therapy with a combination of active agents. Given the non-curative nature of myeloma, patients with relapsed disease typically continue on one drug/regimen until relapse or toxicity and then try the next option. The regimens discussed in untreated patients (Thal/Dex, Len/Dex, Vel/Dex, VTD, MPT, VMP, and MPR) can all be used in relapsed/refractory patients.

Thalidomide and thalidomide-based regimens

The finding of increased angiogenesis in myeloma and the antiangiogenic properties of thalidomide led to the investigation of thalidomide in myeloma (Singhal et al. 1999). As a single agent, thalidomide produces response rates in about 25–35% of patients with relapsed/refractory MM. The median duration of response is approximately 1 year. Thalidomide is usually given in a dosage of 100–200mg daily. After a response is achieved, the dose should be adjusted to the lowest dose that can achieve and maintain a response in order to minimize long-term toxicity. High response rates can be achieved by combining thalidomide with dexamethasone, or with three-drug combinations such as cyclophosphamide, thalidomide, dexamethasone (CTD), or VTD.

Thalidomide is a teratogenic agent. Its use in pregnancy is absolutely contraindicated. Most countries have programmes in place to prevent teratogenicity through strict restrictions for women of child-bearing potential.

Bortezomib and bortezomib based regimens

Bortezomib is a novel proteasome inhibitor approved for the treatment of patients with relapsed and refractory multiple myeloma. In patients with relapsed/refractory myeloma, approximately one-third respond to single-agent bortezomib therapy, with an average response duration of 1 year (Richardson et al. 2003, 2005). The starting dose of bortezomib is 1.3mg/m^2 given twice weekly on days 1, 4, 8, and 11 every 21 days. Dosage may need to be decreased to 1.0mg/m^2 or 0.7mg/m^2 based on toxicity.

Bortezomib can be combined with dexamethasone or liposomal doxorubicin to improve response rates.

Lenalidomide

Lenalidomide belongs to a class of thalidomide analogues termed immunomodulatory drugs (ImiDs). Two large phase III trials have shown significantly superior time to progression with Len/Dex compared to placebo plus dexamethasone in relapsed myeloma (Dimopoulos et al. 2007; Weber et al. 2007). Typical dosing of lenalidomide for myeloma is 25–30mg per day on days 1–21 of a 28-day cycle, with dose adjustments based on toxicity.

Other options

Several other options exist for relapsed/refractory disease. High-dose pulsed dexamethasone or intravenous methylprednisolone are reasonable options, particularly in patients with severe cytopenias and poor PS. Conventional combination chemotherapy regimens can be effective in relapsed/refractory disease. Intravenous melphalan at a dose of 25mg/m^2 is another active regimen, but usually requires transfusion and growth factor support. Liposomal doxorubicin in combination with bortezomib, Vel/Dex or Thal/Dex is also effective in relapsed/refractory disease.

There is a continued search for other active agents based on advances in myeloma biology. CC-4047 (another thalidomide analogue) and carfilzomib (a novel proteasome inhibitor) have shown early signs of clinically meaningful activity in myeloma.

Supportive care and treatment of complications

Hypercalcaemia
Hydration plus a single dose of pamidronate, 60–90mg intravenously over 2–4 hours, or zoledronic acid 4mg intravenously over 15 minutes, will normalize the calcium levels within 24–72 hours in most patients.

Skeletal lesions
Surgical fixation of fractures or impending fractures of long bones may be needed. Local radiation should be limited to patients with disabling pain due to a myeloma lesion that has not responded to conventional therapy, and patients with spinal cord compression.

Bisphosphonates are recommended as secondary prophylaxis in patients with multiple myeloma who have one or more lytic lesions on skeletal X-rays. Such therapy can reduce the incidence of osteolytic bone lesions. Pamidronate is favoured over zoledronic acid. Avascular osteonecrosis of jaw (ONJ) is a risk with bisphosphonate therapy. The standard recommendation is 1–2 years of monthly bisphosphonate therapy following diagnosis in patients with myeloma bone disease.

Vertebroplasty or kyphoplasty are helpful in patients with vertebral fractures to decrease pain and help restore height.

Renal insufficiency
Non-steroidal anti-inflammatory agents, dehydration, infection, and radiographic contrast may contribute to acute renal failure in myeloma. Patients with acute or subacute renal failure due to light-chain cast nephropathy should be treated with VTD, Vel/Dex, or Thal/Dex to reduce the tumour mass as quickly as possible. A trial of plasmapheresis should be considered in these patients in an attempt to prevent irreversible renal damage.

Anaemia
Iron, folate, or B–12 deficiency must be recognized and treated. Treatment of the underlying disease and renal failure often leads to improvement in the haemoglobin level. Transfusions, erythropoietin (40,000U subcutaneously weekly) or darbepoietin (200mcg subcutaneously every 2 weeks) are useful in patients with persistent symptomatic anaemia despite antimyeloma therapy.

Infections
Newly diagnosed patients should receive prophylaxis with antibiotics such as ciprofloxacin, levofloxacin, or trimethoprim–sulfamethoxazole to prevent infections in the first months of corticosteroid-based therapy. Trimethoprim-sulfamethoxazole should, however, be avoided in patients receiving thalidomide or lenalidomide since concomitant use may increase the risk of serious skin rash.

Hyperviscosity syndrome
Infrequently patients with multiple myeloma develop hyperviscosity syndrome. Plasmapheresis promptly relieves the symptoms and should be done regardless of the viscosity level if the patient has signs or symptoms of hyperviscosity.

Further reading
Attal M, Harousseau JL, Stoppa AM, et al. A prospective, randomized trial of autologous bone marrow transplantation and chemotherapy in multiple myeloma. Intergroupe Français du Myélome. N Engl J Med 1996; **335**:91–7.

Attal M, Harousseau JL, Facon T, et al. Double autologous transplantation improves survival of multiple myeloma patients: final analysis of a prospective randomized study of the 'Intergroupe Francophone du Myélome' (IFM 94). Blood 2002; **100**:5a

Barlogie B, Kyle R, Anderson K, et al. Comparable Survival in multiple myeloma (MM) with high dose therapy (HDT) employing MEL 140 mg/m2 + TBI 12 Gy autotransplants versus standard dose therapy with VBMCP and no benefit from interferon (IFN) Maintenance: Results of Intergroup Trial S9321. Blood 2003; **102**:42a.

Bruno B, Rotta M, Patriarca F, et al. A comparison of allografting with autografting for newly diagnosed myeloma. N Engl J Med 2007; **356**:1110–20.

Cavo M, Cellini C, Zamagni E, et al. Superiority of double over single autologous stem cell transplantation as first-line therapy for multiple myeloma. Blood 2004; **104**:155a (A536).

Child JA, Morgan GJ, Davies FE, et al. High-dose chemotherapy with hematopoietic stem-cell rescue for multiple myeloma. N Engl J Med 2003; **348**:1875–83.

Dimopoulos M, Spencer A, Attal M, et al. Lenalidomide plus dexamethasone for relapsed or refractory multiple myeloma. N Engl J Med 2007; **357**:2123–32.

Facon T, Mary JY, Hulin C, et al. Major superiority of melphalan-prednisone (MP) + thalidomide (THAL) over MP and autologous stem cell transplantation in the treatment of newly diagnosed elderly patients with multiple myeloma. Blood 2005; **106**:230a (A780).

Facon T, Mary JY, Hulin C, et al. Melphalan and prednisone plus thalidomide versus melphalan and prednisone alone or reduced-intensity autologous stem cell transplantation in elderly patients with multiple myeloma (IFM 99-06): a randomised trial. Lancet 2007; **370**:1209–18.

Garban F, Attal M, Michallet M, et al. Prospective comparison of autologous stem cell transplantation followed by dose-reduced allograft (IFM99-03 trial) with tandem autologous stem cell transplantation (IFM99-04 trial) in high-risk de novo multiple myeloma.. Blood 2006; **107**:3474–80.

Hulin C, Virion J, Leleu X, et al. Comparison of melphalan-prednisone-thalidomide (MP-T) to melphalan-prednisone (MP) in patients 75 years of age or older with untreated multiple myeloma (MM). Preliminary results of the randomized, double-blind, placebo controlled IFM 01-01 trial. J Clin Oncol (Meeting Abstracts) 2007a; **25**:8001.

Hulin C, Facon T, Rodon P, et al. Melphalan-Prednisone-Thalidomide (MP-T) demonstrates a significant survival advantage in elderly patients >=75 years with multiple myeloma compared with melphalan-prednisone (MP) in a randomized, double-blind, placebo-controlled trial, IFM 01/01. ASH Annual Meeting Abstracts 2007b; **110**:75.

Kyle RA, Rajkumar SV. Multiple myeloma. N Engl J Med 2004; **351**:1860–73.

Myeloma Trialists' Collaborative Group. Combination chemotherapy versus melphalan plus prednisone as treatment for multiple myeloma: An overview of 6,633 patients from 27 randomized trials. J Clin Oncol 1998; **16**:3832–42.

Palumbo A, Bringhen S, Caravita T, et al. Oral melphalan and prednisone chemotherapy plus thalidomide compared with melphalan and prednisone alone in elderly patients with multiple myeloma: randomised controlled trial. Lancet 2006; **367**:825–31.

Rajkumar SV, Hayman SR, Lacy MQ, et al. Combination therapy with lenalidomide plus dexamethasone (Rev/Dex) for newly diagnosed myeloma. Blood 2005; **106**:4050–3.

Rajkumar SV, Kyle RA. Multiple myeloma: diagnosis and treatment. Mayo Clin Proc 2005; **80**:1371–82.

Rajkumar SV, Blood E, Vesole DH, et al. Phase III clinical trial of thalidomide plus dexamethasone compared with dexamethasone alone in newly diagnosed multiple myeloma: a clinical trial coordinated by the Eastern Cooperative Oncology Group. *J Clin Oncol* 2006; **24**:431–6.

Rajkumar SV, Jacobus S, Callander N, *et al.* A randomized trial of lenalidomide plus high-dose dexamethasone (RD) versus lenalidomide plus low-dose dexamethasone (Rd) in newly diagnosed multiple myeloma (E4A03): A Trial Coordinated by the Eastern Cooperative Oncology Group. *ASH Annual Meeting Abstracts* 2007; **110**:74.

Rajkumar SV, Rosiñol L, Hussein M, *et al.* A multicenter, randomized, double-blind, placebo-controlled study of thalidomide plus dexamethasone versus dexamethasone as initial therapy for newly diagnosed multiple myeloma. *J Clin Oncol* 2008; **26**:2171

Richardson PG, Barlogie B, Berenson J, *et al.* A phase 2 study of bortezomib in relapsed, refractory myeloma. *N Engl J Med* 2003; **348**:2609–17.

Richardson PG, Sonneveld P, Schuster MW, *et al.* Bortezomib or high-dose dexamethasone for relapsed multiple myeloma. [see comment]. *N Engl J Med* 2005; **352**:2487–98.

San Miguel JF, Schlag R, Khuageva N, *et al.* MMY-3002: A Phase 3 study comparing bortezomib-melphalan-prednisone (VMP) with melphalan-prednisone (MP) in newly diagnosed multiple myeloma. *ASH Annual Meeting Abstracts* 2007; **110**:76.

Singhal S, Mehta J, Desikan R, *et al.* Antitumor activity of thalidomide in refractory multiple myeloma. *N Engl J Med* 1999; **341**:1565–71.

Weber DM, Chen C, Niesvizky R, *et al.* Lenalidomide plus Dexamethasone for relapsed multiple myeloma in north america. *N Engl J Med* 2007; **357**:2133–42

Internet resources

International Myeloma Foundation: http://www.myeloma.org

Multiple Myeloma Research Foundation: http://www.multiplemyeloma.org

Mayo Stratification for Myeloma and Risk Adapted therapy. http://www.msmart.org

Solitary plasmacytoma

Epidemiology and aetiology

Solitary plasmacytomas are uncommon relative to multiple myeloma, with an incidence that is approximately one-tenth of myeloma. The aetiology and epidemiology are similar to multiple myeloma. In over half of the cases, a solitary plasmacytoma is a precursor to myeloma.

Solitary plasmacytoma may be confined to bone (solitary bone plasmacytoma) or occur in extramedullary sites (extramedullary plasmacytoma) (Dimopoulos et al. 1999). Patients with solitary plasmacytoma are at risk for progression to multiple myeloma. Increased microvessel density detected in the initial diagnostic tissue specimen has been associated with an increased risk of progression to multiple myeloma, suggesting that the evolution to systemic disease may be dependent on an angiogenic switch (Kumar et al. 2003).

Solitary plasmacytoma of bone

Solitary bony plasmacytomas may occur anywhere in the axial or appendicular skeleton. Common sites of involvement include the spine, ribs, femur, humerus, and skull.

Solitary extramedullary plasmacytoma

Extramedullary plasmacytoma is localized to the upper respiratory tract (nasal cavity and sinuses, nasopharynx, and larynx) in >80% of cases, but can also occur in the GI tract, CNS, urinary bladder, thyroid, breast, testes, parotid gland, or lymph nodes.

Clinical features

Pain is the most common clinical symptom of solitary bone plasmacytoma. In general, clinical symptoms depend on the site of involvement. For example, a solitary bone plasmacytoma in the spine can manifest as back pain, or can cause spinal cord compression and extremity weakness. Similarly symptoms related to extramedullary plasmacytomas reflect the region of involvement.

In over half the patients, solitary plasmacytoma is a precursor to multiple myeloma, but in many the lesion is truly solitary and curable. Over 50% of patients with a solitary bone plasmacytoma are alive at 10 years, and DFS at 10 years ranges from 25–50% (Dimopoulos et al. 1999). Progression to myeloma, when it occurs, usually appears within 3 years, but patients must be followed indefinitely. Prognosis is better in patients with solitary extramedullary plasmacytoma, with 10 year DFS rates of approximately 70–80% (Dimopoulos et al. 1999).

Diagnosis

Diagnostic criteria are listed in the box (Rajkumar et al. 2006). A skeletal survey is essential to ensure that the lesion is solitary. In addition, an MRI of the spine and pelvis should be performed since approximately one-third of patients may have additional occult lesions that will be missed on skeletal survey. Serum and urine protein electrophoresis and immunofixation must be done, and may reveal a small monoclonal protein. By definition, bone marrow does not show evidence of a clonal plasma cell disorder.

Diagnostic criteria for solitary plasmacytoma

- Biopsy proven solitary lesion of bone or soft tissue with evidence of clonal plasma cells, and
- Normal bone marrow with no evidence of clonal plasma cells, and
- Normal skeletal survey and MRI of spine and pelvis, and
- Absence of end-organ damage such as anaemia, hypercalcaemia, renal failure or additional lytic bone lesions that can be attributed to a plasma cell proliferative disorder

---

Treatment

Treatment consists of radiation to a dose of 40–50Gy to the involved site (Dimopoulos et al. 2000). Patients who meet the criteria for solitary plasmacytoma except for evidence of clonal involvement of the bone marrow are treated identically, and then observed until disease progression is similar to monoclonal MGUS (<10% bone marrow plasma cells) or SMM (≥10% plasma cells).

Prognosis

Patients with a baseline serum M protein >1g/dL have a high risk of persistent M protein following radiation therapy to the involved site (Dimopoulos et al. 1992). Persistence of an M protein 1 year or more after radiation therapy has been associated with an increased probability of progression to multiple myeloma in patients with solitary bone plasmacytoma. The 10-year myeloma-free survival was 29% in patients with a persistent serum or urinary M protein compared to 91% in those in whom the M protein was not detectable following radiation therapy. An abnormal serum free light chain ratio at baseline is a risk factor for progression to multiple myeloma (Dingli et al. 2006).

Further reading

Dingli D, Kyle RA, Rajkumar SV, et al. Immunoglobulin free light chains and solitary plasmacytoma of bone. *Blood* 2006; **108**:197–83.

Dimopoulos MA, Goldstein J, Fuller L, et al. Curability of solitary bone plasmacytoma. *J Clin Oncol* 1992; **10**:587–90.

Dimopoulos MA, Kiamouris C, Moulopoulos LA. Solitary plasmacytoma of bone and extramedullary plasmacytoma. *Hematol Oncol Clin North Am* 1999;. **13**:1249–57.

Dimopoulos MA, Moulopoulos LA, Maniatis A, et al. Solitary plasmacytoma of bone and asymptomatic multiple myeloma. *Blood* 2000; **96**:2037–44.

Kumar S, Fonseca R, Dispenzieri A, et al. Prognostic value of angiogenesis in solitary bone plasmacytoma. *Blood* 2003; **101**:1715–7.

Rajkumar SV, Dispenzieri A, Kyle RA. Monoclonal gammopathy of undetermined significance, Waldenström macroglobulinemia, AL amyloidosis, and related plasma cell disorders: diagnosis and treatment. *Mayo Clinic Proc* 2006; **81**:693–703.

Monoclonal gammopathy of undetermined significance

Almost all patients with multiple myeloma and Waldenström macroglobulinaemia evolve from a premalignant stage termed monoclonal gammopathy of undetermined significance (MGUS), although in most patients this is unrecognized clinically due to the asymptomatic nature of the condition.

Epidemiology and aetiology

MGUS is an asymptomatic premalignant disorder characterized by limited monoclonal plasma cell proliferation in the bone marrow and absence of end-organ damage (Kyle et al. 2002). It is the most common plasma cell dyscrasia, prevalent in approximately 3% of the general population 50 years of age and older (Kyle et al. 2006). The prevalence increases with age; 1.7% in those 50–59 years of age, and >5% in those >70 years. Age-specific incidence is higher in males than females. MGUS is also twice as common in African-Americans compared with Caucasians.

MGUS is associated with a lifelong risk of progression to multiple myeloma or a related disorder. The rate of progression of MGUS to multiple myeloma or related malignancy is 1% per year (Kyle et al. 2002). However, the true lifetime probability of progression is substantially lower when competing causes of death are taken into account, approximately 11% at 25 years (Rajkumar et al. 2005). The risk of progression with MGUS does not diminish with time.

The aetiology of MGUS is not known. MGUS is characterized by evidence of genomic instability on molecular genetic testing. The trigger for this genomic instability is not well understood, but current evidence suggests that in many cases antigenic stimulation or immunosuppression may be a key factor. Thus the current hypothesis for the pathogenesis of MGUS is that infection or immunosuppression triggers proliferation of plasma cells, and cytogenetic errors at this time (either immunoglobulin heavy chain translocations or hyperdiploidy) contribute to the development of MGUS.

Diagnosis

Since MGUS is asymptomatic, its identification is usually incidental, and occurs when serum and urine electrophoresis and immunofixation studies are performed during the investigation of patients with a wide variety of medical conditions, including suspected myeloma, hypercalcaemia, neuropathy, renal failure, etc.

MGUS is defined by a serum M-protein concentration <3g/dL, <10% plasma cells in the bone marrow, and absence of lytic bone lesions, anaemia, hypercalcaemia, and renal insufficiency that can be attributed to a monoclonal plasma cell disorder (see Chapter 4, Multiple myeloma, Table 4.10.18, p.502).

Serum protein electrophoresis and immunofixation

Agarose gel serum protein electrophoresis (SPEP) and immunofixation are the preferred methods of detection of serum monoclonal (M) proteins. M proteins appear as a localized band on SPEP. After recognition of a localized band suggestive of an M protein on SPEP, immunofixation is necessary for confirmation, and to determine the heavy- and light-chain class of the M protein. In addition, immunofixation is more sensitive than SPEP, and allows detection of smaller amounts of M protein.

Quantitative immunoglobulin studies

Quantitation of serum immunoglobulins is performed by nephelometry and is a useful adjunct to protein electrophoresis in patients with MGUS, SMM and other plasma cell disorders.

24-hour urine protein electrophoresis and immunofixation

Urine studies are needed when evaluating suspected monoclonal plasma cell disorders since a subset of patients with myeloma and amyloidosis may have an M protein restricted to the urine and absent on serum studies.

Serum free light chain assay

The serum free light-chain (FLC) assay allows quantitation of free kappa (κ) and lambda (λ) chains. An abnormal

Table 4.10.22 Risk-stratification model to predict progression of monoclonal gammopathy of undetermined significance to myeloma or related disorders*

Risk group	No. of patients	Relative risk	Absolute risk of progression at 20 years	Absolute risk of progression at 20 years accounting for death as a competing risk
Low-risk (serum M protein <1.5g/dL, IgG subtype, normal FLC ratio (0.26–1.65)	449	1	5%	2%
Low-intermediate-risk (any 1 factor abnormal)	420	5.4	21%	10%
High-intermediate-risk (any 2 factors abnormal)	226	10.1	37%	18%
High-risk (all 3 factors abnormal)	53	20.8	58%	27%

*Rajkumar SV, Kyle RA, Therneau TM, et al. Serum free light chain ratio is an independent risk factor for progression in monoclonal gammopathy of undetermined significance (MGUS). *Blood* 2005; **106**:812–17. © The American Society of Hematology.

kappa/lambda FLC ratio indicates an excess of one light chain type over the other, and is interpreted as a surrogate for presence of monoclonal light chains. The FLC assay can eliminate need for urine studies when evaluating a patient with a suspected monoclonal plasma cell disorder. It is also useful in assessing prognosis in MGUS, SMM, myeloma, plasmacytoma, and light chain amyloidosis.

Risk-stratification of MGUS

A risk stratification system can be used to predict the risk of progression of MGUS based on three risk factors: size of the serum M protein, the type of immunoglobulin, and the serum FLC ratio (Table 4.10.22) (Rajkumar et al. 2005). Patients with three adverse risk factors, namely an abnormal serum FLC ratio, non-IgG MGUS, and a high serum M protein level (≥15g/L), had a risk of progression at 20 years of 58% (high-risk MGUS) compared to 37% in patients with any two of these risk factors present (high-intermediate-risk MGUS), 21% with one risk factor present (low-intermediate risk MGUS) and 5% when none of the risk factors were present (low-risk MGUS). In fact, the low-risk MGUS subset (constituting almost 40% of the cohort) had a lifetime risk of only 2% when competing causes of death are taken into account.

Treatment

The current standard of care for MGUS is observation alone, without therapy (Kyle et al. 2004). Patients with MGUS may benefit from risk-stratification as discussed earlier to guide follow-up. Patients with low-risk MGUS can be rechecked in 6 months, and then once every 2–3 years (Rajkumar et al. 2005). All other subsets of patients need to be rechecked in 6 months and then yearly thereafter.

Further reading

Kyle RA, Therneau TM, Rajkumar SV, *et al*. A long-term study of prognosis of monoclonal gammopathy of undetermined significance. *N Engl J Med* 2002; **346**:564–69.

Kyle RA, Rajkumar SV Multiple myeloma. *N Engl J Med* 2004; **351**:1860–73.

Kyle RA, Therneau TM, Rajkumar SV, *et al*. Prevalence of monoclonal gammopathy of undetermined significance. *N Engl J Med* 2006; **354**:1362–9.

Rajkumar SV, Kyle RA, Therneau TM, *et al*. Serum free light chain ratio is an independent risk factor for progression in monoclonal gammopathy of undetermined significance (MGUS). *Blood* 2005; **106**:812–17.

Smouldering myeloma

Introduction

In almost all patients, multiple myeloma evolves from the premalignant stage termed MGUS. In some patients, an intermediate asymptomatic but more advanced premalignant stage referred to as smouldering multiple myeloma (SMM) is recognized clinically. Both MGUS and SMM represent asymptomatic plasma cell disorders, but the latter needs to be differentiated from MGUS in the clinical setting because progression to myeloma or related malignancy is markedly higher, approximately 10% per year in SMM compared with 1% per year in MGUS (Kyle et al. 2007). However, a separate biological stage of SMM with a unique pathogenetic mechanism probably does not exist. The classification of MGUS and SMM is done only for clinical purposes. In fact, patients clinically diagnosed as SMM are most likely a mix of patients with biological premalignancy (MGUS) and early myeloma.

SMM accounts for approximately 15% of all cases with newly diagnosed multiple myeloma. The prevalence estimates for SMM are not reliable since some studies include asymptomatic patients with small lytic bone lesions on skeletal survey and/or abnormalities on MRI.

As for MGUS and active myeloma, almost all patients with SMM appear to have evidence of genomic instability manifested as IgH translocations or hyperdiploidy on molecular genetic testing.

Diagnosis

SMM is defined by the presence of an IgG or IgA M-protein level >3g/dL in the serum or >10% plasma cells in the bone marrow in the absence of anaemia, renal insufficiency, hypercalcaemia, or skeletal lesions that can be attributed to the underlying plasma cell disorder. Often, a small amount of M protein is found in the urine, and the concentration of normal immunoglobulins in the serum is decreased.

Testing to differentiate SMM from multiple myeloma is as described for MGUS (see Chapter 4, Monoclonal gammopathy of undetermined significance, p.512)

Note that patients with serum IgM monoclonal protein ≥3g/dL and/or bone marrow lymphoplasmacytic infiltration ≥10%, and no evidence of end-organ damage such as anaemia, constitutional symptoms, hyperviscosity, lymphadenopathy, or hepatosplenomegaly that that can be attributed to a plasma cell proliferative disorder are considered to have smouldering Waldenström's macroglobulinaemia (also referred to as indolent or asymptomatic Waldenström's macroglobulinaemia), an asymptomatic condition similar to SMM, but associated with a risk of progression to Waldenström's macroglobulinaemia rather than multiple myeloma.

Treatment

No therapy is indicated. The standard of care is observation alone until evidence of progression to myeloma (Kyle et al. 2004). Patients with SMM need more frequent follow-up than those with MGUS, at least every 3–4 months. Two small randomized trials have shown no benefit with early therapy compared with therapy at the time of symptomatic progression (Hjorth et al. 1993; Grignani et al. 1996).

There is preliminary data that thalidomide may delay time to progression, but data are needed from randomized trials before such therapy can be recommended, particularly given the adverse effects associated with the drug. Outside a clinical trial, therapy with bisphosphonates is not recommended. With the increasing availability of novel targeted therapies for myeloma, clinical trials are ongoing to determine if the early use of new agents or bisphosphonates can delay progression in SMM.

Prognosis

The risk of progression of SMM to multiple myeloma is approximately 10% per year for 5 years, 3% per year for the next 5 years, and 1.5% per year thereafter (Kyle et al. 2007). Thus the risk decreases with time in contrast to MGUS where the risk of progression does not change with time.

The presence of occult bone lesions on MRI increases the risk of progression in patients otherwise defined as having SMM. The median time to progression is significantly shorter with an abnormal MRI compared with normal MRI, 1.5 years versus 5 years, respectively.

Risk-stratification

A risk-stratification model is useful in assessing prognosis of SMM using three risk factors: bone marrow plasmacytosis ≥10%; serum M spike ≥3g/dL; and FLC ratio <0.125 or >8 (Dispenzieri et al. 2008). The cumulative probability of progression at 10 years is 50% in patients with one risk factor; 65% in those with two risk factors; and 84% in those with three risk factors

Further reading

Dispenzieri A, Kyle RA, Katzmann JA, et al. Immunoglobulin free light chain ratio is an independent risk factor for progression of smoldering (asymptomatic) multiple myeloma. *Blood* 2008; **111**:785–9.

Grignani G, Gobbi PG, Formisano R, et al. A prognostic index for multiple myeloma. *Br J Cancer* 1996; **73**:1101–17.

Hjorth M, Hellquist L, Holmberg E, et al. Initial versus deferred melphalan-prednisone therapy for asymptomatic multiple myeloma stage I – a randomized study. Myeloma Group of Western Sweden. *Eur J Haematol* 1993; **50**:95–102.

Kyle RA, Rajkumar SV. Multiple myeloma. *N Engl J Med* 2004; **351**:1860–73.

Kyle RA, Remstein ED, Therneau TM, et al. Clinical course and prognosis of smoldering (asymptomatic) multiple myeloma. *N Engl J Med* 2007; **356**:2582–90.

Waldenström's macroglobulinemia

Epidemiology and aetiology

Waldenström's macroglobulinaemia is a clonal IgM monoclonal protein secreting lymphoid/plasma cell disorder, which currently also includes the entity referred to previously as lymphoplasmacytic lymphoma.

Clinical features

The median age at diagnosis is approximately 65 years, with a slight male predisposition. The typical symptoms at presentation are weakness and fatigue due to anaemia. Other clinical manifestations include constitutional symptoms (fever, night sweats, and weight loss), hepatosplenomegaly, lymphadenopathy, hyperviscosity, cryoglobulinaemia, and sensorimotor peripheral neuropathy. Patients with hyperviscosity may present with headaches, epistaxis, blurred vision, somnolence, and seizures. Unlike multiple myeloma, osteolytic bone lesions and immunoglobulin heavy chain translocations are not seen in Waldenström's macroglobulinaemia.

Diagnosis

The diagnostic hallmark is the presence of an IgM monoclonal protein on serum immunofixation. The serum protein electrophoresis often reveals a fairly large spike, but in some patients the M spike may be small despite significant tumour burden. Anaemia is a major presenting symptom, and is normochromic, normocytic. The erythrocyte sedimentation rate is typically very high. Bone marrow biopsy reveals infiltration by clonal lymphoplasmacytoid cells. Serum viscosity may be elevated, usually in proportion to the size of the serum monoclonal protein.

Criteria for diagnosis of Waldenström's macroglobulinaemia

The diagnostic criteria for Waldenström's macroglobulinaemia require IgM monoclonal gammopathy (regardless of the size of the M protein), 10% or greater bone marrow infiltration (usually intertrabecular) by small lymphocytes that exhibit plasmacytoid or plasma cell differentiation and typical immunophenotype (e.g. surface IgM+, CD5+/−, CD10−, CD19+, CD20+, CD23−) that satisfactorily excludes other lymphoproliferative disorders including chronic lymphocytic leukaemia and mantle cell lymphoma (Table 4.10.23).

Differentiation from IgM MGUS and smouldering Waldenström's macroglobulinaemia

The presence of <10% lymphoplasmacytic infiltration in the absence of end-organ damage represents IgM MGUS and not Waldenström's macroglobulinaemia; such patients have a risk of progression to symptomatic disease at a rate of 1.5% per year (Baldiniet al. 2005; Gobbi et al. 2005; Rajkumar et al. 2006). On the other hand, patients with serum IgM monoclonal protein ≥3g/dL and/or bone marrow lymphoplasmacytic infiltration ≥10%, and no evidence of end-organ damage such as anaemia, constitutional symptoms, hyperviscosity, lymphadenopathy, or hepatosplenomegaly that can be attributed to a plasma cell proliferative disorder are considered to have smouldering Waldenström's macroglobulinaemia (also referred to as indolent or asymptomatic Waldenström's macroglobulinaemia), an asymptomatic condition similar to SMM, but which is associated with a risk of progression to Waldenström's macroglobulinemia.

Waldenström's macroglobulinaemia and lymphoplasmacytic lymphoma

Historically, patients with an IgM M protein <3g/dL meeting criteria for Waldenström's macroglobulinaemia were once classified as 'lymphoplasmacytic lymphoma with an IgM M protein'. However, except for hyperviscosity, the clinical picture, therapy, and prognosis in these patients is no different from that of patients classified as having Waldenström's macroglobulinaemia who have an IgM protein level ≥3g/dL (Gertzet al. 2000). By the current definition, such patients are considered to have Waldenström's macroglobulinaemia regardless of the size of the serum M protein.

Treatment

Patients with Waldenström's macroglobulinaemia who are asymptomatic do not need immediate therapy. The indications for therapy are anaemia (haemoglobin <10g/dL) or

Table 4.10.23 Diagnostic criteria

Disorder	Diagnostic criteria
IgM MGUS	1 Serum IgM monoclonal protein <3g/dL, and
	2 <10% clonal bone marrow lymphoplasmacytic infiltration, and
	3 No evidence of anaemia, constitutional symptoms, hyperviscosity, lymphadenopathy, or hepatosplenomegaly that can be attributed to a lymphoproliferative disorder
Smouldering (asymptomatic) Waldenström's macroglobulinaemia	1 Serum IgM monoclonal protein ≥3g/dL and/or bone marrow lymphoplasmacytic infiltration ≥10%, and
	2 No evidence of end-organ damage such as anaemia, constitutional symptoms, hyperviscosity, lymphadenopathy, or hepatosplenomegaly that can be attributed to a lymphoproliferative disorder
Waldenström's macroglobulinaemia	1 IgM monoclonal gammopathy (regardless of the size of the M protein), and
	2 >10% bone marrow lymphoplasmacytic infiltration (usually intertrabecular) by small lymphocytes that exhibit plasmacytoid or plasma cell differentiation and a typical immunophenotype (surface IgM+, CD10−, CD19+, CD20+, and CD23−)
	3 Evidence of end-organ damage such as anaemia, constitutional symptoms, hyperviscosity, lymphadenopathy, or hepatosplenomegaly that that can be attributed to a lymphoproliferative disorder

thrombocytopaenia (platelet count <100,000) which are thought to be related to Waldenström's macroglobulinaemia; constitutional symptoms such as weakness, fatigue, night sweats, or weight loss; hyperviscosity; symptomatic cryoglobulinaemia; and significant hepatosplenomegaly or lymphadenopathy.

Initial therapy

There are four options for initial therapy: rituximab, purine nucleoside analogues, alkylators, and combination chemotherapy. Unfortunately there are no randomized data to determine the best option; therapy is typically decided based on the age of the patient and the aggressiveness of the presentation. Patients should where possible be treated in clinical trials.

Single agent therapy with rituximab, a chimeric anti-CD20 monoclonal antibody, produces a response in approximately 50% of untreated patients. Responses to rituximab can delayed and may occur months after initial therapy. An initial increase in IgM levels (flare) has been reported. The usual dose is 375mg/m^2 administered intravenously weekly for 4 weeks (Gertz et al. 2004), with consideration given to further doses or maintenance depending on response. Rituximab is particularly useful in patients with low tumour burden.

Purine nucleoside analogues, fludarabine or cladribine, are effective as initial therapy (Dimopoulos et al. 1994; Dhodapkar et al. 2001). Response rates are approximately 50–80%. Cladribine at a dose of 5mg/m^2 intravenously over 2 hours for 5 days, repeated once after 28 days if needed, is an excellent choice particularly for patients with high tumour burden. The need for further cycles is determined by extent of response to the first two cycles as well as observed toxicity.

Alkylators such as chlorambucil are preferred as initial therapy in older patients. Chlorambucil is administered orally in a dosage of 6–8mg/day with dose adjustments based on blood counts. Patients are treated until the disease has reached a plateau state; the treatment can then be discontinued and patients observed closely.

The role of combination chemotherapy is not well defined. Preliminary results of several combination chemotherapeutic approaches suggest high response rates of >75%. Examples of active combinations include fludarabine plus rituximab, fludarabine plus cyclophosphamide, cladribine plus cyclophosphamide plus rituximab, and R-CHOP (rituximab, cyclophosphamide, doxorubicin, vincristine, prednisone).

Relapsed disease

Options listed for initial therapy discussed previously can be tried at the time of relapse, if there is an adequate interval between cessation of therapy and relapse. Other agents useful in relapsed disease include thalidomide, lenalidomide,

and bortezomib. Selected patients may be candidates for autologous stem cell transplantation.

Supportive care

Patients with refractory anaemia or anaemia during chemotherapy will benefit from erythropoietin and/or red cell transfusions. Plasmapheresis is indicated for the treatment of hyperviscosity syndrome. Plasmapheresis may need to be continued on an intermittent basis until a therapeutic response is achieved with one of the treatment options discussed earlier.

Prognosis

The median survival is approximately 5 years. Adverse prognostic factors include age >70 years, haemoglobin <9g/dL, weight loss, and cryoglobulinaemia. The risk-stratification model proposed by Morel and colleagues is useful in determining prognosis. It is based on a set of three adverse prognostic factors: age 65 or higher, albumin <4.0g/dL, and cytopenias. Cytopenia restricted to one haematopoietic lineage is scored as one risk factor, while two or more cytopenias are scored as two risk factors. Patients with 0–1 risk factors (low-risk), 2 risk factors (intermediate-risk) and 3–4 risk factors (high-risk) have 5-year survival rates of 87%, 62%, and 25%, respectively

Further reading

Baldini L, Goldaniga M, Guffanti A, et al. Immunoglobulin M monoclonal gammopathies of undetermined significance and indolent Waldenström's macroglobulinemia recognize the same determinants of evolution into symptomatic lymphoid disorders: proposal for a common prognostic scoring system. J Clin Oncol 2005; **23**:4662–8.

Dhodapkar MV, Jacobson JL, Gertz MA, et al. Prognostic factors and response to fludarabine therapy in patients with Waldenström macroglobulinemia: results of United States intergroup trial (Southwest Oncology Group S9003). Blood 2001; **98**:41–8.

Dimopoulos MA, Kantarjian H, Weber D, et al. Primary therapy of Waldenström's macroglobulinemia with 2-chlorodeoxyadenosine. J Clin Oncol 1994; **12**:2694–8.

Gertz MA, Fonseca R, Rajkumar SV. Waldenström's macroglobulinemia. Oncologist 2000; **5**:63–7.

Gertz MA, Rue M, Blood E, et al. Multicenter phase 2 trial of rituximab for Waldenström macroglobulinemia (WM): an Eastern Cooperative Oncology Group Study (E3A98). Leuk Lymphoma 2004; **45**:2047–55.

Gobbi PG, Baldini L, Broglia C, et al. Prognostic validation of the international classification of immunoglobulin M gammopathies: a survival advantage for patients with immunoglobulin M monoclonal gammopathy of undetermined significance? Clin Cancer Res 2005; **11**:1786–90.

Rajkumar SV, Dispenzieri A, Kyle RA. Monoclonal gammopathy of undetermined significance, Waldenström macroglobulinemia, AL amyloidosis, and related plasma cell disorders: diagnosis and treatment. Mayo Clinic Proc 2006; **81**:693–703.

Amyloidosis

Epidemiology and aetiology

Amyloid is the term given to a fibrillar proteinaceous material deposited in various tissues that is detected with Congo-red staining showing a characteristic apple-green birefringence under polarized light (Rajkumar and Gertz 2007). It consists of rigid, linear, non-branching fibrils, 7.5–10nm in width, aggregated in a β-pleated sheet conformation. There are several distinct types of amyloidosis classified based on the protein composition of the amyloid material (Table 4.10.24) (Rajkumar et al. 2006).

AL (immunoglobulin light chain) amyloidosis refers to the type of amyloidosis derived from the variable portion of a monoclonal light chain and occurs as a result of a clonal plasma cell proliferative disorder. AL amyloidosis may be localized (a benign disorder) or systemic. Systemic AL amyloidosis is commonly referred to as primary systemic amyloidosis or primary amyloidosis. The pathogenesis of AL amyloidosis is not well understood. It involves aberrant *de novo* synthesis and abnormal proteolytic processing of light chains.

Clinical features

The median age at diagnosis of systemic AL amyloidosis is 65 years. The clinical manifestations vary greatly, and depend on the dominant organ involved. Nephrotic syndrome, restrictive cardiomyopathy, and peripheral/autonomic neuropathy are common presenting syndromes. Patients may also have associated macroglossia, carpal tunnel syndrome, and purpura involving the neck, face and eyes. Immunofixation reveals an M protein in the serum or urine in almost 90% of patients at diagnosis. Regardless of the number of bone marrow plasma cells in the bone marrow, the syndrome is referred to as 'AL' or 'primary' as long as the amyloid fibrils are composed of immunoglobulin light chain. Approximately 10% of patients with systemic AL amyloidosis have myeloma, and vice versa, but usually one of the two disorders dominates the clinical picture.

The clinical features of other forms of amyloidosis depend on the type of organ involvement (Table 4.10.24).

Diagnosis

The diagnosis of systemic AL amyloidosis requires documentation of positive amyloid staining on a tissue biopsy as well as supporting evidence that the amyloid is derived from immunoglobulin light chains (see Table 4.10.25 in 'POEMS syndrome' section, p.520). AL amyloidosis should be suspected when patients with nephrotic syndrome, axonal neuropathy, or restrictive cardiomyopathy display evidence of a plasma cell proliferative disorder and/or a serum or urine monoclonal protein. It should be differentiated from localized amyloidosis which can be derived from immunoglobulin light chains in many patients. Localized amyloidosis, unlike systemic AL amyloidosis is typically benign, and is treated primarily for symptom relief as needed.

Treatment

Systemic AL amyloidosis

The standard treatment for systemic AL amyloidosis is melphalan and high-dose dexamethasone. Melphalan is administered in a dose of 0.22mg/kg per day orally on days 1–4 with high dose dexamethasone 40mg/day orally on the same 4 days. Cycles are repeated every 28 days for about 9 months (Palladini et al. 2004). Selected patients may be treated with ASCT in specialized centres with significant experience with the procedure. A recent randomized trial found that stem cell transplantation was not superior to melphalan and high-dose dexamethasone (Jaccard et al. 2007). However, interpretation of this trial is confounded by the high treatment-related mortality observed in the transplant arm. Second-line treatment options include thalidomide plus dexamethasone, lenalidomide plus dexamethasone, and bortezomib. Patients with amyloidosis require significant supportive care based on the nature of organ involvement such as treatment of nephrotic syndrome, malabsorption, neuropathy, and heart failure.

Other forms of amyloidosis

Treatment for other forms of amyloidosis varies depending on the type of amyloidosis (Table 4.10.24)

Table 4.10.24 Classification and treatment of common forms of amyloidosis

Type of amyloidosis	Constituent amyloid protein	Treatment
AL (primary) amyloidosis	κ or λ immunoglobulin light chain	Melphalan plus dexamethasone; autologous stem cell transplantation in selected patients
AA (secondary) amyloidosis	Protein A	Treat underlying infection or inflammation
Transthyretin (ATTR) amyloidosis:		
• Familial ATTR	Mutant transthyretin	Liver transplantation for selected patients
• Senile amyloidosis	Wild-type transthyretin	No specific therapy

Prognosis

Survival varies greatly depending on the type of amyloidosis. In systemic AL amyloidosis, survival is greatly dependent on the dominant organ involved. Cardiac amyloidosis has the worst outcome. The number of major organs involved is another major factor that influences outcome. Patients not eligible for stem cell transplantation have an estimated median survival of 18 months, compared with >40 months for those eligible for transplantation

(Dispenzieri et al. 2001). Elevated levels of cardiac troponin T levels and N-terminal pro-brain natriuretic peptide (NT-proBNP) levels are associated with an adverse prognosis.

Further reading

Dispenzieri A. POEMS syndrome. *Hematology (Am Soc Hematol Educ Program)* 2005; **1**:360–7.

Dispenzieri A, Lacy MQ, Kyle RA, *et al.* Eligibility for hematopoietic stem-cell transplantation for primary systemic amyloidosis is a favorable prognostic factor for survival. *J Clin Oncol* 2001; **19**:3350–6.

Dispenzieri A, Kyle RA, Lacy MQ, *et al.* POEMS syndrome: definitions and long-term outcome. *Blood* 2003; **101**:2496–506.

Jaccard A, Moreau P, Leblond V, *et al.* High-dose melphalan versus melphalan plus dexamethasone for AL amyloidosis. *N Engl J Med* 2007; **357**:1083–93.

Palladini G, Perfetti V, Obici L, *et al.* Association of melphalan and high-dose dexamethasone is effective and well tolerated in patients with AL (primary) amyloidosis who are ineligible for stem cell transplantation. *Blood* 2004; **103**:2936–8.

Rajkumar SV, Gertz MA. Advances in the treatment of amyloidosis. *N Engl J Med* 2007; **356**:2413–5.

Rajkumar SV, Dispenzieri A, Kyle RA. Monoclonal gammopathy of undetermined significance, Waldenström macroglobulinemia, AL amyloidosis, and related plasma cell disorders: diagnosis and treatment. *Mayo Clinic Proc* 2006; **81**:693–703.

POEMS syndrome

POEMS syndrome (polyneuropathy, organomegaly, endocrinopathy, monoclonal protein, skin changes) is defined by the criteria listed in Table 4.10.25 (Dispenzieri et al. 2006; Rajkumar et al. 2006). It is a rare, atypical, plasma cell proliferative disorder variously referred to in the literature as osteosclerotic myeloma, Crow–Fukase syndrome, PEP (plasma cell dyscrasia, endocrinopathy, polyneuropathy) syndrome, and Takatsuki syndrome.

Clinical features

The median age at presentation is approximately 50 years. Almost all patients have either osteosclerotic lesions or Castleman's disease. The major clinical features are a predominantly motor chronic inflammatory demyelinating polyneuropathy, sclerotic bone lesions, and a varying number of associated abnormalities such as hepatomegaly, hyperpigmentation, hypertrichosis, gynaecomastia, testicular atrophy, clubbing, polycythaemia, thrombocytosis, and Castleman's disease. Biopsy of an osteosclerotic lesion may be necessary for the diagnosis. In almost all cases the immunoglobulin light chain type is lambda.

Treatment

If the lesions are in a limited area, radiation therapy (40–50Gy) is the treatment of choice. For patients with widespread osteosclerotic lesions, treatment is similar to myeloma.

Prognosis

POEMS syndrome may have an indolent or a fulminant course. In one study of 99 patients, median survival was 13.8 years (Dispenzieri et al. 2003). If unchecked, the clinical course is characterized by progressive disabling neuropathy, inanition, anasarca, and pulmonary demise.

Further reading

Dispenzieri A. POEMS syndrome. *Hematology (Am Soc Hematol Educ Program)* 2005; **1**:360–7.

Dispenzieri A, Kyle RA, Lacy MQ, et al. POEMS syndrome: definitions and long-term outcome. *Blood* 2003; **101**:2496–506.

Rajkumar SV, Dispenzieri A, Kyle RA. Monoclonal gammopathy of undetermined significance, Waldenström macroglobulinemia, AL amyloidosis, and related plasma cell disorders: diagnosis and treatment. *Mayo Clinic Proc* 2006; **81**:693–703.

Table 4.10.25 Diagnostic criteria for systemic AL amyloidosis and POEMS syndrome

Disorder	Disease definition
Systemic AL amyloidosis	1 Presence of an amyloid-related systemic syndrome (such as renal, liver, heart, GI tract, or peripheral nerve involvement), and
	2 Positive amyloid staining by Congo red in any tissue (e.g., fat aspirate, bone marrow, or organ biopsy), and
	3 Evidence that amyloid is light-chain related established by direct examination of the amyloid (immunoperoxidase staining, direct sequencing, etc.), and preferably
	4 Evidence of a monoclonal plasma cell proliferative disorder (serum or urine M protein, abnormal free light chain ratio, or clonal plasma cells in the bone marrow)
POEMS syndrome	1 Presence of a monoclonal plasma cell disorder, and
	2 Peripheral neuropathy, and
	3 At least 1 of the following 7 features: osteosclerotic myeloma, Castleman's disease, organomegaly, endocrinopathy (excluding diabetes mellitus or hypothyroidism), oedema, typical skin changes, and papilloedema, and
	4 The features should have a temporal relationship to each other and no other attributable cause.

Heavy chain disease

The heavy-chain diseases (HCDs) are characterized by the presence of an M protein consisting of a portion of the IgH chain in the serum or urine or both, and are classified based on the type of heavy chain that is involved.

Gamma heavy chain disease (γ-HCD)

Patients with γ-HCD often present with a lymphoma-like illness. The electrophoretic pattern often shows a broad-based band more suggestive of a polyclonal increase than an M protein. Treatment is indicated for symptomatic patients and consists of chemotherapy similar to myeloma or NHL.

Alpha heavy chain disease (α-HCD)

This is the most common form of HCD, and occurs in patients from the Mediterranean region or Middle East. Most commonly, the GI tract is involved, resulting in severe malabsorption with diarrhoea, steatorrhoea, and loss of weight. The usual treatment is with antibiotics. Patients who do not respond adequately to antibiotics are treated with chemotherapy similar to that used to treat NHL.

Mu heavy chain disease (μ-HCD)

This disease is characterized by the demonstration of a monoclonal μ-chain fragment in the serum. Treatment is with corticosteroids and alkylating agents.

Histiocyte disorders

Introduction

The primary histiocyte disorders are rare conditions that occur most often in children. They remain incompletely defined both in terms of phenotype and biological behaviour, and pose a significant challenge from the standpoint of nosology. The clinical presentation is variable and ranges from self-limiting to lethal disease. The central controversies relate to whether the individual histiocyte disorders represent malignant or inflammatory conditions; identification of the cell of origin within the context of normal histiocyte development (ontogeny); and correlation of biological behaviour with aspects of histiocyte morphology, immunophenotype, and clonality. The primary focus of this review is Langerhans cell histiocytosis (LCH), which is discussed within the framework of other histiocyte disorders.

Epidemiology

Many patients with LCH are children, with a peak between 1–3 years of age, and a predilection for males (male: female ratio 3–4:1). The annual incidence in children <15 years has been estimated to range from 0.5–1 cases per 100,000 children. In adults, LCH is probably underdiagnosed given the heterogeneous clinical presentation, and the variety of specialists involved in patient care. The prevalence in adults is estimated at one to two cases per one million population. In one study of 274 adult patients, 52% were men, and the median age at diagnosis was 35 years. Although familial LCH has been reported, most cases are sporadic in nature.

Aetiology

The aetiology of primary histiocyte disorders remains unknown. Clonality studies indicate that in most LCH cases, the pathological cell (Langerhans cell; LC) is clonally derived. However, the frequent spontaneous regression of LCH lesions, and the inability to propagate LC in ex vivo culture or in immune-deficient mice, support the view that LCH is not a conventional neoplasm. The most well accepted environmental risk factor is cigarette smoking which is virtually universally associated with the pulmonary form of adult LCH, which in contrast to other forms of systemic LCH, represents a reactive polyclonal proliferation of LC. Although human herpes virus-6 (HHV-6) has been identified in LCH lesions, its role in LCH pathogenesis remains controversial. LCH has also been proposed to result from an abnormal cytokine microenvironment, wherein immune cells such as macrophages and T-lymphocytes produce cytokines (tumour necrosis factor-alpha, various interleukins) that inhibit normal maturation of LC. This cytokine dysregulation may explain several features, including presence of eosinophils within LCH lesions, elevated erythrocyte sedimentation rate (ESR), and thrombocytosis, that are often associated with active disease.

Classification

The classification of malignant tumours derived from histiocytes remains controversial, apart from classical LCH. On the basis of morphological, ultrastructural, and functional features, two major categories of histiocytes are recognized: 1) dendritic cells (DC) that play a key role in antigen presentation to lymphocytes, and include LC (skin, bronchial, and gut epithelium), interstitial DC/dermal dendrocytes (IDC; counterpart of LC in parenchymal organs), and follicular DC (FDC; germinal centre of lymph nodes); and 2) phagocytes, which may be freely mobile, such as circulating monocytes, or fixed within tissues, such as Kupffer cells of the liver or alveolar macrophages of the lung. There exists a close relationship between histiocytes that results in phenotypic and functional overlap, with specific cell characteristics being governed by the stage of development as well as the cytokine micro-environment. The histological classification is based on the dominant histiocyte involved; consequently, histiocyte disorders are broadly grouped into DC-related and macrophage/phagocyte-related histiocytoses (Favara et al. 1997), a classification that has been facilitated by recent advances in histiocyte immunophenotyping in both snap-frozen and paraffin-embedded tissue sections. LCH and juvenile xanthogranuloma (JXG) are examples of the former group, while Rosai–Dorfman disease (sinus histiocytosis with massive lymphadenopathy) and the haemophagocytic syndromes (primary haemophagocytic lymphohistiocytosis [HLH] and secondary haemophagocytic syndromes) represent the latter. LC exhibit low levels of lysozyme and are CD14−, CD1a+, S-100+, Langerin+, and factor XIIIa−. In contrast, IDC which represent the putative precursor cell for most non-LCH histiocytoses (JXG family of cutaneous histiocytoses, xanthoma disseminatum, Erdheim–Chester disease), are typically CD14+, Factor XIIIa+, CD68+, Fascin+, CD1a−, and S-100−. Histiocyte disorders derived from polyclonal activated macrophages such as Rosai–Dorfman disease exhibit lesional cells that are CD14+, CD68+, CD163+, Fascin+, S-100+, and CD1a−. Rare histiocyte disorders lack markers for LC, IDC, and macrophages, but clearly originate from DC (e.g. indeterminate cell histiocytosis).

Clinical features

LCH presents as several overlapping syndromes: unifocal disease, most often involving bone (lytic lesions involving skull, ribs, pelvis, or femur) which present as a painless isolated lesion, or cause pain, fracture, deformity, dental problems, or hearing loss; extension into adjacent soft tissue may compromise vital structures (e.g. spinal cord, optic nerve). Less common sites of unifocal involvement include skin (seborrhea-like or papular rash), lymph node, or lung—in adults isolated pulmonary involvement is a distinct condition and is considered a LCH-variant. Multfocal LCH can affect a single system (most often bone), or multiple systems—the latter is subclassified into two groups, based on whether there is 'risk organ' involvement (spleen, liver, lungs, and bone marrow). Risk organ compromise (<15% of paediatric cases) may be accompanied by hypoalbuminaemia, oedema, ascites, jaundice, and/or coagulopathy (liver); tachypnoea, dyspnoea, and/or chest pain from pneumothorax (lung); and cytopaenias (bone marrow involvement and/or hypersplenism). Between 15–50% of cases have pituitary/hypothalamic involvement, presenting as diabetes insipidus (DI) or growth retardation that may predate the LCH diagnosis—risk factors for DI include multisystem disease and involvement of craniofacial bones. CNS involvement (cerebellum, brainstem) may be seen late in the disease, with ataxia, dysarthria, or visual problems. Poor prognosis features include 'risk organ' involvement, multisystem disease, CNS involvement, and/ or poor early (6 weeks) response to therapy—a 30–50% mortality has been reported in the presence of such features, as compared to <10% in their absence. In addition, >50% of children with multisystem involvement suffer from late sequelae of the disease (DI, short stature, orthopaedic deformities, cognitive dysfunction, pulmonary fibrosis, etc.). Survival of adults with isolated pulmonary LCH has been reported to be significantly shorter than that of age- and sex-matched control subjects. The non-LCH histiocyte disorders can be distinguished into three groups based on clinical presentation: those that predominantly affect skin (e.g. JXG, benign cephalic histiocytosis, solitary reticulohistiocytoma, progressive nodular histiocytosis); those that affect skin but have a major systemic component (e.g. xanthoma disseminatum, multicentric reticulohistiocytosis); and those that primarily involve extracutaneous sites (e.g. Erdheim–Chester and Rosai– Dorfman diseases).

Diagnosis

The diagnosis of histiocyte disorders rests on pathological examination of the involved organ or tissue. The use of criteria set forth by the Histiocyte Society is strongly recommended to definitively diagnose LCH. Recognition of characteristic histiocyte cytomorphology, as displayed by haematoxylin & eosin (H&E) stain, may allow for a presumptive diagnosis of this condition. A definitive diagnosis however additionally requires demonstration of characteristic tennis racket-shaped Birbeck granules in lesional cells by electron microscopy (present in 1–75% of LC), and is considered the 'gold standard'. The CD1a antigen is a more convenient but less specific marker, and also allows for definitive diagnosis of LCH when detected in lesional cells by immunostaining. The frequency of positive tests varies according to the specific organ or tissue examined. For instance, it may be difficult to demonstrate Birbeck granules or positive staining for the CD1a antigen in CNS lesions. Staining for S-100 is also commonly employed in the evaluation of histiocyte disorders, but its presence is not specific for LC; other cell types (e.g. interstitial or indeterminate histiocytes), reactive activated macrophages, and naeval cells and chondrocytes are also S-100+. Langerin, a novel C-type lectin specific to LC cells, is an endocytic receptor that induces the formation of Birbeck granules. Langerin expression, as detected by immunohistochemistry, appears to be a highly sensitive and relatively specific marker for LCH. It is virtually uniformly coexpressed with CD1a in LCH lesions, and in contrast, is rarely expressed in proliferative disorders involving non-LC histiocytes. The diagnosis of non-LCH histiocyte disorders is similarly made on the basis of morphology and immunophenotype.

Treatment

Treatment of LCH is individualized and based upon patient age, risk group, number of lesions, and site(s) of involvement. Treatment options range from a 'wait-and-see' approach, to local approaches (curettage, intralesional steroids, radiation, topical steroids, or nitrogen mustard), to corticosteroids in combination with single- or multiagent chemotherapy (vinblastine and etoposide are mainstays; other active agents include 6-mercaptopurine, and 2-chlorodeoxyadenosine), to myeloablative therapy with allogeneic stem cell rescue. Several randomized multicentre clinical trials have been conducted under the auspices of the Histiocyte Society, with the recent LCH II study demonstrating improved survival of patients with 'risk organ' involvement with intensification of treatment.

Further reading

Favara BE, Feller AC, Pauli M, et al. Contemporary classification of histiocytic disorders. The WHO committee on histiocytic/reticulum cell proliferations. Reclassification working group of the histiocyte society. *Med Pediatr Oncol* 1997; **29**(3):157–66.

Gadner H, Grois N, Pötschger U, et al. Improved outcome in multisystem Langerhans cell histiocytosis is associated with therapy intensification. *Blood* 2008; **111**(5):2556–62.

Henter JI, Tondini C, Pritchard J. Histiocyte disorders. *Crit Rev Oncol Hematol* 2004; **50**(2):157–74.

Pileri SA, Grogan TM, Harris NL, et al. Tumours of histiocytes and accessory dendritic cells: an immunohistochemical approach to classification from the International Lymphoma Study Group based on 61 cases. *Histopathology* 2002; **41**(1):1–29.

Weitzman S, Jaffe R 2005; Uncommon histiocytic disorders: the non-Langerhans cell histiocytoses. *Pediatr Blood Cancer.* **45**(3):256–64.

Internet resource

Histiocytosis Society: http://www.histio.org

Thyroid cancer: introduction

Epidemiology
Malignancies of the thyroid gland are the commonest endocrine malignancy but comprise <1% of cancer incidence overall (Coleman et al. 1999). The incidence is increasing slowly. The highest incidence is seen in North and Central America, and Australasia, with the lowest incidence in Africa.

Histological types
Classification is according to the cell of origin. Of those of epithelial cell origin, the differentiated papillary and follicular carcinomas are the most common; anaplastic or undifferentiated thyroid carcinomas are less frequent. Medullary carcinomas originate from the parafollicular C cells. Finally, primary thyroid lymphomas can occur which are discussed elsewhere (see p.462). Reporting of histopathology should be performed by a histo/cytopathologist with a special interest in thyroid malignancy (RCP 2005).

Molecular profiles are being established for thyroid cancers and many genetic abnormalities have been identified. At present this has clinical relevance for medullary carcinoma but may become increasingly important for other tumour types.

Aetiology
Papillary:
- Majority are idiopathic
- Radiation exposure particularly during childhood (Thompson et al. 1987)
- Inherited conditions:
    Familial adenomatous polyposis (FAP)
    Cowden's disease
    Gardner's syndrome
- As an isolated inherited syndrome

Follicular:
- Endemic goitre associated with iodine deficiency
- RAS mutations are common

Medullary carcinoma thyroid:
- 80% are sporadic
- Inherited conditions:
    MEN2 syndromes (Mulligan et al. 1994)
    Familial medullary thyroid cancer (FMTC) syndrome (Mulligan et al. 1994)
- RET mutations are common

Anaplastic carcinoma thyroid:
- History of other thyroid pathology
    Differentiated thyroid cancer (20%)
    Multinodular goitre (50%)
- BRAF mutations are seen as abnormalities in RAS/RAF signalling pathways

Clinical features
Well-differentiated carcinoma thyroid
This typically affects females in their fourth decade. Most commonly presents with a slow growing or pre-existing enlarging solitary nodule. Lymphadenopathy is unusual with follicular tumours and is more common in papillary tumours. Symptomatic metastases at presentation are uncommon.

Medullary carcinoma thyroid
These patients are typically older than those with differentiated cancer with a mean age of 50–60 years. A solitary thyroid nodule is the commonest presenting feature. Cervical lymphadenopathy is common. There may be symptoms of local invasion such as hoarse voice, or dysphagia. Diarrhoea and flushing can occur as a result of calcitonin secretion. Rarely Cushing's syndrome may be seen.

Anaplastic carcinoma thyroid
Patients are older than those with other forms of thyroid malignancy. Mean age is 65 years. Presentation is with a rapidly growing thyroid mass. Symptoms and signs of local invasion are common, including dysphagia, stridor, hoarse voice due to paralysis of the vocal cords, and evidence of SVC obstruction. There may be skin involvement with erythema or ulceration. Pain is a common feature. The mass may be fixed to underlying structures. Lymphadenopathy is often seen. There may be symptoms of metastatic disease and systemic symptoms such as fever, weight loss, and lethargy. The important differential diagnosis is that of thyroid lymphoma.

Diagnosis
Initial thyroid function tests should be performed. Elevated thyroid hormones make a malignant diagnosis extremely unlikely, as it is rare for any form of thyroid malignancy to be associated with over-secretion of thyroid hormones. FNA with or without ultrasound guidance is the investigation of choice. Anaplastic thyroid cancer and lymphomas may require a core biopsy. It should be noted that the diagnosis of follicular thyroid cancer cannot be made on a biopsy since it requires evidence of capsular or vascular invasion (Sclabas et al. 2003). All follicular lesions diagnosed by FNA require further evaluation with a hemithyroidectomy; 15% will prove to be malignant (Sclabas et al. 2003).

Additional investigations will depend on the clinical presentation and may include:
- Three-dimensional imaging with CT or MRI, particularly if there is clinical evidence of local invasion. MRI may be preferred as it avoids the use of iodine containing contrast, which may cause thyroid stunning and prevent effective use of radioiodine for at least 3 months subsequently.
- Thyroid auto-antibodies if underlying Hashimoto's thyroiditis is suspected.
- Calcitonin in suspected medullary carcinoma.
- Flow volume loop if there is evidence of airway obstruction.

Staging
The recommended pathological staging is by the TNM staging system (Sclabas et al. 2003). There are a number of other postoperative staging systems in use for differentiated thyroid cancers which are used for assessing prognosis. The TNM and MACIS have been shown to be the best

predictors of outcome in validation studies (Sobin and Wittekend 2002; D'Avanzo et al. 2004).

AJCC/UICC TNM Classification (6th edition)
Primary
- pT1: intrathyroidal tumour ≤2cm in greatest dimension
- pT2: intrathyroidal tumour >2–4cm in greatest dimension
- pT3: intrathyroidal tumour >4cm in greatest dimension
- pT4: tumour of any size extending beyond the thyroid capsule
- pTX: primary tumour cannot be assessed

Regional lymph nodes (cervical and upper mediastinal)
- N0: no nodes involved
- N1: regional nodal involvement
  N1a: ipsilateral cervical nodes
  N1b: bilateral, midline or contralateral cervical nodes, or mediastinal nodes
- NX: nodes cannot be assessed

Distant metastases
- M0: no distant metastases
- M1: distant metastases
- MX: distant metastases cannot be assessed

Staging of epithelial thyroid carcinomas
- *Stage I:*
  Aged 45 or younger with any pT, any N M0
  Aged 45 or older with pT1N0M0
  20-year overall survival approximately 98% (5th edition data)
- *Stage II:*
  Aged 45 or younger with any pT any N M1
  Aged 45 or older with pT2N0M0 or pT3N0M0
- *Stage III:* aged 45 or older with pT4N0M0 or any pT, N1M0
- *Stage IV:*
  Aged 45 or older with any pT, any N, M1
  Anaplastic thyroid carcinoma any age or stage
  5-year survival approximately 10–20% (5th edition data)

Other staging/prognostication systems in use
- *MACIS:* Metastasis, Age, Completeness of resection, Invasion, Size:

Composite scoring system for 20-year survival probability
Score = 3.1 (age <40 years) or age × 0.08 (age 40 years or more):
      + 3 if metastasis
      +1 if incomplete resection
      +1 if invasion seen
      + 0.3 × size in cm

Score:	<6	6–6.99	7–7.99	>8
20-year survival:	99%	89%	56%	24%

- *AMES:* Age Metastasis Extent Size
- *AGES:* Age Grade Extent Size
- *De Groot:* Thyroid limited disease, nodal disease, extra-thyroidal extension, metastases.
- *EORTC:* Age, Sex, Histology, Invasion, Distant metastases
- *NTCTS:* Age, Size, Multicentricity, Invasion, Nodal metastases. Distant metastases.

Further reading
Coleman PM, Babb P, Damiecki P, *et al. Cancer survival trends in England and Wales 1971–1995: deprivation and NHS region.* Series SMPS No. 61, pp.471–8. London: Stationery Office, 1999.

D'Avanzo A, Ituarte P, Treseler P, *et al.* Prognostic scoring systems in patients with follicular thyroid cancer: a comparison of different staging systems in predicting the patient outcome. *Thyroid* 2004; **14**:453–8.

Mulligan LM, Eng C, Healey CS, *et al.* Specific mutations of the RET proto-oncogene are related to disease phenotype in MEN 2A and FMTC. *Nat Genet* 1994; **6**:70–4.

Royal College of Pathologists. Standards and datasets for reporting cancers: datasets for histopathology reports on head and neck carcinomas and salivary neoplasms, 2nd edition. London: RCPath, 2005—available at: www.rcpath.org/resources/pdf/HeadNeckDatasetJun05.pdf

Sclabas GM, Staerkel GA, Shapiro SE, *et al.* Fine-needle aspiration of the thyroid and correlation with histopathology in a contemporary series of 240 patients. *Am J Surg* 2003; **186**:702–9.

Sobin LH and Wittekend C (eds). *TNM classification of malignant tumours,* 6th edn. New York: Wiley-Liss, 2002.

Thompson DE, Mabuchi K, Ron E, *et al.* Cancer incidence in atomic bomb survivors. Part II: Solid tumours, 1958–1987. *Radiat Res* 1994; **137**:S17–67.

Thyroid cancer: management of differentiated cancer

The care of patients with thyroid cancer should be under-taken within the context of a specialist MDT (see 'Internet resource'). The surgeon(s) should have a special training in thyroid surgery (DOH 2004).

Surgery

Thyroid
The majority of patients will require total or near total thy-roidectomy with complete removal of virtually all thyroid tissue, preserving the recurrent laryngeal nerve.

Those defined as low risk may be treated with lobectomy. Low risk includes:
• Papillary thyroid cancer diameter <1cm and no evidence of nodal involvement.
• Follicular thyroid cancer, diameter <1cm with minimal capsular invasion.
• Follicular thyroid cancer in females <45 years old with tumour diameter <2cm.

In addition to these patients there is an intermediate group of patients (those without additional risk factors with tumours of diameters 2–4cm) for whom it may be appropriate to perform a lobectomy after MDT and patient discussion.

Parathyroid glands should be conserved where possible. It is recommended that where the vascular supply is com-promised they may be reimplanted into muscle.

Lymph nodes
As for thyroidectomy, the extent of surgery depends on assessment of the risk of metastatic spread. Those patients with high-risk disease should undergo elective dissection of level VI (anterior compartment) nodes. Risk factors for nodal involvement include:
• Males >45 years of age.
• Tumour diameter >4cm.
• Evidence of extracapsular spread or extrathyroid disease.

Patients with palpable level VI nodes should have dissec-tion of central compartment nodes. If there is evidence of lateral compartment (levels II–V) involvement this should be confirmed with FNA or frozen section and a modified radical neck dissection should be performed.

Postoperative management

All patients should have serum calcium measured postop-eratively as profound transient hypocalcaemia may occur. Triiodothyronine (T3), 20mg twice daily should be com-menced as thyroid hormone replacement. Thyroglobulin is a protein secreted both by normal thyroid tissue and by differentiated thyroid carcinomas. It is used as a tumour marker. Serum thyroglobulin should be measured at least 6 weeks postoperatively. In patients who have undergone total thyroidectomy and who are free of disease, thy-roglobulin should be undetectable.

Radioiodine ablation
After thyroidectomy some residual thyroid tissue may remain, making thyroglobulin unreliable as a tumour mark-er. Radioiodine ablation eliminates residual thyroid tissue. It also allows identification and possible elimination of occult micrometastatic disease, and in intermediate and high-risk patients several retrospective studies have shown a survival advantage. The current recommendations for radioiodine ablation are for those with differentiated

tumours >1–1.5cm, in diameter, where there is a reduced local and, distant relapse rate and cancer death rate in those >45 years and tumours >1.5cm in diameter (Mazzaferri and Jhiang 1994). The benefit may be less for low-risk disease and therefore it is also important to con-sider the risk of radioiodine causing second malignancies (Sandeep et al. 2006). Decision-making for radioiodine administration should be within the MDT setting and the British Thyroid Association guidelines aim to assist this process (see 'Internet resource'). A summary of this sec-tion of the guidelines is shown in the box.

Indications for radioiodine ablation

Absolute indications
• Metastatic disease
• Incomplete excision—unsuitable for further excision
• Extracapsular spread
• Tumour diameter >1.5–2cm

Probable indications
• Less than total thyroidectomy
• Unknown lymph node status
• Diameter >1cm with other high-risk factors
• Multifocality

Radioiodine ablation unnecessary
Providing **all** of the following:
• Total thyroidectomy
• Favourable histology
• Unifocal tumour without vascular invasion
• Absence of extracapsular extension
• Diameter <1cm

Procedure for ablation
In order to ensure maximal uptake of radioiodine, patients are rendered hypothyroid prior to administration. This is achieved by commencing a low iodine diet, and by avoiding other sources of iodine, e.g. contrast from CT imaging. Amiodarone may need to be discontinued for 2–3 months before radioiodine administration. Thyroxine (T4) replace-ment is withdrawn. Initially 4–6 weeks before treatment T4 is stopped and replaced with shorter-acting T3. Two weeks before therapy, replacement is discontinued com-pletely. In some circumstances withdrawal may be danger-ous, for example, in patients with a history of myxoedema psychosis, severe cardiac disease, or high-volume meta-static disease. In these situations recombinant human TSH (rhTSH) may be used, avoiding the need to induce a hypothyroid state. 0.9mg rhTSH is given by intramuscular injection once daily for 48 hours before administration of radioiodine.

Patients are admitted to a specialist facility with appro-priate lead shielding and sanitation. Consent is confirmed (see box) and pregnancy is excluded. Stimulated TSH and thyroglobulin are measured. 3.7GBq of radioiodine is administered orally as a drink or capsule. Patients remain in isolation until safe levels are measured by medical physics staff. During isolation patients are advised to keep hydrat-ed, empty the bladder frequently, and to take prescribed laxatives to avoid constipation. These measures minimize absorbed dose of radiation. An uptake scan using a gamma scintillation camera is performed 3–10 days after radioiod-ine administration.

Consent for radioiodine: information for patient

Early effects
- Symptoms of hypothyroidism for 4–6 weeks
- Sialoadenitis and taste changes
- Nausea
- Neck pain and swelling
- Radiation cystitis, gastritis

Late effects
- Dry mouth and taste changes
- Dry eyes due to lachrymal gland dysfunction
- Epiphora due to nasolacrimal duct stenosis
- Risk of second malignancy <1%—leukaemia, bladder, breast, salivary glands
- Pulmonary fibrosis—miliary pulmonary disease and multiple doses of I [131]
- Male infertility—rare with cumulative doses <5.5GBq
- Increase in miscarriage rate in first year after treatment

Postablation measurement of thyroglobulin and the uptake scan are useful in the diagnosis of residual disease. In these patients, with elevated TG and positive uptake scans, management is according to the site of disease. If residual neck disease is found, consideration should be given to further surgery. If the residual disease is not amenable to surgery, a therapy dose of radioiodine (5.5MBq) is administered.

Follow-up and further management

Six months after radioiodine ablation a stimulated thyroglobulin is measured and in all but very low-risk cases a radioiodine uptake scan is performed to guide further management. Those with undetectable stimulated thyroglobulin and satisfactory uptake scan appearances are routinely followed-up. These patients are followed-up lifelong, both because of the risk of curable late relapses and to monitor and manage the toxicity of supraphysiological thyroid replacement. Patients are initially reviewed to ensure satisfactory T4 dose. When levels are stable they are seen 6–12-monthly. At review, apart from clinical examination, thyroid function tests, serum thyroglobulin (TG) and serum calcium are estimated. Assessment of toxicity of T4 replacement is made and in some cases dose may be reduced despite unsuppressed TSH levels depending on the risk and toxicity. Baseline DEXA scan for bone mineral density is performed and follow-up imaging and bisphosphonates are prescribed as necessary. Patients who have had calcium abnormality requiring long-term replacement should be assessed by an endocrinologist.

In patients with elevated stimulated TG but no evidence of residual disease, a repeat stimulated TG is performed after 6 months and often the TG level will have fallen. In these patients it is important to ensure that the uptake scan is not spuriously negative as a result of inadequate TSH stimulation or iodine contamination. If the TG level is rapidly rising, it is suggestive of occult metastatic disease and hence further assessment with other imaging modalities is required. FDG-PET may be helpful in those with elevated TG. If no disease is identified, management options lie between expectant or empirical use of therapy doses of radioiodine. In patients who are initially disease-free but develop recurrent disease this usually manifests as elevated unstimulated thyroglobulin (5% will relapse

without elevation in TG and 25% of patients will have antithyroglobulin antibodies making serum TG levels unreliable). A stimulated TG and whole-body uptake scan are performed to identify the site of recurrence. As for residual disease, local recurrence is managed by surgery where possible. In patients with inoperable or soft tissue metastatic disease, a therapy dose of radioiodine is administered in the same way as an ablation dose. A dose of 5.5MBq is usually given. (Lower doses are used in renal impairment.) Following treatment an uptake scan is performed as per ablation scan. In those with uptake, further doses of radioiodine are given every 6 months. Treatment is continued until uptake ceases or there are concerns regarding bone marrow suppression or lung fibrosis. In patients with skeletal metastases, radioiodine can be less effective and may require additional treatment with EBRT. Patients with solitary brain metastases should be considered for surgical excision if of good PS and with otherwise controlled disease. Otherwise whole-brain radiotherapy is used. In some cases stereotactic boosts may be employed.

Role of external beam radiotherapy
Radiotherapy is not commonly used in differentiated thyroid cancer because the majority take up radioiodine. The evidence for the use of EBRT is unclear. The majority of studies are retrospective and surgical procedures, use of radioiodine, and TSH suppression are variable. It is therefore difficult to draw conclusions. Many studies show no benefit. However, this may reflect the inclusion of many low-risk patients diluting the benefits to those at high risk of relapse. There does appear to be reduction in local recurrence in those with high-risk features such as older age, gross extrathyroidal extension, and extensive extranodal spread. EBRT should therefore be considered in patients with tumours that do not take up radioiodine, those with gross microscopic residual tumour, and patients >60 years of age with pT4 disease (even when completely excised) and extensive extranodal disease.

The target volume includes the entire thyroid bed, and draining lymph nodes (levels III–VI); this may be adjusted depending on the operative findings and pathology results. Sixty Gy in 30 fractions is delivered ideally using a conformal IMRT plan.

Medical management
TSH is thought to stimulate tumour growth. Retrospective data has shown improvements in relapse-free survival when TSH levels are undetectable. This is achieved by administration of T4 in supraphysiological doses which both replaces endogenous thyroid hormones and suppresses TSH release from the pituitary by negative feedback on the hypothalamus. T4 dose is adjusted by 25mcg every 6 weeks until a TSH level of <0.1MiU/L is achieved. Most patients require a T4 dose of 175–200mcg.

Role of chemotherapy
There is no role for chemotherapy in the adjuvant setting. It may be used as palliative therapy in patients with symptomatic progressive disease for whom there are no further surgical or radiotherapeutic options. Numerous agents have been used, none of which have shown dramatic activity or prolonged responses. Single agents include doxorubicin and cisplatin. Combination regimens include doxorubicin, cisplatin, and bleomycin. Thyroid tumours are commonly extremely vascular and much research activity is investigating antiangiogenic agents, although none are in routine clinical use to date.

Prognosis

Overall the prognosis is excellent with long-term survival >90%.

Further reading

DOH. *Head and neck specific measures.* London: Department of Health, 2004—available at: http://www.dh.gov.uk/assetRoot/04/13/55/91/04135591.pdf

Mazzaferri EL, Jhiang SM. Long-term impact of initial surgical and medical therapy on papillary and follicular thyroid cancer. *Am J Med* 1994; **97**:418–28.

Sandeep TC, Strachan MW, Reynolds RM et al. Second primary cancers in thyroid cancer patients: a multinational record linkage study. *J Clin Endocrinol Metab* 2006; **91**:1819–25.

Internet resource

British Thyroid Association: http://www.british-thyroid-association.org/guidelines

Thyroid cancer: medullary carcinoma

Evaluation

The management of these patients is complex and should be undertaken within a team with experience of the management of medullary thyroid cancer (MTC). The biology of MTC has unique implications for the development and structure of clinical services and management. Twenty-five per cent of MTC is familial, inherited in an AD fashion, necessitating a comprehensive and integrated approach to both patient and their family. When MTC arises within a familial syndrome, assessment and management of other endocrine tumours is required.

Up to 20% of patients will have metastatic disease at presentation. This does not preclude extensive neck surgery since retrospective series have demonstrated a survival advantage for surgery even in the face of advanced disease. Baseline serum calcitonin should be measured. Calcitonin is almost invariably elevated. Neck disease should be evaluated with ultrasound and CT. Staging of the chest and abdomen is with CT. Even in the absence of obvious familial disease, MEN2 syndromes should be considered. Screening for phaeochromocytoma with 24-hour urinary catecholamines and metanephrines should be undertaken and serum calcium should be measured in order to exclude hyperparathyroidism.

Surgery

Thyroid

The optimum procedure is total thyroidectomy. In all inherited and one-third of sporadic MTCs the disease is multifocal. There is no role for more conservative surgery. Surgery is recommended even in the presence of advanced metastatic disease Effective treatment of the primary tumour limits the risk of aerodigestive tract compromise, and may assist in the control of calcium levels.

Lymph nodes

There is high risk of nodal involvement in all forms of MTC. Up to 50% of patients will have metastases to level VI nodes. Elective dissection of level VI and VII nodes is standard practice. This approach appears to reduce the risk of relapse and probably improves survival. The management of the rest of the neck is more controversial. The risk of metastasis to the ipsilateral and contralateral neck nodes ranges from 20–60%. Bilateral selective neck dissection of levels IIa–Vb is recommended if palpable nodes are identified, in the clinically normal neck either routine modified neck dissection or sampling followed by dissection for positive nodes is undertaken. If there is suspicion of upper mediastinal nodal involvement, sternotomy and dissection may be considered.

Postoperative management

There is high risk of hypocalcaemia secondary to hypoparathyroidism so serum calcium should be closely monitored and replaced intravenously or orally as necessary. T4 should be commenced with the intention of rendering the patient euthyroid.

Postoperative baseline levels of calcitonin should be measured. It is recommended that serum calcitonin measurement is delayed until 4–6 months postoperatively as this appears to be the most predictive level.

Role of external beam radiotherapy

The role of adjuvant radiotherapy is controversial. There are no randomized studies investigating the value of radiotherapy in medullary carcinoma of the thyroid. Most retrospective studies have shown a prolongation in time to relapse after radiotherapy. However, others have shown no benefit. In patients who are unable to undergo complete resection, postoperative radiotherapy may improve relapse-free survival. A dose of 50–60Gy in 25–30 fractions may be delivered to the thyroid bed, bilateral cervical and upper mediastinal nodes using conformal planning techniques.

There is no role for radioiodine as parafollicular cells do not demonstrate iodine uptake.

Follow-up

Follow-up should be lifelong as late relapse can occur and those with inherited genetic mutations are at risk of new malignancies. Patients who undergo complete resection and who have undetectable calcitonin postoperatively are at low risk of relapse and persisting disease is unlikely. They are reviewed 6-monthly with clinical examination, with particular reference to the thyroid bed. Serum calcitonin levels are measured at each visit and assessment of adequacy of T4 replacement is made.

Prognosis

Overall the 10-year survival is 50–69%. Patients may survive for many years even with a significant tumour burden. This makes the risk–benefit decisions for additional intervention for persistent or recurrent disease difficult. A number of factors affect prognosis.

- *Stage at presentation*: using the AJCC/UICC system, a study with median follow up of 4 years showed risk of death is 0 for stage I disease and rises to 13%, 56%, and 100% for stage II, III, and IV respectively.

- *Preoperative calcitonin levels*: levels above 500ηg predict for failure to achieve biochemical remission after surgery due to occult metastatic disease.

- *Postoperative serum calcitonin*: those with normalization of calcitonin levels postoperatively have a 5-year recurrence rate of 5%.

- *Age at diagnosis*: age over 40 years confers a poorer DFS (95% vs. 60%). Risk of dying rises by 5% for each year of age.

- *MEN2B*: the MEN2B genotype has a more aggressive pattern of disease and as such a worse prognosis than sporadic or other inherited forms of the disease.

- Other factors:
  Exon 16 mutations
  Elevated CEA levels
  Low levels of tumour calcitonin staining
  Male gender

Recurrence and management

Persistently elevated calcitonin or CEA postoperatively is highly suggestive of persistent disease. Calcitonin levels rise in proportion to disease extent. As outlined previously, complete surgical excision appears to predict for good outcome. Patients with elevated postoperative calcitonin should be carefully reassessed for evidence of metastatic disease and residual neck disease. This may require high-resolution ultrasound of the neck, conventional three-dimensional imaging, FDG-PET (although this is only shown to have adequate sensitivity when calcitonin levels are >500ηg). In some cases selective intravenous calcitonin measurements with or without pentagastrin stimulation can be helpful in identifying site of residual disease, particularly in the neck. In patients with isolated residual disease in the neck or mediastinum or no evidence of disease, further neck dissection should be considered. This may result in biochemical cures of up to 35%.

In patients relapsing with elevated calcitonin at a later date a similar approach is employed. Where possible, further surgery is attempted. Surgical excision of metastatic disease is also appropriate in solitary or small volume metastatic disease as this can be helpful in the control of hypercalcaemia and symptoms from calcitonin secretion.

EBRT is used in patients with inoperable recurrence. There is some data to suggest it may delay progression. Radiotherapy is also utilized in the palliation of symptoms of pain, particularly in the case of bony metastatic disease.

The management of disseminated disease must be tailored to the individual. Often the pace of disease may be slow and in the absence of symptoms systemic therapy may be inappropriate. Systemic therapy should be reserved for patients with rapidly progressive disease or those with symptoms uncontrolled by other palliative measures.

Radiolabelled somatostatin analogues and or ^{131}I-MIBG therapy may be useful in a small subgroup of patients

Agents targeting the RET kinase mutations are also under investigation. Agents including vadetinib, motesanib, and sorafenib have shown disease stabilization for prolonged periods in up to 50% of patients in clinical trial settings.

Palliative measures

Diarrhoea may be managed with the use of loperamide or codeine. Patients with severe flushing or diarrhoea found to have large liver metastases may benefit from embolization procedures.

Genetic counselling

The RET mutation is a proto-oncogene causing constitutive activation of the RET tyrosine kinase which results in uncontrolled downstream signalling. A number of cysteine mutations at 10q22 have been identified including those at exons 10, 11, 13, and 16.

An underlying familial RET mutation is identified in 25% of patients. In some there may be no obvious family history despite the presence of a germline mutation. The presence of an inherited RET mutation predicts for early development of C-cell hyperplasia and of MTC. This can occur before the age of 5 in MEN 2A and before 18 months in MEN2B.

The early identification of germline mutations allows the possibility of prophylactic thyroidectomy at a young age preventing the development of thyroid malignancy. It is therefore advocated that all patients with a diagnosis of MTC are referred for genetic screening. The counselling process should include discussion that in MEN2 families prophylactic thyroidectomy will not negate the risk of other associated malignancies although screening for these can be undertaken. Furthermore rare kindreds of MEN2 do not have any known RET mutation. Therefore a negative result does not entirely exclude a heritable form of MTC. In these patients if there is a clear family history it may be possible to perform annual screening with stimulated calcitonin and neck ultrasound in relatives of the index case.

Prophylactic surgery should be in the form of thyroidectomy in disease-free relatives. This should be performed before 1 year in MEN2B (central lymphadenectomy should also be undertaken), between 5–10 years in MEN2A and after age 10 in carriers of familial thyroid cancer. Lymph node dissection is not routinely recommended except in MEN2B unless there is risk of occult disease. As more information becomes available from individual mutation phenotypes this will help in management of unaffected carriers.

Further reading

Jiménez C, Hu MI, Gagel RF. Management of medullary thyroid carcinoma. *Endocrinol Metab Clin North Am* 2008; **37**(2):481–96.

Hoff AO, Hoff PM. 2007. Medullary thyroid carcinoma. *Hematol Oncol Clin North Am* 2007; **21**(3):475–88.

Internet resource

Department of Health: information about cancer—www.dh.gov.uk/en/policyandguidance/healthandsocialcaretopics/cancer/dh41355

Thyroid cancer: anaplastic carcinoma

Role of surgery

The majority of patients present with locally advanced or metastatic disease. The disease is usually rapidly progressive and so surgery only has a role in a minority of patients. Those with small tumours not yet invading adjacent structures are best served by complete excision (Haigh et al. 2001). Surgery also has a role in airway management in advanced disease. Over half of patients have airway compromise and this may be palliated in some cases with procedures such as tracheostomy.

Role of radiotherapy

Radiotherapy is the mainstay of treatment of this disease. It does not confer a survival advantage. The majority of patients will initially respond to treatment but local relapse typically occurs within weeks or months of completing treatment. Some patients will demonstrate rapid disease progression during radiotherapy. Attempts to accelerate treatment with hyperfractionated schedules of radiotherapy have not improved survival rates or had a dramatic impact on rates of local control. Although not expected to cure disease, radical doses are required in order to achieve the best rates of local control. Typically doses of between 50–60Gy are delivered in fractions of 2Gy daily over approximately 6 weeks.

Anaplastic tumours do not concentrate radioiodine and there is no role for radioiodine therapy in these patients.

Role of chemoirradiation

Attempts have been made to improve outcome by combining radiation with chemotherapy. Various combinations have been reported as individual cases or small series. The majority of other reports are using hyperfractionated accelerated schedules. All of these regimens are associated with significant grade 3 and 4 toxicities. Another approach has been to add full dose systemic therapy. After surgery, patients received 2 cycles of doxorubicin 60mg/m^2 with cisplatin 120mg/m^2 followed by accelerated radiotherapy to a dose of 55Gy using 1.25Gy twice daily fractionation. This was followed with a further 4 cycles of full dose chemotherapy. This approach gave an overall survival of 27% at 3 years and a median survival of 10 months (De Crevoisier et al. 2004). However, significant grade 3 or 4 toxicity was seen with haematological toxicity in >70%.

Follow-up

These patients are followed-up regularly in a multidisciplinary clinic. The rapidly progressive nature of this disease means they should have clinic access at short notice. Routine review includes assessment of neck and airway together with examination for evidence of metastatic disease.

Prognosis

The outcome in this patient group is very poor. Median survival is usually <6 months and 5-year survival <10%. Factors predicting for poorer outcome include:
- Disease extending beyond the thyroid
- Tumour diameter >6cm
- Older age
- Male gender
- Dyspnoea at presentation
- Incomplete excision
- Single modality treatment strategies

Progression and management

Local progression is often inevitable despite aggressive initial local treatment. This often proves difficult to manage and early involvement of the palliative care team is vital. Systemic therapy does not seem to improve survival but may induce initial response. Single-agent or combination regimens may be considered for palliation.

Palliative radiotherapy may be used for treatment of symptomatic localized metastases.

In the majority of cases, death results from airway obstruction and unless carefully managed can be especially distressing for patients and family. Tracheostomy and endotracheal stenting can have a role although do not always prevent this mode of death.

Heliox can be helpful and some advocate nebulized epinephrine.

Opiates and short-acting benzodiazepines are helpful in reducing the symptoms and anxiety associated with terminal airway obstruction.

Further reading

De Crevoisier R, Baudin E, Bachelot A, et al. Combined treatment of anaplastic thyroid carcinoma with surgery, chemotherapy, and hyperfractionated accelerated external radiotherapy. Int J Radiat Oncol Biol Phys 2004; **60**:1137–43.

Haigh PI, Ituarte PH, Wu HS, et al. Completely resected anaplastic thyroid carcinoma combined with adjuvant chemotherapy and irradiation is associated with prolonged survival. Cancer 2001; **91**:2335–42.

Primary thyroid lymphoma

Introduction

Primary thyroid lymphomas (PTLs) constitute 1–5% of thyroid malignancies and <2% of extranodal lymphomas. The usual age of occurrence is 50–80 years and females are affected more than male (3–4:1).

Hashimoto's thyroiditis appears to be the only known risk factor (60 times higher).

Pathology

PTL are almost always NHL. Two most common subtypes are diffuse large B-cell lymphoma (DLCL) and mucosa-associated lymphoid tissue (MALT) lymphoma. DLCL (50–70%) are positive for CD5, CD10, CD23, CD43, CD30, and bcl-2 oncogene whereas MALT lymphomas (30%) are positive for CD5, CD10 and CD23 Rarely Hodgkin lymphoma and Burkitt's lymphoma can occur.

Clinical features

Rapidly enlarging neck mass is the most common (70–90%) presentation followed by pressure symptoms (30%) such as dysphagia, stridor, and hoarseness. Ten per cent of patients have associated B symptoms and up to 10% can have hypothyroidism. Occasionally lymphoma can present as solitary nodule.

Investigations

Ultrasound of the thyroid with needle biopsy or excision biopsy is needed to confirm diagnosis. CT scan and MRI scan are helpful in local staging. Other investigations include full blood count, biochemistry including serum LDH and β2 microglobulin, thyroid function tests, CT scan of the chest, abdomen, and pelvis, and bone marrow biopsy. PET should be interpreted cautiously as it can be falsely negative in MALT lymphoma and can show diffuse uptake (false positive) in Hashimoto's thyroiditis. However, SUV (standardized uptake value) in large cell lymphomas tends to be >6 whereas in inflammatory conditions it is usually <6. Some centres advise gastroscopy in MALT lymphoma to exclude gastric involvement.

Staging

- IE: disease localized within the thyroid (50% of patients)
- IIE: disease localized within the thyroid and regional nodes (45% patients)
- IIIE: lymph nodes involving both sides of diaphragm (<5%)
- IVE: disseminated disease (<5%)

Treatment

Treatment of PTL depends on the histological subtype and stage. These tumours are both radio- and chemo-sensitive. It is not clear where a single-modality treatment or combined treatment is better.

Based on experience from other extranodal B-cell lymphomas, localized DLCL is treated with combination chemotherapy (CHOP–rituximab for 3–4 courses) and radiotherapy. Some suggest 6–8 courses of CHOP–R alone. However, a retrospective study showed that combined modality treatment results in fewer relapses than with single modality treatment (<10% vs 37–43%). It should be noted that the role of rituximab is not fully evaluated in PTL.

Advanced stage DLCL is treated mainly with chemotherapy. Some advocate local radiotherapy to all patients irrespective of stage.

Since MALT lymphomas are indolent, localized disease is treated with EBRT. However, bulky IE and stages IIE–IVE are treated with chemoradiotherapy or chemotherapy alone.

Surgery

There is no role for radical surgery as a single-modality treatment and it is likely to result in increased morbidity. It may have a role for palliation of obstructive symptoms developing while on chemotherapy and radiotherapy.

Prognostic factors and survival

Stage is the important prognostic factor. Stagewise 5-year survivals are 80% for IE, 50% for stage IIE, and <36% for stages IIIE and IVE. Other reported poor prognostic factors include tumours of >10cm size, presence of pressure symptoms, mediastinal involvement, and rapid tumour growth. MALT lymphoma presents at an early stage, and has an indolent behaviour.

Relapse

Relapse is common with DLCL and principles of management are similar to any recurrent DLCL. If feasible, high dose chemotherapy with autologous transplantation is considered.

Further reading

Mack LA, Pasieka JL. An evidence-based approach to the treatment of thyroid lymphoma. *World J Surg* 2007; **31**(5):978–86.

Parathyroid cancer

Epidemiology
These are extremely rare tumours, with an incidence of 0.015 per 100,000 in the USA. They may occur slightly more frequently in Japan than elsewhere. They affect males and females equally and are commonest in the fourth and fifth decades. They account for <1% of all hyperparathyroidism.

Aetiology
Aetiology is largely unknown; the majority are probably sporadic. A minority occurs as part of familial hyperparathyroidism, either within the MEN1 complex or as an autosomal dominant condition comprising benign and malignant parathyroid tumours. Mutation in the hyperparathyroidism 2 gene (HRPT2) which encodes C1 parafibromin has been identified in these patients (Carpten et al. 2002). The role of C1 parafibromin is unclear but may be involved in transcription control. Sporadic parathyroid malignancies also commonly show mutations of HRPT2. Absence of expression of retinoblastoma protein and overexpression of Cyclin D1 has also been identified. Other factors implicated included radiation exposure to the neck, and pre-existing parathyroid adenomas.

Pathology
The differential lies between carcinoma and adenoma. The distinction may not be easy to make. Macroscopically malignant tumours are typically hard lobulated structures often enclosed in a fibrous capsule while benign tumours are softer and reddish in colour without a capsule. Microscopically chief cells are seen, arranged in sheets in a uniform lobular pattern, separated by fibrous trabeculae. Occasionally transitional cells may be identified or a mixed picture is seen. The differentiation from adenoma relies on the presence of mitoses and evidence of capsular or vascular invasion although these may been seen in adenomas.

Clinical features
The vast majority of tumours are functioning and patients present with symptoms of hypercalcaemia, including fatigue, weakness, nausea, vomiting, dehydration, polyuria, polydipsia, and confusion. Neck masses are seen in 30–70%. Local invasion may cause voice changes due to involvement of the recurrent laryngeal nerve causing vocal cord palsy. Lymphadenopathy is rare. Renal disease, including renal colic, nephrolithiasis, and renal failure are common. Bone disease may manifest as pain or pathological fracture. Less commonly recurrent pancreatitis and peptic ulcer disease are seen.

Diagnosis
Diagnosis may be difficult as tumours are often small. The condition may be mistaken for primary hyperparathyroidism. A number of factors make malignancy more likely.
- Age <60 years.
- Palpable neck mass.
- Elevated parathyroid hormone—typically 3–10 times the upper limit of normal compared to 1–2 times the upper limit of normal in primary hyperparathyroidism.
- Elevated serum calcium, ALP, α and βHCG.
- Presence of neck mass or vocal cord palsy.

Neck ultrasound may be required to identify a parathyroid mass. CT may be required to investigate evidence of local invasion. Metastatic disease occurs in <1% at presentation so routine screening for metastatic disease is not required. Skeletal survey will demonstrate features of bone disease including osteopenia.

In patients with suspected recurrent disease thallium-201 technetium scanning may be helpful in identifying sites of recurrence.

Staging
There is no universally accepted staging system. Commonly the distinction between localized disease and metastatic (lymphatic or distant) is the only system used.

Treatment
Surgical treatment
The mainstay of treatment in these patients is en bloc excision of parathyroid mass and any invaded tissues, with a wide margin, including the ipsilateral thyroid gland and isthmus. It is important to maintain the integrity of the tumour capsule to reduce the risk of tumour spillage. Often the diagnosis is made after surgery in which case further surgery may be indicated particularly if the calcium remains elevated. The role of lymph node dissection is unclear. Any clinically involved lymph nodes should be dissected and many advocate prophylactic ipsilateral neck dissection in view of the difficulties in managing recurrent disease. However the risk of lymph node involvement at diagnosis is <5% and there may be considerable morbidity attached to neck dissection.

Postoperatively calcium levels may drop precipitously requiring large replacement doses for prolonged periods.

In cases of recurrent hypercalcaemia some time after surgery, careful reassessment of the neck with ultrasound or MRI should be undertaken with a view to re-excision of locally recurrent disease which may be curative.

Surgery also has a role in metastatic disease. Persistently elevated calcium, uncontrolled by other means may justify metastatectomy even in the face of advanced disease.

Radiotherapy
The paucity of controlled trials in this rare condition means that the role of radiotherapy is uncertain. It has been shown in case series to reduce the risk of local recurrence in the adjuvant setting. The presence of vascular or capsular invasion may predict for local recurrence and these may be used as an indication for postoperative radiotherapy. There are case reports of its use as primary therapy in patients unfit for surgical intervention. It is also used palliatively in the control of symptomatic metastases.

Medical treatment
The main difficulty in patients with metastatic disease is control of hypercalcaemia and this is usually the cause of death rather than extensive metastatic disease. Measures to control serum calcium include hydration, diuretics, and bisphosphonates although care may be required in the face of renal impairment. Endocrinology input is invaluable.

Chemotherapy has been used for metastatic disease. Agents shown to have activity include dacarbazine, either as single agent or in combination with 5-FU and cyclophosphamide. In a non-functioning parathyroid carcinoma, prolonged partial response was reported with a combination of methotrexate, cyclophosphamide, doxorubicin, and lomustine.

Genetic screening

Referral for genetic screening should be considered in all patients with parathyroid carcinoma. The presence of a mutation would make a second primary more likely in the setting of apparent disease recurrence which would underline to need to reassess the neck. Relatives found to be carriers of HRPT2 may be surveyed with serum calcium and parathyroid hormone levels. However, during the counselling process it should be noted that surveillance in this manner is not infallible since not all tumours are functioning.

Prognosis

The prognosis is very variable, with 10-year survival rates of 49–77% reported. The rule of thirds applies; with one-third cured by aggressive surgical management. One-third has slowly progressive disease, relapsing many years after the original presentation. The final third sadly develop aggressive, rapidly progressive disease and fail to receive significant benefit from medical interventions.

Further reading

Carpten J, Robbins C, Villablanca A, et al. HRPT2 encoding para-fibromin is mutated in hyperparathyroidism-jaw tumours syndrome. Nat Genet 2002; **32**:676–80.

Lang B, Lo CY. Parathyroid cancer. Surg Oncol Clin N Am 2006; **15**(3):573–84.

Rao SR, Shaha AR, Singh B, et al. Management of cancer of the parathyroid. Acta Otolaryngol 2002; **122**(4):448–52.

Adrenocortical carcinoma

Introduction

Adrenocortical carcinoma (ACC) is a rare malignancy with heterogenous manifestations and poor prognosis. The estimated prevalence is 4–12 per million adults. The age distribution is bimodal with a first peak at 3.5 years and second peak at 57 years of age. There are no proven aetiological factors. ACC is rarely reported in MENI, Li–Fraumeni and Wiedemann–Beckwith syndromes.

Clinical features

Approximately 60% of patients present with features of adrenal steroid hypersecretion. Benign adrenocortical tumours secrete a single class of steroid whereas ACC can secrete various steroids. Rapidly progressing Cushing's syndrome with or without virilization is the most common presentation. Androgen secreting tumours in women can lead to features of virilization whereas oestrogen secreting tumours in males lead to gynaecomastia and testicular atrophy. Aldosterone producing tumours present with hypertension and hypokalaemia.

Non-secreting tumours present with abdominal discomfort or back pain due to mass effect. Rarely patients can present with fever, weight loss, and anorexia.

Diagnosis

Initial investigations include imaging (CT chest and abdomen) and hormonal workup. Size of tumour on CT scan remains one of the best indicators of malignancy. Tumours >6 cm are highly suspicious for malignancy. On CT scan, ACCs are irregularly enhancing non-homogenous masses. Apart from size of the adrenal mass, imaging characteristics are also helpful in distinguishing benign from malignant lesions. Measurement of Hounsfield units (HU) in unenhanced CT may be useful in distinguishing benign from malignant lesions. A value of >10HU (indicating low fat content) has a sensitivity of 71% and specificity of 98% to diagnose ACC. On MRI scan, ACCs present as iso-intense to liver on T1-weighted and intermediate to increased intensity on T2-weighted images. MRI is also useful in identifying invasion of adjacent organs and the inferior vena cava, and hence in planning surgery. Recent studies suggest ACC has a high uptake on FDG-PET.

All patients should have endocrine assessment prior to surgery. This helps to:
- Establish the steroid secretory profile
- Plan surgery and postoperative management
- Establish tumour markers for follow-up
- Exclude a pheochromocytoma

Biopsy of adrenal tumour is controversial because of the theoretical risk of needle tract metastases. However, it may be acceptable if primary surgical management is not feasible and diagnosis cannot be established with non-invasive measures.

Pathological assessment

Differentiation between benign and malignant tumour is based on macroscopic and microscopic features. Nuclear atypia, atypical and frequent mitoses (>5 per 50 HPF), vascular and capsular invasion, and necroses are suggestive of malignancy.

Staging

WHO (2004) staging for ACC is as follows:
- Stage I: localized tumour of ≤5cm
- Stage II: localized tumour of >5cm
- Stage III: locally invasive or tumours with regional lymph node metastases
- Stage IV: tumour invading adjacent organs or distant metastases

Management

Multidisciplinary management involves surgeons, oncologist, and endocrinologist.

Surgery

Complete removal of tumour offers the best chance for cure in patients with stage I–III tumours. Peroperatively, it is important to remove the tumour with intact capsule to avoid tumour spillage to reduce the risk of local recurrence. Presence of tumour thrombus in the IVC or renal vein does not preclude a complete excision.

Limited experience shows that laparoscopic adrenalectomy results in higher risk of recurrence (up to 40%) and intraperitoneal dissemination. Hence it is not advisable except in a prospective trial setting.

Role of tumour debulking in the presence of metastatic disease is not established. It may have a role in selected patients to control hormonal excess and to facilitate other therapies.

Surgery may have a role in surgical removal of limited metastatic disease. Radiofrequency thermal ablation is an alternative to surgery for lung and liver metastases.

Radiotherapy

Radiotherapy has an established role in the palliation of bone and brain metastases. Role of primary radiotherapy in inoperable adrenocortical tumour is not well established. Adjuvant tumour bed radiotherapy in completely resected stage III and high-risk stage II adrenocortical cancer may reduce local recurrence, though not proven in a randomized trial setting.

Chemotherapy

Mitotane (o,p'-DDD) is a specific drug for the treatment of adrenocortical cancer. It is cytotoxic to adrenocortical cells and inhibits steroidogenesis. It was approved for clinical use by FDA in 1970 and by the European Medicine Agency in 2004. It leads to an objective response in 25% of cases and control of hormonal hypersecretion in the majority. A mitotane blood level of at least 14mg/L seems to improve the tumour response rate. However, >80% patients experience some side effects. The main side effects are GI (nausea, vomiting, diarrhoea, anorexia, and mucositis) or CNS (lethargy, somnolence, depression, dizziness, polyneuropathy). It also induces adrenal insufficiency and increased metabolic clearance of glucocorticoids. Hence all patients need high-dose gluococorticoid replacement (e.g. 50mg hydrocortisone daily) which helps to minimize mitotane-induced side effects.

The starting dose of mitotane is 2g/daily in 4 divided doses. Dose is increased by 1g by day every 1–2 weeks until maximum tolerated dose is reached or serum level of 14–20mcg/dL. The dose limiting toxicities are anorexia and nausea.

There has been no randomized trial of the benefit of adjuvant mitotane.

Combination chemotherapy
Several combinations have been tried with dismal results. Cisplatin with or without etoposide appears to have activity in ACC. A combination of mitotane with streptozotocin has yielded a response rate (partial and complete) of 36%.

The commonly used combination regimes are cisplatin, etoposide and doxorubicin (EDP) with mitotane (Berruti regimen) and EDP with streptozocin (Khan regimen). The ongoing FIRM-ACT trial is comparing the efficacy of these two combination regimes in patients with inoperable stage III–IV disease.

General medical management
Patients with Cushing's syndrome need medical treatment to control symptoms and complications of Cushing's syndrome. Ketoconazole is commonly used and it can be combined with mitotane. Other agents include etomidate, metyrapone, and aminoglutethimide.

Survival and prognosis
Overall outcome depends on the tumour stage as well as completeness of resection. Tumours of >12 cm in spite of complete resection have a poor prognosis. Other reported prognostic factors include high mitotic rate, atypical mitoses, tumour necrosis, and tp53 mutation. The reported 5-year survival is 60% for stage I, 58% for stage II, 24% for stage III, and 0% for stage IV. Median survival of stage IV patients is <12 months. Cortisol secreting tumours are associated with worse prognosis, partially attributable to morbidity associated with Cushing's syndrome.

Follow-up
Patients with hormonal markers need 3-monthly hormonal assays to detect a tumour recurrence. Since surgical salvage of a local or metastatic recurrence is feasible, all patients need imaging of abdomen and chest for at least 5 years.

Further reading
Allolio A, Fassnacht M. Adrenocortical carcinoma: clinical update. *J Clin Endocrinol Metab* 2006; **91**(6):2027–37.

Schteingart DE, Doherty GM, Gauger PG, *et al.* Management of patients with adrenal cancer: recommendations of an international consensus conference. *Endocr Relat Cancer* 2005; **12**:667–80.

Internet resources
Adrenal Cancer Support: http://www.adrenalcancersupport.org

European Network for the study of adrenal tumours: http://www.ensat.org/

FIRM ACT trial: http://www.firm-act.org

Orphanet: the portal for rare diseases and orphan drugs: http://www.orpha.net

Neuroendocrine tumours

Epidemiology

Neuroendocrine tumours (NETs) account for only 0.5% of all malignancies. The main primary sites are the GI tract and the lung. Carcinoid tumours represent >50% of all NETs but are still uncommon with an incidence rate of approximately 1 per 100,000 per year in the UK. They can occur at any age, with a mean of 50–60 years. In the last decades, the incidence has been rising. This might be due to more awareness and improved diagnostic tools.

Aetiology

Little is known about the aetiology of NETs. Most commonly NETs are sporadic (aetiology unknown). There are a few known associations:
• Chronic atrophic gastritis
• Pernicious anaemia
• MEN1 syndrome (up to 10% of NETs are associated with this)
• Neurofibromatosis type 1 (Von Hippel–Lindau disease)

Pathology

NETs arise from neuroendocrine cells that are located widely throughout the body. Carcinoid tumours are NETs derived from enterochromaffin (or Kulchitsky) cells, which are also widely distributed throughout the body.
NETs can be classified according to:
• Primary site
• Histopathological status
• Immunohistochemistry
• Type of neuropeptide secreted

WHO classification estimates malignant potential based upon stage- and grade-related criteria. Poorly differentiated neuroendocrine carcinomas have a characteristic small cell undifferentiated appearance by light microscopy. These are high-grade malignancies, such as SCLC.

Another group of NETs that mainly involve the GI tract have variable behaviour and well-differentiated histological features. This group includes carcinoid tumours, pancreatic islet cell tumours, and pheochromocytomas. Carcinoid tumours may arise anywhere in the GI tract, in the bronchi, and occasionally elsewhere. Metastatic carcinoid tumours are sometimes found without an obvious primary site. The metastases most often involve the liver.

Clinical features

Clinical features are highly variable and patients can remain asymptomatic for years with the more indolent tumours. Commoner features of gastroenteropancreatic NETs include vague abdominal pain, acute appendicitis (if primary site is the appendix) and rectal symptoms—bleeding, pain, change in bowel habit. Patients can present with symptoms from bulky secondary disease in the liver.

Patients with functioning hormone secretory tumours can present with symptoms specific to the hormone. The secretion of serotonin and other vasoactive substances cause the carcinoid syndrome in patients with carcinoid tumours with metastatases in the liver. The liver inactivates the bioactive products of carcinoid tumours, explaining why patients who have GI carcinoid tumours have the carcinoid syndrome only if they have liver metastases. Symptoms of the carcinoid syndrome include:
• Flushing (35%)
• Abdominal pain (70%)
• Diarrhoea (60%)
• Bronchospasm
• Peripheral oedema
• Heart lesions (up to 50% of patients in postmortem studies)

Carcinoid heart lesions are characterized by plaque-like, fibrous endocardial thickening that involves the right side of the heart, resulting in right-sided heart failure in the majority of cases.

Diagnosis

Many NETs are diagnosed incidentally, during radiographic, endoscopic, or surgical procedures. Once detected, clarification may be needed as to the site of the primary tumour and whether the tumour is functional. There are various blood tests, urine tests, and imaging tests that can aid in this diagnosis. Ultimately a biopsy should be performed and certain immunostains should be used to pathologically diagnose the tumour correctly.
Specifics blood tests that are useful include:
• Fasting gut hormones
• Serotonin (5 hydroxytryptamine) levels
• Chromogranin A
• ACTH
• Cortisol
• Calcitonin
• Pituitary hormone screen

These are not offered in all hospitals, although samples can be sent away for testing.

Perhaps the most useful initial test to perform is 24-hour urinary 5-hydroxyindoleacetic acid (5-HIAA-breakdown product of serotonin). This has a specificity of almost 100% but a lower sensitivity (35%). Errors can occur due to the ingestion of certain drugs and foods. These include substances such as caffeine, bananas, ethanol, and certain nuts. Diet should always be checked prior to performing the test. Urinary catecholamine may also be measured.

If the tumour has been confirmed biochemically it must still be localized. The main imaging techniques used for this purpose are;
• CT (or MRI) of chest/abdomen/pelvis with contrast
• Somatostatin receptor scintigraphy (Octreoscan®)
• Barium studies/endoscopy/colonoscopy (if intestinal problems)
• Cardiac evaluation

Gastroenteropancreatic NETs often contain high concentrations of somatostatin receptors; these can be radiolabelled using a somastatin analogue, octreotide (indium-111 pentetreotide), which can then be imaged by an Octreoscan®. These have also been shown to be predictive of clinical response to treatment with somatostatin analogues.

Once a site for biopsy has been established, tissue should be sent for specific immunostains including:
- CD56 (neuroendocrine marker, including small cell)
- Chromogranin
- Synaptophysin
- Gastrin 9/other gut hormones
- Ki67 (MIB1) marker of proliferation

Treatment

Surgical treatment
Surgery is the treatment of choice for patients with localized non-metastatic tumours. The extent of surgery depends on the primary site of the tumour. Unfortunately the majority of patients with NETs present with metastatic disease. Potentially curative surgery can still be offered to the uncommon patient with resectable nodal or isolated brain/local metastasis. Valve surgery can be performed in those with symptomatic carcinoid heart disease

There is a role for debulking surgery, in particular hepatic resection, in patients with adequate liver function and no extensive extrahepatic disease. Hepatic resection can provide symptom relief and, in some cases, prolong survival.

Medical treatment
There are multiple ways of managing metastatic NETs medically and summaries of each are given here.

Embolization of liver metastases
This can be performed alone or with intra-arterial chemotherapy. Response rates can be >50% but duration is variable. The commonest agents used are 5-FU, doxorubicin, and mitomycin. Mortality used to be as high as 7% although recently this has improved.

Radiofrequency ablation/cryoablation
Only useful for smaller lesions and no evidence of long-term efficacy.

Somatostatin analogues
These interfere with the release of hormones and neurotransmitters through activation of membrane receptors. There are various types in use:
- Octreotide (short acting)
- Sandostatin LAR (longer acting)
- Lanreotide SR (longer acting form of octreotide)

These can control hypersecretion in NETs that express somatostatin receptors. There are side effects that occur with these treatments. About a third of patients will initially develop nausea, abdominal discomfort, and loose stools. These effects generally wear off after the first few weeks, although there is a later risk of developing cholesterol gallstones. Despite this, symptomatic relief is usually achieved in >60% of patients. Actual radiological regression following treatment with somatostatin analogues has been reported to occur <5% of cases.

Interferon alpha
This has been used with somatostatin analogues but side effects limit its use in the metastatic setting.

Systemic chemotherapy
This is used first-line for highly proliferating tumours, i.e. metastatic disease with angio/invasion and proliferation index >10%. Combination treatment has been shown to have higher response rates than single agent, 63% versus 36% (streptozocin/5FU vs. streptozocin alone). Other agents that have been used are doxorubicin, temozolamide, and platinum-based regimens (better results in poorly differentiated tumours). There is no standard regimen and the role continues to be debated. There is a lack of large randomized trials in this area.

Molecular targeted therapy
There have been some encouraging results from small phase 2 trials thus far using agents such as small molecule tyrosine kinase inhibitors (e.g. imatinib, sunitinib, and sorafenib) and monoclonal antibodies (such as the anti-VEGF bevacizumab) in patients with advanced NETs. They are not used as part of standard care and are expensive.

Radiolabelled somatostatin
Relatively new directed treatment, examples include:
- High-dose indium-111
- Yttrium-90-labelled somatostatin analogues
- MIBG pentetreotide

There are encouraging early results.

Carcinoid crisis
This is a life-threatening form of the carcinoid syndrome. It can be triggered by tumour manipulation, anaesthesia, chemotherapy, or radionuclide therapy in patients who have extensive tumour bulk. Symptoms include flushing, diarrhoea, arrhythmias, altered blood pressure, and bronchospasm. Octreotide should be ready during any surgical procedure and can be given intravenously alongside an infusion of plasma.

Prognosis
The prognosis of patients with NETs varies widely due to the variety of tumours patients can present with. Prognosis generally depends upon the following factors:
- Site of origin
- Size of tumour
- Histology
- The presence/extent of metastases
- The presence/absence of carcinoid syndrome

NETs of the small bowel, resected early, have an excellent prognosis. Histological features that predict reduced survival include depth of tumour invasion, vascular and lymphatic invasion, areas of focal necrosis, and an increased mitotic index and proliferative index (Ki67).

Patients with carcinoid syndrome have a worse prognosis than those with metastatic disease without carcinoid syndrome; however, it is not usual for patients to survive past 5 years. Individuals with severe carcinoid heart disease have a lower 5-year survival, around 30%.

Further reading
Cheng PN, Saltz LB. Failure to confirm major objective antitumour activity for streptozocin and doxorubicin in the treatment of patients with advanced islet cell carcinoma. *Cancer* 86:944–8

Fjallskog ML, Granberg DP, Welin SL, *et al*. Treatment with cisplatin and etoposide in patients with neuroendocrine tumours. *Cancer* **92**:1101–7.

Kwekkeboom DJ, Teunissen JJ, Bakker WH, *et al*. Radiolabelled somatostatin analog in patients with endocrine gastroenteropancreatic tumours. *J Clin Oncol* 2005; **23**:2754–62.

Lamberts SW, van der Lely AJ, de Herder WW, *et al*. Octreotide. *N Engl J Med* 1996; **334**:246–54.

Moertel CG, Hanky JA, Johnson LA, *et al*. Streptozocin alone compared with streptozocin plus fluorouracil in the treatment of advanced islet-cell carcinoma. *N Engl J Med* 1980, **303**:1189–94.

Oberg K, Norheim I, Lind E, *et al*. Treatment of the malignant carcinoid syndrome: Evaluation of a long acting somatostatin analogue. *N Engl J Med* 1986; **315**:663–6.

Leukaemia

Leukaemia is the commonest cancer (accounting for >40% of cases) in children. It is a clonal proliferation of stem cells which leads to bone marrow failure and tissue infiltration.

Epidemiology

Incidence/100,000 under 16

- Acute lymphoblastic leukaemia (ALL): 4/100,000
- Acute myeloid leukaemia (AML): 0.7/100,000
- Chronic myeloid leukaemia (CML): 0.2/100,000
- Myelodysplastic syndromes (MDS)/proliferative disorders: 0.3/100000

Peak incidence of ALL is 2–5 years. T cell-ALL is commoner in adolescence. AML, CML, MDS occur at all ages.

Aetiology

Genetic predisposition

Chromosome fragility Increased incidence in children with Fanconi's (10–15% will develop AML), Bloom's syndrome (ALL), and ataxia telangiectasia (ALL). DNA repair defects including Li–Fraumeni syndrome, BRCA, and MSH2 mutations are associated with increased familial risk of leukaemias and solid tumours; the child may be index case.

Trisomy 21 (Down's syndrome) predisposes to ALL (15 times risk) and AML. Transient abnormal myelopoeisis (TAM) a myeloproliferative disorder with circulating megakaryoblasts, variable cytopenia, and organomegaly occurs in at least 10% of children with Down's syndrome. The majority of cases resolve spontaneously within 3 months although progressive hepatic or respiratory impairment may require therapy. Trisomy 21 results in disturbed foetal haemopoiesis in the liver and acquisition of GATA1 mutations which are present in blast cells of TAM and in the blasts of myeloid leukaemia of Down's syndrome (ML-DS), which may develop in up to 20% of children, post TAM.

Therapy related

Topoisomerase II inhibitors (particularly VP16 (etoposide) and VM26 (teniposide) cause secondary MDS and AML characterized by an 11q23 rearrangement within 2 years of exposure. Alkylator exposure is associated with development of MDS/AML with partial or whole deletions of chromosome 7 within 4 years of exposure.

Sporadic

There is 100% concordance of clonally identical 11q23 infant ALL in monozygotic twins consistent with prenatal origin and metastasis in placental circulation. Guthrie cards confirm prenatal origin of t12: 21 but limited concordance in identical twins and high incidence of t12:21 in non-leukaemic Guthrie cards suggest the need for a second hit. Likely candidates include viral infection through population mixing although no specific virus has been identified. There is no proof of a role of radon, electromagnetic fields, or parental radiation exposure.

Clinical features

History and symptoms

Acute leukaemia has a short (2–4 week) history, CML often presents with hyperviscosity.

Symptoms of marrow failure:
- Poor feeding, lethargy, bleeding, infection

Symptoms of organ infiltration:
- Bone pain, limping, fracture
- Headache and (rarely) meningism
- Cough, stridor from mediastinal mass, (T-ALL)
- Confusion, dyspnoea, deafness, visual disturbance are signs of hyperviscosity

Examination

- Pallor, bruising
- Lymphadenopathy and hepatosplenomegaly
- Gum infiltration, signs of SVC obstruction
- Papillloedema, cranial nerve palsy
- Chloroma present in 10% of AML patients

Diagnosis

- Full blood count and blood film
- Clotting screen with fibrinogen
- Renal profile and urate
- CXR to exclude mediastinal mass
- Bone marrow aspirate and trephine
- Immunophenotyping and cytogenetics
- Save material for minimal residual disease (MRD) (see later)
- Diagnostic lumbar puncture

Management

Supportive care

Treatment of infection

Neutropenic sepsis is the commonest cause of non-leukaemic death. Prompt intervention with broad-spectrum antibiotics and circulatory support and liaison with a specialist paediatric haematology unit is essential. Early empirical therapy of fungal infection is common practice. Non-neutropenic fever is often caused by central venous line infections.

Treatment of bleeding

Platelet transfusions may be required and clotting abnormalities should be corrected with fresh frozen plasma and cryoprecipitate.

Treatment of anaemia

Blood transfusion is usually necessary and is required in most children when Hb <7g/dL. Caution must be taken in children with high white cell count (WCC) due to risk of hyperviscosity.

Prevention of tumour lysis

Hyperhydration with $3L/m^2$ of fluid and reduction of urate with either allopurinol or for bulk disease, rasburicase, a potent urate oxidase that converts urate to allantoin (a readily excreted soluble metabolite) should be employed.

Treatment of hyperviscosity

Hyperhydration and aggressive chemotherapy will usually result in resolution of hyperviscosity. Coagulation support is often necessary. Leucopheresis is rarely indicated and if used must be accompanied by chemotherapy (steroid in ALL, anthracycline in AML) to prevent rebound leucostasis.

Curative therapy: risk-directed protocols

Multiagent chemotherapy is very effective for acute leukaemia: 88% 5-year EFS in ALL, 62% 5-year EFS in AML.

Prognostic factors (see Table 4.12.1) are widely used in risk-directed protocols in which the most intensive therapy is reserved for those at highest risk of relapse. It is now clear that for children receiving homogeneous therapy, cytogenetics and response to treatment as measured by MRD are the strongest prognostic indicators.

In acute leukaemia, BMT is reserved for very high risk disease in CR1 (first complete remission) and treatment of

Table 4.12.1 Prognostic factors of childhood acute leukaemia

Acute lymphoblastic leukaemia

	% of patients	5-year EFS
Clinical features		
NCI standard risk (age 1–10, WCC < 50 x 10^9/L)	62%	88%
NCI high risk (age < 1or >10, and/or WCC > 50 x 10^9/L)	38%	80%
Cytogenetics		
Tel AML	25%	94%
High hyperdiploidy	25%	85%
Hypodiploidy <44 chromosomes	2%	40%
iAMP 21	2%	35%
Philadelphia positive	3%	55%
Response to therapy		
Day 8/15 marrow >25% blasts	14%	70%
No CR day 35	2%	40%
MRD < 0.01% day 28	35%	95%

Acute myeloid leukaemia

	% of patients	5 year OS
Cytogenetics (MRC classification)		
Favourable {t8:21, t 15:17 inv 16}	31%	76%
Intermediate {11q23, normal}	61%	52%
Poor {–7,–5, del3q, complex}	7%	40%
Response to therapy		
Day 35 marrow > 15% blasts	16%	23%

Outcomes for ALL are illustrative and are derived from composite outcomes of recent, UK, US, and European trials. AML outcomes are based on UKAML X

relapse. Stem cell transplant (SCT) remains the only proven curative option for CML and MDS.

Treatment of acute lymphoblastic leukaemia
Treatment is divided into 4 phases:
- *Induction*: 4 weeks of corticosteroid, vincristine, asparaginase, and anthracycline achieves remission in 98% of cases.
- *CNS prophylaxis* through regular intrathecal methotrexate and/or high-dose systemic methotrexate.
- *Intensification/re-induction*: at present all risk groups benefit from intensive re-induction.
- *Maintenance*: oral 6MP/methotrexate for up to 3 years from diagnosis is required. The benefit of pulses of vincristine and steroid during maintenance is unclear.

Subgroup-specific therapy
Infant ALL
This has a unique biology with MLL rearrangement, a pro-B immunophenotype. The relatively poor prognosis seen in

the past has improved with a protocol based on high-dose cytarabine. The value of additional AML chemotherapy is now to be trialled. Very high-risk patients (age <6 months, MLL rearrangement and WCC >300 x 10^9/L) proceed to SCT in CR1.

Philadelphia-positive ALL
Associated with a poorer prognosis and these patients are treated with imatinib with intensive chemotherapy and in the UK most proceed to SCT in CR1.

Relapse
Prognosis depends on site and timing of relapse. Re-induction chemotherapy is followed by bone marrow transplant in those with an early relapse (<6 months from end of treatment) or high levels of minimal residual disease at week 5 of re-treatment. Full systemic therapy is required for isolated extramedullary relapse. Up to 50% of relapses are cured.

Treatment of acute myeloid leukaemia
Involves up to five courses of anthracycline and cytarabine-based intensive chemotherapy. In the UK BMT is no longer offered to children in CR1.

Subgroup-specific therapy
Downs's syndrome-TAM spontaneously resolves in the majority of cases but low-dose cytarabine may be necessary to treat symptomatic children. Twenty per cent of children with TAM will develop AML within 3 years. AML of DS is uniquely sensitive to cytarabine. Relapse is very rare but toxicity leads to an EFS of 85%. Consequently, anthracycline is now reduced in induction and high-dose cytarabine is given in consolidation to reduce toxicity and infective complications.

AML M3 (acute promyelocytic leukaemia/APML) is treated with ATRA (all-transretinoic acid) and chemotherapy. ATRA causes selective proteolytic degradation of PML-RARA and allows normal differentiation of promyelocytes. Serial MRD monitoring allows identification of molecular relapse, which can be treated with arsenic trioxide. Bone marrow transplant is considered in those with persistent MRD.

Relapse
All relapsed patients will undergo re-induction and those who remit are considered for bone marrow transplantation. Patients who relapse within 1 year of diagnosis have a very poor outcome (20% EFS).

Treatment of chronic myeloid leukaemia
Children with CML often present with symptoms of hyperviscosity and leucopheresis may be indicated. Cytoreduction with hydroxyurea followed by introduction of a signal transduction inhibitor (STI) is now routine. STIs are well tolerated in children. A significant minority of children present in lymphoid blast crisis. They respond well to simple ALL induction and then should be treated as for chronic phase CML until SCT.

Most authorities agree that SCT from a well-matched donor remains the treatment of choice in children with CML. As in adults, a minority of patients will enter a molecular remission after STI and the role of SCT for these patients is more controversial. Ultimately it is likely that algorithms similar to those used in adults will be used to guide SCT in CML. The strong graft-versus-leukaemia effect seen after donor lymphocyte infusions in adults is also seen in children, suggesting a role for reduced intensity conditioning in SCT.

Myelodysplasia/myeloproliferative disorders

MDS in children is rare and the diagnosis should be made with caution in those without a clonal cytogenetic abnormality. MDS is commonly seen in Down's syndrome, Fanconi anaemia, Diamond–Blackfan, neurofibromatosis and Schwachmann–Diamond syndrome.

Juvenile myelomonocytic leukaemia is analogous to adult CMML. It is characterized by a monocytosis >1 x 10^9/L, < 20% blasts, high HbF, WCC >10 x 10^9/L, hypersensitivity to GM CSF, clonal abnormality including monosomy 7. Massive hepatosplenomegaly and skin rashes are also a feature. There is an association with neurofibromatosis and Noonan's syndrome and two-thirds of patients will have defects in the RAS signalling pathways (inactivation of NF1, mutations in PTPN11). Treatment is with bone marrow transplantation, sometimes preceded by AML type chemotherapy for cytoreduction.

Refractory anaemia with ring sideroblasts is not seen in children. The presence of ring sideroblasts indicates either X linked ALA synthase deficiency or a mitochondrial cytopathy.

Further reading

Hasle H, Niemeyer CM, Chessels JM, et al. A pediatric approach to the WHO classification of MDS and myeloproliferative diseases. Leukemia 2003; 2:277–82.

Kaspers GJ, Creutzig U. Pediatric acute myeloid leukemia: international progress and future directions. Leukemia 2005; 12:2025–9

Koike K, Matsuda K. Recent advances in the pathogenesis and management of juvenile myelomonocytic leukaemia. Brit J Haem 2008; 141(5):567–75.

Millot F, Guilhot J, Nelken B, et al. Imatinib mesylate is effective in children with chronic myelogenous leukemia in late chronic and advanced phase and in relapse after SCT. Leukemia 2006; 20(2):187–92.

Moorman AV, Richards SM, Martineau M, et al. Outcome heterogeneity in childhood high-hyperdiploid acute lymphoblastic leukemia. Blood 2003; 102(8):2756–62.

Moorman AV, Richards SM, Robinson HM, et al. Prognosis of children with acute lymphoblastic leukemia (ALL) and intrachromosomal amplification of chromosome 21. Blood 2007; 109(6):2327–30.

Pui CH, Evans WE. Treatment of acute lymphoblastic leukemia. N Engl J Med 2006; 354(2):166–78.

Lymphoma

Lymphomas account for 8–10% of all childhood cancers. NHL in children is aggressive often leading to symptoms from tissue infiltration or compression of vital structures. Classification and incidence/100,000 population:
- Hodgkin lymphoma (HD): 0.3/100,000
- Non Hodgkin lymphoma (NHL): 0.6/100,000

NHLs are aggressive, high-grade malignancies of B and T lymphocytes, often pathologically indistinguishable from leukaemia but do not diffusely involve the bone marrow. In practice only three WHO NHL categories of NHL are seen: mature B cell lymphoma (55%) including Burkitt's and diffuse large B cell lymphoma (DLBCL); lymphoblastic lymphoma (B and T cell) (25%); and anaplastic large cell lymphoma (5%).

Aetiology

Genetic predisposition
- *Chromosome fragility*: increased incidence in children with Bloom's syndrome and ataxia telangiectasia (T-NHL).
- *Congenital immune deficiency/dysregulation*: increased incidence in Wiskott–Aldrich syndrome and autoimmune lymphoproliferative syndrome.
- *X-Linked lymphoproliferative disease (XLP)*: defects in expression of SAP (SLAM associated protein) lead to failed T and NK cell control of EBV and the development of EBV positive lymphoma.
- *Infection*—endemic Burkitt lymphoma
  Epstein–Barr virus: 100% of endemic African BL is EBV genome positive. Endemic BL is restricted to areas in which malaria is holoendemic, supporting a role for chronic immune stimulation by *Plasmodium falciparum*. The role of EBV in sporadic Burkitt's lymphoma is much less clear.
- *Immune suppression*: advances in transplant technology revealed the central role of T-cell immunity in the control of EBV. EBV post-transplant lymphoproliferative disorder (PTLD) is an increasing feature of alternative donor BMT and solid organ grafts.

Clinical features

History and symptoms
- Lymphadenopathy, especially cervical in HD
- Abdominal pain and distension secondary to abdominal mass. Occasional jaundice due to cholestasis
- Cough, wheeze, shortness of breath and signs of SVC obstruction secondary to mediastinal mass
- Fever, weight loss, night sweats
- CNS symptoms and cranial nerve palsy

Examination
- Large 'rubbery' lymph nodes, especially cervical
- Hepatosplenomegaly
- Abdominal mass (B cell Lymphoma)
- Signs of SVC obstruction
- Cranial nerve palsies

Investigation
- Full blood count and blood film
- Renal profile and urate /ESR/LDH

- EBV serology and PCR
- CXR/chest CT/baseline PET
- Abdominal US/CT
- Lymph node biopsy
- Bone marrow aspirate and trephine
- Diagnostic lumbar puncture

NB Invasive diagnostics are potentially very dangerous in those with mediastinal tumours. In this situation empirical therapy with steroids is appropriate.

Classification
Based on morphology, immunochemistry, and cytogenetics.

Immunohistochemistry
- Pre-B- and T-lymphoblastic lymphoma are TDT positive and express CD19, CD79a (B markers), and cytoplasmic CD3 (T marker).
- Burkitt's and DLBCL are TDT negative and express CD 19, CD20, CD79a, often surface immunoglobulin and CD10.
- Anaplastic lymphoma may express T-cell markers and CD30 and Alk 1 in 80% which confers a better prognosis.

Cytogenetics
In all cases of Burkitt's lymphoma, C-MYC at 8q24 is translocated to proximity with an immunoglobulin enhancer. The t (8;14)(q24;q32) is seen in 80% and t(2;8)(p11;q24), t(8;22)(q24;q11) are less common.

Translocation of ALK and NPM is seen t(2;5)(p23;q35) and t(1;2)(q25;p23) are present in anaplastic lymphoma.

Management

Supportive care
- Supportive care (see p.540).
- Prevention of tumor lysis is particularly important in abdominal B-NHL and T-NHL (see p.540).

Curative therapy: risk directed protocols
Multiagent chemotherapy directed by histological subtype is very effective for NHL in childhood. Broadly three different 'disease specific' approaches are used.

Mature B-cell lymphoma
B-NHL has a very high proliferative index and a propensity for CNS involvement. Consequently the most effective regimens maintain dose and schedule intensity. CHOP based regimens with additional high-dose methotrexate and intensive intrathecal chemotherapy are highly effective. It is important to note that cranial irradiation is not required even if there is CNS involvement. High-dose cytosine and etoposide are also of value in higher risk groups.

As in all childhood cancer the aim is to reserve the most intensive regimens for those at highest risk of relapse. Stratification is based on resection of the tumor and stage. Treatment regimen and outcomes by stage are shown in Table 4.12.2.

Relapse of B-NHL is often rapid and rarely curable. In those who respond to further therapy, allogeneic BMT is recommended but there is no evidence of a graft-versus-lymphoma effect.

Table 4.12.2 Treatment regimen and outcomes by stage

Treatment regimen	Stage	EFS (%)
Euro LB-02 for T-NHL	1–3	91
	High risk (visceral ± mediastinal ± skin)	61
	Low risk	87
	1	99.3
	2	90.8
	3	89.2
	4 (marrow or CNS)	83

Lymphoblastic lymphoma

T-lymphoblastic lymphoma is treated similarly to ALL. Comparison of data from the BFM and MRC suggest that use of a block of 4 cycles of high methotrexate optimizes systemic and CNS control. Maintenance treatment is required, though several groups are trialling whether the duration of this could be reduced. Cranial radiation is largely reserved for those with CNS disease at diagnosis. Stage 3 T-NHL has over 90% EFS with BFM chemotherapy.

B lymphoblastic lymphoma is optimally treated as ALL with full maintenance chemotherapy. Outcomes are as for B-cell precursor ALL.

Anaplastic large cell lymphoma. Optimal therapy for ALCL is less well defined than its commoner counterparts.

Most regimes rely on B-NHL type therapy. The risk of CNS disease is less than that seen in other NHL and CNS relapse can be prevented with moderate dose systemic methotrexate. Overall 5 year EFS rates of 65% are reported.

EBV driven lymphoproliferative disorder (LPD) This should be staged as for other NHL. In X-linked proliferative syndrome, disease should be cytoreduced with low-dose chemotherapy and/or rituximab. This should be followed by BMT from an unaffected donor.

Where LPD arises in the context of immune suppression, therapy is guided by staging and cytogenetics. Limited stage disease without marrow involvement may respond to withdrawal of immune suppression and/or rituximab. Rapid development of bulky disease, marrow involvement, or clonal cytogenetics are indications for consideration of full B-NHL therapy. Third-party cytototoxic lymphocytes may be of value in LPD.

Further reading

Cairo MS, Gerrard M. Results of a randomized international study of high risk central nervous system B NHL and B ALL. *Blood* 2007; **109**:2736–43.

Okano M, Gross TG. Advanced therapeutic and prophylactic strategies for Epstein-Barr virus infection in immunocompromised patients. *Expert Rev Anti Infect Ther* 2007; **5**(3):403–13.

Reiter A. Diagnosis and treatment of childhood non-Hodgkin lymphoma. *Hematology Am Soc Hematol Educ Program* 2007; 285–96.

Reiter A, Schrappe M, Ludwig WD, et al. Intensive ALL-type therapy without local radiotherapy provides a 90% event-free survival for children with T-cell lymphoblastic lymphoma: a BFM group report. *Blood* 2000; **95**(2):416–21.

Paediatric central nervous system tumours

Introduction

CNS tumours are the most common group of solid tumours in childhood and comprise 20–25% of all childhood neoplasms (about 400 cases per year in the UK). However, mortality for CNS tumours is on a par with that from leukaemia (35% of tumours). Diagnosing brain and spinal cord tumours may be difficult, particularly in young children as the symptoms may be non-specific or misleading.

In survivors, the morbidity caused by the tumour or its treatment may be devastating. In many cases, a clear and frequently very difficult balance must be struck between giving effective therapy and avoiding severe sequelae particularly in young children with immature CNS development.

Incidence

The incidence of CNS tumours is about 3.3 cases per 100,000 children.

Current survival rates

Unlike other childhood malignancies, improvements in survival for CNS tumours have been modest. Some tumours such as the hemispheric low-grade gliomas have always had very good survival rates and prognosis has recently improved for tumours such as medulloblastoma. On the other hand, very little progress has been made in improving the outcome for patients with supratentorial high-grade glioma and survival remains poor. Patients with high-grade gliomas of the brainstem continue to have an almost universally fatal outcome.

Classification/types of tumours

WHO have developed a classification and grading of CNS tumours. A simplified version of this classification is presented in Table 4.12.3, listing only the more common types that occur in childhood. This histological grading of tumours from I to IV is based on the amount of atypia, cellularity, vascularity, mitoses, and necrosis in the tumour and reflects broadly the prognosis, i.e. the higher the grade the poorer the prognosis. There are anomalies in this grading for children, particularly for infants.

Aetiology and biology

The precise cause of most brain tumours is unknown. The only proven aetiological association is ionizing radiation. Fewer than 10% are associated with an inherited syndrome (see p.26).

Over recent years, however, there has been an explosion in our understanding of the molecular biology of CNS tumours. This includes definition of the pathways involved in tumours such as medulloblastoma and glioma and the recognition of the biological heterogeneity of these and other tumour types. This offers the potential for improved disease stratification and/or the identification of novel therapeutic targets.

Clinical presentation

Brain tumours in childhood frequently present with hydrocephalus due to blockage of CSF flow, for example, by obstruction at the level of the fourth ventricle or the aqueduct, leading to symptoms and signs of raised intracranial pressure such as headache and vomiting. Unsteadiness and visual difficulties are also common. The range of presenting

Table 4.12.3 Brain tumour types in childhood

Types of tumours (% incidence)	WHO Grade
Astrocytic tumours (32%)	
Pilocytic astrocytoma	I
Pilomyxoid astrocytoma	II
Pleomorphic xanthoastrocytoma	II
Diffuse astrocytomas	
Fibrillary, gemistocytic, and protoplasmic	II
Anaplastic astrocytoma	III
Glioblastoma multiforme	IV
Oligodendroglial tumours (2.8%)	
Oligodendroglioma	II
Anaplastic oligodendroglioma	III
Oligoastrocytic tumours (4.7%)	
Oligoastrocytoma	II
Anaplastic oligoastrocytoma	III
Ependymal tumours (5.5%)	
Ependymoma—classic	II
Ependymoma—anaplastic	III
Neuronal and mixed neuronal-glial tumours (7%)	
Desmoplastic infantile astrocytoma/ganglioglioma	I
Ganglioglioma	I
Neurocytoma (central and extraventricular)	II
Tumours of the pineal region (1.4%)	
Pineocytoma	I
Pineoblastoma	IV
Embryonal tumours (19.4%)	
Medulloblastoma	IV
Supratentorial PNET	IV
Atypical teratoid rhabdoid tumour (ATRT)	IV
Tumours of cranial and paraspinal nerves (1%)	
Schwannoma	I
Neurofibroma	I
Malignant peripheral nerve sheath tumour (MPNST)	II–IV
Tumours of the meninges (2.8%)	
Meningioma	I
Germ cell tumours (5.3%)	
Germinoma	
Non-germinomatous germ cell tumours	
Tumours of the sellar region (6.7%)	
Craniopharyngioma	I

symptoms is, however, protean and many children present with features such as educational and behavioural difficulties, seizures, focal weakness, increased head circumference, growth, and endocrine abnormalities and others.

General principles of management

The management of CNS tumours in childhood requires a dedicated MDT of professionals dealing with the patient's management, psychosocial problems, side effects of treatment, and other important issues.

Imaging

CT is often the initial investigation leading to diagnosis and usually reveals the presence of the tumour and frequently evidence of hydrocephalus with ventricular dilatation. MRI which gives very detailed anatomical information has, however, completely revolutionized management with respect to both diagnosis and treatment. MRI is becoming increasingly sophisticated with techniques such as tractography and diffusion weighted imaging. The use of functional imaging such as PET and magnetic resonance spectroscopy MRS shows promise and is currently under investigation.

Surgery

Surgery is vital in most cases because it provides tumour for histological diagnosis, either from tumour resection or by open or closed (stereotactic) biopsy. For patients presenting with hydrocephalus, surgery is used to relieve intracranial pressure either by removal of the tumour itself or by CSF diversion techniques such as insertion of a shunt or an external ventricular drain or by an endoscopic third ventriculostomy.

For several tumour types such as hemispheric low-grade gliomas, surgery alone is curative and for malignant tumours such as high-grade glioma, medulloblastoma, and ependymoma, many studies have shown a correlation between the degree of resection and survival.

Perioperative mortality is now ≤1%. This is attributable to factors such as the use of dexamethasone, improved paediatric intensive care units (PICU) and high dependency unit (HDU) facilities and improved surgical technique.

Tumours are usually resected using the Cavitron ultrasonic surgical aspirator (CUSA) to gently and steadily remove the tumour. In addition, neuronavigation has become a standard of care. This links the digital data from the patient's MRI or CT scan images with a neuronavigation pointer so that the surgeon is able to define intraoperative anatomy and orientation. The use of endoscopy for procedures within the third and lateral ventricles has also become routine. Intraoperative MRI is being gradually introduced and is likely to become standard practice.

Radiotherapy

Radiotherapy has a vital role in treatment of several tumour types and is curative for lesions such as medulloblastoma, germinoma, and ependymoma. It is, however, especially in young children, associated with long-term side effects, such as neuropsychological damage, learning difficulties, and abnormalities of growth and endocrine function. Such sequelae occur particularly when whole CNS radiotherapy is used or when radiotherapy is given locally to midline structures. Although the late effects of radiotherapy are greatest in young children, there is clear recent evidence that difficulties with learning and short-term memory affect even adults.

There have been major recent advances in radiotherapy. Three-dimensional planning and conformal delivery of radiotherapy has become increasingly sophisticated with the aim of focusing the radiotherapy to the tumour as much as possible and limiting the radiotherapy dose to normal tissues. In addition, there is increasing interest in the use of intensity modulated radiation therapy (IMRT) that uses multiple fields defined by a computer-generated planning system to optimize dose to the tumour and reduce dose to normal tissues. In a few centres, principally in North America, proton beam therapy has been introduced to exploit the unique physical nature of proton beams which have a finite range in tissue that allows extremely tight dose distributions. Proton beam radiation is not associated with an exit dose so that as well as a potential reduction in damage to normal CNS structures, there is theoretically a reduced risk of induction of second tumours.

For radiosensitive malignant tumours, there is a theoretical radiobiological improvement in therapeutic index with hyperfractionated (twice a day) radiotherapy using a lower dose per fraction to spare normal tissues. This has been the subject of a number of European clinical trials.

Chemotherapy

Chemotherapy has much less impact in CNS tumours than in paediatric solid tumours elsewhere in the body. Trials of chemotherapy have been used to attempt to improve survival but also to try to reduce the radiotherapy dose or volume.

The limitations of chemotherapy in brain tumours are principally due to the relative resistance of some tumours such as malignant gliomas, and to the so called blood–brain barrier (BBB) caused by tight brain capillary endothelial junctions. Thus early trials of chemotherapy focused on the use of small lipophilic unionized drugs such as the nitrosoureas that were considered more likely to be able to cross directly into the brain. We now recognize that in many cases the barrier is disrupted around tumours which allow classical chemotherapy drugs to enter tumours. Thus the majority of drugs now used in children comprise agents such as the classical alkylators, platinum derivatives, and others such as etoposide.

Chemotherapy clearly has a role in the treatment of medulloblastoma and CNS germ cell tumours but also in low-grade gliomas where it has some benefit in delaying or avoiding radiotherapy.

Various ways of overcoming drug resistance and the problem posed by the BBB have been studied. High-dose chemotherapy with stem cell rescue has been investigated to deliver higher doses of drug to brain tumours. There is as yet no evidence for a benefit of high-dose chemotherapy in the initial treatment of tumours in older children, although some evidence exists for efficacy in infants and for some patients with relapsed tumours.

Radiosensitization agents have been explored without, at present, any good evidence for efficacy and with concern about possibly increased neurotoxicity.

Other attempts to overcome the BBB include using osmotic or chemical BBB disruption or direct intra-arterial injection of agents. Again benefit is limited and there is clear concern about increased toxicity.

Regional intrathecal therapy, widely used in leukaemia and lymphoma, offers promise and may be particularly beneficial for young patients with disseminating tumours such as medulloblastoma as a way of replacing or reducing radiotherapy. Encouraging results were noted in the German HIT SKK 92 study in which IT methotrexate was added to systemic chemotherapy in the treatment of infantile medulloblastoma. A number of other intrathecal agents are currently being explored in phase I/II studies.

Individual tumour types

Low-grade gliomas

Low-grade gliomas make up about 30–40% of childhood brain tumours. Most occur in the first decade of life with the most common age of onset at 6–9 years. There is a male predominance and an association with neurofibromatosis type I (NF1).

The great majority of low-grade gliomas in childhood are pilocytic astrocytomas (WHO grade I). Others include fibrillary astrocytomas, oligoastrocytomas, and oligodendrogliomas. A newly described variant of the pilocytic astrocytoma is the pilomyxoid astrocytoma (WHO Grade II) which tends to occur in younger children, often affects the optic pathway/hypothalamus and has a poorer prognosis.

The most common location is cerebellar hemisphere followed by the cerebral hemispheres, deep midline structures, and then the optic pathway. Leptomeningeal dissemination may occur in up to 5% of cases.

Optic pathway gliomas (OPG) may involve the optic nerves, the chiasm, the hypothalamus, and optic radiations and may extend into adjacent structures. They represent 5% of childhood brain tumours and 60–70% occur in the first 5 years of life. Up to 50% of patients with optic pathway glioma have NF1 and around 15% of NF1 patients will develop OPGs. Most OPGs are pilocytic astrocytomas; pilomyxoid and fibrillary astrocytomas are less common.

Clinical presentation

The pattern of clinical presentation is related to the location of the tumour. Cerebellar astrocytomas usually present with hydrocephalus. For supratentorial tumours, the duration of symptoms before diagnosis is frequently long, reflecting the slow-growing nature of these tumours.

OPGs may present with raised intracranial pressure, altered vision, squint, cranial nerve abnormalities, diencephalic syndrome or occasionally with symptoms suggestive of hypothalamic or endocrine dysfunction. For tumours of the optic nerve the diagnosis is made radiologically without the need for biopsy, although biopsy is generally indicated for chiasmatic tumours.

Treatment

Standard treatment for most tumours is an attempt at complete surgical excision. This is achievable in the majority of both cerebral and cerebellar hemispheric tumours and in these cases the surgery is usually curative (>90% survival).

In other locations, total excision is generally not possible and the management of low-grade gliomas after biopsy only or incomplete resection is dependent on tumour location, age, severity of neurological symptoms, and risk to neighbouring structures, (e.g. optic pathway and hypothalamus). Stable disease, sometimes for prolonged periods, is often seen after biopsy or incomplete resection, and therefore some patients may be observed only, with serial imaging.

For OPGs, indications to start treatment include severely affected vision bilaterally in which there is a significant threat to remaining vision, progressive visual loss, severe or progressive neurological dysfunction, documented progression of tumour radiologically, or diencephalic syndrome.

If treatment is necessary, radiotherapy (total 54Gy in 1.8Gy per fraction) has been the standard therapy for many years. However, there is now an established role for chemotherapy in low-grade gliomas. It is the treatment of choice in younger children (<8–10 years old) in whom the use of radiotherapy may be delayed or avoided; in patients with NF in whom radiotherapy is associated with an increased risk of second tumours; in those patients whose tumours progress after radiotherapy; and in those with leptomeningeal dissemination. An established multiagent drug combination commonly used is vincristine and carboplatin.

Supratentorial high-grade gliomas

Although high-grade gliomas are the predominant tumour type in adults, they only constitute about 10% of childhood brain tumours outside the brainstem. Median age at diagnosis is 9–10 years. Histologically, the main entities are glioblastoma multiforme (WHO IV), anaplastic astrocytoma (WHO III), and anaplastic oligoastrocytoma and oligodendroglioma (WHO III). Excluding brainstem tumours, around 25% occur in the deep midline structures (thalamus, hypothalamus, and third ventricle), 15% occur in the cerebellum, and the rest in the cerebral hemispheres.

Clinical presentation

The pattern of presentation and duration of symptoms before diagnosis is more dependent on location rather than on histological grade. MRI is likely to show a heterogeneous space-occupying lesion with diffuse margins, contrast enhancement, and surrounding oedema. Areas of necrosis, haemorrhage, and cystic change may occur although calcification is rare. Leptomeningeal dissemination may occur at diagnosis or relapse.

Management

Gross or near-total resection (>90%) together with tumour grade (III–IV) are the principal prognostic factors in children. Radiation therapy to a dose of 54–59.5Gy to the tumour bed is given postoperatively. Despite the addition of single or multiagent chemotherapy drugs in numerous phase II or phase III trials, there is no convincing evidence that the use of chemotherapy has been associated with an improvement in survival which ranges from 0–40%. The current UK treatment guidelines do, however, incorporate the use of temozolamide which has been shown to be of benefit in a subpopulation of adults.

Brainstem gliomas

Tumours of the midbrain, pons, and medulla account for around 10% of CNS tumours in children. The commonest radiological pattern on MRI (brainstem lesions are poorly defined on CT scan) is the diffuse intrinsic pontine glioma (DIPG). It is probably useful to consider brainstem tumours as either diffusely infiltrating tumours or focal tumours. Until recently, there has been a reluctance to biopsy these lesions but it is now known that within the spectrum of diffuse lesions, gliomas of all grades occur (WHO I to IV) although it would appear that lower grades make up only about one-fourth of biopsied cases. Focal tumours are particularly associated other histologies including PNET, ependymoma, and atypical teratoid rhabdoid tumour (ATRT). Focal tumours at the very top (tectum) and bottom (cervicomedullary junction) are most likely to be low-grade gliomas.

Clinical presentation

These tumours commonly present with cranial nerve abnormalities, ataxia, or limb weakness. The history is usually short, although longer symptom duration may suggest lower grade histology.

Treatment

Surgical resection should be performed for tumours at the cervicomedullary junction and dorsally exophytic tumours, and may be considered for other focal tumours. There is no role for surgery in the cases of indolent tectal plate tumours which are usually low-grade tumours and need to be observed only. Other low-grade tumours demonstrated at surgery may also be observed.

For DIPGs, radiotherapy remains the mainstay of therapy. Although rarely resulting in cure, radiation therapy is often an effective palliative measure resulting in a temporary improvement in neurological status. Median survival times for DIPGs are about 12 months with around 5% survival at 2 years.

Medulloblastoma

Medulloblastoma is the most common malignant brain tumour in childhood, accounting for between 15–20% of all childhood primary CNS neoplasms and around 80% of PNETs. The large majority occur within the first decade of life with a peak incidence at 5 years. There is a 2:1 male to female ratio. By definition, medulloblastoma arises in the posterior fossa, usually from the cerebellar vermis in the roof of the fourth ventricle. As with other PNETs, medulloblastomas have a marked propensity to seed within the CSF pathways, with evidence of such metastatic spread occurring in up to 35% of cases at diagnosis.

Histologically, the majority of medulloblastomas (about 80%) are described as having a classical phenotype composed of sheets of malignant small round cells with frequent mitoses. Various degrees of glial or neuronal differentiation may be seen. Other histological types include desmoplastic/nodular medulloblastoma and medulloblastoma with extensive nodularity, both predominantly occurring in very young children, and anaplastic medulloblastoma and large-cell medulloblastoma which are both associated with a poorer outcome than with the classic phenotype.

Recent research has shown a number of types of medulloblastoma associated with distinct molecular characteristics. For example, the Wnt/Wingless (Wnt/Wg) and Sonic hedgehog (SHH) developmental cell signalling pathways become aberrantly activated in subsets of medulloblastomas. Wnt/Wg pathway activation can be identified by expression of β-catenin on immunohistochemistry and it has been clearly shown that β-catenin positive tumours have a good prognosis. On the other hand, tumours with amplification of the MYC oncogene are associated with an adverse outcome.

Clinical presentation

The majority of patients with medulloblastoma present with signs and symptoms of raised intracranial pressure due to hydrocephalus. Other presenting features include ataxia due to cerebellar involvement and diplopia, cranial nerve palsies, and long tract signs as a result of pressure on, or infiltration of, the brainstem. Occasionally, patients may present with manifestations of spinal metastases such as back pain or lower limb weakness.

Treatment

Staging should include MRI of the head and spine, and postoperative MRI of the head and a lumbar puncture to examine for residual disease and CSF infiltration respectively.

The therapeutic approach for medulloblastoma consists of complete or near complete surgical resection followed by postoperative craniospinal radiotherapy (CSRT) followed by chemotherapy. Standard risk patients are those aged at least 3–5 years of age with no evidence of metastatic spread and with <1.5^2cm of post-surgical residual disease. In these patients a CSRT dose of 23.4Gy is used with a boost to the posterior fossa or tumour bed (total tumour dose 54Gy). For high-risk cases (e.g. metastatic disease) the CSRT dose is around 36Gy, again with a tumour boost.

Both standard and high-risk cases are given postradiation chemotherapy, with the most widely used regimen consisting of eight courses of a combination of cisplatin, CCNU (lomustine), and vincristine (or modifications thereof).

Survival is around 75–80% for standard risk patients and around 50% for those with metastatic disease.

Supratentorial PNET

This group comprises around 2–3% of CNS tumours in childhood. The majority arise in the cerebral hemispheres principally in the frontal, parietal and temporal lobes. About 20% arise in the pineal region, where they are known as pineoblastomas.

Clinical presentation

Supratentorial PNETs (StPNETs) usually present with symptoms and signs associated with the mass effect of the tumour including headaches, seizures and hemiplegia Pineoblastoma usually presents with symptoms and signs of hydrocephalus and sometimes Parinaud's syndrome.

Treatment

Staging investigations are similar to those for medulloblastoma. Non-pineal StPNETs are usually large at presentation with around half being >5cm in diameter at diagnosis.

Because of the rarity of supratentorial PNETs, there have been no large multicentre studies specifically for StPNETs; instead, they are generally treated with protocols designed for children with high-risk medulloblastoma. Thus the generally accepted standard therapy is to remove the tumour as completely as possible, although this may be difficult, and complete resection rates are lower than with medulloblastoma. CSRT is delivered with doses of 35–36Gy with a boost to the primary tumour that is a particular concern in terms of the potential for severe neurological damage. Chemotherapy is generally administered according to high-risk medulloblastoma protocols.

Several studies have shown an improved outcome for patients with pineoblastomas with survival of around 65–70% compared with those with non-pineal supratentorial PNETs of whom only around 40% survive.

Ependymoma

Ependymomas arise from the ependymal lining of the ventricles or central canal of the spinal cord. Ninety per cent are intracranial of which around 65% arise in the posterior fossa from the fourth ventricle. They make up about 6–10% of childhood brain tumours and they tend to occur in younger children under the age of 7.

There are two principal histological grades, namely classic (grade II ~80%) and anaplastic (grade III ~20%). In children with ependymoma, the impact of grading on prognosis is at present unclear. Grade I myxopapillary and sub-ependymal ependymomas occur rarely in children.

Clinical presentation

As with most other CNS tumours in childhood, the presenting features principally reflect tumour location. MRI will show a tumour in the ventricular system or less commonly periventricularly. Calcification, haemorrhage, and cysts are common and most ependymomas will show a degree of gadolinium enhancement. Posterior fossa lesions frequently infiltrate into and around the brainstem and may extend down the cervical spinal cord. Leptomeningeal dissemination occurs in up to 10% of cases at diagnosis.

Treatment

One of the more significant and consistent prognostic factors in ependymoma is the extent of surgical resection. Every attempt should be made to achieve a complete resection although this may be difficult, particularly with fourth ventricular lesions. A postoperative MRI should be performed within 72 hours of surgery and if there is residual disease the original neurosurgeon should be involved in a decision as to whether second-look surgery is feasible. A lumbar puncture performed 15 days after surgery to assess CSF for malignant cells is mandatory.

Local radiation therapy is standard postoperative treatment. The usual dose is 54Gy, although there is interest in using higher doses of radiation. Craniospinal radiotherapy has ceased to be indicated except in metastatic cases. The role of chemotherapy has been the subject of numerous trials and for older children and adults there appears to be no benefit to date, although chemotherapy will continue to be investigated in future clinical trials. There does appear to be a role for chemotherapy in infants when chemotherapy has been used to delay giving radiotherapy and in some to avoid radiotherapy completely. Most recurrences are local. Five-year overall survival rates for ependymoma are about 65%.

Germ cell tumours

Intracranial germ cell tumours (GCTs) are a rare (around 3% of childhood CNS tumours) and heterogeneous group of tumours that share a common cellular origin with their extracranial counterparts, the primordial germ cell.

GCTs include benign teratoma and the malignant subtypes, namely germinoma, embryonal carcinoma, yolk-sac tumour, and choriocarcinoma. Mixed types do occur and immature or benign teratomas may contain malignant elements.

Non-germinomatous malignant types are characterized by the secretion of tumour markers detected in both blood and CSF; for yolk-sac tumour—AFP, and for choriocarcinoma—beta human choriogonadotrophin. For yolk-sac tumours a high level of AFP is an adverse prognostic factor.

Teratoma may present as a neonatal tumour, but with increasing age malignant types become more common, with germinoma being a tumour of teenagers and young adults. GCTs mainly arise in the suprasellar region or the pineal area or metachronously in both areas. Malignant types have a propensity to spread locally within the ventricular system with a small proportion of cases metastasizing distally within the CNS.

Clinical presentation

The duration of symptoms prior to diagnosis is variable and relates to tumour location and the rate of tumour growth. Suprasellar tumours typically present with endocrine abnormalities such as diabetes insipidus, hypopituitarism, and visual impairment including visual field defects. Pineal lesions generally present with a short history, with the majority associated with acute hydrocephalus due to cerebral aqueduct obstruction. Visual changes, particularly Parinaud's syndrome, are also common.

Treatment

For treatment purposes, the malignant GCTs are subdivided into either germinoma or non-germinomatous types (also referred to as secreting GCTs).

Recent studies have emphasized the importance of complete staging including MRI of the whole CNS axis, lumbar

CSF examination for both tumour markers and malignant cells and also blood sampling for markers.

Germinoma is exquisitely sensitive to radiotherapy and until recently standard treatment has been with craniospinal radiotherapy (24Gy CSRT dose) with a boost to the tumour (40Gy total tumour dose). Surgical excision is not necessary as initial treatment. Using CSRT, the prognosis for germinoma is excellent, with survival of at least 90%.

More recently there has been interest in exploiting the chemosensitivity of germinoma to enable a reduction in the volume and possibly dose of radiation. Thus the next European study recommends the use of two courses of initial chemotherapy followed by whole ventricular radiotherapy (24Gy) with or without a tumour boost, depending on the chemotherapy response.

Non-germinomatous malignant GCTs are more challenging and have a less favourable outcome than germinoma. Standard treatment consists of platinum and ifosfamide-based chemotherapy followed by local radiotherapy for non-metastatic disease. Although surgery is not necessarily required, it is clear that prognosis is related to the degree of residual tumour after treatment. In this respect, surgical excision before radiotherapy should generally be undertaken in patients with significant residual disease after chemotherapy. OS for non-germinomatous malignant GCTs is around 70%.

Craniopharyngioma

Craniopharyngiomas are the commonest tumour in the pituitary area in children. In childhood the peak age of onset is between 5–10 years and there is a slight male predominance. Despite being classified as low-grade tumours (WHO grade I) and being slow growing, they may often have a very 'malignant' course because of their invasive nature, their tendency to recur locally, and their ability to cause very significant visual, pituitary, and hypothalamic morbidity.

Clinical presentation

Childhood craniopharyngiomas may present with endocrine symptoms (short stature and delayed puberty), raised intracranial pressure (due to hydrocephalus), visual dysfunction (e.g. visual field defects), and behavioural problems. CT and MRI scans are helpful in making a radiological diagnosis, typically showing a mixed solid and cystic tumour with calcification.

Treatment

Involvement of specialist paediatric endocrinology and neurosurgery services is vital for the management of this tumour with a detailed endocrinological assessment being performed at diagnosis and perioperatively. The role of radical surgery is controversial although it should be considered for the patients (around 50%) with small tumours and in whom other factors indicating more extensive invasion such as hydrocephalus, hypothalamic involvement or breach of the third ventricular floor are absent. In patients not suited for resection, particularly when the risk of damage to the hypothalamus is high, partial resection followed by radiotherapy is the accepted standard approach in the UK. In very young patients (e.g. <5 years old), a period of close observation with conservative management may be followed before radiotherapy will usually become necessary. No role for chemotherapy has been proven for craniopharyngiomas. For recurrent craniopharyngiomas after radiotherapy there may be a role for surgery or intracystic instillation of chemotherapeutic agents or radio-isotopes.

Intramedullary spinal tumours

Intrinsic spinal cord tumours in childhood are rare, comprising <5% of CNS tumours in childhood. Seventy per cent of them are astrocytomas (mostly low grade), 10% ependymomas, and the rest comprise other glial tumours such as oligodendrogliomas, gangliogliomas, and PNETs. Leptomeningeal spread often accompanies higher grade tumours. Histologically these tumours are indistinguishable from their intracranial counterparts.

Clinical presentation

Spinal tumours in children most often present with persistent back pain, abnormal gait, and neurological deficits in the lower or upper limbs. Abdominal pains may complicate the picture in younger children and bladder and bowel dysfunction may be present.

Treatment

A histological diagnosis is always necessary. Paediatric neurosurgeons with experience of operating on the spinal cord should be consulted. Ependymomas are often amenable to complete resection. Complete resections for astrocytoma are achieved much less often (<50%) because of difficulties finding a clear cleavage plane. Consideration of chemotherapy or radiotherapy is given as for intracranial counterparts although the total dose of radiotherapy achievable is limited by spinal cord tolerance. The prognosis for these tumours varies but is mostly poorer than for their intracranial counterparts and morbidity is often significant.

Infant tumours

A third of all childhood brain tumours will occur in infants <3 years old. Tumour types include low-grade (predominantly midline) gliomas, high-grade gliomas, ependymomas, medulloblastomas, ATRT, choroid plexus carcinoma (CPC), and teratoma.

Tumour types such as ATRT and CPC are predominantly tumours of 'infants', and are particularly challenging to treat, with a poor prognosis.

There is, however, evidence that the biology and natural history of 'infant tumours' may differ from their counterparts in older children. For example, the outlook for high-grade glioma in infants appears better than in individuals >3–5 years of age.

Clinical presentation

Brain tumours occurring in babies <6 months old are termed congenital tumours and indeed some of them are discovered on antenatal scans. Common presentations thereafter are with increasing head circumference, visual abnormalities (particularly roving nystagmus or squint), delayed acquisition or regression of developmental milestones, seizures or abnormal behaviour. Classical symptoms and signs of raised intracranial pressure may be obscured by the inability of the infant to self-report and the ability of the head to expand.

Management

Infant tumours have generally been considered separately from the older age groups principally because the side effects of treatment, particularly radiotherapy, are greatest in very young children. This necessitates different approaches to therapy, which generally aim to delay or avoid the use of radiation therapy, particularly to the whole CNS or supratentorial structures.

For two decades from the 1970s a number of 'baby brain' protocols were developed internationally where all infants were given the same treatment regimens whatever the histology, using chemotherapy in an attempt to delay or avoid radiotherapy and improve the often dismal prognosis. More recently it has become clearer that disease specific infant protocols are required, with different treatment approaches for individual tumour types.

The increased ability to deliver precise conformal radiotherapy has led to renewed recent interest in using posterior fossa radiotherapy in upfront strategies for very young children, particularly for posterior fossa tumours such as medulloblastoma and ependymoma.

Late effects

Children with brain tumours are at risk of developing significant long-term sequelae which may be devastating. These children are likely to require a longer period of MDT follow-up than their counterparts with haematological malignancies or other solid tumours.

Principal late effects include neuropsychological impairment with cognitive defects, short-term memory loss, learning and behavioural difficulties. More specific abnormalities include growth and endocrine dysfunction, and motor defects and visual impairment.

The aetiology of late effects is frequently multifactorial, and may be due to the effect of the tumour itself, including the effect of hydrocephalus, or be related to treatment. With regard to surgery, a particular postoperative problem is the so called 'posterior fossa syndrome' ('akinetic mutism') occurring in up to 20% of patients and characterized by mutism, limb weakness, cranial nerve palsies, personality changes, and involuntary movements. Chemotherapy may lead to specific late effects such as infertility, hearing loss, and nephrotoxicity.

However, the most important factor predisposing to severe late effects, particularly neuropsychological impairment, is the use of radiation therapy. It is clear that these adverse effects are most marked in very young children, aged <5–7 years old, in whom the brain is particularly immature. Radiotherapy is also particularly damaging when the whole CNS is irradiated, as in the treatment of medulloblastoma, or when it is given to midline structures for tumours such as chiasmatic gliomas.

A systematic evaluation of late effects is a prominent feature of current and proposed North American and European clinical trials in CNS tumours.

Further reading

Giangaspero F, Eberhart CG, Haapasalo H, et al. Medulloblastoma. In: Louis DM, Ohgaki H, Wiestler OD, et al. (eds) WHO Classification of Tumors of the Central Nervous System, 4th edition, pp.132–140. Lyon: IARC Press, 2007.

Gottardo HG, Gajjar A. Chemotherapy for malignant brain tumors of childhood. J Child Neurol 2008; **23**(10):1149–59.

Hargrave DR, Zacharoulis S. Pediatric CNS tumors: current treatment and future directions. Expert Rev Neurother 2007; **7**(8):1029–42.

Packer RJ. Childhood brain tumors: accomplishments and ongoing challenges. J Child Neurol 2008; **23**(10):1122–7.

Pizer B, Clifford S. Medulloblastoma: new insights into biology and treatment. Arch Dis Child Educ Pract Ed 2008; **93**(5):137–44.

Walker DA, Perilongo G, Punt JAG, et al. (eds). Brain and spinal tumours of childhood. London: Arnold, 2004.

Wechsler-Reya R, Scott MP. The developmental biology of brain tumors. Annu Rev Neurosci 2001; **24**:385–428.

Wilne S, Collier J, Kennedy C, et al. Presentation of childhood CNS tumours: a systematic review and meta-analysis. Lancet Oncol 2007; **8**(8):685–95.

Paediatric solid tumours and kidney tumours

Introduction

Children with solid tumours require multidisciplinary care from paediatric: oncologists, radiologists, histopathologists, pharmacists, chemotherapy-trained nurses, radiotherapists, and surgeons. Children should be clinically stabilized and then referred to a paediatric oncology centre for diagnostic work-up and treatment. Decision making should take place in a multidisciplinary setting. Useful websites to connect to international treatment programmes are given at the end of the chapter in 'Internet resources'.

Where possible all children should be treated in a clinical trial. Children should have access to paediatric intensive care, and the paediatric specialties such as endocrinology, nephrology, ophthalmology, and audiology. Painful procedures and the placing of central lines should be done under general anaesthesia. For imaging, sedation may be adequate and young infants may be able to be fed and wrapped if left in a safe position.

Chemotherapy guidelines should be carefully adhered to. Weight and age define how the dose is prescribed. Many chemotherapy agents need to be administered with hydration fluids in order to reduce toxicity and careful adjustment of total fluid load and electrolytes is required.

Follow-up after treatment should be assured for a minimum of 5 years with guidance from a specialist in late effects. In addition, the supportive care of children who have become myelosuppressed as a result of chemotherapy is vital. Particularly crucial is the early treatment with antibiotics of children susceptible to severe infections when neutropenic. This care tends to be delivered in local hospitals close to the patient.

Kidney tumours

Introduction

Kidney tumours account for 6–8% of childhood cancer. The most common form of kidney tumour is Wilms' tumour named after Max Wilms, a German surgeon. Wilms' tumour was the first tumour to be found to be sensitive to radiotherapy and to the first chemotherapeutic agents, vincristine and actinomycin D, which were discovered in the 1950s. A rarer form of kidney tumour, which occurs in very young children, called mesoblastic nephroma, is benign. This is genetically different from Wilms' tumour. Wilms' tumour sometimes develops from nephrogenic rests which are difficult to distinguish pathologically from Wilms' tumour.

Clear cell sarcoma is a rare form of kidney tumour occurring in older children—this used to be called 'bone metastasizing Wilms' tumour'. Rhabdoid tumours can also occur in the kidney as well as in the brain and other organs.

Diagnosis and staging

Children with Wilms' tumour often present with an abdominal mass which has been found incidentally by the carer.

The tumour is sometimes easily palpable or becomes palpable by gently lifting the tumour with the left hand under the flank and palpating with the right hand. It can usually be mobilized in this way and is therefore distinguishable from a mass in the liver or spleen. The child may also present with haematuria. If the tumour has bled, pressure on the capsule of the kidney may cause pain and there may be a fall in haemoglobin, and in severe cases an increase in the girth of the abdomen may result in respiratory difficulties.

Investigations

The first investigations include urinanalysis, full blood count, ultrasound of the abdomen, and CXR, as Wilms' tumour metastasizes to the lung. If a kidney mass is confirmed on ultrasound, further imaging of the primary tumour with MRI or CT scan is necessary. The chest should be imaged with spiral CT scan to detect smaller lung metastases.

Biopsy

The diagnosis should be confirmed by histological examination following biopsy of the tumour. This can be done as percutaneous core needle biopsy or open biopsy under general anaesthesia. FNA is a useful tool in resource challenged nations and can be diagnostic; however, the architecture of the tumour is lost.

Histopathology, cytogenetics, and molecular biology

Wilms' tumour is commonly a triphasic tumour consisting of blastemal, stromal, and tubular elements. Some tumours are predominantly blastemal in composition and some may contain areas of anaplasia or diffuse anaplasia which increases the risk status of the disease. Cytogenetics will often show abnormalities of the WT1 (Wilms' tumour 1) tumour suppressor gene which can also be found using molecular biological techniques exposing the presence of an abnormal WT1 transcript.

Treatment

Treatment consists of a combination of chemotherapy and surgery, the extent of which is defined by both stage and pathology. In North America primary surgery is preferred to permit surgical staging. In Europe, preoperative chemotherapy is preferred and imaging is used to identify image-defined risk factors (IDRFs). Initially the diagnosis of Wilms' tumour, whether metastatic (stage IV) or non-metastatic (stages I–III) and uni- or bilateral (stage V), is sufficient to start treatment. Unilateral non-metastatic tumours receive a short course of preoperative chemotherapy according to the current SIOP Wilms' tumour protocol using a combination of two drugs, vincristine and actinomycin D. For metastatic disease, three drugs may be used as primary therapy with the addition of doxorubicin.

Non-metastatic unilateral disease

In the case of unilateral, non-metastatic disease, surgery is currently performed at week 5, allowing for full histopathological examination of the resected specimen. Postoperative treatment is guided by the histopathological and surgical stage. The postoperative chemotherapy regimen depends on whether or not anaplasia, a poor prognostic factor, is found on careful histopathological examination, and will consist of further vincristine/actinomycin D chemotherapy or three drugs with the addition of doxorubicin. The surgical stage of the tumour is described as: stage I—complete resection; stage II—resection but with microscopical residual disease; and stage III—resection leaving macroscopic residual or nodal disease. In the latter case flank radiotherapy will be required.

Bilateral Wilms' tumour

In the case of bilateral Wilms' tumour the surgical intervention is usually delayed by a few weeks and isotope imaging performed to discover the amount of functioning kidney remaining on each side. Around week 7 or later the tumours will be surgically removed leaving a functioning kidney on one side where possible. Postoperative chemotherapy will depend on the highest surgical stage designated separately for each kidney.

Metastatic Wilms' tumour

In the case of metastatic Wilms' tumour, clearance of lung disease, which may involve surgical metastatectomy, is aimed at by week 7. Postoperative chemotherapy with three agents, and where appropriate additional lung radiotherapy, is given. Radiotherapy is also given to the area of the primary tumour if it is surgical stage III. A radiotherapy dose ranging from 12–15Gy is used which gives few sequelae to the lungs and is relatively well tolerated by the kidney.

Follow-up

Follow-up is with regular CXR and abdominal ultrasound. All children who have received doxorubicin should have an echocardiogram at 6 months after ending treatment and, if normal, every 5 years lifelong.

Prognostic factors and survival

Prognosis and survival are dependent on appropriate treatment, stage, and histopathology. Higher stage, presence of blastemal Wilms' tumour or anaplasia confers a poorer prognosis. Overall survival at 5 years ranges from 70% for stage IV tumours to >95% for stage I disease and risk categories and directed treatment continue to be refined in the current SIOP trial.

Further reading

Lemerle J, Voûte PA, Tournade MF, *et al.* Effectiveness of pre-operative chemotherapy in Wilms' tumour: results of an International Society of Paediatric Oncology (SIOP) clinical trial. *J Clin Oncol* 1983; **1**:604–9.

Mitchell C, Morris-Jones P, Kelsey A, *et al.* The treatment of Wilms' tumour: results of the United Kingdom children's cancer study group (UKCCSG) second Wilms' tumour study. *Br J Cancer* 2000; **83**:602–8.

Sarcomas

Introduction

Whereas the majority of childhood solid tumours are embryonal in nature and carcinomas are extremely rare, sarcomas do occur at all ages and in most parts of the body. Infants and children develop PNETs and fibrosarcoma. Rhabdomyosarcoma is a childhood sarcoma arising from striated muscle elements, while older children may develop clear cell sarcoma of the kidney, Ewing sarcoma of bone and soft tissue, as well as osteosarcoma.

There are also rarer forms of sarcoma occurring in the liver, embryonal sarcoma and smooth muscle leiomyosarcoma. We will deal here with the most common form of childhood sarcoma, rhabdomyosarcoma, which occurs in two main forms: embryonal and alveolar. Embryonal rhabdomyosarcoma is the most common type and carries a better prognosis.

Diagnosis and staging

Presentation

Presentation is a function of the organ of origin of the tumour and includes pain, visible swelling, palpable mass, lump, proptosis, airway obstruction, visible protrusion/bleeding of tumour through nasal, anal, oral, or vaginal orifices, urinary retention, or symptoms of raised intracranial pressure. In the rare case of widespread medullary metastatic alveolar rhabdomyosarcoma, presenting symptoms can mimic those of leukaemia. The presenting mass may be regional lymph node disease and careful examination of the area of lymph drainage to that region is essential. It is particularly important, when inguinal nodes are found, to examine and image the whole leg including the foot, as well as palpating the foot carefully. The extent of nodal involvement is an important prognostic factor and in uncertain cases lymph node biopsy is necessary, before initiating treatment.

Investigations

Cross-sectional imaging of the primary tumour as well as all areas of regional lymph node drainage should be obtained if possible with gadolinium contrasted MRI. Complete staging includes CXR, spiral CT scan of the chest, technetium bone scan, bilateral bone marrow aspirates, and trephine biopsies. There is no specific serum tumour marker for rhabdomyosarcoma; however, the full blood count will give an indication of bleeding into the tumour or bone marrow invasion. A high level of serum LDH, above the normal for age, is a non-specific marker of high cellular turnover and a very high level is indicative of a poorer prognosis. Serum urea and creatinine and liver function tests will guide on the general well-being of the child and any organ failure due to compression. Children with

fever should have appropriate cultures and an infectious disease screen. Abdominal ultrasound is useful in assessing liver, kidney, and bladder function. In prostatic or bladder rhabdomyosarcoma, cystourethroscopic examination under general anaesthesia, both at diagnosis and before surgery, is useful. Diagnostic work-up, staging, stabilizing the child, and optimizing organ function should be completed before treatment. Exceptions are where there is spinal cord compression or airway obstruction which demands urgent chemotherapy reduction. In these cases, full staging can be done after the start of chemotherapy.

Biopsy

Tru-cut or open biopsy needs to be planned so that the biopsy scar and trajectory can be excised at the time of definitive surgery. Freshly obtained biopsy material is needed for immunohistochemistry and biology. Frozen sections at the time of surgery, for diagnostic purposes, are not useful.

Histopathology and molecular biology

The differential diagnosis between embryonal and alveolar rhabdomyosarcoma can be made from morphology and immunohistochemistry in most cases. Molecular biological techniques can be used to detect the abnormal PAX3 (Paired Box 3, a family of transcription factors) or PAX7 (Paired Box 7) fusion transcript which distinguish the alveolar subtypes.

Prognostic factors and survival

The location of the tumour in the head and neck or limbs, alveolar pathology, size >5cm, advanced stage, and age >10 years are poor prognostic factors.

Treatment

The current European Paediatric Soft tissue Sarcoma study Group (EpSSG) trial treats children in four categories; low, intermediate, high, and very high risk. The treatment is with multiagent chemotherapy and local surgery. Children who have unresectable tumours or parameningeal tumours will require radiotherapy. The role of maintenance chemotherapy in rhabdomyosarcoma is currently being assessed.

Further reading

Asmar L, Gehan EA, Newton WA, et al. Classification of rhabdomyosarcomas and related sarcomas. Pathological aspects and proposal for a new classification-an Intergroup Rhabdomyosarcoma Study. Cancer 1995 76:1073–85.

Stevens MC, Rey A, Bouvet N, et al. Treatment of non-metastatic rhabdomyosarcoma in childhood and adolescence: third study of the International Society of Paediatric Oncology-SIOP Malignant Mesenchymal Tumor 89. J Clin Oncol 2005; 23(12):2618–28.

Neuroblastoma

Introduction

Neuroblastoma is a malignant tumour of neural crest cells and commonly occurs in the midline or in the adrenal glands. Differentiation into benign ganglioneuroma can occur. Some tumours are mixed ganglioneuroblastomas. If they are intermixed they carry a good prognosis; but if there are nodules of undifferentiated neuroblastoma, called nodular ganglioneuroblastoma, they carry a poor prognosis. Age has always been a clear prognostic factor in neuroblastoma, with young age conferring a better prognosis. Older children and adolescents tend to have more indolent but prognostically poor disease, whereas infants, even with stage 4 disease, have a good prognosis if treated appropriately.

Neuroblastoma was the first solid tumour in paediatric practice to have treatment stratified according to molecular markers. Tumours carrying multiple copies of the Myc-N oncogene tend to be aggressive and metastasize. They initially respond well to treatment, but recur early, developing multidrug resistance and making therapy for relapse extremely difficult.

Diagnosis and staging

Infants may present with stage 4 S disease (S stands for special) where a relatively small primary tumour metastasizes to the liver, skin, and occasionally bone marrow. The liver can be diffusely infiltrated and become large enough to fill the abdominal cavity. This can compromise respiration and may be accompanied by intravascular coagulopathy.

Infants and children may also present with signs of spinal cord compression. An urgent MRI scan of the spine should be performed and chemotherapy initiated the same day, even before biopsy, if the imaging is typical. A rare subgroup of patients present with opsoclonus myoclonus (dancing eye syndrome). These children require whole body MRI scanning to exclude neuroblastoma. Ultrasound of the abdomen may show an adrenal primary tumour and aid diagnosis. Most neuroblastomas secrete catecholamine metabolites HVA (homovanillic acid) and VMA (vanillyl-mandelic acid). A spot urine test for VMA can aid diagnosis. Staging uses an isotope scan with MIBG as well as bone marrow aspirates and trephine biopsies. Imaging of the primary tumour should be with MRI. Neuroblastoma rarely metastasizes to the lungs and so CT scan of the chest is not necessary. If the MIBG scan is positive at the primary tumour site, a bone scan is not necessary. If the primary tumour does not take up MIBG, a CT scan of the head with bony windows is advised to exclude bony metastases of the skull and base of skull. A skeletal survey or bone scan is adequate for the rest of the body.

Biopsy

Wherever possible, core needle or open biopsy under GA should be performed. Fresh tissue should be analysed for immunohistochemistry and Myc-N amplification as well as other structural chromosomal abnormalities such as 1p deletion, 17q gain, 11q deletion, etc.

The International Neuroblastoma Risk Grouping (INRG) has put together the data from thousands of patients treated by different national and international groups and has developed criteria to divide patients into low-, intermediate-, and high-risk groups. In order to group the patients successfully, age at diagnosis, operability defined by the presence (L2) or absence (L1) of image-defined risk factors, histopathology, cytogenetics, and molecular biology all need to be considered. Myc-N amplified patients at any stage or age are considered high risk (exceptions may be made for young children with resected stage 1 tumours). Patients <18 months of age carry a better prognosis than those >18 months. An infant with an isolated congenital adrenal tumour carries an excellent prognosis and may require no treatment. A child with a tumour carrying any cytogenetic structural abnormality will have an intermediate prognosis. Survival ranges from <20% to >90% depending on all of these factors. Adolescents carry the worst prognosis and congenital low stage tumours have the best prognosis. The majority of children present with stage 4 disease and are high risk.

Treatment

Treatment should be according to a clinical trial. All children with high-risk disease require induction chemotherapy, surgery to the primary tumour, high-dose chemotherapy with stem cell rescue, radiotherapy to the preoperative site of the primary tumour, and differentiation therapy with 13 cis-retinoic acid. In Europe treatment protocols are driven by the SIOPEN (Europe neuroblastoma) group and contacts can be found on the SIOPEN-R-NET website listed under 'Internet resources' at the end of this chapter. The UK neuroblastoma society website also carries useful information.

Follow-up

Follow-up should take all the side effects of therapy into consideration. After therapy for high-risk disease, hearing loss, kidney problems, and infertility are the most common.

Further reading

Brodeur GM. Neuroblastoma: biological insights into a clinical enigma. *Nat Rev Cancer* 2003; **3**:203–16.

Matthay KK, Villablanca JG, Seeger RC, *et al*. Treatment of high-risk neuroblastoma with intensive chemotherapy, radiotherapy, autologous bone marrow transplantation, and 13-cis-retinoic acid. Childrens Cancer Group. *N Engl J Med* 1999; **341**:1165–73.

Other paediatric tumours and Langerhans cell histiocytosis

Hodgkin lymphoma

Hodgkin lymphoma is described in Chapter 4, Hodgkin disease, p.434. Classical Hodgkin can occur in children, usually no younger than 5 years of age. The prognosis is good and where possible chemotherapy alone should be used. A negative PET scan at the end of treatment is a good prognostic sign. Lymphocyte predominant Hodgkin lymphoma is now considered a different entity to classical Hodgkin lymphoma and can be treated by surgery alone.

Germ cell tumours

Germ cell tumours are described in Chapter 4, p.356. In neonates sacrococcygeal teratomas must be recognized; they can be diagnosed prenatally and affected children may need to be delivered by Caesarean section to prevent complications. These are benign tumours but need to be removed before the age of 2 months to prevent degeneration to malignancy. The coccyx must be removed in its entirety to prevent recurrence. AFP and β-hCG are serum markers of malignant germ cell tumours. However, the serum levels of AFP are raised from birth to the age of 8 months and so levels in children with tumours must be compared with normal levels for age.

Liver tumours

Liver tumours are described in Chapter 4, Hepatocellular cancer, p.192. In young children hepatoblastoma (HB) is the most common primary liver malignancy. HB usually secretes AFP but the levels must be compared with normal levels for age. HBs are staged by the PRE-TEXT system (PRE-Treatment EXTent of disease), with MRI imaging of liver and spiral CT of chest. Treatment and management can be found on the SIOPEL website, the International Society of Paediatric Oncology epithelial liver tumour treatment strategy group (see 'Internet resources').

Langerhans cell histiocytosis

Langerhans cell histiocytosis is a neoplastic disorder affecting CD1a positive dendritic Langerhans cells. Patients present with a wide variety of symptoms, the most common being lytic bony lesions in the skull. In young children the presentation can mimic leukaemia.

Further reading

Mann JR Germ cell tumours of childhood. In: Souhami RL, Tannock I, Hoehenberger P, et al. (eds) *Oxford Textbook of Oncology*, 2nd edition, pp.2638–55. Oxford: Oxford University Press, 2002.

Perilongo G, Shafford E, Maibach R, et al. Risk adapted treatment for childhood hepatoblastoma. Final report of the second study of the International Society of Paediatric Oncology-SIOPEL 2. *Eur J Cancer* 2004: **40**:411–21.

Internet resources

https://www.cure4kids.org/ums/home/
http://www.mrc.ac.uk/index.htm
http://www.histiocytosissociety.org
http://www.histiocytosisresearchtrust.org
http://www.siop.nl/
http://siopel.org/
https://www.siopen-r-net.org/
http://www.ukccsg.org/

Kaposi's sarcoma

Kaposi's sarcoma (KS) is a low-grade multifocal vascular tumour associated with human herpesvirus 8 (HHV8)/ Kaposi's sarcoma herpes virus (KSHV) infection.

KS lesions of all epidemiological forms are similarly comprised of HHV8-positive (LNA-1 immunoreactive) spindle-shaped tumour cells, vessels, and chronic inflammatory cells. Lesions evolve from early patch, to plaque, and later tumour nodules.

Epidemiology

KS affects patients of all ages, with a predilection for men. Epidemiological forms include:
* Classic KS affecting mainly elderly men of Mediterranean or Jewish origin.
* African KS endemic in central Africa, affecting both young patients and adults.
* AIDS-associated KS arising in HIV-infected persons (considered an AIDS-defining illness).
* Iatrogenic KS associated with immunosuppression from drugs or following solid organ transplantation.

Incidence

* Classic KS has the highest rates in Mediterranean countries.
* KS rates in Africa are markedly increased because of the AIDS epidemic.
* KS is the most common tumour arising in HIV-infected persons. AIDS-KS without highly active antiretroviral therapy (HAART) is 20,000 times more common than in the general population. In the post-HAART era (after 1996) this has diminished markedly to 3500 times compared to the general population.
* Post-transplant KS is at least 500 times more common than in the general population.

Prognosis

* Classic KS has an indolent course with a median survival of years to decades. Rapid disease with visceral involvement is infrequent.
* African KS has a more aggressive course with a median survival of months to years. The lymphadenopathic form seen in children has a fulminant course and poor prognosis.
* HIV coinfection results in more aggressive and widespread KS disease. Without antiretroviral therapy the median survival is months.
* Transplant-associated KS has a protracted but aggressive course with a median survival of months to years. Visceral, especially pulmonary involvement portends a poor prognosis.

Clinical variants

KS regression can occur spontaneously (rare), following appropriate therapy or after removal of immunosuppressive therapy.

KS flare (exacerbation) can occur with immune reconstitution inflammatory syndrome (IRIS) following HAART, after corticosteroids, and with rituximab therapy.

Clinical approach
History
* Patients may be asymptomatic, as skin lesions are usually painless and non-pruritic.
* Intraoral KS lesions may cause pain, bleeding, ulceration, and affect mastication, speech, and swallowing.
* Conjunctival KS can cause red eyes, discharge, or visual disturbance.
* GI tract KS can cause weight loss, abdominal pain, nausea and vomiting, ileus, upper or lower GI bleeding, malabsorption, intestinal obstruction, or diarrhoea.
* Pulmonary KS can present with shortness of breath, fever, cough, haemoptysis, chest pain, and effusions.
* There may be associated psychosocial stress due to HIV stigma or cosmetic concerns.

Examination
* Document all KS mucocutaneous lesions including the soles, face, genitalia, conjunctiva, oral cavity, and pharynx.
* Skin lesions are multifocal, asymmetrically distributed, vary in size and colour (pink, red, purple, brown to blue), and may be papular, plaque-like, bullous-like, indurated (woody) with a verrucous appearance, or fungating with ulceration and secondary infection.
* Lymphoedema of the legs, genitalia and face may be painful, extensive, and can mask underlying KS.
* Primary visceral KS, without mucocutaneous lesions, is uncommon and can involve lymph nodes, the GI tract and respiratory system. Virtually no organ is spared from involvement.

Staging
Unique staging systems available for classic and AIDS-associated KS (e.g. AIDS Clinical Trials Group staging classification) are used mainly for patients on trials.

Specific investigations
* HIV test (and if positive a CD4 cell count and HIV viral load).
* Chest imaging may show nodular, interstitial and/or alveolar infiltrates, pleural effusion, hilar and/or mediastinal lymphadenopathy, and only rarely a solitary nodule. Concomitant pulmonary infection must be excluded.
* Bronchoscopy can be used to identify pulmonary KS lesions.
* FOBT is useful to screen for GI tract KS disease.
* GI endoscopy in symptomatic individuals can be helpful.
* CT scan, MRI, and PET may be helpful for evaluating deep nodal and visceral KS.
* Bone lesions which frequently go undetected on plain X-ray or bone scans are better detected by CT scan and MRI.
* Biopsy of a suspected KS lesion is encouraged to confirm the diagnosis. Laryngeal and pulmonary KS lesions may bleed significantly.
* Evaluate patients requiring systemic chemotherapy for hepatic, renal, and bone marrow function.

Differential diagnosis

KS can clinically mimic dermatofibromas, other vascular entities, melanocytic lesions, bruising, haematomas, cutaneous lymphoma, or gouty tophi.

On biopsy, KS can resemble bacillary angiomatosis (associated with *Bartonella* infection), pyogenic granuloma, angioma, acroangiodermatitis, pigmented purpuric dermatoses, kaposiform haemangioendothelioma, and angiosarcoma.

Treatment

- Treatment is aimed at symptom palliation, preventing progression, cosmetic improvement, and abatement of oedema, organ compromise, and psychological stress.
- Local therapy can be considered to manage bulky lesions and for cosmetic reasons.
- Surgical excision should be restricted for cosmetically disturbing lesions, to alleviate discomfort or control local tumour growth such as conjunctival KS obscuring vision.
- Indications for systemic chemotherapy include widespread skin involvement (>25 lesions), extensive oral KS, marked symptomatic oedema, rapidly progressive disease, symptomatic visceral KS, and KS flare.

Local therapy

- External beam radiation (8–12Gy)
- Laser therapy
- Cryotherapy
- Photodynamic therapy
- Topical panretinin gel (alitretinoin 0.1%)
- Intralesional vinblastine (0.2–0.3mg/mL solution with a volume of 0.1mL per 0.5cm^2 of lesion)

Systemic therapy

Liposomal anthracyclines including:
- Pegylated liposomal doxorubicin 20 mg/m^2 every 3 weeks.
- Liposomal daunorubicin 40 mg/m^2 every 2 weeks.

Taxanes including:
- Paclitaxel 100 mg/m^2 every 2–3 weeks. Reduced steroid premedication should be used and in HIV-infected persons toxicity related to possible antiretroviral drug interaction must be monitored.

AIDS-associated KS patients should receive HAART. KS flare alone following HAART should not be considered as treatment failure or warrant change in antiretroviral regimen.

Alternative therapy

- Vinorelbine may be effective for AIDS-related KS in patients who have failed other therapies.
- Interferon-alpha, for patients with a robust immune system, has limited use due to toxicity.
- Thalidomide, COL-3, antiherpes therapy, and imatinib have shown therapeutic efficacy.
- For iatrogenic KS consider adjusting immunosuppressive therapy and use of sirolimus (rapamycin) in post-transplant KS.

References

Antman K, Chang Y. (2000) Kaposi's sarcoma. *N Engl J Med* **342**:1027–38.

Bower M, Nelson M, Young AM, *et al.* (2005) Immune reconstitution inflammatory syndrome associated with Kaposi's sarcoma. *J Clin Oncol* **23**:5224–8.

Dezube BJ, Pantanowitz L, Aboulafia DM. Management of AIDS-related Kaposi sarcoma: advances in target discovery and treatment. *AIDS Read* 2004; **14**:236–53.

Dhillon T, Stebbing J, Bower M. Paclitaxel for AIDS-associated Kaposi's sarcoma. *Expert Rev Anticancer Ther* 2005; **5**:215-9.

Di Lorenzo G, Konstantinopoulos PA, Pantanowitz L, *et al.* Management of AIDS-related Kaposi's sarcoma. *Lancet Oncol* 2007; **8**:167–76.

Krown SE, Northfelt DW, Osoba D, Stewart JS. Use of liposomal anthracyclines in Kaposi's sarcoma. *Semin Oncol* 2004; **31**:36–52.

Lebbé C, Euvrard S, Barrou B, *et al.* Sirolimus conversion for patients with posttransplant Kaposi's sarcoma. *Am J Transplant* 2006; **6**:2164–8.

Non-AIDS defining cancers

Definition

HIV-associated neoplasms not included in the case definition of AIDS. It excludes AIDS-defining cancer (KS, NHL, cervical cancer).

General overview

- Increased overall relative risk (1.9) in the HIV population.
- Reported increased incidence may be attributed to true increased prevalence, greater screening, enhanced detection with imaging work-up, augmented reporting, and/or improved patient survival (longevity).
- Accountable for increased mortality in the HAART era.
- Tumours occur at a younger age than in HIV-negative counterparts.
- Tumours commonly exhibit more aggressive behaviour, atypical pathology, and higher grade.
- Presentation with advanced cancer is common.
- High risk for metastatic disease.
- Overall poor outcome is related to an aggressive course, rapid progression, and frequent relapse.

Potential risk factors

- Immunodeficiency (low CD4 count) is not always essential.
- Chronicity (duration) of HIV immunosuppression.
- Longevity (age >40 years).
- Interrupted antiretroviral therapy.
- Lifestyle habits (smoking, sun exposure).
- Oncogenic viruses (HPV, EBV, HCV, HBV).
- Familial cancer history.
- Increased genomic instability (microsatellite alterations)

Management issues

- Preferable to confirm an HIV-related cancer diagnosis with pathological evaluation to exclude infections and reactive conditions. Submit procured tissue for microbiologic study.
- Treatment decisions require consideration be given to comorbid disease, Karnofsky PS, and potential surgical suitability.
- Avoid overstaging cancer due to reactive lymphadenopathy or unrelated imaging abnormalities.

Treatment related complications may include:
- Chemotherapy-enhanced immunosuppression.
- Additive cytotoxicity.
- Drug interactions with antiretroviral therapy.
- Severe radiation adverse effects.
- Postoperative infection.

Regularly monitor CD4 count during and 1 month after chemotherapy.

Control of HIV viraemia is key to improve overall patient survival. HAART should always be provided.

Provide prophylaxis for opportunistic infections.

Contemplate haematopoietic growth factor support.

Specific neoplasms

Anal cancer

Overview

HIV infected persons are at increased risk for anal intraepithelial neoplasia (AIN) and invasive anal cancer. At-risk groups include:
- Patients who practice receptive anal intercourse.
- Men who have sex with men.
- Anal coinfection (e.g. HPV, syphilis, gonococcus).

Progression from low- to high-grade AIN is associated with immunosuppression and multiple HPV types. AIN may not regress with HAART alone.

Clinical
- Symptoms may include pruritis, pain, bleeding, discharge, irritation, constipation, incontinence, tenesmus, warts, or anal mass.
- Clinical staging requires primary tumour biopsy, groin palpation, abdomen and pelvis imaging.
- Anal canal cancer arises from mucosa, unlike anal margin cancer which arises from perianal skin and is therefore staged differently.

Treatment
- AIN can be treated with topical agents (acetic acid), infrared coagulation, laser ablation or surgery.
- Invasive carcinoma is treated with standard combined chemotherapy and radiation.
- Chemotherapy regimens include cisplatin and 5-FU.
- For high-grade AIN, invasive anal margin cancer, and patients with severe drug toxicity refer to an anal surgeon for surgical management.

Outcome
- Response to multimodal therapy is equivalent to non-HIV patients.
- Radiotherapy related toxicity may warrant diverting colostomy or resection.

Breast cancer
- Possible decreased incidence reported in HIV patients.
- Propensity for bilateral disease, poorly differentiated cancer, and early metastases.
- Recommended treatment is similar to HIV negative counterparts.

Colorectal cancer
Reported increased prevalence of colonic adenomas and aggressive adenocarcinoma.

Conjunctival cancer
Overview
- Risk factors include age >50 years, high solar ultraviolet radiation exposure, and geography (sub-Saharan Africa).
- Majority of lesions occur at the limbus (transition zone).

Clinical
- Presentation includes eye irritation, erythema, mass (plaque, nodular), orbit involvement, and/or metastasis.
- Aggressive histological variants may develop (e.g. spindle cell carcinoma).
- Biopsy is required to distinguish leukoplakic lesions ranging from pinguecula, to intraepithelial carcinoma (dysplasia, carcinoma *in situ*), and invasive SCC.
- Evaluate patients for eyelid infiltration, intraocular and orbital invasion, and metastatic disease.

Treatment
- Treatment is mainly surgical.
- Potential non-invasive therapies include photodynamic therapy and topical mitomycin-C.

Gestational trophoblastic disease
- HIV is not an apparent risk factor for molar pregnancy.
- Choriocarcinoma has a dismal outcome in AIDS.
- Chemotherapy is required for afflicted patients.
- Surgery should be considered for bulky disease, resistant malignancy, or complications (e.g. bleeding).

Head and neck cancer
- Common sites that require evaluation include the oral cavity, tonsillar area, and larynx.
- Dental caries may hamper radiation therapy.
- Treatment for early stage and locoregionally advanced disease is surgery or radiation.
- Radiation side effects may include severe mucositis, xerostomia, oral infection, and malnutrition.
- For metastatic disease systemic chemotherapy may be of palliative benefit.

Hepatocellular carcinoma
Overview
- Documented increased risk (8-fold) in HIV-infected population.
- Occurs with chronic liver disease (viral hepatitis) and cirrhosis.
- Hepatitis (HBV, HCV) coinfection results in accelerated progression to carcinoma. The interval between HCV exposure and carcinoma development is shortened.
- Tumours tend to be more symptomatic, advanced at presentation (higher AFP levels), infiltrating, with an aggressive behaviour.
- Extrahepatic metastases are common.

Treatment
- For early stage cancer, resection or liver transplantation is feasible.
- For large tumours (>5cm), multiple tumours, or extrahepatic metastases, systemic chemotherapy is required.

Outcome
- Poor prognosis is associated with severity of liver disease (e.g. Child–Pugh stage), high platelet count ($\geq$100,000/mm^3), large tumour size, inoperable location, and extrahepatic metastases.
- Reduced survival rate is not influenced by CD4 count.

Hodgkin lymphoma
Overview
- Presently the most common non-AIDS defining cancer.
- Increased risk of 5–15-fold in patients with AIDS.
- Develops early in HIV infection.
- High rate of EBV coinfection (75–100%).
- Frequent unfavourable subtypes are common (mixed cellularity, lymphocyte depleted, sarcomatous pattern).

Clinical
B symptoms are commonly reported in afflicted patients. Patients present with frequent extranodal disease with 40–50% bone marrow involvement, as well as liver, spleen, GI tract, and intracerebral lymphoma. Mediastinal involvement is infrequent.

Treatment
- No separate standard of care is available.
- Chemoradiotherapy regimens include:
- Stanford V regimen
- BEACOPP
- ABVD

Table 4.13.1 Comparison of Hodgkin lymphoma chemotherapy regimens

	ABVD	**Stanford V**	**BEACOPP**
CR (%)	87	81	100
EFS/DFS (%)	71 (at 5 years)	68 (at 3 years)	83 (at 2 years)
OS (%)	76 (at 5 years)	51 (at 3 years)	83 (at 2 years)

(CR = complete response rate, EFS = event free survival, DFS = disease free survival, OS = overall survival)

Outcome
Median overall survival around 12–18 months.

Leukaemia
- Increased incidence of AML has been noted, mainly of B-cell origin and monocytic lineage.
- Clinical presentation and biological features are similar to HIV negative persons.
- Patients can experience complete stable remission with standard therapy.
- Poor prognosis has been reported with CD4 count <200 cells/mm^3.

Lung cancer
Overview
- There is an increased incidence of 4–14-fold with HIV infection, but no particular association with prior opportunistic infections.
- Expected male predominance.

Clinical
The most common presentation is a lung mass (80–100%). Non-small cell cancer (80–95%) is more common than small cell cancer (5–15%). Histological subtypes likely to be encountered include adenocarcinoma (30–50%) and SCC (20–50%).

Treatment
- Surgery is the treatment of choice for localized disease in patients with good pulmonary function and general health status, regardless of immune status.
- Systemic chemotherapy is used for small cell cancer, metastatic disease, and with radiotherapy for locally advanced disease.

Outcome
Poor prognostic factors include comorbid disease, poor PS, advanced tumour stage, and non-squamous cancers. Average 1-year survival is around 0–15%.

Plasma cell neoplasia
HIV infected patients can develop paraproteinaemia, amyloidosis, light chain deposition disease, plasmacytomas, multiple myeloma, and plasma cell leukaemia. These may occur at an earlier than expected age.

Paraproteinaemia (monoclonal gammopathy)
- Overall slightly increased incidence (2.5%).
- Up to 5% of HIV-infected patients may have serum monoclonal bands, which can be transient or persistent.
- Monoclonal bands are associated with higher HIV viral load, higher CD4 count, and HBV/HCV coinfection.
- Many (50%) bands may decrease while receiving HAART.
- Patients on follow-up may develop myeloma, plasmacytoma, or lymphoma.

Plasmacytoma
- In the setting of HIV infection these may be multiple and present in unusual locations.
- Tumours with anaplastic features need to be differentiated from plasmablastic lymphoma.

Multiple myeloma
- Extramedullary disease is a common feature.
- Patients may be at risk for renal failure, marked cytopaenia, intractable hypercalcaemia, and hyperviscosity.

Treatment
Treatment should be similar to HIV negative patients, including stem cell transplantation if indicated.

Prostate cancer
- Risk factors include increased age, black race, familial history of prostate cancer, androgen use, and prostatitis.
- HIV status does not appear to influence PSA levels, clinical presentation, management, nor the outcome of treated cancer.
- Afflicted patients are amenable to cure of their cancer with standard therapy.

Skin cancer
Excludes KS (see Chapter 4.13, Kaposi's sarcoma, p.558).

Overview
Documented increased incidence of:
- Basal cell carcinoma
- Merkel cell carcinoma
- HPV-associated penile and vulvar *in situ* and invasive SCC
- Possibly non-genital SCC
- Possibly dysplastic nevi and melanoma

Risk factors include fair skin, excessive sun exposure, HPV anogenital infection, and family history of skin cancer.

Clinical
Atypical presentation due to young patient age, multiple synchronous tumours, and involvement of areas unexposed to sun. Melanoma may be atypical (e.g. nevoid appearance) with only a sparse lymphocytic inflammatory response.

Treatment
- Ensure wide excision to avoid recurrence, which may be up to 20% with SCC.
- For high-risk cancers treatment may require:
  Local or regional adjunctive radiation
  Sentinel lymph node biopsy and/or lymphadenectomy
  Chemotherapy
- For genital carcinoma *in situ* consider surgical ablation or topical 5-FU.
- For invasive genital carcinoma consider radical surgical resection and possible inguinal lymphadenectomy.

Smooth muscle tumours
Overview
- Increased incidence of benign (leiomyoma) and malignant (leiomyosarcoma) smooth muscle tumours in HIV infected individuals.
- They occur mainly with low CD4 count (<200 cells/mm^3).
- There is a strong association with EBV infection.

Clinical
- These tumours may arise in HIV infected children.
- Smooth muscle tumours are frequently multiple.
- Locations may include lung, spleen, brain, GI tract, pleura, epidural space, adrenal glands, orbit, lymph nodes, liver, and heart.
- Malignant tumours tend to behave in an aggressive fashion.

Treatment
First-line therapy includes:
- Complete local excision
- Radiation therapy
- Chemotherapy with doxorubicin or interferon-alpha

Outcome
Aggressive tumours tend to recur despite therapy. Malignant tumours are associated with poor survival.

Testicular germ cell tumours
- Seminoma is more common in HIV positive men, unlike non-seminomatous tumours.
- Stage at presentation is not affected by HIV status.
- The natural history is similar to HIV negative patients.
- Standard therapy is recommended.
- There is no convincing evidence that outcome is poorer.

Prevention and screening
Earlier diagnosis and risk-adapted therapy can improve survival. Assertive preventive strategies should include:

Avoidance of risk factors
- Excessive sun exposure (promote sunscreen).
- Smoking cessation.
- Exposure to HPV (promote safe sexual practice).
- Exposure to HCV (intravenous drug use).
- Alcohol and hepatotoxic drugs in cirrhotics.

Examination and tests
- Regular and careful examination of skin, anogenital region, and conjunctiva with biopsy of suspicious lesions.
- Anal cancer screening including anal Pap test, HPV detection, anoscopy and/or anal colposcopy.
- Monitor cirrhotics and/or those with chronic viral hepatitis frequently (at least every 6 months) for hepatocellular carcinoma with serum AFP and/or imaging studies like ultrasound.
- Regular breast examination and mammography.
- For CRC screening colonoscopy.
- For plasma cell neoplasia serum protein electrophoresis.
- For prostate cancer DRE and PSA.

Early treatment
- Initiation of uninterrupted HAART.
- Vaccinate if not immune to HBV.
- For viral hepatitis coinfection (HBV, HCV) maintenance therapy is recommended.
- Consider HPV vaccination in the appropriate population.

Further reading

Aboulafia DM, Meneses M, Ginsberg S, et al. Acute myeloid leukemia in patients infected with HIV-1. *AIDS* 2002; **16**:865–76.

Bernardi D, Salvioni R, Vaccher E, et al. Testicular germ cell tumors and human immunodeficiency virus infection: a report of 26 cases. Italian Cooperative Group on AIDS and Tumors. *J Clin Oncol* 1995; **13**:2705–11.

Bräu N, Fox RK, Xiao P, et al.; North American Liver Cancer in HIV Study Group. Presentation and outcome of hepatocellular carcinoma in HIV-infected patients: a U.S.-Canadian multicenter study. *J Hepatol* 2007; **47**:527–37.

Burgi A, Brodine S, Wegner S, et al. Incidence and risk factors for the occurrence of non-AIDS-defining cancers among human immunodeficiency virus-infected individuals. *Cancer* 2005; **104**:1505–11.

Cadranel J, Garfield D, Lavolé A, et al. Lung cancer in HIV infected patients: facts, questions and challenges. *Thorax* 2006; **61**:1000–8.

Cheung MC, Pantanowitz L, Dezube BJ. AIDS-related malignancies: emerging challenges in the era of highly active antiretroviral therapy. *Oncologist* 2005; **10**:412–26.

Cooley TP. Non-AIDS-defining cancer in HIV-infected people. *Hematol Oncol Clin North Am* 2003; **17**:889–99.

Dezube BJ, Aboulafia DM, Pantanowitz L. Plasma cell disorders in HIV-infected patients: from benign gammopathy to multiple myeloma. *AIDS Read* 2004; **14**:372–9.

Gewurz BE, Dezube BJ, Pantanowitz L. HIV and the breast. *AIDS Read* 2005; **15**:392–402.

Grulich AE, Li Y, McDonald A, et al. Rates of non-AIDS-defining cancers in people with HIV infection before and after AIDS diagnosis. *AIDS* 2002; **16**:1155–61.

Haigentz M Jr. Aerodigestive cancers in HIV infection. *Curr Opin Oncol* 2005; **17**:474–8.

Hartmann P, Rehwald U, Salzberger B, et al. Current treatment strategies for patients with Hodgkin's lymphoma and HIV infection. *Expert Rev Anticancer Ther* 2004; **4**:401–10.

Lim ST, Levine AM. Non-AIDS-defining cancers and HIV infection. *Curr HIV/AIDS Rep* 2005; **2**:146–53.

McClain KL, Joshi VV, Murphy SB. Cancers in children with HIV infection. *Hematol Oncol Clin North Am* 1996; **10**:1189–201.

Pantanowitz L, Schlecht HP, Dezube BJ. The growing problem of non-AIDS-defining malignancies in HIV. *Curr Opin Oncol* 2006; **18**:469–78.

Panther LA, Schlecht HP, Dezube BJ. Spectrum of human papillomavirus-related dysplasia and carcinoma of the anus in HIV-infected patients. *AIDS Read* 2005; **15**:79–91.

Powles T, Bower M, Shamash J, et al. Outcome of patients with HIV-related germ cell tumours: a case-control study. *Br J Cancer* 2004; **90**:1526–30.

Puoti M, Bruno R, Soriano V, et al.; HIV HCC Cooperative Italian-Spanish Group. Hepatocellular carcinoma in HIV-infected patients: epidemiological features, clinical presentation and outcome. *AIDS* 2004; **18**:2285–93.

Remick SC. Non-AIDS-defining cancers. *Hematol Oncol Clin North Am* 1996; **10**:1203–13.

Roland JT Jr, Rothstein SG, Mittal KR, et al. Squamous cell carcinoma in HIV-positive patients under age 45. *Laryngoscope* 1993; **103**:509–11.

Suankratay C, Shuangshoti S, Mutirangura A, et al. Epstein-Barr virus infection-associated smooth-muscle tumors in patients with AIDS. *Clin Infect Dis* 2005; **40**:1521–8.

Yegüez JF, Martinez SA, Sands DR, et al. Colorectal malignancies in HIV-positive patients. *Am Surg* 2003; **69**:981–7.

Cancer of unknown primary site

Introduction
Cancer of unknown primary (CUP) site is one of the 10 most frequent cancers, accounting for approximately 3–5% of all malignant tumours. Patients with CUP present with disseminated metastatic lesions for which a laboratory and clinical work-up fail to identify the primary site.

CUP represents a heterogeneous group of mainly epithelial tumours with more or less unique clinical and biological behaviour.

Definition
The definition of CUP includes patients who present with histologically confirmed metastatic cancer in whom a detailed medical history, complete physical examination, full blood count, biochemistry, urinalysis and stool occult blood testing, histopathological review of biopsy with the use of immunohistochemistry, chest radiography, CT of the abdomen and pelvis, and in certain cases mammography or FDG-PET scan, fail to detect the primary tumour.

Pathology
CUP consists of several clinicopathological subsets of favourable or unfavourable prognosis.

Histologically, 80% of CUP patients are diagnosed with an adenocarcinoma type, 50% of which are well to moderately differentiated and 30% poorly differentiated or undifferentiated adenocarcinomas. Squamous cell histology accounts for 15% of the cases and of the rest 5% are undifferentiated neoplasms such as not specified carcinomas, neuroendocrine tumours, lymphomas, germ cells tumours, melanomas, sarcomas, or embryonal malignancies.

Clinical approach
Clinical picture and special investigations
The clinical picture and physical examination as well as the diagnostic investigations of CUP patients are related to the specific clinicopathological entity.

Recently an algorithm with a diagnostic panel of 10 immunohistochemical markers for CUP patients with adenocarcinomas has been suggested. These include CA-125, CDX2, cytokeratins 7 and 20, oestrogen receptor, gross cystic disease fluid protein 15, lysozyme, mesothelin, prostate-specific antigen, and thyroid transcription factor-1.

Favourable subsets
Women with adenocarcinoma involving only axillary lymph nodes
These are mostly female patients presenting with lymph node enlargement isolated to one axillary area. Breast examination remains within normal limits. Median age is 52 years and histopathology shows an invasive ductal adenocarcinoma. Metastatic disease is observed only in 5% of the patients. Mammography and/or sonography and recent MRI of the breast are highly recommended.

Women with papillary adenocarcinoma of peritoneal cavity
These patients present with ascites and peritoneal masses without evidence of primary tumour in the ovaries. Median age is 60 years old. Diagnosis is usually made by exploratory laparotomy. Serum CA-125 level is very often raised and is useful for monitoring the disease.

Poorly differentiated carcinoma with midline distribution (extragonadal germ cell syndrome)
These are mostly male patients of relatively young age <50 years old. Clinically presentation is with midline involvement of mediastinal and retroperitoneal lymph nodes with or without lung metastases and rapidly progressive disease. Histologically, it is characterized by undifferentiated or poorly differentiated carcinoma. CT scans are useful imaging methods to establish disease extension. Serum β-HCG or AFP are elevated in almost 20% of the patients.

Squamous cell carcinoma involving cervical or supraclavicular lymph nodes
These patients are most commonly males of median age of around 60 years. The main clinical feature is cervical and/or supraclavicular lymphadenopathy of squamous histology without primary detectable site. This subset accounts for 1–2% of head–neck malignancies.

FDG-PET scan is useful in detecting the primary tumour in the head–neck area. In patients with supraclavicular nodal metastases, lungs are the most probable hidden primary site.

Poorly differentiated neuroendocrine carcinomas
These are rapidly growing tumours with disseminated metastases. They are rarely associated with clinical signs or symptoms produced by tumour secretion of bioactive substances. Patients predominantly present with lymphadenopathy and some patients have nodal enlargement in midline distribution. Immunohistochemically, they express neuroendocrine markers, i.e. chromogranin, synaptophysin or neurospecific enolase.

Men with osteoblastic bone metastases and elevated PSA with adenocarcinoma histology
These patients with have either solitary or multiple blastic bone metastases and an increased serum PSA. Histology is compatible with an adenocarcinoma of various differentiations. Immunoperoxidase staining with PSA is mandatory. Bone scintigraphs, CT scans, and bone plain films are helpful imaging investigations.

Isolated inguinal lymphadenopathy from squamous cell carcinoma
A rare subset in which primary tumours in the genital (vulva, vagina, cervix, penis, or scrotum) or anorectal areas should always be ruled out.

Patients with a single metastatic site
A rare subset of CUP patients presented with a solitary site of metastases in lymph nodes or in splanchnic organs.

Unfavourable subsets
Metastatic disease primarily to the liver or to multiple other sites.
It is one of the most frequent subset of CUP accounting for almost 25% of all patients. The median age approaches the seventh decade of life. The most common clinical presentation is multiple liver metastases on imaging, an enlarged palpable liver on physical examination, and biochemical abnormalities of liver function tests. Metastatic lesions to other organs are not uncommon at the time of diagnosis. Histologically, adenocarcinoma of various differentiations

is the usual diagnosis. Investigations including CT scan, endoscopies, or epithelial tumour markers are not usually helpful in detecting the primary site.

Malignant ascites of unknown origin with non-papillary serous adenocarcinoma histology
The median age of these patients is around 65 years and they present with abdominal masses and ascites. They could be either males or females and they carry a histological diagnosis of adenocarcinoma. If a mucinous adenocarcinoma is present with signet ring cells appearance, a GI cancer should be suspected.

Metastatic CUP to the lungs either as parenchymal metastases or isolated malignant pleural effusion
Symptoms and signs are associated with lung involvement, i.e. dry cough, dyspnoea, haemoptysis or thoracic pain. Imaging investigations with CXR or CT scan show lung lesions or pleurisy, whereas bronchoscopy is unable to detect the primary site. The most common histology is adenocarcinoma.

Patients with multiple brain metastases
They present with a diverse variety of neurological symptoms and signs, while brain biopsy shows a metastatic adenocarcinoma or a SCC.

Patients with multiple metastatic bone lesions
This is not a very common CUP subset and patients manifest with bone pain or fracture. Adenocarcinoma is the most common histology. Investigational work-up should rule out breast or prostate cancer.

Natural history and further management
The natural history of CUP patients is unique and different from patients with known primary tumours. The fundamental characteristics of CUP are: the aggressiveness of the disease, the early dissemination, the absence of primary site, and the unpredictable metastatic pattern. More than 50% of patients present with multiple metastatic lesions and carry an unpredictable pattern of metastatic spread which differs from those with known primary carcinomas, i.e. lung cancer presenting as CUP involves the bones in 4%, while when diagnosed as a known primary the predilection to bones is 30–50%.

The therapeutic management of CUP patients is based on the specific clinicopathological entity.

Favourable subsets
Women with adenocarcinoma involving only axillary nodes
The treatment of these patients is similar to stage II or III breast cancer patients. The recommendation for N1 disease with mobile nodes is axillary clearance followed by radiotherapy or simple mastectomy. In addition, for premenopausal patients with positive oestrogen receptors, adjuvant chemotherapy followed by tamoxifen is the treatment of choice. However, for postmenopausal patients with positive receptors tamoxifen or aromatase inhibitor is recommended. The recommendations for N2 disease with fixed nodes is neoadjuvant chemotherapy following the guidelines for stage III breast cancer. In chemoresistant cases or in elderly women, radical radiotherapy is recommended with tamoxifen continuation if oestrogen receptors are positive. The 5- and 10-year OS rates are 75% and 60%, respectively.

Women with papillary adenocarcinoma of peritoneal cavity
These patients are treated as FIGO stage III ovarian cancer with surgical cytoreduction and postoperative intravenous taxane/platinum-based chemotherapy. Response rates range from 32–66% with 10–40% complete responses. A median survival of 15–20 months and a median long-term survival of 16% have also been observed.

Poorly differentiated carcinoma with midline distribution
This subgroup of CUP patients should be managed as poor prognosis germcell tumours with platinum-based systemic chemotherapy. Objective responses are >50% with 15–25% complete responses, whereas 10–15% of the cases are long-term disease-free survivors.

Squamous cell carcinoma involving cervical or supraclavicular lymph nodes
This CUP entity should be treated similarly to locally advanced head and neck cancer with surgery and radiotherapy. Radiotherapy following surgery has been reported to improve the risk of locoregional relapse and survival and hence combined modality treatment is considered as standard treatment in this subset of patients. The 5-year survival rates range from 35–50% with some long term disease-free survivors. The role of chemotherapy in this subset remains unclear, although in locally advanced head–neck cancer, patients showed a beneficial effect especially those with N2 or N3 disease.

Poorly differentiated neuroendocrine carcinomas
Systemic chemotherapy with platinum-based or taxane/carboplatin regimens is recommended. Responses are as high as 50–70% with 25% complete responders and some 10–15% long-term survivors.

Men with osteoblastic bone metastases and elevated PSA with adenocarcinoma histology
These patients should be considered as having disseminated prostate cancer and therapeutic management with endocrine treatment is recommended.

Isolated inguinal lymphadenopathy from squamous cell carcinoma
Nodal dissection with local radiotherapy is the treatment of choice in most of the cases. Long-term survivors have been observed.

Unfavourable subsets
The majority of these patients belong to the unfavourable subset with predominantly liver metastases. Unfortunately, most of these CUP patients are relatively unresponsive to chemotherapy although some responses ranging from 10–40% have been reported with almost no complete responders. The most common drug combination consists of platinum-based or taxane/platinum regimens. In general, median survival is around 8–9 months. Currently, chemotherapy is recommended for younger patients with good PS, while older patients with a poor performance could be managed with mainly supportive care.

References
Pavlidis N, Briasoulis E, Hainsworth J, *et al.* Diagnostic and therapeutic management of cancer of an unknown primary. *Eur J Cancer* 2003; **39**(14):1990–2005.

Pavlidis N. Forty years' experience of treating cancer of unknown primary. *Acta Oncol* 2007; **46**(5):592–601.

Pentheroudakis G, Briasoulis E, Pavlidis N. Cancer of unknown primary site: missing primary or missing biology? *Oncologist* 2007; **12**(4):418–25.

Oncological emergencies

Tumour lysis syndrome

Aetiology

Tumour lysis syndrome is a constellation of metabolic disturbances resulting from the initiation of anticancer therapy and the subsequent destruction of malignant cells.

It is characterized by hyperkalaemia, followed by hyperuricaemia, hyperphosphataemia, hypocalcaemia, and acute renal impairment. Tumour lysis syndrome becomes evident 12–72 hours after starting cancer treatment. It is most commonly seen in malignancies that have a large tumour bulk, high proliferative rate, and are highly sensitive to therapy. It is therefore most frequently reported in the treatment of acute lymphoblastic leukaemia and high grade NHL, especially Burkitt's lymphoma, but is also seen with solid tumours, e.g. small cell carcinoma. Further risk factors for tumour lysis syndrome include pre-existing dehydration or renal impairment and an elevated lactate dehydrogenase.

Tumour lysis syndrome is often but not exclusively a side effect of systemic chemotherapeutic agents. It can arise spontaneously and has also occurred after the administration of steroids, monoclonal antibodies, hormonal agents, bisphosphonates, and radiotherapy. It does not only occur with systemic administration and mass cell lysis has occurred after intrathecal chemotherapy and chemotherapeutic embolization.

The syndrome is prompted by the rapid release of nucleic acids, proteins, intracellular ions, and metabolites into the circulation which overwhelm native buffering and excretion mechanisms.

Hyperkalaemia and hyperphosphataemia are the immediate consequences of cell lysis and the release of these ions. Purine nucleic acids are metabolized to uric acid. The kidney is the major route of excretion for potassium, phosphate, and uric acid. Uric acid crystallization in the kidney tubules is a major cause of the acute renal failure that is part of the tumour lysis syndrome. Hypocalcaemia occurs as a response to hyperphosphataemia as calcium phosphate deposits in soft tissues to correct phosphate levels. This includes nephrocalcinosis which can exacerbate acute renal failure.

Clinical features

This condition can present with multiple non-specific symptoms that reflect the metabolic disturbances. These include nausea, vomiting, malaise, confusion, oliguria, and anorexia. Symptoms of hyperkalaemia include paraesthesiae, weakness, chest pain, and palpitations. Marked hypocalcaemia can manifest with paraesthesiae, tetany, and bronchospasm. High uric acid levels may result in arthralgia. Evidence of fluid overload, such as shortness of breath and oedema, can develop as a result of renal failure.

Diagnosis

Routine blood tests will show the metabolic derangements that occur in tumour lysis syndrome and will reveal a metabolic acidosis. Hyperkalaemia is usually the first metabolic abnormality that appears. An electrocardiogram may show the characteristic changes of hyperkalaemia or lengthening of the QT interval as a result of hypocalcaemia. Urine pH needs to be monitored as an acidic pH will further encourage uric acid deposition in the renal tubules.

Cairo and Bishop have classified tumour lysis syndrome into laboratory tumour lysis syndrome or grades of clinical tumour lysis syndrome. Laboratory tumour lysis syndrome is defined when uric acid, potassium, phosphate, and calcium levels are either 25% increased from baseline or exceed a defined value. Clinical tumour lysis syndrome is graded on the presence or absence of laboratory tumour lysis syndrome, cardiac arrhythmias and seizures, and serum creatinine level.

Treatment

Prompt supportive care is the mainstay of treatment. If metabolic disturbances do not respond to initial acute management, haemodialysis must be considered. Aggressive rehydration is required to maintain urine output, aid excretion of metabolites, and prevent uric acid deposition. Hyperkalaemia and hyperphosphataemia can be managed initially with short-term measures such as insulin and dextrose until more long-term treatment is in place, such as potassium exchange resins, phosphate binders, or haemodialysis. Hypocalcaemia should not be corrected until phosphate levels have normalized to prevent further calcium deposition, unless there is evidence of neuromuscular irritability.

Allopurinol is given to prevent conversion of nucleic acids to uric acid by xanthine oxidase. Rasburicase, a recombinant form of urate oxidase, can be given if uric acid levels remain high despite allopurinol. It converts uric acid to water-soluble metabolites that can be excreted more easily. Urinary alkalinization with intravenous bicarbonate or acetazolamide is controversial and requires very close monitoring as it can worsen the magnitude of hypocalcaemia. Diuretics are also not a key part of early management as the patient is likely to be volume depleted on presentation.

Persistent hyperkalaemia, hyperphosphataemia, and hyperuricaemia, uraemia, and symptomatic hypocalcaemia are all indications for haemodialysis. Haemodialysis is preferred to peritoneal dialysis as uric acid and phosphate clearance is better. Critical care support may be required.

Prevention

An important part of the management of this potentially lethal syndrome is to recognize those at risk before they begin cytotoxic therapy and initiate prophylactic measures.

High-risk patients, such as those with a large tumour burden or baseline renal impairment, should receive 24–48 hours of pre-hydration before therapy and up to 72 hours of hydration after therapy. These patients should be monitored very closely for metabolic derangements at all times. If there is any evidence of tumour lysis syndrome before therapy is started, cytotoxics should be withheld until this is corrected.

Further reading

Locatelli F, Rossi F. Incidence and pathogenesis of tumour lysis syndrome. *Contrib Nephrol* 2005; **147**:61–8.

Zojer N, Ludwig H. Haematological emergencies. *Ann Oncol* 2007; **18**:i45–i48.

Hypercalcaemia

Aetiology

Hypercalcaemia is a recognized complication of malignancy and occurs in up to 30% of cancer patients at some stage in their disease. It is most commonly seen in breast, renal, multiple myeloma, lymphoma, and non-small cell cancers of the lung.

There are three main mechanisms that contribute to a rise in calcium levels. The first, and most common, is the secretion of parathyroid hormone-related peptide (PTHrP) by the tumour cells, termed humoral hypercalcaemia of malignancy. PTHrP simulates many of the actions of PTH such as stimulation of osteoclasts, calcium reabsorption from the distal renal tubules, and increased intestinal uptake of calcium. The effects of PTHrP may be systemic in patients with high serum PTHrP levels or limited to the local tissues. PTHrP production is more often found in solid tumours such as renal cell carcinoma and breast adenocarcinoma.

Hypercalcaemia in multiple myeloma and other haematological malignancies is often the result of secreted cytokines like tumour necrosis factor, interleukins 1 and 6, and macrophage inflammatory factor 1. These cytokines stimulate macrophages to differentiate into osteoclasts causing increased bone resorption and release of calcium.

Vitamin D overproduction or production of vitamin D analogues, including calcitriol, by tumour cells also contributes to hypercalcaemia in malignancy. This third mechanism is more common in HD, NHL, and adult T-cell lymphoma.

Clinical features

The early symptoms of hypercalcaemia are vague and include anorexia, nausea and vomiting, constipation, nonspecific abdominal pain, fatigue, and muscle weakness. Polyuria and polydipsia are more specific early symptoms of increasing calcium levels. Patients will also be very dehydrated. As calcium levels rise further, there may be neurological manifestations such as decreased conscious level, hallucinations, and psychosis. Renal function will also deteriorate.

Diagnosis

High ionized calcium levels, corrected for calcium bound to albumin, can be measured in a peripheral blood sample. Renal function, alkaline phosphatase, and PTH levels should also be evaluated simultaneously. An electrocardiogram may show signs of hypercalcaemia such as shortening of the QT interval or ventricular arrhythmias.

PTHrP levels can be measured to assess the mechanism of hypercalcaemia but are not essential for a diagnosis of hypercalcaemia of malignancy. High PTHrP levels have been reported, however, to be associated with a poorer response to bisphosphonate therapy and a higher risk of recurrent hypercalcaemia and so PTHrP levels may be useful in guiding treatment.

Treatment

Hypercalcaemic patients are usually profoundly hypovolaemic and the first step in management is aggressive rehydration with intravenous saline, as appropriate to the individual patient's cardiovascular status. Sources of calcium should be eliminated as should medications such as vitamin D and thiazide diuretics, which could increase calcium levels. Loop diuretics should be avoided in the early stages of treatment as they can exacerbate renal hypoperfusion as a result of hypovolaemia and further impair renal calcium excretion.

Once the patient is adequately hydrated, bisphosphonates are the first-line agent for normalizing calcium levels. Intravenous pamidronate or zolendronic acid effectively inhibit osteoclast activity and restore normocalcaemia in 5 days in 80% of patients. There is emerging evidence that zolendronic acid is the more potent bisphosphonate but the clinical relevance of this is uncertain. It is also more renal toxic than pamidronate and so the dose must be altered according to creatinine clearance.

Life threatening hypercalcaemia can be treated with intravenous calcitonin which causes a rapid but unsustained fall in calcium levels. Haemodialysis may be ultimately needed for patients especially when severe hypercalcaemia is accompanied by renal failure or congestive cardiac failure.

Hypercalcaemia that is caused by elevated vitamin D levels, as occurs in HD and other types of lymphomas can be effectively treated with corticosteroids.

Treatment of the underlying tumour burden with the appropriate chemotherapy or radiotherapy can help prevent recurrence of hypercalcaemia.

Further reading

Coleman R. Clinical features of metastatic bone disease and risk of skeletal morbidity. *Clin Cancer Res* 2006; **12**(20 Suppl):6243s–49s.

Halfdanarson TR, Hogan WJ, Moynihan TJ. Oncologic emergencies: Diagnosis and treatment. *Mayo Clin Proc* 2006; **81**(6):835–48.

Zojer N, Ludwig H. Haematological emergencies. *Ann Oncol* 2007; **18**:i45–i48.

Hyponatraemia

Aetiology

Hyponatraemia, defined as a serum sodium concentration of <136mmol/L, is a common finding in both hospital in-patients and cancer patients. Mild degrees of hyponatraemia cause symptoms that decrease the QoL of a cancer patient and a more significant and rapid decrease in sodium levels can cause cerebral oedema and other ensuing neurological complications.

Electrolyte and body fluid balance is controlled by anti-diuretic hormone (ADH) secreted from the posterior pituitary. The osmolarity of the blood is tightly maintained at around 285mOsm/kg. If the osmolarity increases, ADH secretion increases. It binds to receptors in the collecting ducts of the kidney and stimulates the production and insertion of aquaporins into the collecting duct membrane, increasing water reabsorption. A fall in serum osmolality has an inverse effect on ADH secretion.

Oncology patients are at risk of developing hyponatraemia for a variety of reasons. Many chemotherapeutics are known to stimulate ADH release such as cyclophospha-mide, cisplatin, and vincristine. Chemotherapy-induced nausea and vomiting increase ADH production and vomit-ing also increases enteral sodium loss. Abdominal radio-therapy and analgesics such as morphine and carbamazepine also promote ADH secretion. In addition, aggressive hydration to prevent the sequelae of anticancer treatment may exacerbate hyponatraemia, e.g. tumour lysis syndrome or haemorrhagic cystitis. Interferon, monoclonal antibod-ies, and other therapies targeting immune function have also been shown to cause hyponatraemia.

In addition to increased central ADH secretion as a result of malignancy or treatment, around 30% of cases of hyponatraemia in an oncological setting are caused by ectopic ADH secretion from tumour cells, also known as SIADH, the syndrome of inappropriate antidiuretic hor-mone. The patient is euvolaemic and has an inappropri-ately high urine osmolality and sodium excretion in the setting of hyponatraemia and low plasma osmolality. The commonest cancer by far associated with SIADH is SCLC but it has been reported in many other types of cancer including oesophageal, pancreatic, adrenal, bladder, breast, brain, and head and neck cancers.

Clinical features

Symptoms of hyponatraemia are vague and become more severe with the degree of sodium loss and the faster the onset of hyponatraemia. A reduction in intracerebral sodium results in an increase in intracellular water. Organic acids and other solutes diffuse out to limit the possibility of cer-ebral oedema but if the onset of hyponatraemia is too rapid, these adaptive mechanisms can be overwhelmed and oedema can result.

Mild hyponatraemia or more severe hyponatraemia of slow onset can be asymptomatic. At lower serum sodium levels, patients can present with headache, anorexia, depression, behavioural changes, lethargy, and mild nau-sea. Serum sodium levels <115mmol/L can result in psy-chosis, confusion, coma, respiratory arrest, brain stem herniation, and death.

Diagnosis

A diagnosis of hyponatraemia can be easily made on a venous or arterial blood sample. The volume status of the patient must then be assessed to diagnose the possible cause of the hyponatraemia. Hypervolaemic patients can be overloaded with fluid as a result of renal, liver, or car-diac failure. Hypovolaemic patients may have lost sodium through vomiting or diarrhoea or through the kidneys as a result of aggressive diuresis, adrenal insufficiency, or neph-ropathy. Cerebral salt wasting can occur as part of CNS malignancy or after neurosurgery. If the patient is euvolae-mic, a diagnosis of SIADH may be made if the appropriate criteria are met.

Treatment

Hyponatraemia associated with malignancy is best treated by treating the underlying cause. A study has shown that 80% of cases of hyponatraemia associated with SCLC resolved within 3 weeks of beginning chemotherapy. If, however, the malignancy is not amenable to treatment or drugs that may contribute to the hyponatraemia cannot be stopped, other strategies can be used.

The first-line treatment for euvolaemic patients with hyponatraemia is fluid restriction. If this method meets with little success, desmocycline can be used. Desmocycline prevents the kidney responding to circulating ADH. It may take up to 3 weeks for detectable response to desmo-cycline, however, and possible side effects include photo-sensitivity, nephrotoxicity, and GI intolerance. In severe hyponatraemia, infusion of hypertonic saline under close monitoring may be appropriate. Increasing the serum sodium level too rapidly carries a risk of cerebral dehydra-tion and central pontine demyelination. Serum sodium levels should initially rise by no more than 1mmol/L per hour and not rise >10mmol/L in the first 24 hours of the infusion.

ADH receptor antagonists are being developed as pos-sible new agents to treat hyponatraemia. These antago-nists act directly on ADH receptors in the kidney and so increase water excretion whilst sparing electrolytes. One agent of this group of antagonists, conivaptan, is now licensed for use in hyponatraemic patients in the USA. It is yet to be shown whether ADH receptor antagonists will be efficacious in the treatment of malignancy associated hyponatraemia.

Further reading

Raftopoulos H. Diagnosis and management of hyponatremia in cancer patients. *Support Care Cancer* 2007; **15**:1341–47.

Hyperkalaemia

Aetiology

Hyperkalaemia in oncology patients often occurs in the context of renal failure or as part of tumour lysis syndrome. There are multiple possible causes:

Pre-renal causes of renal impairment include:
- Hyperviscosity in haematological malignancy
- Neutropenic or non-neutropenic sepsis with accompanying hypovolaemia and vasodilatation
- Hyperuricaemia
- Hypercalcaemia

Renotoxic agents such as cisplatin, contrast media, antibiotics, and NSAIDs directly damage the kidneys and impair function.

Renal function can also be compromised by:
- Direct tumour invasion
- Radiation nephritis
- Renal infections

Urinary tract obstruction by intrinsic or extrinsic malignancy is the commonest postrenal cause of impairment in this setting. Hyperkalaemia may also occur as a result of multiple transfusions of packed red blood cells.

High levels of serum potassium prevent repolarization of cardiac and skeletal muscle. Treatment is essential to prevent cardiac arrhythmias, respiratory arrest, and death.

Clinical features

Hyperkalaemia is often asymptomatic. Symptoms that can occur include paraesthesiae, weakness, chest pain, and palpitations.

Diagnosis

A diagnosis of hyperkalaemia can be easily made on a non-haemolysed venous or arterial blood sample.

Renal function should be checked simultaneously. Uric acid, calcium and phosphate levels, and an arterial blood gas will help diagnose tumour lysis syndrome if this is suspected. An electrocardiogram may show the classical signs of hyperkalaemia, namely tented T waves, flattened P waves, and widening of the QRS complex. At high potassium concentrations, the QRS complex may appear as a sinusoidal wave.

Treatment

The first priority is to protect the cardiac action potential and prevent arrhythmias. If any changes are apparent on the electrocardiogram, an intravenous bolus of 10% calcium gluconate must be given. Short-term effective measures can be employed to lower serum potassium levels. An infusion of short-acting insulin and 10% dextrose will drive potassium into cells and this effect can be supported with salbutamol nebulizers. Sodium bicarbonate can be given in hyperkalaemia in the presence of an acidosis but this approach is not universally adopted due to the poor reduction in potassium levels when this agent is given alone. Potassium excretion then needs to be increased to provide a more long-term correction of hyperkalaemia. Diuretics that increase potassium excretion can be used in a patient with normal renal function. Otherwise, a cation exchange resin may be given orally or rectally. In severe hyperkalaemia or hyperkalaemia-resistant to conservative intervention, haemodialysis can be used.

Further reading

Halfdanarson TR, Hogan WJ, Moynihan TJ. Oncologic emergencies: Diagnosis and treatment. *Mayo Clin Proc* 2006; **81**(6):835–48.

Kim GH, han JS. Therapeutic approach to hyperkalaemia. *Nephron* 2002; **92**(Suppl 1):33–40.

Hypoglycaemia

Aetiology

Hypoglycaemia can be described as a fall in blood glucose that causes glycopenic and adrenergic symptoms, which can be resolved with the restoration of a normal blood glucose level. Varying absolute figures are used to define hypoglycaemia. In guidelines published by the American Diabetic Association, the threshold for hypoglycaemia is set at a blood glucose of <3.9mmol/L, but a recent study suggested that 3.1mmol/L would be a more relevant threshold clinically.

Hypoglycaemia in oncology patients can be related to neuroendocrine tumours such as insulinomas or as a result of hyperglycaemic treatment in pancreatic insufficiency after removal of pancreatic tumours. Retroperitoneal and mediastinal malignant mesenchymal tumours can secrete an aberrant form of insulin like growth factor (IGF) which binds IGF-1 receptors and causes hypoglycaemia. Primary or secondary adrenal insufficiency due to adrenal or pituitary tumours should also be considered. Hypoglycaemia in oncology patients can also be due to management of diabetes and unrelated to malignancy.

Clinical features

Adrenergic symptoms usually precede glycopenic symptoms in hypoglycaemia. The sympathetic nervous system has been shown to respond to the absolute level of glucose in the blood. Sympathetic stimulation manifests as sweating, shaking, anxiety, hunger, and palpitations. Glycopenic symptoms reflect the decrease in the amount of glucose available to the brain and include confusion, hallucinations, irritability, coma, and eventually death. Patients who are recurrently hypoglycaemic can become physiologically unaware of falling blood glucose levels and do not suffer any adrenergic symptoms to alert them to the impending glycopenia.

Diagnosis

Blood glucose can be easily and rapidly checked on a blood glucose meter but these can be inaccurate at very low measurements. If hypoglycaemia is suspected, a blood sample should be laboratory tested for insulin and glucose levels. Simultaneous C-peptide levels will distinguish between exogenous and endogenous hyperinsulinaemia. The diagnosis of hypoglycaemia can be further proved by reversal of symptoms on administration of glucose and restoration of normal blood glucose levels. A short synacthen test can diagnose primary adrenal insufficiency. Plasma cortisol and ACTH levels may suggest a diagnosis of secondary adrenal insufficiency, which can be confirmed with ACTH stimulation tests.

Treatment

The aim of treatment in the short term is to restore blood glucose levels as quickly as possible to prevent any permanent glycopenic damage. This can be achieved by oral intake of sugary foods and drink, or if the patient is unconscious with oral dextrose gel or intravenous dextrose. A more long-term strategy then needs to be considered to prevent the recurrence of hypoglycaemia.

Prevention

Patients with metastatic or inoperable insulinoma may need long-term medical therapy to prevent hypoglycaemia. Diazoxide and octreotide prevent peripheral glucose metabolism and can be effective in these cases. Other measures such as a continuous glucose monitor have been reported to be successful if medical therapy fails. Oncology patients with pancreatic insufficiency or diabetes can prevent hypoglycaemia with alterations to their insulin regimen, oral intake, and exercise levels.

Further reading

Sawyer AM, Schade DS. Use of a continuous glucose monitor in the management of inoperable metastatic insulinoma: a case report. *Endocr Pract* 2008; **14**(7):880–3.

Swinnen SG, Mullins P, Miller M, et al. Changing the glucose cut-off values that define hypoglycaemia has a major effect on reported frequencies of hypoglycaemia. *Diabetologia* 2009; **52**(1):38–41.

Hyperuricaemia

Aetiology

Tumour cell death in malignancy can occur spontaneously or after administration of chemotheraputics, steroids, radiotherapy, or other agents. The subsequent release of intracellular contents includes purine nucleic acids, which are metabolized by xanthine oxidase to form uric acid. Hyperuricaemia can occur alone, but if it occurs on a massive scale and is accompanied by hypocalcaemia, hyperphosphataemia, hyperkalaemia, and acute renal impairment, a diagnosis of clinical or laboratory tumour lysis syndrome is more appropriate.

Clinical features

Hyperuricaemia is often asymptomatic. Chronically raised uric acid levels can result in crystal deposition in joints causing painful arthralgia and under the skin as painless gouty tophi. Deposition of uric acid or its metabolites in the kidney tubules can cause renal impairment with accompanying oliguria and fluid overload. The clinical features of more acute hyperuricaemia as part of tumour lysis syndrome are described elsewhere.

Diagnosis

A raised baseline uric acid level is a well-recognized risk factor for tumour lysis syndrome and so detection of hyperuricaemia is important in oncology patients. Uric acid levels can be easily quantified in a venous blood sample.

Treatment

Hyperuricaemia in the context of malignancy needs to be treated to prevent progressive metabolic derangement should further cell lysis occur. Aggressive hydration appropriate to renal and cardiovascular function should be attempted with the aim of a urine output of at least 80–100mL/hour. If the patient is euvolaemic and there is no evidence of renal failure, diuretics may be used to sustain urine output. Urinary alkalinization to encourage solubility of uric acid in the urine is no longer recommended as it promotes xanthine crystal deposition in the renal tubules. Hyperuricaemic patients at low risk of developing tumour lysis syndrome may be managed with hydration and careful monitoring alone.

Patients at higher risk of tumour lysis syndrome, e.g. those with a high tumour burden, will benefit from administration of rasburicase, a recombinant form of urate oxidase. Rasburicase promotes the breakdown of uric acid and rapidly and effectively lowers serum uric acid levels. It has been shown to be more efficacious than allopurinol, the urate oxidase inhibitor that was the treatment of choice in hyperuricaemia in this setting until recent years.

Prevention

The main strategy for prevention of hyperuricaemia in oncology patients is to detect those most likely to develop the condition and those who may be at risk of progression to tumour lysis syndrome. Risk factors include the extent of disease, the cell turnover rate, tumour type, and the modality of treatment planned. Close monitoring of patients at risk and appropriate interventions, such as delaying the onset of therapy if hyperuricaemia is detected, are central to prevention.

Further reading

Coiffier B, Altman A, Pui CH, et al. Guidelines for the management of paediatric and adult tumor lysis syndrome: an evidence based review. *J Clin Oncol* 2008; **26**(16):2767–78.

Febrile neutropenia

Definition

The diagnosis of FN requires that the following two criteria are met:

- A single oral temperature measurement of 38.3°C or higher or two measurements of >38°C 1 hour apart.
- A neutrophil count of <0.5 x 10^9/L or a neutrophil count of <1 x 10^9/L with a projected decrease to <0.5 x 10^9/L over the next 48 hours.

Aetiology

FN is the cause of considerable morbidity and mortality in patients with cancer. The development of neutropenia following cytotoxic chemotherapy has been recognized as a predisposing factor for infections in cancer patients for more than four decades. The frequency and severity of infections are influenced by the depth of the nadir in neutrophil counts, the duration of neutropenia, and the rate of the neutrophil count decline. Infections are particularly frequent and severe when the neutrophil count is <0.1 x 10^9/L.

Many other factors may compound the effect of neutropenia on the risk of infection. Haematological malignancies such as chronic lymphocytic leukaemia and multiple myeloma are associated with immunodeficiency due to absolute or functional hypogammaglobulinaemia and increased risk of infection with Gram-positive cocci. Extensive marrow infiltration by tumours causes marrow failure and accentuates chemotherapy myelotoxicity.

Disruption of anatomical barriers by the tumour also contributes to the risk of infection. For example, lung carcinomas can obstruct large bronchi and predispose to postobstructive pneumonias. Obstruction of the ureters or the biliary tree by tumours increases the risk of pyelonephritis or biliary sepsis. Perforating bowel tumours are associated with the development of peritonitis. Spontaneous or treatment-induced necrosis of the tumour mass also increases the risk of superadded infection. The mucosal toxicity of many chemotherapy agents further adds to the risk of infection due to disruption of epithelial mucosal barriers and impaired mucosal immune function.

The adverse effects of cancer treatments on the risk of infection are not limited to neutropenia. Agents such as fludarabine and alemtuzumab cause profound lymphopenia and are associated with the development of *Pneumocystis jiroveci (carinii)* and cytomegalovirus (CMV) infections in the absence of suitable prophylaxis. High-dose corticosteroids cause immunosuppression and can mask signs of infection. Splenectomy or functional asplenia following irradiation predisposes patients to infections with encapsulated bacteria.

Patients undergoing bone marrow transplantation merit special consideration. The prolonged initial neutropenia leads to frequent bacterial, viral, and fungal infections. Following marrow reconstitution, infective risk is mediated by functional phagocytic defects and the need for immunosuppression for chronic graft-versus-host disease.

Gram-negative bacteria such as enterobacteriaceae and *Pseudomonas* were the predominant causes of FN in the 1960s and 1970s. Since then, there has been a shift towards Gram-positive cocci, mainly staphylococci and streptococci, as the principal causative agents. The reasons for this shift are multiple and include the increasing use of indwelling vascular access devices and prophylactic quinolones. Most recent reports of bacteraemia causes in neutropenic patients show approximately equal contributions from Gram-negative and Gram-positive organisms. Local patterns of infection vary and should be taken into account when designing empirical antibiotic treatment strategies. Fungal infections are mainly due to *Candida* and *Aspergillus* spp., but are uncommon causes of fever when the duration of neutropenia is short (i.e. <7–10 days).

Outside of bone marrow transplantation, the risk of FN varies greatly among chemotherapy regimens. FN rates of >20% have been reported with many regimens. Examples include TAC and AT for breast cancer, CAV and topotecan for SCLC, ESHAP and DHAP for relapsed NHL, and VeIP for relapsed germ cell tumours (Smith et al. 2006).

Clinical features

Fever is a very sensitive but non-specific sign of infection in neutropenic patients. Localizing symptoms and signs such as sputum production or purulent drainage are commonly absent but, when present, can point to the likely source of infection. The presence of diarrhoea may point towards a GI source of infection but may also constitute unrelated chemotherapy toxicity. Patients often complain of non-specific symptoms such as shivering, rigors, malaise, and myalgias.

Certain medications such as corticosteroids and paracetamol may mask or blunt infection-associated fever and heightened clinician awareness is paramount in ensuring prompt diagnosis. Any report of rigors or fever when accessing an indwelling catheter should be investigated urgently.

Septic shock manifests as:

- Tachycardia
- Tachypnoea
- Hypotension
- Confusion
- Diaphoresis
- Presence of fever while the extremities are usually paradoxically warm
- Oliguria is frequently present

Diagnosis

FN is a true oncological emergency and empirical antibiotic administration, as detailed in the next section, should not be delayed while an extensive diagnostic evaluation is carried out.

A meticulous physical examination with particular attention to common sites of infection is essential. Assessment of the oral cavity may be difficult due to the presence of mucositis that can mask signs of superadded infection with agents such as HSV. Careful examination of the skin, including the nails, may reveal a portal of entry for pathogenic bacteria or cutaneous signs of systemic infection such as the *Pseudomonas aeruginosa*-associated ecthyma gangrenosum. Catheter sites should be carefully evaluated. The examination should include the paranasal sinuses, ears, lungs, groin, and perivaginal and perirectal areas. It should be noted that, whereas inspection of the perineum is important, PR examination is contraindicated in the setting of profound neutropenia as it is thought that it can promote bacteraemia by pathogenic gut bacteria.

Additional historical information should be sought, including the presence of comorbidities, exposure history, the time since the last chemotherapy administration and the regimen used, any recent prophylactic or therapeutic antibiotic use, and any prior documented infections and colonizations with bacteria such as meticillin resistant *Staphylococcus aureus* (MRSA).

Initial laboratory evaluation includes the determination of the full blood and neutrophil count and assessment of renal and hepatic function. Obtaining two sets of blood cultures from different sites is recommended. In the presence of a venous access catheter, cultures should be taken both from the catheter and a peripheral site. Some authors, however, dispute the need for a peripheral site blood culture in this situation and patient acceptance of peripheral venipuncture can be low. Bacteraemia is documented in approximately 20% of cases of uncomplicated FN. A urine culture and a chest radiograph are also recommended, although their diagnostic yield is typically low in the absence of localizing signs. The presence of diarrhoea should prompt examination of a stool sample for *Clostridium difficile* toxin.

It should also be kept in mind that infection is not the only cause of fever in neutropenic patients; blood transfusions, drugs, CSFs, and the tumour itself are common causes of pyrexia.

Treatment

The treatment of FN is a true emergency. In the UK, the Department of Health has stated that all patients undergoing chemotherapy should receive written information regarding the appropriate course of action should signs of neutropenic sepsis develop. All hospitals that admit patients with chemotherapy-related complications should have written policies to ensure prompt and appropriate management (Department of Health 2004). Although randomized trial data are lacking, it is reasonable to recommend that the first dose of empirical antibiotics should be administered within 30 minutes of diagnosis.

Empirical antibiotics

There are three main strategies for initial empirical antibiotic treatment (Segal et al. 2003).
- Monotherapy
- Combination therapy without vancomycin
- Combination therapy that includes vancomycin

Local protocols should take into account the susceptibility patterns of local isolates and the possibility of infection with antibiotic-resistant organisms such as MRSA or vancomycin-resistant enterococci (VRE). Prior antibiotic exposure, drug allergies, and the clinical stability of the patient also have a bearing on the choice of initial treatment.

Monotherapy with an extended spectrum antipseudomonal agent is a reasonable initial treatment option and avoids the use of an aminoglycoside with the attendant nephrotoxicity. Suitable agents include: piperacillin/tazobactam (4.5g IV, four times daily), imipenem/cilastatin (500mg IV, four times daily), meropenem (1g IV, three times daily), cefepime (2g IV, three times daily), and ceftazidime (2g IV, three times daily) (NCCN 2008). It should be noted that ceftazidime has limited activity against Gram-positive organisms and that cefepime was inferior to piperacillin/tazobactam in a randomized trial (Segal et al. 2005).

A meta-analysis of 29 trials has confirmed that initial monotherapy has similar efficacy to aminoglycoside-containing combinations (Furno et al. 2002).

The addition of an aminoglycoside to an extended spectrum β-lactam is a commonly employed strategy particularly for unstable patients and in institutions with frequent isolation of multiresistant organisms. Once-daily aminoglycoside dosing (e.g. gentamicin 5–7mg/kg) is less nephrotoxic than schedules utilizing more frequent dosing. Aminoglycoside monotherapy has unacceptably high failure rates and is not recommended. An alternative strategy is the combination of an extended spectrum penicillin such as piperacillin with a quinolone such as ciprofloxacin.

Considerable debate surrounds the incorporation of vancomycin into empirical antibiotic regimens. The addition of vancomycin did not improve survival in a large trial and was associated with more nephrotoxicity and hepatotoxicity (EORTC 1991). However, the increasing frequency of fulminant Gram-positive infections supports the empirical addition of vancomycin. The National Comprehensive Cancer Network (NCCN) recommends adding vancomycin in the following situations: intravenous-catheter associated infections, soft tissue infections, known MRSA colonization, presence of septic shock, Gram-positive cocci grown in blood cultures before susceptibility information becomes available and in the presence of risk factors for viridans group streptococcal infection (NCCN 2008).

Rapid stabilization is critical in the patient with septic shock. Initial antibiotic therapy includes a combination of an antipseudomonal agent, aminoglycoside, and vancomycin. Supportive measures include high-flow oxygen, intravenous fluids, and vasopressor support. Stress dose corticosteroids (e.g. hydrocortisone IV 50mg, four times daily) have been shown to improve survival but the role of activated protein C products is controversial. Invasive haemodynamic monitoring and nursing in a high-dependency unit environment may be necessary.

Changes in initial treatment

The median time to defervescence in patients receiving appropriate initial antibiotic treatment is 5 days. Therefore a change of antibiotic regimen in a clinically stable patient based solely on the persistence of fever is not indicated. However, new physical examination findings, signs of clinical instability, and radiographic or blood culture results should prompt re-evaluation of the antibiotic regimen being used.

Signs of clinical instability should prompt a careful re-examination of the patient. Localizing symptoms and signs such as right iliac fossa tenderness suggesting typhlitis or tenesmus suggesting a perirectal abscess may become apparent with time. The development of respiratory symptoms is best investigated by CT scanning which is more sensitive than plain radiographs. Repeating blood cultures after 48 hours if the patient is still febrile is a reasonable strategy.

If the patient is being treated with monotherapy, clinical deterioration should prompt the addition of an aminoglycoside and vancomycin. In the presence of signs suggesting a GI tract infection, the addition of metronidazole (500mg IV, four times daily) is recommended. The presence of mucosal or cutaneous lesions suggestive of HSV should prompt treatment with acyclovir (5mg/kg IV, three times daily). If *P. jiroveci* infection is suspected, treatment with high-dose trimethoprim/sulfamethoxazole (120mg/kg IV in 2–4 divided doses) is indicated. Close liaison with a microbiologist or infectious disease specialist is invaluable in ensuring that appropriate regimens are utilized.

Clinical fungal infections are uncommon in FN of <7 days duration. However, clinical examination and cultures lack sufficient sensitivity and empirical antifungal therapy is usually initiated if fever persists >4–7 days. Although fluconazole has proven utility as a prophylactic agent, its lack of activity against filamentous fungi renders it unsuitable for empirical antifungal treatment of FN. Options for empirical antifungal treatment include liposomal amphotericin B, voriconazole, posaconazole, and caspofungin. Laboratory markers of fungal infection such as serum galactomannan have low sensitivity and their value in guiding empirical antifungal treatment is limited.

Broad-spectrum intravenous antibiotic treatment should continue until the neutropenia resolves (neutrophil count >0.5 x 10^9/L) and the patient has been afebrile for 24 hours. Documented bacteraemia necessitates continuation of intravenous treatment for at least 7–10 days and up to 21 days for complicated intra-abdominal infections. If *S. aureus* is isolated from the blood cultures, transoesophageal echocardiogram can help determine the duration of intravenous treatment. In the absence of valvular vegetations, a 14-day course is considered sufficient; their presence should lead to treatment prolongation for up to 4–6 weeks.

Outpatient management of FN

The recognition that a substantial proportion of patients have an uncomplicated clinical course and that inpatient treatment of FN is associated with significant costs prompted the evaluation of the feasibility of outpatient management of FN. Talcott identified a subgroup of patients characterized by the absence of comorbidities, controlled cancer, and outpatient status at the onset of the febrile episode that experienced a very low level of infection-related morbidity (Talcott et al. 1988). The Multinational Association for Supportive Care in Cancer (MASCC) has also developed a risk stratification index (Klastersky et al. 2000).

Patients from the low-risk Talcott group, who are not receiving prophylactic antibiotics, have a short expected duration of neutropenia and timely access to emergency care, are suitable for outpatient treatment after a short period of observation (2–12 hours) to ensure that there is no rapid clinical deterioration. A combination of ciprofloxacin (500mg, two to three times daily) and amoxicillin–clavulanate (625mg, three times daily) appears to be efficacious with very low complication rates. Close telephone and face-to-face follow-up is advised for timely intervention if complications occur. A further option is daily outpatient intravenous treatment. Although once daily ceftriaxone is frequently used in this setting, it should be noted that many *Peudomonas* strains exhibit high levels of resistance.

Prevention

Antibiotic prophylaxis has been utilized as a means to prevent FN. Fluoroquinolones such as ciprofloxacin are the commonest used prophylactic agents and have been shown to decrease infection-related and all-cause mortality in hospitalized neutropenic patients with predominantly haematological malignancies.

A recently published trial showed a reduction in episodes of fever (10.8% vs. 15.2%) and hospitalization (15.7% vs. 21.6%) with levofloxacin compared to placebo in outpatients receiving chemotherapy for solid tumours or lymphomas (Cullen et al. 2005).

The use of prophylactic antibiotics is not without controversy. The main concerns revolve around the possibility of promoting the emergence of drug-resistant organisms, the poor coverage of Gram-positive organisms such as viridans group streptococci by the fluoroquinolones, and their association with the development of *C. difficile* diarrhoea. Also, it is not clear that prophylactic administration is more advantageous than outpatient treatment of uncomplicated febrile episodes.

Antifungal prophylaxis is not routinely recommended to reduce the risk of invasive fungal infections during neutropenia. However, prophylaxis with fluconazole or posaconazole is recommended for patients undergoing bone marrow transplantation or intensive chemotherapy for acute leukaemias. Routine prophylaxis against HSV, CMV, and *P. jiroveci* is only indicated for this same, high-risk, group of patients as well as patients receiving alemtuzumab.

Isolation and the use of high-efficiency particulate air (HEPA) filtration are not necessary for the majority of patients with short-lived neutropenia but are of proven benefit in the setting of bone marrow transplantation.

Secondary prevention after an episode of FN begins with an assessment of the therapeutic goals. If treatment is given with curative intent, it is reasonable to attempt to maintain dose intensity through the use of CSFs (see next section) and prophylactic antibiotics. For palliative treatments, though, a reduction in the chemotherapy dose is often more appropriate.

Role of colony-stimulating factors

The benefit from the use of granulocyte or granulocyte-macrophage colony stimulating factors (G-CSF, GM-CSF) in the treatment of established FN is limited. The published evidence suggests that CSFs have no impact on infection-related mortality but modestly shorten the duration of neutropenia and antibiotic treatment. The American Society of Clinical Oncology (ASCO) recommends that G-CSF use should be considered for high-risk patients such as those with severe, prolonged neutropenia and septic shock or organ dysfunction (Smith et al. 2006).

In the preventive setting, the use of G-CSF reduces the incidence of FN by at least 50%. Primary G-CSF prophylaxis is recommended by ASCO when the risk of FN exceeds 20% or in the presence of factors such as age >65 years, poor PS, extensive prior chemotherapy, open wounds, or active infection (Smith et al. 2006). G-CSF administration is an integral component of dose-dense chemotherapy schedules.

The recommended doses for lenograstim and filgrastim are 19.2MU/m^2/day subcutaneously and 0.5 MU/kg/day subcutaneously respectively, starting at least 24 hours after chemotherapy and continuing until granulocyte recovery. A pegylated formulation exists (pegfilgrastim) which is administered as a once-only dose of 6mg subcutaneously approximately 24 hours after chemotherapy. It should be noted that there are very limited data regarding the efficacy of commonly used G-CSF schedules such as 3 or 4 doses every other day starting 6–10 days after chemotherapy. Data from the GEPARTRIO study of neoadjuvant TAC chemotherapy for breast cancer showed that pegfilgrastim was more effective in reducing the incidence of FN than a 6-day course of lenograstim or filgrastim starting on day 5 post-chemotherapy (von Minckwitz et al. 2008).

Further reading:

Cullen M, Steven N, Billingham L, et al. Antibacterial prophylaxis after chemotherapy for solid tumours and lymphomas. *N Engl J Med* 2005; **353**:988–98.

Department of Health (2004). *Manual for cancer services.* Available online at: http://www.dh.gov.uk/en/Healthcare/NationalServiceFrameworks/Cancer/DH_4135595.

European Organization for Research and Treatment of Cancer – the National Cancer Institute of Canada. Vancomycin added to empirical combination antibiotic therapy for fever in granulocytopenic cancer patients. *J Infect Dis* 1991; **163**:951–8.

Furno P, Bucaneve G, Del Favero A. Monotherapy or aminoglycoside-containing combinations for empirical antibiotic treatment of febrile neutropenic patients: a meta-analysis. *Lancet Infect Dis* 2002; **2**:231–42.

Klastersky J, Paesmans M, Rubenstein E. The Multinational Association for Supportive Care in Cancer risk index: a multinational scoring system for identifying low-risk febrile neutropenic cancer patients. *J Clin Oncol* 2000; **18**:3038–51.

NCCN clinical practice guidelines in oncology (2008): Prevention and treatment of cancer-related infections v1. Available online at: http://www.nccn.org/professionals/physician_gls/PDF/infections.pdf

Segal B, Walsh T, Gea-Banacloche J, et al. Infections in the cancer patient. In: DeVita VT, Hellman TS, Rosenberg SA (eds) *Cancer: Principles & Practice of Oncology*, 7th edition, pp. 2461–514. Philadelphia, PA: Lippincott Williams & Wilkins, 2005.

Smith T, Khatcheressian J, Lyman G, et al. 2006 update of recommendations for the use of white blood cell growth factors: an evidence-based clinical practice guideline. *J Clin Oncol* 2006; **24**:3187–205.

Talcott J, Finberg R, Mayer R, et al. The medical course of cancer patients with fever and neutropenia. Clinical identification of a low-risk subgroup at presentation. *Arch Intern Med* 1988; **148**:2561–8.

von Minckwitz G, Kummel S, du Bois A, et al. Pegfilgrastim +/− ciprofloxacin for primary prophylaxis with TAC (docetaxel/doxorubicin/cyclophosphamide) chemotherapy for breast cancer. Results from the GEPARTRIO study. *Ann Oncol* 2008; **19**:292–8.

Thrombocytopenia

Aetiology

Thrombocytopenia generally results from decreased platelet production in the bone marrow or increased peripheral destruction or sequestration. In patients with cancer it is most often secondary to widespread marrow infiltration by haematological malignancies or solid tumours.

Bone marrow suppression by cytotoxic chemotherapy can result in significant thrombocytopenia, which, however, is usually of short duration. Prolonged thrombocytopenia occurs after myeloablative chemotherapy in haematological malignancies. Treatment-induced thrombocytopenia is graded using the Common Terminology Criteria for Adverse Events (CTCAE v.3) as follows:

- Grade 1: 75×10^9/L–LLN (institutional lower limit of normal)
- Grade 2: $50–75 \times 10^9$/L
- Grade 3: $25–50 \times 10^9$/L
- Grade 4: $<25 \times 10^9$/L

Nutritional factors as well as extensive bone marrow irradiation can also result in acute and chronic thrombocytopenia.

Platelet sequestration can occur in the presence of massive splenomegaly, but this is rarely the only cause of thrombocytopenia in advanced leukaemias or lymphomas.

Immune-mediated platelet destruction is seen in chronic lymphocytic leukaemia and lymphomas and has been rarely associated with solid organ tumours such as breast, lung, or GI cancer as a paraneoplastic phenomenon (Arnold et al. 2005).

Treatment with unfractionated or low-molecular-weight heparin is common in patients with malignancy. Rarely (in 1–3% of exposed patients) it is associated with the development of antibodies against platelet factor 4 (PF4)–heparin complexes and subsequently thrombocytopenia (HIT).

Non-immunologic platelet destruction occurs in the setting of disseminated intravascular coagulation (DIC) complicating advanced malignancy. Haemolytic-uraemic syndrome and microangiopathic haemolytic anaemia with development of thrombocytopenia has been reported after treatment with mitomycin C.

It should also be noted that massive red blood cell transfusion can cause or exacerbate thrombocytopenia due to loss of platelet viability in stored blood.

Clinical features

Although bleeding time can be prolonged when the platelet count drops below 100×10^9/L, clinical episodes of bleeding do not seem to increase until the platelet count drops below 50×10^9/L. Minor trauma can lead to excessive bleeding when the platelet count is $20–50 \times 10^9$/L, whereas spontaneous bleeding generally does not occur unless the platelet count is $<20 \times 10^9$/L. Even with platelet counts $<10 \times 10^9$/L, a substantial proportion of patients remain asymptomatic.

Thrombocytopenia causes a characteristic pattern of bleeding with prominent petechiae and small ecchymoses as well as mucosal bleeding (epistaxis, GI bleeding, and haematuria). Haemarthoses and soft tissue haematomas are rare and suggest a coexisting coagulopathy.

Diagnosis

A full blood count and coagulation studies (PT and APTT) are usually adequate for the patient with solid tumour and extensive bone marrow involvement or recent cytotoxic chemotherapy. A peripheral blood smear, bone marrow examination, and detailed platelet function studies are indicated if the cause of the thrombocytopenia is uncertain.

DIC is characteristically associated with prolonged PT and APTT, increased levels of thrombin degradation products, low levels of fibrinogen, thrombocytopenia, and schistocytes on the blood film.

If HIT is suspected, testing for heparin-dependent antibodies is indicated. Currently available commercial immunoassays have high sensitivity but relatively low specificity. Positive predictive values range from 10–93% whereas negative predictive values are high (>95%) (Arepally et al. 2006).

Treatment

Platelet transfusion has been the mainstay of thrombocytopenia management in patients with malignancy. Active bleeding in the setting of thrombocytopenia necessitates transfusion, although there is little evidence on which to base recommendations regarding optimum platelet target levels.

Medications that impair platelet function such as aspirin, clopidogrel, and NSAIDs should be discontinued once thrombocytopenia develops.

Guidelines regarding the use of prophylactic platelet transfusions for thrombocytopenia have been published by the British Committee for Standards in Haematology (2003) and the American Society of Clinical Oncology (Schiffer et al. 2001). Prophylactic platelet transfusion is recommended for platelet counts $<10 \times 10^9$/L. A higher threshold of 20×10^9/L should be adopted in patients with sepsis, coagulopathy, rapid fall in platelet count or acute promyelocytic leukaemia. ASCO recommends a threshold of 20×10^9/L for patients receiving aggressive therapy for bladder tumours and those with necrotic tumours due to an increase in bleeding risk.

Platelet transfusion should be used to bring the platelet count above 50×10^9/L prior to invasive procedures such as lumbar puncture, biopsy, or indwelling line insertion. However, experienced practitioners can perform these procedures safely even in patients with severe thrombocytopenia. A platelet count of $>100 \times 10^9$/L is recommended prior to ophthalmologic or intracranial surgery.

It should be remembered that platelet transfusions are not risk-free. Minor allergic reactions occur frequently during administration and may necessitate pre-medication with antihistamines or corticosteroids. Alloimmunization, acute lung injury, and transmission of infections can also occur. Platelet transfusions are contraindicated, except in the presence of life-threatening haemorrhage, in patients with thrombotic thrombocytopenic purpura or HIT as there is an increased risk of thrombotic complications. Furthermore, platelet transfusion will be ineffective in immune-mediated platelet destruction. The latter, when it occurs as a paraneoplastic syndrome, can respond to splenectomy or high dose corticosteroids.

Tranexamic acid has been shown to reduce platelet requirements during consolidation therapy for acute myeloid leukaemia (Shpilberg et al. 1995). Adoption of even more stringent transfusion thresholds (e.g. $<5 \times 10^9$/L) has also been advocated in an attempt to reduce transfusion frequency.

Treatment of DIC is directed towards the underlying cause if feasible. Infection is a common precipitating factor and broad-spectrum antibiotics are indicated. Cryoprecipitate or fresh frozen plasma is administered to correct the clotting abnormality whereas platelet transfusion is relatively contraindicated.

Treatment of HIT involves discontinuation of the heparin product and alternative anticoagulation with either a direct thrombin inhibitor (e.g. bivalirudin or argatroban) or a factor Xa inhibitor (danaparoid) until platelet recovery. HIT is a prothrombotic state and anticoagulation with warfarin is recommended for at least 4 weeks after resolution of the thrombocytopenia (Arepally et al. 2006).

The development of thrombopoietic growth factors is the subject of intense research efforts and has the potential to ameliorate cancer associated thrombocytopenia and reduce the need for platelet transfusions. Further along clinical development is interleukin-11 (oprelvekin) which is licensed in the USA for the prevention of thrombocytopenia and reduction in need for platelet transfusions in patients receiving myelosuppressive chemotherapy for nonmyeloid malignancies.

Further reading

Arepally G, Ortel T. Heparin-induced thrombocytopenia. N Engl J Med 2006; **355**:809–17.

Arnold S, Lieberman F, Foon K (2005). Paraneoplastic syndromes. In: DeVita VT, Hellman TS, Rosenberg SA (eds) Cancer: Principles & Practice of Oncology, 7th edition, pp. 2189–210. Philadelphia, PA: Lippincott Williams & Wilkins, 2005.

British Committee for Standards in Haematology. Guidelines for the use of platelets transfusion. Br J Haematol 2003; **122**:10–23.

Schiffer C, Anderson K, Bennett C, et al. Platelet transfusion for patients with cancer: clinical practice guidelines of the American Society of Clinical Oncology. J Clin Oncol 2001; **19**:1519–38.

Shpilberg O, Blumenthal R, Sofer O, et al. A controlled trial of tranexamic acid therapy for the reduction of bleeding during treatment of acute myeloid leukaemia. Leuk Lymphoma 1995; **19**:141–4.

Catheter associated infections

Aetiology

Vascular access devices (VADs) are frequently used in cancer patients to ensure prolonged intravenous access for treatment delivery. Catheters with an external component are simpler to insert and include peripherally inserted central catheters (PICCs) and tunnelled catheters such as the Hickman or Groshong designs. Completely implanted devices are accessed percutaneously; their main advantages are durability and a low device profile.

Infection is the most serious complication associated with the presence of a VAD. Infection rates are lower with completely implanted devices compared to tunnelled lines.

The main causative agents are Gram-positive cocci, mostly coagulase-negative staphylocci and *S. aureus*. Early postinsertion infections follow the pattern of postoperative cellulitis, whereas later infections are mostly related to colonization of the catheter tunnel or hub. The incidence of Gram-negative infections, including those caused by *P. aeruginosa* and *S. maltophilia*, is rising.

Clinical features

Catheter related infections can be subdivided into:
• Exit site infections
• Tunnel or port infections
• Septic thrombophlebitis
• Catheter-associated bacteraemia

Exit site infections may be associated with purulent discharge. However, in immunosuppressed or neutropenic patients signs of infection may be minimal and difficult to differentiate from sterile inflammation. Pyrexia or rigors following catheter manipulation are strongly suggestive of catheter-associated bloodstream infection.

Diagnosis

The diagnostic evaluation of the febrile neutropenic patient is described in Chapter 5.2, Febrile neutropenia, p.574. Swabs taken from the exit site as well as blood cultures obtained from both a peripheral site and all catheter lumens are essential.

Determining the role of a VAD in documented bacteraemia is complicated in the absence of obvious tissue inflammation. Various methods have been described, including determining the differential time to positivity of central and peripheral blood cultures and quantitative assessment of organism recovery from central and peripheral culture sites. However, the clinical utility of such assessments is limited.

Treatment

Initial antibiotic treatment of catheter-related infections should include vancomycin to provide adequate cover against Gram-positive cocci including MRSA. Most uncomplicated exit site infections can be treated successfully without necessitating catheter removal.

In contrast, tunnel or port infections are difficult to eradicate using only antibiotics and catheter removal is often necessary. Immediate catheter removal is advised if fungi or non-tuberculous mycobacteria are isolated in blood cultures as well as in the presence of clinical instability or septic thrombophlebitis. Opinion is divided as to whether immediate catheter removal is necessary in infections with bacillus species, *Acinetobacter*, *P. aeruginosa*, *S. maltophilia*, enterococci, or *S. aureus* (NCCN 2008). If an attempt is made to treat the infection with the catheter in situ, repeat blood cultures after 48–72 hours of antibiotic treatment can assist decision making. If blood cultures remain positive or recurrent bacteraemia with the same organism occurs, catheter removal is recommended.

Prevention

Meticulous attendance to aseptic techniques when accessing the catheter is paramount in preventing VAD-associated infections. The Dacron cuff of Hickman and Groshong catheters acts as a barrier to propagation of skin organisms and reduces infection rates compared to short-term catheters. Contrary to the established role of chlorhexidine and silver impregnation in reducing infection rates with short-term catheters, evidence supporting their use with long-term catheters is lacking.

Antibiotic lock therapy with vancomycin is used to sterilize long-term catheter lumens and has been shown in randomized trials to reduce infection rates (Ferretti et al. 2003). However, there are concerns that their routine use will promote the emergence of vancomycin resistant strains and the Centers for Disease Control (CDC) advises against the practice.

Further reading

Ferretti G, Mandala M, Di Cosimo C et al (2003). Catheter related bloodstream infections Part II: Specific pathogens and prevention. *Cancer Control* **10**:79–91.

NCCN clinical practice guidelines in oncology (2008): Prevention and treatment of cancer-related infections v1. Available online at: http://www.nccn.org/professionals/physician_gls/PDF/infections.pdf.

Raised intracranial pressure

Aetiology

Both primary and metastatic malignancies can cause raised intracranial pressure. Expansion of the tumour in combination with accompanying cerebral oedema within the confines of the skull can only be tolerated temporarily. Pathological elevation of intracranial pressure above 20mmHg can damage neurons and compromise cerebral perfusion and so sustained raised intracranial pressure requires urgent treatment.

The commonest forms of primary brain tumours in both adults and children are astrocytomas and these can often present with symptoms of raised intracranial pressure.

Up to a quarter of adult cancer patients develop intracranial metastatic disease and the incidence may be increasing, due to both improved detection of small metastases by MRI and better control of extracerebral disease resulting from improved systemic therapy. Lung cancer is the most common cancer to metastasize to the brain, closely followed by melanoma, renal cell carcinoma and breast cancer. Eighty-five per cent of metastases are to the cerebrum and are often located at the watershed between the white and grey matter as a result of haematogenous spread. In some cases, cerebral metastases are the first sign of disseminated malignancy of unknown primary.

Clinical features

Symptoms of raised intracranial pressure in this setting are often part of a subacute presentation. The classic description is of a headache that is worse in the morning and on performing the Valsalva manoeuvre. This may be accompanied by nausea and vomiting, also more prevalent in the morning. The subtle development of intracranial malignancy, however, means that only about half of patients report headaches as a presenting symptom. Other generalized symptoms include lethargy, weight loss, confusion, and seizures. Focal neurological signs such as gait disturbance, motor weakness, and personality changes can develop depending on the site of the malignancy. Double vision can also be a presenting symptom. This can be due to focal neural compression due to the tumour mass or a false localizing sign of raised intracranial pressure.

Diagnosis

The most sensitive and specific imaging modality for cerebral malignancy with raised intracranial pressure is MRI. CT is less sensitive, especially for posterior fossa lesions.

If the intracerebral lesion is the first manifestation of malignancy, further imaging such as CT or diffusion weighted MRI is necessary. In some cases a biopsy or excision biopsy of the lesion may be necessary.

Treatment

Treatment strategies depend on the patient's overall PS, the volume of active extracerebral malignancy, the primary site of the malignancy, and the number and volume of the cerebral lesions.

Raised intracranial tension can be treated with high-dose steroids, whole brain or stereotactic radiotherapy, or with neurosurgical decompression. Excision of a single lesion is appropriate for suspected primary brain tumours and should also be considered for oligometastatic disease, particularly if there is raised intracranial tension. Whole-brain radiotherapy (WBRT) can be used as an adjuvant to

surgery and has been shown to improve recurrence-free survival. Three randomized clinical trials have compared surgery plus WBRT to WBRT alone. Two of these demonstrated a survival benefit and provided an indication of those patients who can benefit from this combined approach (Patchell et al. 1990; Vecht et al. 1993).

Postoperative WBRT following surgery in patients with brain metastases has the potential to eliminate residual cancer cells, thereby reducing the recurrence rate. Retrospective studies suggested that the addition of WBRT reduced the rate of recurrence and possibly prolonged survival.

In a randomized multicentre trial, 95 patients who had undergone complete resection of a single brain metastasis were randomly assigned to either postoperative WBRT or observation. WBRT significantly decreased the incidence of relapse in the brain, both at the site of original resection and remotely. Patients receiving postoperative WBRT were less likely to die of neurological causes, but there was no difference in overall survival or the duration of functional independence (Patchell et al. 1998).

Multiple cerebral metastases are most commonly treated with WBRT which improves symptoms and increases survival, although for most patients, OS is likely to be determined by the activity and extent of extracranial disease. Around 30Gy in 10 fractions is a standard dose, although 20Gy in 5 fractions is also used commonly. Various different fractionation regimens have not shown superior effects on OS, neurological impairment, or symptom control. The final choice of fractionation schedule depends upon the severity of CNS symptoms, the extent of systemic disease, and doctor preference. The role of neurosurgery in this situation is controversial.

Stereotactic radiotherapy lends itself in theory to the treatment of oligometastatic disease. It reduces the side effects associated with WBRT and the risks of neurosurgery, whilst having the advantage of reaching more anatomically difficult sites. Trials have shown that it is effective in patients with good PS and limited intracranial disease, but in patients with multiple cerebral metastases there is no survival advantage with WBRT and stereotactic radiotherapy over WBRT alone.

Corticosteroids remain an important part of the treatment of metastatic cerebral disease with raised intracranial tension. Dexamethasone is the steroid of choice as it can easily penetrate the blood–brain barrier and has less of an effect on cognitive function. It reduces cerebral oedema effectively and so provides symptomatic control and a marginal improvement in survival. It should also be given to asymptomatic patients before stereotactic radiotherapy.

Prognosis

Raised intracranial tension as a result of cerebral malignancy generally has a poor prognosis. The response of primary brain tumours to treatment is dependent on several factors including the type of tumour and will not be discussed here. Metastatic cerebral disease is often the end-stage of disseminated malignancy but only 40% of patients who present with multiple cerebral metastases die from the cerebral disease. Untreated metastatic intracranial malignancy has a median survival of 1–2 months. This can be increased by around a month with corticosteroids and up to 6 months with radiotherapy. Oligometastatic lesions that are amenable to surgery and radiotherapy have a slightly better prognosis with a median survival of 10–16 months. In the light of the marginal survival benefits, treatment strategies must be carefully evaluated to maximize symptomatic relief as well as improving prognosis.

Further reading

Patchell RA, Tibbs PA, Walsh JW, *et al.* A randomized trial of surgery in the treatment of single metastases to the brain. *N Engl J Med* 1990 **322**(8):494–500.

Patchell RA, Tibbs PA, Regine WF, *et. al.* Postoperative radiotherapy in the treatment of single metastases to the brain: a randomized trial. *JAMA* 1998; **280**(17):1485–9.

Tsao MN, *et al.* Whole brain radiotherapy for the treatment of brain metastases. *Cochrane Database Syst* Rev 2006; **3**: CD003869.

Vecht CJ, Haaxma-Reiche H, Noordijk EM, *et al.* Treatment of single brain metastasis: radiotherapy alone or combined with neurosurgery? *Ann Neurol* 1993; **6**:583–90.

Spinal cord compression

Aetiology

Malignant spinal cord compression is a well-recognized oncological emergency. It is estimated to occur in 2.5–6% of patients with malignancy. The risk of spinal cord compression varies depending on cancer type. Nearly two-thirds of cases are due to breast, lung, and prostate cancer (Loblaw et al. 2004). Spinal cord compression is very uncommon with other tumour types such as pancreatic or ovarian cancer. Most cases of spinal cord compression are due to vertebral body metastases, most commonly in the thoracic spine (Klimo and Schmidt 2004), that extrinsically compress or directly invade the spinal cord. Indirect venous or arterial obstruction by malignancy can also result in compression from the resulting cord oedema (Prasad and Schiff 2005). More than 80% of patients with metastases to the vertebra have lesions that involve more than one vertebral body.

Diagnosis

Localized vertebral or radicular pain is a presenting symptom of spinal cord compression in 90% of cases. These are not from the cord compression but rather from involvement of the vertebral structures and nerve roots at the level of compression. Other common symptoms are gait disturbance, sphincter disturbance, and motor weakness. Physical signs of neuronal compression such as spastic paraparesis and a sensory level may be present. Permanent neurological dysfunction may develop after the initial presentation of back pain, so there must be a high index of suspicion for spinal cord compression in oncology patients. Eighty per cent of cases are in those already diagnosed with malignancy. There may be compression simultaneously at several levels from multiple metastatic deposits.

Studies have shown that the imaging modality of choice for detecting spinal cord or cauda equina compression is MRI. If this is contraindicated or unavailable, CT myelography can be used (Loblaw et al. 2005).

Treatment

Steroids

The mainstay of treatment for spinal cord compression is traditionally corticosteroids and radiotherapy. Dexamethasone is the steroid most frequently prescribed and studies have shown that although higher doses improve neurological outcome, there is a higher incidence of adverse effects. This should be continued throughout radiotherapy and can be reduced afterwards.

Radiotherapy

Radiotherapy is an important part of the management of spinal cord compression secondary to malignancy and has been shown to be effective in relieving symptoms and improving neurological and ambulatory function. There is yet to be a consensus on the ideal radiotherapy regimen. In a phase 3 randomized trial comparing different fractionation schedules in patients with unfavourable histology or an estimated poor survival, there was no difference in outcomes between patients receiving 16Gy in 2 fractions and 30Gy in 8 fractions (Maranzano et al. 2005). There are no trials comparing radiotherapy doses, schedules, or techniques in patients with a good prognosis and hence, no

conclusions can be drawn regarding the optimal radiotherapy dose for such patients (George et al. 2008).

Surgery and radiotherapy

The combination of radiotherapy and decompressive spinal surgery has been evaluated in a study of a single site of cord compression (Patchell et al. 2005). This study revealed a significant increase in ambulation, pain control, and survival in comparison to radiotherapy alone. Although there is some benefit in carefully selected patients there can be significant morbidity and mortality associated with the surgery. These operations should be performed in large regional centres, with expertise in this type of surgery. Complication rates are higher for vertebral body resection than for laminectomy. Patients with preoperative paraparesis seem to benefit less from surgical intervention.

Carefully selected patients with a single site of cord compression, who are fit for surgery and have not been paraplegic for >48 hours should be considered for decompressive surgery before radiotherapy. A surgical opinion should also be sought in the following cases;

- Worsening neurological symptoms
- New neurological findings during radiotherapy
- Vertebral collapse at presentation
- Disease recurrence within a prior radiation site
- Spinal instability

Prognosis

Development of spinal cord compression confers a poor prognosis, with a median overall survival of 3 months irrespective of therapy (Loblaw et al. 2004). Factors that influence outcome include rate of symptom development, neurological impairment at diagnosis, certain tumour types, and response to therapy. Studies have shown, however, that radioresistant tumours do not have a significantly reduced response to medical therapy. Thus there is yet to be reliable evidence for the recommendation of spinal surgery in the management of spinal cord compression caused by these tumour types.

Further reading

George R, Jeba J, Ramkumar G, et al. Interventions for the treatment of metastatic extradural spinal cord compression in adults. *Cochrane Database Syst Rev* 2008; 4:CD006716.

Klimo P Jr, Schmidt MH. Surgical management of spinal metastases. *Oncologist* 2004; 9:188–96.

Loblaw DA, Laperriere NJ, Mackillop WJ. A population-based study of malignant spinal cord compression in Ontario. *Clin Oncol (R Coll Radiol)* 2004; 15:211–17.

Loblaw DA, Perry J, Chambers A. Systematic review of the diagnosis and management of malignant epidural spinal cord compression: the Cancer Care Ontario Practice Guidelines Initiative's Neuro-Oncology Disease Site Group. *J Clin Oncol* 2005; 23:2028–37.

Maranzano E, Bellavita R, Rossi R, et al. Short-course versus split-course radiotherapy in metastatic spinal cord compression: results of a phase III, randomized, multicenter trial. *J Clin Onc* 2005; 15:3308–10.

Patchell RA, Tibbs PA, Regine WF, et al. Direct decompressive surgical resection in the treatment of spinal cord compression caused by metastatic cancer: a randomised trial. *Lancet* 2005; 366:643–8.

Prasad D, Schiff D. Malignant spinal-cord compression. *Lancet Oncol* 2005; 6:15–24.

Cardiac arrest: introduction

Cardiac arrest in a cancer patient can be an unexpected event related to potentially reversible causes or the end result of irreversible functional decline in the setting of extensively metastatic disease. There is no evidence to suggest that the pathophysiology and clinical features of cardiac arrest differ in the presence of malignancy and the diagnostic and treatment algorithms are the same as for the general population. Overall survival-to-discharge rates for hospitalized patients with cancer who undergo cardio-pulmonary resuscitation are comparable to those of unselected hospitalised patients (Reisfield et al. 2006).

Decision not to resuscitate

Whereas resuscitation may be appropriate in the presence of a reversible precipitant, it is clearly inappropriate in a large number of patients with end-stage disease. Careful and sensitive discussion of end-of-life issues with patients and their families and timely institution of Do Not Attempt Resuscitation (DNAR) orders can help prevent inappropriate interventions at the terminal disease phase.

Cardiac tamponade

Aetiology

Malignant pericardial disease is found at autopsy in approximately 5–10% of cancer patients; breast, lung, leukaemias, and lymphomas are the commonest primaries. Pericardial involvement by the tumour is the commonest cause of effusion and tamponade. However, other causes include acute inflammatory or chronic effusive post-radiotherapy pericarditis and drug toxicity. Chemotherapeutic agents that are known to cause pericarditis, and occasionally tamponade, include the anthracyclines, bleomycin, cyclophosphamide, cytarabine, and all-transretinoic acid.

Tamponade develops when pericardial fluid accumulation causes the intrapericardial pressure to rise sufficiently to impair right ventricular diastolic filling.

Clinical features

Malignant pericardial effusion almost always occurs in the setting of previously diagnosed advanced malignancy. The presence of pericardial effusion can be associated with relatively non-specific symptoms of dyspnoea, cough, chest pain, and oedema. The development of tamponade depends to a great extent on the rate of accumulation of pericardial fluid and the underlying cardiac function; large volumes of pericardial fluid can be tolerated if the rate of accumulation is slow.

Tamponade presents with the clinical features of cardiogenic shock:
• Dyspnoea
• Orthopnoea
• Diaphoresis
• Low blood pressure
• Tachycardia
• Signs of low cardiac output (peripheral vasoconstriction, clammy extremities and poor capillary refill).

The neck veins are distended, cardiac sounds are muffled, and there is pulsus paradoxus.

Diagnosis

A pericardial effusion in an asymptomatic patient can be detected on chest radiograph as an enlarged globular cardiac silhouette. Asymptomatic effusions are also commonly visualized on routine CT scans.

In tamponade the electrocardiogram usually shows low voltage complexes and electrical alterans but these findings lack sensitivity and specificity. The investigation of choice is two-dimensional echocardiography to confirm the presence of pericardial fluid and its haemodynamic effects. This should be done as an emergency, within minutes, as tamponade causing cardiogenic shock can be rapidly fatal.

Treatment

Medical management

Emergency bedside pericardiocentesis, preferably under echocardiographic guidance, can be lifesaving when patients are acutely haemodynamically compromised. Under local anaesthetic, a needle is inserted at either side of the xiphoid process, at a 45° angle, aiming towards the left scapula. Removal of as little as 50mL of pericardial fluid can result in haemodynamic improvement (Nguyen et al. 2005).

Surgical management

Simple pericardiocentesis is associated with very high recurrence rates and, therefore, definitive surgical management is indicated. Various surgical techniques, such as partial pericardiectomy or 'pericardial window', percutaneous tube pericardiostomy, and pericardial sclerotherapy, have been described. However, the procedure of choice appears to be subxiphoid pericardiostomy. A review of the clinical experience with this technique showed very low procedural morbidity and mortality with a pericardial effusion recurrence rate of 3.5% (Nguyen et al. 2005).

Further reading

Nguyen D, Schrump P (2005). Malignant pleural and pericardial effusions. In: DeVita VT, Hellman TS, Rosenberg SA (eds) *Cancer: Principles & Practice of Oncology*, 7th edition, pp. 2387–92. Philadelphia, PA: Lippincott Williams & Wilkins, 2005.

Reisfield G, Kish Wallace S, Munsell M, *et al.* Survival in cancer patients undergoing in-hospital cardiopulmonary resuscitation: a meta-analysis. *Resuscitation* 2006; **71**:152–60.

Venous thromboembolism (deep venous thrombosis and pulmonary embolism)

Aetiology

VTE, which encompasses both DVT and PE, occurs in up to 20% of cancer patients. Conversely, up to 20% of community VTE cases are associated with the presence of active malignancy.

A population-based case–control study showed that the odds ratio for development of a first lifetime VTE was 4.1 in patients with malignancy who were not receiving chemotherapy, increasing to 6.5 during treatment with chemotherapy (Heit et al. 2008). These numbers are likely to underestimate the total burden of VTE, as postmortem studies have consistently shown that only a minority of events are diagnosed antemortem. As is the case in the general population, Virchow's triad describes the factors that contribute to VTE:

• Venous stasis

• Endothelial injury

• Hypercoagulability

Risk factors such as obesity, immobilization, and prothrombotic mutations are common to patients with and without malignancy. However, the presence of malignancy can accentuate the impact of such traditional risk factors. For example, the risk of fatal postoperative PE has been reported to be 3-fold higher in cancer patients compared to patients undergoing similar surgery for a non-malignant diagnosis (Gallus 1997).

The primary site of malignancy influences the risk of VTE. It seems to be particularly high for pancreatic, ovarian, and brain primaries, whereas renal, lung, gastric, and haematological cancers are also associated with above-average risk. VTE risk is also higher in the period immediately following a new diagnosis of malignancy, even if successfully treated. The development of metastatic disease markedly influences the risk of VTE as evidenced by reports of 5–20-fold increased risk compared to patients with localized disease.

Cancer treatments also have an impact on the risk of VTE. As mentioned earlier, chemotherapy has been associated with increased risk, over and above the risk conferred by the malignancy itself. Particularly high risks of VTE have been reported with the use of thalidomide and lenalidomide-based combinations in the treatment of multiple myeloma, with VTEs affecting up to 28% of patients in one study (Bennett et al. 2006). The anti-VEGF antibody bevacizumab has also been shown to increase the risk of VTE as well as causing arterial thromboembolism and bleeding.

Hormonal manipulations have been implicated in increasing VTE episodes. Treatment with tamoxifen and diethylstilboestrol increases VTE risk in breast and prostate cancer patients respectively.

Additional risk factors in cancer patients include the frequent presence of central venous access catheters and the use of erythropoiesis-stimulating agents. The latter, when used for the treatment of chemotherapy-associated anaemia, carry a 1.6-fold increase in VTE risk.

Clinical features

The vast majority of DVTs affect the lower limbs where they usually present with pain, tenderness, erythema, and oedema. A difference in calf circumference of >3cm is strongly predictive of DVT whereas Homan's sign (calf tenderness on ankle dorsiflexion) is neither sensitive nor specific. Swelling of the whole leg can be a sign of pelvic or femoral DVT.

Approximately 10% of DVTs affect the upper limb, where they present with similar symptoms. The frequency of upper limb DVT appears to be increasing, probably reflecting the increasing use of central venous catheters.

The clinical features of PE can vary depending on the extent of thrombosis and the underlying lung function. Moderate and large PE commonly causes dyspnoea, pleuritic chest pain, cough, and haemoptysis. Massive PE is a frequent cause of circulatory collapse and cardiac arrest. The commonest clinical signs of PE are hypoxia, tachypnoea, and tachycardia; a pleural rub may be audible if pulmonary infarction develops. Massive PE causes signs of acute right ventricular failure with hypotension, distended jugular veins, loud P2, S3, or S4 gallop and a pansystolic murmur of acute tricuspid regurgitation.

It should be kept in mind that the majority of VTE events are asymptomatic. This is supported by studies of DVT development in the postoperative setting that have shown that only a small proportion of the ultrasound-detected cases were clinically apparent. Similarly, whereas it is thought that almost all PEs are the consequence of a lower limb or pelvic DVT, clinically apparent DVT is present in only 20% of cases. In addition, the clinical use of multi-detector high resolution CT scanning for staging and response assessment purposes in cancer patients has resulted in increased detection of PE in otherwise asymptomatic patients.

Diagnosis

Despite the progress in imaging technologies, the diagnosis of VTE remains challenging. As symptoms and signs can be minimal, heightened clinical awareness is paramount. Various clinical decision rules, such as the Wells score, are in use, but it should be noted that, although cancer patients were included in the rule derivation studies, they usually constituted a small minority. None of the clinical decision rules have been specifically validated in a population comprised exclusively of patients with malignancy. The use of D-dimer testing as a screening tool prior to imaging studies is not recommended in patients with malignancy.

Duplex ultrasonography is the investigation of choice for suspected DVT. It has high sensitivity (>90%) and specificity (>95%) for femoral or popliteal DVT, particularly if assessment of venous compressibility is carried out. However, the accuracy of the test is lower for calf or pelvic vein DVT. Repeat examination a week later is recommended if the clinical suspicion of DVT is moderate or high but the initial ultrasonography is negative.

CT with intravenous contrast administration is the preferred method for diagnosing thrombi in the pelvic veins or the IVC. Invasive venography is less commonly used, but can still be of value particularly in diagnosing upper extremity DVT. Catheter-associated DVT can be diagnosed with contrast administration via the catheter ('linogram'). However, it should be kept in mind that neither clot inside the catheter, nor the presence of a fibrin sheath constitutes a DVT.

Non-specific electrocardiographic abnormalities such as tachycardia or ST–T wave changes are common in PE. An $S_1Q_3T_3$ pattern or development of a new right bundle branch block is very specific but insensitive, as it occurs in only 5% of patients. Similarly, the value of a plain chest radiograph is limited, although it can aid V/Q scan interpretation.

CT pulmonary angiogram (CTPA) is the investigation of choice for diagnosing PE. In addition to demonstrating any emboli, it allows evaluation of the lung parenchyma and mediastinal structures revealing any additional or alternative pathology. The PIOPED II trial showed that multidetector CT had a sensitivity of 83% and specificity of 96% for the diagnosis of PE. The positive predictive value was 96% when the clinical probability, derived by the Wells score, was concordant with the scan result. However, a negative CTPA could not reliably exclude PE when the clinical probability was high, as the negative predictive value in that setting was only 60% (Stein et al. 2006). Most of the CT scanners used in that study were 4-slice machines; whether modern 16- or 64- slice scanners can overcome these limitations is not known.

V/Q scan is associated with less radiation exposure and is an alternative to CTPA, particularly when renal insufficiency precludes intravenous contrast administration and in pregnant patients. However, it has lower sensitivity and specificity than CTPA and is non-diagnostic when the clinical probability is discordant with the scan results or when the scan shows an intermediate or low probability of PE. Invasive pulmonary angiography, while still considered the 'gold standard' for diagnosing PE, is rarely used clinically.

Treatment

Both ASCO (Lyman et al. 2007) and NCCN (2008) have issued guidelines for the prevention and management of VTE in patients with cancer. It should be noted that the consensus is that incidental PE requires the same treatment as clinically apparent PE. In fact, many 'asymptomatic' patients notice clinical improvement once treatment is initiated.

Low-molecular-weight heparin (LMWH) is the preferred anticoagulation modality in patients with cancer and VTE. The recommendation is based on the results of multiple randomised trials that have shown that LMWH therapy administered subcutaneously for 3–6 months is associated with significantly lower rates of recurrent VTE and similar rates of bleeding complications compared to vitamin K antagonists. This has been confirmed by a recent Cochrane review that showed a HR for recurrence of 0.47 (95% CI 0.32–0.71) in favour of LMWH (Akl et al. 2008). The choice of the specific LMWH (e.g. enoxaparin 1.5 mg/kg SC once daily, tinzaparin 175U/kg SC once daily, dalteparin 200U/kg SC once daily) is usually dependent on institutional preference; there is no evidence to suggest that one is more effective or safer than the other. Similarly, multiple studies have confirmed the equivalence of LMWH and unfractionated heparin (UFH) in the initial (first 5–10 days) treatment of VTE. However, the former is much easier to administer and does not require routine monitoring of coagulation parameters. Fondaparinux, a factor Xa inhibitor, is also recommended as an alternative to LMWH.

Warfarin can be used for the chronic treatment of VTE if patient preference or cost issues dictate so. However, an initial period of heparin therapy for at least 5–7 days and until the INR has been >2 for at least 48 hours is recommended. A target INR of 2–3 is reasonable in this setting.

Warfarin is subject to many pharmacokinetic interactions and concomitant medications, including chemotherapy, can affect drug levels, necessitating frequent INR monitoring to ensure efficacy and safety.

The optimum duration of anticoagulant therapy in not defined. Generally, treatment for at least 3–6 months is recommended for DVT and 6–12 months for PE. Both ASCO (Lyman et al. 2007) and the NCCN (2008) recommend that indefinite treatment should be considered for selected patients such as those with metastatic disease or patients on chemotherapy. Randomized trial data, though, are lacking.

Contraindications to anticoagulant therapy in cancer patients include recent major surgery, recent intracranial bleed, active major bleeding, thrombocytopenia, and platelet or coagulation abnormalities. Placement of an IVC filter should be considered in this situation.

Failure of anticoagulation treatment is defined as extension of a known DVT/PE or development of a new DVT/PE while on treatment. In the first instance measurement of INR, APTT, and anti-Xa activity is recommended to ensure adequate drug exposure. Therapeutic manoeuvres include placement of an IVC filter, switching from warfarin to LMWH, increasing the dose of LMWH, moving to a twice-daily schedule of LMWH administration, or switching to a factor Xa inhibitor (NCCN 2008).

Removal of the catheter, if feasible, is the preferred option for catheter-related DVT. Anticoagulation with LMWH is recommended while the catheter is still *in situ* and for 1–3 months afterwards. A small pilot study has demonstrated the feasibility of a strategy of dalteparin and warfarin administration without removing the catheter (Kovacs et al. 2007).

Catheter-directed or intravenous thrombolytic therapy is an option for the treatment of massive PE causing haemodynamic compromise. Thrombolysis has been shown to significantly reduce the risk of death or recurrent PE in these patients compared to heparin treatment alone. However, careful consideration of the risks and benefits of the procedure is important as the risk of major bleeding approaches 15%. There is no evidence to suggest that catheter-directed thrombolysis (with catheter placement in the pulmonary artery) is superior to intravenous thrombolysis or that one agent (e.g. streptokinase, alteplase, reteplase) is superior to another. Surgical or percutaneous transcatheter embolectomy is an option in massive PE when thrombolysis is contraindicated. Thrombolysis should also be considered for patients with massive or non-resolving ileofemoral DVT threatening limb viability.

Prevention

Prophylactic treatment is recommended for all hospitalized patients with cancer, unless there are specific contraindications to anticoagulant use. The recommendation is based on the results of three randomized trials that have shown a reduction in VTE events with prophylactic LMWH (Lyman et al. 2007). However, patients with cancer constituted only a small minority of the enrolled subjects. Suitable options include enoxaparin 40mg SC once daily, dalteparin 5000U SC once daily, or UFH 5000U SC once daily

Patients undergoing surgery require VTE prophylaxis perioperatively. Mechanical devices alone appear to be insufficient and LMWH or UFH should be added for at least 7–10 days following major surgery. Recent randomized trials have shown that extending prophylactic treatment with LMWH for 4 weeks following major abdominal or pelvic surgery for cancer is more effective at preventing VTE than a 7-day course.

Routine VTE prophylaxis is not recommended for cancer patients receiving chemotherapy. However, prophylactic treatment should be considered for patients receiving thalidomide or lenalidomide based combinations for multiple myeloma in view of the extremely high incidence of VTE in this setting.

Post hoc and subgroup analyses of anticoagulant trials have suggested improved survival in cancer patients receiving anticoagulation. At present however, anticoagulant therapy in not recommended when used with the express goal of improving survival, in the absence of confirmed VTE, outside of clinical trials.

Further reading

Heit J, Silverstein M, Mohr D, et al. Risk factors for deep vein thrombosis and pulmonary embolism: a population-based case-control study. Arch Intern Med 2000; 160:809–15.

Gallus AS. Prevention of post-operative deep vein leg thrombosis in patients with cancer. Thromb Haemost 1997; 78:126–32.

Bennett C, Angelotta C, Yarnold P, et al. Thalidomide- and lenalidomide-associated thromboembolism among patients with cancer. JAMA 2006; 296:2558–60.

Stein P, Fowler S, Goodman L, et al. Multidetector computed tomography for acute pulmonary embolism. N Engl J Med 2006; 354:2317–27.

Lyman G, Khorana A, Falanga A, et al. American Society of Clinical Oncology Guideline: Recommendations for venous thromboembolism prophylaxis and treatment in patients with cancer. J Clin Oncol 2007; 25;5490–505.

NCCN clinical practice guidelines in oncology. Venous thromboembolic disease v2, 2008—available online at: http://www.nccn.org/professionals/physician_gls/PDF/vte.pdf.

Akl E, Barba M, Rohilla S, et al. Anticoagulation for the long term treatment of venous thromboembolism in patients with cancer. Cochrane Database Syst Rev 2008; 16:CD006650.

Kovacs M, Kahn S, Rodger M, et al. A pilot study of central venous catheter survival in cancer patients using low molecular weight heparin (dalteparin) with warfarin without catheter removal for the treatment of upper extremity deep vein thrombosis (the Catheter Study). J Thromb Haemost 2007; 5:1650–3.

Stridor and airway obstruction

Aetiology

Stridor is a high-pitched musical breathing sound predominantly heard on inspiration. It results from obstructed airflow in the upper extrathoracic airways and the intrathoracic trachea and major bronchi.

There are multiple benign causes of stridor some of which can be related to previous surgery for malignancy such as bilateral vocal cord palsy following cervical or thyroid surgery or post-tracheostomy tracheal stenosis.

Malignant causes of stridor can be subdivided into extrinsic and intrinsic. Extrinsic causes include:
- Direct invasion by primary pulmonary neoplasms or aggressive thyroid carcinomas
- Involvement of the airways by enlarged lymph nodes in tumours such as lymphomas
- Involvement by metastases from a distant site

Metastases that directly invade the major airways most commonly originate from renal, colon, breast or melanoma primaries and account for 2–5% of all lung metastases.

Intrinsic obstruction is usually due to bulky primary tumours originating from the hypopharynx, larynx, trachea, or proximal large bronchi.

Clinical features

The timing of the stridor in relation to the respiratory cycle can help determine the level of obstruction. Supraglottic lesions cause inspiratory stridor whereas glottic and subglottic tumours cause biphasic stridor with both an inspiratory and an expiratory component. Intrathoracic lesions can cause a predominantly expiratory stridor that can easily be confused with wheezing.

Depending on the severity of obstruction there may be signs of respiratory compromise such as dyspnoea, tachypnoea and cyanosis. Cough and haemoptysis may be present. Careful auscultation of the neck and chest can help locate the site of obstruction. In addition, physical examination may reveal clues as to the likely aetiology such as thyroid masses, gross cervical lymphadenopathy, clubbing, or pleural effusions. Note that physical examination of the neck is contraindicated if there is a suspicion of epiglottitis.

Diagnosis

The diagnosis of stridor is clinical. Patients who present with severe respiratory compromise require emergency management of their airway. Fibreoptic-assisted intubation in this setting provides both immediate relief and diagnostic information.

Pulse oximetry and arterial blood gas analysis aid in the initial evaluation of the patient. Plain X-rays of the chest and neck can assist in the diagnosis by revealing lymphadenopathy or a lung primary. More detailed anatomical information is provided by CT of the neck and thorax. Spirometry with flow-volume loops can help differentiate between extrathoracic and intrathoracic obstruction. Rigid bronchoscopy may facilitate therapeutic interventions and provide tissue for histological diagnosis.

Treatment

Initial treatment depends on the severity of obstruction. Severe respiratory compromise necessitates emergency intubation or tracheostomy. Helium–oxygen gas mixtures (Heliox®) or non-invasive positive pressure ventilation can aid in the stabilization of the acutely unwell patient. High-dose dexamethasone (16mg daily) can help reduce peritumoral oedema and partially relieve the obstruction.

Definitive treatment depends on the diagnosis and extent of disease. Urgent surgery is the preferred option for resectable primary tracheal tumours. A variety of techniques can be used for unresectable endoluminal tumours. These include;
- Endoluminal resection ('core out') at rigid bronchoscopy
- Nd: YAG laser vaporisation of the tumour
- Brachytherapy with ^{125}I or ^{192}Ir
- Photodynamic therapy or
- Cryotherapy

Insertion of a tracheal stent can relieve extrinsic compression. Small case series indicate that symptomatic relief is achieved in the majority of patients, but all these techniques require specialized personnel and equipment and are not widely available (Biller 2006).

External beam radiotherapy is widely available and is usually the first treatment option for airway obstruction from relatively chemotherapy-resistant tumours such as NSCLC. Radiotherapy can initially exacerbate peritumoral oedema and therefore corticosteroid pre-medication is advisable. Initial chemotherapy is advised for chemotherapy-sensitive tumours such as SCLC or lymphomas; the role of radiotherapy is limited in these situations.

Further reading

Biller J (2006). Airway obstruction, bronchospasm and cough. In: Berger A, Shuster A, Von Roenn A (eds) *Palliative Care and Supportive Oncology* 3rd edition, pp. 297–308. Philadelphia, PA: Lippincott Williams & Wilkins, 2006.

Superior vena caval obstruction

Aetiology
The superior vena cava (SVC) provides venous drainage for the upper half of the body. It is a thin-walled, easily compressible vessel surrounded by a dense lymphatic network, rendering it vulnerable to malignant processes involving the middle or anterior mediastinum, particularly to the right of the midline.

Obstruction is commonly the result of extrinsic compression with or without associated thrombosis. Isolated thrombosis can also occur and is a common cause of non-malignant obstruction.

Malignancy accounts for approximately 80% of cases of SVC obstruction. Lung cancer is the commonest cause and is implicated in almost 75% of cases, with NSCLC causing twice as many cases as SCLC. Rarer causes include (Wilson et al. 2007):
- Lymphomas (10–15%)
- Metastatic disease (primarily breast cancer 10%)
- Germ cell tumours (3%)
- Thymomas (2%)

Clinical features
Obstruction of the SVC leads to extensive collateral venous circulation redirecting blood flow to the azygos vein or the inferior vena cava. This collateral network develops over a period of several weeks and can result in improvement of symptoms and signs.

The commonest symptoms are dyspnoea (60%) and various degrees of facial or limb oedema (40–80%). Other complaints include:
- Cough (20–50%)
- Chest pain (15%)
- Headache (10%)
- Dizziness or syncope (10%)

The classic physical finding is of fixed engorgement of the neck and chest wall veins (50–60%) with visible cutaneous collaterals, plethora (20%), and cyanosis (20%). Papilloedema can be a late development. Rare but potentially life-threatening presentations include cerebral or upper respiratory tract oedema. Respiratory compromise is rarely the result of SVC obstruction per se; it usually reflects direct involvement of the major airways by the malignant process (Yahalom 2005).

Diagnosis
The diagnosis is usually evident clinically and subsequent investigations aim to establish the underlying cause, as 60% of cases of SVC obstruction occur without a prior diagnosis of malignancy (Yahalom 2005).

The chest radiograph is abnormal in >85% of cases with superior mediastinal widening and pleural effusion being the commonest findings. CT with intravenous contrast material provides anatomical information and allows the examination of other critical structures such as the trachea and spinal canal. Depending on the distribution of the disease, histological confirmation can be provided by sputum or pleural fluid cytology, lymph node or CT-guided biopsy, or at bronchoscopy. The diagnostic yield of these procedures is in the order of 50–75%. Mediastinoscopy has a higher diagnostic yield (>90%) and it seems to be safe in the hands of an experienced operator.

Prognosis
There are no data to suggest that the presence of SVC obstruction adversely affects prognosis beyond the obvious staging implications.

Treatment
Management aims both at the relief of symptoms and treating the underlying cause.

Medical management
Elevation of the patient's head to reduce hydrostatic pressure is a useful therapeutic manoeuvre. Corticosteroids (e.g. dexamethasone 4mg four times daily) are frequently prescribed but there are limited data to support their efficacy. It can, however, result in tumour response in lymphomas and thymomas. Similarly, there is no evidence to support the administration of loop diuretics.

Radiotherapy and chemotherapy
The use of radiotherapy or chemotherapy requires a histological diagnosis. In the rare case where immediate relief is required, stent placement is preferable to proceeding to radiotherapy without available histology. Radiotherapy provides symptomatic relief in 60–80% of patients with NSCLC or SCLC; improvement is usually noted within 72 hours. However, autopsy series show that the rate of SVC re-canalization is low, suggesting that collateral development contributes to the symptomatic improvement. In fit patients without distant metastases the radiation field should encompass all gross disease with a total dose of 30–50Gy in 2–3-Gy fractions. In the palliative setting a small study showed improved symptom control with three, compared to two, weekly 8Gy fractions. Systemic chemotherapy can result in rapid relief of symptoms and is the preferred modality of treatment for chemotherapy-sensitive tumours. Reported rates of complete symptomatic relief range from 40–80% for patients with lymphoma or SCLC.

Anticoagulation and thrombolysis
Thrombolytic therapy has been used in the setting of catheter-associated thrombosis. The benefit of either short or long term anticoagulation is uncertain (Yahalom 2005).

Stent
Stent placement can result in immediate symptomatic relief while diagnostic investigations are carried out. It is the preferred option for treatment resistant tumours such as mesothelioma.

Further reading
Wilson L, Detterbeck F, Yahalom J (2007). Superior vena cava syndrome with malignant causes. *N Eng J Med* 2007; **356**:1862–9.

Yahalom J. Superior vena cava syndrome. In: DeVita VT, Hellman TS, Rosenberg SA (eds) *Cancer: Principles & Practice of Oncology*, 7th edition, pp. 2273–9. Philadelphia, PA: Lippincott Williams & Wilkins, 2005.

Pleural effusion

Aetiology

Malignant pleural effusion (MPE) is common in advanced malignancy and can be the initial manifestation of cancer in 10–50% of cases. The commonest primary sites include lung (35%), breast (25%), and lymphoma (10%). MPE of unknown primary accounts for approximately 10% of cases.

MPE commonly results from diffuse subpleural lymphatic involvement disrupting the delicate lymphatic system that underlies normal pleural fluid dynamics. Pulmonary tumours can directly disrupt the integrity of the visceral pleura and spill cells in the pleural space, whereas pleural deposits can also result from haematogenous spread from distant sites (Nguyen and Schrump 2005).

Clinical features

Dyspnoea is the commonest presenting symptom, followed by cough and pleuritic chest pain. Up to 25% of patients are asymptomatic on presentation, the pleural effusion being an incidental finding on physical examination or the chest radiograph.

Physical findings include decreased expansion and breath sounds in the affected hemithorax with diminution of vocal resonance and tactile fremitus. Mediastianal structure displacement towards the contralateral side can occur with massive effusions, unless there is associated pulmonary collapse.

Diagnosis

The diagnosis of pleural effusion is usually straightforward on physical examination and chest radiograph. Subsequent investigations are aimed at identifying the cause of the effusion and staging the disease.

CT of the chest can identify fluid loculations and associated parenchymal masses as well as mediastinal or hilar lymphadenopathy.

Thoracentesis can provide immediate symptomatic relief and aid in the diagnosis. Typically MPEs fulfil Light's criteria for an exudate (fluid to serum protein ratio >0.5, fluid to serum LDH ratio >0.6, and fluid LDH level >2/3 the upper limit of normal serum values). Frequently the fluid is haemorrhagic or blood-tinged and in up to one-third of cases acidic; the latter is associated with poorer prognosis. As much fluid as possible should be sent for cytological examination. Initial cytology is positive in approximately 50% of MPEs.

If initial cytology is negative, further diagnostic options include either repeat thoracentesis or thoracoscopy. VATS has a diagnostic yield that approaches 100% in malignant pleural involvement (Antunes et al. 2003).

Treatment

The management of MPE depends on the fitness of the patient and the overall disease prognosis, with lung primaries or mesothelioma being associated with worse outcomes than breast or ovarian primaries.

Medical management

Observation is a reasonable treatment strategy for patients who are asymptomatic or if there is no recurrence of the MPE following initial thoracentesis. Chemotherapy for sensitive tumours such as breast carcinomas or lymphomas can result in resolution of the MPE; repeated thoracentesis may be required until satisfactory disease response occurs.

Patients with very poor life expectancy can be managed by repeated thoracentesis alone. It must be noted though, that the 1-month recurrence rate after aspiration alone approaches 100%.

Surgical management

Intercostal tube insertion and pleurodesis with intrapleural sclerosant instillation is the commonest surgical procedure. There is randomized evidence that small-bore (10–14F) tube insertion is as efficacious as traditional large-bore tubes and is associated with less patient discomfort. Following intercostal tube insertion, drainage of pleural fluid should proceed in a controlled fashion, approximately 500mL/hour, to minimize the risk of re-expansion pulmonary oedema (Antuneset al. 2003).

The commonest sclerosing agents in use are tetracyclines, bleomycin, and talc, either as slurry or as poudrage. Talc appears to be more efficacious but has been rarely associated with acute respiratory distress syndrome (ARDS). However, a recent study involving 558 patients reported no cases of ARDS with the use of large particle talc poudrage (Janssen et al. 2007).

Surgical methods that can be used if initial pleurodesis fails include repeat attempts, long-term indwelling catheters, pleuroperitoneal shunts or surgical pleurectomy.

Further reading

Antunes G, Neville E, Duffy J, et al. BTS guidelines for the management of malignant pleural effusions. *Thorax* 2003; **58**(suppl II) ii29–38.

Janssen J, Collier G, Astoul P, et al. Safety of pleurodesis with talc poudrage in malignant pleural effusion: a prospective cohort study. *Lancet* 2007; **369** 1535–9.

Nguyen D, Schrump P (2005). Malignant pleural and pericardial effusions. In: DeVita VT, Hellman TS, Rosenberg SA (eds) *Cancer: Principles & Practice of Oncology*, 7th edition, pp. 2381–7. Philadelphia, PA: Lippincott Williams & Wilkins, 2005.

Gastrointestinal bleeding

Aetiology
GI bleeding can originate anywhere in the GI tract from the mouth to the anus. Chronic GI tract blood loss is a common presenting symptom of gastric, small bowel, and colonic malignancy.

Acute GI bleeding as an oncological emergency usually occurs in the setting of an advanced, incurable disease and can be a terminal event. It is commonly the result of direct involvement of luminal blood vessels by tumour. Other potential mechanisms include rupture of highly vascularized tumours such as gastrointestinal stromal tumours (GIST) or variceal bleeding in the setting of extensive hepatic disease and portal hypertension.

GI bleeding may be compounded by coagulopathy. Clotting factor abnormalities, thrombocytopenia and DIC are often present in advanced malignancy, especially in the setting of extensive hepatic metastases.

GI bleeding can also be a consequence of anticancer treatments. Most cytotoxic chemotherapy agents cause a degree of myelosuppression and thrombocytopenia is especially pronounced with drugs such as carboplatin or gemcitabine. Novel compounds targeting cancer angiogenesis such as bevacizumab have a distinct toxicity profile that includes both bleeding and thrombotic events. Furthermore, the increasing use of indwelling vascular access devices as well as the easier diagnosis of venous thromboembolism afforded by modern imaging techniques result in an ever increasing proportion of cancer patients being treated with antiplatelet or anticoagulant agents.

Clinical features
The clinical features depend on the site and severity of bleeding. Common presentations include haematemesis, melaena, and haematochezia. Loss of large blood volumes leads to hypovolaemic shock presenting with lethargy, diaphoresis, pale, cool, and clammy extremities, and prolonged capillary refill. Tachycardia, hypotension, and decreased urinary output are usually present.

Diagnosis
The diagnosis of major acute GI bleeding is clinical. Further investigations depend on the clinical situation and generally aim to assess either the severity of bleeding or the potential site of origin. Determining the site of bleeding can be accomplished by upper or lower GI endoscopy, CT, or angiography in selected cases.

Treatment
Treatment is guided by an initial assessment of the severity of bleeding and the overall patient prognosis.

If it is thought that the bleeding represents a terminal event then active resuscitation measures are inappropriate. The patient should be preferably nursed in a sideroom. Sedation with midazolam and diamorphine is helpful for alleviating pain, anxiety, and distress. Dark towels should be used to cover areas of active bleeding as this has been shown to reduce patient and relative distress.

Immediate fluid resuscitation using crystalloid or colloid solutions is the first management step if active treatment is deemed appropriate. Blood transfusions are used to maintain adequate haemoglobin levels and platelet and coagulation abnormalities are corrected with platelet, fresh frozen plasma, or prothrombin complex concentrate infusions.

Endoscopy can be used as both a diagnostic and therapeutic procedure. GI bleeding originating from relatively immobile structures, such as the rectum or the oesophagus, can be effectively controlled in many instances with palliative radiotherapy. Palliative surgery also has a role in removing a troublesome primary even in the presence of metastatic disease.

Intestinal obstruction

Aetiology

Intestinal obstruction in cancer patients can be mechanical or functional. Upper GI obstruction is usually mechanical in origin due to luminal involvement or compression by oesophagogastric or pancreatic neoplasms. Twenty-five per cent of patients with unresectable pancreatic tumours eventually develop gastroduodenal obstruction.

Mechanical small bowel obstruction can be due to non-malignant causes, such as adhesions, in up to 25–30% of cases. Although obstruction may result from primary small bowel tumours, it is more commonly due to peritoneal metastases from ovarian, gastric, or colorectal primaries. These three tumour sites account for approximately 75% of cases of malignant mechanical small bowel obstruction. Melanoma can cause luminal metastases with obstruction due to intussusception. Primary colorectal tumours account for the vast majority of mechanical large bowel obstruction.

Constipation is a common cause of non-mechanical obstruction. It can be secondary to chemotherapeutic agents such as vincristine, medications such as opioids, anticholinergics and HT_3 antagonists, or dehydration and electrolyte abnormalities such as hypercalcaemia.

Other causes of bowel obstruction include late radiation enteritis with stricture formation which predominantly affects the small bowel, and autonomic denervation by the tumour (Ogilvie's syndrome) (Schwartzentruber et al. 2006)

Clinical features

Upper GI obstruction at the level of the pylorus presents with large volume projectile vomiting soon after eating. Typically bile is absent and in complete obstruction severe dehydration ensues. A succussion splash may be elicited.

Mechanical small bowel obstruction presents with colicky abdominal pain and tenderness, vomiting, constipation, and abdominal distention. Bowel sounds are characteristically high-pitched and hyperactive. Paralytic ileus is associated with diffuse, and typically non-colicky, pain as well as absent bowel sounds. Large bowel obstruction produces similar symptoms and signs, although they tend to develop more gradually. Vomiting can be faeculent and an obstructing colonic primary may be palpable. Complete bowel obstruction results in an empty rectum on rectal examination.

Dianosis

Plain abdominal radiographs are usually the first investigation in suspected bowel obstruction. They can show dilated small or large bowel loops and any associated constipation. CT of the abdomen can provide additional diagnostic information, especially if the aetiology is unclear or surgical intervention is planned. CT was more sensitive and specific than plain radiographs in diagnosing intestinal obstruction in a small study involving 32 patients (Suri et al. 1999).

Barium follow-through or enema studies are also useful in determining the level of obstruction. It should be noted, however, that barium studies are absolutely contraindicated if there is suspicion of perforation.

Treatment

Treatment depends on the level of obstruction and the general condition of the patient. As a rule, patients with bowel obstruction are dehydrated and hence intravenous fluid administration is indicated.

Nasogastric tube placement can help decompress the stomach in upper GI obstruction. Resectable tumours are best managed by definitive surgery. Palliative procedures can include endoscopic stent placement, gastroduodenal bypass, or feeding tube placement.

Small bowel obstruction often resolves with conservative management. Surgical intervention is usually impossible due to the presence of extensive abdominal disease and multiple levels of obstruction, but should be considered if a single level of obstruction is present or for adhesiolysis. In contrast to small bowel obstruction, mechanical large bowel obstruction rarely resolves spontaneously and tumour resection or decompressive surgery is indicated.

Conservative management aims to alleviate pain, nausea and vomiting, decrease bowel secretions, and increase bowel motility if constipation is the precipitant. Medications are preferably administered intravenously, subcutaneously or per rectum, as oral absorption is generally impaired.

Buscopan or hyoscine butylbromide via a subcutaneous syringe driver are useful for alleviating colic; opioids can be added if pain control is unsatisfactory. The choice of antiemetic depends on the presence or not of colic and complete bowel obstruction. If they are present, cyclizine or haloperidol is the antiemetic agent of choice. For partial bowel obstruction without colic, a prokinetic agent such as metoclopramide is useful.

Octreotide reduces bowel secretions and has been shown in randomized trials to provide superior symptom relief in inoperable bowel obstruction. Although corticosteroids (e.g. dexamethasone 4–16mg/day) are frequently prescribed to reduce bowel wall oedema, the evidence regarding their efficacy is limited.

In most cases the agents discussed here need to be used in various combinations to provide adequate symptomatic relief. Laxatives are added in cases of incomplete bowel obstruction and constipation.

Further reading

Schwartzentruber D, Lublin M, Hostetter R. Bowel obstruction. In: Berger A, Shuster A, Von Roenn A (eds) *Palliative Care and Supportive Oncology* 3rd edition, pp. 177–85. Philadelphia, PA: Lippincott Williams & Wilkins, 2006.

Suri S, Gupta S, Sudhakar PJ, *et al*. Comparative evaluation of plain films, ultrasound and CT in the diagnosis of intestinal obstruction. *Acta Radiol* 1999; **40**:422–8.

Genitourinary bleeding

Aetiology

Genitourinary bleeding can be a manifestation of malignancy. Eighty per cent of bladder cancers present with painless gross haematuria. Postmenopausal vaginal bleeding is the commonest presenting feature of endometrial malignancy. Vaginal bleeding can also result from other malignancies such as cervical cancer and rarer malignancies such as invasive trophoblastic disease.

In addition, oncology patients can develop haemorrhagic cystitis as a result of infection or treatment. Those undergoing chemotherapy are more prone to develop infective interstitial cystitis. Haemorrhagic cystitis can become a dose-limiting toxicity when giving cyclophosphamide or ifosfamide chemotherapy and is particularly noted in the paediatric population. Acrolein, a metabolite of these nitrogen mustard-derived alkylating agents, is toxic to the urothelium.

Pelvic radiotherapy can also cause acute haemorrhagic cystitis after treatment, but symptoms can develop up to months and years later. End arteritis results in mucosal ischaemia, ulceration, and bleeding.

Alternatively, genitourinary bleeding in an oncology patient can be a reflection of bone marrow depression or dysfunction and a bleeding diathesis as a result of the primary disease or of treatment.

Clinical features

Painless gross haematuria is the commonest presentation of bladder carcinoma. The haematuria can be complicated by clot retention and urinary incontinence. Haemorrhagic cystitis presents with symptoms of bladder irritation such as urgency, frequency, dysuria, and suprapubic discomfort. There can be microscopic or gross haematuria.

Postmenopausal bleeding due to endometrial malignancy is painless and is often the only symptom. Unlike bladder carcinoma, however, only about 20% of postmenopausal bleeding represents uterine cancer. Cervical malignancy typically causes postcoital bleeding which may be accompanied by vaginal discomfort and abnormal vaginal discharge.

Diagnosis

The method of diagnosis is dependent on the suspected cause of bleeding. All patients should have blood counts, clotting screens, and renal function evaluated. Cystoscopy is the key investigation for suspected bladder carcinoma but it contributes very little to the management of haemorrhagic cystitis. All patients with haematuria should also have a renal and urinary tract ultrasound unless there is a clear precipitant, for example, recent cyclophosphamide therapy. If infective haemorrhagic cystitis is suspected, urine cultures are indicated.

Suspected endometrial carcinoma is diagnosed by hysteroscopy and endometrial biopsy. Cervical carcinoma is evident on cervical smear samples and colposcopy and endocervical biopsy. For evaluation of more widespread cervical or endometrial disease, pelvic MRI, PET scan, or staging CT is appropriate.

Treatment

Treatment is dependent on the severity of genitourinary haemorrhage. Significant bleeding must be treated with fluids, packed cells, platelets, and clotting factors as required to stabilize the patient. Large volume frank haematuria and clot retention can be treated with three-way large-bore catheterization and irrigation. Intravenous hydration also helps to prevent clots reforming. If the haematuria persists, cystoscopy with diathermy of identified bleeding points can be helpful. Diffuse haemorrhage may be stopped by injecting intravesical therapy such as prostaglandins, alum, or 1% silver nitrate whilst closely monitoring renal function. Intravesical formalin is reserved for severe haemorrhagic cystitis. Intractable haematuria may require surgical intervention.

Prophylactic treatment to prevent haemorrhagic cystitis as a result of cyclophosphamide therapy is recommended. Mesna is a compound that binds the acrolein metabolite of cyclophosphamide and its related compounds, thus reducing their urotoxicity. It is routinely administered with cyclophosphamide therapy. Pentosan polysulfate sodium is also known to decrease the risk of haemorrhagic cystitis, though its mechanism is less clear.

Vaginal bleeding is usually less profuse and so can be conservatively managed. As with haematuria, all patients should have blood counts, clotting screens, and renal function evaluated. Treatment is often definitive treatment of the underlying cause. Bleeding in advanced disease where the aim is palliation can be treated with pelvic radiotherapy.

Urinary tract obstruction

Aetiology

Urinary tract obstruction can occur in the cancer patient for a variety of reasons, ranging from the underlying primary disease or complications of treatment to unrelated benign prostatic disease.

Advancing pelvic or abdominal malignancy causes obstruction via direct invasion or extrinsic compression of the ureters. Cervical, colorectal, or prostatic cancer can locally invade the urinary tract whilst retroperitoneal malignancies such as sarcoma encroach on the ureters from the outside. Malignant abdominal lymphadenopathy can also extrinsically compress the ureters. Previous pelvic radiotherapy can contribute to retroperitoneal fibrosis and induce urethral strictures.

Ureteral obstruction secondary to malignancy confers a poor prognosis, with a median survival of 3–7 months. This therefore must be taken into account when exploring treatment options.

Clinical features

Urinary tract obstruction secondary to malignancy often has a much more insidious presentation than the acute urinary obstruction that occurs with urinary tract infection or benign prostatic hypertrophy. Patients may present with obstruction of only one ureter and gradually deteriorating renal function. Symptoms are vague such as lethargy, nausea, vomiting, and abdominal or flank discomfort. If the obstruction develops more rapidly, patients may present with considerable abdominal distension and discomfort accompanied by nausea. In some cases, symptoms of superadded urinary tract infection may be the only indication of underlying obstruction.

Diagnosis

Localization of the obstruction and the resulting dilatation of the proximal urinary tract can be well documented by ultrasound. More detailed imaging of the abdomen and pelvis by CT or MRI will illustrate the cause of the obstruction and the extent of underlying malignant disease. Urine microscopy and culture will accurately diagnose any urinary tract infection. It is important that renal function is also considered as this may alter subsequent management.

Treatment

The variable success of the management options available to those with urinary tract obstruction secondary to malignancy, along with the poor prognosis that it entails, makes it imperative that the management of the condition is tailored to the individual patient and the underlying diagnosis.

Decompression of ureteral obstruction is necessary to prevent hydronephrosis, renal failure, and urinary tract infections. It can be achieved using retrograde or anterograde techniques. Endoscopic insertion of an indwelling stent is usually more successful for intrinsic ureteral blockages such as strictures than for extrinsic ureteral compression, particularly in the presence of hydronephrosis. Studies have shown that stent insertion can work better for some types of malignancy, such as bladder and cervical cancer, and less well for others, such as colorectal cancer. Stent failure is attributed to ureteral peristaltic dysfunction, irritation of the urothelium, and stent encrustation. Ureteral obstruction at the pelvic brim and direct invasion of the urothelium at the time of stent placement are highly predictive of stent failure. Drug-eluting stents and stents made of stronger materials to better resist extrinsic compression are being developed to provide further interventional options.

Anterograde relief of ureteral obstruction by percutaneous nephrostomy is an alternative method of treating urinary tract obstruction. This method also has variable success with patients experiencing problems with recurrent urinary tract infections, tube dislodgement, and readmission to hospital. Nephrostomies can be well suited to some patient groups, however, such as those with intractable flank pain that benefit from renal decompression and those who can be removed from haemodialysis as a result of nephrostomy insertion. Patients with urethral stents often report ongoing lower urinary tract symptoms and even if the stent is a success, it requires changing at intervals. Studies have shown, however, that there is no significant statistical difference in quality of life between ureteral stent insertion and percutaneous nephrostomy.

Medical therapy may also add symptomatic relief in the treatment of obstruction. The role of prostaglandins, angiotensin II, and calcium channel blockers in urothelial spasm is currently being investigated. Transdermal oxybutynin has few systemic anticholinergic side effects but can help relieve lower urinary tract symptoms. Analgesia remains an important part of symptom control regardless of whether any mechanical intervention takes place.

Further reading

Kouba E, Wallen EM, Pruthi RS. Management of ureteral obstruction due to advanced malignancy: optimizing therapeutic and palliative outcomes. *J Urol* 2008; **180**(2):444–50.

Wolf S Jr. The undoing of ureteral obstruction from malignancy—who and how? *J Urol* 2008; **180**(2):435–6.

Impending and pathological fractures

Aetiology

Metastatic disease in the skeleton causes a wide range of clinical presentations ranging from bone pain and hypercalcaemia to pathological fractures and spinal cord compression.

The destruction of the cortex is mediated by humoral and paracrine substances secreted by the metastatic deposit as well as the direct effect of skeletal metastasis. Osteoclast activity and bone turnover are greatly increased. Once >50% of the cortex has been destroyed, there is an 80% chance of pathological fracture especially if the lesion is lytic and in a weight-bearing bone. The commonest sites of pathological fracture are the ribs and the vertebrae.

The commonest solid cancers that metastasize to bone are breast and prostate, with around 70% of patients showing evidence of bony involvement at postmortem. Renal, thyroid, and lung cancer also commonly present with skeletal disease. Lytic skeletal destruction is common in myeloma.

Clinical features

Both impending and completed pathological fractures can present with bone pain at the site of the fracture. A number of pain syndromes can also occur depending on the site of cortical destruction, for example, neuralgia and headache secondary to base of skull metastases.

Hypercalcaemia is present in 10–15% of patients with metastatic skeletal deposits. This is often as a result of bone destruction. The hypercalcaemia is further exacerbated by humoral factors secreted by the tumour cells such as PTHrP, intact parathyroid hormone, and rarely 1-α hydroxylase. PTHrP secretion has been noted in renal cell carcinoma, squamous cell carcinoma, breast adenocarcinoma, bladder carcinoma, and more rarely in melanoma and pancreatic neuroendocrine tumours. It contributes to hypercalcaemia by increasing calcium reabsorption from the renal tubules.

Hypercalcaemia can present with vague symptoms such as constipation, fatigue, muscle aches, and anorexia. Confusion, nausea, and vomiting can develop, and at its most extreme hypercalcaemia can cause renal failure, coma, and cardiac arrhythmias.

Pathological fractures can also present with symptoms of spinal cord or conus medullaris compression due to vertebral fracture. Spinal metastases are most common in the thoracic region, followed by the lumbar region, with cervical spine involvement being uncommon. Spinal cord compression most commonly presents with motor weakness or paralysis. Bone pain over the site of the fracture is also very common and is characteristically worse at night or with increase in intradural pressure, e.g. when coughing. Sensory symptoms distal to the level of the lesion develop later as do autonomic symptoms. In comparison, autonomic manifestations appear much earlier with in conus medullaris compression.

Diagnosis

The likelihood of pathological fracture increases with the proportion of cortical destruction. Plain radiographs of the affected bone can aid diagnosis of a metastatic deposit but alone are an unreliable guide to the probability of pathological fracture and as an indication of the optimal timing of intervention. The recommended scoring system is Mirels' scoring system for metastatic bone disease (Table 5.22.1) which encompasses the site and type of lesion, the severity of symptoms and the maximum degree of cortical damage.

The rate of cortical destruction and bone resorption by osteoclasts can also be measured in other ways that have been shown to predict morbidity. Markers such as the bone resorption marker n-telopeptide of type 1 collagen (NTX) are under development as markers of the extent of metastatic bone disease, the probability of pathological fracture, and as a guide to timing intervention.

Diagnosis of spinal column compression is most accurately illustrated with MRI. This imaging modality also provides enough detail to plan spinal surgery and radiotherapy as appropriate.

Treatment

Survival with skeletal metastases carries a significantly better prognosis than with visceral metastases. Multiple trials have illustrated the significant improvement in morbidity with long-term bisphosphonate therapy, although few studies have evaluated the utility of bisphosphonates for metastatic cancers other than multiple myeloma, breast, and prostate cancer. Recent trials show that zolendronic acid is equally as effective as pamidronate. Ibandronate is also being studied as an alternative. There are no clear data to indicate when it is best to initiate bisphosphonate treatment, the most appropriate intervals between treatments, and the duration of treatment.

Hormone therapy is proven to be effective at prolonging survival in hormone-sensitive prostate cancer with skeletal metastases. Androgen deprivation using a GnRH agonist confers the same survival benefit as orchiectomy. Hormone therapy can be used in combination with other treatment options in these patients to minimise morbidity and mortality from skeletal disease.

External beam radiotherapy has been used to treat bone pain from metastatic skeletal disease for >50 years and a single-fraction of 8Gy remains the gold standard of treatment in the UK. It is as effective as multiple treatments for symptomatic relief, but whether retreatment is more frequently required after a single treatment rather than multiple treatments is yet to be ascertained. Other forms of radiotherapy, e.g. stereotactic and radioisotope treatment, are also being developed.

Surgery for both impending and pathological fractures is also an important part of the management of skeletal disease. Patients with a Mirels score of ≥8 should be

Table 5.22.1 Mirels' scoring system for metastatic bone disease

Variable	Score		
	1	2	3
Site	Upper limb	Lower limb	Peritrochanteric
Pain	Mild	Moderate	Functional
Lesion	Blastic	Mixed	Lytic
Size*	<1/3	1/3–2/3	>2/3

*Indicates maximal cortical destruction as seen on plain X-ray in any view.

referred for prophylactic orthopaedic fixation. This may be even more pertinent for patients with primary tumours that are radioresistant, e.g. renal cell carcinoma and for patients with a primary tumour that suggests a longer life expectancy with skeletal metastasis than with other types of primary tumour, e.g. breast cancer. Recent guidelines recommend radical excision of solitary bone metastases in renal cell carcinoma.

Surgical repair of non-axial pathological fractures can be achieved by a variety of different methods that ensure stabilization and continuing function of the limb. Spinal surgery to repair pathological fractures, stabilize the spine, and restore neurological function in spinal cord compression has been shown to affect morbidity dramatically but no trial has reliably shown it to be preferential to radiotherapy as yet. Currently spinal surgery is reserved for those with neurological deficit of <24 hours, radioresistant tumours, progressive neurological deficit despite radiotherapy,

spinal instability secondary to fracture, and for those patients who have a life expectancy of ≥3 months.

Further reading

Bartels RH, van der Linden YM, van der Graaf WT. Spinal extradural metastasis: Review of current treatment options. *CA Cancer J Clin* 2008; **58**(4):245–59.

Body J. Breast cancer: bisphosphonate therapy for metastatic bone disease. *Clin Cancer Res* 2006;**12**(20 Pt 2):6258s–6263s.

Coleman R. Clinical features of metastatic bone disease and risk of skeletal morbidity. *Clin Cancer Res* 2006; **12**(20 Pt 2):6243s–6249s.

Tammela T. Endocrine treatment of prostate cancer. *J Steroid Biochem Mol Biol* 2004; 92(4):287–95.

Internet resource

British Orthopaedic Association: *Metastatic bone disease: a guide to good practice*—available at: http://www.boa.ac.uk

Special situations in oncology

Cancer in the elderly

Epidemiology
The incidence of cancer increases with increasing age, and in the UK a third of all cancers arise in those aged >75 years. In the USA, 60% of diagnoses and 70% of deaths from cancer occur in those aged >65. For a man aged 75, life expectancy is now 8.5 years, and for a woman 11.1 years so that long-term survival after successful cancer treatment may be obtained.

The profile of cancer types differs from those in the younger age group, where tumours such as those arising from germ cells are associated with a particularly good prognosis. The most prevalent cancers are those of breast, colon, prostate, and lung. There is some evidence that biologically favourable histological subtypes are more common in the elderly with breast cancer than in younger age groups and good treatment outcomes are therefore to be expected. However, access to treatment is poorer in this age group and treatment outcomes overall are significantly worse than in younger age groups. Many screening programmes have upper age limits which exclude most patients >65 years. The elderly cannot be considered as a homogeneous group, as there are very wide variations in health and function between people of the same age.

Factors affecting access to treatment
Many factors other than those relating to the cancer and its treatment alone may be significant in determining whether elderly patients receive the same treatment as those in the younger age group.

It is known that fewer diagnoses are made and less treatment undertaken in the elderly group than in younger patients although there is no clear evidence that outcome of treatment is affected by age per se.

A lower referral rate for treatment by primary care physicians may reflect concern about toxicity of any possible treatment or therapeutic nihilism. Problems with transportation, particularly in geographically isolated areas, may also restrict access to hospital treatment.

Social support is of critical importance. As many as 30% or more elderly cancer patients may live alone, and up to 40% do not have children living near enough to help them.

A study of mental attitudes in the elderly to cancer treatment have shown that some feel that treatment would not be worthwhile for them but that many are anxious to prolong good-quality life for as long as possible.

There is much evidence to show that entry to clinical trials improves outcomes, but there are very few trials which are open to those over the age of 65. There is therefore a relatively poor evidence base on which to make decisions about cancer treatment in the elderly, as well as less evidence of improvement in outcomes in recent years than in younger groups.

Concern about affordability for intensive treatment in this patient group is unlikely to influence individual decisions, but is likely to become more of an issue as this elderly population increases, and affordability of treatment by the individual may have to be considered with some healthcare systems.

Factors affecting choice of treatment
Comorbidities
Abnormalities of major organ function become increasingly common with age and may limit some of treatment options.

There is an age-related decline in renal function which may limit use of drugs excreted through the kidneys, and the fluid loading needed, for example, for treatment with cisplatin may not be possible in those with impaired cardiac function. Liver blood flow may be impaired, with low serum albumin levels and reduction in cytochrome P450, which is involved in metabolism of many chemotherapeutic agents. Polypharmacy may also alter the pharmacokinetics and dynamics of chemotherapeutic agents.

There is evidence of decrease in DNA mismatch repair processes in haemopoietic stem cells with increasing age, which may lead to the elderly experiencing more myelosuppression than in younger patients.

Impaired mobility and sensation or specific deficits, such as deafness, may make use of some drugs such as cisplatin inadvisable. Poor nutritional status may decrease the tolerability of some chemotherapy regimens and specific situations such as dementia, depression, and other illnesses may need to be taken into consideration. Consent may be difficult to obtain in a meaningful way. Movement disorders such as benign tremor or Parkinson's disease may make it difficult to maintain the precision of radiotherapy treatment. Kyphoscoliosis and other deformities may make it difficult for the patient to lie comfortably during treatment. Vascular disease and diabetes may lead to poorer outcomes of surgery and other cancer treatments, with delays in healing. The Karnofsky/ECOG scales for PS alone are not sensitive enough to be useful in this patient group and a Comprehensive Geriatric Assessment using a standard tool such as that devised by the Society of Geriatric Oncology is recommended. This considers many factors including age, ECOG status, independence for activities of daily living (self care), instrumental activities of daily living (independence in the community), social support, geriatric syndromes (osteoporosis, dementia, depression, falls), numbers of comorbidities, nutrition, and polypharmacy. Using such scales, treatment decisions are made on the basis of physiological rather than chronological age, remembering that there may be very considerable differences in treatment possibilities between patients of similar age.

Chemotherapy in the elderly
There is no direct evidence that chemotherapy is less effective in the treatment of cancer than in younger patients. Reduction in dose, however, may be unavoidable, because of poor haemopoietic tolerance, and this will certainly lead to reduced efficacy. Every attempt should be made to maintain drug intensity by using G-CSF support when appropriate although dose reductions may be necessary. Treatment with neurotoxic drugs may result in more neurotoxicity than expected if there are abnormalities before treatment starts. The Cockcroft formula (see Chapter 9.3, Glomerular filtration rate, p.701) which incorporates an age function should be used to estimate renal capacity. Doxorubicin is known to produce more cardiotoxicity in this age group and bleomycin more lung toxicity and these agents must therefore be used with care. Mucositis may be more marked and oral drugs such as capecitabine may be less well tolerated if there is a reduced healthy area of gut for absorption.

With time it is hoped that there will be more data from controlled trials in this age group to facilitate treatment decisions, and developments with new drugs such as biological agents, and use of biomarkers to individualize treatment may produce a more favourable toxicity/efficacy ratio.

Radiotherapy and surgery

Shortened recovery times following surgery, and improved healing rates may be achieved through the use of laparoscopic surgery which will also help to minimize the risk of complications such as venous thrombosis and embolism. The use of increasingly conformal radiotherapy may reduce normal tissue side effects with particular benefit in this group. However, the current schedules for radical radiotherapy extending over 4–6 weeks may pose particular problems for the very elderly because of fatigue and difficulty with transportation. Stereotactic body radiotherapy with hypofractionated radiotherapy regimens (e.g. lung cancer) is shorter and the available outcome results are favourable. The efficacy of single fraction radiotherapy treatments for palliation of troublesome symptoms means that few patients should be denied this approach.

Appropriate treatments for individual tumour types are discussed in articles in 'Further reading'.

In summary, treatment in this age group must be individualized on the basis of information about the likely biological behaviour of the tumour, taking account of the available treatments and any comorbid factors in the patient which would alter the cost–benefit ratio. In particular, attention should be paid to conducting trials of new agents and approaches which do not exclude this group in which cancer is commonest. Particular attention should be paid to prevention and early diagnosis of disease so that simpler treatment approaches such as limited surgery may be used.

Further reading

Ausili-Cefaro G, Olmi P. The role of radiotherapy in the management of elderly cancer patients in light of the GROG experience *Crit Rev Oncol/Hematol* 2001; **39**:313–17.

Balducci L. Supportive care in elderly cancer patients. *Curr Opin Oncol* 2009; **21**:310–17.

Balducci L, Colloca G, Cesari M, *et al.* Assessment and treatment of elderly patients with cancer. *Surg Oncol* 2010; **19**:117–123.

Extermann M, Hurria A. Comprehensive geriatric assessment for older patients with cancer. *J Clin Oncol* 2007; **25**:1824–31.

Jones R, Leonard RC. Treating elderly patients with breast cancer *Breast Cancer Online* 2005; **8**(4):e21.

Kristjansson SR, Farinella E, Gaskell S, *et al.* Surgical risk and postoperative complications in older unfit cancer patients. *Cancer Treat Rev* 2009; **35**:499–502.

Lichtman SM, Wildiers H, Chatelut E, *et al.* International Society of Geriatric Oncology Chemotherapy Taskforce: evaluation of chemotherapy in older patients—an analysis of the medical literature. *J Clin Oncol* 2007; **25**:1832–43.

Pallis A.G, Gridelli C, van Meerbeeck JP, *et al.* EORTC Elderly Task Force and Lung Cancer Group and International Society for Geriatric Oncology (SIOG) experts' opinion for the treatment of non-small-cell lung cancer in an elderly population. *Ann Oncol* 2010; **21**(4):692–706.

Papamichael D, Audisio R, Horiot J-C, *et al.* Treatment of the elderly colorectal cancer patient: SIOG expert recommendations. *Ann Oncology* 2009; **20**:5–16.

Syrigos KN, Karachalios D, Karapanagiotou EM, *et al.* Head and neck cancer in the elderly: An overview on the treatment modalities. *Cancer Treat Rev* 2009; **35**:237–45.

Wildiers H. Mastering chemotherapy dose reduction in elderly cancer patients 2007; *Eur J Cancer* **43**:2235–41.

Internet resource

International Society of Geriatric Oncology: http://www.siog.org

Cancer in pregnant women

Epidemiology
The incidence of pregnancy-associated cancer is low, complicating 1:1000 gestations. However, the tendency to delay pregnancy to later reproductive age as well as the age-dependent increase in the incidence of malignancy are likely to result in higher incidences of gestational cancer in the next decades. Cancer is the second leading cause of death among women of reproductive age in Western countries. The diagnosis of cancer during pregnancy poses challenging dilemmas for patient, family, and physicians. Invasive carcinomas of the uterine cervix, breast, and melanomas are the malignancies most commonly encountered during pregnancy, followed by lymphomas, leukaemias, genitourinary, and GI tract cancers (Table 6.2.1).

The parameters that modulate the risk of development of cancer during pregnancy are the genetic and environmental factors that define the risk of cancer in the age-matched general population. Hallmarks of pregnancy-associated cancer that are distinct from cancer affecting non-pregnant women are:
- Earlier diagnosis of cervical cancer due to frequent gynaecological examinations, and later diagnosis of most other solid tumours, mostly due to symptom/sign misinterpretation as physiological changes due to pregnancy.
- Frequent occurrence of poorly differentiated, HR-negative (HR-hormone receptor), HER2-overexpressing breast adenocarcinomas, occasionally with genetic background (BRCA1/2 mutations).
- Predominance of high-grade histology among gestational lymphomas.
- Uncommon metastatic spread seen for some malignancies (lymphomas, GI tract cancer).
- Predominance of rectal primaries in gestational colorectal cancer.

Interaction of pregnancy with cancer
Most available data show that pregnancy causes a diagnostic delay of 3–7 months, resulting in presentation of cancer at more advanced stages. However, pregnancy has not been associated with adverse maternal prognosis in comparison to non-pregnant patients when matched for stage and age. Only a few gestational melanoma series pointed to decreased maternal survival. Accordingly, current evidence does not establish a significant detrimental effect of pregnancy on the prognosis of cancer patients.

The impact of cancer on pregnancy varies with the stage, site, and bulk of tumour. Published cases show that birth of healthy infants is achieved in three-quarters of patients, with a small increase in the rate of still birth, low birth weight, premature delivery, and myelosuppression. Absolute indication for chemotherapy/abdominal radiotherapy administration during the first trimester, poor maternal life expectancy, poor maternal general condition due to metastatic disease, or presence of locally advanced invasive cervical cancer usually necessitate pregnancy termination and antineoplastic therapy. Metastases to placenta and fetus are extremely rare, malignant melanoma being the tumour most often responsible. Placental histological examination should always take place and in the presence of placental involvement, neonates should be considered high risk and be carefully monitored.

Modifications of investigations and treatment
Physical examination, including examination of the pelvis, rectum, skin, breasts, and lymph nodes, should be thorough. Most biopsy or cytological procedures can be safely performed during pregnancy under local anaesthesia, though the histopathologist should be informed about the presence of pregnancy in order to avoid false positive results. Foetal radiation exposure at doses >10–20cGy should be avoided, especially during the first trimester (organogenesis) and second trimester (continuing development of eyes, teeth, brain). Estimated foetal average doses per radiographic examinations are shown in Table 6.2.2. Radiographic and staging procedures should offer all necessary and relevant information for assigning a treatment plan while minimizing the risk of untoward effects for mother and foetus. CXR and ultrasound of thorax, abdomen/pelvis, and breasts are safe to perform. MRI of the brain, or abdomen/pelvis is both sensitive and safe, though gadolinium enhancement should be avoided during the first trimester. Radioisotope scans, abdominopelvic CT and 18-FDG-PET scans should be avoided. With modern surgical and anaesthetic techniques, surgery can be safely performed throughout pregnancy, with only a slight increase of the risk of foetal loss (3–10%) seen for abdominal operations during the first trimester. Oesophagogastroscopy, bronchoscopy, lumbar puncture and bone marrow aspiration/biopsy are

Table 6.2.1 Cancer incidence in pregnancy

Malignancy	Incidence per 100,000 pregnancies
Cervical cancer	10–1000
Breast cancer	10–40
Melanoma	15–100
Lymphomas	10–50
Leukaemias	1–2
Gastrointestinal cancer	5–10
Ovarian cancer	1–10

Table 6.2.2 Estimated average foetal dose per radiographic examination

CXR	<0.005mGy
Abdominal/pelvic X-ray	2–2.5mGy
Chest CT	0.2mGy
Abdominal CT	20mGy
Mammography	0.1–1mGy
Thoracic spine X-ray	0.1mGy
Lumbar spine X-ray	2–7mGy
Barium enema	9mGy
Head X-ray	<0.005mGy
Bone scan	2–5mGy

quite safe and should be done when clinically indicated, with appropriate caution to avoid excessive use of intravenous sedatives and opioids drugs. Pulse oximetry monitoring should be implemented to avoid maternal/fetal hypoxia.

Radiation exposure during organogenesis (weeks 2–8) can cause abortion or congenital malformations at a threshold dose of 10cGy, while during weeks 8–25 it may result in mental retardation above doses of 10–20cGy. Moreover, prenatal radiation has been linked to second tumours during childhood or later adult life. However, radiation therapy is not absolutely contraindicated during pregnancy, if the distance of radiation fields from the uterus is such as to keep fetal exposure below 10–20cGy (e.g. of head, neck, extremities, and chest). This is especially true in the presence of medical/medical physics expertise or after the 25th week of pregnancy.

Pharmacokinetic effects of pregnancy on cytotoxic drugs are not known, but administration of chemotherapy seems to be feasible after the first trimester. Chemotherapy during the first trimester has been associated with a 17–25% risk of malformations or foetal death and should be avoided. Absolute indication for chemotherapeutic treatment during the first trimester usually necessitates pregnancy termination. Antimetabolites and alkylators seem to have the most potent teratogenic effect, while vinca alkaloids, anthracyclines, and cyclophosphamide have been less often incriminated in causing malformations. Chemotherapy may be administered during the second and third trimesters relatively safely, with a 5–7% incidence of intrauterine growth retardation, premature delivery, or myelosuppression and a 3–5% incidence of foetal death. After administration of chemotherapy, postponement of delivery for 2–3 weeks allows for placental drug elimination from the foetus and resolution of maternal and foetal myelosuppression. There are no data on the impact of novel targeted therapies (small molecule inhibitors, antibodies) on pregnancy. Current evidence does not seem to show increased risk of neurocognitive disorders, second cancers, sexual malfunction, or impaired reproductive ability in humans exposed to chemotherapy *in utero*. Cancer chemotherapy is incompatible with breastfeeding.

Specific cancer management

Cervical cancer

The majority of pregnant patients are asymptomatic, diagnosed by abnormal cytology at early stages of disease (80% IA–IIA). Atypical cytological findings are common during pregnancy and should be interpreted with caution. Colposcopic examination with biopsy of suspicious lesions should be performed when cervical pathology is suspected. Conization, or loop excision, is associated with increased risks of bleeding, abortion, premature delivery, and residual disease. Cervical intraepithelial neoplasia is safe to manage with follow-up by means of cytology and colposcopy until delivery. Radical treatment of invasive cervical cancer cannot be performed with preservation of foetal life. Second- or third-trimester pregnant patients with stage IA disease may be amenable to treatment deferral until delivery, followed by radical hysterectomy. For patients in the first or second trimester of pregnancy and invasive cervical cancer (stage IB–IVA), pregnancy termination and immediate institution of therapy is traditionally advised. Third-trimester pregnant patients with invasive disease may opt for deferral of therapy and week 32–36 delivery, as retrospective case series did not show an adverse impact on prognosis.

In such a setting, neoadjuvant chemotherapy for stage IB–IVA disease may be given during the second and third trimesters of pregnancy so as to buy time for delivery of a viable fetus and enable postpartum radical treatment.

Breast cancer

In contrast to other tumours, gestational breast cancer is defined as a tumour diagnosed during pregnancy and up to 12 months postpartum. Delayed diagnosis ranges from 2–15 months and may be seen in up to 78% of pregnant patients who develop breast tumours. FNA or core-needle biopsy and in dubious cases, an open surgical biopsy, establish the diagnosis. For lactating women, stopping milk production with ice packs, breast binding, and bromocryptine 1 week prior to biopsy reduces the risk of haematoma and fistula. The majority of tumours are high-grade malignancies, with axillary nodal involvement seen in 60–90% and hormone-negative status in 40–70% of pregnant patients. Recent data suggest that pregnancy does not modify the natural course of breast cancer, nor does it adversely affect patient outcome, despite high circulating oestrogen levels. Modified radical mastectomy with axillary node dissection is the treatment of choice for patients with stage I–II and selected stage III breast cancer patients during the first two trimesters of pregnancy. Patients with localized disease diagnosed in the third trimester may be managed with breast-conserving surgery and postpartum breast irradiation. Patients in need of adjuvant chemotherapy can relatively safely have it administered after the first trimester. CMF or anthracycline-based regimens (AC, CAF) have been administered with only 1.3% risk of malformations after week 12. The administration of hormonal therapy and trastuzumab should be avoided throughout gestation. Patients with metastatic disease may be managed preferably with palliative combination chemotherapy (AC, CAF) rather than newer agents (taxanes, vinorelbine) beyond the first trimester of pregnancy.

Melanoma

A diagnostic delay has been demonstrated in several reviews, resulting in disease presentation with thicker primary lesions and nodal metastases, without any difference observed in site, ulceration, vascular invasion, or distant spread. Excisional biopsy is warranted for diagnosis and assessment of risk factors with thorough physical examination and laboratory work-up. Superficial spreading melanoma accounts for 74% of gestational cases, followed by nodular melanoma (16%). Wide surgical excision with 1–3-cm margins according to the thickness of the primary is the treatment of choice for localized melanomas. Regional lymphadenectomy of involved nodes should be performed and although interferon has been safely administered in pregnant women with viral hepatitis, myeloma, and haematological disorders, adjuvant regimens for resected high-risk melanoma employ higher doses and should be avoided. Management of metastatic melanoma is at best palliative.

Lymphomas

The median age of pregnant patients at diagnosis of Hodgkin disease (HD) is 32 years, while that of patients with non-Hodgkin lymphomas (NHL) is 37–42. Recent data show that stage I–II HD at presentation is seen in 70% of both pregnant and non-pregnant women; there is no diagnostic delay during gestation. In contrast, pregnant women present with stage III–IV NHL in 70–80% of cases, with >40% experiencing a diagnostic delay >30 days. Combination chemotherapy is imperative as most HD and NHL patients need treatment with curative intent. When the diagnosis is made in the first trimester, pregnancy termination with prompt institution of chemotherapy is advisable, especially in the presence of B symptoms, bulky stage I–II disease, advanced stage III–IV disease, or evidence of fulminant course of the lymphoma. In the absence of these or upon refusal of abortion by the mother, single-agent vinblastine may be given or treatment may be deferred until the second trimester. During the second and third trimesters, the relative safety of chemotherapy administration has been demonstrated in several retrospective series, for both mother and foetus. ABVD is preferred for HD and CHOP for most high-grade NHL in pregnant women. Alternatively, third trimester pregnant patients may be managed expectantly with 32–35th week delivery and postpartum chemotherapy.

Limited-field supradiaphragmatic radiotherapy has been advocated for stage IA lymphocyte predominant HD, but most physicians would defer any ionizing radiation therapy until after delivery. Rituximab administration during pregnancy is not advised due to lack of safety data. The rare patients with low-grade lymphomas may be managed expectantly, receive second or third trimester single-agent chemotherapy or limited-field radiotherapy, according to preferences and expertise.

Further reading

Aviles A, Neri N. Hematological malignancies and pregnancy: a final report of 84 children who received chemotherapy in utero. *Clin Lymphoma* 2001; **2**(3):173–7.

Cardonick E, Iacobucci A. Use of chemotherapy during human pregnancy. *Lancet Oncol* 2004; **5**:283–91.

Garel C, Brisse H, Sebag G, et al. Magnetic resonance imaging of the foetus. *Pediatr Radiol* 1998; **28**:201–11.

Kal HB, Struikmans H. Radiotherapy during pregnancy: fact and fiction. *Lancet Oncol* 2005; **6**:328–33.

Pavlidis NA, Pentheroudakis G. The pregnant mother with breast cancer: Diagnostic and therapeutic management. *Cancer Treat Rev* 2005; **31**(6):439–47.

Nicklas A, Baker M. Imaging strategies in pregnant cancer patients. *Semin Oncol* 2000; **27**:623–32.

Pentheroudakis G, Pavlidis N. Cancer and pregnancy: poena magna, not anymore. *Eur J Cancer* 2006; **42**:126–40.

Smith LH, Dalrymple JL, Leiserowitz GS, et al. Obstetrical deliveries associated with maternal malignancy in California, 1992 through 1997. *Am J Obstet Gynecol* 2001; **184**(7):1504–12.

Sadurai E, Smith LG. Hematologic malignancies during pregnancy. *Clin Obstet Gynecol* 1995; **38**:535–46.

Van Calsteren K, Vergote I, Amant F. Cervical neoplasia during pregnancy: Diagnosis, management and prognosis. *Best Pract Res Clin Obstet Gynecol* 2005; **5**:1–20.

Internet resources

ESMO Clinical Recommendations on Cancer, Fertility and Pregnancy—available at http://www.esmo.org

Motherisk: http://www.motherisk.org

Fertility and cancer

Although the average age of a patient with cancer is >60 years, approximately 4% of cancers occur in those aged 15–40. These patients may still want to complete a family and yet their treatment could have a significant effect on their fertility. This section concerns the risks and strategies available for managing infertility related to cancer.

Significance

Infertility as a consequence of cancer or its treatment remains a significant issue for young people who have not yet completed their families. The risk depends on the gender of the patient and the type of therapy administered as well as the type of cancer. In the UK, guidelines have been developed by a working party to highlight possible management strategies and risks of infertility with different cancer treatments.

Overall the fertility of childhood cancer survivors when compared with their siblings is 0.76 for men and 0.93 for women. In a study which examined birth of children to those aged up to 35 years, the probability of fathering a child as a cancer survivor (63%) was similar to that of the general population (64%). Carrying a pregnancy to full term was, however, significantly different for female cancer survivors (66%) when compared with the general population (79%).

Patients require information about their risks of infertility, possible options, and risks to future pregnancy as part of their discussions about their cancer treatment. Some hospitals provide an acute fertility service linked to their oncology service.

Male infertility

Infertility in men commonly occurs after use of alkylating agents or radiotherapy to the gonadal region, or after total body irradiation for conditioning for stem cell transplant. For this reason, all men who are capable of producing sperm should be offered sperm banking. Sperm production is rarely effective under the age of 13 but semen should be examined if the patient is capable of ejaculation. Sperm aspiration may be considered for those unable to ejaculate.

Some men will retain or recover their fertility. This can occur up to 2 years after treatment is completed. It is possible to have semen reassessed for sperm production and quality.

Retrograde ejaculation can occur in men who have had bilateral retroperitoneal lymph node dissection.

Testosterone production may be impaired if the patient has received gonadal radiotherapy. This should be assessed after treatment is completed.

Female infertility

Premature ovarian failure can occur in response to pelvic (or spinal) radiotherapy or certain (but not all) chemotherapy agents. The risk of menopause is associated with the type of therapy rather than the type of cancer. The highest risk is for women aged between 21–25 years, who had infradiaphragmatic radiotherapy combined with alkylating agents. High-dose treatments (including total body irradiation) and alkylating agents will usually render a woman infertile. Even in those cases where fertility is preserved after treatment, the timing of the menopause is likely to be several years earlier than for their peers.

Some women do retain their fertility so it is important they continue contraception until a decision is made about future fertility or pregnancy.

Fibrosis of the uterus (often associated with impaired blood supply) can occur following pelvic radiotherapy and cause foetal growth restriction (<2.5kg birth weight), placental complications, and a greater risk of midterm miscarriage. Such pregnancies should be closely monitored with regular ultrasound.

Fertility-sparing surgery should now be considered (where possible) in ovarian germ cell tumours. In one study, 83% who had fertility-sparing surgery plus combination chemotherapy had restored menstrual function. Of 61 survivors who had fertility sparing surgery, 24 went on to have a total of 37 children between them. There were no increased risks of congenital abnormalities.

Female fertility strategies

Ovarian suppression with LHRH agonists such as goserelin acetate (Zoladex®) with HRT (for non-oestrogen-containing tumours) or hormonal treatment (for oestrogen-sensitive tumours) may preserve fertility for some women.

Frozen embryos can be stored but the woman needs to be able to defer her treatment for an *in vitro* fertilization (IVF) cycle and egg retrieval which may not be possible for some malignancies, e.g. acute leukaemias. For this option the woman needs to have a long-term partner and according to the current UK regulations, if the partner later withdraws consent, the embryos must be destroyed.

Oocyte removal after an IVF cycle has been tried but again requires the delay of an IVF cycle and is currently far less successful than a frozen embryo in producing a full-term pregnancy.

Freezing or vitrification (slow freezing) of an immature egg is now in development and has resulted in up to a 5% successful pregnancy rate in experienced centres.

Research has been undertaken in freezing a strip of ovary and there have been some case reports which suggest that this can be successful. However as some women retain their fertility despite intensive treatment and no fertility intervention, it is not possible to state whether these few cases are due to the implanted ovarian tissue.

Other options include surrogacy, egg donation, and adoption.

Risks for the offspring of survivors

Women are most concerned not only about retaining their fertility but also about possible risks to their future children of congenital abnormalities or cancer. Several large studies have shown no increased risks of congenital abnormalities after chemotherapy or radiotherapy nor of cancer in the offspring unless there is an underlying genetic predisposition e.g. Li–Fraumeni syndrome or retinoblastoma.

Timing of future pregnancy

Young women diagnosed with cancer will often ask when they can become pregnant and whether it will affect the risk of cancer returning. In general, patients are advised to wait at least 2 years from diagnosis (particularly breast cancer patients) as this represents the time within which recurrence is most likely. With the exception of high-risk (node positive, local recurrence, and >35 years) breast cancer there has been no increased incidence of breast cancer at the time of pregnancy. This has also been shown for melanoma.

Monitoring in future pregnancy

Ultrasound to monitor growth and placental blood flow is recommended for those who have had uterine radiation.

In those patients who received anthracyclines during treatment or mediastinal radiation, pregnancy may place an additional strain on cardiac output and cardiac assessment with an echocardiogram may be recommended before and during pregnancy.

Further reading

Byrne J, Rasmussen S, Steinhorn S, et al. Genetic disease in offspring of long-term survivors of childhood and adolescent cancer. *Am J Hum Genet* 1998; **62**:45–52.

Critchley H, Wallace W. Impact of cancer treatment on uterine function. *J Natl Cancer Inst Monogr* 2005; **34**:64–8.

Georgescu E, Goldberg J, du Plessis S, et al. Present and future fertility preservation strategies for female cancer patients. *Obst Gynaecol Surv* 2008; **63**:725–32.

Gershenson D, Miller A, Champion V, et al. Reproductive and sexual function after platinum-based chemotherapy in long-term ovarian germ cell survivors. *J Clin Oncol* 2007; **25**(19):2792–7.

Magelssen H, Melve K, Skjaeverven R, et al. Parental probability and pregnancy outcome in patients with a cancer diagnosis during adolescence and young adulthood. *Human Reprod* 2008; **23**:178–86.

Maltaris T, Beckmann MW, Dittrich R. Fertility preservation for young female cancer patients. *In Vivo* 2009, **23**:123–30.

Mulvihill J, Myers M, Connolley R, et al. Cancer in the offspring of long-term survivors of childhood and adolescent cancer. *Lancet* 1987; **2**:813–17.

Royal College of Radiologists, Royal College of Obstetricians and Gynaecologists, *The effects of cancer treatment on reproductive functions: guidance and management.* Report of a Working Party. London: RCP, 2007.

Sonmezer M, Oktay K. Assisted reproduction and fertility preservation techniques in cancer patients. *Curr Opinion Endocrinol Diabetes Obes* 2008; **15**:514–22.

Velentgas P, Daling J, Malone K, et al. Pregnancy after breast carcinoma: outcomes and influence on mortality. *Cancer* 1999; **85**:2424–32.

Internet resource

The UK guidelines from The Royal College of Radiologists which include patient information are available at http://www.rcr.ac/publications.aspx?PageID=149&PublicationID=269

Late effects

The long-term effects of cancer can affect the medical, psychological, and social well-being of an individual and their carers. This section concerns the medical effects: infertility and other aspects of cancer survivorship are discussed elsewhere.

Medical late effects
Late effects are dependent upon the original cancer, its treatment, the family genetics, and the developmental stage of the individual when treated for cancer.

Lessons learned from paediatrics
The median age of diagnosis of cancer in the general population is 70 years but the most significant increase in survival rates in the past 30 years has been in the area of paediatric oncology. Many of these young people were treated in the context of a clinical trial and the initial survivorship data was gained from paediatric patients. The medical sequelae of cancer treatment as a child have profound consequences given the current average life expectancy. The medical consequences can include development of a second malignancy, infertility, and potential abnormalities within any organ system of the body. These are described in the rest of this section but it should be noted that current paediatric treatment regimens have been modified to minimize or prevent some of these medical sequelae, such as deafness or second malignancies.

Second malignancy
The risk of second malignancy is increased with the combination of chemotherapy and radiotherapy. The increased risk of breast cancer in patients treated with mantle radiotherapy for HD has led to the omission of radiotherapy in the majority of cases for these patients. In historical series the cumulative incidence of any second malignancy increased from 10.6% at 20 years to 26.3% at 30 years following treatment for HD.

In survivors of NHL, the overall risk of second malignancy was raised (RR 1.3). Specifically there was a significantly increased risk of leukaemia (RR 8.8, 95% CI 5.1–14.1) and lung cancer (RR 1.6, 95% CI 1.1–1.6) (Mudie 2006). The relative risk of second malignancy was greatest at younger age at time of diagnosis and decreased with older age at the time of treatment. The risk of leukaemia was associated with chemotherapy treatment, regardless of whether or not radiotherapy was given.

Lung cancer risk was associated with radiotherapy. The 15-year cumulative risk of a second malignancy was 11.2% overall, with the greatest number of cases with lung cancer (2.8%), leukaemia (1.5%), colorectal cancer (1.5%), and breast cancer (1.2%). The cumulative risk of second cancer was greater for men and was greater in patients who were treated at or after 50 years of age.

Infertility
Infertility as a consequence of cancer or its treatment remains a significant issue for young people who have not yet completed their families and is discussed in detail in Chapter 6, Fertility and cancer, p.608.

Osteoporosis and osteonecrosis
Bone growth is affected by steroids, given to support chemotherapy or as part of the regimen, and by chemotherapy or radiotherapy itself. Osteopenia occurs frequently at the end of treatment with combination chemotherapy and for some patients bone recovery will be permanently affected. An extreme example of this is in ER-positive breast cancer where patients may have chemotherapy followed by an aromatase inhibitor. The hormonal treatment compounds the osteoporotic effect of the chemotherapy and calcium supplementation or bisphosphonates may be required to prevent fractures.

Osteonecrosis is a known complication of treatment for leukaemia, lymphoma, or bone marrow transplantation and is thought to be due to high-dose steroids. It tends to occur most in weight-bearing bones. Arthroplasty of the hip joint may be required in up to 20% of patients with femoral head osteonecrosis. Given that many of these patients are young, the joints are likely to require further replacements throughout life.

Neurological toxicity
Neurological damage can occur either centrally to the brain itself or to the peripheral nerves depending on the tumour and treatment given. The risk of neurocognitive deficit is greatest amongst survivors of ALL and CNS tumours. Many of these patients are treated at a young age so the impact of neurocognitive impairment reduces their opportunities in further education or employment.

For those with CNS tumours, cranial radiotherapy is sometimes given in combination with chemotherapy which can produce combined peripheral and central neurological deficits.

The treatment of ALL previously used cranial radiotherapy to prevent or treat CNS disease but there has been a move towards using intrathecal methotrexate and high-dose chemotherapy to reduce neurocognitive impairment (Packer 2003).

Certain chemotherapeutic agents such as platins and vinca alkaloids are known to be neurotoxic. The risk is greater with increasing age, particularly over the age of 50, and unless specifically and carefully monitored during treatment, the damage may be permanent and debilitating.

Adult patients suffer greater neurological side effects and sequelae from cranial radiotherapy with neurotoxic chemotherapy. Alternative chemotherapy or biological therapies may reduce this in the future.

Cardiac toxicity
Cardiac toxicity can take several forms following treatment including cardiac failure, arrhythmias, and increased risk of myocardial infarction. The major risk factors are mediastinal or left chest wall radiotherapy, anthracyclines, and vincristine. Asymptomatic arrhythmias are common. Cardiac failure is associated with use of anthracyclines in children but occurs rarely in adults if total doses are restricted.

Children treated with anthracyclines have reduced left ventricular wall thickness and reduced left ventricular function which can continue to deteriorate many years after treatment. This can lead to congestive cardiac failure. Treatment with ACE inhibitors has been shown to improve left ventricular function in the short term but did not prove effective in symptomatic patients in the longer term (Lipschultz 2002).

In a British cohort study of survivors of HD compared with aged-matched controls, supradiaphragmatic radiotherapy, treatment before age 55, anthracyclines, and vincristine were all associated with an increased risk of death from myocardial infarction (standardized mortality ratio [SMR] of 2.5 overall) (Swerdlow 2007). The greatest risk was for those who received supradiaphragmatic radiotherapy with vincristine but no anthracyclines (SMR 14.8, 95% CI 4.8–34.5). The chemotherapy regimen with doxorubicin, bleomycin, vinblastine, and darcarbazine was associated with a SMR of 9.5 (95% CI 3.5–20.6).

A screening study of 294 HD survivors who had received at least 35Gy radiotherapy to the mediastinum showed that 21.4% had abnormal left ventricular function at rest and 14% developed perfusion defects on scintigraphy during physical stress. Almost 10% of the patients had had a myocardial infarction during a median follow up of 6.5 years and two patients had died as a result. Of the 40 patients who underwent angiography as a result of the screening, 55% had significant coronary artery stenosis, 22.5% had <50% stenosis, and the remainder had no stenosis (Heidenreich 2007).

Pulmonary toxicity
Long-term pulmonary toxicities include fibrosis (from radiotherapy or bleomycin), pneumonitis (radiotherapy, gemcitabine), asymptomatic abnormalities of lung function tests (radiotherapy and combination chemotherapy), or lung cancer (especially after radiotherapy and chemotherapy). Patients given hemithorax radiotherapy for metastatic Wilms' tumours in childhood are at particular risk. The long-term consequences of asymptomatic lung function test abnormalities are currently unknown.

Endocrine toxicity
Endocrine abnormalities can occur in those who have received radiotherapy close to the pituitary or thyroid. Abnormalities do not occur immediately after treatment so they should be screened for starting at least 1 year post-treatment or earlier if there are symptoms. Abnormalities of gonadal dysfunction are discussed in Chapter 6, Fertility and cancer, p.608. Hormonal replacement may be necessary for these patients.

Chronic health conditions
In addition to specific toxicities, the overall health of an individual is likely to be affected after treatment for cancer. Chronic health conditions, especially for those who have complications of treatment graded as severe by common terminology criteria for adverse events (CTCAE), are significantly higher in survivors compared with siblings or controls. In a study of childhood survivors, chronic health conditions occurred in almost all patients, with 27.5% experiencing severe or life-threatening health effects. Multiple chronic conditions were also more frequent, with 37.6% experiencing at least two and 23.8% experiencing at least three significant comorbidities.

Follow-up
Many centres run late effects clinics to monitor for these and other sequelae of cancer treatment.

Causes of death after cancer treatment
The main cause of death following a diagnosis of cancer is the cancer itself even after surviving 5 years from diagnosis. This was confirmed in a childhood cancer survivor study of 20,227 patients who had survived 5 years from diagnosis (Mertens 2001). Overall the survivors had a 10.8 times excess mortality compared with age- and sex-matched controls. Sixty-seven per cent of deaths were due to recurrence. After recurrence, the greatest risk of death was from a second malignancy, followed by cardiac and then pulmonary problems. The SMR was 19.4 for second malignancy, 8.2 for cardiac death, and 9.2 for pulmonary death with other causes at 3.3. The risk of death was greatest for females, particularly those diagnosed before age 5 and those with an initial diagnosis of leukaemia or CNS tumour. Second malignancies reflect not only risks from treatments for cancer but also the underlying genetic make-up of the individual. Other risks, especially cardiac and pulmonary, reflect more closely the treatments given (as detailed in their respective chapter headings). It is hoped that many of the treatment-related complications may reduce as treatments are changed to try to minimize late effects. This is particularly the case in HD.

In patients treated for HD who do not relapse with their disease, second malignancy is the most common cause of death followed by cardiovascular disease. Fifteen years after diagnosis, 64% of deaths were from second malignancy and 21% from cardiac disease. Given the recent change in treatment to reduce mediastinal radiotherapy, both these side effects could be expected to reduce in the future.

Health behaviours
Since cancer survivors are at increased risk of second malignancy, cardiac, and other medical problems, it is important to encourage them to live a healthy lifestyle after treatment is completed. Smoking, exercise, and reducing risk-taking behaviours such as alcohol consumption or substance abuse all contribute to future health. A review of health behaviours of childhood cancer survivors (Clarke 2007) showed that they were less likely to be smokers or plan to take up smoking than their peers. Binge drinking and heavy drinking were lower in incidence than in age-matched controls. However, continued cancer screening, dental care, and follow-up clinics were attended less frequently than deemed optimal. Eating balanced meals and exercising for >1 hour a week occurred in approximately 75% of survivors. Education to minimize future health problems should be a priority in long-term survivorship care.

Treatment summaries and care plans
Many centres produce a treatment summary giving the doses of chemotherapy and radiotherapy administered during treatment and guidelines for further follow-up based on the risks not only of recurrence but also of secondary medical late effects.

Further reading
Clarke S-A and Eiser C. Health behaviours in childhood cancer survivors: A systematic review. *Eur J Cancer* 2007; **43**:1373–84.

Heidenreich P, Schnittger I, Strauss W, *et al.* Screening for coronary artery disease after mediastinal irradiation for Hodgkin's disease. *J Clin Oncol* 2007; **25**:43–9.

Lipschultz S, Lipsitz S, Sallan S, *et al.* Long-term enalapril therapy for left ventricular dysfunction in doxorubicin-treated survivors of childhood cancer. *J Clin Oncol* 2002; **20**:4517–22.

Mertens A, Yasui Y, Neglia J, *et al.* Late mortality in five-year survivors of childhood and adolescent cancer: The childhood cancer survivor study. *J Clin Oncol* 2001; **13**:3163–72.

Mudie N, Swerdlow A, Higgins C, et al. Risk of second malignancy after non-Hodgkin's lymphoma: A British cohort study. *J Clin Oncol* 2006; **24**:1568–74.

Packer R, Gurney J, Punyko J, et al. Long-term neurologic and neurosensory sequelae in adult survivors of a childhood brain tumour: childhood cancer survivor study. *J Clin Oncol* 2003; **21**:3255–61.

Swerdlow A, Higgins C, Smith P, et al. Myocardial infarction mortality risk after treatment for Hodgkin disease: a collaborative British cohort study. *J Natl Cancer Inst* 2007; **99**:206–14.

Internet resource

National Cancer Institute: SEER survival data—available at http://seer.cancer.gov/csr/1975_2005/

Cancer survivorship

The term cancer survivorship has many meanings depending on geography, job description, and whether you are a patient or a relative. In the context of this book it is meant to describe the medical, psychological, and social consequences of a diagnosis of cancer. The Lance Armstrong Foundation, which has been a major worldwide advocate for cancer patients, includes the time from diagnosis, recognizing that the diagnosis itself has significant consequences for the patient and their family.

In the UK the Cancer Reform Strategy included survivorship issues. In the USA the National Action Plan for Cancer Survivorship has been developed to tackle these issues in collaboration with the Lance Armstrong Foundation.

The long-term medical effects of cancer survivorship and their follow-up have been discussed elsewhere. This section concerns the psychological, social, and economic issues which can significantly contribute to a patient's quality of life after a diagnosis of cancer. It also touches on the effects on the immediate family.

Prevalence

In the UK the estimated numbers of people living after a cancer diagnosis range from 1–1.5 million. With increasing cancer incidence and survival it is thought that this will rise to represent 1.5–2.5% of the adult population.

In the USA, >11 million people were living with a diagnosis of cancer in 2004, representing about 4% of the population. The 5-year survival for children diagnosed with cancer is now 79% and for adult cancers is 64%.

The survival rates reflect not only the primary diagnosis but also the availability of healthcare provision, but are increasing in most areas of the world.

Lessons learned from paediatrics

Given the dependence of children upon their parents and the developmental needs of a growing child, some of their psychosocial survivorship issues are different from those of adults. In addition, the families of children treated for cancer are significantly affected and many parents of childhood survivors suffer long-lasting psychological and social consequences, even when the clinical outcome has been good.

Psychological consequences

Following a diagnosis with cancer, patients and their families make psychological adjustments to cope with the treatment and potential outcome. Stress is, not surprisingly, very common and occurs in >95% of patients. The majority of these will have anxiety and mild depression which may not require treatment. However, some will have more significant psychological symptoms and needs including depression, post-traumatic stress disorder (PTSD), suicidal ideation, and various psychoses.

Most psychological studies have been undertaken in patients with breast cancer, haematological malignancy, or childhood cancers. More recently those with colorectal cancer and prostate cancer have been included in such studies due to their improved survival. Men with prostate cancer are also undergoing androgen deprivation for many years even when the disease is advanced.

There is conflicting evidence about the impact of psychological well-being and its effect on outcome in breast cancer. A meta-analysis has, however, shown that stress-related psychosocial factors were associated with a worse prognosis in cancer patients (Chida 2008).

In breast cancer patients with stage IIA–IIIB disease, psychological intervention in addition to health assessment improved survival compared with health assessment alone (HR 0.44, p = 0.016) at a median of 11 years after diagnosis, even when known predictors of prognosis were taken into account (Anderson 2008).

In survivors of childhood cancer there is a greater degree of some aspects of psychological distress in the parents than in the patients themselves. Parents were more concerned about their child's health and thought more often of the cancer and its diagnosis than the patient.

PTSD has been described in survivors of childhood cancer and NHL specifically. The incidence varies from <5% to 80% depending on the type of cancer, age at diagnosis, and degree of PTSD. In one USA study of NHL survivors 10 years after diagnosis, only 8% fulfilled all criteria for PTSD, although 39% showed some signs of PTSD. PTSD was associated with treatment intensity, problems with employment or insurance, less social support, and negative appraisals of life threat (Smith 2008).

In survivors of childhood cancer, features of PTSD (intrusion, avoidance, and arousal) have been recorded in approximately up to 12% of parents >5 years following their child's diagnosis (Norberg 2005). These features occurred in up to 30% of parents within the first 3 months of diagnosis and fathers were as affected as mothers. Levels of anxiety and depression were also 1.8–2.01 times those of parents with healthy children even 5 years after diagnosis.

Suicidal ideation and previous attempts at suicide have been shown to be present in up to 12.8% of childhood cancer survivors (Recklitis 2006). Standardized mortality ratios for suicide deaths in cancer patients are in the order of 1.35–2.9 compared with the general population. Risk factors include male sex, older age, higher disease stage, poor prognosis, poor PS, alcoholism, other psychiatric illness, fatigue, pain, loss of function, and previous or family history of suicide attempts. Lack of family or social support also correlates with increased suicide risk.

Relationships

The long-term impact of a cancer diagnosis on the ability to form lasting relationships is of particular concern in those treated as young adults who have not yet formed strong bonds with a partner. On average, cancer survivors are less likely to be married and have a higher incidence of divorce than their peers but there is also more positive evidence. In one study of survivors after treatment for germ cell tumours, there were more single women among survivors than controls but the married survivors reported better relationships with their partners than their age-matched controls (Gershenson 2007; Monahan 2008).

Social consequences

On average, cancer survivors have a lower income than their age-matched controls. They are more likely to have difficulties obtaining life and health insurance or a mortgage after surviving cancer. In the USA, a significantly reduced proportion of cancer survivors have health insurance.

In the UK, cancer survivors are 1.4 times more likely to be unemployed than the general population and one in five survivors say that their working life deteriorated following the diagnosis of cancer. Doctors are poorly qualified to address these financial and social problems of their patients but they are being addressed now through the National Cancer Survivorship Initiative in the UK and the USA National Action Plan for Cancer Survivorship.

Further reading

Anderson B, Yang H, Farrar W, *et al.* Psychologic intervention improves survival for breast cancer patients. *Cancer* 2008; **113**:3450–8.

Chida Y, Hamer N, Wardle J, *et al.* Do stress-related psychosocial factors contribute to cancer incidence and survival? *Nat Clin Pract Oncol* 2008; **5**:466–75.

Earle C. Failing to plan is planning to fail: Improving the quality of care with survivorship care plans. *J Clin Oncol* 2006; **24**:5112–16.

Ganz P. *Cancer survivorship. Today and Tomorrow.* New York: Springer Press, 2007.

Gershenson D, Miller A, Champion V, *et al.* Reproductive and sexual function after platinum-based chemotherapy in long-term ovarian germ cell survivors. *J Clin Oncol* 2007; **25**(19):2792–7.

Monahan P, Champion V, Zhao Q, *et al.* Case-control comparison of quality of life in long-term ovarian germ cell tumour survivors. *J Psychosocial Oncol* 2008; **26**(3):19–42.

Norberg A, Boman K. Parent distress in childhood cancer: A comparative evaluation of posttraumatic stress symptoms, depression and anxiety. *Acta oncologica* 2005; **30**(1):99–113.

Recklitis C, Lockwood R, Rothwell M, *et al.* Suicidal ideation and attempts in adult survivors of childhood cancer. *J Clin Oncol* 2006; **24**:3852–7.

Rowland J. Foreward: Looking beyond cure: Pediatric cancer as a model. *J Pediatric Psychology* 2005; **30**(1):1–3.

Smith S, Zimmerman S, Williams C, *et al.* Post-traumatic stress outcomes in Non-Hodgkin's Lymphoma survivors. *J Clin Oncol* 2008; **26**:934–41.

Internet resources

The USA National Action Plan for Cancer Survivorship: http://www.cdc.gov/cancer/survivorship/pdf/plan.pdf

Lance Armstrong Foundation: http://www.livestrong.org/site/c.khLXK1PxHmF/b.2660611/k.BCED/Home.htm

The National Cancer Survivorship Initiative: http://www.macmillan.org.uk

National Cancer Institute: SEER survival data—available at http://seer.cancer.gov/csr/1975_2005/

Travel

For people who have cancer, travelling may raise a number of issues, such as whether they are fit to travel, how to get travel insurance, vaccinations, and other preventive measures, and getting help abroad if needed. This section aims to give an overview of the travel-associated issues for cancer patients.

Pre-travel preparation

The 'Yellow Book' from the Center for Disease Control and Prevention recommends that the pre-travel preparations of an immunosuppressed person must address the following concerns:

- The travellers need to contact their healthcare provider for an overall assessment of their medical condition, to assess whether their illness is stable, and to verify what drugs are needed and the correct doses.
- The doctor should assess whether the disease or its treatments contraindicate or decrease the effectiveness of any disease prevention measures such as vaccination, and malaria chemoprophylaxis recommended for the proposed travel.
- The doctor must consider whether any of the disease prevention measures present a risk for the underlying medical condition. Any specific health hazards at the destination that would be likely to exacerbate the underlying illness or be more severe in an immunocompromised traveller must be considered with any interventions which would mitigate such a risk.

All patients intending to travel are advised to have a medical consultation at least 4–8 weeks before to assess the need for any vaccination and/or malarial chemoprophylaxis as well as to order any other medical items the traveller may require. Patients who intend to be away for a long time may also need to think about regular appointments such as dental and gynaecological check-ups.

Issues associated with mode of travel

Air travel

The health problems of air travel are associated with hypoxia, gas expansion, cabin humidity, dehydration, motion sickness, exposure to infection, and risk of deep vein thrombosis (DVT). For people with cancer, air travel may normally be contraindicated in the following situations due to the effects of disease itself, treatment, or commonly associated medical comorbidities:

- When there are features of increased intracranial pressure.
- After recent surgery where trapped air or gas may be present—abdominal or GI surgery, craniofacial or ocular surgery, and brain surgery.
- If there is breathlessness at rest or unresolved pneumothorax.
- If the person has angina or chest pain at rest.

Fitness to air travel

Prolonged air flight can lead to an increased risk of oxygen desaturation due to the progressive fall in cabin PO_2 and acute mountain sickness, which usually occurs 6–18 hours after exposure to altitudes of >7000 feet (2130 metres). Hence a pre-flight assessment is necessary in cancer patients with respiratory or cardiovascular symptoms.

Lung cancer per se is not a contraindication to fly. People with a baseline SpO_2 >95% or SpO_2 of 92–95% with no risk factors (see later) do not require supplemental oxygen. However, those with SpO_2 92–95% with at least one risk factor need a proper evaluation to assess the need for supplemental oxygen during the flight. The risk factors include hypercapnia, FEV1 <50% predicted, lung cancer, restrictive lung disease involving the parenchyma (fibrosis,) abnormalities of the chest wall (kyphoscoliosis) or respiratory muscles, previous history of ventilator support, cerebrovascular or cardiac disease, discharge <6 weeks previously for an exacerbation of chronic lung or cardiac disease. Those with SpO_2 of <92% generally need in-flight oxygen supplementation.

One practical method to assess fitness to fly is to see whether the person can walk 50 yards/metres at a normal pace or climb one flight of stairs without severe dyspnoea. If this can be accomplished, it is likely that most people will tolerate the normal aircraft environment.

Another method is the hypoxic challenge test. It uses a oxygen–nitrogen mix to simulate the cabin environment. If it results in a PaO_2 of <55, medical oxygen is indicated.

A number of guidelines are available for assessment for fitness for air travel (see'Internet resources').

Deep vein thrombosis

Cancer patients have an increased risk of venous thromboembolism (VTE), and the risk is likely to increase further with air travel. Other risk factors for DVT include previous DVT or PE, history of DVT or PE in a close family member, and recent surgery or trauma particularly to the abdomen, pelvic region, or legs. Tamoxifen is also known to increase the risk of VTE.

The results of the WHO Research into Global Hazards of Travel (WRIGHT) study have shown that the risk of VTE approximately doubles after a long-haul flight (>4 hours). The risk increases with the duration of the travel and with multiple flights within a short period. However, the additional risk posed for cancer patients is unknown.

All cancer patients with active disease and/or with any of the other risk factors are advised to seek medical advice regarding prevention of DVT during air travel.

General measures such as avoiding dehydration, moving around the cabin during long flights to reduce the period of immobility (e.g. regular trips to the bathroom every 2–3 hours), calf muscle exercise (most airline cabin leaflets explain this), wearing loose and comfortable clothes and leg stockings can reduce the risk of thrombosis. It is also advised to avoid excessive alcohol or sleeping tablets. A recent systematic review suggested that travellers on flights of <6 hours and with no known risk factors may not need any DVT prophylaxis. However, patients with known risk factors and/or on flights of >6 hours need risk-based DVT prophylaxis.

There are no evidence-based guidelines on specific DVT prophylaxis. Current evidence suggests no benefit from prophylactic aspirin. In cancer patients with a history of DVT or PE or a perceived high risk of VTE, a single injection of low-molecular-weight heparin (enoxaparin 1000IU per 10kg of body weight) 2–4 hours before departure may be considered, especially for flights >4–6 hours.

Travel by sea

The most common health problems due to sea travel are respiratory tract infections, injuries, motion sickness, and GI illnesses. Outbreaks of infection can be a particular problem in immunosuppressed cancer patients.

Before travel it is important to get a letter from the treating physician detailing medical conditions, treatment, and prescription doses.

Specific measures include vaccinations, including influenza and destination-specific vaccinations and other prophylactic measures (e.g. malaria chemoprophylaxis)

Medical kit for a traveller

The medical kit should contain basic medicines to treatment common illnesses, first-aid articles, and other specific drugs and items (e.g. syringes) which the individual needs. A physician's letter stating the medical conditions and treatment, details of medications, and prescribed doses is necessary as it may be required to clear customs.

Disability and travel

Physical disability is not a contraindication for travel for an otherwise healthy person. Since there are specific airline regulations, necessary information should be obtained in advance and wheelchairs or other aids booked with the airport authority.

Patients who are unable to look after their own needs during the flight need an escort as the cabin crew is not permitted to provide such a service.

Further reading

Philbrick JT, Shumate R, Siadaty MS, *et al.* Air travel and venous thromboembolism: A systematic review *J Gen Intern Med* 2007 **22**:107.

Internet resources

General travel advice

British Foreign Office Safety Information for Travellers: http://www.fco.gov.uk/travel

Centers for Disease control and prevention: Yellow Book—available at http://wwwnc.cdc.gov/travel/

Frontier Medical: http://www.frontiermedical.co.uk/

Health Advice for Travellers from the UK Departments of Health: http://www.dh.gov.uk/PolicyAndGuidance/HealthAdviceForTravellers/fs/en

International Association for Assistance for Travellers: http://www.iamat.org/

International Society of Travel Medicine (ISTM): http://www.istm.org

Mobility International: http://www.miusa.org/

National Travel Health Network and Centre (NaTHNaC): http://www.nathnac.org/

Royal Society for the Prevention of Accidents: http://www.rospa.co.uk/

Travel Medicine and Vaccination Centres (TMVC) Australia: http://www.tmvc.com.au/

World Health Organization International Travel: http://www.who.int/ith/

Fitness to fly

British Thoracic Society: http://www.brit-thoracic.org.uk/

International Civil Aviation Organizations: http://icao.int

UK Civil Aviation Authority: http://www.caa.co.uk/docs/923/FitnessToFlyPDF_FitnesstoFlyPDF%20Feb%2009.pdf

Sea travel

International Council of Cruise Lines: http://www.iccl.org/policies/medical.cfm

International Maritime Health Association: http://www.imha.net/

Insurance

Travel insurance

Obtaining travel insurance with appropriate cover for cancer patients has become increasingly difficult. This may reflect the increasing cost of healthcare and the different standards of care worldwide. Cancer patients therefore have to shop around or get advice from an insurance broker (see 'Internet resources'). Several insurance companies have been established recently that specialize in offering insurance to cancer patients (see 'Internet resources'). However obtaining travel insurance, particularly during treatment, can be expensive or may not even be possible.

The cost of an insurance premium depends on the destination of travel and on the healthcare system of destination.

Reciprocal arrangements between countries

It is important to seek information on possible reciprocal healthcare arrangements between the country of residence and the destination country. To be eligible for treatment under such an arrangement, it is important to obtain the necessary documentation from the country of residence prior to travel. When a reciprocal arrangement does not exist, or does not cover all the possible health risks, it is important to obtain the necessary special insurance.

Residents of the UK travelling to the Europe can obtain a European Health Insurance card (see 'Internet resources') which covers any medical treatment due to an accident or illness within the European Economic Area and Switzerland. This also covers chronic or pre-existing illness treatments which would normally be covered by the state. However, the EHIC alone may not always be sufficient. The UK also has reciprocal healthcare arrangement with non-EEA countries details of which can be found on the NHS website (see 'Internet resources').

Life insurance and mortgages

Life insurance is usually needed to take out a mortgage. Cancer survivors, especially children and young adults, can be in a difficult position due to either refused insurance cover or an offer of insurance under specific conditions. Most often it also involves paying a high premium.

Approaching a large insurance company or an independent financial advisor can be useful in finding appropriate life insurance cover. Every case will be considered individually based on the prior cancer, its treatment, and the time elapsed since treatment.

Driving and car insurance

Most cancer patients can continue to drive without any problem. In the UK, the Driver and Vehicle Licensing Authority (DVLA) should be notified in the following situations:
• Tumours of the CNS
• Treatment or weakness preventing normal daily activities
• Medications which are likely to affect safe driving

In these situations, patients are advised not drive with immediate effect and to inform the DVLA, who will then send the patient a medical questionnaire and get relevant information from the doctor, if necessary, before making a decision about fitness to drive.

Car and motor cycle

In patients with brain tumours, depending on the grade and treatment, the following driving restrictions may apply:
• Benign tumours: can drive after recovery.
• Grade 1–2 tumours: 1 year off driving from the date of completion of treatment.
• Grade 3–4 and metastatic brain tumour: 2 years off driving after treatment.
• Completely excised solitary metastasis: may be considered for licensing 1 year after completion of treatment provided there is no evidence of local or systemic spread.
• In patients who suffer fits as part of their illness, 2 years free from fits (with or without medication) must pass before driving can be resumed.

Large goods vehicle and passenger carrying vehicle

Diagnosis of a brain tumour, except of a benign tumour leads to a permanent refusal or revocation of a licence to drive in the UK. Permission to drive after treatment of a benign tumour is made after individual assessment.

Motor insurance

Insurance companies cannot refuse cover based on a time-restricted licence. However, they can increase the premium or policy excess due to the new disability or condition. Patients have to disclose the details of the medical condition as soon as possible to their motor insurance company. Further details on motor insurance are available from the Cancer Help website (see 'Internet resources')

Internet resources

Cancer Help—gives the details of insurance companies and insurance brokers: http://www.cancerhelp.org.uk

Driver and Vehicle Licensing Authority (DVLA), UK: www.dft.gov.uk/dvla

European Health Insurance card—available at http://www.ehic.org/

Macmillan Cancer support—provides details on travel insurance and travel advice: http://www.macmillan.org.uk/

NHS—Travelling outside the European Economic Area (EEA): http://www.nhs.uk/NHSEngland/Healthcareabroad/Pages/NonEEAcountries.aspx

Some of the insurance companies for cancer patients (A detailed list of insurance companies is available from http://www.macmillan.org.uk for UK residents):

http://www.cancertravelinsurance.com/

http://www.insurecancer.com/

Vaccination

Cancer and its treatment result in varying degrees of immunosuppression. The highest degree of immunosuppression is seen after haematopoietic stem cell transplantation (HSCT), in active leukaemia and lymphoma, in active generalized malignancies, and during chemotherapy. Immunosuppression will persist after chemotherapy for leukaemia and lymphoma for 6–12 months, 3 months after chemotherapy for other cancers, and 2 years after SCT.

For the purposes of vaccination and immunization, the following groups of patients are considered as immunosuppressed:
- Patients receiving chemotherapy and up to 6 months after chemotherapy
- Patients who had treatment for leukaemia and lymphoma in the previous 2 years
- Patients after allogeneic HSCT, not on immunosuppressant drugs, for 2 years after transplant
- Patients after autologous HSCT for 1 year post-transplant

Vaccines

Killed vaccines

Indications for inactivated vaccines (Table 6.8.1) in cancer patients are the same as for the general population. Killed vaccine can also be administered during cancer treatment. However, due to weakened body immunity, these may be less effective than in the general population.

Routine vaccinations in cancer patients are modified based on their individual risk for any particular infection. Patients with chronic cardiovascular and/or respiratory conditions or diabetes mellitus are at high risk of influenza and hence need annual vaccination. Patients with absent spleen function (e.g. after splenectomy or with asplenia) are recommended to have *Haemophilus influenza* type b (Hib), meningococcal (conjugate C or quadrivalent conjugate vaccine), and pneumococcal vaccine (with booster every 5 years) in addition to the influenza vaccine.

Patients who are likely to need blood products are advised to have hepatitis B vaccine along with other routine vaccines. Malaria can be severe in splenectomised patients which necessitates special precautions (see later)

Live vaccines

Administration of live vaccines in immunosuppressed patients can lead to a high risk of severe complications due to the live organisms in the vaccine. Hence live vaccines (Table 6.8.1) are contraindicated in all cancer patients who had total body radiotherapy or chemotherapy (including high dose) in the past 6 months. Live vaccines should also be avoided for 3 months after steroid therapy. Live vaccines may be avoided for the rest of life in lymphoma, leukaemia, and HIV-related cancer.

Vaccination of family members

In the UK, all vaccines are given by injection and hence cancer patients are not at risk of getting an infection from a vaccinated family member, even after live vaccine. However, in some countries, some live vaccines are given orally (e.g. oral polio), or nasally (e.g. intranasal influenza). After oral polio vaccine, a person can shed the viruses from their bowel for up to 3 weeks after the vaccination which rarely may be infective. Hence these vaccines are contraindicated for family members of immunocompromised cancer patients. Intranasal and smallpox vaccines also pose a similar risk. It is also important to avoid contact with anyone outside the family who has recently had a live vaccine by mouth.

Live vaccines which are less likely to be transmitted (measles, mumps, rubella [MMR], yellow fever, oral salmonella, and varicella) may be administered to family members. If the varicella vaccine recipient develops a rash, direct contact with the immunocompromised cancer patient should be avoided until the rash resolves.

Family members should receive all other recommended vaccines to reduce the risk of exposure of the

Table 6.8.1 Types of vaccines and immunization

Live vaccines	Killed vaccines	Passive immunization
MMR	Tetanus/diphtheria	Measles
Oral polio	Killed polio	Hepatitis A and B
BCG	Hepatitis A and B	Varicella
Varicella	Hib	Rabies
Varicella zoster	Meningococcal polysaccharide and conjugate	
Salmonella typhi Ty21a	Salmonella—Typhim Vi®	
Intranasal—influenza	Parenteral—influenza	
	Pneumococcal polysaccharide	
	HPV	
	Rabies	
	Yellow fever	
	Oral cholera	
	Swine flu (H1N1)	

immunocompromised patient. Immunization recommendations differ in different countries.

Travel vaccination

Principles of travel vaccination in cancer patients

Indications for vaccination in cancer patients are similar to those for non-immunocompromised people. However, a number of exceptions occur (Kotton 2008).

- Cancer patients should have vaccinations several months prior to travel to allow for serological evaluation and additional booster doses if needed.
- Passive immunization should be used if available and emergency travel presents a potential high risk situation (e.g. hepatitis A immunoglobulin).
- To obtain an optimal immunological response, cancer patients should be vaccinated during periods of no or low immunosuppression.
- Cancer patients are likely to have less immunoresponse to vaccination and any response can be short lived.

The vaccination needs of cancer patients during travel depend on the destination(s). Inactivated vaccines such as hepatitis A and B, inactivated polio, Japanese encephalitis, meningococcal polysaccharide and conjugate, typhim Vi®, and rabies vaccines are safe if needed. Table 6.8.2 gives recommendations for individual travel vaccines.

Re-vaccination

After HSCT, recipients lose immunological memory of previous exposure to infectious agents and vaccines. Hence all patients who have had high-dose chemotherapy and a stem cell transplant need revaccination 6 months after treatment. The recommended vaccinations in this group include diphtheria/tetanus toxoid,

pertussis vaccine, Hib conjugate, inactivated influenza and polio vaccine, live attenuated MMR, pneumococcal and other vaccines.

The ACIP suggest that patients vaccinated while on chemotherapy should be considered unimmunized and be revaccinated. An adequate immune response usually occurs 3–12 months after cessation of chemotherapy. There are no definite recommendations on revaccination with live or inactivated vaccines for individuals vaccinated prior to undergoing treatment with immunosuppressive therapy. The options are booster dose and individualized vaccination based on serological testing for antibody.

Passive immunization

Passive immunization with immunoglobulins, if available, should be considered prior to emergency travel to countries with a high risk of infection or when travelling to an area at high risk of disease when live vaccines are contraindicated. Immunoglobulins are available for measles, hepatitis A and B, rabies, and varicella. Passive immunization should also be considered for immunosuppressed patients exposed to the above infections.

Timing and administration of vaccines (Table 6.8.2)

It is preferable to administer vaccines at least 2 weeks before the start of chemotherapy or SCT, during maintenance chemotherapy (for acute lymphatic leukaemia) or when the peripheral neutrophil and lymphocyte counts are $>1.0 \times 10^9$/L. Re-vaccination can be deferred until completion of treatment and immune recovery.

Inactivated vaccines do not generally interfere with other vaccines and can therefore be given with other vaccines or separately at any time.

Table 6.8.2 Recommendations on individual vaccines for immunosuppressed patients

Vaccine	Recommendation
Tetanus	Routine booster for all
Diphtheria	Indicated if antibody titre is <0.1IU/mL or last injection >10 years prior to travel
Influenza	Annually
Pneumococcal	Before travel
Hepatitis B	Indicated in those with new sexual partners while travelling and those likely to need blood products or medical procedures (including injections) during travel
Hepatitis A	Indicated when travelling to high-risk destinations. At least two doses, 6–12 months apart are needed. Otherwise consider intramuscular immunoglobulin, which offers protection for 3–6 months.
Inactivated polio	Consider if travelling to a destination with a polio outbreak (e.g. Haiti, Dominican Republic, Philippines) or with circulating wild-type polioviruses. Recommend a booster dose if >10 years after previous dose.
Meningococcal	Indicated when travelling to destinations with known outbreaks, meningitis belt of sub-Saharan Africa and travelling to Saudi Arabia for Muslim pilgrimages.
Salmonella	Indicated when travelling to endemic areas. Inactivated vaccine (Typhim Vi®) is the choice in immunocompromised patients.
Rabies	Indicated if intense contact with animals is expected or in those who plan to be far from medical care. An adequate response after vaccination (antibody titre >0.5 IU/ml) is unlikely in immunocompromised patients and hence immunoglobulin is advised after all risk exposures
Japanese encephalitis	When travelling to endemic Asian destinations.
Swine flu (H1N1)	Recommended for cancer patients and family members

Table 6.8.3 Summary of recommendations for vaccination in cancer patients

During and within 6 months of chemotherapy/total body irradiation	Routine vaccines: • Live vaccines are contraindicated • Killed vaccines are recommended according to national guidelines: Give killed vaccines >2 weeks before start of chemotherapy or total body radiotherapy. Some vaccines (e.g. varicella zoster) need to be given at least 1–3 months prior to undergoing immunosuppressive treatments. If vaccines cannot be given during this time scale, they should be given when the neutrophil and lymphocyte count is >1.0 x 10^9/L • Travel vaccines and chemoprophylaxis: Live vaccines are contraindicated; consider passive immunization if urgent travel is contemplated Killed vaccines are recommended as indicated based on the destination(s) Malaria chemoprophylaxis is advised if indicated
6 months after chemotherapy/total body irradiation	• All vaccines can be given provided there is no active cancer • Routine and travel vaccinations as indicated
Bone marrow and STC patients	• Re-vaccination: All patients should receive vaccination for tetanus, diphtheria, polio, HiB (2 doses at 4th and 12th month), pneumococcal, influenza (seasonal, can start after 6 months), hepatitis A and hepatitis B 12 months after transplantation • Travel vaccination: Live vaccines if indicated can be considered if patients are not on immunosuppressant drugs, have no active disease, and are at least 24 months after transplantation. Otherwise passive immunization should be considered
Vaccination of family members of cancer patients	Oral polio, intranasal influenza and smallpox vaccines are contraindicated in family members of the cancer patients with immunosuppression to prevent cross infection

Live vaccines are given simultaneously and if they cannot be given on the same day should be separated by an interval of at least 4 weeks.

A number of combination vaccines are available now which are convenient for travellers.

Assessment of success of vaccination

Measurement, if available, of antibody titres following immunization is helpful to assess the need for booster doses. A 4-fold increase in the antibody titre is generally considered as evidence of seroconversion. The specific titres for seroprotection depend on the individual vaccines. In immunocompromised patients the immunological response is often partial and of short duration.

Malaria chemoprophylaxis

Cancer patients travelling to malaria-endemic areas should receive malaria chemoprophylaxis and advice on avoiding mosquito bites. Appropriate clinical assessment should be performed to address the potential possibilities of:
• Malaria chemoprophylaxis drugs interacting with treatment of cancer.
• Risk of acquiring serious malarial infection in certain subgroups (e.g. after splenectomy).
• Impact of malaria infection and its treatment on the course of malignancy.

Enteric infections

Enteric infections can be severe in immunocompromised cancer patients. These infections can be either water- or food-borne.

To avoid water-borne infections, patients are advised to avoid swallowing water during swimming and to avoid swimming in possibly contaminated water.

Frequent and thorough hand washing is the best way to prevent gastroenteritis.

Further reading

Kotton CN. Vaccination and immunization against travel-related diseases in immunocompromised hosts. *Expert Rev Vaccines* 2008; **7**:663.

Internet resources

Advisory committee on Immunization Practices (ACIP): http://www.cdc.gov/vaccines/recs/ACIP/default.htm

UK Immunisation against infectious disease: the Green Book—available from: http://www.immunisation.nhs.uk

Lifestyle choices after cancer

Historically, the link between cancer and lifestyle was highlighted by an increased incidence of cancer in Asian men and women following migration to North America and Europe and the adoption of stereotypical Western habits; high fat and red meat consumption, low intake of fresh vegetables and fruit, and low levels of exercise (Wilkinson 2003; Thomas 2007). Obesity, for example, from latest estimates could account for 14% of male and 20% of female cancer deaths in the UK (Haydon 2006). Regular physical activity lowers the risk of colorectal cancer in the order of 40–50% compared to those with a sedentary lifestyle (Haydon 2006). The benefits of lifestyle are not, however, confined to prevention. After a diagnosis of cancer a positive change can reduce side effects and risks during therapy, slow the progression of an established cancer, reduce the incidence of relapse; and improve overall survival following initial therapy.

As oncologists are now frequently involved in lifestyle discussions, a knowledge of the evidence and its underlying mechanisms is now a fundamental aspect of routine clinical practice.

Summary of the benefits of lifestyle modification after cancer

Good nutritional status, stopping smoking, and regular exercise have been shown to help the following (Thomas 2007):
- Cancer- and treatment-related fatigue
- Risk of thromboembolism
- Chemotherapy-associated weight gain
- Muscle strength and walking distance
- Constipation
- Bone mineral density
- Bowel adhesions
- Urinary continence
- Secondary malignancy
- Psychological well-being
- Reduces progression rate of indolent prostate cancer (Ornish 2005; Pantuck 2006)
- Improves survival after adjuvant chemotherapy for breast and colorectal cancer (Chlebowski 2005; Meyerhardt 2005; Dignam 2006; Gross 2006; Haydon 2006; Kroenke 2006)

Mechanisms of the interaction between lifestyle factors and cancer

Overweight women have higher oestrodiol which can stimulate oestrogen receptors in breast and endometrial cancer (Chlebowski 2005) although a high-fat diet may also influence hormone production and metabolism by a direct action, and not via obesity.

Oily fish via the ratio of long-chain marine omega-3: omega-6 fatty acid can modulate the COX2 pathway, a potential route for cancer development and progression.

Dietary carcinogenic chemicals such as tars found in cigarette smoke and polycyclic aromatic hydrocarbons and aromatic amines, found in superheated, processed or fried foods, are converted to products which can directly or indirectly oxidize water or oxygen via short-lived but highly energetic free radicals. These cause double or single DNA strand breaks allowing cancer-promoting genes to escape from the influence of their suppressor gene guardians (Wilkinson 2003; Haydon 2006). Although patients with established cancer have already sustained the DNA damage in order to mutate from benign to malignant cells, avoiding further DNA insult may avoid further mutation of indolent malignant or premalignant cells into more aggressive phenotypes (Wilkinson 2003). The US Food and Drug Association (FDA) now regularly publish a list of foods containing high levels of acrylamides and other potential carcinogens (see 'Internet resources') such as:

Xenoestrogens chemicals which have harmful oestrogenic properties including pesticides, herbicides, aluminium salts, some cosmetic preservatives, fuel pollution and plastic products.

Antioxidants wield their anticancer properties by directly or indirectly counterbalancing superoxide free radicals. Most dietary antioxidants originate from plant chemicals known as polyphenols, including the phenolic acids namely benzoic acid (hydroxybenzoic acid, gallic acid) and cinnamic acid (caffeic and quinic acid), together with the non-oestrogenic flavanoids including anthocyanidins, the flavanols (catechins and proanthocyanidins), kaempferol, lignans, and stilbens (Wilkinson 2003).

Carotenoids such as lycopene and beta-carotene, found in tomatoes and chillies. As well as being antioxidants, they also wield their anticancer properties by preventing cell dedifferentiation and proliferation.

Phytoestrogens are polyphenols which also have weak oestrogenic properties and include the flavones, isoflavones and flavanones, which are derived, in human diet, mainly from soybeans, legumes, including peas, lentils, and beans, genistein, daidzein, and equaol (Wilkinson 2003). Dietary intake could potentially create a more favourable hormonal milieu for prostate cancer by inhibiting 5-alpha-reductase, the enzyme responsible for converting testosterone to the more active metabolite dihydrotestosterone. Although foods containing phytoestrogens are generally healthy with high antioxidant properties, there are concerns about phytoestrogenic supplements and breast cancer, and hence supplements should be discouraged.

Trace elements such as manganese, copper, and zinc are essential for the production of superoxide dismutase (SOD) and selenium is essential for glutathione peroxidase (Wilkinson 2003). Together with catalase these form an enzymic defence against carcinogenic oxygen reduction metabolites. Deficiencies in these essential metals have been linked to a greater risk of cancer. The FDA publish league tables relating to foods' ability to induce these defence enzymes, known as their Oxygen Radical Absorbance Capacity (ORAC) score (see 'Internet resources').

Vitamin C has been shown to prevent the inhibition of gap-junction intercellular communication induced by toxic products such as hydrogen peroxide, thereby facilitating DNA repair.

Vitamin D is converted to the active metabolite calciferol in the kidney. Calciferol exposure of cancer cell lines reduces proliferation, promotes differentiation, inhibits invasion and loss of adhesion. It has also been shown in interact with the androgen signalling pathway *in vivo*, inhibiting angiogenesis.

Exercise helps prevent colon cancer by increasing bowel transit time, reducing the time that potentially carcinogenic substances are in contact with the bowel wall. Exercise and diet also help control obesity, serum lipids, and cholesterol (Meyerhardt 2005). Physical activity results in higher levels of insulin-like growth factor 1 (IGF-1) and C peptide, and lower levels of insulin-like growth factor binding protein 3 (IGFBP-3) levels, which has cellular anticancer properties (Giovannucci 2001; Meyerhardt 2005; Haydon 2006).

COX2 overexpression correlates with a more aggressive tumour phenotype and resistance to hormonal therapies. *In vitro*, inhibitors of COX2, such as NSAIDs, have been shown to induce apoptosis, inhibit proliferation, impair adhesion and signal angiogenesis in prostate cancer cell lines and xenographs. People with diets rich in fruit and vegetables, particularly vegetarians, have serum salicylate levels equivalent to a dose of 80mg a day—more than enough to initiate COXs conversion of arachidonic acid to prostaglandins (Blacklock 2001).

Acrylamide concentrations in common foods (FDA 2004 survey)

Often >1000mcg/kg

- Burnt barbecued meat
- Grilled sweet potato crisps (chips)
- Veggie chips potato snacks
- Sweet potato crisps (chips)
- Roasted oat bran crackers
- Veggie crisps (chips)

Usually between 500–1000mcg/kg

- French fries
- Pretzels
- Processed baked potatoes
- Ginger snap cookies
- Toasted corn
- Kettle crunch potato chips
- Hash browns
- Pitted ripe olives
- Tortillas original tostadas
- Low fat bruschetta vegetable crackers
- Sesame snacks
- Dried soup mix

Usually between 200–500mcg/kg

- Butter flavoured popcorn
- Crackers with peanut butter
- Frozen potato skins
- Corn flaked cereals
- Corn chips
- Cream crackers
- Processed prune juice
- Pepper toast
- Coffee

How can clinicians guide patients to improve their lifestyle?

Although dietary supplements seem convenient, long-term use of alpha tocopherol, zinc, calcium, selenium, and antioxidants may have some detrimental effects. Whereas studies have demonstrated that correction of a specific deficit has resulted in a decreased incidence of cancer, adding supplements to groups of individuals with normal or high serum levels actually increased the risk of cancer (Omenn 1996; Rodriguez 2004). Furthermore, those with underlying risks such as smoking, diabetes, or hypertension had a higher rate of heart disease and cerebral haemorrhage. These data suggest that unless detailed analysis and monitoring of the individual components of food is undertaken, lifestyle advice should concentrate on a broad, balanced, and healthy diet combined with regular exercise, stopping smoking, avoiding excess alcohol, regular low-intensity sun exposure without burning, and a sensible sleep pattern.

Basic lifestyle advice—summary

Smoking cigarettes or other substances should stop immediately—most GPs offer smoking cessation clinics or numerous helpful gadgets and books, and independent counselling groups can be found on the Cancernet-UK website (see 'Internet resources').

Alcohol is best avoided following breast cancer or otherwise limited to <14 units per week for women, <21 units per week for men. A premium pint of lager or beer (5% vol.) contains 3 units. A standard 175mL glass of wine (11–12% vol) contains 2 units. A double 35mL shot of spirits contains 3 units. It is also best to have days off alcohol and avoid binge drinking.

Exercise should aim to be regular, at least 30 minutes every day at a level where the individual is hot, breathless, and sweating. To achieve this in the long term, it has to be fun and convenient. There are numerous exercise groups throughout the UK and online services (see 'Internet resources') can be used to search for a range of activities by postcode, ranging from swimming, ballroom, line and salsa dance lessons, aerobics, yoga and fitness classes, local walking and cycling groups through to gyms, sport centres, tennis and badminton courts, Pilates and personal trainers, with times, contact numbers, and locations.

Nutrition—provided a specific nutritional problem has arisen, the following general tips may be helpful:
- *Saturated fats*: avoid processed fatty foods, cream, and fried foods. Check serum cholesterol and discuss taking a statin, if it is elevated.
- *Meat intake*: use meat for its taste, preferably not more than once a day. Excess fat should be removed, and the meat gently grilled rather than fried to further reduce the fat content and to avoid burning. If extra oil needs to be used in cooking, use olive oil rather than animal fat.
- *Fish intake*: increase all fresh fish, particularly the oily varieties such as mackerel and sardines. Fresh water fish such as trout have the advantage of avoiding the potential heavy metal contamination of tuna and sword fish, which some suggest should not be eaten more than twice a week.
- *Antioxidant intake*: non-oestrogenic polyphenols including carotenoids in the skin of colourful foods such as cherries, strawberries, blackcurrants, blackberries; lycopene in tomatoes, tomato source, chilli, carrots; green vegetables and other phytochemicals in dark green salads, prunes, gogi berries, dates, cranberries, red grapes,

white button mushrooms, onions, leeks, broccoli, blueberries, tea, apricots, pomegranates, plums, cherries, parsley, celery, mint and other herbs; phytoestrogens in soybeans, other legumes, including peas, lentils, pinto beans, other beans and nuts (caution is recommended for breast cancer patients and supplements not recommended); lignans and stilbens in flaxseed, linseeds, hemp nuts, grains.

- *Dietary vitamins*: increase intake via fresh ripe fruit, raw and calciferous vegetables, grains, oily fish, nuts, and salads.
- *Trace element and metal intake*: aim for a broad and balanced diet to ensure sufficient intake. Dietary selenium can be increased by eating Brazil nuts, sardines, prawns, and shellfish. Supplements should be avoided, but if required, restrict selenium to 60–75mcg/day, and certainly no more than 200mcg/day. Avoid excessive calcium (>1500mg/day) and zinc (>11mg/day). Unless prescribed for other reasons avoid supplements which give more calcium and zinc per day.
- *Avoid carcinogenic chemicals*: acrylamides, polycyclic or aromatic hydrocarbons in high temperature cooking of carbohydrates, smoked, burnt, grilled, or barbecued foods; N-nitroso compounds in red meat, allylaldehyde (acrolein), butyric acid, and other nitrosamines in heated oils; Pesticides, fertilizers, herbicides, water, unwashed crops and vegetables (consider buying organic if you can afford it).
- *Avoid oestrogenic chemicals*: petrol and diesel fumes; excessive aluminium- or paraben-containing deodorants and antiperspirants, use glass rather than polycarbonate plastic bottles where possible; rinse soap and detergents thoroughly from cups and dishes after they are washed. Avoid storing food in plastic food containers, including plastic film.

Further reading

Blacklock CJ, Lawrence JR, Wiles D, *et al.* Salicylic acid in the serum of subjects not taking aspirin. Comparison of salicylic acid concentrations in the serum of vegetarians, non-vegetarians and patients taking low dose aspirin. *J Clin Pathol* 2001; **54**:553–5.

Chlebowski RT, Blackburn GL, Elashoff RE, *et al.* (2005) Dietary fat reduction in post menopausal women with primary breast cancer. *J Clin Oncol* 2005; **24**(10):3s.

Dignam JJ, Polite B, Yothers P, *et al.* Effect of body mass index on outcome in patients with Dukes B and C colon cancer: An analysis of NSABP trials. *J Clin Oncol* 2006; **3533**:254s.

Giovannucci E. Insulin, insulin-like growth factors and colon cancer: a review of the evidence. *J Nutrit* 2001; **131**(suppl 11):3109–20S.

Gross M, Jo D, Huang J, *et al.* Obesity, ethnicity and surgical outcome for clinically localized prostate cancer. *J Clin Oncol* 2006; **5**(9615 suppl):865.

Haydon AM, MacInnis RJ, English DR, *et al.* The effect of physical activity and body size on survival after diagnosis with colorectal cancer. *Gut* 2006; **55**:62–7.

Kroenke CH, Fung TT, Hu FB, *et al.* Dietary patterns and survival after breast cancer diagnosis. *J Clin Oncol* 2005; **23**(36):9295–303.

Meyerhardt JA, Heseltine D, Niedzwiecki D, *et al.* The impact of physical activity on patients with stage III colon cancer: Findings from Intergroup trial CALGB 89803. *Proc Am Soc Clin Oncol* 2005; **24**:abstract 3534.

Omenn GS, Goodman GE, Thornquist MD, *et al.* Risk factors for lung cancer and for intervention effects in CARET, the beta-carotene in retinol efficacy trial. *J Natl Cancer Inst* 1996; **88**:1550–9.

Ornish D, Weidner G, Fair WR, *et al.* Intensive lifestyle changes may affect the progression of prostate cancer. *J Urol* 2005; **174**:1065–70.

Pantuck AJ, Leppert JT, Zomorodian N, *et al.* Phase 11 study of pomegranate juice for men with rising PSA following surgery or RXT for prostate cancer. *Clin Cancer Res* 2006; **12**(13):4018–26.

Rodriguez C, Jacobs EJ, Mondul AM, *et al.* Vitamin E supplements and risk of prostate cancer in U.S. men. *Cancer Epidemiol Biomarkers Prev* 2004; **13**(3):378–82.

Thomas R, Davis N. Lifestyle during and after cancer treatment. *Clin Oncol* 2007; **19**:616–27.

Thomas R, Woodward C. Diet, salicylates and prostate cancer. *Br J Cancer Manage* 2006; **3**(1):5–9.

Wilkinson S, Chodak GW. Critical review of complementary therapies for prostate cancer. *J Clin Oncol* 2003; **21**(11):2199–210.

Internet resources

Cancernet-UK: http://www.cancernet.co.uk

http://www.cancernet.co.uk.smoking.htm

http://www.cancernet.co.uk/exercise.htm

http://www.cancernet.co.uk/carcinogens.htm

Oxygen Radical Absorbance Capacity (ORAC) score: http://cancer-net.co.uk/antioxidants.htm

The internet and oncology

Online access is now regarded as a basic tool for routine oncology practice. Although the majority of us will have already established a portfolio of useful websites which suit our individual clinical needs, this section offers some further suggestions for reputable web-based resources which may help doctors and patients make informed treatment decisions.

Patient information online

Not all patients have the ability, resources, or motivation to browse the internet for information about their disease, treatments, clinicians, and hospitals, but in an audit of Bedford and Cambridge Hospital patients in late 2007, over half do. The attraction for patients and their relatives or close friends is considerable; electronic mailing lists, online support groups, and websites devoted to their specific cancers can provide valuable information as well as a degree of emotional support (Kadan-Lottick 2005). It improves a consumer's sense of control as well as their ability to participate actively in healthcare decisions (Thomas 2000).

The ability for anyone in the world to freely and easily add information onto a website is clearly the secret of its success, but likewise it is the key to its dangers. As there is no control of quality and quantity, much of the information is inaccurate or misleading, and it is difficult for patients to make judgements on the relevance of the advice offered. Inaccurate information could have serious consequences. An over optimistic view of medical treatment could foster demand for inappropriate intervention, leading to iatrogenic harm and unnecessary cost. Furthermore, there is no protection from unscrupulous or bogus websites preying on the vulnerability of newly diagnosed and terminally ill patients—persuading them to buy 'remedies' of unproven benefit.

Although patients relish the freedom to search for what they like, there is still sound evidence that they take guidance from their clinicians (Thomas 1999). Providing patients and their relatives with a number of useful and reliable patient information sites would be a good first step. In our organization, like many others, we have worked with national organizations to produce a patient information website (http://www.cancernet.co.uk), which contains a list of websites which have been reviewed by a panel of patients and carers, and hence help steer patients towards reliable resources. This practical site also contains peer reviewed, concise information sheets on the common chemotherapy, immunotherapy, radiotherapy, and hormone therapy treatments which can be downloaded by the patients themselves, or by clinical staff, and given to the patients in a hand-held file. Following user demands, it also contains information on lifestyle and environmental issues which may empower patients to help themselves alleviate the side effects, or reduce the risks, associated with cancer or its treatments, such as fatigue, thromboembolism, hot flushes, indigestion, constipation, weight gain, and osteopenia, as well as practical advice on travelling and insurance (Pinto 2003). CancerBACUP is the most comprehensive UK patient information resource; as well as internet access it also provides a free helpline staffed by specialist nurses who can give information over the telephone and by sending helpful booklets and factsheets. The nurses can also provide medical, social, psychological, and financial information and put callers in touch with other support groups (http:www.cancerbacup.org.uk, telephone 0808 800 1234). Other charities, such as Macmillan Cancer Support, produce websites which specialize in important practical issues which physically and emotionally affect patients following the disruption of a cancer diagnosis, such as where to find local specialized nurses, emotional support, financial guidance and grants, help with holidays and disability allowances. A list of US hospital websites, which include patient information, can be found on http://www.onco.net/usa.htm. With >10,000 patient information sites to choose from it is difficult to produce a comprehensive list in this chapter but well-known examples include:

- American Cancer Society: http://www.cancer.org
- Bowel Cancer Help: http://www.bowel-cancer.org
- Bowel Cancer UK: http://www.bowelcanceruk.org.uk
- Breast Cancer Care: http://www.breastcancercare.org.uk
- Breast Cancer UK: http://www.breast-cancer.net.uk
- Cancernet UK: http://www.cancernet.co.uk
- Kidney Cancer UK: http://www.kcuk.org
- Lymphoma Association: http://www.lymphoma.org.uk
- Macmillan: http://www.macmillan.org.uk
- Memorial Sloan–Kettering Hospital: http://www.mskcc.org
- Prostate Cancer Charity: http://www.prostate-cancer.org.uk
- Prostate Cancer Options: http://www.prostate-cancer.co.uk
- Roy Castle Lung foundation: http://www.roycastle.org
- Royal College of Radiologists: http://www.rcr.org.uk
- Royal London Homoeopathic Hospital: http://www.uclh.nhs.uk
- USA National Cancer Institute: http://www.cancer.gov

Clinician's online resources

A range of useful websites are now freely available to help oncologists with decision making, to keep up to date, and access best practice guidelines. All major oncology journals now have online pages, requiring subscription for the full issue, where data are often released before the paper versions (e.g. *British Journal of Cancer*—http://www.nature.com/bjc; *Journal of Clinical Oncology*—jco.ascopubs.org; *Clinical Oncology*—http://www.rcr.ac.uk; *European Journal of Cancer*—http://www.intl.elsevierhealth.com/journals/ejca; *Annals of Oncology*—http://www.annonc.oxfordjournals.org/).

Many journals also supply information free of charge such as abstracts, but then ask for payment for a second tier of more detailed information. There is an emerging trend towards purely online journals such as *Focus on Cancer Medicine* (http://www.rila.co.uk). Google remains the most popular search engine as it is free and specificity can be improved by using the *academic* option. One of the most useful publication search tools is *Pubmed*, a facility developed by the US National Library of Medicine in conjunction with the National Institute of Health (http://www.pubmed.gov). UK sources include the British Library (http://www.bl.uk) who tend to charge for information, and the Bevan Library which is popular with UK hospital post-graduate centres, and hence free to those employed by that hospital trust.

Management guidelines

Most UK cancer networks have their own websites housing their local tumour specific guidelines, most of which require registration usernames and passwords, but thereafter are free. A particularly well-established comprehensive network site is the West Anglia Cancer Network (http://www.wacn.org.uk). National guidelines can be downloaded from the NICE site (http://www.nice.org). Internationally, the American Society of Clinical Oncology (http://www.asco.org), the National Cancer Institute (http://www.cancer.gov), the European Society of Medical Oncology (http://www.esmo.org), and the Memorial Sloan–Kettering sites are well respected, although not necessary applicable to UK practice.

A very useful online breast cancer guideline resource has been set up by Professor Jonat from Hamburg. After entering the patient's demographics and tumour profile, including size, stage, grade, vascular invasion, HER and ER status, it provides the adjuvant treatment recommendations according to the St Gallen consensus guidelines (http://www.adjuvantconsensus.com). The University of Sheffield's Metabolic Bone Disease Unit has developed an eloquent web resource to predict the risk of osteoporosis and fracture and advise whether patients should be investigated and treated. This is particularly relevant for patients postchemotherapy or those taking AIs (http://www.shef.ac.uk/frax).

Clinical trials

Internationally the NCI produces a comprehensive list of ongoing clinical trials (http://www.cancer.gov). In the UK, the National Cancer Research Network (http://www.ncrn.org.uk) and the Medical Research Council (http://www.mrc.ac.uk) both have excellent sites providing portfolio lists of ongoing studies, information on clinical governance, sponsorship, the European Directive, and ethical issues.

Prognostic (decision aide) tools

By far the most commonly used online resource is Adjuvant! Online (http://www.adjuvantonline.com). It helps clinicians and patients consider and discuss the risks and benefits of adjuvant chemotherapy or hormone therapy (or both), after surgery or radiotherapy. It derives its predictive information from the San Antonio database of adjuvant trials (Ravdin 2001). As well as breast cancer, it now includes colon and lung tumours, and provides information on relapse and survival rates, with or without various adjuvant scenarios. The site requires registration but is then free. The fields for breast include age, sex, comorbidities, histology, stage, and ER status but it must be remembered it is only an approximate guide as it does not take into account other predictive variables such strength of ER status (Allred score), progesterone receptors, vascular invasion, and HER2 status. It does, however, include a genomic signature score section for node-positive and ER-positive tumours. The colon cancer section uses age, sex, comorbidities, depth of invasion, number of positive nodes, number of nodes examined, histological grade, and chemotherapy type for predictive analysis. The non-small-cell lung cancer analysis uses age, sex, comorbidities, tumour, and nodal stage.

Further reading

Kadan-Lottick NS, Vanderwerker LC, Block SD, *et al.* Psychiatric disorders and mental health service use in patients with advanced cancer. *Cancer* 2005; **104**(12):2872–81.

Pinto, BM, Trunzo J, Rabin C, *et al.* Moving Forward: A randomized trial of home-based physical activity among breast cancer patients. Paper presented at the 24th Annual Society of Behavioral Medicine Meeting, Salt Lake City, UT, 2003.

Ravdin PM, Siminoff LA, Davis GJ, *et al.* Computer program to assist in making decisions about adjuvant therapy for women with early breast cancer. *Journal of Clinical Oncology*, 2001; **19**(4):980–91.

Thomas R, Thornton H. Patient Information materials in Oncology: Are they needed and do they work? *Clin Oncol* 1999; **11**:225–31.

Thomas R, Daly M, Perryman B, *et al.* Forewarned is forearmed - Randomised evaluation of a preparatory information film for cancer patients. *Eur J Cancer* 2000; **36**:1536–43.

Negligence and risk management in oncology

Introduction
This section will analyse the commonest issues giving rise to claims of negligence in oncology and suggest how these can best be avoided by risk management.

What constitutes medical negligence and leads to claims?
The practice of medicine centres on the relationship of trust which is established between the doctor and patient. This special relationship carries with it a duty of care, a duty to behave professionally in accordance with the guidelines now codified by the General Medical Council.

Medical negligence comprises three components. In proving negligence there must first be established that there was a doctor/patient relationship and therefore a duty of care on the part of the doctor towards the particular patient. Secondly there must be demonstrated a failure of that duty and thirdly that damage to the patient has flowed directly from the failure of duty.

To substantiate a claim in negligence certain key stages are necessary in the doctor/patient interaction:

To establish a claim in negligence a patient (plaintiff/claimant) must show:
- Not only that there was a duty owed by the doctor to the patient and
- That there was a breach of this duty. And
- That damage was caused but also
- That the damage flowed *directly* from that specific breach of duty.

Commonest sources of claim in oncology
- Delay in diagnosis
- Toxicity of treatment (surgery, irradiation, or chemotherapy)

Other issues of possible dispute:
- Diagnostic errors
- Cancer wrongly diagnosed or wrong communication of diagnosis of cancer
- Problems of consent or failure of communication
- Chemotherapy and other treatment mistakes
- Underlying issues, inability to come to terms with diagnosis

Scope of litigation in oncology
In 1995 the National Health Service Litigation Authority (NHSLA) was established. This authority covers all hospital practice under the NHS whereas the individual medical insurance companies, Medical Defence Union (MDU), and the Medical Practitioners' Society continue to have responsibility for risk management in general practice and in private practice.

The scope of the problem
Information concerning the proportion of negligence cases that involve oncology has been obtained from the NHSLA and the MDU.

Data obtained from the NHSLA comprise figures taken from claims submitted under their 'Clinical Negligence Scheme for Trusts', i.e. claims of clinical negligence relating to incidents which took place on or after 1 April 2002.

As a proportion of all cases recorded, 4.22% concerned patients with a diagnosis of cancer (1032 out of 24,428). The most frequent alleged cause of claims was delay in diagnosis amounting to 46.84% of all cancer claims. Claims concerning

failure of communication or improper consent however, only amounted to 1.55%. Poor communication appears to be a frequent contributor to other complaints but rarely amounts to a claim of itself. Complaints about breast reconstruction after mastectomy amounted to 1.8% of all cancer cases but formed an important group among breast cancer cases (9.3%). Reflecting similar findings by the MDU, the commonest diagnoses associated with complaints would appear to be breast cancer 19.2%, cervical cancer 11.5%, and bowel cancer 7.3%.

Medical Defence Union
An analysis of MDU primary care claims shows that a delay or failure to diagnose conditions continues to be the number one cause of claims involving compensation payments on behalf of GP members.

In a recent 5-year period the MDU settled 620 such claims. Of these, 148 claims or 24% related to delayed diagnosis in malignancy. It is important to point out that delay in diagnosis is not necessarily negligent. It can be possible to defend doctors successfully if the clinical management is shown to be competent and reasonable.

Malignancy is the most frequently occurring condition that GPs miss or delay diagnosing. This may not be surprising given that cancers are common diseases and that symptoms and signs can be difficult to distinguish from other less serious conditions. However, looking at past MDU studies of claims in this area that were settled, there has been an increase in the proportion of cases arising from diagnostic problems with malignancy. For example, between 1990 and 2002 there were 19% of delayed diagnoses related to malignancy.

To put this in context the current figure of 24% compares with 13% of cases with delayed diagnosis of meningitis or other infections and 13% in delay of diagnosis over trauma or orthopaedic problems.

The commonest type of cases from the 148 cases arising from failure to diagnose malignancy are those of:
- Breast cancer—38 claims
- Bowel cancer—19 claims
- Skin cancer—17 claims

In the MDU analysis the highest award for delay in diagnosing malignancy was £500,000 for a claim settled following failure to diagnose a malignant melanoma. This 'quantum' as it is called refers to the factors such as the age of the claimant and the working life lost, especially if there are dependants.

The average compensation paid to claimants was £62,000 plus legal costs.

Total oncology cases involved in claims
NHSLA 2002–2006 (hospital cases)
- Total 1032 claims
- Approx. 206 per year
- (Only 4.22% of all cases, 24428)

MDU (GP and private case)
In general practice over 5 year period
- 620 settled claims
- 24% of claims related to delay, failure, or incorrect diagnosis
- 11% diagnostic problems
- 5% relate to delayed, inappropriate, or failure of referral

Among MDU settled claims involving delay in diagnosis.
- 19% relate to malignancy
- 16% relate to orthopaedics
- 13% relate to general medicine
- 12% relate to general surgery

Commonest diagnosis in settled claims
MDU
- 21% breast cancer
- 14.5% cervical cancer
- 13.5% bowel cancer

Commonest diagnosis in recorded cases
NHSLA 1995–2003
- 19.2 % breast cancer
- 11.5% cervical cancer
- 7.3% bowel cancer

Legally important issues in the management of malignant disease

1. Delay in diagnosis
Unnecessary delay in the diagnosis of any cancer can deprive the patient of an opportunity for cure or result in the need for more aggressive and combined treatments than would otherwise have been necessary. Delay can occur at any level and mistakes can occur at each stage of diagnosis and treatment.

The GP who fails to examine patients adequately or to take seriously the anxieties expressed by patients may deprive the patient of the opportunity either for immediate diagnosis or for referral to an appropriate Assessment Centre where the proper diagnosis could have been established.

Surgeons may accept the evidence of benign cytology and, for example, apparently benign mammographic appearances and decide against removal of a single breast lump, which ultimately proves in fact to contain malignant cells. Again the opportunity for timely diagnosis and intervention is missed.

Faults in the *referral process* may equally lead to delay. Failure on the part of the GP to alert hospital staff to the urgency of the referral or failure on the part of these staff to respond appropriately to delay may form the basis of a complaint.

Delay in the diagnosis of breast cancer (the commonest disease site in cancer claims)
- GP fails to listen to or examine patient
- GP fails to refer
- Mammography error
- Surgeon accepts benign cytology/ fails to excise mass
- Faults in referral process: GP or Breast Unit

2. Complaints arising from toxicity of treatment for cancer
Toxicity may arise following surgery, irradiation, or chemotherapy. Frequently it is the combination of two or more of these treatment modalities which together cause unfortunate sequelae.

Examples of radiotherapy toxicity which have led to legal action include damage to the brachial plexus and to the lymphatic drainage of the arm resulting in lymphoedema following radiotherapy for breast cancer, and these problems are more likely following prior axillary surgery. Claims have also followed the inclusion of excessive volumes of lung tissue in radiotherapy fields or excessive cardiac dose.

Toxicity claims in breast cancer: surgery
- Inappropriate selection of procedure—mastectomy vs WLE
- Inappropriate or failed cosmetic procedure

Toxicity claims in breast cancer: radiotherapy
- Arm lymphoedema
- Brachial plexus damage
- Lung damage
- Cardiac damage

Another important group of cases have concerned the long-term effects of irradiation to the pelvis, especially for cervical cancer. The late effects of treatment such as bowel and bladder damage have been devastating for some patients and even though they have been cured of their disease and have achieved long-term survival their quality of life has been very severely reduced as a result of treatment. Many of these patients would have chosen a greater risk of recurrence had they been warned of the crippling effects of therapy aimed at cure.

3. Negligence claims arising from diagnostic mistakes
The principal issue that has given rise to complaints of diagnostic negligence concerns the faulty interpretation of cervical smears. False reassurance arising from failure to report abnormal cells can afford the opportunity for disease to develop unrecognized.

However, cytopathology work is both intensive and repetitive and the scope for human error is unfortunately considerable.

A further large group of claims concerns the missed diagnosis of breast cancer at mammography. *Radiologically* identifiable cancers have been missed and lead to unfortunate delay in diagnosis. As a result great efforts have been made to create and monitor safe procedures combining clinical findings with radiology and cytology to minimize both false negative and false positive diagnoses.

4. Cancer wrongly diagnosed or wrongly communicated
Occasionally the diagnosis of cancer is made in error. The circumstances may seem to be an emergency, for example, when a serious infection mimics the rapid evolution of cancer and early treatment is considered essential (e.g. osteomyelitis vs osteosarcoma). The unintended sequelae may be devastating for the patient. One case, for example, which was widely reported in the press, concerned a man in whom advanced bladder cancer was diagnosed. As a result this patient was given a very adverse prognosis and decided to sell his property and use his savings to travel around the world in what he thought were the last few weeks of his life. On his return it became evident that his disease was in fact non-malignant with a much better prognosis than expected. The patient sued his professional advisers in negligence on the basis that he would not have spent his life savings had he been given the correct information. This case was settled out of court but serves as a timely reminder for practising oncologists to verify the pathological diagnosis of cancer before proceeding to treatment.

In recent years the MDU reports that inappropriate diagnoses among settled hospital claims have totalled 44 of which 14 were false negative and 30 false positive cases (MDU 2003).

5. Failure of communication and consent

Problems of communication are not infrequent in oncology. Most malignant disease carries a serious prognosis with far reaching implications for work, family, or fertility, and the potential for severe emotional distress. The working environment in busy wards or clinics where time is at a premium is not conducive to the private, sympathetic communication of bad news which is the ideal. Patients who perceive that the doctor is uninterested in their welfare, unsympathetic, or poorly informed in the subject can become irritated, angry, and alienated. The patient's perception that he/she has no control over their situation and no access to information about the disease and its consequences can lead to a sense of dissatisfaction and grievance.

Until now doctors have not been trained in communication skills and patients' accounts of rude, hasty, and unsympathetic consultations remain all too common. In addition, the detailed concepts of treatment options, survival statistics, risks and benefits, and randomized clinical trials are difficult to convey in an understandable way to a lay person.

Misunderstandings are not uncommon and if handled unhelpfully can lead on to complaint and the legal process.

Similarly in the process of obtaining informed consent the complexities of treatment, and especially the anticipated side effects, need very careful explanation and patients frequently pursue a complaint when they feel that they were not given adequate information, especially information on which to decline a treatment which subsequently caused damage.

Failure of communication
- Serious diagnosis
- Poor working environment, lack of privacy
- Rushed, unsympathetic consultation
- Fear of loss of control
- Complexity of information: complex treatment options, survival statistics, risks and benefits, randomized trials

6. Chemotherapy mistakes

Claims involving chemotherapy may arise from inappropriate selection or overdosage of treatment drugs, inadequate information concerning treatment toxicity which would have enabled the patient to decline such treatment, administration of the wrong agent, wrong route of administration, and damage caused by faulty intravenous administration with local tissue damage (extravasation).

The improper provision and supervision of safe procedures, monitoring, and safety checks form a further possible basis of negligence claims. Very often when mistakes occur they result not from a single error but from a whole series of incidents which although not inherently serious themselves add up eventually to a disaster.

One such case concerned the sequence of events in 1999 that resulted in the mistaken intrathecal injection of the drug vincristine into the spinal cord of a 12-year-old patient with leukaemia by a specialist registrar in paediatric anaesthesia. This event followed a series of departures from normal practice and it was ultimately realized that 'significant systems failures within the hospital administration' were important factors in the boy's death (Ferner 2003) Despite the 'Report of an expert group on learning from adverse events in the NHS' chaired by the chief medical officer the same mistake was unfortunately repeated at the Queen's Medical Centre, Nottingham in 2003 (Editorial 2003) This mistake was the 23rd incident, and the 14th in 15 years in the UK in which this drug had been mistakenly and fatally injected into the spine.

Many oncological treatments are both complicated and risky and the possibility of mistakes is considerable. *When things go wrong* the patient or their family can very quickly feel aggrieved and litigious if an explanation and expression of regret are not speedily forthcoming. Expressions of sympathy and regret at any suffering should be speedy and sincere but it is wiser to keep an 'apology' in the sense of acceptance of blame to await the results of investigation. Often a sequence of errors is revealed each of which may have been negligible on its own but which together lead to serious consequences. And sometimes errors occur for which no person is to blame and no personal negligence is found.

Thorough and open investigation is essential when things go wrong. Patients and their families frequently assert that if they had gained confidence that every member of the medical team had been made aware of the mistake and had learned the lesson then further complaint might well have been unnecessary. It means a great deal to a family to know that they have been heard and that no-one else is likely to experience the same problem.

Toxicity claims in chemotherapy
- Inappropriate choice of drugs
- Overdosage
- Inadequate information and consent
- Extravasation

7. Negligence in oncology: broader issues

Because cancer is known to progress with time the perceived negligence of doctors in failing to deal correctly and urgently with cancer investigation and referral is a recurring theme in oncology. Experienced oncologists, however, observe that underlying a complaint of delay in diagnosis there frequently lies the patient's or family's inability to come to terms with the fact of a diagnosis of cancer. This failure to come to terms with the situation creates a sense of agitation and injustice. The patient may feel 'it must be someone's fault' and pursue a claim in negligence as a result.

In reality there are mixed messages concerning the influence of time on cancer survival. On the one hand, government guidelines stress the importance of reduced waiting times for cancer referral and treatment and screening programmes claim to saves lives by early diagnosis. On the other hand an expert witness analysing the individual case will frequently assert that although delay did occur, the impact of this delay on survival was in fact negligible. For the layman this discrepancy between the general and the particular case is difficult to rationalize. The explanation lies either in the fact that the disease was inherently aggressive and untreatable whenever the diagnosis was made or that the delay occurred during a stage which was not critical to future prognosis.

Risk management recommendations

- Take careful notes not only of positive but also of negative findings on examination.
- Take careful contemporaneous notes of what was said during phone calls as well as in clinic

- Ensure your practice or multidisciplinary team has a safe system for following-up test results and for reporting adverse incidents so that the team can analyse and learn from any mistakes or 'near misses'.
- Ensure that patients know of any serious symptom or sign which should be reported urgently, e.g. weakness in the legs in metastatic disease of bone.
- Explain and apologize to patients if things go wrong and ensure that you take steps to deal with the consequences and arrange appropriate treatment and follow-up.

Further reading

Editorial. The criminalisation of fatal medical mistakes *BMJ* 2003; **327**:1118–19.

Ferner RE. Medication errors that have led to manslaughter charges. *BMJ* 2000; **321**:1212–16.

Haie-Meder C, Kramar A, Lambin P, *et al*. Analysis of complications in a prospective randomised trial comparing two brachytherapy low dose rates in cervical carcinoma. *Int J Radiat Oncol Biol Phys* 1994; **29**:1195.

Complementary therapies

Complementary therapy is an umbrella term for a heterogeneous array of interventions which are not part of mainstream medicine. Table 6.12.1 provides an overview of some of the most popular modalities. Even though the treatments differ in many respects, they have in common that certain claims are regularly made for them by their proponents:

- The interventions are holistic
- They are natural and hence safe
- They are highly individualized
- They maximize the self-healing properties of the human body

Essentially, these are claims which require evidence. Many complementary therapies are furthermore characterized by the fact that they have a long history of usage and, in most countries, constitute private medicine.

The reason why complementary medicine is an important topic in oncology is obvious: at least one-third of all cancer patients employ some type of complementary therapy (Ernst and Cassileth 1998). Prevalence figures vary hugely and depend on a range of factors, for instance, a precise definition of what is a complementary therapy. Many patients do not tell their oncological team about their use of complementary medicine. It seems to follow that any thorough medical history must include questions about complementary medicine usage.

The reasons why so many cancer patients are tempted to try complementary therapies are diverse and include:

- Desperation
- Hope for a cure
- Incessant media-hype

- The wish to leave no stone unturned
- Irresponsible marketing of some interested parties
- The fact that many patients can afford the extra cost

Disappointment with conventional oncology is, contrary to what is sometimes argued, not a prominent reason; only very few cancer patients abandon conventional oncological treatments altogether. By and large, complementary therapies are used in addition to mainstream healthcare.

In order to assess the value of complementary therapies, it is helpful to differentiate between i) interventions claimed to change the natural history of the disease, e.g. 'curative treatments'; ii) preventative measures; and iii) supportive or palliative approaches. In the following, I will address these three areas in turn asking which complementary therapies demonstrably generate more good than harm. In doing so, I will rely on the evidence of rigorous clinical trials and systematic reviews of such studies. This body of evidence has recently summarized in more detail elsewhere (Ernst et al. 2006, 2007).

Curative treatments

It is in this area where patients' interest is keenest. Several surveys have shown that a sizable part of cancer patients' reason for trying complementary therapies is their claim to change the natural history of the disease, i.e. offer a cure, a reduction of tumour burden, or a prolongation of life (e.g. Trevena and Reeder 2005). A simple Google search (18 Sept 2007) for 'cancer, alternative medicine' generated 32.2 million hits. Patients are thus bombarded with promises that this or that alternative remedy will cure their cancer, and the daily press does its share in promoting the

Table 6.12.1 Some of the most important complementary therapies

Therapy	Description
Acupuncture	Insertion of a needle into the skin and underlying tissues in special sites, known as points, for therapeutic or preventive purposes
Aromatherapy	The use of plant essences for medicinal purposes
Biofeedback	The use of apparatus to monitor, amplify, and feed back information on physiological responses so that a patient can learn to regulate these responses. It is a form of psychophysiological self-regulation
Chiropractic	A system of healthcare which is based on the belief that the nervous system is the most important determinant of health and that most diseases are caused by spinal subluxations which respond to spinal manipulation
Herbal medicine	The medical use of preparations that contain exclusively plant material
Hypnotherapy	The induction of a trance-like state to facilitate the relaxation of the conscious mind and make use of enhanced suggestibility to treat psychological and medical conditions and effect behavioural changes
Massage	A method of manipulating the soft tissue of whole body areas using pressure and traction
Osteopathy	Form of manual therapy involving massage, mobilization, and spinal manipulation
Reflexology	The use of manual pressure on reflex zones usually on the soles of the feet to prevent or treat illness
Relaxation therapy	Techniques for eliciting the 'relaxation response' of the autonomic nervous system

myth that 'alternative cancer cures' exist (Milazzo et al. 2007).

Evaluating the evidence for such claims is, however, a sobering task indeed. Data from clinical trials are available for at least 18 different modalities; in no case is it convincing or even promising (Ernst et al. 2006) (Table 6.12.2).

On closer inspection, the concept of an 'alternative cancer cure' turns out to be inherently absurd. It presupposes that reasonably good evidence exists that a treatment is effective and, at the same time, rejected by the conventional oncological community for the sole reason of not originating from conventional medicine. Even though this type of conspiracy theory is very much alive in the field of complementary medicine (it seems to be a precondition for selling quackery to unsuspecting, vulnerable patients), there is no evidence that oncologists behave in this way. In my experience, they would be more than delighted to add another effective curative method to the existing therapeutic options. Thus 'alternative cancer cures' is and will remain a contradiction in terms.

Preventative measures

Several 'natural' approaches have shown considerable promise in reducing cancer risks (Ernst et al. 2006). Modalities for which the evidence is encouraging include:
- Regular consumption of allium vegetables (e.g. garlic)
- Regular consumption of green tea
- Regular consumption of tomato-based products (lycopene)
- Regular exercise

Arguably all of these approaches are entirely mainstream lifestyles or nutritional habits based on the evidence from conventional epidemiological and other research. Even if we initially considered them to be complementary therapies, they would rapidly become conventional cancer prevention, once the evidence is promising.

Supportive and palliative care during chemotherapy

In this area, complementary therapies have an important role to play. Many of the modalities have the potential to increase well-being and quality of life of cancer patients by alleviating the symptoms of the disease or by reducing the adverse effects of conventional treatments.

Table 6.12.2 Treatments that have been tested as 'alternative cancer cures'

Aloe vera	Melatonin
Asian mixtures	Mistletoe
Beta glucan	PC-SPES
Di Bella therapy	Reishi
Essiac	Shark cartilage
Gerson	Support group therapy
Hydrazine sulfate	Thymus extracts
Laetrile	Ukrain
Macrobiotic	'714-x'

For instance, several complementary therapies have been shown to reduce cancer pain (Ernst et al. 2007).
- Exercise (arguably a conventional intervention)
- Hypnotherapy
- Massage
- Reflexology

Other complementary treatments have been demonstrated to reduce other symptoms (Ernst et al. 2006):
- Acupuncture and acupressure reduce nausea and vomiting after chemotherapy.
- Aromatherapy improves psychological well-being of cancer patients.
- Music therapy enhances quality of life and mood of cancer patients.
- Specific relaxation programs reduce fatigue and improve quality of life of cancer patients.

One could argue that the level of proof does not need to be as high for palliation as for curative treatments. If a dying cancer patient feels in any way better after an aromatherapy massage, for instance, few clinicians would insist on irrefutable evidence before administering it? On the other hand, we have to concede that the trial evidence for those treatments may be promising but it is certainly not compelling. The studies are usually designed in such a way that it is impossible to tell whether a specific or a non-specific effect was the cause of the observed outcome. Finally one should stress that conventional methods of care do, of course, also generate benefit, and it is usually unclear whether the orthodox or the heterodox approach yields a greater effect size or is better value for money.

Conclusion

Complementary therapies are popular with cancer patients. Oncologists should therefore know the essentials about them. The evidence is vastly different depending on whether we are dealing with cancer 'cures', prevention or supportive/palliative care. Alternative cancer 'cures' turns out to be a contradiction in terms. The most important role of the oncological team in this setting may well be to show empathy and prevent serious harm. Some 'natural' therapies have shown promise in cancer prevention. It is, however, debatable whether these are complementary or conventional approaches. In the area of supportive/palliative care, complementary therapies could find a truly beneficial role. Several of the modalities in question can improve the quality of life of cancer patients either through alleviating some of the symptoms of the disease or through reducing the adverse effects of the treatment.

Further reading

Ernst E, Cassileth BR. The prevalence of complementary/alternative medicine in cancer: a systematic review. *Cancer* 1998; **83**:777–82.

Ernst E, Pittler MH, Wider B, Boddy K. The desktop guide to complementary and alternative medicine, 2nd edition. Edinburgh: Mosby/Elsevier, 2006.

Ernst E, Pittler MH, Wider B, et al. Complementary therapies for pain management. Edinburgh: Mosby/Elsevier, 2007.

Milazzo S, Lejeune S, Ernst E. Laetrile for cancer: a systematic review of the clinical evidence. Support Care Cancer 2007; June:583–95.

Trevena J, Reeder A. Perceptions of New Zealand adults about complementary and alternative therapies for cancer treatment. *N Z Med J* 2005; **16**:U1787.

Supportive care during chemotherapy

Nausea and vomiting

This may occur in up to 70% of patients receiving cancer chemotherapy and is of three types:

- Acute nausea and vomiting within the first 12–24 hours after chemotherapy.
- Delayed nausea and vomiting occurring up to 5 days after chemotherapy.
- Anticipatory nausea and vomiting which is a conditioned response because the patient expects to experience nausea and vomiting.

Drugs vary in their emetogenic potential as shown in Table 6.13.1.

Appropriate antiemetic regimens for each group are shown in Table 6.13.2.

Myelosuppression

Myelosuppression is a potentially serious consequence of cancer chemotherapy. Chemotherapy-induced febrile neutropenia often leads to hospital admission for administration of parenteral antibiotics and has a considerable impact on quality of life. It is also a major cause of treatment delays and dose reductions which may result in poorer tumour control rates.

Colony stimulating factors

Recombinant human granulocyte colony stimulating factors, G-CSF or granulocyte-macrophage colony stimulating factors (GM-CSFs) can be used to minimize or prevent neutropenia and its associated complications and support dose-dense and dose-intense chemotherapy regimens. Febrile neutropenia is commonest with aggressive chemotherapy regimens and international guidelines advocate routine G-CSF support in patients with solid tumours and lymphomas, where there is an estimated risk of 20%. Chemotherapy regimens commonly associated with high risk (>20%) of febrile neutropenia (FN) are listed in Table 6.13.3. Factors associated with risk of FN are age >65 years, advanced stage of disease, previous episodes, and lack of antibiotic prophylaxis. Previous chemotherapy, use of high-intensity regimens, and diagnosis of haematological malignancies also increase the risk of FN. G-CSF may reduce the

duration of FN and hospitalization if given during the episode but its use should be limited to those patients who are not responding to appropriate antibiotic management. Clinical evidence so far suggests similar efficacy of all the available preparations, although there is some evidence of superior effectiveness with pegfilgrastim compared with filgrastim or lenograstim. Pegfilgrastim also has the advantage of once per cycle administration compared with daily injections of other forms of G-CSF. ESMO guidelines suggest administration of G-CSF from 24–72 hours after chemotherapy continuing until recovery of neutrophil counts. Doses of filgrastim used are 5mcg/kg by daily subcutaneous injections starting on day 2 for up to 14 days or ANC of 10 x 10^9/L and of pegfilgrastim 100mcg/kg on day 2 of each cycle as a single subcutaneous injection.

Erythropoietin

Maintenance of good haemoglobin levels is important for patients with cancer both for general well-being and to ensure efficacy of treatment. A target haemoglobin level of 12g/dL is recommended. For many years, studies of erythropoiesis stimulating agents (ESAs) have been carried out and have shown that it is possible to reduce the need for blood transfusion in patients receiving chemotherapy. Epoietin alpha, beta and darbepoietin are equally effective and can be used in patients for whom blood transfusion is contraindicated or where there is symptomatic anaemia. However, a recent Cochrane meta-analysis of studies of the role of ESA in cancer patients has concluded that these agents are associated with an increased mortality and decreased overall survival rate. These effects were less marked in patients receiving chemotherapy, but an adverse effect could not be excluded, and care is therefore needed in the use of ESA, which may stimulate tumour growth and increase the risk of thromboembolic episodes.

Mouth care

Mucositis is a troublesome side effect of neutropenia. Patients should be advised to avoid spirits and spices. Good mouth care is essential with use of a soft toothbrush and mouthwashes with saline, 0.15% benzydiamine 3-hourly, or chlorhexidine. Soluble aspirin or paracetamol may help pain. Protective gels such as Orobase® or Gelclair® may be used. Oral candidal infections may be treated with topical nystatin 100,000 units four times daily after food or in the immune suppressed patient with oral fluconazole 50–100mg daily for 14 days. Herpetic ulcers may be treated with topical acyclovir 5% cream five times a day for 5 days, or widespread infection with oral acyclovir 400mg five times a day for 5 days.

Preventing hair loss

Use of scalp cooling with a cold cap can reduce blood flow to the scalp and therefore dose of chemotherapy to the hair follicles. It should not be used if there is a risk of scalp metastasis or for haematological malignancies and it is only effective for some chemotherapy schedules such as single agent anthracyclines, regimens including Adriamycin® or epirubicin in combination with other cytotoxic drugs which cause minimal hair loss, and the taxanes. It must be applied at least 30 minutes before administration of chemotherapy and remain in place for 60–90 minutes after completion. It may cause discomfort or headaches.

Table 6.13.1 Emetogenic potential of various drugs

Mildly emetic treatment (risk <10%)	Fluorouracil
	Etoposide
	Methotrexate (<100mg/m²)
	Vinca alkaloids
	Gemcitabine
	Taxanes
Moderately emetic treatment (30–90% risk)	Doxorubicin
	Cyclophosphamide (low and intermediate doses)
	Mitoxantrone
	Methotrexate (high does: 0.1–1.2g/m²)
	Oxaliplatin
	Irinotecan
Highly emetic treatment (>90% of patients)	Cisplatin
	Dacarbazine
	Cyclophosphamide (high doses)

Table 6.13.2 First-line antiemetic therapy for chemotherapy

Chemotherapy	Antiemetic combination
Highly emetic regimens	Dexamethasone 12 mg orally day 1, 8mg orally daily days 2–4 Granisetron 2 mg orally (1 mg intravenously) *or* ondansetron 24 mg orally (8 mg intravenously) *or* dolasetron 100 mg orally (or intravenously) *or* palonosetron 0.25 mg intravenously day 1 Aprepitant 125 mg orally day 1, 80mg orally days 2–3
Moderately emetic regimens	Dexamethasone 12mg orally day 1, 4mg orally daily days 2–3 Granisetron 2 mg orally (1 mg intravenously) *or* ondansetron 8 mg orally twice daily (8mg intravenously) *or* dolasetron 100mg orally (or intravenously) *or* palonosetron 0.25mg intravenously day 1 Aprepitant 125mg orally day 1, 80mg orally days 2–3
Low emetic risk	Dexamethasone 10mg intravenously, or 4mg orally twice daily days 2–3 (for low-dose cisplatin: 10mg intravenously for at least 3 days) Granisetron 2mg orally (1mg intravenously) *or* ondansetron 8mg orally twice daily (8mg intravenously) *or* dolasetron 100mg orally (or intravenously) *or* palonosetron 0.25mg intravenously

Table 6.13.3 Common chemotherapy regimens associated with high risk of febrile neutropenia

Malignancy	Regimen
Breast cancer	AC followed by docetaxel Paclitaxel followed by AC TAC Doxorubicin with taxanes
Non-small-cell lung cancer	Docetaxel/carboplatin Cisplatin/etoposide
Small-cell lung cancer	ACE Topotecan ICE
Ovarian cancer	Docetaxel Paclitaxel
Urothelial cancer	Carboplatin/paclitaxel MVAC
Germ cell tumours	BOP→VIP VeIP
Gastric cancer	LVFU LVFU-cisplatin LVFU-irinotecan ECF TCF
Other cancers	Irinotecan (colon cancer) TIC (head and neck cancer)
	Cisplatin/paclitaxel
Hodgkin lymphoma	BEACOPP
Non-Hodgkin lymphoma	DHAP ESHAP CHOP-21 HyperCVAD+rituximab ICE

Preservation of fertility during chemotherapy (see Chapter 6, Fertility and cancer, p.608)

There is as yet no means of preventing the gonadal toxicity of chemotherapy in men, and sperm storage before treatment starts is the only option. Gonadal toxicity of chemotherapy occurs in up to 60% of girls and women. The risk of premature ovarian failure increases with increasing age, and with cumulative drug dose. Options for preservation of fertility include IVF and embryo cryopreservation, unfertilized ova cryopreservation, or use of GnRH agonists. The first two options necessitate delay in starting treatment, whereas hormonal treatment can start immediately.

Goserelin 3.6mg is given subcutaneously, 1 week before chemotherapy and then 4-weekly throughout the course of treatment. Side effects are minimal with only a small decrease in bone mineral density. The mode of action is uncertain. There may be a direct effect on the ovary, or it may break the cycle of follicle depletion with chemotherapy followed by a rise in FSH and consequent accelerated recruitment of more follicles with further damage.

LHRH analogues given during treatment can decrease the rate of ovarian failure. Using the agent goserelin, various groups have shown a reduction in premature ovarian failure from approximately 55% to 11% as indicated by return of menses and FSH level of <40IU/L within 12 months of the last cycle of chemotherapy.

In survivors of childhood cancer there is an 8% risk of premature ovarian failure before the age of 40 compared with an incidence of <1% in the general population. Several large clinical trials of goserelin are recently completed or are still continuing, including the German ZORO trial and the SWOG S0230 Phase III trial of LHRH analogue administration during chemotherapy to reduce ovarian failure following chemotherapy in early stage or receptor-negative breast cancer. There is some evidence that use of goserelin may also decrease recurrence rate and death from recurrence in breast cancer.

References

Feyer P, Jordan K. Update and new trends in anti-emetic therapy: the continuing need for novel therapies. *Ann Oncol* 2011; Vol **22**(1):30–38.

Aapro M, Lyman GH, 2009 update of EORTC guidelines for the use of granulocyte colony stimulating factors to reduce the incidence of chemotherapy induced febrile neutropenia in adult patients with lymphomas and solid tumours. *Eur J Cancer* (in press).

Bohlius J, Schmidlin K, Brillant C, *et al.* Erythropoietin or darbepoetin for patients with cancer – meta-analysis based on individual patient data. *Cochrane Database Syst Rev* 2009; **3**:CD007303.

Devon KM, McLeod RS. Pre and peri-operative erythropoietin for reducing allogeneic blood transfusions in colorectal cancer surgery. *Cochrane Database Syst Rev* 2009; 1:CD007148.

Del Mastro L, Catzeddu. T, Boni L, *et al.* 2006; Prevention of chemotherapy-induced menopause by temporary ovarian suppression with goserelin in young, early breast cancer patients. *Ann Oncol* 2006; **17**(1):74–8.

Cuzick J, Ambroisine L, Davidson N, *et al.* LHRH-agonists in Early Breast Cancer Overview group. Use of luteinising-hormone-releasing hormone agonists as adjuvant treatment in premenopausal patients with hormone-receptor-positive breast cancer: A meta-analysis of individual patient data from randomised adjuvant trials. *Lancet* 2007; **369**:1711–23.

Internet resource

Goserelin acetate study for ovarian function in patients with primary breast cancer—available at http://clinicaltrials.gov/ct2/show/NCT00429403

Palliative care

Pain management

Pharmacological Interventions

In general, cancer pain management should be focused on the three-step WHO analgesic ladder for cancer pain relief (Ventafridda et al. 1997) (Fig. 7.1.1) This strategy should, however, be integrated with other methods, as appropriate, of cancer pain control. This includes tumoricidal therapy, radiotherapy, palliative surgery, physiotherapy, occupational therapy, anaesthetic interventions, psychosocial care, and any other care which adds to pain relief. It can be more appropriate with some patients to miss step two of the ladder and simply prescribe low-dose step three (strong opioid) which can mean fewer drug changes. In specialist units, the WHO ladder will relieve up to 80% of cancer pain.

Step one: non-opioid analgesia

The most common non-opioid analgesic used is paracetamol, usually prescribed 1g four times daily. The side effects of paracetamol are minimal and it is generally effective in mild pain. As paracetamol works differently from opioids, it is usual to continue it even on the second and third steps of the analgesic ladder. Non-steroidal anti-inflammatory drugs (NSAIDs) are an alternative or addition to paracetamol at each step.

Step two: weak opioid

The most commonly used weak opioid is codeine. This has a potency of approximately one-tenth of morphine. It often exists in combination with paracetamol; codeine 60mg/paracetamol 1g prescribed four times daily. Although other weak opioids are available, there is no evidence to suggest any benefit over codeine. Codeine remains the weak opioid of choice in stage two of the analgesic ladder. Tramadol is another weak opioid which is often prescribed; however, this can cause confusion in elderly patients.

Step three: strong opioids

These should be prescribed at low doses and titrated as described in the following section. Patients often have preconceptions regarding strong opioids and thus they should be counselled fully regarding their use and any concerns explored.

Strong opioid titration

- An immediate release strong opioid should be prescribed orally on a regular basis, typically 4-hourly.

- Breakthrough (rescue) analgesia, at the same dose as the regular dose, should also be available.
- After a period of 48–72 hours the daily analgesic dose can be calculated.
- A controlled release preparation can be commenced at the equivalent required daily dose
- Breakthrough medication, usually with the same opioid, should be available and this is usually one-sixth of the total daily dose of regular opioid.

Strong opioids

Morphine

- Remains the gold standard opioid.
- Available by oral route or by injection (SC, IM, IV).
- Half-life of 2–3.5 hours.
- Duration of analgesia 4–6 hours.
- Metabolized to M-6-G (morphine-6-glucuronide) which is active and M-3-G (morphine-3-glucuronide) which is not analgesic but is thought to cause neuro-excitation.
- Metabolites are eliminated by the kidney and accumulate in renal insufficiency.
- Starting dose from 2.5–10mg (orally, four times daily) depending on patient
- Commonly available preparations: sustained release e.g. MST (lasts 12 hours), immediate release e.g. Sevredol® (tablets) or Oramorph® (liquid)

Diamorphine (di-acetylmorphine)

- Prodrug of morphine but more soluble.
- Only available in UK and Canada.
- Potency ratio 3:1 with oral morphine.
- Generally only available as a parenteral preparation.

Oxycodone

- Semi-synthetic opioid.
- Metabolized in the liver and excreted in the urine.
- Fewer hallucinations, less confusion/itch than morphine.
- Oral preparations are immediate release (oxynorm) and sustained release (oxycontin) in UK.
- Injection (oxynorm) also available.

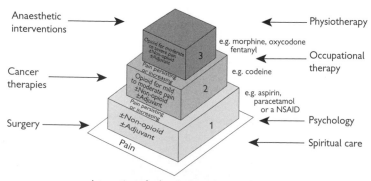

Integration of other interventions to the
WHO 3-step or 2-step analgesic ladder

Fig. 7.1.1 World Health Organization analgesic ladder for cancer pain relief. From WHO Pain Relief and Palliative Care, http://www.searo.who.int/linkfiles/publications_ch11.pdf, with permission from the World Health Organization.

Hydromorphone
- Available in oral or injectable form.
- Common preparations: sustained release; Palladone® SR (lasts 12 hours); immediate release; Palladone®.

Fentanyl
- Short half-life when used sublingually or intravenous or subcutaneous.
- Transdermal patches available for cancer pain deliver 12–100 mcg/h over 3 days.
- Transmucosal, buccal, and nasal preparations are becoming available and may be beneficial in breakthrough pain.
- Elimination half-life after patch removal is almost 24 hours, compared with 3–4 hours after IV injection.
- May take 48 hours to reach steady state when first applied.
- Patches used only for *stable* pain.
- Breakthrough opioid should be used at appropriate dose.
- Relatively safer in renal failure than renally excreted drugs such as morphine.

Alfentanil
- Injection or buccal spray only, short half-life.
- Like fentanyl—often used perioperatively, however becoming more commonly used in palliative care.
- Relatively safe in renal failure.

Buprenorphine
- Opioid with agonist and antagonist action—effects are only partly reversed by opioid antagonist naloxone.
- Exists in the UK as transdermal patches.
- Relatively safe in renal failure.

Methadone
- N-methyl-D-aspartate acid (NMDA) antagonist—useful in neuropathic pain.
- Plasma half-life 24 hours on average.
- Duration of analgesia often only 4–8 hours.
- Can take 5–28 days to reach steady state.
- More potent by oral route than subcutaneous.
- Morphine equivalent dose varies according to prior morphine dose—when using methadone, specialist advice is advised.
- Potentially of use in renal failure.

Transdermal buprenorphine
New transmucosal buccal and nasal fentanyl preparations are the latest additions to the opioid armamentarium.

Choice of strong opioid
In general, morphine is the strong opioid of choice. The greatest amount of evidence exists for morphine, thus unless a specific reason exists, this should be prescribed in preference to other opioids. It is available in both oral and parenteral preparations.

Transdermal opioids
If a transdermal route is indicated, fentanyl or buprenorphine patches may be of use. Transdermal opioids are only indicated when the pain is stable and are not advised in the acute pain setting. A transdermal fentanyl patch of 12mcg/h equates to a daily morphine dose of approximately 40mg, so caution is advised.

Opioid toxicity (Fig. 7.1.2)
Opioid toxicity can carry a 50% mortality rate in its severe form, and it is therefore important to identify early. Opioid toxicity can occur when the patient has reached the maximum tolerated dose of a specific opioid. It can also be

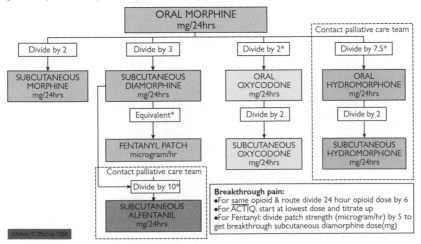

Fig. 7.1.2 Opioid conversion chart. (Courtesy of Dr J Adam and Carolyn Mackay, Marie Curie Hospice Glasgow.)

caused by dehydration, causing an accumulation of opioid metabolites. Toxicity can occur with any opioid and has a spectrum of clinical features.

Clinical features of opioid toxicity

- Pseudo-hallucinations—shadows at the peripheries of the field of vision.
- Myoclonic jerks—rapid involuntary jerks of muscle groups.
- Cognitive impairment—can range from mild to severe. Often confused with distress or terminal agitation.
- Hallucinations—both auditory and visual hallucinations can exist and may be frightening for the patient.

Management of opioid toxicity

- Early recognition is important as it can often be reversed easily.
- Rehydration.
- Reduction of opioid dose.
- Occasionally a switch of opioid.
- Treatment of cognitive impairment—haloperidol (1.5–3mg orally—as needed).

When a patient is opioid toxic, but still has not attained sufficient analgesia, general reassessment of pain, biochemistry (urea and electrolytes and corrected calcium in particular), and general drug review should be the first step. Once this has been done, if the patient still has insufficient analgesia and is opioid toxic, then a switch to another opioid may be indicated.

Opioid switching

If the situation exists where toxicity occurs but adequate analgesia does not exist, then, assuming a history of opioid responsiveness, the ceiling dose of that particular opioid has been reached and a switch to another opioid is indicated. There is little evidence to support the use of any particular opioid over another. Oxycodone or hydromorphone are alternative opioids which may be used if morphine toxicity exists. When converting from one opioid to another it is usual to calculate the total daily dose of morphine—morphine equivalent daily dose (MEDD). In general the equi-analgesic dose is calculated, and then this figure is reduced further, usually by one third (Fig. 7.1.2).

This should be done with specialist guidance in the complex situation of opioid toxicity.

Adjuvant analgesics

Adjuvant analgesics are drugs whose primary function is not analgesia but which can have an analgesic effect (Table 7.1.1). Examples include anti-inflammatory, anticonvulsive, and antidepressant medications. In neuropathic pain, amitriptyline or gabapentin are commonly used. These should be started at low doses and titrated to reach the desired effect. As sedation may occur, it is helpful to commence treatment at night, as any sedation should then be less pronounced.

Non-steroidal anti-inflammatory drugs

NSAIDs are particularly useful analgesics and are usually prescribed for metastatic bone pain, although they are also used for other indications. Coprescription of a proton pump inhibitor is advised to reduce the incidence of GI side effects. While interesting preclinical data support the role of the COX-2 inhibitors, particularly in malignant bone pain (antiangiogenesis role), clinical superiority remains unclear. For practical purposes, etirocoxib can be used for patients at high risk of GI side effects.

Neuropathic pain

Malignant neuropathic pain remains a significant clinical challenge and the reasons are twofold. Firstly, it is one of the most common symptoms in patients with cancer and some studies have suggested that 50% of all difficult to manage cancer pain is neuropathic (Caraceni et al. 1999). Secondly, neuropathic pain can be poorly responsive to opioids because higher doses of opioids are often required, increasing the likelihood of unacceptable side effects which limit dose escalation.

Adjuvant analgesics are an important part of our neuropathic pain armamentarium. Most commonly used adjuvant analgesics have a number-needed-to-treat of about three (NNT = 3). This means that of every three patients treated, one is likely to get pain relief. The choice of adjuvant analgesic is based on an individual's predicted sensitivity to a specific side-effect profile, e.g. postural hypotension with amitriptyline and the usefulness of the adjuvant in dealing with more than one symptom, e.g. duloxetine for neuropathic pain and depression.

Table 7.1.1 Adjuvant analgesics

Drug	Dosage	Indications	Side effects
NSAIDs (COX 2 inhibitors can be used if high risk of GI side effects)	E.g. diclofenac 50mg TDS Orally, 100mg OD par rectum	Bone metastases, hepatic pain, inflammatory pain, soft tissue infiltration	Gastric irritation, headache, fluid retention. Use with caution in renal impairment
Steroids	E.g. dexamethasone 8–16mg daily, best used in the morning. Titrate down to the lowest dose which controls pain	Raised intracranial pressure, nerve compression, soft tissue infiltration, hepatic pain	Hyperglycaemia, cushingoid appearance, confusion, gastric irritation if used with a NSAID
Gabapentin	100–300mg (nocte). Titrate to 600mg TDS. Higher doses may be needed.	Nerve pain of any cause	Mild sedation, confusion, tremor.
Amitriptyline	Starting dose 25mg (nocte). In elderly start at 10mg.	Nerve pain of any cause	Sedation, dizziness, confusion, dry mouth, constipation, urinary retention. Avoid in cardiac disease
Carbamazepine	Starting dose 100–200mg (nocte)	Nerve pain of any cause	Vertigo, sedation, constipation, rash

Anticonvulsants

Currently gabapentin and pregabalin are commonly used as adjuvant analgesics on the basis of easier titration. However, so far they have not been shown to have a lower NNT than the older anticonvulsants (Finnerup et al. 2005).

Antidepressants

A Cochrane review provided a valuable summary of the current evidence for the use of antidepressants in non-malignant neuropathic pain (Saarto et al. 2007). Tricyclic antidepressants have been shown to provide at least moderate pain relief (NNT = 3.6). More recently, data from three studies have supported the use of venlafaxine (NNT = 3.1) A newer dual uptake inhibitor, duloxetine, also shows early evidence of a possible benefit in neuropathic pain. At present there is insufficient evidence to support the use of selective serotonin reuptake inhibitors (SSRI).

The advantage of venlafaxine and duloxetine is that they can serve a useful therapeutic role for clinical depression. Venlafaxine has more side effects than duloxetine.

Ketamine

The NMDA receptors within the spinal cord have been shown to have a significant role in the pathophysiology of neuropathic pain. Ketamine is an NMDA antagonist which has been studied in neuropathic pain and evidence exists for its use, either orally or parenterally (Mercadante et al. 2000; Mitchell et al. 2002). It can be useful in neuropathic pain where there are clinical indicators of central wind-up such as pain on light touch and increased pain to any painful stimulus. In addition, if opioid doses are escalating with reduced response, ketamine can be considered to achieve renewed opioid response.

Topical lignocaine

There is supporting evidence advocating the use of topical lignocaine in patients with postherpetic neuralgia and patients with localized peripheral neuropathic pain. It is available either as a patch or as a topical gel. It has a good side-effect profile and has a NNT of 4 and can be used either alone or in combination with other medications. Lignocaine patches have been used in cancer-related neuropathic pain where allodynia (sensitivity to light touch) exists.

Neuropathic cancer pain—treatment strategy

The commonly-used drugs in cancer-related neuropathic pain have been studied extensively in non-malignant neuropathic pain. It is reasonable to extrapolate these findings to neuropathic cancer pain.

A suggested treatment strategy is as follows. This is based on a combination of available evidence and clinical experience in the UK (Finnerup et al. 2005; Dworkin et al. 2007).

All steps are in conjunction with the WHO analgesic ladder. Titrate individual drugs to effect.
- Start amitriptyline. If patient is already taking amitriptyline, then
- Add in or replace amitriptyline with either gabapentin or pregabalin.
- Trial of ketamine—either orally or via parenteral route.
- Anaesthetic interventions, e.g. nerve block, epidural or intrathecal.

Cancer-induced bone pain

Cancer-induced bone pain (CIBP) is a major cause of morbidity in patients with cancer. Up to 85% of patients with bone metastases have pain and CIBP is a common cause of hospital or hospice admission. Commonly occurring malignancies such as cancers of the breast and prostate frequently metastasize to bone. In addition, advances in treatment have led to patients living longer with advanced cancer and symptoms of bone metastases.

Palliative radiotherapy remains the most effective anti-cancer treatment for CIBP. Systematic reviews show 41% of patients achieve 50% pain relief within 4 weeks of treatment (McQuay et al. 2000). While this is an excellent response for any analgesic method, for individual patients, other methods are required.

Treatment of CIBP
- The treatment of CIBP involves a combination of analgesia (as per the WHO ladder), NSAIDs, and appropriate short-acting opioids.
- Rest pain responds well to conventional analgesic regimens.
- CIBP is often worsened by movement-related pain.
- Movement-related CIBP often responds poorly to opioid analgesia because it can be sudden and of short duration. This means that opioid-related adverse effects will be more common.
- Use short-acting oral opioids (fentanyl lozenges, alfentanil spray) prior to movement.
- Short acting opioids briefly increase analgesic levels during movement so minimizing unwanted opioid side effects at rest.

Bisphosphonates

Bisphosphonates have been shown to be effective in reducing the incidence of skeletal events and time to skeletal events. Their use as analgesics is less clear. They do have some analgesic effect, but the NNT to achieve 50% pain relief at 4 weeks was 11 (Wong et al. 2002). At present there is insufficient evidence to support the use of bisphosphonates in the acute pain setting, but the evidence base is likely to evolve. It is clear that some patients do achieve acute analgesia.

Anaesthetic interventions

In the majority of cases, cancer pain can be controlled using conventional analgesics. The WHO ladder can be thought of as the central pillar of analgesic management, but additional therapies such as radiotherapy and chemotherapy, surgery, physiotherapy and TENS can be used alongside the WHO ladder.

If, however, standard systemic analgesia has been either ineffective or side effects have prevented adequate doses being reached, then anaesthetic interventions may be necessary. Anaesthetic interventions are often regarded as step four of the WHO ladder but can be implemented at any stage of the ladder as clinical need dictates.

Methods include regional nerve blocks (commonly coeliac plexus block for upper abdominal pain) and neuro-destructive blocks. The latter are often reserved for cases when other measures have failed. Neuraxial analgesia (epidural and intrathecal—also known as spinal) are often used in the management of malignant pelvic pain (Table 7.1.2).

Whether or not an anaesthetic intervention is indicated is influenced by:
- Underlying pain and pathology
- Patients' expectations
- Prognosis
- Required duration of analgesia
- Availability of specialist staff

Table 7.1.2 Factors affecting choice of neuraxial analgesia

Epidural	Intrathecal (spinal)
Prognosis	
Short term use only—where prognosis is limited	Long-term use—both external or implantable pumps can be used
As a trial of analgesia prior to intrathecal	
Other treatment planned e.g. radiotherapy	
Procedure	
Usually local anaesthetic ± sedation	Sedation or general anaesthetic usually required
Fixation may be difficult	Deep fixation when inserted
Catheters may migrate to intrathecal space—potential for overdose	Catheters can only migrate back to epidural space
Drug distribution may be limited if there is epidural tumour or radiotherapy scarring	Drug distribution is determined by lipid solubility and spreads within CSF
Catheters short-term use only	Catheters designed for long-tem use
Drug dose	
One tenth of systemic dose	One-hundredth of systemic dose

If the choice of route is appropriate and the technique undertaken and managed by trained staff, neuraxial analgesia can provide effective analgesia. Often a trial of epidural analgesia is done to determine effect. If this is successful then intrathecal analgesia may follow on from this. Intrathecal catheters are often tunnelled subcutaneously to reduce the risk of infection and dislodgement. A trial of an external pump is usually done before an implantable pump is inserted.

Choice of drug

Usually a combination of local anaesthetic (levobupivicaine) and strong opioid (morphine or diamorphine) is effective. For the intrathecal administration, opioid doses are usually in the region of one hundredth of the systemic dose. This allows much smaller doses to be administered, minimising side effects and toxicity.

Clonidine, ketamine and midazolam can also be delivered via the intrathecal route.

Non-pharmacological interventions

Non-pharmacological interventions are an important adjunct in the management of cancer pain with, a very low risk of side effects. TENS, acupuncture, relaxation techniques, and massage may all be of benefit. Appropriate review and intervention by both physiotherapists and occupational therapists may improve pain through rehabilitation and functional aids.

Further reading

Caraceni A, Portenoy R. An international survey of cancer pain characteristics and syndromes. IASP Task Force on Cancer Pain. International Association for the Study of Pain. *Pain* 1999; **82**: 263–74.

Dworkin RH, O'Connor AB, Backonja M, *et al*. Pharmacologic management of neuropathic pain: evidence-based recommendations. *Pain* 2007; **132**:237–51.

Finnerup NB, Otto M, McQuay HJ, *et al*. Algorithm for neuropathic pain treatment: an evidence based proposal. *Pain* 2005; **118**:289–305.

McQuay HJ, Collins SL, Carroll D, Moore RA. Radiotherapy for the palliation of painful bone metastases. *Cochrane Database Syst Rev* 2000; CD001793.

Mercadante S, Arcuri E, Tirelli W, Casuccio A. Analgesic effect of intravenous ketamine in cancer patients on morphine therapy: a randomized, controlled, double-blind, crossover, double-dose study. *J Pain Symptom Manage* 2000; **20**:246–52.

Mitchell AC, Fallon MT. A single infusion of intravenous ketamine improves pain relief in patients with critical limb ischaemia: results of a double blind randomised controlled trial. *Pain* 2002; **97**:275–81.

Saarto T, Wiffen PJ. Antidepressants for neuropathic pain. *Cochrane Database Syst Rev* 2007; CD005454.

Ventafridda V, Tamburini M, Caraceni A, *et al*. A validation study of the WHO method for cancer pain relief. *Cancer* 1987; **59**:850–6.

Wong R, Wiffen PJ. Bisphosphonates for the relief of pain secondary to bone metastases. *Cochrane Database Syst Rev* 2002; CD002068.

Nausea and vomiting

The most common symptoms in advanced cancer, nausea and vomiting, can be difficult to palliate unless treatment is directed in a logical and specific way. To this end an understanding of the pathophysiology of nausea and vomiting is required (Fig. 7.2.1).

Vomiting is the result of stimulation of the vomiting centre. The vomiting centre is not an anatomical area per se but rather acts as a coordinating centre from various neurogenic inputs.

Knowledge of the pathophysiology of nausea and vomiting, in combination with history and examination findings, will assist in recognizing the pathway affected. The receptors in this specific pathway should then be targeted by the appropriate antiemetic (Fig. 7.2.2).

Clinical approach

History: key points

- Nature of vomitus, e.g. bile stained vomiting may suggest a more proximal cause and help to rule out gastric outlet obstruction; faecally stained vomit suggests a more distal cause or the presence of a fistula between the large and small bowel.
- Volume of vomitus—large volume may suggest gastric stasis or bowel obstruction.
- Timing of vomiting—early morning vomiting may be a sign of raised intracranial pressure. Vomiting late in the day may be due to bowel obstruction.
- Query triggering/alleviating factors.
- Frequency of vomiting (high frequency can lead to dehydration).
- Vomiting related to movement may suggest an inner ear cause.

Examination: key points

- Assess for hydration state.
- Abdominal examination; including careful observation looking for peristalsis, testing for a succussion splash, auscultation.
- Rectal examination—to exclude constipation.

Investigations

Investigations are tailored to the individual and can include the following:
- Plasma urea and electrolytes, glucose
- Serum corrected calcium—hypercalcaemia commonly causes constipation
- Abdominal X-ray—presence of air-fluid levels suggests obstruction

Possible causes of nausea and vomiting in cancer

- Bowel obstruction—secondary to underlying disease or constipation
- Chemotherapy
- Radiotherapy
- Pain
- Drug-induced, e.g. opioids, antibiotics
- Electrolyte imbalance, e.g. uraemia, hypercalcaemia
- Paraneoplastic causes

Table 7.2.1 Common causes of nausea and vomiting and first-line treatments

Cause of nausea and vomiting	Treatment: first-line antiemetic
Chemotherapy	Granisetron 1mg BD PO Dexamethasone 4–8mg OD PO Metoclopramide 20mg QDS PO
Radiotherapy	Granisetron 1mg BD PO Haloperidol 1.5mg OD or BD PO
Raised intra-cranial pressure	Cyclizine 50mg tds PO
Delayed gastric emptying	Metoclopramide 10–20mg QDS PO or domperiodone 10–20mg QDS PO
Drug induced	Haloperidol 1.5mg OD or BD PO.
Metabolic, eg uraemia or hypercalcaemia	Haloperidol 1.5mg OD or BD PO.

- Brain metastases
- Psychological factors e.g. anxiety

Management

- Ascertain the likely cause(s) of nausea and vomiting through history and examination.
- Use appropriate non-pharmacological measures.
- Identify the specific pathway(s) involved and receptors.
- Use the most potent drug for the pathway identified (Table 7.2.1).
- Use the most appropriate route of administration.
- In established nausea and vomiting, parenteral administration is needed in the initial stages—to ensure drug absorption.
- Titrate the dose and monitor clinical effect.
- If symptoms do not improve, consider additional antiemetics or use another antiemetic.

Non-pharmacological measures

- Remove any nausea stimuli from the environment.
- Use palatable food and drinks.
- Offer frequent small amounts of food and drink.
- Cognitive therapy may be helpful in anticipatory nausea.
- TENS can enhance pharmacological measures.
- Acupuncture (P6 point, midpoint palmar aspect of each wrist).

First-line antiemetics

Haloperidol
- Antipsychotic.
- Acts on the dopamine (D_2) receptors in the chemoreceptor trigger zone.
- Effective in nausea and vomiting associated with drugs and metabolic disturbance.
- Dose: usually 1.5mg at night by mouth which can be increased to 3mg if needed.

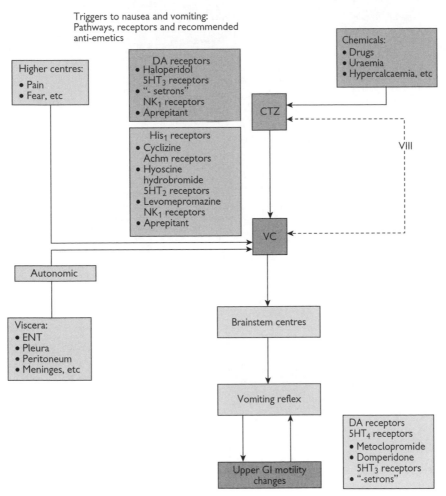

Fig. 7.2.1 Pathophysiology of nausea and vomiting.

- Long half-life so a single daily dose is usually sufficient. Parenteral doses are usually between 2.5–5mg subcutaneously over 24 hours.
- Can cause sedation in high dose (generally >20mg daily).

Cyclizine
- Antihistamine.
- Acts on the H_1 receptors in the cerebral cortex, vomiting centre, and inner ear.
- Antiemetic of choice in complete bowel obstruction.
- Effective in nausea associated with cerebral irritation e.g. cerebral metastases. Usual dose is 25–50mg three times daily (PO)
- Can be given parenterally, 75–150mg over 24 hours.
- Can cause sedation.

Metoclopramide
- Prokinetic.
- Acts mainly on $5HT_4$ and D_2 receptors and is effective in gastric stasis.

- Has been shown to be beneficial in incomplete bowel obstruction but should be avoided in cases of complete obstruction as colic may occur.
- In early satiety associated with delayed gastric emptying, metoclopramide is usually effective.
- Dose: usually 10mg four times daily (PO) but can also be given parenterally 40–80mg over 24 hours
- Domperidone is an alternative to metoclopramide which has less central activity and therefore is less likely to cause extrapyramidal side effects

5-HT₃ antagonists
- E.g. ondansetron, granisetron.
- 5-HT₃ receptor antagonist.
- Useful in nausea and vomiting secondary to chemo- or radiotherapy.

Second-line antiemetics
Levomepromazine
- Broad spectrum; acts on Ach, H_1, $5HT_2$, and D_2 receptors.
- Effective in most cases of nausea and vomiting.

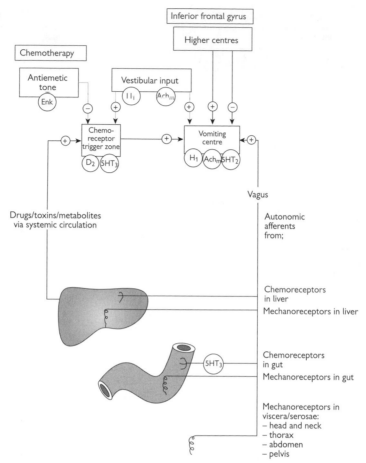

Fig. 7.2.2 Receptors involved in nausea and vomiting. Courtesy of Kathryn Mannix (2009).

- Can cause sedation so in general it is started at low doses and increased as needed.
- Usual dose is 6.25–25mg subcutaneously per 24 hours.
- An oral preparation is available (6mg tablet) administered once per day, usually at night.

Dexamethasone
- No specific receptor affinity.
- Mechanism of action is unclear. It is often used in addition to first-line antiemetics.

- Dose 4–8mg once daily (PO) with equivalent doses parenterally (often given as a single daily dose)

Further reading

Mannix KA. Palliation of nausea and vomiting. In: Hanks G, Cherney NI, Christakis NA, *et al.* (eds) *Oxford Textbook of Palliative Medicine*, 4th edition. 2010 Oxford: Oxford University Press.

Malignant bowel obstruction

Malignant bowel obstruction (MBO) is one of the common complications of both abdominal and pelvic cancers, especially colorectal and ovarian cancer. Treatment depends on various factors from level of obstruction to underlying disease. MBO can be a clinical challenge and surgery, if appropriate, is the treatment of choice. Often surgery is not appropriate due to poor clinical condition and thus conservative management is the mainstay of treatment in these cases.

Clinical approach: key points

The clinical approach is very much dependent on the level of the obstruction. However the following symptoms and signs are often present:
- Abdominal pain: frequently colicky in character prior to vomiting.
- Nausea: usually relieved to varying degrees after a vomit.
- Vomiting: this is often bile stained if the obstruction is proximal. If the obstruction is distal it is more likely to be faecally stained.
- Constipation: if complete obstruction is present, the patient is unable to pass flatus. In the early stages of constipation, diarrhoea can occur.
- Abdominal distension.
- Succussion splash.
- Increased bowel sounds (borborygmi) often 'tinkling' in nature.

Investigations
- Plasma urea and electrolytes: patients often uraemic.
- Abdominal x-rays show dilated loops of bowel and can assist in locating the level of the obstruction.
- CT of abdomen is useful to determine if there are multiple levels of obstruction which would normally preclude surgery.

Management
While, if possible, surgery is the treatment of choice, in most cases treatment is conservative.

Steroids
- Although the evidence is limited, a trial of steroids is worthwhile (Laval et al. 2000).
- Dexamethasone is the usual prescribed steroid in MBO.
- Doses range from 8–16mg per day.
- Best administered parenterally (usually subcutaneously) to ensure absorption.

Somatostatin analogue (octreotide)
- Reduces GI secretions (Mystakidou et al. 2002).
- Promotes water reabsorption from the bowel lumen and slows bile flow.

- Decreases intestinal motility and colic.
- Dose: 600–800mcg per day administered SC over 24 hours.
- Sustained release formulation of octreotide. (administered intramuscularly once every 4 weeks (20mg) equates to a dose of approx 1mg per day).

Antiemetics
- Incomplete obstruction; metoclopramide is the antiemetic of choice providing there is no colic present.
- Complete obstruction; cyclizine is the antiemetic of choice.

Venting gastrostomy
- Useful in proximal GI obstruction.
- Inserted relatively easily by endoscopy.
- Often better tolerated than nasogastric tubes and complications are far less frequent.

Nasogastric intubation
- Decompresses the stomach and upper GI tract.
- Patients often find nasogastric tubes uncomfortable and this can limit their use.
- Blocking or dislodgement can complicate their use.

Malignant bowel obstruction: a strategy
A multi-faceted approach is often needed. Parenteral drug administration (usually subcutaneous) is usually needed to ensure absorption:
- Pain: managed according to the WHO analgesic ladder. Patients will often require strong opioids.
- Nausea and vomiting: in incomplete obstruction, metoclopramide can be used. If complete obstruction develops, cyclizine is the antiemetic of choice.
- Steroids can be beneficial to control nausea, and reduce gut wall oedema and extrinsic compression. This may assist in resolution of an incomplete obstruction.
- Nasogastric tube: consider this on an individual basis.
- Octreotide: helpful in reducing intestinal secretions and may be beneficial in patients with vomiting as a symptom.

Further reading
Laval G, Girardier J, Lassauniere JM, et al. The use of steroids in the management of inoperable intestinal obstruction in terminal cancer patients: do they remove the obstruction? *Palliat Med* 2000; **14**:3–10.

Mystakidou K, Tsilika E, Kalaidopoulou O, et al. Comparison of octreotide administration vs conservative treatment in the management of inoperable bowel obstruction in patients with far advanced cancer: a randomized double-blind controlled clinical trial. *Anticancer Res* 2002; **22**:1187–92.

Constipation

Constipation is a common problem and some studies suggest that up to 50% of cancer patients will develop constipation. A far greater proportion will require drugs to prevent this.

Causes

* Opioid-induced bowel syndrome—opioids cause a reduction in peristalsis, increasing sphincter tone, increasing smooth muscle tone, and tone in the anal sphincter.
* Decreased mobility leading to decreased frequency of peristalsis.
* Dehydration and subsequent electrolyte abnormalities, e.g. hypercalcaemia.
* It can also be the due to intestinal obstruction secondary to the underlying malignancy.
* Neurological—spinal cord compression will leave the anocolic reflex intact—thus rectal intervention will stimulate bowel emptying. In cauda equina lesions the colon will be lax.

Clinical approach: key points

* History: frequency and consistency of stools, nausea, abdominal discomfort, bloating and abdominal distension, flatulence, tenesmus. Overflow diarrhoea can occur in some cases.
* Examination: abdominal examination; faecal loading, rectal examination. Dehydration.
* Investigation: abdominal x-ray—faecal loading or, in extreme cases, dilatation of the colon and bowel obstruction.

Management

* Ensure adequate fluid intake.
* Ensure patient has privacy and ease of access to toilet facilities.
* The mainstay of management is prevention and it is important that any patient commenced on an opioid has access to a prophylactic laxative.
* If the current laxative regimen is sufficient, continue.
* In advanced cancer, a combined stimulant/softener is preferred, e.g. co-danthramer (2 capsules once or twice daily) or movicol is usually effective.
* Osmotic diuretics (e.g. lactulose) can be helpful. Sufficient oral intake is essential to ensure they work correctly.
* Rectal administration of drugs is advised if oral measures fail. Rectal examination should be performed prior to this, as the stool softening preparations will only be effective if they come into direct contact with faeces.
* Bisacodyl suppositories work by stimulating the rectum whilst glycerol suppositories soften stools.
* Enemas (e.g. arachis oil or phosphate enemas) may be needed in more severe cases.
* New approaches, such as peripherally-acting opioid, opioid antagonist preparations and opioid antagonist alone are becoming available.

Diarrhoea

Common causes
- Cancer: producing irritation and inflammation of the bowel mucosa.
- Faecoliths or tumour obstructing the bowel resulting in overflow diarrhoea.
- Chemotherapy, e.g. irinotecan, capecitabine, 5-FU.
- Radiotherapy.
- Infection e.g. *Clostridium difficile*
- Medical conditions, e.g. autonomic neuropathy, Crohn's disease.

Clinical approach: key points
- History: particularly recent bowel habit and medication.
- Examination: should include rectal exam.
- Abdominal X-ray: may show obstruction or toxic colon.
- Electrolytes: dehydration may be present.

Management
Supportive
Rehydrate as appropriate. Oral hydration is preferred.

Loperamide
Reduces secretion of digestive agents into the bowel. Approximately 50 times more potent than codeine for treatment of diarrhoea. Dose usually 4mg (four times daily). This can be reduced to twice-daily dosing once diarrhoea has responded to treatment.

Octreotide
Useful in severe diarrhoea. It is given via subcutaneous infusion in doses from 200–1200mcg per 24 hours.

Antibiotics
If an infective cause has been identified, appropriate antibacterial treatment is indicated.

Opioids
Act by reducing peristalsis in the gut. Loperamide should be used in preference to opioids as first-line treatment. If the patient requires opioid analgesics this may negate the need for any additional antidiarrhoeal agents.

Hiccups

Hiccups are a reflex spasm of the diaphragm causing sudden movement of the glottis. Although rarely a source of severe distress, hiccups can be troublesome and a challenge to treat at times.

Common causes

- Gastric distension
- Gastro-oesophageal reflux disease (GORD)
- Raised intra-abdominal pressure, e.g. ascites, hepatomegaly
- Steroids
- Electrolyte imbalance (e.g. hyponatraemia, uraemia)

Management

(Depends on treating the underlying cause.)

Gastric distension and GORD

- Prokinetic drugs such as metoclopramide (10mg qds PO). Dimethicone which is an antifoaming agent which eases flatulence and distension (Asilone® 5mL four times daily) can be effective.

Smooth muscle relaxants

- Baclofen and nifedipine may also be effective and act by relaxing smooth muscle. Baclofen (5mg three times daily PO) or nifedipine can be used either PRN (5mg) or regularly (5mg three times daily).

Central hiccup reflex suppression

- Chlorpromazine is often effective but should only be used when other measures have failed due to its sedating side effects. Usual dose (12.5–25mg daily)

In severe intractable hiccups if the patient becomes exhausted, a trial of midazolam by continuous sub-cutaneous infusion may be appropriate.

Depression

Depression is common in patients with advanced cancer, occurring four times more frequently than it does in the general population (Derogatis et al. 1983). It is often underdiagnosed in patients with cancer and antidepressants are used fairly infrequently (Block et al. 2000). Depression is often easily treated and this can improve quality of life and also physical symptoms such as pain.

There are many reasons why depression is underdiagnosed and undertreated. It is often assumed that patients with advanced malignancy will be depressed. It is reasonable to assume that patients will have a low mood at times, but persistent low mood warrants further assessment. There may be a stigma associated with depression and this can result in patients being reluctant to commence treatment.

Clinicians may also be less likely to diagnose depression. This can be due to lack of experience or even prejudice. Clinical depression can and does frequently exist and is a real clinical problem that should be considered as important as other symptoms.

Diagnosis

In the physically well patient, the main symptoms used to diagnose depression are poor appetite, weight loss, and even fatigue. These are less reliable in patients with advanced cancer as the symptoms can often be due to the underlying cancer.

It is impossible to diagnose depression if there is cognitive impairment present. In particular hypoactive delirium is often misdiagnosed as depression and therefore it is essential to ensure the patient has no cognitive impairment before assessing for depression.

The Endicott Criteria (Table 7.7.1) are a modified version of the DSM (Diagnostic and Statistical Manual) criteria which replaces symptoms which may be attributable to cancer (Endicott 1984).

Some studies have used the question 'Are you depressed?' as a tool for diagnosing depression. Whilst this showed good sensitivity in North America, this question was less reliable in the UK. This demonstrates that the term 'depression' means different things in different cultures and thus should be interpreted with caution.

The Hospital Anxiety and Depression Scale (HADS) was designed to assist in diagnosing anxiety and depression. It has been shown to be effective at diagnosing depression in patients with advanced cancer. This has a maximum score of 42 (encompassing both anxiety and depression scores) A combined anxiety and depression score of 20 or above makes a diagnosis of depression highly likely.

Principles of management

Once the diagnosis has been made, appropriate treatment is essential. Some studies have shown that depression may affect survival so appropriate treatment is paramount (Fawzy et al. 1993).

* Counselling is effective in mild to moderate depression.
* Spiritual support and appropriate psychological intervention are often helpful either alone or in combination with pharmacological therapy.
* Traditional antidepressants, e.g. amitriptyline and other tricyclics, are used less frequently due to the side-effect profile.
* Treatment with newer antidepressants is more desirable.
* There is little evidence of the superiority of one antidepressant over another—the side-effect profile is often the discriminating factor.

Drug treatments

Citalopram
* SSRI as first-line treatment of depression (Laird et al. 2005).
* Dose: 20mg daily is often effective; however this can be increased if necessary to 40mg daily

Mirtazapine
* Noradrenaline and specific serotonin antagonist (NaSSA).
* Dose: 15mg daily, increased to 45mg daily if needed. Paradoxically, lower doses can be more sedating.
* May be effective in nausea (action on the $5HT_3$ receptor).

Venlafaxine
* Serotonin–noradrenergic reuptake inhibitor (SNRI). Effective in depression with lack of noradrenergic drive.
* Starting dose 75mg daily.

Once an antidepressant is chosen it is important to start at a therapeutic dose and monitor response. If a patient does not begin responding within 4 weeks of treatment then it is appropriate to change to another class of antidepressant either an SNRI (venlafaxine) or a NaSSA (mirtazapine).

Psychostimulants, e.g. methylphenidate
* Used with effect for depression in patients near the end of life (Rozans et al. 2002).
* Quick onset of action, usually within a few days, is the main advantage,
* Can improve mood and energy,
* Dose usually 5mg morning and lunchtime with usual total daily dose of 30mg.

Table 7.7.1 Endicott Criteria for diagnosing depression in advanced cancer

1	Depressed mood, subjective or observed
2	Marked diminished interest or pleasure in most activities, most of the day
3	Fearful or depressed appearance
4	Social withdrawal or decreased talkativeness
5	Psychomotor agitation or retardation
6	Brooding, self-pity, or pessimism
7	Feelings of worthlessness, or excessive or inappropriate guilt
8	Mood is non-reactive to environmental events
9	Recurrent thoughts of death or suicide

For a diagnosis of depression to be present, 5 out of 9 symptoms must be present most of the time most days for a 2-week period

Further reading

Derogatis LR, Morrow GR, Fetting JM, et al. The prevalence of psychiatric disorders among cancer patients. *JAMA* 1983; **249**:751–7.

Block SD. Assessing and managing depression in the terminally ill patient. ACP-ASIM End-of-Life Care Consensus Panel. American College of Physicians – American Society of Internal Medicine. *Ann Intern Med* 2000; **132**:209–18.

Endicott J. Measurement of depression in patients with cancer. Cancer 1984; **53**:2243–9.

Fawzy FI, Fawzy NW, Hyun CSm, et al. Malignant melanoma. Effects of an early structured psychiatric intervention, coping, and affective state on recurrence and survival 6 years later. *Arch Gen Psychiat* 1993; **50**:681–9.

Laird BJ, Mitchell J. The assessment and management of depression in the terminally ill. *Eur J Palliat Care* 2005; **12**: 4.

Rozans M, Dreisbach A, Lertora JJ, et al. Palliative uses of methylphenidate in patients with cancer: a review. *J Clin Oncol* 2002; **20**:335–9.

Delirium

Delirium is also known as acute confusional state and is the second most common psychiatric disorder in cancer patients (Massie et al. 1987). Epidemiological data regarding delirium have shown a prevalence of delirium in hospitalized cancer patients of 38% (Bond et al. 2006). This increases with age with the elderly most at risk. Patients with delirium are often more unwell prior to admission and have an increased level of functional impairment. Delirium is also associated with increased morbidity.

It is important to be able to distinguish between dementia and delirium. Both can be due to a number of underlying conditions, but dementia is usually chronic and irreversible. It is possible to have an acute delirium on a background of a dementing illness. In such scenarios detailed discussion with carers and psychogeriatric review may be needed.

There are many subtypes of delirium ranging from pseudo-delirium to hypoactive delirium and the classical manic delirium. The underlying pathophysiology is unclear although various theories have been postulated. From a clinical point of view it is often best to determine the likely causes.

Causes of delirium in cancer patients

- Metabolic disturbances (hyponatraemia, hypercalcaemia)
- Opioid toxicity can cause delirium and has a wide range of presentations
- Benzodiazepines and steroids can cause drug induced delirium
- Cancer treatments, e.g. cranial radiotherapy
- Direct effects of cancer, e.g. brain metastases
- Indirect effects of cancer, e.g. para-neoplastic syndromes
- Substance abuse—alcohol and illicit drug use and withdrawal
- Infection, e.g. urinary tract, respiratory

Diagnosis of delirium

Informal methods

- Fluctuating symptoms—at some points of the day patients may appear lucid.
- Inability to focus on a subject or conversation
- Hallucinations
- Nocturnal agitation, daytime somnolence

Formal methods

- Mental state examination
- Confusion assessment method (Inouye et al. 1990) (Table 7.8.1)

Table 7.8.1 Confusion assessment method

1	*Acute onset and fluctuating course* Evidence of a change in the patient's mental status from its baseline. Does this fluctuate during the day?
2	*Inattention* Does the patient have difficulty focusing attention?
3	*Disorganized thinking* Is the patient's thinking incoherent, have an illogical flow, or rambling?
4	*Altered level of consciousness* This can range from a coma to a hyper-alert state.

To diagnose delirium features 1 and 2 plus either 3 *or* 4 are required to be present

Treatment of delirium

- General measures such as adequate lighting, a calm environment, and familiar staff are useful.
- Suspected cause should be treated.
- Antipsychotic medications: the challenging aspect is managing symptoms of delirium whilst the treatment takes effect. Antipsychotic medications are often needed.
- Haloperidol is a commonly used antipsychotic medication. It can be administered either orally or parenterally. Doses of between 5–30mg daily are usually required. Howeaver this should be started at the lower end of this dose range and titrated. Sedation rarely occurs unless doses exceed 30mg per day.
- Other antipsychotics are often used; however these are only of benefit if haloperidol has been ineffective or is contraindicated.
- Benzodiazepines may also be required if there is marked patient distress. These should be used *in addition* to antipsychotic medications as benzodiazepines used alone will not correct any underlying biochemical disturbance.
- Oral or parenteral benzodiazepines will often be required in the early stages of delirium management.

Further reading

Bond SM, Neelon VJ, Belyea MJ. Delirium in hospitalized older patients with cancer. *Oncol Nurs Forum* 2006; **33**:1075–83.

Inouye S, van Dyck C, Allessi C, *et al.* Clarifying confusion: the confusion assessment method. *Annals Intern Med* 1990; **113**:941–8.

Massie MJ, Holland JC. The cancer patient with pain: psychiatric complications and their management. *Med Clin North Am* 1987; **71**:243–58.

Oral care

Oral care is an extremely important aspect of care for the cancer patient. A healthy oral cavity protects the body from infections whilst being crucial for eating, drinking, and communication. Cancer treatments, drugs, dehydration, and localized disease all affect the normal function of the oral cavity.

Xerostomia

This is the feeling of a dry mouth with or without a decrease in saliva. It affects most cancer patients at some point during the course of their illness. Causes include:
- Radiotherapy: treatment for head and neck cancers if the parotid or submandibular glands are affected. This leads to a decrease in saliva production and is related to the amount salivary gland irradiated.
- Surgery
- Drugs
- Localized cancer spread
- Chemotherapy—causing erosion of buccal mucosa
- Dehydration
- Oxygen therapy
- Systemic or localized infection

Treatment
Treatment depends on the underlying cause. Radiotherapy-induced xerostomia causes reduced salivary flow as treatment progresses. This can then recover to some extent but in some cases it may persist. Drug-induced xerostomia usually improves when the causal agent is removed or dose reduced.
- Treatment of infections, e.g. oral candida
- Saliva substitutes, e.g. water, glycerine preparations
- Saliva stimulants, e.g. chewing gum, pilocarpine, anethole-trithione

Oral infections
General principles of management
First-line antimicrobial therapy should be commenced with treatment directed at the likely causal organism.

Good oral hygiene will minimize the risk of infection and will aid resolution.
Fungal
- In patients with malignancy, fungal infections are the commonest oral infections. Immunosuppression, antibiotics, and reduced saliva production are all thought to be predisposing factors.
- *Candida albicans* is the most common fungus in oral infections although other candidal strains are becoming increasingly prevalent. Clinically, this appears as white-yellow plaques. In atrophic cases, however, it may exist as redness of the oral cavity, with contact bleeding and pain.
- Oral swabs are not indicated in the first instance but if the patient fails to respond to standard antifungal therapy with nystatin, amphotericin or miconazole, mouth swabs should be taken.

Bacterial
- Although less common than fungal infections, oral bacterial infection is prevalent and can be distressing and severely compromise the immunosuppressed patient. Good oral hygiene and appropriate systemic antibiotic treatment are important. As these infections are often extremely painful, systemic opioid analgesia (often parenteral due to oral pain) is usually needed. In contrast to fungal infections, oral swabs should be taken when bacterial infection is suspected, to direct treatment appropriately.

Viral
- The most common cause is HSV which presents as painful, yellow lesions on the oral mucosa. These may be associated with vesicles on the lips. Systemic antiviral agents (acyclovir) are usually needed and in some cases high-dose intravenous antiviral drugs are required. Pain is often severe with such infections and systemic strong opioid analgesics are usually needed.

Cancer-related fatigue

Cancer-related fatigue has been defined as a 'a persistent subjective sense of tiredness related to cancer or cancer treatment that interferes with usual functioning' (Mock et al. 2000). It is disproportionate to the feeling of being tired.

Epidemiology
- Prevalence varies from 39–90% (Prue et al. 2006).
- Increases in prevalence as disease progresses.
- Patients are more likely to have fatigue when undergoing cancer treatment.

Causes
Multifactorial:
- Inactivity
- Psychological distress
- Anaemia
- Possible role of inflammatory response: interleukin 6 (IL-6), interleukin 1 receptor antibody, and neopterin may have a role in the aetiology (Stone et al. 2008)

Treatment
- Treat possible contributing factors, e.g. psychological distress, insomnia, anaemia.

- Exercise: there is some evidence to suggest that regular, moderate exercise may help.
- Psychological interventions: cognitive behavioural, supportive, and educational therapies have been shown to be of benefit.
- Pharmacological: haemopoietic growth factors (e.g. erythropoietin) improve fatigue associated with anaemia. Methylphenidate has been shown to be helpful in small trials. Steroids and antidepressants have not been shown to be of benefit.

Further reading
Mock V, Atkinson A, Barsevick A, et al. NCCN Practice Guidelines for Cancer-Related Fatigue. *Oncology (Williston Park)* 2000; **14**:151–61.

Prue G, Rankin J, Allen J, et al. Cancer-related fatigue: A critical appraisal. *Eur J Cancer* 2006; **42**:846–63.

Stone PC, Minton O. Cancer-related fatigue. *Eur J Cancer* 2008; **44**:1097–104.

Cancer cachexia

Cachexia has been defined as an involuntary weight loss of >5% of premorbid weight in the previous 6 months, although this definition is over simplistic. It is now recognized that cancer cachexia is a triad of the following (Fearon 2008):
• Weight loss >10%
• Reduced food intake (<1500kcal/day)
• Systemic inflammation (CRP >10mg/L)

Anorexia is the absence or loss of appetite. Asthenia is a syndrome of fatigue (physical and mental) and generalized weakness. Anorexia, asthenia, and cachexia will often coexist in the cancer patient.

Cachexia results in the loss of both lean and fatty tissue. It is associated with psychological distress, altered body image, and reduced physical function. It adversely affects survival, quality of life, and the response to tumouricidal therapies.

Epidemiology

Epidemiology is difficult to determine due to lack of consistent definitions. Approximately 50% of cancer patients will lose weight and 20% will die directly as a result of cachexia. Cachexia is more common in tumours of the GI tract and lung than in breast or prostate cancer. Cachexia increases in prevalence towards the end of life.

Cachexia is a complex condition which is a combination of anorexia and an altered metabolism. When anorexia exists as a sole entity, nutritional supports may allow some weight gain. However as anorexia commonly exists as a component of cachexia, treatment is less straightforward.

Pathophysiology

The following are thought to be implicated in the underlying mechanisms of cachexia (Fearon 2008):
• Systemic inflammation resulting from tumour–host interaction—fat reserves utilized in the acute phase response.

• Tumour producing 'pro-cachectic factors' which cause protein and fat degradation.
• Negative nitrogen balance in cancer cachexia results in wasting of skeletal muscle.
• Hypermetabolism results from activation of neuroendocrine pathways.
• Altered protein metabolism.
• Lack of physical activity may exacerbate muscle wasting.

Treatments

• Reversible causes should be identified and treated, e.g. treat psychological distress. Use enzyme supplements where needed (e.g. in pancreatic cancer).
• Nutritional support: supplements containing at least 1.5kcal/mL are effective in preventing further weight loss.
• Progestogens: e.g. megestrol acetate (160–320mg/day) or medroxyprogesterone acetate (200mg three times daily). These will improve appetite and increase body fat mass. Onset of action is usually 2 weeks and there is no benefit from using doses >800mg per day
• Steroids: although these will improve appetite and give a sense of well-being, they do not have any effect on weight gain. Adverse effects limit their use.
• Fish oils: there is evidence that some patients respond but further characterization of responders is required.

Further reading

Fearon KC. Cancer cachexia: developing multimodal therapy for a multidimensional problem. *Eur J Cancer* 2008; **44**:1124–32.

Breathlessness

Breathlessness is the subjective experience of discomfort in breathing that consists of qualitatively distinct sensations that vary in intensity (Cachia and Ahmedzai 2008). It can be very distressing for patients and is very subjective. It can occur in cancer due either to direct effects of the tumour or indirect effects.

Epidemiology

It varies in prevalence from 40–80% and can occur at any stage of the cancer illness. It commonly occurs in lung, lymphoma, head and neck, genitourinary and breast cancers (Cachia and Ahmedzai 2008).

Pathophysiology

Normally, breathing is maintained by a physiological pathway controlled by the respiratory centre in the brain stem. Various factors including oxygen and carbon dioxide levels, lung mechanoreceptors, and arterial chemoreceptors all help regulate respiration. In cancer, distortion of mechanoreceptors (through disease), fatigue, muscle weakness, disease bulk, and anxiety can all impede the normal breathing process. Usually oxygen levels are maintained in cancer patients who are breathless.

Common causes

- Lung metastases
- Primary tumour site, e.g. lung
- Co-existing conditions e.g. COPD
- Pulmonary thromboembolism
- Pleural effusions
- Anaemia
- Increased intra-abdominal pressure, e.g. ascites
- Anxiety
- Cachexia resulting in muscle weakness
- Cardiac failure

Management

General principles

As breathlessness can be very distressing for patients, it is important to reassure both patients and family members. A multidisciplinary approach is often needed with physiotherapists available to offer techniques for managing dyspnoea. Advice on breathing exercises, management of anxiety attacks, posture, and expectoration can often be beneficial.

A stream of air, either from a fan or through an open window, will often provide symptomatic relief.

Correct reversible causes

- Treat respiratory infections with antimicrobial treatment.
- Manage coexisting disease (e.g. COPD, cardiac failure) in the usual manner.
- Treat anaemia.

Cancer specific treatment

- Radiotherapy to large tumour bulk.
- Endobronchial disease can be treated by stenting or removed by laser treatment.

- Lymphangitis carcinomatosis can be treated with high-dose steroids, (dexamethasone 16mg daily PO).

Drainage of effusions

- Drainage of large pleural effusions may lead to relief of symptoms. If they recur consider pleurodesis
- If symptomatic drain pericardial effusions

Oxygen therapy (Booth et al. 2004)

- Hypoxic respiratory drive usually only occurs when SaO_2 <90%. In cases where SaO_2 is >90%, oxygen is less likely to be of any benefit.
- Short-burst oxygen therapy (intermittent use of oxygen for the relief of dyspnoea either before or after exercise) may be useful in some cases. Each case must be assessed on an individual basis and the response monitored.
- Ambulatory oxygen therapy (use of oxygen during exercise or activities of daily living) may be of use in those who desaturate on exertion.
- In those patients with COPD, assessment should be made on an individual basis.

Opioids

The exact mechanism of effect in dyspnoea is unclear but opioids may work in several ways. They reduce pain, cough, the ventilator reaction to hypercapnia, and also pre- and postcardiac load.

There is no inherent benefit of one opioid over another in managing dyspnoea. The opioid most commonly used is morphine. This is usually commenced orally at a dose of 5mg four times daily and the effect subsequently assessed. This can be titrated upwards as effect dictates. If the patient is already taking opioids for pain then it may be that the opioid dose prescribed to be given as required can be increased by 25–50% to be used as needed for dyspnoea.

Respiratory depression is very rare, provided treatment of opioid naïve patients is commenced with low doses and titrated upwards slowly.

Benzodiazepines

Benzodiazepines are particularly useful when there is an associated anxiety component to breathlessness. Usually short-acting oral benzodiazepines are preferred (e.g. lormetazepam 0.5mg sublingually) prescribed as needed for dyspnoea. At the end of life, a continuous infusion of parenteral benzodiazepine may be needed. In such cases midazolam (5–20mg over 24 hours) is effective.

Further reading

Cachia E, Ahmedzai SH. Breathlessness in cancer patients. *Eur J Cancer* 2008; **44**:1116–23.

Booth S, Wade R, Johnson M, *et al.* The use of oxygen in the palliation of breathlessness. A report of the expert working group of the Scientific Committee of the Association of Palliative Medicine. *Respir Med* 2004; **98**:66–77.

Cough

Although cough is a normal physiological mechanism, it is more common in malignant disease. There are a number of causes which can be due to the underlying malignancy or due to coexisting non-malignant conditions (Table 7.13.1).

Management
Depends on the type of cough and underlying cause.

General principles
• Physiotherapy will aid expectoration.
• Repositioning (lying on same side as pleural effusion) may palliate cough.
• Treat any underlying infection.
• Drain pleural effusions if thought to be causal.
• Treat stridor secondary to central airway tumour with steroids.
• Remove any drugs thought to be causing the cough.
• In patients who are generally weak and unable to cough, repositioning, suction and the use of drugs to manage respiratory secretions are advised.

Expectorants
Stimulate cough reflex or reduce viscosity of mucus aiding expectoration, e.g. nebulized saline.

Cough suppressants (antitussives)
• Most potent are opioids.
• Work on opioid receptors centrally (cough centre) and in the airways.

Table 7.13.1 Common causes of cough

Malignant	Non-malignant
Airway obstruction	Infection (acute or chronic)
Lymphangitis	COPD
Pulmonary metastases	Asthma
Radiotherapy related pneumonitis	Recurrent aspiration
Pleural effusions	Drug related, e.g. ACE inhibitors
Hilar disease affecting vocal cord	

• Usually start with codeine linctus (unless taking strong opioid for another reason).
• If ineffective, use strong opioids—no evidence to suggest any benefit of one over the other.
• Methadone (low dose) may be helpful—due to long half-life which allows daily dosing.
• Nebulized local anaesthetics may be helpful in endo-bronchial malignancy.

Haemoptysis

Haemoptysis may have been the presenting symptom in the cancer patient and can be worrying for the patient and family. In mild haemoptysis the patient should be reassured. The use of oral haemostatic agents (e.g. tranexamic acid) and cough suppressants may be needed.

Massive haemoptysis (>200mL of blood in 24 hours) should be considered an emergency. Studies suggest this is usually more prevalent in non-malignant disease than lung cancer.

In such cases families (and occasionally patients if appropriate) should be informed of management principles. The use of opioids and anxiolytics given parenterally (even intravenously if warranted clinically) is indicated. These should be titrated to relieve any anxiety and reduce conscious level if needed. The aim of such treatment is not to make the patient unconscious but to sedate to appropriate levels to relieve distress. In such cases, support for the patient, family, and other members of staff is of paramount importance.

Symptom clusters

Although the aforementioned symptoms are discussed individually, in the cancer patient these symptoms rarely exist in isolation. A symptom cluster has been defined as 'three or more concurrent symptoms that are related to each other' (Dodd et al. 2001). Relationship does not imply causality or a common underlying mechanism. There has been increasing interest in symptoms with a common underlying pathophysiology.

At present, a firm evidence base, which defines clearly specific symptom clusters, is lacking. Studies have shown that fatigue, pain, and drowsiness tend to occur together (Chow et al. 2008). Other clusters suggested include poor appetite, nausea, anxiety, and low mood. It has also been demonstrated that pain, fatigue, low mood, and function may cluster together.

Currently there is a lack of consistently validated symptom clusters and work in this field is ongoing.

Nevertheless, clinical experience would support the dictum that symptoms often coexist.

It is important, therefore, to note that in the optimal symptom management of the cancer patient, treating a single symptom in isolation may not achieve resolution. The approach should be adopted where several symptoms are treated in unison, e.g. the patient who has pain and depression should be treated for both. By addressing several symptoms at once, the individual symptoms may respond better to treatment.

Further reading

Chow E, Fan G, Hadi S et al. Symptom clusters in cancer patients with brain metastases. *Clin Oncol* 2008; **20**:76–82.

Dodd M, Miaskowski C, Paul S. Symptom clusters and their effect on the functional status of patients with cancer. *Oncol Nurs Forum* 2001; **28**:465–70.

End of life care

End of life care of the cancer patient can be one of the most rewarding aspects of care. It can also be the most challenging as it is the end of the cancer journey for the patient, the family, and the health professionals involved in their care. It is important that care at this stage is tailored to the patient and the family. As death approaches there will be increased physical and psychological needs. Greater nursing needs and increased symptoms often necessitate 'intensive' care. The physician should accept that the primary illness is no longer the priority and the focus of care should move to physical and psychological symptom control. Patient and family anxiety is often high so a thoughtful, sensitive approach is needed.

Recognition of end of life

Perhaps one of the most difficult aspects is to recognize, and subsequently acknowledge, that someone has entered the terminal phase of their illness. If the oncologist has cared for the patient for a considerable length of time it can be challenging to decide that treatment should be stopped or that further active treatment is unlikely to confer a benefit. Decisions are best made following consultation with the patient, family, and members of the oncology team. It is important that the realization that the patient is dying is understood and accepted by all involved parties. Only then can care be directed towards patient comfort and family support, as the primary aim.

Signs of dying

The following signs and symptoms (in the context of the patient's disease state) are suggestive that the patient is dying (Adam et al. 1997):
• Usually bedbound or immobile
• Difficulty managing medication
• Confusion
• Marked generalized weakness
• Drowsy or comatose
• Poor appetite and decreased fluid intake

General principles of end of life care

The Liverpool Care Pathway for the Dying Patient (LCP) is a 'continuous quality improvement framework for the care of the dying patient' (Bennett et al. 2002). This pathway emphasizes the fundamental principles that should be employed in end of life care. It can be used in either malignant or non-malignant disease and in either a primary or secondary care setting. The general principles adopted in the LCP are the foundations to end of life care and are as follows:
• Discontinue any inappropriate interventions. This includes blood tests, antibiotics, and intravenous fluids or parenteral nutrition.
• Document that the patient is not to receive cardiopulmonary resuscitation. Ensure that any implantable defibrillators have been deactivated.
• Stop any inappropriate nursing interventions. Regular observations of vital signs should be stopped. Blood glucose monitoring should be undertaken if clinically indicated. Patients should only be repositioned for comfort rather than on a routine basis.
• Required medications (analgesics and anxiolytics) should be given by syringe driver and this should be started within 4 hours of prescribing.
• Assess that communication is not an issue, particularly if English is not the first language. Interpreters may be needed.
• Assess insight of condition of patient (if patient requests this) and family.
• Assess any religious/spiritual needs and involve appropriate clergy at patient's request.
• Give appropriate information to relevant hospital professionals and general practice.
• Ensure that the plan of care (if the LCP is being utilized explain the nature of this) has been understood.
• Following death, the patient's body should be managed according to local policy. Any religious requirements should be adhered to.
• The GP should be informed of the patient's death.
• Appropriate information regarding arranging a funeral and death registration should be given to the family in written format.
• Information on bereavement support should be given to the family.

(Adapted from the principles suggested by Professor John Ellershaw.)

Principles of drug use in end of life care
• Use the minimum amount of medications to treat the patient and ease distress and pain.
• Use of parenteral routes of medication—as condition deteriorates and conscious level decreases, the ability to swallow effectively declines. Medication should change to parenteral routes. A subcutaneous infusion via syringe driver is preferred.
• Assess pain and other symptoms regularly.
• Continue with medications even if the patient is in a coma as pain and other symptoms may be present and cause distress, indicated through non-verbal means.
• Often other drugs can be administered parenterally in combination with the strong opioid. This should be checked on an individual basis.
• Stop non-essential medications, e.g. those for hypertension, diabetes, etc., as the potential benefit is likely to be very low

Specific symptom control
Pain
Pain should be managed according to the basic principles of the WHO analgesic ladder. Thorough assessment of pain through history and examination should be followed by appropriate treatment. Analgesic requirements may increase so regular review of pain should be undertaken. Particular care should be taken of the unconscious patient as they will not be able to complain of pain but pain may still exist.
• Convert oral analgesia (usually a strong opioid) to a parenteral route (SC) via syringe driver.
• Opioid conversions should be done as indicated previously.
• Long-acting opioids such as analgesic patches should not be stopped at this stage due to the delay in reaching peak plasma levels.
• Adjuvant analgesics and NSAIDs should still be used when appropriate.
• Pain may also be helped by non-drug measures such as repositioning, TENS, etc.

Dyspnoea

Breathlessness may be due to a number of causes including pre-existing disease and manifestations of malignancy, e.g. lung metastases, pleural effusions, lymphangitis carcinomatosis.

- Reversible causes should be treated when appropriate. Use of diuretics (cardiac failure) and bronchodilators (bronchospasm) are indicated where appropriate (Adam 1997).
- Supportive measures such as positioning, assistance with expectoration, and the use of cool air (via fan or open window) will relieve the sensation of breathlessness.
- Oxygen has been shown to be helpful in some patients with dyspnoea. Often patients find face masks restrictive and uncomfortable and nasal cannulae are often preferred. Oxygen can be delivered effectively up to 28% (4L) via this route.
- Nebulized saline may help to expectorate secretions if present.
- The use of opioids and benzodiazepines in patients with dyspnoea is often helpful.
- As the conscious level deteriorates, changes in the breathing pattern occur. Cheyne–Stokes breathing is frequently observed and consists of alternating periods of rapid breathing followed by spells of apnoea.

Anxiety/restlessness

Anxiety and restlessness can be due to angst regarding death and the plethora of accompanying emotions. It can also be due to symptoms and should be managed as a priority. Exploration of fears, discussion, and reassurance should be undertaken in the first instance. Often however, pharmacological interventions are needed to manage this. Even in small doses, drugs can alleviate the symptoms of anxiety without causing sedation. Low-dose anxiolytics (e.g. benzodiazepines) are usually used in these situations and can be administered concurrently with strong opioids in a syringe driver. In the UK, the commonly used benzodiazepine in this setting is midazolam, usually starting at doses of 5–10mg via subcutaneous syringe driver over 24 hours. As required doses of one-sixth of the total daily dose should be prescribed concurrently.

Delirium/acute-confusional state (Table 7.16.1)

When delirium occurs at the end of life it is often referred to as terminal agitation and can be very distressing for the patient and the family. It can affect cognition and thus affect the emotional issues that require to be worked through at the end of life. There can be many causes including biochemical disturbance, hypoxia, hepatic and renal failure, cerebral disease, infective sources, and drugs, e.g. steroids or opioids.

Treatment of the underlying source is important but in many cases the cause is unknown and treatment has to be given 'blind'. Use of antipsychotic medications, such as haloperidol, is helpful and can usually be given in a syringe driver with opioids and anxiolytics.

Haloperidol is of particular use in cases of opioid toxicity at the end of life. At this point, switching to another opioid to combat toxicity is not advised. Thus controlling side effects appropriately is the ideal. If the patient is markedly distressed, the use of midazolam for anxiety/distress and haloperidol (to treat psychosis) is the normal practice in the UK. The lowest dose should be used to achieve the desired effect.

In cases of severe terminal agitation where escalating doses of midazolam and haloperidol have been unsuccessful, second-line agents should be used. Methotrimeprazine is

helpful and should be titrated to achieve effect. Where terminal agitation exists, frequent review is needed as this will be a very distressing time for both patients and family members.

Respiratory secretions

As the patient becomes increasingly weak and exhausted, respiratory secretions gather in the posterior pharynx. The sound produced is often referred to as the 'death rattle'. However this term is best avoided as its use can be distressing for patients and family members.

Marked respiratory secretions at the end of life are present in approximately 50% of deaths (Bennett et al. 2002). These usually occur when the patient is comatose so that they are often unaware of them. It could be argued that as the patient is unaware of the symptom it is not necessary to treat it. However, family members can find this disturbing and often concerns are expressed that the patients is either choking or drowning. It is accepted practice that respiratory secretions should be treated and antimuscarinic agents such as hyoscine hydrobromide, hyoscine butylbromide, and glycopyrronium are used (Table 7.16.2). There is insufficient evidence to indicated superiority of any one over the other.

In some cases oral pharyngeal suction is needed. This is best used in patients who are comatose as it can be distressing if patients are conscious.

Mouth care

Mouth care is extremely important at the end of life. Patients are likely to be dehydrated and if conscious level is impaired, their oral hygiene and intake may have been compromised. It is important that regular mouth care is undertaken throughout the dying phase. The principles are the same as those discussed previously (see p.657). The use of mouth swabs soaked in cool water can be used to hydrate the oral mucosa and improve mouth care. Family members can be instructed to do this in addition to healthcare staff.

Fluids and parenteral nutrition

Patients who have undergone intensive hospital treatment may have intravenous fluids and parenteral nutrition in place. As the dying process is acknowledged and the focus of care changes to symptom control, dealing with fluids and parenteral nutrition can be challenging. These are highly visible, intensive treatments and withdrawing them carries much meaning. In these cases, careful, thoughtful discussions with the patient and family members should be undertaken. Concerns are often raised that the patient will starve or be thirsty. Abrupt cessation of these may be perceived as lack of care or abandonment.

In the end of life setting, intravenous fluids and nutritional support are unlikely to provide any benefit. This information should be imparted to the patient/family and the negative effects of these interventions highlighted. Sites for fluids may become inflamed and, due to peripheral oedema that often exists at the end of life, absorption is likely to be impaired. As conscious level deteriorates, nasogastric or PEG feeding may lead to an increased likelihood of developing aspiration pneumonia which may accelerate death.

In some cases withdrawing fluids or feeding may improve symptoms. The resulting dehydration may relieve the oedema resulting from end-stage liver failure. In patients with brain metastases, the improvement in oedema may improve the neurological symptoms associated with raised intracranial pressure. It is, however, always important to

Table 7.16.1 Drug treatment for terminal agitation and distress

Drug	Route	Indication	Usual starting dose	Dose range over 24 hours (continuous infusion)
Haloperidol	SC	Delirium	2.5mg	5–30mg
Midazolam	SC	Distress	2.5–5mg	10–80mg
Methotrimeprazine*	SC	Delirium	25mg	25–250mg

*Usually used when standard doses of haloperidol and midazolam have been ineffective

keep an open mind and individualize decisions, in particular about fluids.

Psychological aspects of end of life care

Ideally a good death should be free from distress. Symptoms, both physical and psychological, should be addressed appropriately. Whilst we often have at our disposal a variety of drugs to treat physical symptoms, addressing psychosocial aspects can be more challenging. An important psychological issue is patient dignity (Chochinov et al. 2002). Dignity is a triad of honour, self-esteem, and respect, and is a key area that should be addressed in end of life care.

Dignity has been examined in patients who are terminally ill (Chochinov et al. 2002): 46% of patients had some loss of dignity, whilst 7.5% considered loss of dignity a serious issue. In the hospital setting patients were more likely to suffer a loss of dignity as opposed to patients in primary care. There does not appear to be any relationship between prognosis and loss of dignity. Patients who feel their dignity has not been compromised are less likely to suffer from depression, anxiety, and even a feeling of hopelessness. Also, as sense of dignity increases, there is an increase in quality of life. In contrast, loss of dignity is positively correlated with a desire for hastened death.

Dignity therapy

The concept of dignity therapy was devised by Chochinov et al. (2002). It builds on the foundations of dignity conserving care which should occur in the management of every patient. Dignity therapy is based on the concept of generativity with the aim of bringing meaning to the life lost.

Dignity therapy can be undertaken by trained therapists. Through careful discussion, the patient is interviewed about their life and how they feel they would like to be remembered. Areas are explored such as life history, key events, and accomplishments. If the patient wants to impart any specific messages, these can also be documented.

Conversations are recorded and are then transcribed to meaningful narrative form. Following this and after the patient is happy with the end result, the patient is given the finished document. The patient is free to give this

to whomever they choose, but these are often given to young ones.

Although dignity therapy is best done by those who have had formal training, it can also be done less formally. Through the use of a question based format, health professionals or even family members can discuss these issues.

Care should be taken if the patient is very near dying and in particular has cognitive impairment. If records of conversations or thoughts are not recorded accurately, false information may be imparted. In the scenario of end of life there may be no opportunity to address this.

How long?

This question is commonly asked by patients and families and may be a source of anxiety for the health professional who has to answer this. It may be very difficult to estimate and there is a dearth of research within this area. As a result, physicians are often very bad at estimating prognosis. Patients and families will however request this information. If a likely timescale is known, this allows for business and emotional issues to be addressed. It may also be necessary if family members are overseas and wish or are requested by the patient to be seen. It can be very useful for the patient to know how close death is and if this is the patient's wish, it should be discussed.

It is often very difficult to predict death and usually it is best to give estimates in the region of 'days', 'weeks', 'days to weeks', etc. Often a useful predictor is the rate of decline over a set time period. If patients have deteriorated very quickly in a short spell then it is likely that their decline will continue at this rate and death is likely to be sooner. Frequent discussions with patients and more often family members will be of great comfort. Changes such as marked decrease in urine output, deterioration in conscious level or Cheyne–Stokes breathing are likely to signify that few days are left.

In some cases, if the dying process is slow some patients and families feel it is taking too long. This is a particular issue if families are caring for a patient at home on the basis that they can cope for a short time. This too can be a real challenge to deal with. There should be regular review and discussions with patients and their families. Although these patients may not require much in the way

Table 7.16.2 Drug treatment for respiratory secretions at the end of life

Drug	Route	Initial dose	Review response after	Dose over 24 hours (continuous infusion)—if initial dose effective
Hyoscine hydrobromide	SC	400mcg	30 minutes	1.2–2mg
Glycopyrronium	SC	200mcg	60 minutes	1.2–2mg
Hyoscine butylbromide	SC	20mg	30 minutes	200mg

of medical or nursing support (particularly when they are in a coma) they should still have regular review. It is important in these times that families feel supported and not abandoned.

The bitter or angry patient

This is an area which can be very difficult to manage. As a result of the intense psychological stresses the dying patient is under, there may be bitterness and anger. Lack of independence and increased level of care can cause frustration which can lead to anger, often directed at loved ones, causing distress. Delirium may cause anger and should be addressed.

It is important to try to address any issues and in some cases spiritual and psychological support may be required. The physician should explore tactfully any concerns or anxieties and address as many issues as possible. It should be acknowledged that in some cases this may be very difficult or impossible for the doctor to correct. In these cases ongoing support for the patient and family should continue, despite any hostility.

Post-death care

The death certificate should be issued with appropriate advice on the necessary legal requirements and process of arranging a funeral. It is often helpful to meet with the family to explain this and answer any questions or address any concerns. Depending on religion or beliefs there may be certain requirements or rituals that should be adhered to and all efforts should be made to deal with these.

Following death, bereavement care is often offered either actively or passively to family members. If the patient died in a hospice, this is generally done as standard. In some cases the family may want to meet with the medical team some time following the death. This will often deal with unanswered questions and may ease the process of bereavement.

Conclusion

End of life care is one of the most rewarding aspects of care. It can also be one of the most challenging. Despite best efforts, in some cases patients do not have a good death. In these cases it is important to remember that we may not be able to fix all symptoms but we should continue to offer our support and be there for the patient and family at this distressing time.

Further reading

Adam J. ABC of palliative care. The last 48 hours. *BMJ* 1997; **315**:1600–3.

Bennett M, Lucas V, Brennan M, *et al.* Using anti-muscarinic drugs in the management of death rattle: evidence-based guidelines for palliative care. *Palliat Med* 2002; **16**:369–74.

Chochinov HM, Hack T, Hassard T, *et al.* Dignity in the terminally ill: a cross-sectional, cohort study. *Lancet* 2002; **360**:2026–30.

Internet resource

Liverpool Care Pathway for the Dying Patient: http://www.mcpcil.org.uk/liverpool_care_pathway

Clinical management of cancer: flowcharts

Bladder cancer

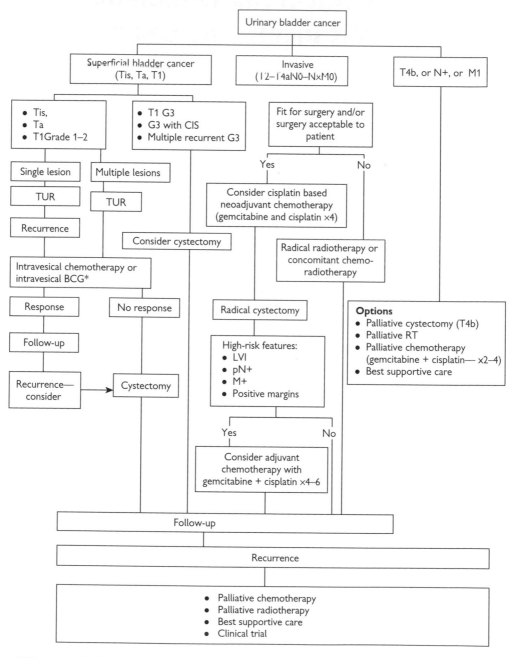

TUR—transurethral resection

* See p.269 for details of intravesical treatment and chemotherapy and p.268–9 for radiotherapy details

Fig. 8.1.1

Breast cancer

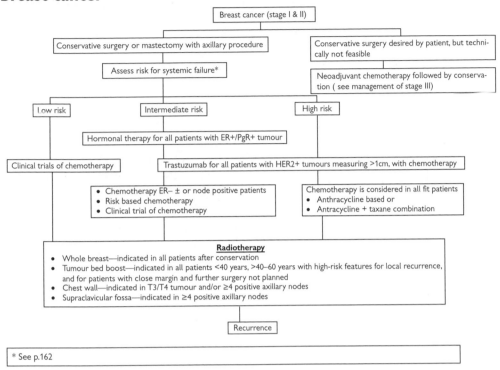

* See p.162

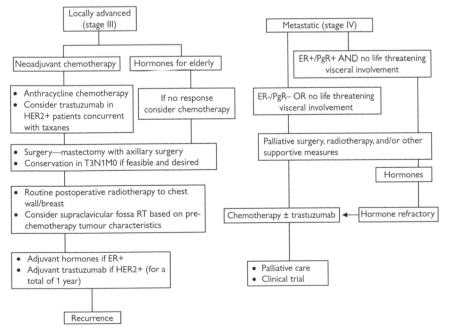

Fig. 8.2.1

Cervical cancer

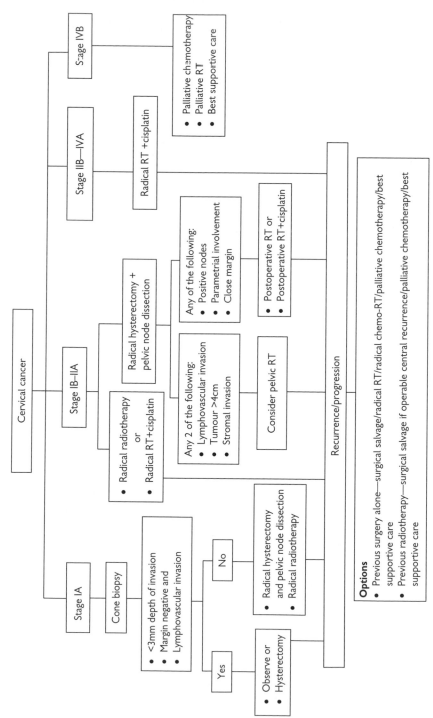

Fig. 8.3.1

Colon cancer

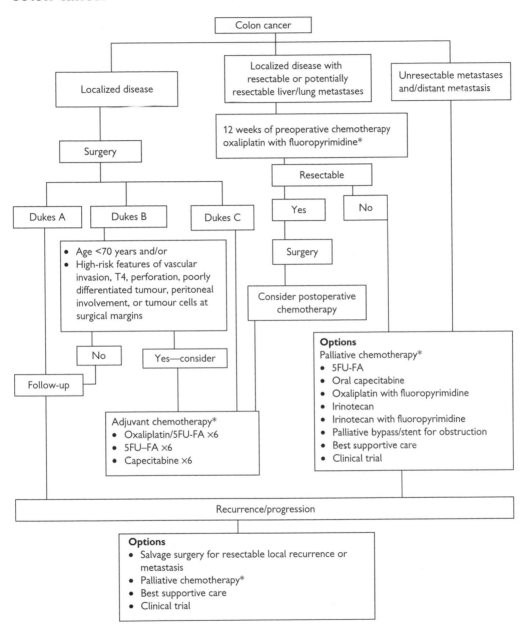

Fig. 8.4.1

Endometrial cancer

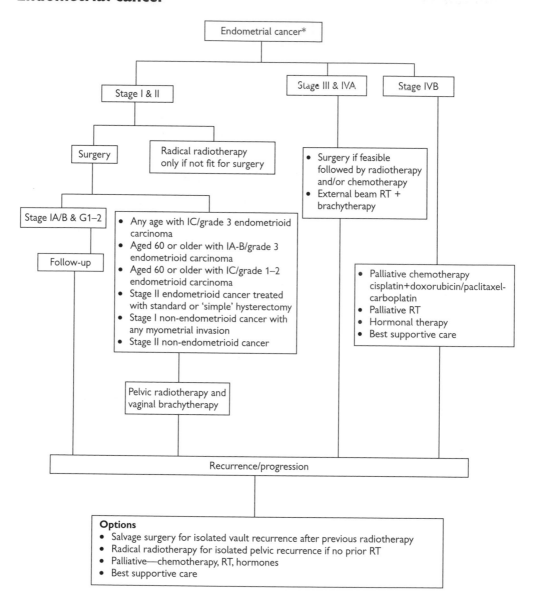

Fig. 8.5.1

Epithelial ovarian cancer

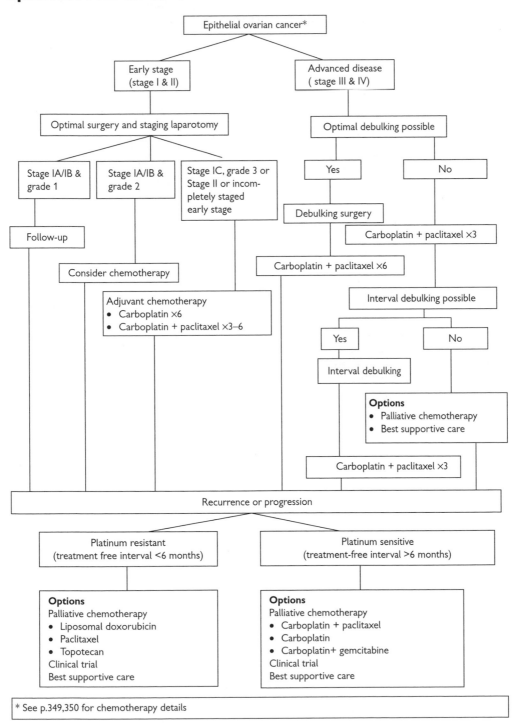

Fig. 8.6.1

Hepatocellular cancer

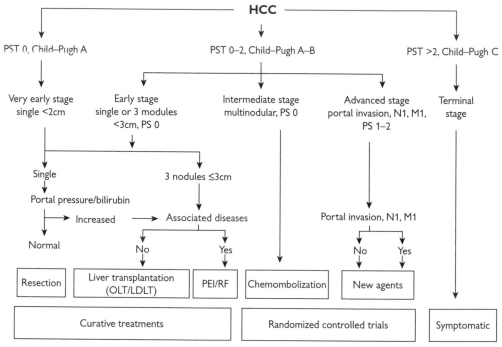

Fig. 8.7.1 Strategy for staging and treatment in patients diagnosed with HCC according to the BCLC protocol (Bruix and Sherman 2005). RF, Radiofrequency ablation; LDLT, living donor liver transplantation; OLT, orthotopic liver transplantation; PS, performance status.

Small-cell lung cancer

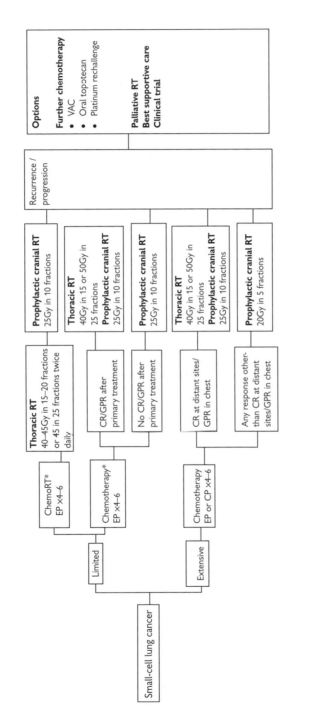

Fig. 8.8.1

* For details of chemotherapy radiotherapy regimens—see p.134–5

Non-small cell lung cancer

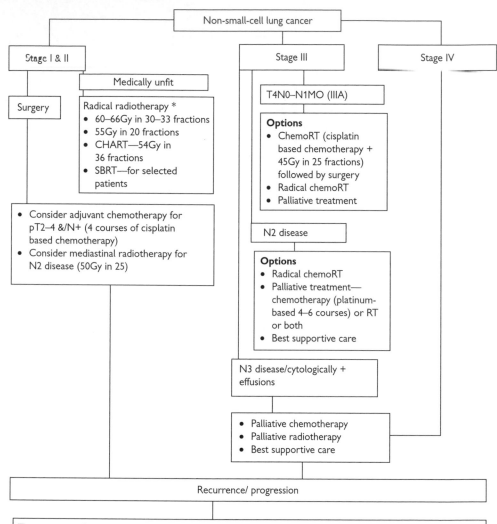

```
                        ┌──────────────────────────────┐
                        │  Non-small-cell lung cancer   │
                        └──────────────────────────────┘
```

Stage I & II

Medically unfit

Surgery

Radical radiotherapy *
• 60–66Gy in 30–33 fractions
• 55Gy in 20 fractions
• CHART—54Gy in
  36 fractions
• SBRT—for selected
  patients

• Consider adjuvant chemotherapy for
  pT2–4 &/N+ (4 courses of cisplatin
  based chemotherapy)
• Consider mediastinal radiotherapy for
  N2 disease (50Gy in 25)

Stage III

T4N0–N1M0 (IIIA)

Options
• ChemoRT (cisplatin
  based chemotherapy +
  45Gy in 25 fractions)
  followed by surgery
• Radical chemoRT
• Palliative treatment

N2 disease

Options
• Radical chemoRT
• Palliative treatment—
  chemotherapy (platinum-
  based 4–6 courses) or RT
  or both
• Best supportive care

N3 disease/cytologically +
effusions

• Palliative chemotherapy
• Palliative radiotherapy
• Best supportive care

Stage IV

Recurrence/ progression

Treatment options
Isolated local recurrence with no previous RT
• Radical radiotherapy/radical chemoRT/palliative RT/best supportive care
Previous RT/metastatic recurrence
• Palliative chemotherapy (platinum-based chemotherapy if no previous chemotherapy/docetaxel
  or erlotinib® if had previous platinum)/palliative radiotherapy/best supportive care

Selection of treatment based on performance status
• Radical treatment is only considered in patients with PS 0–1
• All patients with PS2 should be carefully evaluated prior to palliative chemotherapy
• Patients with PS 3–4—palliative chemotherapy should not be given

* see p125

Fig. 8.9.1

Oesophageal cancer

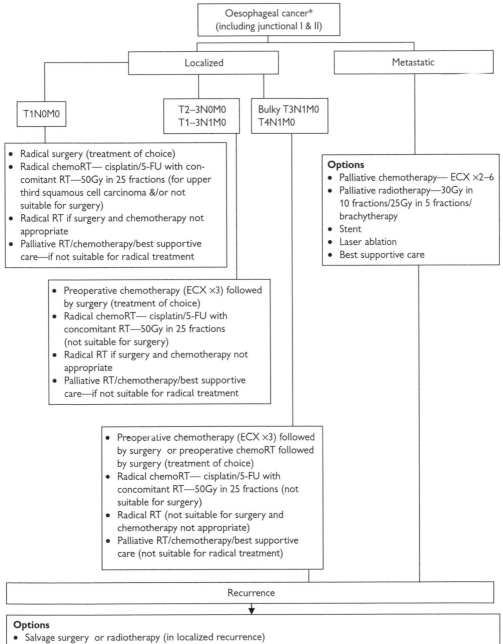

Oesophageal cancer*
(including junctional I & II)

Localized

Metastatic

T1N0M0

T2–3N0M0
T1–3N1M0

Bulky T3N1M0
T4N1M0

- Radical surgery (treatment of choice)
- Radical chemoRT— cisplatin/5-FU with concomitant RT—50Gy in 25 fractions (for upper
  third squamous cell carcinoma &/or not
  suitable for surgery)
- Radical RT if surgery and chemotherapy not
  appropriate
- Palliative RT/chemotherapy/best supportive
  care—if not suitable for radical treatment

Options
- Palliative chemotherapy— ECX ×2–6
- Palliative radiotherapy—30Gy in
  10 fractions/25Gy in 5 fractions/
  brachytherapy
- Stent
- Laser ablation
- Best supportive care

- Preoperative chemotherapy (ECX ×3) followed
  by surgery (treatment of choice)
- Radical chemoRT— cisplatin/5-FU with
  concomitant RT—50Gy in 25 fractions
  (not suitable for surgery)
- Radical RT if surgery and chemotherapy not
  appropriate
- Palliative RT/chemotherapy/best supportive
  care—if not suitable for radical treatment

- Preoperative chemotherapy (ECX ×3) followed
  by surgery or preoperative chemoRT followed
  by surgery (treatment of choice)
- Radical chemoRT— cisplatin/5-FU with
  concomitant RT—50Gy in 25 fractions (not
  suitable for surgery)
- Radical RT (not suitable for surgery and
  chemotherapy not appropriate)
- Palliative RT/chemotherapy/best supportive
  care (not suitable for radical treatment)

Recurrence

Options
- Salvage surgery or radiotherapy (in localized recurrence)
- Palliative chemotherapy (taxanes or platinum or 5-FU based) /radiotherapy/ best supportive care

* See p.180–181 for chemotherapy regimens and p.180,182 for radiotherapy

Fig. 8.10.1

Pancreatic cancer

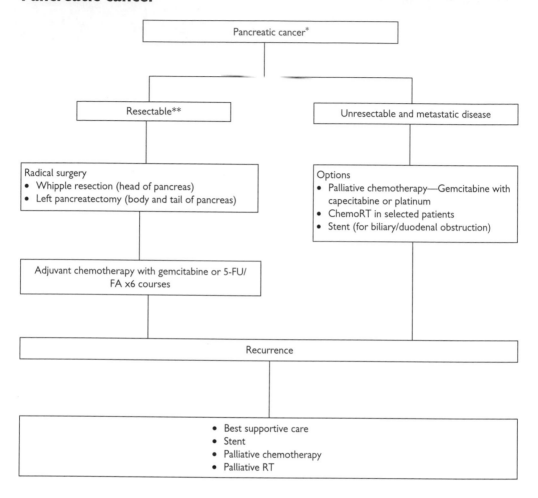

* See p.217 for chemotherapy regimens

**Definition of resectable disease:
- No coeliac, hepatic, or superior mesenteric artery involvement
- A patent superior mesenteric-portal venous confluence
- Portal venous involvement of not >2cm in length or >50% circumference
- No liver, peritoneal, or other distant metastases
- Absence of portal hypertension and cirrhosis
- No severe comorbidity to exclude surgery

Fig. 8.11.1

Prostate cancer

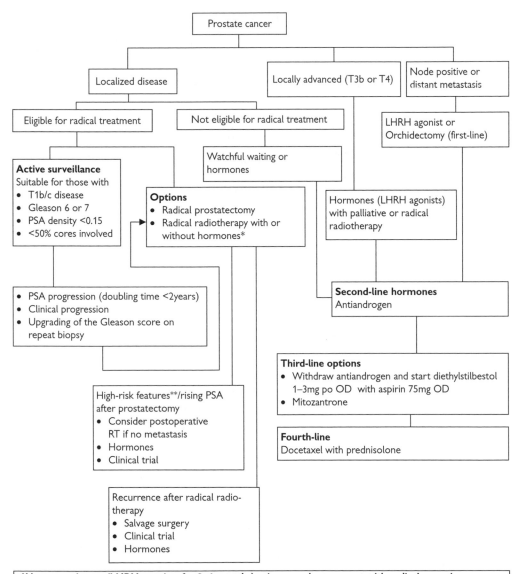

Active surveillance
Suitable for those with
• T1b/c disease
• Gleason 6 or 7
• PSA density <0.15
• <50% cores involved

• PSA progression (doubling time <2years)
• Clinical progression
• Upgrading of the Gleason score on repeat biopsy

High-risk features**/rising PSA after prostatectomy
• Consider postoperative RT if no metastasis
• Hormones
• Clinical trial

Recurrence after radical radio-therapy
• Salvage surgery
• Clinical trial
• Hormones

Options
• Radical prostatectomy
• Radical radiotherapy with or without hormones*

Watchful waiting or hormones

Hormones (LHRH agonists) with palliative or radical radiotherapy

Second-line hormones
Antiandrogen

Third-line options
• Withdraw antiandrogen and start diethylstilbestol 1–3mg po OD with aspirin 75mg OD
• Mitozantrone

Fourth-line
Docetaxel with prednisolone

*Hormone therapy(LHRH agonists for 3–6 months) prior to and concurrent with radiotherapy is considered if:
• pT1b/c
• CT2a-c
• Gleason <8
• PSA≤ 30
Patients with the following high-risk factors for systemic disease may be considered for adjuvant hormones (LHRH agonists) for 3 years
• cT3/4a
• Gleason ≥8
• PSA >30
** Positive surgical margins and/or PSA fails to suppress

Fig. 8.12.1

Rectal cancer

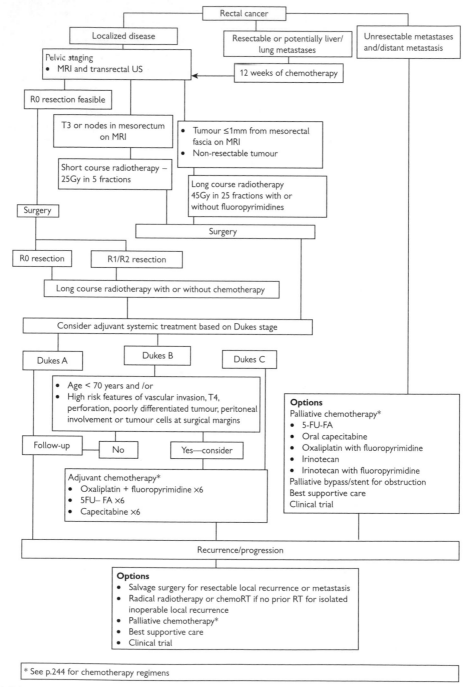

Fig. 8.13.1

Stomach cancer

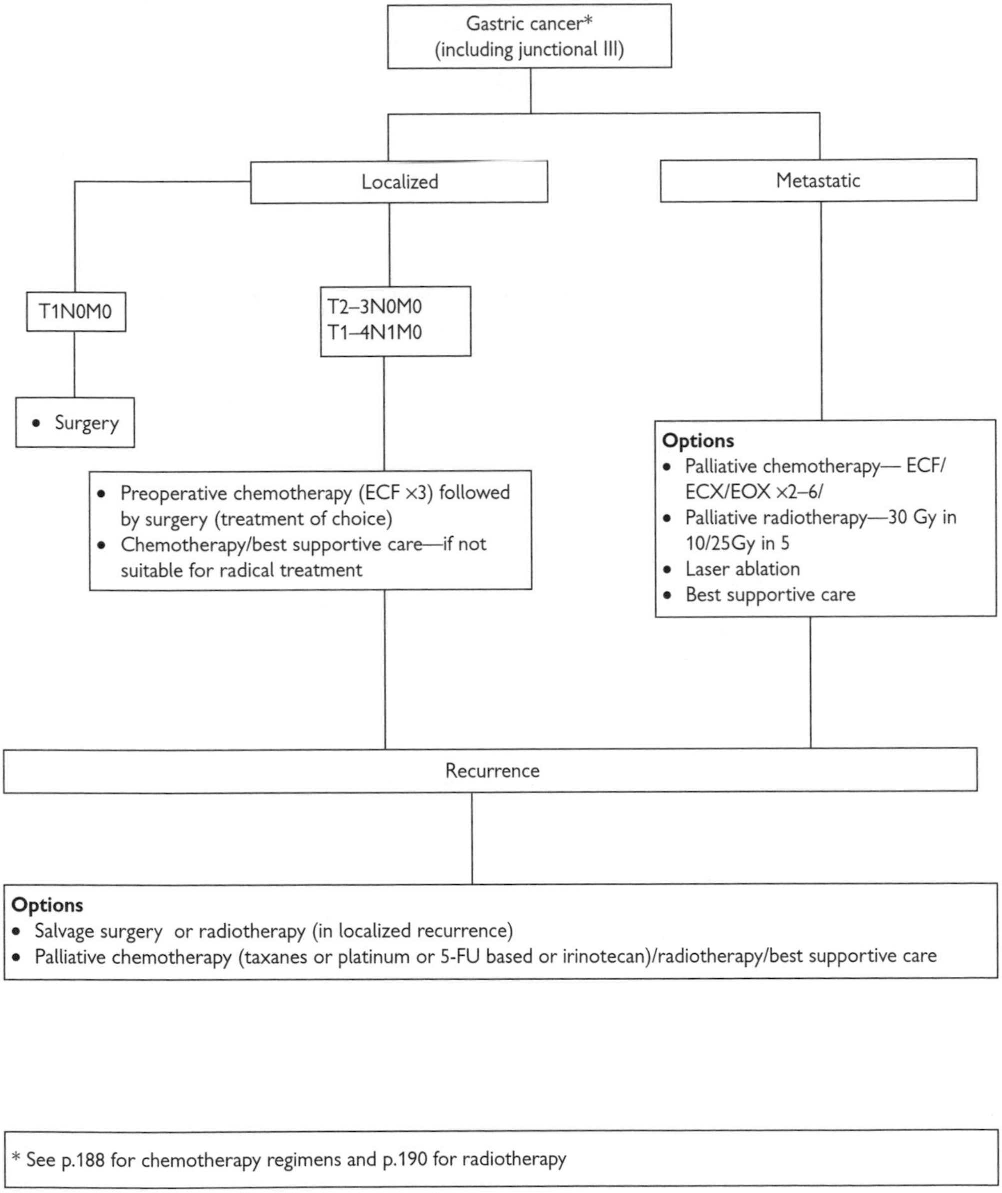
Gastric cancer*
(including junctional III)
Localized
Metastatic
T1N0M0
T2–3N0M0
T1–4N1M0
• Surgery
• Preoperative chemotherapy (ECF ×3) followed by surgery (treatment of choice)
• Chemotherapy/best supportive care—if not suitable for radical treatment
Options
• Palliative chemotherapy— ECF/ ECX/EOX ×2–6/
• Palliative radiotherapy—30 Gy in 10/25Gy in 5
• Laser ablation
• Best supportive care
Recurrence
Options
• Salvage surgery or radiotherapy (in localized recurrence)
• Palliative chemotherapy (taxanes or platinum or 5-FU based or irinotecan)/radiotherapy/best supportive care
* See p.188 for chemotherapy regimens and p.190 for radiotherapy

Fig. 8.14.1

Testicular cancer: seminoma

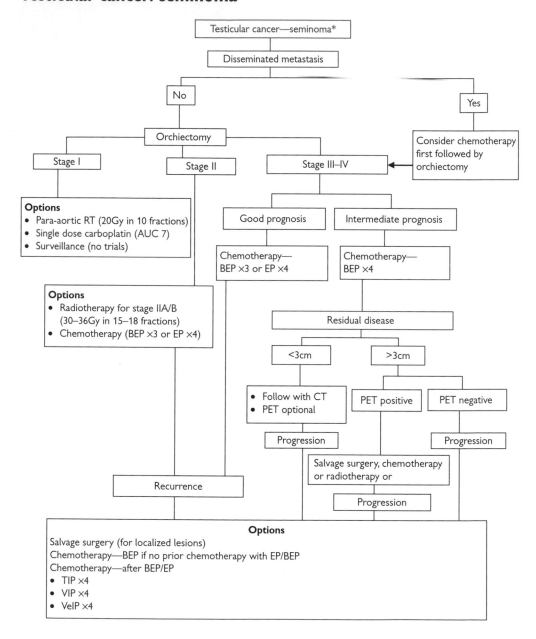

* See p.697 for radiotherapy details and p.296,302 for chemotherapy details

Fig. 8.15.1

Testicular cancer: non-seminoma

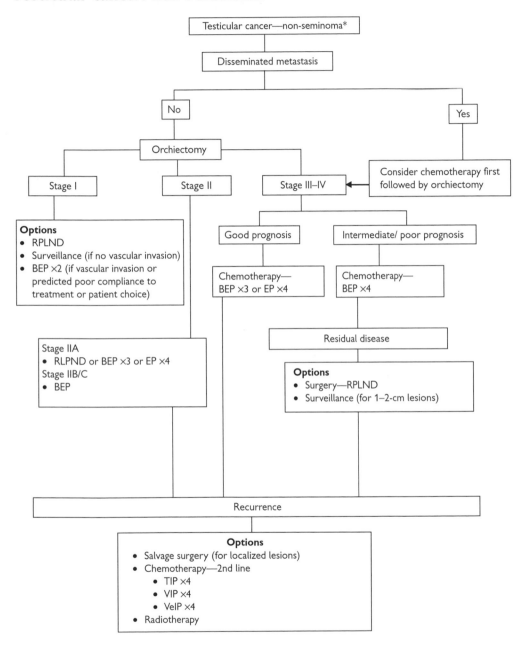

Fig. 8.16.1

Thymic cancer

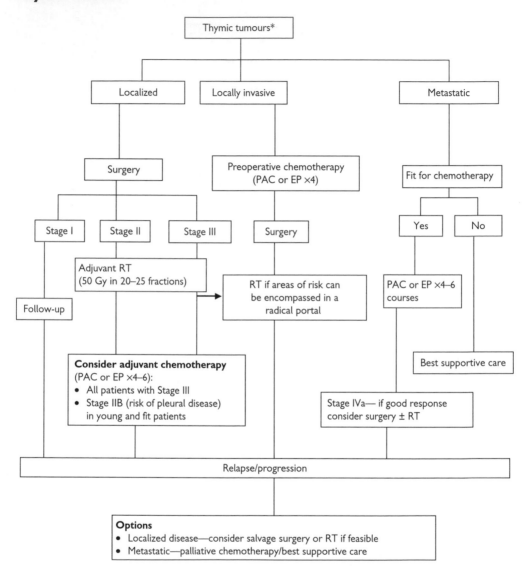

* See p.696 for radiotherapy details and p.692 for chemotherapy details

Fig. 8.17.1

Vaginal cancer

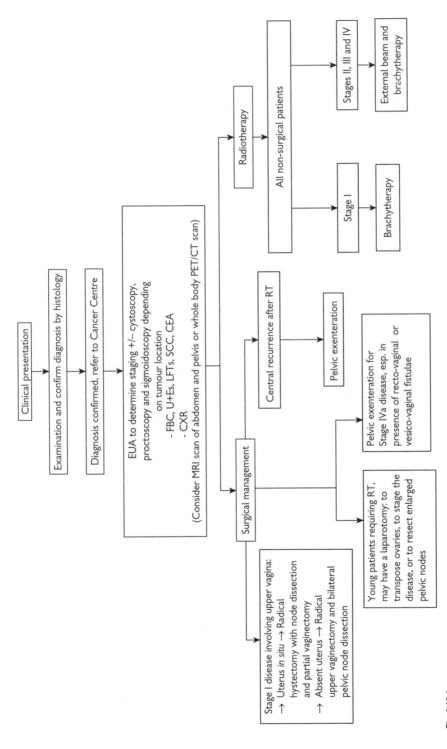

Fig. 8.18.1

Vulval cancer

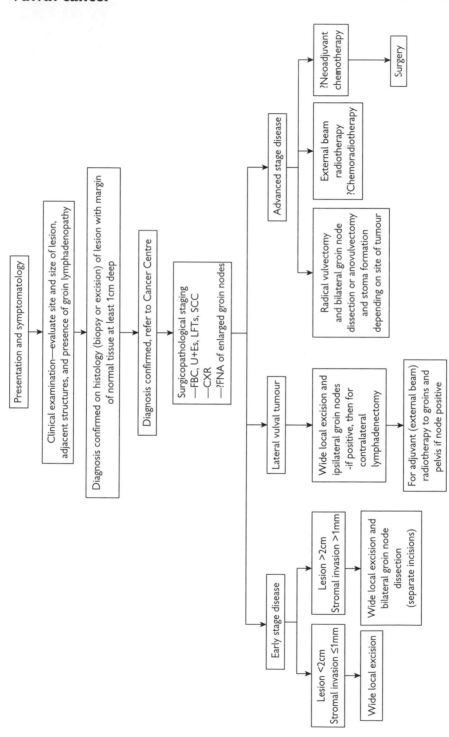

Fig. 8.19.1

Unknown primary

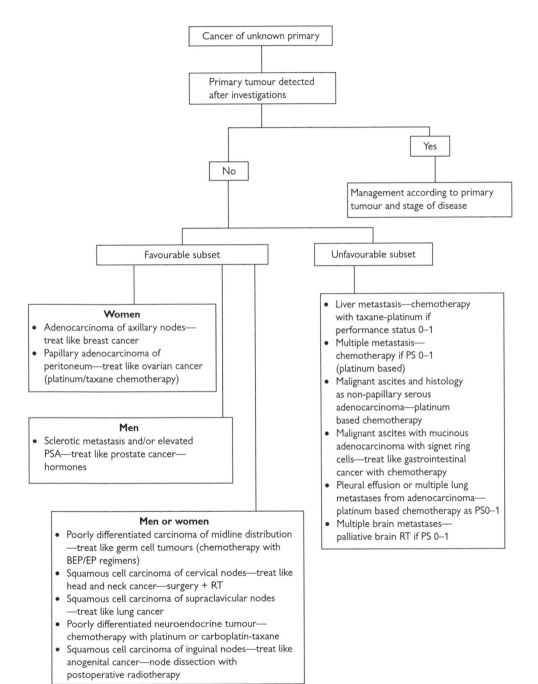

Fig. 8.20.1

Appendix

Systemic therapy regimens

Tumours of head and neck
Cisplatin–5-fluorouracil
- Cisplatin 80–100mg/m^2 IV infusion Day 1
- 5 FU 1g/m^2 24-hour infusion Days 1–5
- 3-week cycle

Tumours of nervous system
Temozolomide
Concomitant
- 75mg/m^2 for 42 days starting on the first day of radio-therapy. Give 1 hour prior to radiotherapy and morning at weekend

Adjuvant and palliative
- 150mg/m^2 first course and if well tolerated increase to 200mg/m^2 for a total of 6 courses. 4-week cycle

PCV
- Procarbazine 100mg/m^2 oral Days 1–10
- CCNU 100mg/m^2 oral Day 1
- Vincristine 1.4mg/m^2 (max. dose 2mg) IV Day 1
- 6 week cycle

Thoracic tumours
Non-small cell lung cancer
Cisplatin–vinorelbine
- Cisplatin 80mg/m^2 IV Day 1
- Vinorelbine 30mg/m^2 IV Days 1 and 8
- 3-week cycle—adjuvant 4 cycles, palliative 4–6 cycles

Gemcitabine–carboplatin
- Gemcitabine 1000mg/m^2 IV Days 1 and 8
- Carboplatin (AUC 5) IV Day 1
- 3-week cycle, 4–6 cycles

Carboplatin–paclitaxel
- Carboplatin AUC 6 Day 1
- Paclitaxel 225mg/m^2 IV Day 1
- 3- week cycle

Docetaxel
- Docetaxel 75mg/m^2 Day 1
- 3-week cycle

Vinorelbine
- Vinorelbine 30mg/m^2 (max 60mg) Days 1, 8—3-week cycle
- Oral vinorelbine 60mg/m^2 Day 1—weekly. Increase to 80mg/m^2 if no grade 4 neutropenia after third cycle

Small-cell lung cancer
Carboplatin–etoposide
- Carboplatin AUC 5 IV Day 1
- Etoposide 100mg/m^2 IV Days 1–3 (day 2–3 can be substituted with oral etoposide 100mg/m^2 twice daily)
- 3-week cycle

VAC
- Vincristine 1.4mg/m^2 (max 2mg) IV Day 1

- Adriamycin 40mg/m^2 IV Day 1
- Cyclophosphamide 600mg/m^2 Day 1
- 3-week cycle

Oral topotecan
- Topotecan 2.3mg/m^2 Days 1–5
- 3-week cycle

Oral etoposide
- Oral etoposide 50mg PO twice daily Days 1–5
- 3-week cycle

Mesothelioma
Cisplatin–pemetrexed
- Cisplatin 75mg/m^2 Day 1 (carboplatin AUC 5)
- Pemetrexed 500mg/m^2 Day 1
- 3-week cycle

Thymoma
PAC
- Cisplatin 50mg/m^2 Day 1
- Adriamycin 50mg/m^2 Day 1
- Cyclophosphamide 500mg/m^2 Day 1
- 3-week cycle

Cisplatin–etoposide
- See above

Breast cancer
AC
- Adriamycin 60mg/m^2 IV Day 1
- Cyclophosphamide 600mg/m^2 IV Day 1
- 3-week cycle for 4–6 courses

Epi-CMF
- Epirubicin 100mg/m^2 Day 1, 3-week cycle for 4 courses followed by 4 cycles of CMF
- Cyclophosphamide 100mg/m^2 PO Days 1–14
- Methotrexate 40mg/m^2 IV (max. 50) Days 1, 8
- 5-FU 600mg/m^2 IV (max. 1g) Days 1, 8
- 4-week cycle

FEC
- 5-FU 600mg/m^2 IV bolus Day 1
- Epirubicin 60mg/m^2 IV bolus Day 1
- Cyclophosphamide 600mg/m^2 IV bolus Day 1
- 3-week cycle for 6 courses

FEC-T
- 3 courses of FEC (100mg/m^2) followed by 3 courses of T (docetaxel)
- Docetaxel 100mg/m^2 IV—3-week cycle

TAC
- Docetaxel 75mg/m^2 IV
- Adriamycin 50mg/m^2 IV
- Cyclophosphamide 500mg/m^2 IV
- 3-week cycle for 6 courses

Docetaxel
- 75mg/m^2 IV infusion Day 1
- 3-week cycle for 6 courses

Capecitabine
- 1000–1250mg/m^2 PO Days 1–14
- 3-week cycle until progression or intolerable toxicity

Vinorelbine
- 25–30mg/m^2 IV (max 60mg) Days 1, 8
- 3-week cycle for 6 courses

Oral vinorelbine
- 60mg/m^2 (increase dose to 80mg/m^2 in second cycle if no neutropenia) Day 1, 8
- 3-week cycle

Paclitaxel
- 175mg/m^2 3-hour infusion Day 1; 3-week cycle or
- 80mg/m^2 1-hour infusion Day 1, 8, 15; 4-week cycle

Hormones
- Tamoxifen 20mg PO daily
- Letrozole 2.5mg PO daily
- Anastrazole 1mg PO daily
- Exemestane 25mg PO daily
- Megesterol 160mg PO daily

Trastuzumab
Loading dose 8mg/kg 90-minute infusion followed after 3 weeks by 6mg/kg IV infusion—3-week cycle. Total 17 cycles for adjuvant setting and until disease progression for metastatic disease

Trastuzumab–docetaxel
Trastuzumab followed by 30 minutes to 1 hour observation followed by docetaxel

Cancers of gastrointestinal system
Oesophageal and gastric cancer
Cisplatin–5-fluorouracil
- Cisplatin 100mg/m^2 Day 1
- 5-FU 1000mg/m^2 Days 1–4 IV infusion
- 3-week cycle

ECX
- Epirubicin 50mg/m^2 Day 1
- Cisplatin 60mg/m^2 Day 1
- Capecitabine 625mg/m^2 twice daily Days 1–21
- 3-week cycle

ECF
- Epirubicin 50mg/m^2 Day 1, repeat 3-weekly
- Cisplatin 60mg/m^2 Day 1, repeat 3-weekly
- 5-FU 200mg/m^2 IV 24-hour continuous infusion for 18–24 weeks

EOX
- Epirubicin 50mg/m^2 Day1
- Oxaliplatin 130mg/m^2 Day 1
- Capecitabine 625mg/m^2 Day 1
- 3-week cycle

Pancreatic cancer
- Gemcitabine 1000mg/m^2 weekly for 7 weeks followed by 1 week's rest

Colorectal cancer
Oxaliplatin–5 Fluorouracil/FA
- Oxaliplatin 85mg/m^2 IV infusion Day 1
- 5-FU 400mg/m^2 bolus Days 1 and 2
- 5-FU 600mg/m^2 22-hour infusion Days 1 and 2
- Folinic acid 200mg/m^2 infusion Days 1 and 2
- 2-week cycle

5-Fluorouracil–folinic acid (Mayo regimen)
- 5-FU 425mg/m^2 IV (325mg/m^2 when given with radiotherapy) Days 1–5
- Folinic acid 20mg/m^2 IV Days 1–5
- 4-week cycle

Capecitabine
- Capecitabine 1250mg/m^2 twice daily Days 1–14
- 4-week cycle

Irinotecan
- Irinotecan 300–350mg/m^2 IV Day 1
- 3-week cycle

Irinotecan–5-fluorouracil/folinic acid
- Irinotecan 125mg/m^2 IV infusion Day 1
- Folic acid 20mg/m^2 IV bolus Day 1
- 5-FU 500mg/m^2 bolus Day 1
- 3-week cycle

There are modifications of the above regimen with infusional 5-FU/FA.

Anal cancer
Mitomycin C–5-fluorouracil
- Mitomycin C 10mg/m^2 IV Day 1
- 5-FU 750mg/m^2 24-hour infusion Days 1–5 repeated at week 5

Cancers of genitourinary system
Urinary bladder
Gemcitabine–cisplatin
- Gemcitabine 1000mg/m^2 IV infusion Days 1, 8, and 15
- Cisplatin 70mg/m^2 IV infusion Day 1
- 4-week cycle

MVAC
- Methotrexate 30mg/m^2 IV Days 1, 15, 22
- Vinblastine 3mg/m^2 IV Days 1, 15, 22
- Doxorubicin 30mg/m^2 IV Days 1
- Cisplatin 70mg/m^2 IV infusion Day 1
- 4-week cycle

Testicular cancer
BEP (3-day)
- Bleomycin 30mg Day 2, 8, 15
- Etoposide 120mg/m^2 Days 1–3
- Cisplatin 50mg/m^2 Days 1, 2
- 3-week cycle

BEP (5 day)
- Bleomycin 30mg Days 2, 8, 15
- Etoposide 100mg/m^2 Days 1–5
- Cisplatin 20mg/m^2 Days 1–5
- 3-week cycle

Carboplatin
- AUC 7 Day 1—one course

TIP
- Paclitaxel 175mg/m^2 Day 1
- Ifosfamide 1.2 gm/m^2 Days 2–6 with mesna
- Cisplatin 20mg/m^2 Days 2–6
- 3-week cycle

VIP
- Vinblastine 0.11mg/kg Days 1, 2
- Ifosfamide 1.5 gm/m^2 Days 1–4 with mesna
- Cisplatin 20mg/m^2 Days 1–5
- 3-week cycle

Prostate cancer
Mitozantrone–prednisone
- Mitozantrone 12mg/m^2 Day 1
- Prednisone 10mg daily
- 3-week cycle

Docetaxel–prednisone
- Docetaxel 75mg/m^2 Day 1
- Prednisone 10mg daily
- 3-week cycle

Cancers of female genital system
Cervical cancer
Cisplatin (concurrent with radiotherapy)
- Cisplatin 40mg/m^2 IV weekly for 4–5 courses

PMB
- Cisplatin 60mg/m^2 IV Day 2
- Methotrexate 300mg/m^2 IV Day 1

- Bleomycin 30 units IV Day 1
- 3- week cycle

Endometrial cancer
Cisplatin–doxorubicin
- Cisplatin 50mg/m^2 IV Day 1
- Doxorubicin 50mg/m^2 Day 1
- 3- week cycle

Paclitaxel–carboplatin
- See 'Epithelial ovarian cancer'

Epithelial ovarian cancer
Paclitaxel–carboplatin
- Paclitaxel 175mg/m^2 3-hour infusion Day 1
- Carboplatin (AUC 5) 1-hour infusion Day 1
- 3-week cycle

Carboplatin
- AUC 5—3-week cycle

Paclitaxel
- 175mg/m^2 Day 1, 3-week cycle *or*
- 90mg/m^2 Day 1, 1-week cycle for 18 weeks

Liposomal doxorubicin
- Liposomal doxorubicin 50mg/m^2 IV Day 1
- 4-week cycle

Topotecan
- Topotecan 1.5mg/m^2 Days 1–5
- 3-week cycle

Carboplatin–gemcitabine
- Carboplatin AUC 5 IV
- Gemcitabine 1000mg/m^2 Days 1, 8
- 3-week cycle

Ovarian germ cell tumour
- See 'Testicular cancer'

Radiotherapy fractionation

See Tables 9.2.1–11.

Table 9.2.1 Tumours of head and neck

Indication	Dose fractionation
Locally advanced	66–68Gy in 33–34 fractions
Accelerated radiotherapy	66–70Gy in 33–35 fractions
Chemoradiotherapy	55Gy in 20 fractions/60Gy in 30 fractions
Concomitant boost	64–70Gy in 32–35 fractions
Adjuvant (postoperative) radiotherapy	60–66Gy in 30–33 fractions to high risk sites
	44Gy in 22 fractions (to potential microscopic nodal disease)
	55Gy in 20 fractions/50Gy in 16 fractions (stage I& II)
Glottic larynx—stage I & II	70Gy in 35 fractions (advanced)

Table 9.2.2 Tumours of nervous system

Indication	Dose fractionation
Glioma	
Low grade glioma—radical	54Gy in 30 fractions
High grade glioma—radical	60Gy in 30 fractions over 5 weeks
High grade glioma—palliative	40Gy in 15 fractions (PS0–1) or 30Gy in 6 fractions over 2 weeks (>70 years or PS 2)
Ependymoma	
Cranial	54Gy in 30 fractions or 55Gy in 33 fractions
Spinal—localized	50.4Gy in 28 fractions if localized
Spinal—metastasis to spinal cord	Craniospinal RT 35Gy in 21 fractions followed by boost to the sites of disease to a total dose of 50.4Gy
Craniospinal RT—medulloblastoma	Craniospinal RT 35Gy in 21 fractions followed by posterior cranial fossa RT 19Gy in 12 fractions
Primary CNS lymphoma	40Gy in 20 or 45Gy in 25 fractions
Germinoma	24Gy in 15 fractions (after chemotherapy complete response)
	40Gy in 25 fractions (after partial response)
Non-germinoma	24Gy in 15 fractions to whole ventricle followed by 25.2Gy in 14 fractions to primary tumour
Germ cell tumour with CNS dissemination	30Gy in 15 fractions to craniospinal axis followed by 25.2Gy in 14 fractions to primary tumour
Pituitary adenoma	45Gy in 25 fractions over 5 weeks
Craniopharyngioma	50Gy in 30 fractions over 6 weeks
Meningioma	50–55Gy in 30–33 fractions
Acoustic neuroma	50Gy in 30 fractions

(Continued)

Table 9.2.2 (Cont'd.)

Indication	Dose fractionation
Brain metastasis	
Metastases—solitary	30Gy in 10 fractions (PS 0–1)
Metastases—multiple	20Gy in 5 fractions (PS 0–1)
	12Gy in 2 fractions (PS 2)
Spinal cord compression	
Impending or evolving compression	20Gy in 5 fractions or 30Gy in 10 fractions
Postoperative	20Gy in 5 fractions or 30Gy in 10 fractions
Established paraplegia	8Gy in 1 fraction (for pain control)
Retreatment	8Gy in 1 or 20Gy in 8

Table 9.2.3 Thoracic tumours

Indication	Dose fractionation
Non-small cell lung cancer	
Radical radiotherapy	54Gy in 36 fractions over 12 days (CHART)
	60–66Gy in 30–33 fractions
	52.5–55Gy in 20 fractions
Postoperative	60Gy in 25–30 fractions
	50Gy in 20–25 fractions
Palliative	36–39Gy in 12–13 fractions (36Gy if spinal cord in the field)—PS 0–1
	20Gy in 5 fractions—PS 0–1
	27Gy in 6 fractions (3 fractions per week)—PS 0–1
	17Gy in 2 fractions (PS 2)
	10Gy single (PS>2)
Small-cell lung cancer	
Localized	50Gy in 25 fractions/45Gy in 20 fractions
	45Gy in 30 fractions over 3 weeks
	36–39Gy in 12–13 fractions (36Gy if spinal cord in the field)—PS 0–1
Extensive	20Gy in 5 fractions—PS 0–1
	27Gy in 6 fractions (3 fractions per week) –PS 0–1
	17Gy in 2 fractions (PS 2)
	10Gy single (PS>2)
Prophylactic cranial RT	
Limited stage	24–30Gy in 8–10 fractions (25Gy in 20)
Extensive	20Gy in 5 fractions
Thymus	
Postoperative	50Gy in 25 fractions or 60Gy in 30 fractions
Primary radiotherapy	60Gy in 30 fractions
Mesothelioma	
Drain site –prophylactic	21Gy in 3 fractions
Palliative	20Gy in 5 or 8Gy single

Table 9.2.4 Breast cancer

Indication	Dose fractionation
Whole breast	40Gy in 15 fractions/42.5Gy in 16 fractions
	50Gy in 25 fractions
Boost RT	16Gy in 8 fractions (with 50Gy whole breast RT)
	9–10Gy in 3–5 fractions
Postoperative chest wall	40Gy in 15 fractions
	50Gy in 25 fractions
Supraclavicular fossa	40Gy in 15 fractions
	50Gy in 25 fractions

Table 9.2.5 Cancers of gastrointestinal system

Indication	Dose fractionation
Oesophagus	
Radical chemoradiotherapy	50Gy in 25 fractions
Preoperative chemoradiotherapy	45Gy in 25 fractions
Radical radiotherapy	55Gy in 20 fractions
Palliative	20Gy in 5 or 30Gy in 10 fractions
Stomach	
Adjuvant chemoradiotherapy	45Gy in 25 fractions
Pancreas	
Radical chemoradiotherapy	45–50.4Gy in 25–28 fractions
Palliative	30Gy in 10 fractions
Rectal cancer	
Preoperative—short course	25Gy in 5 fractions
Preoperative—long course	45Gy in 25 fractions
Postoperative	45Gy in 25 fractions
Palliative	45Gy in 25 fractions/30–36 in 5–6 fractions once weekly
Anal cancer	
Two-phase radical or adjuvant	30.6Gy in 17 fractions followed by 19.8Gy in 11 fractions
One-phase radical	50.4Gy in 28 fractions
Palliative	20Gy in 5 or 8Gy single

Table 9.2.6 Cancers of genitourinary system

Indication	Dose fractionation
Prostate cancer	
One-phase radical	74Gy in 37 fractions/50Gy in 16/55Gy in 20
Two-phase radical	56Gy in 28 fractions followed by 18Gy in 9 fractions
3-phase radical (pelvic nodes)	46Gy in 23 fractions followed by 10Gy in 5 followed by 18Gy in 9 fractions
Salvage radiotherapy	66Gy in 33 fractions
Palliative	30Gy in 10 fractions or 36Gy in 6 fractions over 6 weeks
Urinary bladder cancer	
Radical	64Gy in 32 fractions
Palliative	21Gy in 3 fractions on alternate days/36Gy in 6 fractions
Testicular cancer	
Seminoma stage I	20Gy in 10 fractions
Seminoma stage IIA–B	36Gy in 18 fractions
Testicular carcinoma in situ	20Gy in 10 fractions
Palliative	20Gy in 5 fractions/30Gy in 10 fractions
Penile cancer	
Radical	64Gy in 32 fractions to primary and 50Gy in 25 fractions to lymph nodes
Palliative	30Gy in 10 fractions

Table 9.2.7 Cancers of female genital system

Indication	Dose fractionation
Cervical cancer	
Stage IB2–IIA	45Gy in 25 fractions followed by brachytherapy (LDR 27–30Gy to point A or 90% dose covering 100% of high-risk CTV or HDR 21Gy in 3 fractions)
Stage IIB of above	50.4Gy in 28 fractions followed by brachytherapy (LDR 22.5–25Gy to point A or HDR 14Gy in 3 fractions
Central tumour boost when brachytherapy not possible	15Gy in 8 or 20Gy in 11 (total 65Gy)
Boost to residual tumour	5.4Gy in 3 or 10.8Gy in 6 fractions
Adjuvant RT	45Gy in 25 fractions (microscopic disease)
	50.4Gy in 28 fractions (macroscopic disease)
Para-aortic radiotherapy	45Gy in 25 fractions
Vaginal vault brachytherapy	15–20Gy to 0.5cm from the surface of the applicator (LDR) or 8–12Gy in 2–3 fractions (HDR)
Endometrial cancer	
Adjuvant	45Gy–50.4Gy in 25–28 fractions followed by brachytherapy (10–15Gy to 0.5cm from the surface of the applicator using LDR or 8Gy in 2 fractions at 0.5cm from surface of applicator using HDR) or brachytherapy alone
Brachytherapy alone	30Gy at 0.5 cm from the surface of applicator using LDR or 22Gy in 4 fractions using HDR
Primary radiotherapy stage I–II	45Gy in 25 fractions followed by 20Gy to point A (LDR) or 12Gy in 3 fractions (HDR)
	50Gy in 2 fractions using LDR or 33Gy in 5 fractions using HDR
Primary radiotherapy—stage III	50.4Gy in 28 fractions followed by 22.5Gy to point A (LDR) or 14Gy in 2 fractions (HDR)
Palliative	20Gy in 5 fractions/30Gy in 10 fractions
Vaginal cancer	
Radical	45–54Gy in 25–28 fractions followed by brachytherapy (15–20Gy to point A or 0.5cm from the surface of applicator using LDR or 11Gy in 2 fractions using HDR) or external beam radiotherapy boost (15–20Gy in 8–11 fractions)
Brachytherapy alone	65–70Gy in 2 fractions using LDR or 33Gy in 6 fractions using HDR.
Vulval cancer	
Postoperative/radical	45–50.4Gy in 25–28 fractions and if residual tumour, a boost of 15Gy in 8 fractions

Table 9.2.8 Cancers of skin

Indication	Dose fractionation
Basal cell carcinoma	
Lesion <3cm	36Gy in 8 fractions/3 fractions per week
	30–32Gy in 4 fractions/1–2 fractions per week
	18Gy single fraction
Lesion 3–5cm or nose/pinna/poorly vascular area	45Gy in 9 fractions/3 fractions per week
Lesion >5cm	50–54Gy in 20 fractions/4 weeks
	60Gy in 30 fractions/6 weeks
	(consider 10% dose increase when treating with electrons to account for the reduced relative biological dose of electrons)
Squamous cell carcinoma	
Lesion <5cm	45Gy in 9 fractions over 3 weeks
	54Gy in 20 fractions over 4 weeks
Lesion >5cm	54Gy in 20 fractions over 4 weeks
	66Gy in 33 fractions
Brachytherapy (HDR)	45Gy in 10 fractions
Palliative RT	20Gy in 5 fractions
	36Gy in 6 fractions/6 weeks
	8Gy single
Malignant melanoma	
Adjuvant RT after node dissection	48–50Gy in 20 fractions
Cutaneous T cell lymphoma	8Gy in 2 fractions (for patch and plaque)
	12Gy in 3 fractions (nodule)
	20Gy in 10 fractions (mucosal disease)
	30Gy in 15 fractions (lymph node disease)
	30Gy in 20 fractions over 5 weeks (total body electrons)
Cutaneous B cell lymphoma	15Gy in 5 fractions (indolent)
	30Gy in 15 fractions (aggressive)
Kaposi's sarcoma—skin	8Gy single or 15Gy in 3 fractions
Kaposi's sarcoma—mucosal	20Gy in 10 fractions/2 weeks
Merkel cell carcinoma	60Gy in 30 fractions (radical)
	50Gy in 25 fractions (with chemotherapy)
	50Gy in 20 or 45Gy in 15 (adjuvant tumour bed RT)
	50Gy in 25 (adjuvant nodal RT)

Table 9.2.9 Soft tissue sarcoma

Indication	Dose fractionation
Postoperative	66Gy in 33 fractions
Preoperative	50Gy in 25 fractions

Table 9.2.10 Tumours of haemopoietic system

Indication	Dose fractionation
Hodgkin lymphoma	
Adjuvant after complete response	20Gy in 10 fractions
Residual disease after chemotherapy	30Gy in 15 fractions followed by a boost of 6Gy in 3 fractions to bulky disease
Palliative	20Gy in 5 fractions/30Gy in 10 fractions
Non-Hodgkin lymphoma	
Primary RT for low grade	24–30Gy in 12–15 fractions
RT after chemotherapy	30Gy in 15 fractions
Palliative	20Gy in 5 fractions/30Gy in 10 fractions
Splenic irradiation	10–12Gy in 0.5–1.5Gy 3 times per week
Solitary plasmacytoma	45–50Gy in 25 fractions

Table 9.2.11 Palliative radiotherapy

Indication	Dose fractionation
Superior vena caval obstruction	20Gy in 5 fractions or 30Gy in 10 fractions
Choroidal metastasis	20Gy in 5 fractions
Bone pain	20Gy in 5/8Gy single

Further reading

Barrett A, Dobbs J, Morris S, *et al. Practical Radiotherapy Planning*, 4th edition. London: Hodder Arnold, 2009.

Internet resource

Royal College of Radiologists: *Radiotherapy Dose Fractionation*—available at http://www.rcr.ac.uk/publications.aspx?PageID=149&PublicationID=229

Glomerular filtration rate

Calculation of glomercular filtration rate (GFR) is a pre-requisite before prescription of platinum chemotherapy or other agents likely to cause renal dysfunction. It is calculated by one of the following methods:
1. 24-hour urine collection method
2. Using the Cockcroft-Gault formula

Cockcroft-Gault formula

$$\text{Creatinine clearance} = \frac{(140 - \text{age}) \times \text{weight (kg)} \times A}{\text{Serum creatinine}}$$

A = 1.04 in females and 1.23 in males
This method of calculation of GFR is less accurate in:
• Malnourished patients (weight loss of >5kg in the last month)
• Obese patients—needs to be calculated using adjusted ideal body weight
• Patients under 18 years old
• Patients with a rapidly changing creatinine level

Calculation of carboplatin dose (Calvert formula)

Carboplatin dose = AUC x (GFR+25)

Most protocols use AUC of 5 for measured GFR and 6 for calculated creatinine clearance. 120mL/min is the cap on CrCl as this is the maximum physiological GFR. Carboplatin is not given if GFR is <20mL/min. The calculated GFR should be recalculated before each cycle and if there is >25% change from the baseline calculated GFR, Cr Cl should be measured and dose modified accordingly.

Anatomical diagrams

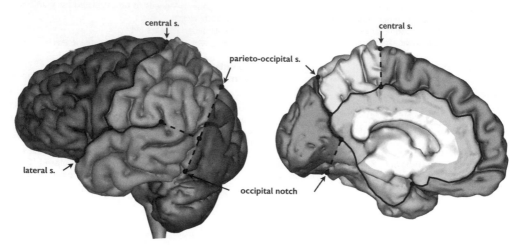

Fig. 9.4.1 Areas and lobes of brain.

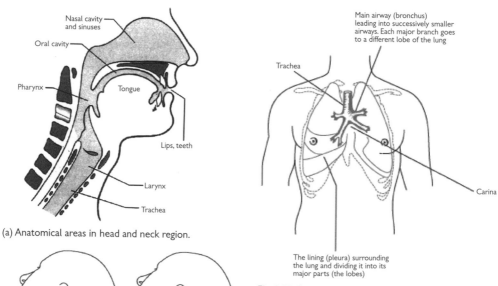

(a) Anatomical areas in head and neck region.

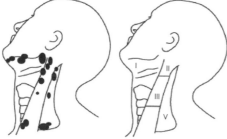

(b) Levels of lymph nodes in the neck.

Fig. 9.4.2 A) Anatomical areas in head and neck region.
B) Levels of lymph nodes in the neck.

Fig. 9.4.3 Anatomy of lung and airways.

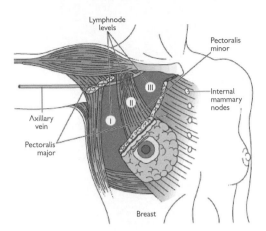

Fig. 9.4.4 Breast and lymphatic area.

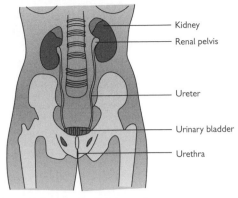

Fig. 9.4.6 Anatomy of genitourinary system.

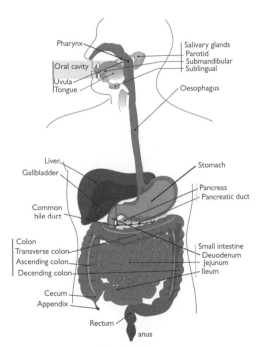

Fig. 9.4.5 Anatomy of gastrointestinal system.

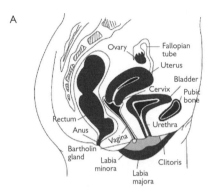

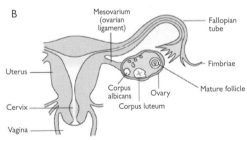

Fig. 9.4.7 A) Anatomy of female genital system. Reproduced from Pattman R et al. *Oxford Handbook of Genitourinary Medicine, HIV, and AIDS.* Oxford: Oxford University Press, 2005. By permission of Oxford University Press. B) Basic coronal view of the female pelvis. Adapted from Pocock G, Richards C. *Human physiology: the basics of medicine,* 2nd edition, Oxford University Press, 2004. By permission of Oxford University Press.

Index

Locators in *italic* refer to figures/diagrams

eye tumours 62
lip/oral cancer 71
nasopharyngeal cancer 68
nose/sinus cancers 66
oropharyngeal cancer 72
radiotherapy fractionation 699
tracheal tumours, primary 118
urothelial cancer 274
vulval cancer 378
St. John's wort 52
staging 2, 33, 33, 38; see also specific cancers by type
standard treatments 2
stem cell transplantation
    Hodgkin disease 444–5
    indications 471
    leukaemia 467, 471–2, 483
    matched unrelated donor transplantations 472
    multiple myeloma 506, 508
    myelodysplastic syndrome 497
    non-Hodgkin lymphoma 458–9
    reduced-intensity conditioning 472
stenting 182, 239, 592
stereotactic radiotherapy 43, 93, 125, 125
steroid synthesis disrupters 48–9
steroid/lipid cell tumours 365
steroids 86, 483, 584, 610, 642, 649
    stomach cancer see gastric cancer
stress 87, 666; see also anxiety; depression
stridor 4, 12, 13, 74, 591
stromal luteomas 365
sunitinib 50, 262–3, 263, 432
superficial X-rays 42
superior vena caval obstruction 4, 592
support sources 2, 35–6
supportive care, chemotherapy 636–8; see also palliative care
supratentorial high-grade gliomas 548
supratentorial PNETs 549
surgery 38–40
    adrenocortical carcinoma 536
    anal cancer 254–5
    basal cell carcinoma 386–7
    biliary tract tumours 208
    brain metastases 108–9, 109
    brain tumours, primary 88–90
    breast cancer 158–9
    cancer prevention 20
    CNS tumours, paediatric 547
    colorectal cancer 238–9, 245
    complications of treatment 325
    ductal carcinoma in situ 156
    elderly patients 603
    endometrial cancer 334–5, 340
    Ewing's sarcomas 414, 415
    gastric cancer 188, 190
    gestational trophoblastic disease 374
    head/neck cancer 58
    hepatocellular cancer 198
    kidney cancer 260–1
    locally advanced breast cancer 166
    lung cancer 124
    malignant pleural mesothelioma 140
    melanoma 398, 400
    neck node management 79
    neuroendocrine tumours 539
    oesophageal cancer 180
    osteosarcoma 410, 412
    ovarian cancer 349, 350, 352–3
    ovarian germ cell tumours 358
    pancreatic cancer 216–17
    penile cancer 310
    prostate cancer 280
    sex cord-stromal tumours 362
    small intestinal tumours 224
    soft tissue sarcomas 424, 426–7
    spinal cord compression 584
    spinal cord tumours 114, 116
    squamous cell carcinoma 390
    thyroid cancer 526, 530, 533, 534
    ureter/pelvic cancers 312

urothelial/bladder cancer 268, 272–3
uterine sarcomas 344
vulval cancer 382
survivorship 614–15
Sutent 50
sweat gland carcinomas 394–5
switch maintenance chemotherapy 132
symptom clusters 663
synovial sarcoma 421
systemic therapy 46–53
    further reading 53
    head/neck cancer 59
    immunotherapy 52–3, 170, 263, 400–1
    molecularly targetted 49–52, 50
    pharmacodynamics/kinetics 46
    regimens 692–4
    see also chemotherapy; hormonal therapy;

T

tamoxifen 10, 19, 39, 163, 170, 328
tamponade, cardiac 586
Tarceva 50
Tasigna 50
taxane 162
T-cell based adoptive therapy 53
temozolamide 96
temsirolimus 50
TENS 644
teratogenesis 361
teratoma 290–1, 356
testicular cancer 6, 290–1
    brain metastases 298
    chemotherapy sensitivity 293
    clinical features 292
    diagnosis 292–3
    fertility/sexuality 306
    follow-up 304–5, 305
    further reading 291, 293–4, 298, 301, 303, 305, 307
    germ cell tumours 562
    internet resources 307
    long-term impacts of treatment 306–7
    metastasis pattern 293
    non-seminoma management 302–3, 304
    prognostic factors 296, 296
    radiotherapy fractionation 697
    rare tumours 305
    recommendations 303
    recurrence management 297–8
    seminoma management 300–1, 304
    staging 293, 293
    systemic therapy regimens 693-4
    treatment flowchart 684, 685
    treatment of advanced disease 296–8
    tumour markers 32
    WHO classification system 291
testicular dysgenesis syndrome 290
testicular intraepithelial neoplasia 291, 293
testicular lymphoma 463
thalidomide 506–7, 508, 559
thecoma 363–4
thoracic tumours
    radiotherapy fractionation 696
    systemic therapy regimens 692
    see also specific cancers by name
thorium dioxide 202
thrombocytopenia 578–9
thromboembolism 624
thrombolysis 592
thrombopoietin 53
thrombosis 19
thymic tumours 142, 142–4
    Masoka staging system 142
    treatment flowchart 686
    WHO classification system 143
thyroid cancer
    aetiology 524, 534
    anaplastic carcinoma 532
    clinical approaches 13
    clinical features 524, 533, 534
    diagnosis 524, 534

epidemiology 524, 534
    further reading 525, 528, 531, 532, 533, 535
    genetics 531
    histological types 524
    internet resources 528, 531
    investigations 533
    management 526–8, 532
    medullary carcinoma 530–1
    palliative care 531
    parathyroid cancer 534
    primary thyroid lymphoma 533
    prognostic factors 528, 530, 532, 533, 535
    radioiodine ablation 526–7
    recurrence management 530–1, 533
    screening 535
    staging 524–5, 533, 534
    treatment 533, 534
    tumour markers 32
thyroid hormone 49
TNM staging system 33, 33
    anal cancer 254
    breast cancer 153, 154
    colorectal cancer 235, 235–6
    head/neck cancer 58
    lung cancer 121
    pancreatic cancer 213
    and surgery 38
    thyroid cancer 524–5
tobacco smoking see smoking
tomatoes 625, 635
topical lignocaine 643
topoisomerase inhibitors 48, 96, 540
Torisel 50
total mesorectal excision 238
toxicity, opioids 641, 641–2; see also neurotoxicity
trace elements 624, 626
tracheal tumours, primary 118
transdermal opioids 641
trastuzumab 51, 106, 163, 168–9
travel, cancer patients 616–17
treatment flowcharts 507
    bladder cancer 670
    breast cancer 671
    cancer of unknown primary 689
    cervical cancer 319, 323, 672
    chronic lymphocytic leukaemia 483
    colon cancer 673
    endometrial cancer 674
    epithelial ovarian cancer 675
    hepatocellular cancer (HCC) 676
    kidney cancer 261
    myelodysplastic syndrome 497
    oesophageal cancer 679
    pancreatic cancer 680
    prostate cancer 681
    rectal cancer 682
    small-cell lung cancer 677
    stomach cancer 683
    testicular cancer 684, 685
    thymic tumours 686
    vaginal cancer 687
    vulval cancer 688
treatment
    impacts see long term impacts
    implementation 34
    options 2
    plans 2, 34
    related mortality 477, 611
triple assessment, breast cancer 152
triple-negative breast cancer 171
TRUS biopsy 276
tubular carcinoma 150
tumour control probability 42
tumour lysis syndrome 568
tumour markers 32, 32, 204, 214, 292
    cervical cancer 326
    ovarian germ cell tumours 357
    sex cord-stromal tumours 362
    urothelial/bladder cancer 266
tumour necrosis factor 53, 569
tumour suppressor genes 24